Thyroid Cancer

Thyroid Cancer

A Comprehensive Guide to Clinical Management

Second Edition

Edited by

Leonard Wartofsky, MD, MPH, MACP
Douglas Van Nostrand, MD, FACP, FACNP

Washington Hospital Center, Washington, DC

Forewords by

E. Chester Ridgway, MD, MACP
University of Colorado Health Sciences Medical Center, Denver, CO

and

Ernest L. Mazzaferri, MD, MACP
University of Florida, Gainesville, FL

HUMANA PRESS ✸ TOTOWA, NEW JERSEY

© 2006 Humana Press Inc.
Softcover reprint of the hardcover 2nd edition 2006
999 Riverview Drive, Suite 208
Totowa, New Jersey 07512
www.humanapress.com

All rights reserved. No part of this book may be reproduced, stored in a retrieval system, or transmitted in any form or by any means, electronic, mechanical, photocopying, microfilming, recording, or otherwise without written permission from the Publisher.

All authored papers, comments, opinions, conclusions, or recommendations are those of the author(s), and do not necessarily reflect the views of the publisher.

Due diligence has been taken by the publishers, editors, and authors of this book to assure the accuracy of the information published and to describe generally accepted practices. The contributors herein have carefully checked to ensure that the drug selections and dosages set forth in this text are accurate and in accord with the standards accepted at the time of publication. Notwithstanding, as new research, changes in government regulations, and knowledge from clinical experience relating to drug therapy and drug reactions constantly occurs, the reader is advised to check the product information provided by the manufacturer of each drug for any change in dosages or for additional warnings and contraindications. This is of utmost importance when the recommended drug herein is a new or infrequently used drug. It is the responsibility of the treating physician to determine dosages and treatment strategies for individual patients. Further it is the responsibility of the health care provider to ascertain the Food and Drug Administration status of each drug or device used in their clinical practice. The publisher, editors, and authors are not responsible for errors or omissions or for any consequences from the application of the information presented in this book and make no warranty, express or implied, with respect to the contents in this publication.

This publication is printed on acid-free paper. ∞
ANSI Z39.48-1984 (American Standards Institute) Permanence of Paper for Printed Library Materials.

Cover illustrations: Figure 3 from Chapter 35; Figure 3 from Chapter 25; Figures 7 and 11 from Chapter 25.

Cover design by Patricia F. Cleary.

For additional copies, pricing for bulk purchases, and/or information about other Humana titles, contact Humana at the above address or at any of the following numbers: Tel.: 973-256-1699; Fax: 973-256-8341; E-mail: orders@humanapr.com; Website: www.humanapress.com

Photocopy Authorization Policy:
Authorization to photocopy items for internal or personal use, or the internal or personal use of specific clients, is granted by Humana Press Inc., provided that the base fee of US $30.00 per copy is paid directly to the Copyright Clearance Center at 222 Rosewood Drive, Danvers, MA 01923. For those organizations that have been granted a photocopy license from the CCC, a separate system of payment has been arranged and is acceptable to Humana Press Inc. The fee code for users of the Transactional Reporting Service is: [978-1-58829-462-3/06 $30.00].

10 9 8 7 6 5 4 3 2 1

eISBN 978-1-59259-995-0
Library of Congress Cataloging-in-Publication Data
Thyroid cancer : a comprehensive guide to clinical management / edited by Leonard Wartofsky and Douglas Van Nostrand ; forewords by E. Chester Ridgway and Ernest L. Mazzaferri.— 2nd ed.
    p. ; cm.
  Includes bibliographical references and index.
  ISBN 978-1-61737-583-5
  1. Thyroid gland—Cancer—Treatment.
  [DNLM: 1. Thyroid Neoplasms. WK 270 T5494 2006] I. Wartofsky, L. II. Van Nostrand, Douglas.
  RC280.T6T527 2006
  616.99'444—dc22   2005029167

Dedicated to the memory of some of the great thyroidologists who have influenced our lives and careers. First and foremost, my mentor and friend, Sidney H. Ingbar, and Clark Sawin, Monte Greer, Ralph Cavalieri, Farahe Maloof, John Dunn, William McConahey, and Robert Volpe.

And to all of our patients who struggle under the cloud of an uncertain future with their malignancies.

LEONARD WARTOFSKY, MD

To my father, Halstead K. Van Nostrand, who paid for the foundation.

DOUGLAS VAN NOSTRAND, MD

Foreword to Second Edition

Cancer remains a major health problem for our society as we enter the new millennium. In 2002 there were approximately 550,000 deaths in the United States from cancer, which remains the second leading cause of mortality in our society behind heart disease. Each one accounts for approximately 25% of the deaths in the United States on an annual basis. The most common cancers to appear in 2005 remain prostate, breast, lung and colon which will generate between 150,000 and 250,000 new cases this year. Likewise, the most common causes of death from cancer during this same period will be lung, colon, breast and prostate which will cause approximately 160,000, 50,000, 40,000, and 30,000 deaths, respectively.

In comparison, thyroid cancer is a relatively uncommon cancer. In 2005 we expect approximately 26,000 new cases and approximately 1500 thyroid cancer deaths will occur in the same period. Interestingly, thyroid cancer is the eighth most common cancer in women, similar in prevalence to ovarian cancer and melanoma. Moreover, American Cancer Society statistics indicate that thyroid cancer is currently the cancer in women with the greatest rate of increased incidence. Fortunately, for most thyroid cancers the five year survival rate has always been outstanding and is continuing to slowly improve. In the 1970s, the five year survival rate for differentiated thyroid cancer was approximately 92% and in 2005 it is expected to be 97%. This is to be compared with 99%, 88%, 63%, and 15% for the five year survival rates of prostate, breast, colon, and lung, respectively. Thus, thyroid cancer is important, not only because it is one of the top 10 cancers in women, but because it is amenable to early diagnosis, accurate and specific therapies, and excellent survival rates. Despite these salutary characteristics of thyroid cancer, it is problematic to both patients and their physicians because of its high, but nonfatal, recurrence rates that approximate 30% for differentiated thyroid cancer over a 40 year followup period. Although not resulting in death, these recurrences result in additional interventions for the patient and the necessity for long-term followup.

In the second edition of *Thyroid Cancer*, Drs. Leonard Wartofsky, Douglas Van Nostrand, and their skilled and expert group of contributing authors have presented a wealth of new information on the problem of thyroid cancer. One would hope that all new editions to existing textbooks would bring as much new information to the subject as Dr. Wartofsky has provided in his new edition. The number of chapters has increased from 52 to 91. The text is again organized according to thyroid cancer type: papillary carcinoma followed by follicular carcinoma, medullary thyroid carcinoma, thyroid lymphomas, and anaplastic cancers. However, new General Considerations sections on Thyroid Cancer and, in particular, on Nuclear Medicine aspects of thyroid cancer, now introduce the entire text with improved organization and wonderfully expanded new information on the molecular pathogenesis, oncogenic determinants and staging of thyroid cancer. This new edition could serve as a textbook for nuclear medicine physicians, with the importance of nuclear medicine in thyroid cancer emphasized and expanded with clearly articulated chapters on radiation exposure, whole-body imaging with iodine isotopes, and on the emergence of important new isotopic imaging techniques such as PET scanning of thyroid malignancies. More and more we are recognizing that one basic standard dose for radioiodine therapy may not be appropriate for all patients, and hence the chapters on "dosimetry" during either thyroxine withdrawal or after recombinant human TSH provide convincing rationale and arguments for this valuable method for determining maximal safe radioactive iodine dosing.

The Thyroid Nodule section has been expanded to emphasize the importance of thyroid ultrasound as a diagnostically critical element for not only the performance of fine needle aspiration biopsy, but also for the diagnosis of thyroid nodules and followup surveillance of thyroid cancer patients for recurrence in cervical lymph nodes. Clearly, the newer ultrasonographic modalities and their use by endocrinologists have been one of the reasons why more thyroid nodules are being detected, which in turn, results in the higher number of thyroid cancer cases seen today than five and ten years ago. Doubtless, the above-mentioned observed improvements in remission and cure rates must relate to this earlier diagnosis.

Recombinant human thyrotropin or Thyrogen®, had just been approved for the diagnostic followup of differentiated thyroid cancer in 1999 at the time of the first edition of this book. In the intervening five years recombinant thyrotropin has emerged as one of the most important discoveries leading to improved diagnosis and followup of thyroid cancer. The new text details and expands our collective experiences in the use of recombinant thyrotropin as well as illuminates the promise for this reagent in remnant ablation treatment of thyroid cancer, and its dramatic potential for augmenting thyroglobulin testing and even its incremental value when utilized prior to PET scanning. Ongoing prospectively designed studies in the United States and Europe are providing intriguing results for these indications that will likely alter our management algorithms for diagnosing and treating thyroid cancer in the future.

Finally, the new edition ends with some very insightful predictions about the future for nuclear medicine as well as genetic and chemotherapeutic approaches to thyroid cancer. I particularly liked the very informative last new section on resources for patients including low iodine diets, and the listings of books, multiple Internet web sites, and recommendations for patients who have recently been treated with radioactive iodine. Drs. Wartofsky, Van Nostrand, and their colleagues should be very proud of this new edition and its formidable amount of new information. The physicians treating thyroid cancer will find this text comprehensive and accurate. The field of thyroid cancer will be enriched and our patients will be the beneficiaries of this new second edition of *Thyroid Cancer*.

E. Chester Ridgway, MD, MACP

Foreword to First Edition

As the 20th century draws to a close, it seems like a propitious time to look back upon the advances we have made in understanding thyroid carcinoma, since our knowledge today will certainly serve to light the path of discovery in the next century. Gazing at the world through a small looking glass focused on thyroid carcinoma seems an appropriate way to begin thinking about the clinical management of this group of diseases. What are the important things that we have learned in recent years that form the basis of our current clinical knowledge? How can we best use that information in the care of our patients? Dr. Leonard Wartofsky's new and sharply focused text, *Thyroid Cancer*, promises to answer this hypothetical set of questions in a succinct and clinically relevant way.

It sometimes seems that thyroid carcinoma is a neglected orphan among human cancers, which is at the root of some important issues. Thyroid carcinomas comprise a diverse group of malignancies ranging from indolent microscopic papillary carcinomas that pose no threat to survival to anaplastic carcinomas that are the most vicious carcinomas afflicting humans. Yet, because of its low incidence, there have been no prospective randomized clinical trials of the treatment of thyroid carcinoma. Furthermore, none are likely to be done, given the prolonged survival and relatively low mortality rates associated with the majority of these cancers. Nonetheless, patients often suffer greatly from this disease: many have serious recurrences and some die from relentlessly progressive and untreatable cancer. This is a disease that knows no boundaries, striking young and old alike. Unfortunately, management paradigms derive from retrospective studies, and few new drugs have been added to our therapeutic armamentarium. One would thus anticipate a deep void in our understanding of these tumors. Despite these shortcomings, the 20th century has seen major advances in our understanding of their etiology, pathophysiology, and management. The good news is that the advances have been rapidly translated into improved outcomes for many patients with thyroid carcinoma. For example, data from the National Cancer Institute shows that, although the incidence of thyroid carcinoma has increased significantly—almost 28%—since the early 1970s in the United States, cancer-specific mortality rates during this same period have dropped significantly—by almost 21%. In my view this results from the earlier diagnosis of the cancer, which allows the full impact of effective therapy, and which I believe has dramatically altered the clinical course of these tumors.

One of the dazzling success stories in medicine in the last half of this century is that with medullary thyroid carcinoma, a truly orphan tumor afflicting relatively few people. First identified in 1959 as a discrete entity, this tumor was identified before calcitonin was known to exist and before the mystery of the multiple endocrine neoplasia syndromes had been completely unraveled. The pieces of the puzzle fell together at lightning speed over a few decades. The *Ret* proto-oncogene mutations recently identified in this tumor will serve as the portal to our eventual complete understanding of its biology and are already the keystone to its diagnosis in members of afflicted kindreds. Now children with this genetic defect can be identified with molecular testing well before medullary thyroid carcinoma becomes clinically manifest or is identifiable by any other test, resulting in thyroidectomy that cures the disease. What a wondrous group of developments to pass on to the patients and physicians of the next century! This work serves as a model for the scientific investigation of malignant tumors.

We are also acquiring a clearer view of the molecular biology of well-differentiated—papillary and follicular—thyroid carcinomas. *Ret* rearrangements found in papillary carcinomas of humans have been shown to produce the tumor in transgenic mice, underscoring the central role of *Ret* in the pathogenesis of papillary carcinoma. Study of familial papillary thyroid carcinoma—now recognized to occur in a small but important subset of patients in whom it may be transmitted as an autosomal dominant trait—undoubtedly will provide important new information. These and other exciting discoveries, such as the identification of the sodium-iodide symporter in laboratory animals and humans, portend more basic discoveries that will generate currently unimaginable diagnostic and therapeutic tools. The latest example of this success in the laboratory is recombinant human TSH, which was recently introduced into clinical practice and already is dramatically improving and simplifying the care of patients with differentiated thyroid carcinoma.

During the past 50 years we have learned much about the important etiologic role of ionizing radiation in thyroid carcinoma. Introduced at the turn of the 20th century by Roentgen, external radiation soon became routine practice in the United States for many benign clinical conditions ranging from "statushymicolymphaticus" to acne. It took over 50 years, however, to understand that the thyroid gland of children is extremely sensitive to the carcinogenic effects of ionizing radiation and that this therapy itself caused papillary thyroid carcinoma, often decades after the exposure. Studies of the Japanese survivors of the atomic bombings of Nagasaki and Hiroshima first documented thyroid carcinoma as a consequence of radioactive fallout. Nonetheless, the notion was long held that internal radiation of the thyroid from ingested radioactive iodine was not a thyroid carcinogen. The outbreak of papillary thyroid carcinoma among children exposed to radioactive iodine fallout from the nuclear reactor accident in Chernobyl, however, abruptly closed the door on this notion. This accident placed a deadly exclamation mark after the statement that small doses of radioiodine indeed are carcinogenic to the thyroid glands of infants and children, and sparked renewed concerns about the above-ground nuclear weapons testing program in Nevada between 1950 and 1960, during which radioactive iodine fallout rained down on nearly the entire continental United States. The National Cancer Institute estimates that a substantial excess of thyroid carcinomas has probably occurred and perhaps will continue to occur as a result of this exposure. How clinicians will deal with this information, including what tests should be done, is under discussion, but national screening studies are not likely to be done.

We also have learned much about the pathology of thyroid carcinoma during the 20th century. The early observations about the prognostic implications of tumor size and invasion through the thyroid capsule are now well accepted. In addition, pathologists now recognize a number of histologic variants of papillary and follicular carcinoma that have important implications that must be carefully factored into the assessment of a tumor's prognosis. Other important advances in our understanding of thyroid pathology have occurred in this decade. What was once considered small-cell anaplastic thyroid carcinoma is now recognized as thyroid lymphoma—known to be a rare complication of Hashimoto's disease—which nevertheless seems to be occurring with increasing frequency. While we were busy discovering thyroid lymphoma, the incidence of anaplastic thyroid carcinoma has been quietly declining, probably as a result of early diagnosis and treatment of well-differentiated tumors that often serve as its forerunner. All of us breathe a quiet sigh of relief at this improvement. Now it is well appreciated that a tumor's prognosis cannot be fully assessed until its final histology has been carefully studied, sometimes both histologically and immunochemically, to uncover the dark secrets of its origin. This has therapeutic implications.

I think much of our success in reducing mortality from thyroid carcinoma stems from early diagnosis. Thirty years ago the main diagnostic tests to identify a malignant nodule were thyroid hormone suppression and radionuclide imaging. Now the standard of care in a clinically euthyroid patient is to perform a fine-needle aspiration biopsy of the nodule before any other tests are done. Though it remains a less than perfect test, the study of fine-needle cytology has prevented unnecessary surgery in many patients while increasing the yield of carcinoma among those undergoing thyroidectomy. I think fine-needle aspiration of nodules has saved more lives than is generally acknowledged—by preventing long periods of thyroid hormone suppression—while malignant nodules sometimes became wildly metastatic. There is evidence that long delays in therapy significantly increase cancer-specific mortality rates of papillary and follicular thyroid carcinoma. The key to fine-needle aspiration diagnosis is to understand the diagnostic details of the cytology report and to act accordingly.

Much of the current debate on thyroid carcinoma has revolved around the extent of initial therapy, both surgical and medical, that is necessary for patients with differentiated thyroid carcinoma. Almost everyone believes that some differentiated thyroid carcinomas require minimal therapy, whereas others require more aggressive management. The problem lies in defining aggressive tumors. Several staging systems and prognostic scoring systems have been devised to discriminate between low-risk patients who are anticipated to have a good outcome with minimal therapy and higher risk patients who require aggressive therapy to avoid morbidity or mortality from thyroid carcinoma. However, most of the prognostic systems do not identify the variants of papillary and follicular carcinoma that have remarkably different behaviors. Most prognostic scoring systems have been created with multiple regression analysis to find predictive combinations of factors, but almost none include therapy in the analysis. Moreover, almost all of them have considered cancer mortality as the endpoint of therapy, ignoring tumor recurrence or disease-free survival. This becomes problematic in defining risk because patients under age 40 typically have low cancer mortality rates, but experience high rates of tumor recurrence. Because most recurrences are in the neck and are easily treated, some clinicians regard them as trivial problems—but my patients find this notion incomprehensible. Most patients are devastated by a recurrence of tumor, regardless of its site. The greatest utility of prognostic scoring systems lies in epidemiological studies and as tools to stratify patients for prospective therapy trials, but they are least useful in determining treatment for individual patients.

In the past few decades most have come to believe that near-total or total thyroidectomy is the optimal treatment for thyroid carcinomas, even for patients at relatively low risk of mortality from their carcinomas. The main reason not to do total thyroidectomy is that it is associated with higher complication rates than those of lobectomy. However, there is now evidence documenting what most of us have known for a long time: surgeons with the most experience have the lowest complication rates, regardless of the extent of the thyroidectomy. Given the low frequency of this disease, a compelling argument can be made to refer patients to centers with highly experienced surgeons for their initial management.

Follow up of differentiated thyroid carcinomas and medullary thyroid carcinoma is greatly facilitated by sensitive serum tests—thyroglobulin and calcitonin—and the use of a variety of scanning techniques. I believe that what we term recurrence of tumor is actually persistent disease that previously fell below the radar of our older, less-sensitive detection tools. With newer sensitive tests including, for example, thyroglobulin measured by messenger RNA, we now have the opportunity to identify and treat thyroid cancers at an earlier and more responsive stage. Perhaps the most vivid example of this is the identification of diffuse pulmonary metastases among patients with high serum thyroglobulin levels and negative diagnostic imaging studies, which are only seen on posttherapeutic whole-body scans done after large therapeutic doses of ^{131}I. Whether this enhances survival continues to be debated, but I think there are compelling reasons to suggest that it does improve outcome.

Thus many relatively new observations and management tools that have largely been developed in the last half of this century are being brought to the bedside to substantially enhance our ability to improve the outcome of most patients with thyroid carcinoma. Many challenges remain, however. More effective therapy is urgently needed for patients with widely metastatic disease that is unresponsive to current therapies. We need to understand more about the molecular predictors of recurrence and death from thyroid cancer. Nonetheless, our present state of knowledge provides clinicians a wide variety of diagnostic and therapeutic modalities to effectively manage this group of cancers. I believe the knowledge contained in *Thyroid Cancer* will give the practicing clinician the necessary information to provide patients with the latest and best diagnostic and therapeutic techniques.

Ernest L. Mazzaferri, MD, MACP

Preface

The second edition of *Thyroid Cancer: A Comprehensive Guide to Clinical Management* marks the publication of a markedly updated and expanded volume that covers all aspects of the etiology, pathogenesis, diagnosis, initial treatment, and long-term management of all varieties of thyroid cancer. Like the first edition, it will serve as a valuable reference source for pathologists, endocrine surgeons, endocrinologists, nuclear medicine physicians, and oncologists. However, the biggest change is that the second edition is significantly enlarged and expanded to encompass important and extensive treatments of more topics related to nuclear medicine. Nuclear medicine physicians and procedures play a key role in the management of thyroid cancer patients and in retrospect, a comprehensive discussion of topics related to that field was somewhat lacking in the first edition. This has been fully remedied with the addition of Dr. Douglas Van Nostrand as co-editor of this second edition. This edition now includes extensive discussion of isotopes, isotope uptake and scanning procedures, radioiodine ablation (with or without recombinant human TSH), stunning, dosimetry (with or without recombinant human TSH), octreotide and FDG-PET scanning and other alternative imaging modalities. There is a valuable reference atlas of scan images and illustrations, and a scholarly summary of the side effects of radioiodine and how to avoid or minimize adverse effects of treatment. In addition to an updated section on ultrasonography of the thyroid gland, new chapters on ultrasonography of cervical lymph nodes and imaging for thyroid cancer employing computerized tomography (CT) and magnetic resonance imaging (MRI) have been added.

When the first edition was published in 2000, it was intended to meet the needs of practicing physicians for up-to-date clinically relevant information concerning the diagnosis and management of patients with thyroid cancer. The book received considerable acclaim and filled a void in the endocrine literature as a guide and reference source on the topics covered. Much has occurred in the field in the past five years that justifies publication of this, an updated and extensively expanded, second edition. The topics of all of the new chapters are too lengthy to list here, and the reader is referred to the Table of Contents. Again, the various chapters are written by highly knowledgeable experts, including many who are new to this edition. The authors provide not only the most current review of their respective areas, but also their own recommendations and approach. The reader is forewarned that in many cases these approaches, albeit rooted in available data, may be empiric rather than based upon clear-cut results of well-controlled clinical trials. Nevertheless, controversial issues are examined and evidence-based recommendations are presented when available.

There are updated chapters on our current state of knowledge of the molecular changes in thyroid cancer, molecular markers, and how targeted therapies are being developed. New therapeutic trials of redifferentiation agents to restore the sodium iodide symporter when lacking and more traditional chemotherapies are discussed, with referral sources listed for entry of patients into Phase 1-3 clinical trials. Happily, most patients with well differentiated thyroid cancer have an excellent prognosis when managed early and appropriately. But contributing authors also present their approaches to the management of more difficult cases, those with extensive bone metastases, those with negative isotope scans but high serum thyroglobulin, and those patients with positive antithyroglobulin antibodies that interfere with measurement of serum thyroglobulin.

Thyroid cancer is fortunately rare in children, but special problems apply to the pediatric population when it does occur. The sections on both differentiated thyroid cancer and medullary thyroid cancer in children have been updated with particular attention to the need for cautious approaches to radioiodine scanning and treatment to minimize radiation exposure. Thyroid cancer occurring under unique circumstances is well covered, such as during pregnancy, in thyroglossal duct cysts, and struma ovarii, as well as the special problem related to radioiodine therapy in the end stage renal patient with thyroid cancer. The rationale and methods for the use of low iodine diets are presented with practical guidelines for the patient, as are radiation safety guidelines (for both physicians and patients) for radioiodine therapy with sample formats and worksheet documents, and a list of resources for more information for patients. And finally, newer such locally ablative techniques to destroy metastatic foci as ethanol instillation and laser and radiofrequency ablation are discussed.

In general, the same format used in the first edition is again employed, that of separating each type of thyroid cancer and having authors separately address clinical presentation, diagnosis, surgery, pathology, followup, treatment, and prognosis for each tumor. This arrangement allows the reader to quickly refer to the specific cancer in his or her patient, with everything and anything that they need to know in one place in a concise, readable format. This format works well in most but not all cases, with some obvious overlap in the management of the two well-differentiated cancers, papillary and follicular, and so some discussions of these two tumors is combined when appropriate. Separate sections deal with Hürthle cell cancer, thyroid lymphoma, and more rare and unusual tumors of the thyroid. Given the publication deadlines for manuscript submission, the most current reference citations possible are provided in the bibliography of each chapter.

I am indebted to the skilled and professional staff of Humana Press, especially Damien DeFrances and Jim Geronimo, and to their executives Thomas Lanigan and Paul Dolgert. I thank our outstanding group of authors for their expert and well written contributions and my coeditor, Doug Van Nostrand, for his invaluable expertise and assistance with this project. We hope that the result will provide useful information to physicians managing patients with thyroid cancer for years to come.

Leonard Wartofsky, MD, MACP

Contents

Foreword to Second Edition by E. Chester Ridgway, MD, MACP vii

Foreword to First Edition by Ernest L. Mazzaferri, MD, MACP ix

Preface xiii

Color Plates xxiii

Contributors xxv

Part I General Considerations I: *Thyroid Cancer*

1. Anatomy and Physiology of the Thyroid Gland: *Clinical Correlates to Thyroid Cancer*
   Nikolaos Stathatos 3

2. Epidemiology of Thyroid Cancer
   James J. Figge 9

3. Molecular Pathogenesis of Thyroid Cancer
   James J. Figge, Nikolai A. Kartel, Dima Yarmolinsky, and Gennady Ermak 15

4. Molecular Aspects of Thyroid Cancer in Children
   Gary L. Francis 33

5. Oncogenes in Thyroid Cancer
   Katherine B. Weber and Michael T. McDermott 41

6. Apoptosis in Thyroid Cancer
   Su He Wang and James R. Baker, Jr. 55

7. Radiation-Induced Thyroid Cancer
   James J. Figge, Timothy Jennings, Gregory Gerasimov,
   Nikolai A. Kartel, Dima Yarmolinsky, and Gennady Ermak 63

8. Classification of Thyroid Malignancies
   Yolanda C. Oertel 85

9. Staging of Thyroid Cancer
   Leonard Wartofsky 87

10. Thyroid Cancer in Children and Adolescents
    Merrily Poth 97

11. Recombinant Human Thyrotropin
    Matthew D. Ringel and Stephen J. Burgun 103

Part II General Considerations II: *Nuclear Medicine*

12 History of the Role of Nuclear Medicine in the Thyroid Gland
and its Diseases: *A Personal Perspective*
Henry N. Wagner, Jr. 117

13 Prophylaxis against Radiation Exposure from Radioiodine
Jacob Robbins and Arthur B. Schneider 129

14 Radioiodine Whole Body Imaging
Frank B. Atkins and Douglas Van Nostrand 133

15 Primer and Atlas for the Interpretation of Radioiodine Whole-Body Scintigraphy
Douglas Van Nostrand, Reetha Bakthula, and Frank B. Atkins 151

16 False-Positive Radioiodine Scans in Thyroid Cancer
*Brahm Shapiro, Vittoria Rufini, Ayman Jarwan, Onelio Geatti, Kimberlee J. Kearfott,
Lorraine M. Fig, Ian D. Kirkwood, John E. Freitas, and Milton D. Gross* 179

Part III The Thyroid Nodule

17. The Thyroid Nodule: *Evaluation, Risk of Malignancy, and Management*
Leonard Wartofsky 201

18 Fine Needle Aspiration: *Technique*
Yolanda C. Oertel 211

19 Thyroid Nodules: *Cellular and Biochemical Markers for Malignancy*
Kathleen A. Prendergast 213

20 Radionuclide Imaging of Thyroid Nodules
Douglas Van Nostrand 223

21 Ultrasonic Imaging of the Neck in Patients with Thyroid Cancer
Manfred Blum 229

22. Thyroid Nodules and Cancer Risk: *Surgical Management*
Orlo H. Clark 247

Part IV Well-Differentiated Thyroid Cancer: *Papillary Carcinoma*
A. Presentation

23 Papillary Cancer: *Clinical Aspects*
Leonard Wartofsky 253

24 Surgical Approach to Papillary Cancer
Orlo H. Clark 261

25 Papillary Carcinoma: *Cytology and Pathology*
Yolanda C. Oertel and James E. Oertel 263

Part IV Well-Differentiated Thyroid Cancer:
B. Initial Management

26 Prescribed Activity for Radioiodine Ablation
Douglas Van Nostrand 273

27 Thyroid Remnant Radioiodine Ablation with Recombinant Human Thyrotropin
R. Michael Tuttle and Richard J. Robbins 283

Part IV Well-Differentiated Thyroid Cancer:
C. Surveillance

28 Follow-Up Strategy in Papillary Thyroid Cancer
Henry B. Burch 289

29 Levothyroxine Therapy and Thyrotropin Suppression
Leonard Wartofsky 293

30 Thyroglobulin and Thyroglobulin Antibodies: *Measurement and Interferences*
D. Robert Dufour 297

31 Diagnosis of Recurrent Thyroid Cancer in Patients with Positive Antithyroglobulin Antibodies
Matthew D. Ringel 305

32 Surveillance Radioiodine Whole-Body Scans
Douglas Van Nostrand 309

33 Radionuclide Imaging and Treatment of Thyroid Cancer in Children
Gary L. Francis 313

34 Positron Emission Tomography in Well-Differentiated Thyroid Cancer
I. Ross McDougall 319

35 Alternative Thyroid Imaging
Anca M. Avram, Karen C. Rosenspire, Stewart C. Davidson,
John E. Freitas, and Milton D. Gross 329

36 The "Stunning" Controversy
A. Stunning: Untoward Effect of ^{131}I Thyroid Imaging Prior to Radioablation Therapy
Hee-Myung Park and Stephen K Gerard 337

B. Stunning Is Not a Problem
I. Ross McDougall 346

C. Stunning: Does it Exist? A Commentary
Douglas Van Nostrand 349

37 Ultrasonic Imaging and Identification of Metastases in Cervical Lymph Nodes
Manfred Blum 351

38 Magnetic Resonance Imaging and Computed Tomography Imaging of Thyroid Cancer
    James J. Jelinek, Kenneth D. Burman, Richard S. Young, and Alexander S. Mark *359*

39 Management of the Patient with Negative Radioiodine Scan and Elevated Serum Thyroglobulin
    Leonard Wartofsky *367*

40 Determinants of Prognosis in Papillary Thyroid Carcinoma
    Henry B. Burch *375*

41 Papillary Cancer: *Special Aspects in Children*
    Andrew J. Bauer and Merrily Poth *377*

42 Special Presentations of Thyroid Cancer in Pregnancy,
    Renal Failure, Thyrotoxicosis, and Struma Ovarii
    Kenneth D. Burman *387*

43 Thyroglossal Duct Carcinoma
    Leonard Wartofsky and Nikolaos Stathatos *393*

Part IV Well-Differentiated Thyroid Cancer
D. Treatment

44 Radiation and Radioactivity
    John E. Glenn *399*

45 Radioiodine Treatment of Distant Metastases
    Douglas Van Nostrand *411*

46 ^{131}I Treatment of Metastatic Thyroid Carcinoma
    Following Preparation by Recombinant Human Thyrotropin
    Richard J. Robbins and R. Michael Tuttle *427*

47 Dosimetry: *Dosimetrically-Determined Prescribed Activity
    of Radioiodine for the Treatment of Metastatic Thyroid Carcinoma*
    Frank B. Atkins, Douglas Van Nostrand, and Leonard Wartofsky *433*

48 Radioiodine Dosimetry with Recombinant Human Thyrotropin
    R. Michael Tuttle and Richard J. Robbins *447*

49 Use of Lithium as an Adjuvant to Radioiodine in the Treatment of Thyroid Cancer
    Monica C. Skarulis, Marina S. Zemskova, and Jacob Robbins *453*

50. Side Effects of ^{131}I for Ablation and Treatment of Well-Differentiated Thyroid Carcinoma
    Douglas Van Nostrand and John Freitas *459*

51 External Radiation Therapy of Papillary Cancer
    James D. Brierley and Richard W. Tsang *485*

Contents

52. A. Chemotherapy of Thyroid Cancer: *General Principles*
    Lawrence S. Lessin 491

    B. Chemotherapy of Well-Differentiated Papillary or Follicular Thyroid Carcinoma
    Lawrence S. Lessin 494

53 Thyroid Carcinoma; *Metastases to Bone*
    Steven P. Hodak and Kenneth D. Burman 497

54 Adjunctive Local Approaches to Metastatic Thyroid Cancer
    Leonard Wartofsky 509

Part V Well-Differentiated Thyroid Cancer: *Follicular Carcinoma*

55 Follicular Thyroid Cancer: *Clinical Aspects*
    Leonard Wartofsky 517

56 Surgical Management of Follicular Thyroid Cancer
    Orlo H. Clark 523

57 Pathology of Follicular Cancer
    Yolanda C. Oertel 527

58 Hürthle Cell Carcinoma
    Kenneth D. Burman and Leonard Wartofsky 531

59 Radionuclide Imaging, Ablation, and Treatment in Follicular Thyroid Carcinoma
    Douglas Van Nostrand 537

60 Follow-Up Strategy in Follicular Thyroid Cancer
    Henry B. Burch 539

61 PET in Follicular Cancer, Including Hürthle Cell Cancer
    I. Ross McDougall 541

62 Follicular Thyroid Cancer: *Special Aspects in Children and Adolescents*
    Andrew J. Bauer 543

63 External Radiation Therapy of Follicular Carcinoma
    James D. Brierley and Richard W. Tsang 545

64 Determinants of Prognosis in Patients with Follicular Thyroid Carcinoma
    Henry B. Burch 549

Part VI Variants of Thyroid Cancer

65. Miscellaneous and Unusual Types of Thyroid Cancer
    Kenneth D. Burman, Matthew D. Ringel, and Barry M. Shmookler 553

66. Pathology of Miscellaneous and Unusual Cancers of the Thyroid
    James E. Oertel and Yolanda C. Oertel 571

Part VII Undifferentiated Tumors: *Medullary Thyroid Carcinoma*

67 Clinical Aspects of Medullary Thyroid Carcinoma
   Douglas W. Ball *581*

68 Pathology of Medullary Thyroid Cancer
   James E. Oertel and Yolanda C. Oertel *591*

69 Medullary Carcinoma of the Thyroid: *Surgical Management*
   Orlo H. Clark *595*

70 Radionuclide Imaging of Medullary Carcinoma:
      Utility of Radiolabeled Somatostatin Analogs and Other Radiotracers
   Giuseppe Esposito *597*

71 PET in Medullary Thyroid Cancer
   I. Ross McDougall *603*

72 External Radiation Therapy of Medullary Cancer
   James D. Brierley and Richard W. Tsang *605*

73 Medullary Carcinoma of the Thyroid: *Chemotherapy*
   Lawrence S. Lessin *609*

Part VIII Undifferentiated Tumors: *Thyroid Lymphoma*

74 Thyroid Lymphoma
   Steven I. Sherman *615*

75 Pathology of Lymphoma of the Thyroid
   Yolanda C. Oertel and James E. Oertel *621*

76 FDG-PET Scanning in Lymphoma and Lymphoma of the Thyroid
   I. Ross McDougall *623*

Part IX Undifferentiated Tumors: *Anaplastic Thyroid Cancer*

77 Anaplastic Carcinoma: *Clinical Aspects*
   Steven I. Sherman *629*

78 Surgical Management of Anaplastic Thyroid Carcinoma
   Orlo H. Clark *633*

79 Pathology of Anaplastic Carcinoma
   James E. Oertel and Yolanda C. Oertel *635*

80 PET Scanning in Anaplastic Cancer of the Thyroid
   I. Ross McDougall *639*

81	External Radiation Therapy of Anaplastic Thyroid Cancer
	James D. Brierley and Richard W. Tsang *641*

82	Chemotherapy for Anaplastic Thyroid Cancer
	Lawrence S. Lessin *643*

83	Anaplastic Carcinoma: *Prognosis*
	Steven I. Sherman *647*

Part X New Frontiers and Future Directions

84	Advances in Radiation Therapy
	James D. Brierley and Richard W. Tsang *653*

85	New Approaches in Nuclear Medicine for Thyroid Cancer
	Douglas Van Nostrand *657*

86	Alternative Options and Future Directions for Thyroid Cancer Therapy
	Matthew D. Ringel *665*

87	Potential Approaches to Chemotherapy of Thyroid Cancer in the Future
	Lawrence S. Lessin *671*

Part XI Resources for Patients with Thyroid Cancer

88	Low Iodine Diets
	Kenneth D. Burman *677*

89	Appendix A: *Books and Manuals*
	Douglas Van Nostrand *683*

90	Appendix B: *Additional Sources of Information: Support Groups, Websites and Additional Information*
	Douglas Van Nostrand *685*

91	Appendix C: *Forms and Instructions for Patients Treated with Radioactivity*
	John E. Glenn *689*

Index *693*

Color Plates

The following illustrations are printed in color in the insert that follows p. 196.

Plate 1   Histology of normal adult thyroid gland (Chapter 1, Fig. 2, p. 5).
Plate 2   Papillary carcinoma invades the normal gland (Chapter 25, Fig. 1, p.264).
Plate 3   Normal thyroid tissue of the papillary carcinoma (Chapter 25, Fig. 2, p. 264).
Plate 4   Small papillae of the papillary carcinoma (Chapter 25, Fig. 3, p. 263).
Plate 5   A psammona body (Chapter 25, Fig. 4, pp. 263–264).
Plate 6   Aspirate showing papillary tissue fragments (Chapter 25, Fig. 5, pp. 263–264).
Plate 7   Aspirate showing neoplastic cells with variation in nuclear sizes (Chapter 25, Fig. 6, pp. 264–265).
Plate 8   Aspirate of papillary carcinoma showing "intranuclear cytoplasmic pseudoinclusion" (Chapter 25, Fig. 7, pp. 264–265).
Plate 9   Aspirate of papillary carcinoma showing "intranuclear cytoplasmic pseudoinclusion" (Chapter 25, Fig. 8, pp. 265–265).
Plate 10 Aspirate showing bubble-gum (chewing gum or ropy) colloid (Chapter 25, Fig. 9, pp. 264–265).
Plate 11 Papillary carcinoma (Chapter 25, Fig. 10, pp. 264–265).
Plate 12 Aspirate of psammoma bodies of the papillary carcinoma (Chapter 25, Fig. 11, pp. 264–265).
Plate 13 Multinucleated histiocyte and neoplastic cells (Chapter 25, Fig. 13, pp. 264–265).
Plate 14 Follicular pattern of papillary carcinoma (Chapter 25, Fig. 13, p. 266).
Plate 15 Follicular pattern of papillary carcinoma (Chapter 25, Fig. 14, p. 266).
Plate 16 Benign adenomatoid nodule with papillae (Chapter 25, Fig. 15, p. 266).
Plate 17 Follicular variant of papillary carcinoma (Chapter 25, Fig. 16, p. 267).
Plate 18 Follicular variant of papillary carcinoma (Chapter 25, Fig. 17, p. 266).
Plate 19 Papillary carcinoma with cystic change (Chapter 25, Fig. 18, p. 267).
Plate 20 Papillary carcinoma of the diffuse sclerosing type (Chapter 25, Fig. 19, p. 268).
Plate 21 Less well-differentiated papillary carcinoma (Chapter 25, Fig. 20, p. 269).
Plate 22 Transaxial scan showing PET, CT, and combined PET and CT (Chapter 34, Fig. 1, p. 320).
Plate 23 Coronal PET scan and PET, CT, and combined PET/CT scans (Chapter 34, Fig. 2, p. 320).
Plate 24 Whole-body ^{99m}Tc sestamibi scan (Chapter 35, Fig. 2A, pp. 330–331).
Plate 25 Demonstrated faint uptake in the left neck area (Chapter 35, Fig. 2B, pp. 330–331).
Plate 26 ^{99m}Tc sestamibi uptake in neck corresponding to papillary thyroid cancer metastasis (Chapter 35, Fig. 3, p. 332).
Plate 27 Longitudinal projections of normal lymph node on sonographic examination (Chapter 37, Fig. 1, pp. 352–353).
Plate 28 Longitudinal view of a narrow, oval normal lymph node showing physiologic vasculature (Chapter 37, Fig. 2, pp. 352–353).
Plate 29 Sonogram of neck of patient who had a total thyroidectomy (Chapter 37, Fig. 3, pp. 353–354).
Plate 30 Sonogram of a plump, heterogeneous lymph node involved with metastatic papillary thyroid cancer (Chapter 37, Fig. 4, p. 354).
Plate 31 Longitudinal view of a lymph node that was plump and therefore deemed suspicious, suggesting benign disease (Chapter 37, Fig. 5, p. 354).
Plate 32 Reduction of thyroglobulin levels with and without embolization (Chapter 53, Fig. 5, pp. 501–502).
Plate 33 CT planning images of a five-field conformal technique (Chapter 84, Fig. 1, pp. 653–654).
Plate 34 3D view of the conformal five-field beam arrangement (Chapter 84, Fig. 2, pp. 635 and 655).

Contributors

FRANK B. ATKINS, PhD • *Nuclear Medicine Physicist, Division of Nuclear Medicine, Washington Hospital Center, Washington, DC*

ANCA AVRAM, MD • *Fellow, Nuclear Medicine, Division of Nuclear Medicine, Department of Radiology, University of Michigan Medical School, Ann Arbor, MI*

JAMES R. BAKER, JR., MD • *Ruth Dow Doan Professor, Department of Medicine, Chief, Division of Allergy, Director, Center for Biologic Nanotechnology, Ann Arbor, MI*

REETHA BAKTHULA, MD • *Division of Nuclear Medicine, Washington Hospital Center, Washington, DC*

DOUGLAS W. BALL, MD • *Associate Professor of Medicine and Oncology, Johns Hopkins University School of Medicine, Baltimore, MD*

ANDREW J. BAUER, MD • *Chief, Pediatric Endocrinology, Department of Pediatrics, Walter Reed Army Medical Center, Washington, DC; Assistant Professor of Pediatrics, Uniformed Services University of Health Sciences, Bethesda, MD*

MANFRED BLUM, MD • *Professor of Medicine and Radiology and Director of Nuclear Endocrine Laboratory, New York University Medical Center, New York, NY*

JAMES D. BRIERLEY, MBBS, MRCP, FRCR, FRCSP(C) • *Associate Professor, Department of Radiation Oncology, University of Toronto, Princess Margaret Hospital, Toronto, Ontario, Canada*

HENRY B. BURCH, MD • *Chief, Endocrinology Division, Department of Medicine, Walter Reed Army Medical Center, and Associate Professor of Medicine, Uniformed Services University of the Health Sciences, Bethesda, MD*

STEPHEN J. BURGUN, MD • *Assistant Professor of Medicine, Division of Endocrinology, Department of Medicine, Ohio State University, Columbus, OH*

KENNETH D. BURMAN, MD, MACP • *Director, Division of Endocrinology, Washington Hospital Center, Professor of Medicine, Georgetown University School of Medicine, Washington, DC, and Uniformed Services University of Health Sciences, Bethesda, MD*

ORLO H. CLARK, MD, FACS • *Professor of Surgery, University of California, San Francisco, School of Medicine, San Francisco, CA*

STEWART DAVIDSON, MBBS, GRAD. DIP. CLIN. EPI. • *Fellow, Nuclear Medicine, Division of Nuclear Medicine, Department of Radiology, University of Michigan Medical School, Ann Arbor, MI*

D. ROBERT DUFOUR, MD • *Chief, Pathology and Laboratory Medicine (Retired), Veterans Affairs Medical Center, Washington, DC, Professor of Pathology, George Washington University Medical Center, Washington, DC, Clinical Professor of Pathology, Uniformed Services University of the Health Sciences, Bethesda, MD*

GENNADY ERMAK, PhD • *Assistant Professor, Division of Molecular and Computational Biology, and Ethel Percy Andrus Gerontology Center, and University of Southern California, Los Angeles, CA*

GIUSEPPE ESPOSITO, MD • *Staff Physician, Division of Nuclear Medicine, Washington Hospital Center, Washington, DC*

LORRAINE M. FIG, MB, ChB • *Nuclear Medicine Service, Department of Veterans Affairs Health System, Ann Arbor, MI*

JAMES J. FIGGE, MD, MBA, FACP • *Adjunct Associate Professor, Department of Biomedical Sciences, School of Public Health, State University of New York; Medical Director, Capital District Physicians' Health Plan and Department of Medicine, St. Peter's Hospital and Albany Medical Center Hospital, Albany, NY*

GARY L. FRANCIS, MD • *Fellowship Program Director, Department of Pediatric Endocrinology, Professor of Pediatrics, Uniformed Services University of Health Sciences, Bethesda, MD*

JOHN E. FREITAS, MD • *Director, Nuclear Medicine Services, Department of Radiology, St. Joseph Mercy Hospital, Ann Arbor, MI; Clinical Professor of Radiology, University of Michigan Medical School, Ann Arbor, MI*

ONELIO GEATTI, MD • *Servizio di Medicina Nucleare, Ospedale Maggiore, Trieste, Italy*

STEPHEN K. GERARD, MD, PhD • *Chief, Nuclear Medicine, Seton Medical Center, Daly City, CA*

GREGORY GERASIMOV, MD • *ICCIDD Regional Coordinator for Eastern Europe and Central Asia, Professor, Endocrinology Research Center, Moscow, Russia*

JOHN E. GLENN, PhD • *Director, Radiation Safety, Georgetown University Hospital, Washington, DC*
MILTON D. GROSS, MD • *Professor, Division of Nuclear Medicine, Department of Radiology, University of Michigan Medical School and Director/Chief, Nuclear Medicine and Radiation Safety Service, Department of Veterans Affairs Health Systems, Washington, DC (field based) and Ann Arbor, MI*
STEVEN P. HODAK, MD • *Division of Endocrinology and Metabolism, University of Pittsburgh School of Medicine, Pittsburgh, PA*
AYMAN JARWAN, MD • *Department of Nuclear Engineering and Radiological Sciences, University of Michigan, Ann Arbor, MI*
JAMES JELINEK, MD, FACR • *Chairman, Department of Radiology, Washington Hospital Center, Washington, DC*
TIMOTHY JENNINGS, MD • *Associate Professor of Pathology, Albany Medical Center, Albany, NY*
NIKOLAI A. KARTEL, PhD • *Professor and Director, Head of the Molecular Genetics Laboratory, Institute of Genetics and Cytology, National Academy of Science of Belarus, Minsk, Belarus*
KIMBERLEE J. KEARFOTT, MD • *Department of Nuclear Engineering and Radiological Sciences, University of Michigan, Ann Arbor, MI*
IAN D. KIRKWOOD, MD, MBBS • *Department of Nuclear Medicine, Royal Adelaide Hospital, North Terrace, Adelaide, Australia*
LAWRENCE S. LESSIN, MD, MACP • *Director, Washington Cancer Institute, Washington Hospital Center, and Clinical Professor of Medicine, George Washington University School of Medicine and Health Sciences, Washington, DC*
ALEXANDER S. MARK, MD • *Director, Magnetic Resonance Imaging, Department of Radiology, Washington Hospital Center, Washington, DC*
ERNEST L. MAZZAFERRI, MD, MACP • *Emeritus Professor of Medicine and Chairman, Department of Medicine, Ohio State University Medical Center, Columbus, OH, Professor of Medicine, University of Florida, Gainesville, FL*
MICHAEL T. McDERMOTT, MD • *Professor of Medicine, Practice Director, S/M Endocrinology/Metabolism/Diabetes Disease, University of Colorado Hospital, Aurora, CO*
I. ROSS McDOUGALL, MD, PhD • *Professor of Radiology and Medicine, Stanford University School of Medicine, Portola Valley, CA*
JAMES E. OERTEL, MD • *Chairman Emeritus, Department of Endocrine Pathology, Armed Forces Institute of Pathology, Washington, DC*
YOLANDA C. OERTEL, MD • *Professor Emerita of Pathology, The George Washington University School of Medicine and Health Sciences; Director, Fine Needle Aspiration Service, Washington Hospital Center, Washington, DC*
HEE-MYUNG PARK, MD • *Professor Emeritus of Radiology, Indiana University, Indianapolis, and Professor of Nuclear Medicine, Kwandong University, Korea*
MERRILY POTH, MD • *Professor, Department of Pediatrics, Uniformed Services University of the Health Sciences, Bethesda, MD; Division of Pediatric Endocrinology, Walter Reed Army Medical Center, Washington, DC*
KATHLEEN A. PRENDERGAST, MD • *Attending Physician, Section of Endocrinology, Department of Medicine, Washington Hospital Center, Washington, DC*
E. CHESTER RIDGWAY, MD, MACP • *Director, Division of Endocrinology and Associate Dean, University of Colorado Health Sciences Medical Center, Denver, CO*
MATTHEW D. RINGEL, MD • *Associate Professor of Medicine, Divisions of Endocrinology and Oncology and Human Cancer Genetics, Ohio State University, Columbus, OH*
JACOB ROBBINS, MD • *Scientist Emeritus, Clinical Endocrinology Branch, National Institute of Diabetes, Digestive and Kidney Diseases, National Institutes of Health, Bethesda, MD*
RICHARD J. ROBBINS, MD • *Professor of Medicine, Cornell University Medical College, Chief, Endocrine Service, Associate Chair of Medicine for Academic Affairs, Memorial Sloan-Kettering Cancer Center, New York, NY*
KAREN ROSENSPIRE, MD, PhD • *Fellow, Nuclear Medicine, Division of Nuclear Medicine, Department of Radiology, University of Michigan Medical School, Ann Arbor, MI*

Contributors

VITTORIA RUFINI, MD • *Instutito di Medicina Nucleare, Universita Cattolica del Sacro Cuore, Rome Italy*
ARTHUR B. SCHNEIDER, MD, PhD • *Chief, Section of Endocrinology and Metabolism, University of Illinois at Chicago, Chicago, IL*
BRAHM SHAPIRO, MB ChB, PhD • *Professor of Radiology (retired), Division of Nuclear Medicine, Department of Radiology, University of Michigan Medical Center, Ann Arbor, MI*
STEVEN I. SHERMAN, MD • *Section of Endocrine Neoplasia and Hormonal Disorders, M. D. Anderson Cancer Center, and Assistant Professor of Medicine, University of Texas-Houston Medical School, Houston, TX*
BARRY M. SHMOOKLER, MD • *Emeritus Director of Endocrine Pathology, Department of Pathology, Washington Hospital Center and Medlantic Research Institute, Washington, DC*
MONICA C. SKARULIS, MD • *Senior Clinical Investigator, Clinical Endocrinology Branch, National Institute of Diabetes, Digestive and Kidney Diseases, National Institutes of Health, Bethesda, MD*
NIKOLAOS STATHATOS, MD • *Division of Endocrinology, Department of Medicine, Washington Hospital Center and Georgetown University Hospital, Washington, DC*
RICHARD W. TSANG, MD, FRCSP(C) • *Associate Professor, Department of Radiation Oncology, University of Toronto, Princess Margaret Hospital, Toronto, Ontario, Canada*
R. MICHAEL TUTTLE, MD • *Associate Professor of Medicine, Cornell University Medical College; Clinical Researcher, Attending Physician, Memorial Sloan-Kettering Cancer Center, Endocrinology Service, New York, NY*
DOUGLAS VAN NOSTRAND, MD, FACP, FACNP • *Director, Division of Nuclear Medicine, Washington Hospital Center, Washington, DC*
HENRY N. WAGNER, JR., MD • *Professor of Environmental Sciences, Bloomberg School of Public Health, Johns Hopkins University, Baltimore, MD*
SU HE WANG, MD • *Research Assistant Professor, Department of Internal Medicine, University of Michigan Medical School, Ann Arbor, MI*
LEONARD WARTOFSKY, MD, MACP • *Chairman, Department of Medicine, Washington Hospital Center, Professor of Medicine, Anatomy, Physiology and Genetics, Uniformed Services University of Health Sciences, Bethesda, MD, and Professor of Medicine, Georgetown University School of Medicine, Washington, DC*
KATHERINE B. WEBER, MD • *S/M Endocrinology/Metabolism/Diabetes Disease, University of Colorado Hospital, Aurora, CO*
DIMA YARMOLINSKY • *Institute of Genetics and Cytology, National Academy of Science of Belarus, Minsk, Belarus*
RICHARD S. YOUNG, MD • *Attending Staff Radiologist, Department of Radiology, Washington Hospital Center, Washington, DC*
MARINA S. ZEMSKOVA, MD • *Clinical Associate, Clinical Endocrinology Branch, National Institute of Diabetes, Digestive and Kidney Disease, National Institutes of Health, Bethesda, MD*

Part I
General Considerations I
Thyroid Cancer

1
Anatomy and Physiology of the Thyroid Gland
Clinical Correlates to Thyroid Cancer

Nikolaos Stathatos

To better understand the biology of thyroid malignancies, it is extremely important to have a thorough understanding of the thyroid's relationship to its surrounding structures, both anatomically and functionally. This would allow a clinician to understand and predict the behavior of such factors as local invasion, regional lymph node, as well as distant metastasis. This short review focuses on some aspects of thyroid anatomy and physiology that are clinically relevant to the diagnosis and management of thyroid cancer.

THYROID ANATOMY, HISTOLOGY, AND EMBRYOLOGY

The thyroid gland is a butterfly-shaped organ located anteriorly to the trachea at the level of the second and third tracheal rings. Its name originates from the Greek term "thyreos," which means shield (named after the laryngeal thyroid cartilage). It consists of two lobes connected by the isthmus in the midline. Its bilaterality is an important clinical fact because the presence of malignant cells on one or both sides can significantly alter the management of the patient, e.g., requiring more extensive surgery, such as bilateral neck dissections if there is local extension of the tumor. Each lobe is about 3–4 cm long, about 2 cm wide, and only a few millimeters thick. Because of its very close anatomic relationship to the rounded trachea, nodules arising from the posterior aspect of the gland are usually inaccessible to the examining fingers and therefore often missed on a routine clinical examination. The isthmus is 12–15 mm high and connects the two lobes. Occasionally, a pyramidal lobe is located in the midline, superior to the isthmus (Fig. 1). It represents a remnant of the thyroglossal duct, as the primitive thyroid gland descends from the base of the tongue to its final location in the neck during embryonic development. Anatomic variations of the thyroid gland occur and are encountered in clinical practice; one of the more common is thyroid hemiagenesis (1), with only one lobe and an isthmus of the gland. Hemiagenetic thyroid lobes are susceptible to the same abnormalities as are normal thyroid glands, including nodules and thyroid cancer.

A fibrous capsule covers the thyroid gland. Nodules within the parenchyma of the gland may also have a capsule or pseudocapsule. Surgical pathology reports may refer to tumor invasion "through the capsule," and for staging purposes, prognosis, and management, it is important to know if this represents extension through the capsule of the gland into the surrounding perithyroidal tissues. Several key structures are located in relation to the capsule and should be considered in the context of surgery on the thyroid gland, such as the parathyroid glands and the recurrent laryngeal nerve. This is particularly significant with total thyroidectomy in patients with thyroid cancer. The small parathyroid glands are located in the posterior aspect of this capsule. Their identification and preservation is critical during surgery and can be particularly difficult with invasive cancers that require extensive surgery for complete resection, including modified lymph node dissections. Also, close monitoring of their function by measurements of serum total and ionized calcium in the early postoperative period is important to avoid or adequately treat surgical hypoparathyroidism in a timely manner.

The recurrent laryngeal nerves are the other notable structures in this regard. These nerves provide an essential part of the innervation of the larynx, and any injury can result in symptoms that range from a hoarse voice to stridor and the need for a tracheostomy. They originate from the vagus nerve at the level of the aortic arch and turn superiorly toward the tracheoesophageal groove. Several anatomic variations have been described, and the recurrent laryngeal nerve runs laterally to the tracheoesophageal groove most commonly on the right side (2,3). It runs close to the inferior thyroid artery and can be found anteriorly, posteriorly, or in between the branches of the blood vessel. Several surgical approaches have been proposed to try to identify and preserve this nerve during surgery of the thyroid gland. Most investigators recommend identifying the nerve before ligating the artery to

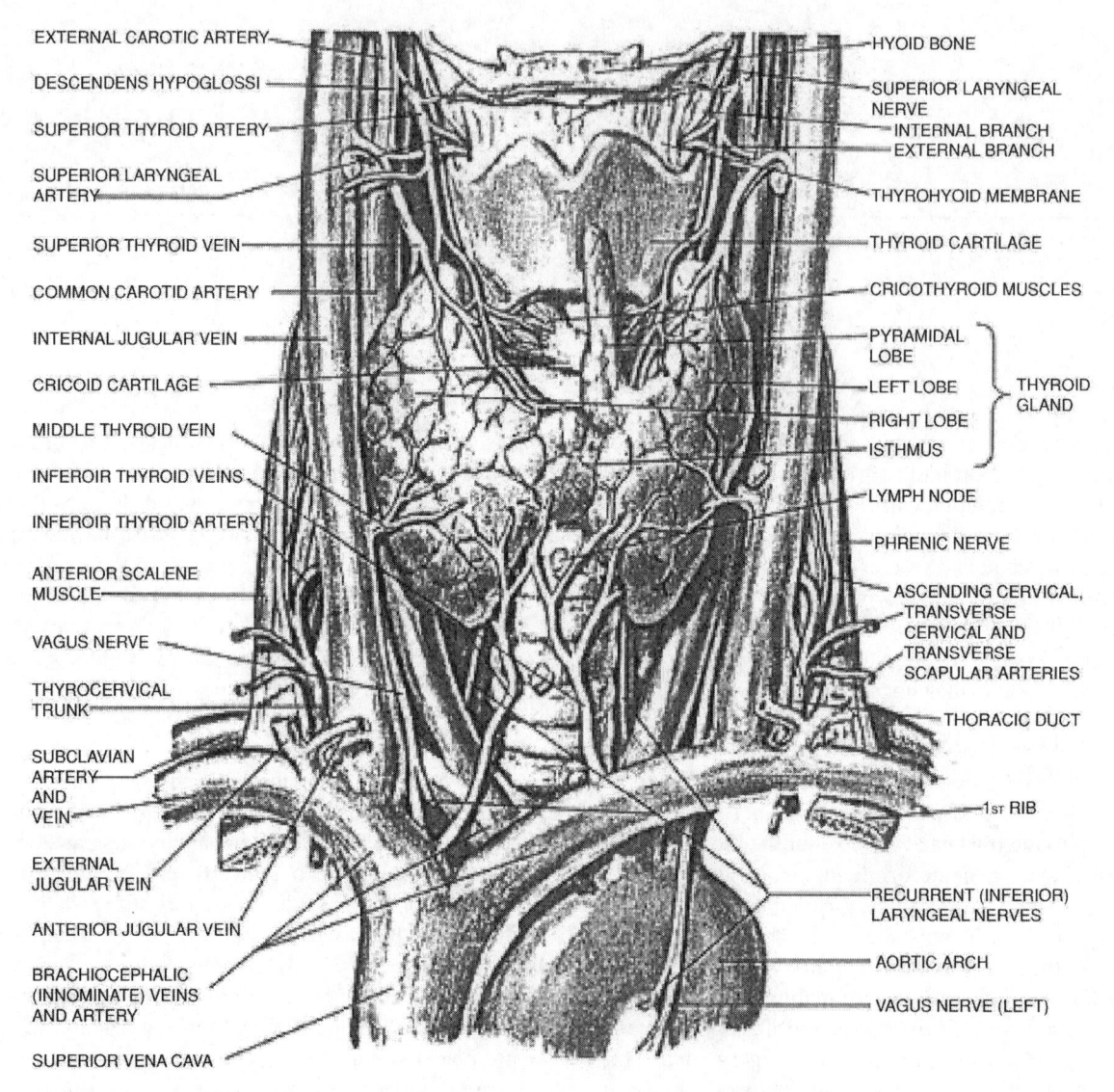

Fig. 1. Thyroid anatomy. Thyroid relations with surrounding cervical structures. (Color illustration is printed in insert following p. 198.)

prevent inadvertent injury to the nerve, but there are variations in the proposed methods to achieve this. As the nerve travels superiorly in or laterally to the tracheoesophageal groove, it is located directly posterior to the thyroid gland itself and can be adherent to it. This requires special attention by the thyroid surgeon to prevent damage to the nerve as the thyroid lobe is removed. Another variation is a division of the recurrent laryngeal nerve before entering the larynx (2,3). In less than 1% of cases, an anomalous non-recurrent nerve has been reported, originating from the cervical potion of the vagus nerve (also called the "inferior laryngeal nerve"), instead of the recurrent laryngeal nerve. This nerve is usually seen on the right side of the neck (4).

The gland's blood supply comes from two sets of arteries bilaterally: the superior thyroid arteries originate from the external carotid arteries. They descend to the superior poles of the thyroid gland and are accompanied by the superior laryngeal nerve. This nerve originates from the inferior vagus ganglion. As it approaches the larynx, it divides into the external and internal branches. The internal branch supplies sensory innervation to the supraglottic larynx, and the external branch innervates the cricothyroid muscle (5). It is usually recommended during a complete thyroidectomy. The surgeon should ligate the superior thyroid artery as close to the thyroid gland as possible to try to avoid damaging any branches of the superior laryngeal nerve.

Clearly, the type of symptoms a patient will develop postoperatively is highly dependent on the experience and skill of the surgeon and the type of nerve injury. Unfortunately, it is not rare that the surgeon may have to sacrifice one of the recurrent laryngeal nerves in an *en bloc* resection because cancer has directly invaded the nerve.

The inferior thyroid artery is a branch of the thyrocervical trunk, and as noted, this artery is in close proximity with the recurrent laryngeal nerve. Occasionally, the thyroidea ima artery also provides blood supply to the thyroid gland, and it originates from either the thyrocervical trunk or the arch of the aorta. The venous drainage of the thyroid gland consists of three sets of veins: the superior, middle, and inferior. The superior and middle thyroid veins drain into the internal jugular veins, and the inferior veins anastomose with each other anteriorly to the trachea and drain into the brachiocephalic vein.

The lymphatic drainage of the thyroid gland mainly involves the deep cervical lymph nodes in the central compartment. This area is usually dissected by the surgeons performing thyroidectomies for malignant disease to minimize the chance of residual malignancy in the neck. A few lymphatic vessels also drain to the paratracheal lymph nodes.

Another important aspect of thyroid anatomy is the potential presence of thyroid tissue at locations that are considered "ectopic." To better understand this, a short description of the embryonic development of the thyroid gland is necessary. The primitive thyroid gland develops in the first month of gestation in the pharyngeal floor and elongates caudally, forming the thyroglossal duct. As the duct descends to its final location in the neck, it comes in contact with the ultimobranchial pouch of the fourth pharyngeal pouch—the origin of the C cells that produce calcitonin. Their final resting place is at the lower part of the upper one third of the adult thyroid gland. Once the thyroid gland reaches its destination at the base of the neck, the thyroglossal duct regresses and usually disappears, leaving a remnant of only the foramen caecum at the base of the tongue. Sometimes, its distal part near the thyroid gland persists and forms the pyramidal lobe of the thyroid gland. Occasionally, the thyroglossal duct remains and presents (most often during childhood) as a neck mass. This mass usually represents a benign thyroglossal duct cyst, but cases of primary thyroid malignancy have been described at any place along the track of the duct's migration (6). In addition to these ectopic sites for thyroid tissue and thyroid malignancy, benign ectopic thyroid tissue has been described in many different parts of the human body. These include the base of the tongue (7–10), intralaryngeal (11), intratracheal (12), submandibular (13), carotid bifurcation (14), intracardiac (15,16), ascending aorta (17), gallbladder (18), porta hepatis (19), intramesenteric (20), and ovarian (21). Thyroid cancer has been described in many of these sites as well, e.g., at the base of the tongue or in the ovary (struma ovarii; 16,22–24), but whether some of these tumors are primary or secondary is a matter of debate.

Another interesting aspect of ectopic thyroid tissue is the presence of benign thyroid tissue in cervical lymph nodes. Significant controversy exists in the literature about whether the thyroid tissue deposits are indeed benign or representative of metastatic disease (25). Nevertheless, the presence of ectopic thyroid tissue—benign or malignant—can confuse the clinical perspective and may require a different therapeutic approach to adequately treat thyroid cancer and to follow the patient optimally.

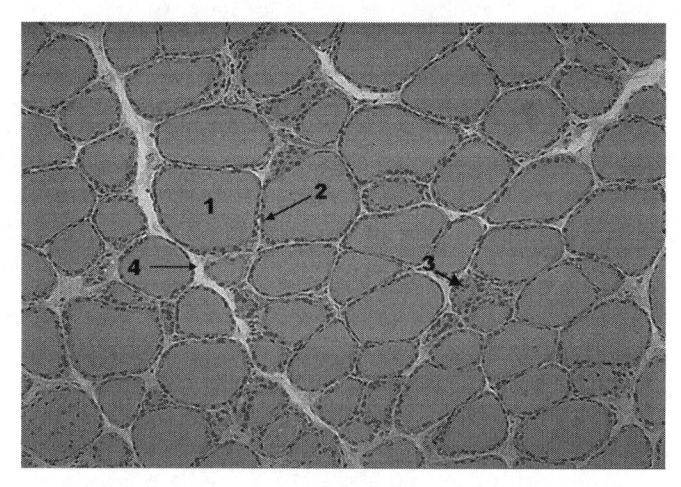

Fig. 2. Histology of normal adult thyroid gland: 1, Colloid of a thyroid follicle; 2, follicular cells. Single layer cells forming a follicle; 3, parafollicular cells (C cells); 4, connective tissue septum.

The thyroid gland has a characteristic histology; because thyroid cancer originates from this tissue and maintains some of its characterists, it is important to have a thorough understanding of this aspect of the thyroid gland. The main histological structure is the thyroid follicle (Fig. 2), which consists of a single layer or epithelial cells—the thyroid follicular cells—surrounded by a basement membrane. The follicle is filled with a colloid material that contains thyroglobulin, the precursor macromolecule and storage protein for the thyroid hormones: thyroxine (T4) and triiodothyronine (T3). The size of these follicles varies significantly, even within a single thyroid gland, but are usually about 200 μm. Every 20–40 follicles are separated from the rest by connective tissue septa. Although most authors believe that the thyroid cells are monoclonal in origin, emerging evidence (26) suggests that different parts of the thyroid originate from different precursors, most interestingly with different malignant potential. These could be reflected by those groups of thyroid follicles separated by the connective tissue septa. Blood vessels and supporting connecting tissue are seen in between the follicles, as well as groups of C cells (also called "parafollicular cells") that produce calcitonin. As mentioned above, these cells are concentrated in the lower part of the upper third of the thyroid gland and the reason why many authors consider nodules in that part of the thyroid gland as more suspicious for medullary thyroid cancer.

THYROID PHYSIOLOGY

The main function of the thyroid gland is to provide adequate amounts of thyroid hormone for the proper regulation

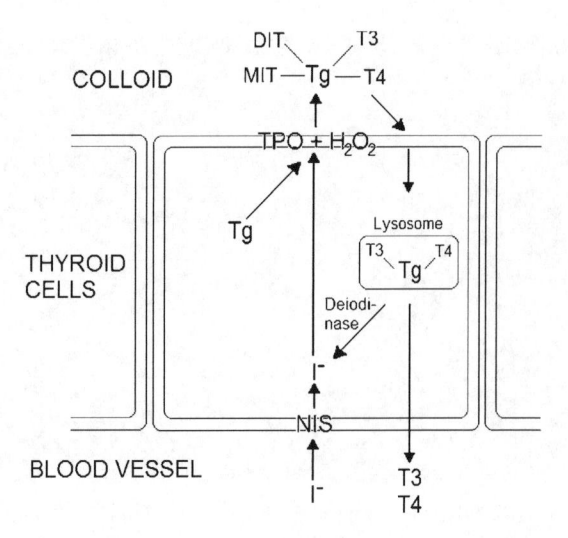

Fig. 3. Organification of iodide, synthesis and release of thyroid hormome. NIS, Sodium–iodide symporter; Tg, thyroglobulin; TPO, thyroid peroxidase; MID, monoiodotyrosine; DIT, diiodotyrosine; H_2O_2, hydrogen peroxide; T3, Triiodothyronine; T4, thyroxine; I^-, iodide.

of a large number of bodily functions, e.g., energy expenditure and metabolic rate. Thyroid hormone is an iodinated hormone and thus requires the ability of the thyroid gland to concentrate iodine from the circulation and organify it for incorporation into the thyroid hormone molecules. The amount of thyroid hormone produced by the thyroid gland is tightly regulated in the human body under normal conditions. This process is very complex and requires several steps, both within and outside of the thyroid gland. Each step may have clinical relevance to thyroid cancer.

First, it should be stressed again that thyroid cancer cells are derived from normal noncancerous thyroid cells and use the same cellular mechanisms to function, depending on their level of dedifferentiation. As a result, these various physiologic functions of thyroid cells are used to identify, characterize, and ultimately treat these malignancies. One of the most critical properties of a thyroid cell is its ability to trap iodine from the circulation, most often against a concentration gradient. This is accomplished by the sodium–iodide symporter (NIS), located at the basal membrane of the thyrocyte (Fig. 3). This active, energy-requiring process can concentrate iodide in the thyrocyte some 20–40-fold above its level in the circulation and is accomplished by the transport of sodium into the cell. Notably, similar iodide transport mechanisms are also present in other tissues, such as the salivary gland. Thus, because salivary tissue will actively transport radioactive iodine when administered, patients may suffer from radiation-induced saliadenitis or xerostomia when treated with radioactive iodine for thyroid cancer.

For organification of the iodide, the enzyme thyroid peroxidase (TPO), together with hydrogen peroxide, are required to organify the inorganic iodide and incorporate it into a tyrosine residue on thyroglobulin. This occurs in the apical membrane of the thyroid cell, facing the colloid (Fig. 3). Each tyrosine molecule can take up to four iodide atoms, forming the different types of thyroid hormone (Fig. 4). Once the thyroid hormone has been synthesized, it is stored in linkage within the thyroglobulin molecule in the colloid of thyroid follicles. Under stimulation by thyrotropin (TSH), the gland receives the signal that thyroid hormone release is needed, and fragments of thyroglobulin enter the thyrocyte (pinocytosis) and are cleaved by endopeptidases in the endosomes and lysosomes. Thyroxine and triiodothyronine are produced and released into the circulation. Under normal conditions, the thyroid gland output consists of mainly thyroxine (~90% or ~75–100 µg/d) and a small amount of triiodothyronine (~10% or 6 µg/d).

Thus, the processes of thyroid hormone synthesis and iodide uptake are largely regulated by TSH, a pituitary hormone that stimulates both of these thyroid functions. As described in detail in the rest of this volume, either endogenous TSH stimulation prompted by thyroid hormone withdrawal or exogenous recombinant human TSH is critical in the diagnosis and treatment of thyroid cancer. On the contrary, as TSH has mitogenic activity, its chronic suppression for thyroxine therapy is critical to the prevention of thyroid cancer growth.

Another important aspect of molecular thyroid physiology is the effect that iodine has on thyroid function. As discussed previously, the thyroid gland actively concentrates iodine from the circulation to synthesize the thyroid hormone. It is a well-known fact that the iodine deficiency causes goiters, and if such patients are given iodine, production of excessive amounts of thyroid hormone and even hyperthyroidism is possible, at least transiently. This result is called the "jod-Basedow phenomenon" (27). The mechanism for this phenomenon is unclear, but it is thought that it is either because of rapid iodination of poorly iodinated thyroglobulin or the "fueling" of a subclinical autonomous functioning thyroid tissue, as in a "hot" nodule or in Graves' disease (28). Alternatively, if there is an excess of iodine present in thyrocytes, the sodium iodide symporter and TPO are inhibited to prevent excessive amounts of thyroid hormone from being synthesized. This inhibition is referred to as "the Wolff-Chaikoff phenomenon" (29). A high concentration of inorganic iodide is needed for this effect. This inhibition of iodide organification is temporary because the inhibition of iodide transport by the NIS depletes intracellular iodine, allowing the system to reset with new iodide organification— this is called the "escape from the Wolff-Chaikoff effect."

Several molecules discussed have significant clinical utility in the daily management of thyroid cancer. Measurement of the TSH receptor, thyroglobulin, antithyroglobulin antibodies, and TPO can be used to determine if a neoplasm is of thyroid origin. Multiple other relevant molecules have been described, such as thyroid transcription factors 1 and 2,

Fig. 4. Thyroid hormones and their precursors.

galectin 3, and oncofetal fibronectin. Assessment of the presence of such proteins may be particularly important in the evaluation of material obtained by fine-needle aspiration of suspected metastatic lesions. See Chapter 19 for a more detailed description of molecular thyroid markers.

REFERENCES

1. Burman KD, Adler RA, Wartofsky L. Hemiagenesis of the thyroid gland. Am J Med 1975; 58:143–146.
2. Monfared A, Saenz Y, Terris DJ. Endoscopic resection of the submandibular gland in a porcine model. Laryngoscope 2002; 112:1089–1093.
3. Moreau S, Goullet de Rugy M, Babin E, et al. The recurrent laryngeal nerve: related vascular anatomy. Laryngoscope 1998; 108: 1351–1353.
4. Abboud B, Aouad R. Non-recurrent inferior laryngeal nerve in thyroid surgery: report of three cases and review of the literature. J Laryngol Otol 2004; 118:139–142.
5. Miller FR, Netterville JL. Surgical management of thyroid and parathyroid disorders. Med Clin N Amer 1999; 83:247–259.
6. Naghavi SE, Jalali MM. Papillary carcinoma of thyroglossal duct cyst. Med Sci Monit 2003; 9:CS67–CS70.
7. Tang ZH, Li WY. Diagnosis of ectopic thyroid in the tongue root by 99mTcO4(-) and 131I radionuclide thyroid imaging: report of one case. Di Yi Jun Yi Da Xue Xue Bao 2003; 23:1041–1042.
8. Thomas G, Hollat R, Daniels JS, et al. Ectopic lingual thyroid: a case report. Int J Oral Maxillofac Surg 2003; 32:219–221.
9. Boer A, Polus K. Lingual thyroid: a rare disease resembling base of tongue neoplasm. Magy Onkol 2002; 46:347–349.
10. Chiu TT, Su CY, Hwang CF, et al. Massive bleeding from an ectopic lingual thyroid follicular adenoma during pregnancy. Am J Otolaryngol 2002; 23:185–188.
11. Jimenez Oliver V, Ruiz Rico R, Davila Morillo A, et al. Intra-laryngeal ectopic thyroid tissue. Report of one case and review of the literature. Acta Otorhinolaryngol Esp 2002; 53:54–59.
12. Byrd MC, Thompson LD, Wieneke JA. Intratracheal ectopic thyroid tissue: a case report and literature review. Ear Nose Throat J 2003; 82:514–518.
13. Ulug T, Ulubil SA, Alagol F. Dual ectopic thyroid: report of a case. J Laryngol Otol 2003; 117:574–576.
14. Hollander EJ, Visser MJ, van Baalen JM. Accessory thyroid gland at carotid bifurcation presenting as a carotid body tumor: case report and review of the literature. J Vasc Surg 2004; 39:260–262.
15. Larysz B, Jedrzychowska-Baraniak J, Nikodemska I, et al. Ectopic thyroid tissue in the heart—a case report. Kardiol Pol 2003; 59:149–151.
16. Chosia M, Waligorski S, Listewnik MH, Wiechowski S. Ectopic thyroid tissue as a tumour of the heart—case report and review of the literature. Pol J Pathol 2002; 53:173–175.
17. Williams RJ, Lindop G, Butler J. Ectopic thyroid tissue on the ascending aorta: an operative finding. Ann Thorac Surg 2002; 73:1642–1647.
18. Ihtiyar E, Isiksoy S, Algin C, et al. Ectopic thyroid in the gallbladder: report of a case. Surg Today 2003; 33:777–780.
19. Ghanem N, Bley T, Altehoefer C, et al. Ectopic thyroid gland in the porta hepatis and lingua. Thyroid 2003; 13:503–507.
20. Gungor B, Kebat T, Ozaslan C, et al. Intra-abdominal ectopic thyroid presenting with hyperthyroidism: report of a case. Surg Today 2002; 32:148–150.
21. Ribeiro-Silva A, Bezerra AM, Serafini LN. Malignant Struma Ovarii: an autopsy report of a clinically unsuspected tumor. Gynecol Oncol 2002; 87:213–215.
22. Perez JS, Munoz M, Naval L, Blasco A, Diaz FJ. Papillary carcinoma arising in lingual thyroid. J Cranio-maxillofac Surg 2003; 31:179–182.
23. Massine RE, Durning SJ, Koroscil TM. Lingual thyroid carcinoma: a case report and review of the literature. Thyroid 2001; 11:1191–1196.
24. Kao SY, Tu H, Chang RC, et al. Primary ectopic thyroid papillary carcinoma in the floor of the mouth and tongue: a case report. Br J Oral Maxillofac Surg 2002; 40:213–215.
25. Meyer JS, Steinberg LS. Microscopically benign thyroid follicles in cervical lymph nodes. Serial section study of lymph node inclusions and entire thyroid gland in 5 cases. Cancer 1969; 24:302–311.
26. Jovanovic L, Delahunt B, McIver B, et al. Thyroid gland clonality revisited: the embryonal patch size of the normal human thyroid gland is very large, suggesting X-chromosome inactivation; tumor clonality studies of thyroid tumors have to be interpreted with caution. J Clin Endocrinol Metab 2003; 88:3284–3291.
27. Stanbury JB, Ermans AE, Bourdoux P, et al. Iodine-induced hyperthyroidism: occurrence and epidemiology. Thyroid 1998; 8:83–100.
28. Ermans AM, Camus M. Modifications of thyroid function induced by chronic administration of iodide in the presence of "autonomous" thyroid tissue. Acta Endocrinol (Copenh) 1972; 70:463–475.
29. Wolff J, Chaikoff I. Plasma inorganic iodide as a homeostatic regulator of thyroid function. J Biol Chem 1948; 147:555.

2
Epidemiology of Thyroid Cancer

James J. Figge, M.D.

INCIDENCE

Thyroid cancer is the most common endocrine malignancy, accounting for 1.9% of all new malignant tumors (excluding skin cancer and *in situ* carcinomas) diagnosed annually in the United States (0.92% of cancers in men; 2.9% in women; *1*). Annual incidence rates vary by geographic area, age, and sex. The age-adjusted annual incidence (from 1996 to 2000) in the United States is 68 new cases per million *(2,3)*, with a higher incidence in women (99/million) than men (36/million) *(2,4)*. Approximately 25,690 new cases of thyroid cancer are now diagnosed annually in the United States with a female : male ratio close to 3 : 1 *(1)*. Worldwide, incidence rates are highest in certain geographic areas, such as Hawaii (119/million women and 45/million men), probably as a result of local environmental influences *(2,5)*. Rates in Poland are among the lowest recorded: 14 per million women and four per million men *(6)*. Thyroid cancer is very rare in children under age 15. The annual U.S. incidence in this population is 2.2 per million girls and 0.9 per million boys *(7)*. The annual incidence of thyroid cancer increases with age, peaking between 100 and 120 per million by the fifth through eighth decades *(2)*.

The incidence of thyroid cancer has increased over a period of several decades in the United States, as well as several other countries, particularly among women *(2–4,8–20)*. For example, in Connecticut, the annual age-standardized incidence in women has progressively increased from 13 per million in 1935–1939, to 36 per million in 1965–1969, to 45 per million in 1985–1989, and reaching 58 per million in 1990–1991. The corresponding figures for men are two per million, 18 per million, 21 per million, and 26 per million, respectively *(4)*. The precise reasons for the increase are not clearly understood but may be related, at least in part, to the introduction of improved diagnostic methodology (e.g., ultrasound, thyroid scans, and fine-needle aspiration biopsy) and improvements in cancer registration *(4,20)*. In the United States, the increased incidence between 1935 and 1975 may also be a consequence of therapeutic radiation treatments administered to the head and neck region of children *(9,21*; see Chapter 7). However, elevations in thyroid cancer incidence were documented in other countries where childhood radiation treatments were never commonly employed *(13,15,19)*; therefore, other factors must also be involved. Exposure to fallout from nuclear weapons testing has been suggested as an influence in Europe, but epidemiological data indicate that there are still more important factors *(14)*. The incidence of thyroid cancer is no longer rising in certain countries, such as Norway and Iceland *(15–17)*, but it continues to rise in the United States *(2)*.

PREVALENCE

Thyroid cancer prevalence rates vary widely by geographic area, patient population, and method of survey. Autopsy rates ranging from 0.03% to over 2% have been reported *(22–26)*. Mortensen and colleagues *(22)* reported on 1000 consecutive routine autopsies and found a 2.8% prevalence rate of thyroid carcinoma. The high cancer prevalence can be attributed to the meticulous histological evaluation protocol *(22)*. On routine clinical assessment, 61% (17/28) of the cancers originated from thyroid glands that were apparently normal *(23)*. Similar prevalence rates (2.3–2.7%) were reported by Bisi and colleagues *(24)* and Silverberg and Vidone *(25)*. The high prevalence rates reported in the latter two studies may have also been influenced by the highly selected inpatient populations studied and may not reflect the prevalence in the general population.

Small foci of papillary thyroid carcinoma, measuring 1 cm or less in diameter, can be classified as "papillary microcarcinomas" *(27)* and occur frequently in autopsy material (reviewed in ref. *28*). Most papillary microcarcinomas measure between 4 and 7 mm *(29)*. These can be subdivided into "tiny" (5–10-mm diameter) and "minute" carcinomas (<5-mm diameter; *27,30–33*). The term "occult"

From: *Thyroid Cancer: A Comprehensive Guide to Clinical Management, 2/e*
Edited by: L. Wartofsky and D. Van Nostrand © Humana Press Inc., Totowa, NJ

carcinoma has no pathological meaning and should be abandoned in favor of these more precisely defined terms, as advocated by LiVolsi (27). Papillary microcarcinomas are usually detected by meticulous sectioning of the thyroid at 2–3-mm intervals, with detailed microscopic examination of each section. The highest prevalence rate of papillary thyroid microcarcinoma (≤1-cm diameter) was reported from Finland (34), with 33.7% of 101 cases harboring this finding. Rates over 20% have been reported from Japan (35,36), whereas the rate of papillary microcarcinoma in Olmsted County, Minnesota, is much lower (5.1%; 37). Minute papillary carcinomas (<5 mm) are rarely detected clinically and are believed to exhibit a relatively benign clinical course. However, there are occasional reports of distant metastases (e.g., pulmonary metastases) that arise from minute papillary carcinomas (38).

Thyroid cancer prevalence rates are significantly greater than incidence figures, reflecting that substantial numbers of patients survive several decades or longer. Data in the Connecticut registry show a prevalence rate of 677 cases per million in women and 237 cases per million in men (39). These data refer only to clinically apparent disease and are therefore lower than the rates in many autopsy series (22–25).

MORTALITY

The annual mortality from thyroid cancer is low—five deaths per million individuals per year (2), presumably reflecting the good prognosis for most thyroid cancers. Mortality rates are lowest in individuals under age 50 and increase sharply thereafter (2). There are about 1490 deaths from thyroid cancer annually in the United States (1), accounting for 0.26% of all cancer deaths (0.21% of cancer deaths in men; 0.31% in women).

Although the incidence of thyroid cancer has been increasing over time in both men and women, mortality has decreased over the past 50 yr (2). The reduced mortality is due to earlier diagnosis, improved treatment, and decreased incidence of anaplastic carcinoma. For example, 5-yr relative survival rates for thyroid cancer have increased from 80% in 1950–1954 to 96% in 1992–1999 (2).

DISTRIBUTION BY HISTOLOGICAL TYPE

The relative proportion of differentiated (follicular and papillary) thyroid cancers in a given geographic area depends on the dietary iodine intake (40). Papillary cancers predominate in iodine-sufficient areas. For example, in Iceland, which has ample iodine intake, the proportions were 85% with papillary and 15% with follicular cancer from 1955 through 1984 (17); in Bavaria, Germany, an iodine-deficient area, the proportions were 35% papillary and 65% follicular during 1960–1975 (40). The introduction of iodine supplementation in an endemic goiter region results in an increased proportion of papillary cancers (41), coupled with an improved outcome relating to life expectancy (42).

In the United States, approximately 80% of thyroid cancers are papillary carcinomas (43). Papillary cancer has a peak incidence in the fourth decade of life and affects women three times more frequently than men. Follicular carcinoma accounts for about 5–10% of U.S. cases (43) and has a peak incidence in the fourth or fifth decade. The tumor is three times more common in women than men.

Medullary carcinomas comprise nearly 5–10% of thyroid carcinomas (44). Of these, 80% are sporadic and 20% are familial, mostly multiple endocrine neoplasia type II (MEN II)-related (44). The sporadic form presents mostly in the fifth and sixth decades of life and affects females 1.5 times more than males (45). MEN IIa-related medullary carcinomas present in the first and second decades, and MEN IIb-associated medullary cancers present during the first decade of life (44). Familial non-MEN medullary thyroid carcinomas present in the sixth decade and beyond (44). Familial forms of medullary carcinoma occur with equal frequency in females and males.

Anaplastic cancers and lymphomas account for the remainder of cases. The incidence of anaplastic cancer has recently declined—a factor that has contributed to the reduction in overall thyroid cancer mortality. The peak incidence of anaplastic cancer is in the seventh decade; the female:male ratio is 1.5:1. Lymphomas represent about 5% of thyroid malignancies, with a mean age of 60–65 at the time of presentation (46,47). Females predominate at all ages: in patients under age 60, the ratio is 1.5:1; in patients over age 60, the ratio ranges from 3 to 8:1 (46,47).

FACTORS ASSOCIATED WITH THYROID CANCER RISK

There are several strong associations between thyroid cancer incidence and certain risk factors.

1. Thyroid cancer incidence increases with age.
2. Thyroid cancer is more common in females than males. The female predominance suggests that hormonal factors may be involved. Some studies suggest that biological changes that occur during pregnancy may increase the risk of thyroid carcinoma (48–50).
3. Several genetic syndromes (e.g., Gardner syndrome, adenomatous polyposis coli, and Cowden's disease) are associated with an increased risk of thyroid cancer (discussed in Chapter 3).
4. Radiation exposure is the only factor that has been shown unequivocally to cause thyroid cancer (discussed in detail in Chapter 7).
5. Strong evidence indicates that individuals with Hashimoto's thyroiditis have an increased chance to develop thyroid lymphoma (51).

In addition to these well-established associations, there are postulated risk factors for thyroid carcinoma that remain unproven. These include iodine deficiency and endemic goiter *(52)*, which may result in prolonged stimulation of thyroid tissue by elevated thyroid-stimulating hormone (TSH) levels. Data on this postulated relationship are inconsistent *(50,52–62)*. A major study comparing goiter prevalence and the effect of iodine supplementation with thyroid cancer rates in the United States failed to support a link between endemic goiter and thyroid cancer *(62)*. Graves' disease has also been postulated to be associated with an increased incidence of thyroid cancer. This hypothesis is of interest because of the TSH-like activity of thyroid-stimulating immunoglobulins. However, the data remain inconclusive *(63–76)*, with reported cancer rates ranging from 0.06% *(66)* to as high as 8.7% *(68)* in glands affected by Graves' disease. Lower rates were reported in older studies *(63–66)*, and several recent studies *(70–72)* show rates in the range of 5.1–7.0%. The possibility that other benign diseases of the thyroid could increase the risk of cancer has also been considered *(50,51,53,57,77–81)*. Given the strong possibility of ascertainment and recall bias, these data are difficult to interpret. Furthermore, it is well established that pathological examinations of thyroid tissue can reveal a high rate of unsuspected microcarcinomas that may be of little clinical significance. Nevertheless, a recent pooled analysis of 14 case-control studies *(82–86)* has provided evidence that a large risk of thyroid cancer is associated with a history of goiter or benign nodules among women. This evidence was validated by a prospective study from Denmark *(87,88)*. Thus, current data tentatively suggest that apart from radiation in childhood, goiter and benign nodules/adenomas are the strongest risk factors for thyroid cancer.

REFERENCES

1. Jemal A, Murray T, Ward E, et al. American Cancer Society. Cancer Statistics, 2005. CA Cancer J Clin 2005; 55:10–30.
2. Ries LAG, Eisner MP, Kosary CL, Hankey BF, Miller BA, Clegg L, et al., eds. SEER Cancer Statistics Review, 1975-2000, National Cancer Institute, Bethesda, MD, 2003. Available at: seer.cancer.gov/csr/1975_2000/.
3. Verby JE, Woolner LB, Nobrega FT, Kurland LT, McConahey WM. Thyroid cancer in Olmsted County, 1935-1965. J Natl Cancer Inst 1969; 43:813–820.
4. Polednak AP. Trends in cancer incidence in Connecticut, 1935-1991. Cancer 1994; 74:2863–2872.
5. Goodman MT, Yoshizawa CN, Kolonel LN. Descriptive epidemiology of thyroid cancer in Hawaii. Cancer 1988; 61:1272–1281.
6. Whelan SL, Parkin DM, Masuyer E. Patterns of cancer in five continents. IARC Sci Publ 1990; 102:1–159.
7. Parkin DM, Stiller CA, Draper GJ, Bieber CA. International incidence of childhood cancer. IARC Sci Publ 1988; 87:1–401.
8. Weiss W. Changing incidence of thyroid cancer. J Natl Cancer Inst 1979; 62:1137–1142.
9. Pottern LM, Stone BJ, Day NE, Pickle LW, Fraumeni JF Jr. Thyroid cancer in Connecticut, 1935-1975: an analysis by cell type. Am J Epidemiol 1980; 112:764–774.
10. Carroll RE, Haddon W Jr, Handy VH, Wieben EE. Thyroid cancer: cohort analysis of increasing incidence in New York State, 1941-1962. J Natl Cancer Inst 1964; 33:277–283.
11. Waterhouse J, Muir C, Correa P, Powell J. Cancer Incidence in Five Continents, vol. 3. Lyon, France: International Agency for Research on Cancer, 1976.
12. Waterhouse J, Muir C, Shanugaratnam K. Cancer Incidence in Five Continents, vol. 4. Lyon, France: International Agency for Research on Cancer, 1982.
13. Pettersson B, Adami H-O, Wilander E, Coleman MP. Trends in thyroid cancer incidence in Sweden, 1958-1981, by histopathologic type. Int J Cancer 1991; 48:28–33.
14. dos Santos Silva I, Swerdlow AJ. Thyroid cancer epidemiology in England and Wales: time trends and geographical distribution. Br J Cancer 1993; 67:330–340.
15. Akslen LA, Haldorsen T, Thoresen SO, Glattre E. Incidence pattern of thyroid cancer in Norway: influence of birth cohort and time period. Int J Cancer 1993; 53:183–187.
16. Glattre E, Akslen LA, Thoresen S, Haldoren T. Geographic patterns and trends in the incidence of thyroid cancer in Norway 1970-1986. Cancer Detect Prev 1990; 14:625–631.
17. Hrafnkelsson J, Jonasson JG, Sigurdsson G, Sigvaldason H, Tulinius H. Thyroid cancer in Iceland 1955-1984. Acta Endocrinol 1988; 118: 566–572.
18. Staunton MD, Bourne H. Thyroid cancer in the 1980's: a decade of change. Ann Acad Med (Singapore) 1993; 22:613–616.
19. Levi F, Franceschi S, Te VC, Negri E, La Vecchia C. Descriptive epidemiology of thyroid cancer in the Swiss canton of Vaud. J Cancer Res Clin Oncol 1990; 116:639–647.
20. Roush GC, Holford TR, Schymura MJ, White C. Cancer Risk and Incidence Trends: The Connecticut Perspective. New York: Hemisphere Publishing, 1987.
21. Sarne D, Schneider AB. External radiation and thyroid neoplasia. Endocrinol Metab Clin North Am 1996; 25:181–195.
22. Mortensen JD, Bennett WA, Woolner LB. Incidence of carcinoma in thyroid glands removed at 1000 consecutive routine necropsies. Surg Forum 1954; 5:659–663.
23. Mortensen JD, Woolner LB, Bennett WA. Gross and microscopic findings in clinically normal thyroid glands. J Clin Endocrinol Metab 1955; 15:1270–1280.
24. Bisi H, Fernandes VS, de Camargo RY, Koch L, Abdo AH, de Brito T. The prevalence of unsuspected thyroid pathology in 300 sequential autopsies, with special reference to the incidental carcinoma. Cancer 1989; 64:1888–1893.
25. Silverberg SG, Vidone RA. Carcinoma of the thyroid in surgical and postmortem material: analysis of 300 cases at autopsy and literature review. Ann Surg 1966; 164:291–299.
26. VanderLaan WP. The occurrence of carcinoma of the thyroid gland in autopsy material. N Engl J Med 1947; 237:221–222.
27. LiVolsi VA. Papillary neoplasms of the thyroid. Am J Clin Pathol 1992; 97:426–434.
28. Ain KB. Papillary thyroid carcinoma. Endocrinol Metab Clin North Am 1995; 24:711–760.
29. Vickery AL Jr, Carcangiu ML, Johannessen JV, Sobrinho-Simoes M. Papillary carcinoma. Semin Diagn Pathol 1985; 2:90–100.
30. Kasai N, Sakamoto A. New subgrouping of small thyroid carcinomas. Cancer 1987; 60:1767–1770.
31. Naruse T, Koike A, Kanemitsu T, Kato K. Minimal thyroid carcinoma: a report of nine cases discovered by cervical lymph node metastases. Jpn J Surg 1984; 14:118–121.
32. Noguchi M, Tanaka S, Akiyama T, Miyazaki I, Michigishi T, Tonami N, et al. Clinicopathological studies of minimal thyroid and ordinary thyroid cancers. Jpn J Surg 1984; 14:110–117.
33. Yamashita H, Nakayama I, Noguchi S, Murakami N, Moriuchi A, Yokoyama S, et al. Thyroid carcinoma in benign thyroid diseases:

an analysis from minute carcinoma. Acta Pathol Jpn 1985; 35:781–788.
34. Harach HR, Franssila KO, Wasenius V-M. Occult papillary carcinoma of the thyroid—a "normal" finding in Finland: a systematic autopsy study. Cancer 1985; 56:531–538.
35. Fukunaga FH, Yatani R. Geographic pathology of occult thyroid carcinomas. Cancer 1975; 36:1095–1099.
36. Sampson RJ. Prevalence and significance of occult thyroid cancer. In DeGroot LJ, editor. Radiation-Associated Thyroid Carcinoma. New York: Grune & Stratton, 1997:137–153.
37. Sampson RJ, Woolner LB, Bahn RC, Kurland LT. Occult thyroid carcinoma in Olmsted county, Minnesota: prevalence at autopsy compared with that in Hiroshima and Nagasaki, Japan. Cancer 1974; 34:2072–2076.
38. Strate SM, Lee EL, Childers JH. Occult papillary carcinoma of the thyroid with distant metastases. Cancer 1984; 54:1093–1100.
39. Feldman AR, Kessler L, Myers MH, Naughton MD. The prevalence of cancer: estimates based on the Connecticut tumor registry. N Engl J Med 1986; 315:1394–1397.
40. Lohrs U, Permanetter W, Spelsberg F, Beitinger M. Investigation of frequency and spreading of the different histological types of thyroid cancer in an endemic goiter region. Verhandl Dtsch Ges Pathol 1977; 61:268–274.
41. Harach HR, Escalante DA, Onativa A, Lederer Outes J, Saravia Day E, Williams ED. Thyroid carcinoma and thyroiditis in an endemic goiter region before and after iodine prophylaxis. Acta Endocrinol 1985; 108:55–60.
42. Farahati J, Geling M, Mader U, Mortl M, Luster M, Muller JG, et al. Changing trends of incidence and prognosis of thyroid carcinoma in lower Franconia, Germany, from 1981-1995. Thyroid 2004; 14:141–147.
43. Mazzaferri EL. Thyroid cancer. In Becker KL, editor. Principles and Practice of Endocrinology and Metabolism, 3rd ed. Philadelphia: Lippincott, Wiiliams & Wilkins, 2001:382–402.
44. Ledger GA, Khosla S, Lindor NM, Thibodeau SN, Gharib H. Genetic testing in the diagnosis and management of multiple endocrine neoplasia type II. Ann Intern Med 1995; 122:118–124.
45. Emmertsen K. Medullary thyroid carcinoma and calcitonin. Dan Med Bull 1985; 32:1–28.
46. Mazzaferri EL, Oertel YC. Primary malignant lymphoma and related lymphoproliferative disorders. In Mazzaferri EL, Samaan NA, editors. Endocrine Tumors. Cambridge, MA: Blackwell Scientific, 1993:348.
47. Anscombe AM, Wright DH. Primary malignant lymphoma of the thyroid-a tumor of mucosa-associated lymphoid tissue: review of seventy six cases. Histopathology 1985; 9:81–97.
48. Kravdal O, Glattre E, Haldorsen T. Positive correlation between parity and incidence of thyroid cancer: new evidence based on complete Norwegian birth cohorts. Int J Cancer 1991; 49:831–836.
49. Glattre E, Kravdal O. Male and female parity and risk of thyroid cancer. Int J Cancer 1994; 58:616–617.
50. Ron E, Kleinerman RA, Boice JD Jr, LiVolsi VA, Flannery JT, Fraumeni JF Jr. A population-based case-control study of thyroid cancer. J Natl Cancer Inst 1987; 79:1–12.
51. Holm LE, Blomgren H, Lowhagen T. Cancer risks in patients with chronic lymphocytic thyroiditis. N Engl J Med 1985; 312:601–604.
52. Wegelin C. Malignant disease of the thyroid gland and its relation to goiter in men and animals. Cancer Rev 1928; 3:297.
53. Franceschi S, Fassina A, Talamini R, Mazzolini A, Vianello S, Bidoli E, et al. Risk factors for thyroid cancer in northern Italy. Int J Epidemiol 1989; 18:578–584.
54. Franceschi S, Talamini R, Fassina A, Bidoli E. Diet and epithelial cancer of the thyroid gland. Tumori 1990; 76:331–338.
55. Kolonel LN, Hankin JH, Wilkens LR, Fukunaga FH, Hinds MW. An epidemiologic study of thyroid cancer in Hawaii. Cancer Causes Control 1990; 1:223–234.
56. Glattre E, Haldorsen T, Berg JP, Stensvold I, Solvoll K. Norwegian case-control study testing the hypothesis that seafood increases the risk of thyroid cancer. Cancer Causes Control 1993; 4:11–16.
57. Preston-Martin S, Jin F, Duda MJ, Mack WJ. A case-control study of thyroid cancer in women under age 55 in Shanghai (People's Republic of China). Cancer Causes Control 1993; 4:431–440.
58. Hallquist A, Hardell L, Degerman A, Boquist L. Thyroid cancer: reproductive factors, previous diseases, drug intake, family history and diet: a case-control study. Eur J Cancer Prev 1994; 3:481–488.
59. Franceschi S, Levi F, Negri E, Fassina A, LaVecchia C. Diet and thyroid cancer: a pooled analysis of four European case-control studies. Int J Cancer 1991; 48:395–398.
60. Correa P, Llanos G. Morbidity and mortality from cancer in Cali, Columbia. J Natl Cancer Inst 1966; 36:717–745.
61. Franssila K, Saxen E, Teppo L, Bjarnason O, Tulinius H, Norman T, Ringertz N. Incidence of different morphological types of thyroid cancer in the Nordic countries. Acta Pathol Microbiol Scand A 1981; 89:49–55.
62. Pendergrast WJ, Milmore BK, Marcus SC. Thyroid cancer and thyrotoxicosis in the United States: their relation to endemic goiter. J Chronic Dis 1961; 13:22–38.
63. Beahrs OH, Pemberton JJ, Black BM. Nodular goiter and malignant lesions of the thyroid gland. J Clin Endocrinol 1951; 11:1157–1165.
64. Pemberton J, Black BM. The association of carcinoma of the thyroid gland and exophthalmic goiter. Surg Clin North Am 1948; 28:935–952.
65. Olen E, Klinck GH. Hyperthyroidism and thyroid cancer. Arch Pathol 1966; 81:531–535.
66. Sokal JE. Incidence of malignancy in toxic and non-toxic nodular goiter. JAMA 1954; 154:1321–1325.
67. Carnell NE, Valente WA. Thyroid nodules in Graves' disease: classification, characterization, and response to treatment. Thyroid 1998; 8:647–652.
68. Shapiro SJ, Friedman NB, Perzik SI, Catz B. Incidence of thyroid carcinoma in Graves' disease. Cancer 1970; 26:1261–1270.
69. Wahl RA, Goretzki P, Meybier H, Nitschke J, Linder M, Roher HD. Coexistence of hyperthyroidism and thyroid cancer. World J Surg 1982; 6:385–390.
70. Farbota LM, Calandra DB, Lawrence AM, Paloyan E. Thyroid carcinoma in Graves' disease. Surgery 1985; 98:1148–1153.
71. Behar R, Arganini M, Wu TC, McCormick M, Straus FH, DeGroot LJ, Kaplan EL. Graves' disease and thyroid cancer. Surgery 1986; 100:1121–1127.
72. Pacini F, Elisei R, Di Coscio GC, Anelli S, Macchia E, Concetti R, et al. Thyroid carcinoma in thyrotoxic patients treated by surgery. J Endocrinol Invest 1988; 11:107–112.
73. Ozaki O, Ito K, Kobayashi K, Toshima K, Iwasaki H, Yashiro T. Thyroid carcinoma in Graves' disease. World J Surg 1990; 14:437–440.
74. Belfiore A, Garofalo MR, Giuffrida D, Runello F, Filetti S, Fiumara A, et al. Increased aggressiveness of thyroid cancer in patients with Graves' disease. J Clin Endocrinol Metab 1990; 70:830–835.
75. Hales IB, McElduff A, Crummer P, Clifton-Bligh P, Delbridge L, Hoschl R, et al. Does Graves' disease or thyrotoxicosis affect the prognosis of thyroid cancer. J Clin Endocrinol Metab 1992; 75:886–889.
76. Cady B. Papillary carcinoma of the thyroid. Semin Surg Oncol 1991; 7:81–86.
77. Goldman MB, Monson RR, Maloof F. Cancer mortality in women with thyroid disease. Cancer Res 1990; 50:2283–2289.
78. Levi F, Franceschi S, La Vecchia C, Negri E, Gulie C, Duruz G, Scazziga B. Previous thyroid disease and risk of thyroid cancer in Switzerland. Eur J Cancer 1991; 27:85–88.
79. Preston-Martin S, Bernstein L, Pike MC, Maldonado AA, Henderson BE. Thyroid cancer among young women related to prior thyroid disease and pregnancy history. Br J Cancer 1987; 55:191–195.

80. Wingren G, Hatschek T, Axelson O. Determinants of papillary cancer of the thyroid. Am J Epidemiol 1993; 138:482–491.
81. McTiernan AM, Weiss NS, Daling JR. Incidence of thyroid cancer in women in relation to previous exposure to radiation therapy and history of thyroid disease. J Natl Cancer Inst 1984; 73:575–581.
82. Negri E, Ron E, Franceschi S, Dal Maso L, Mark SD, Preston-Martin S, et al. A pooled analysis of case-control studies of thyroid cancer. I. Methods. Cancer Causes Control 1999; 10:131–142.
83. Negri E, Dal Maso L, Ron E, La Vecchia C, Mark SD, Preston-Martin S, et al. A pooled analysis of case-control studies of thyroid cancer. II. Menstrual and reproductive factors. Cancer Causes Control 1999; 10:143–155.
84. La Vecchia C, Ron E, Franceschi S, Dal Maso L, Mark SD, Chatenoud L, et al. A pooled analysis of case-control studies of thyroid cancer. III. Oral contraceptives, menopausal replacement therapy and other female hormones. Cancer Causes Control 1999; 10:157–166.
85. Franceschi S, Preston-Martin S, Dal Maso L, Negri E, La Vecchia C, Mack WJ, et al. A pooled analysis of case-control studies of thyroid cancer. IV. Benign thyroid diseases. Cancer Causes Control 1999; 10:583–595.
86. Preston-Martin S, Franceschi S, Ron E, Negri E. Thyroid cancer pooled analysis from 14 case-control studies: what have we learned? Cancer Causes Control 2003; 14:787–789.
87. Mellemgaard A, From G, Jorgensen T, Johansen C, Olsen JH, Perrild H. Cancer risk in individuals with benign thyroid disorders. Thyroid 1998; 8:751–754.
88. From G, Mellemgaard A, Knudsen N, Jorgensen T, Perrild H. Review of thyroid cancer cases among patients with previous benign thyroid disorders. Thyroid 2000; 10:697–700.

Molecular Pathogenesis of Thyroid Cancer

James J. Figge, Nikolai A. Kartel, Dima Yarmolinsky, and Gennady Ermak

CANCERS OF THE THYROID FOLLICULAR EPITHELIUM

Signal Transduction Pathways

The thyroid follicular epithelial cell (thyrocyte) responds to myriad growth-stimulating substances, including hormones, growth factors, cytokines, and other mitogens *(1–15)*, as exemplified in Table 1. Thyrocyte responses to these factors are mediated by distinct signal transduction pathways (Figs. 1–3). Each pathway features a cell surface receptor that is linked to a specific cytoplasmic signal transduction cascade:

1. Receptor tyrosine kinase (RTK)/RAS/RAF/MEK/mitogen-activated protein kinase (MAPK) pathway (Fig. 1).
2. Thyrotropin (TSH) receptor/adenylate cyclase/protein kinase A (PKA) pathway (Fig. 2).
3. Receptor/phospholipase C (PLC)/protein kinase C (PKC) pathway (Fig. 3).

These pathways transmit mitogenic signals from the cell surface through the cytoplasm into the nucleus. Activation of some pathways will increase the concentration of cytoplasmic second messengers, such as cyclic adenosine monophosphate (cAMP) or calcium. The RTK pathway activates a series of protein phosphorylation events involved in signal transduction. All the pathways eventually activate nuclear transcription factors, stimulate or inhibit new protein synthesis, and interact with the cell-cycle machinery of the nucleus. The initial signals generated by each cascade in the cytoplasm are distinct; however, there is considerable (but never complete) convergence of the distal branches of the pathways, particularly within the cell nucleus. Two distinct outcomes occur as a result of pathway activation in the thyrocytes. The TSH receptor/adenylate cyclase/protein kinase A pathway (Fig. 2) stimulates proliferation and maintains thyrocyte differentiation. The other two pathways (Figs. 1 and 3) stimulate proliferation but promote thyrocyte dedifferentiation. These two outcomes result from differential regulatory effects of the pathways on the synthesis of proteins maintaining the normal thyrocyte phenotype (e.g., thyroglobulin, thyroid peroxidase, TSH receptor, sodium iodide symporter [NIS], and cell adhesion molecules, such as E-cadherin).

The Receptor Tyrosine Kinase/RAS/ RAF/MEK/MAPK Pathway

The RTK/RAS/RAF/MEK/MAPK pathway is depicted in Fig. 1 *(16)*. Activation of this pathway stimulates thyrocyte proliferation and loss of differentiation. The epidermal growth factor receptor (EGFR) is a classic example of a RTK that transmits mitogenic signals through this pathway. Ligands for EGFR are epidermal growth factor (EGF) and transforming growth factor-α (TGF-α; Table 1). TGF-α is known to be an autocrine growth stimulator of the thyroid follicular cell in certain proliferative conditions *(17)*. Upon ligand binding, EGFRs dimerize and activate their intrinsic tyrosine kinase function, resulting in autophosphorylation of tyrosine residues in the cytoplasmic domain of the receptor. Phosphotyrosine-containing motifs serve as docking sites for proteins that can complex with the receptor. The adapter protein, growth factor receptor-binding protein 2 (Grb2) contains a single Src homology 2 domain (SH2) flanked by two SH3 domains. The SH2 domain of Grb2 recognizes and mediates binding to specific phosphotyrosine-containing motifs on EGFR. The two SH3 domains of Grb2 bind to SOS, a guanine nucleotide-exchange factor. The mitogenic signal is thereby relayed via Grb2 to SOS, then to a RAS protein *(18)*.

The RAS proteins are a family of 21-kDa guanine nucleotide-binding proteins anchored to the plasma membrane. Three types are known in humans: H-RAS, K-RAS, and N-RAS. Functioning as molecular switches, RAS proteins are central regulators of cellular signal transduction processes. Each type of RAS protein can exist in two forms: an inactive guanosine diphosphate (GDP)-bound form and an activated guanosine triphosphate (GTP)-bound form. The SOS protein facilitates binding of GTP to RAS, causing its

Table 1
Selected Growth-Stimulating Factors for Thyroid Follicular Cells

Growth-Stimulating Substances	Reference
Hormones	
Thyrotropin	2
Human chorionic gonadotropin	3
Growth factors	
Insulin-like growth factor-1	4
Epidermal growth factor	5
Transforming growth factor-α	6
Fibroblast growth factors 1 and 2	7
Hepatocyte growth factor	8
Cytokines	
Prostaglandin E_1	9
Prostaglandin E_2	9
Prostacyclin I_2	10
Interleukin 1	11
Other mitogenic factors	
Agents that increase cyclic adenosine monophosphate	2
Bradykinin	12
Adenosine	13
Acetylcholine	14
Thyroid-stimulating immunoglobulin	15

activation *(18)*. Once activated, RAS passes the mitogenic signal onto the next step in the cascade. Inactivation of RAS occurs by hydrolysis of GTP—a reaction that is catalyzed by the intrinsic GTPase activity of the RAS protein. The rate of GTP hydrolysis is accelerated several orders of magnitude by the binding of a GTPase-activating protein (GAP). Based on X-ray crystallographic data, GAP stabilizes the transition state of the GTPase-catalyzed reaction *(19)*. Arginine-789 of GAP is positioned in the active site of RAS and neutralizes developing charges in the transition state. Glutamine-61 of RAS is essential for GTP hydrolysis, and its orientation is stabilized by the binding of GAP to RAS. Oncogenic mutants of RAS have impaired intrinsic GTPase activity and are unable to switch off the transmitted mitogenic signal. Mutations in the GTP-binding domain of RAS at codons 12 and 13 allow GTP to bind but lock the protein in its active GTP-bound state. Glycine, the native amino acid at position 12, is in close physical proximity to both glutamine-61 of RAS and arginine-789 of GAP. Larger side chains at RAS position 12 would sterically interfere with the arrangement of these critical residues in the transition state, thereby impairing the intrinsic GTPase function. Similarly, mutations in codon 61 of the *RAS* gene inactivate the intrinsic GTPase function and lead to permanent activation of the protein. Either type of mutation will result in the continuous unregulated activation of the downstream signal transduction pathway.

Growth-stimulatory genes (e.g., *RAS*) that can be activated by genetic alterations (e.g., single-base substitutions, gene amplification, or chromosomal rearrangements) are known as *proto-oncogenes*. The activated forms of these genes are called *oncogenes*. Activating mutations in *RAS* genes are frequently found in human thyroid cancers (see the RAS Proteins section). Furthermore, transgenic mice harboring an activated mutant *RAS* gene under control of a thyroglobulin promoter develop papillary thyroid carcinomas, thus demonstrating the role of *RAS* mutations in thyroid oncogenesis *(20)*.

Following activation, RAS can then activate a cascade of kinases that transmit the proliferative signal to the cell nucleus. The first of these kinases is another proto-oncogene product known as RAF. There are three RAF isoforms in mammalian cells: ARAF, BRAF, and CRAF-1, each with different tissue distributions. BRAF appears to be functionally important in thyrocytes (see the BRAF section). RAF proteins are serine/threonine kinases that active MEK (also called MAPK kinase or MAPKK) by phosphorylating target serine or threonine residues within a specific motif. BRAF is more efficient than other RAF isoforms in phosphorylating MEK *(21)*. The mitogenic signal is thereby transmitted from RAF to MEK—the next kinase in the cascade. Once activated, the MEK enzymes are mixed-function serine/threonine/tyrosine protein kinases. MEK, in turn, activates extracellular signal-regulated protein kinase (ERK), also called MAPK, by phosphorylating threonine and tyrosine residues within a consensus sequence. Once activated, ERK can phosphorylate a large number of regulatory proteins in the nucleus. ERK also activates ribosomal S6 kinase (rsk), which can phosphorylate and activate the nuclear transcription factors: c-fos and c-jun *(22,23;* see the Nuclear Transcription Factors section).

Three lines of evidence demonstrate that the expression of an activated mutant RAS protein can induce genomic instability. The first was obtained using the bacterial regulatory elements of the *Escherichia coli lac* operon *(24)*, which was adopted to regulate the expression of an activated mutant *RAS* gene in the NIH 3T3 cell line *(25,26)*. It should be noted that these cells are known to harbor *p53* mutations and are therefore susceptible to genomic damage. Upon treating the cells with the inducing agent, IPTG, a transformed phenotype was induced *(25)*. Furthermore, within the time frame needed for one cell cycle, there was a marked increase in the number of gross chromosomal aberrations noted on karyotype analysis, indicating that the expression of a mutant RAS protein can rapidly induce genomic instability *(26)*. In the second experimental paradigm, the normal *RAS* allele in a rat fibrobast line was replaced by an activated mutant *RAS* gene using homologous recombination *(27)*. Expression of the mutant *RAS* gene under control of its natural promoter increased the rate of spontaneous transformation in these cells, and the mutant *RAS* gene was amplified in the majority of transformed cells. These data indicate that expression of a mutant RAS protein at normal levels is not

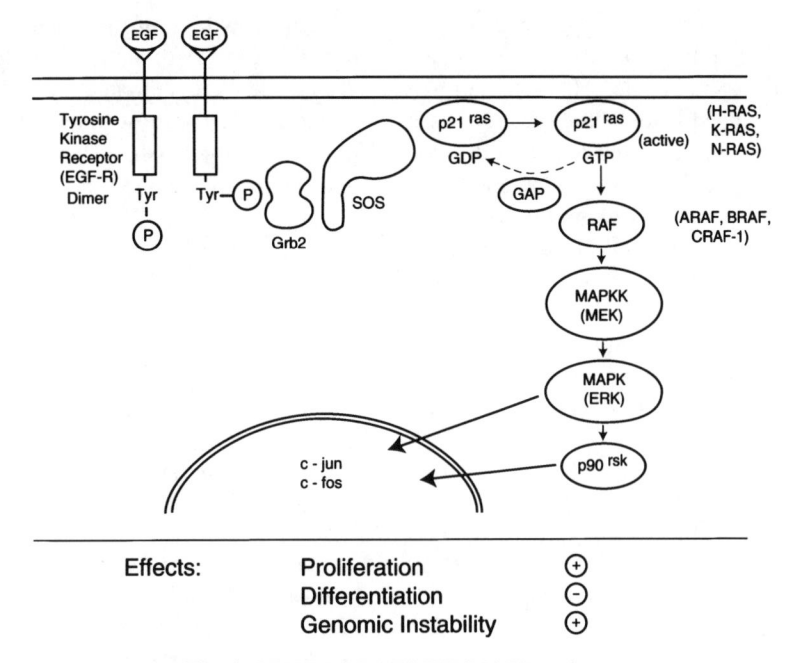

Fig. 1. RTK/RAS/RAF/MEK/MAPK pathway.

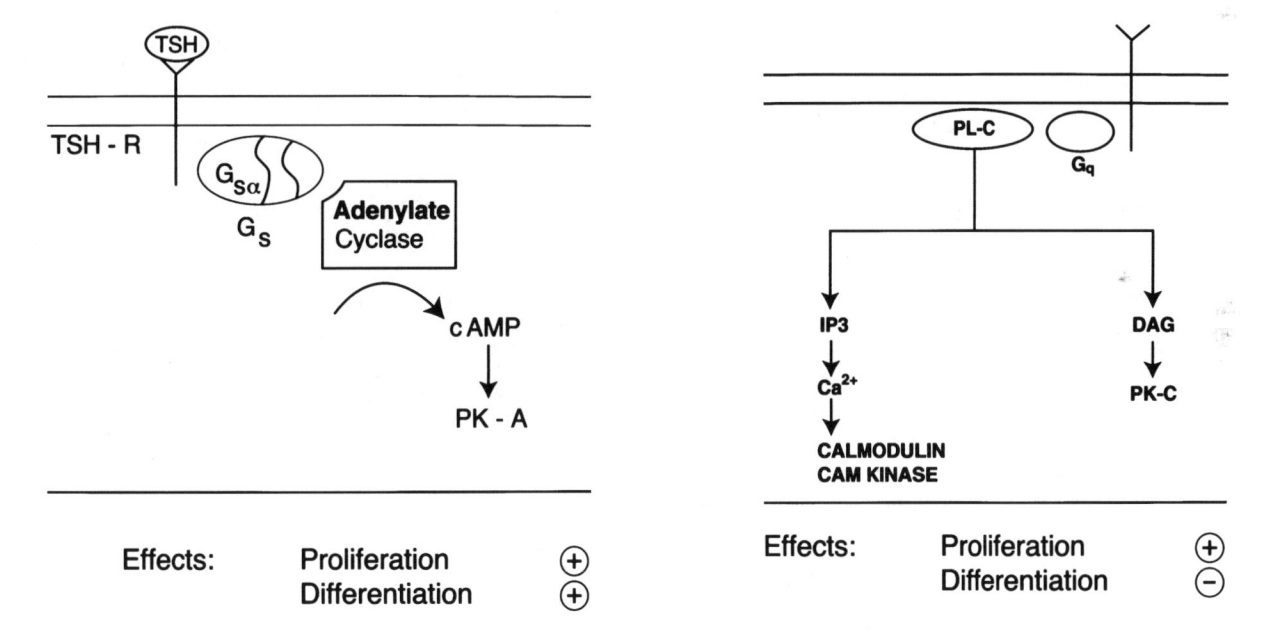

Fig. 2. TSH receptor/adenylate cyclase/PKA pathway.

Fig. 3. Receptor/phospholipase C/PKC pathway.

sufficient to directly transform cells; yet, it is sufficient to induce gene amplification events that eventually result in overexpression of the mutant allele. In the third experimental model, a doxycycline-inducible expression system *(28)* linked to a constitutively activated mutant *RAS* gene was introduced into thyroid PCCL3 cells. Acute expression of the mutant *RAS* gene destabilized the genome of these cells, despite that the sequence of *p53* was confirmed to be wild-type *(29)*.

TSH Receptor/Adenylate Cyclase/PKA Pathway

The TSH receptor/adenylate cyclase/PKA pathway is depicted in Fig. 2 *(30)*. As expected, activation of this pathway stimulates thyrocyte proliferation and maintenance of the differentiated phenotype. Upon TSH binding, the TSH receptor changes its conformation and activates the stimulatory Gs protein. Gs is a heterotrimeric complex that contains an active component (α subunit, Gsα), which is encoded by the *gsp* gene. In the inactive basal state, Gsα is bound to GDP; whereas upon activation, Gsα exchanges GTP for GDP, dissociates from the other two components of the complex, and activates adenylate cyclase—thereby generating cAMP. The increased level of the second messenger, cAMP, then activates PKA, which mediates downstream effects of cAMP. Predictably, activating mutations of both TSH receptor and *gsp* genes are commonly found in toxic (hyperfunctioning) adenomas *(31)*. These adenomas are driven by the constitutive activation of the adenylate cyclase pathway and maintain differentiated function (e.g., thyroid hormone secretion). Surprisingly, mutations in *gsp* are also found occasionally in thyroid cancers (see the G Proteins section); therefore, *gsp* is also classified as a proto-oncogene.

Receptor/PLC/PKC Pathway

The phospholipase C/PKC pathway (Fig. 3) is also active in thyrocytes and stimulates proliferation and loss of differentiation. The pathway can be activated by a number of mitogens, including bradykinin, adenosine, and acetylcholine (Table 1), as well as TSH. Activation of an appropriate receptor can activate another G protein known as Gq. The activated GTP-bound Gqa subunit can activate PLC which then converts phosphatidylinositol 4,5-biphosphate to inositol 1,4,5-triphosphate (IP3) and diacylglycerol (DAG). IP3 acts on receptors in the endoplasmic reticulum and causes the release of calcium stores. This leads to an increased level of cytoplasmic calcium that, upon binding to calmodulin, activates a set of kinases and phosphatases *(32)*. PKC is activated by DAG.

Nuclear Pathways That Control Genomic Integrity

The nuclear protein, p53, is a *tumor suppressor gene product* that functions in cell cycle control and the repair of damaged DNA *(33)*. Tumor suppressor gene products normally function to restrict cell proliferation. Therefore, genetic alterations that inactivate tumor suppressor genes will promote unregulated thyrocyte proliferation. When activated, p53 functions as a transcription factor *(34)* and induces expression of p21$^{CIP1/WAF1}$ and other target gene products that arrest cells at a checkpoint in the late G1 phase of the cell cycle *(35,36)*. In the presence of DNA damage, this p53-mediated pathway allows DNA repair processes to occur before the onset of DNA synthesis (S phase) and mitosis, thus reducing the likelihood that mutations will be passed to daughter cells *(37)*. Under some conditions that are not completely understood, p53 can also trigger apoptosis (programmed cell death) *(38)*.

Cells lacking normal p53 function may develop genomic instability *(39)* because they do not have the normal checkpoint control in late G1—a situation that contributes to the pathogenesis or progression of malignancy. Such cells may accumulate mutations that affect the functioning of other critical growth-controlling genes. For example, germline transmission of a mutant *p53* allele in the Li-Fraumeni syndrome results in a marked increase in cancer risk *(40)*. *p53* mutations are the most frequently observed genetic defects in human cancers *(41)*. There are five known mechanisms that can inactivate p53 function *(35)*.

1. Missense mutations that usually disrupt the specific DNA-binding activity of the p53 protein *(42)*.
2. Nonsense or splice site mutations that result in the expression of a truncated p53 protein.
3. Gene deletion, which eliminates expression of the protein from the affected allele.
4. Complex formation with a viral oncogene product, such as SV40 T antigen, that inactivates the p53 protein.
5. An increased level of the MDM2 protein, which binds to p53 protein and inactivates its transcriptional activation function.

Inactivating p53 mutations are often observed in human anaplastic thyroid carcinomas (see the p53 section). Furthermore, the potential for p53 inactivation to be involved in the pathogenesis of rapidly growing poorly differentiated thyroid carcinomas was demonstrated in transgenic mice experiments *(43)*.

The human *MDM2* gene was initially found to be amplified in sarcomas *(44)*, and it was shown that the MDM2 protein can form a stable complex with the p53 protein *(45)*. The p53 protein can be rendered nonfunctional by complex formation with the MDM2 protein *(35,45,46)*. Specifically, MDM2 binds to the acidic transcriptional activation domain in the amino-terminal portion of p53 *(46,47)*, thereby preventing p53 from interacting with the transcriptional machinery in the cell nucleus. Therefore, overexpression of the MDM2 protein inhibits the ability of p53 to activate the transcription of its target genes, such as p21$^{CIP1/WAF1}$ *(45)*. Notably, the *p53* gene product can also stimulate the transcription of the *MDM2* gene *(48)*. Therefore, an autoregulatory feedback loop involves both p53 and MDM2 *(49)*.

Nuclear Pathways That Control the G1-S Transition of the Cell Cycle

The cell cycle is regulated by a complex system of cyclins and cyclin-dependent kinases *(50)*. D-type cyclins (D1, D2, and D3) act as growth factor sensors and are induced as part of the delayed early response to growth factor stimuli. Cyclin D1 is thought to be most important in the development of thyroid malignancies (see the Cyclin D1 section). An assembly of cyclin D1 with its associated cyclin-dependent kinases (CDK4 and CDK6) facilitates the entry of cells through the G1–S checkpoint of the cell cycle. The cyclin D1–CDK enzyme complex phosphorylates the retinoblastoma (RB) protein, leading to the release and activation of a family of transcription factors known as E2F. The free E2Fs transactivate a set of genes whose products are important for entry into the S phase and subsequent DNA synthesis. The hypophosphorylated form of RB binds to E2F and prevents the transactivation of these same genes. Therefore, cyclin D1 and RB form a crucial regulatory circuit in the regulation of the cell cycle at the G1-S transition. Viral oncoproteins (e.g., SV40 large T antigen, adenovirus E1A, and human papillomavirus E7) each share a consensus motif *(51)* and are able to bind to and functionally inactivate RB *(52,53)*. SV40 T antigen can bind both RB and p53, whereas E1A and E7 are specific for RB. Transgenic mice expressing SV40 T antigen under control of a thyroglobulin gene promoter develop moderately to poorly differentiated thyroid carcinomas *(54)*. Another transgenic mouse model features the expression of SV40 T antigen under control of a major histocompatibility complex gene enhancer *(55)*. Promiscuous expression of T antigen in these mice results in a multiple endocrine neoplasia syndrome, including thyroid tumors. Finally, transgenic mice constructed with the human papillomavirus (type 16) *E7* gene under control of a bovine thyroglobulin gene promoter exhibit goiters that give rise to differentiated thyroid carcinomas in older mice *(56)*.

Multistep Clonal Evolution of Thyroid Neoplasms

Molecular alterations of certain critical genes represent primary oncogenic events *(57)*. These alterations are usually acquired during the individual's lifetime, but in some cases, they can be inherited. Examples include: (1) activation of an oncogene by a gain-of-function point mutation, gene amplification event, or chromosomal rearrangement; (2) inactivation of a tumor suppressor gene by a loss-of-function point mutation or deletion; and (3) perturbation of other genes that control genomic stability, immortalization, apoptosis (programmed cell death), angiogenesis, metastasis, and invasion. According to the "multiple hit" theory of carcinogenesis, thyroid cancer is thought to arise from a series of genetic alterations that cause the sequential activation of oncogenes, inactivation of tumor suppressor genes, and perturbation of other critical genes. Thyrocytes harboring an activated oncogene or an inactivated tumor suppressor gene may derive a growth advantage over normal cells, leading to the clonal expansion of a population of abnormal cells *(58)*. Some of these abnormal cells may acquire additional mutations, resulting in further growth advantage, evasion of apoptosis, or greater susceptibility to genetic damage. Certain genetic lesions (e.g., *RAS* activation and *p53* inactivation) appear to render rapidly dividing cells more susceptible to further genetic damage ("genomic instability"). Hyperplastic thyroid tissue harboring such mutations is susceptible to developing mutations in other critical growth-controlling genes. Cells harboring extensive genetic damage would normally undergo apotosis; however, those tumor cells that can evade apoptosis will continue to proliferate and accumulate genetic damage. Therefore, the multiple hit theory predicts a multistep process of clonal evolution of thyroid neoplasms. The clonality of both benign and malignant thyroid neoplasms has been observed experimentally *(59–61)*.

Specific Molecular Aberrations in Human Thyroid Cancers

A variety of molecular aberrations have been described in human thyroid cancers that involve:

1. DNA methylation.
2. Growth factors.
3. Angiogenic factors.
4. Cell surface receptors (receptor tyrosine kinases and G protein-coupled receptors).
5. Signal transduction proteins.
6. Nuclear transcription factors.
7. Nuclear proteins that control genomic integrity.
8. Nuclear proteins that control cell cycle.
9. Nuclear receptors.
10. Cell surface adhesion molecules.

DNA Methylation

Methylation in vertebrate DNA is controlled by enzymatic processes and is restricted to cytosine nucleotides of cytosine-guanine (CpG) dinucleotide sequences in the cell genome. Aberrant DNA methylation patterns occur frequently in benign and malignant thyroid tumors *(62)*, suggesting that this is an early event in the evolution of thyroid neoplasia. When CpG sequences in the genome are methylated in an unregulated fashion, the expression of various genes may be silenced *(63)*. Methylation-associated transcriptional silencing may result in the inactivation of tumor suppressor genes.

Growth Factors (TGF-α, EGF, IGF-1, FGF-1, and FGF-2)

Some papillary cancers produce TGF-α. As previously noted, TGF-α can bind to EGFRs and may function as a growth-stimulating factor in an autocrine positive-feedback loop *(17,64)*. EGF expression has also been described in malignant thyroid neoplasms *(65)*. The insulin-like growth factor-1 (IGF-1) might also function as an autocrine factor in thyroid neoplasms *(66–68)*. Fibroblast growth factors 1 and 2 (FGF-1 and FGF-2) are known to stimulate thyroid cell proliferation and are overexpressed in benign and malignant thyroid neoplasms *(7)*. Specific mRNA for FGF-2 has been shown to be overexpressed in differentiated thyroid cancers when compared with normal thyroid tissue *(69)*. Growth factor overexpression is likely to be a secondary, not a primary event, in thyroid cancer pathogenesis.

Angiogenic Factors

The vascular endothelial growth factor (VEGF)—an important growth factor for endothelial cells of arteries and veins—has a critical role in angiogenesis. VEGF expression is upregulated in some thyroid cancers *(70–73)*. Abrogation of VEGF activity with an anti-VEGF monoclonal antibody inhibits the growth of anaplastic and papillary thyroid cancer xenografts in nude mice *(74,75)*. It has been demonstrated that VEGF expression correlates with the size of papillary thyroid carcinomas in children and young adults *(76)*.

Cell Surface Receptors: RTKs

ErbB1/HER1 and ErbB2/Neu/HER2

The *ErbB1/HER1* proto-oncogene encodes the EGFR, which binds both EGF and TGF-α. *ErbB2/Neu/HER2*, another member of the *ErbB* gene family, encodes a closely related RTK that is not known to have a direct ligand. The remaining two members of the *ErbB* gene family are *ErbB3/HER3* and *ErbB4/HER4*. Upon ligand binding, members of the ErbB receptor family can form homodimers and heterodimers *(77)*. ErbB2 appears to function primarily as a coreceptor and is the preferred heterodimerization partner for the other ErbB family members. Some papillary carcinomas express mRNA transcripts from *ErbB1* and *ErbB2* genes at two- to threefold higher levels than normal thyroid tissue *(78–80)*, and some anaplastic carcinomas show high levels of specific EGF binding *(81)*. This is a secondary, rather than primary, abnormality. Aberrant activation of EGFR in thyroid malignancies may result in the downstream overexpression and activation of the *MET* proto-oncogene product *(82;* see the *MET* Proto-Oncogene section).

Platelet-Derived Growth Factor Receptor

The receptor for the platelet-derived growth factor is overexpressed in a certain anaplastic cancer cell line *(83)*.

MET Proto-Oncogene

The RTK for hepatocyte growth factor/scatter factor (HGF/SF) is encoded by the *MET* proto-oncogene. Papillary thyroid cancers typically express very high levels of the MET protein *(84–86)*. Furthermore, by Southern blot analysis, the *MET* gene is not amplified or rearranged in thyroid carcinomas *(85)*. Therefore, increased expression of the MET protein is likely owing to transcriptional and/or posttranscriptional regulation. Signaling from mutant *RAS* or *RET/PTC* oncogene products or aberrant activation of EGFR can result in MET overexpression *(82,87)*. HGF is a member of the SF family of related ligands. SFs induce a variety of tissue-specific morphogenic programs in epithelial cells *(88)*, causing epithelial cell dissociation, migration through the exrtracellular matrix, growth, and acquisition of polarity. Evidence demonstrates that HGF can stimulate migration and invasive behavior of thyroid tumor cells that overexpress MET in both primary cell culture and established cell lines *(89–91)*. HGF acts as a chemoattractant for tumor cells and can induce migration of papillary carcinoma cells through Matrigel-coated nucleopore filters *(89,90)*. Taken together, these results suggest that phenotypic properties conferred by activated *RAS* and *RET/PTC* oncogenes may be partly because of the resulting sensitization of tumor epithelium to paracrine (and/or autocrine) HGF *(87,89,90)*. Well-differentiated papillary thyroid cancer cells overexpressing MET may have acquired an HGF-dependent invasive phenotype that underlies intraglandular multifocal dissemination and early lymph node metastasis. Evidence also indicates that the MET protein is not usually overexpressed in poorly differentiated or undifferentiated thyroid cancers *(86,91)*. Papillary thyroid carcinomas with low MET expression are more likely to metastasize to distant sites *(92)*, suggesting that different molecular mechanisms are involved in hematogenous metastasis.

RET and NTRK1

The *RET* and *NTRK1* proto-oncogenes are activated as primary genetic events in papillary carcinomas *(93–153)*. Both encode RTK proteins. In the case of the *NTRK1* proto-oncogene, the encoded receptor is for the nerve growth factor. The ligands for the *RET* proto-oncogene product are glial cell line–derived neurotrophic factor, neurturin, persephin, and artemin. Both receptors are expressed in cells of neuroectodermal origin, and are silent in normal thyrocytes. Activation to oncogene status occurs as a result of a chromosomal rearrangement in thyrocytes. The effect of the rearrangement is to link the tyrosine kinase domain of either RET or NTRK1 to an unrelated protein segment, forming a hybrid fusion protein that is expressed under control of an active promoter in thyroid follicular cells. The unrelated protein segment can be considered to be a "fused activating domain" because it typically contains a dimerization motif (e.g., a leucine zipper or a coiled coil) that mediates dimerization of the hybrid protein and activation of the tyrosine kinase domain in a ligand-independent manner. This results in the expression of a constitutively activated tyrosine kinase domain within the cancer cell. The activated RET and NTRK1 tyrosine kinase domains are each oncogenic and can induce papillary thyroid carcinomas in transgenic mice *(148–150)*.

There are more than 10 known types of *RET* rearrangements, as shown in Fig. 4. The *RET* proto-oncogene (*c-RET*) resides on the long arm of human chromosome 10 (10q11.2). The *RET/PTC1* rearrangement features a fusion between the tyrosine kinase domain of *RET* and a segment of the *H4* (*D10S170*) locus, also on the long arm of chromosome 10 (10q21). With *RET/PTC1*, an intrachromosomal rearrangement known as an inversion, inv(10)(q11.2 q21), has resulted in the fusion between the two genes. The promoter region and 5′ end of the chimeric sequence are derived from the *H4* locus. This places the expression of the tyrosine kinase domain under the control of a heterologous promoter (H4).

RET

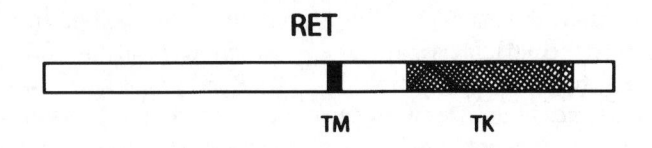

```
       TM     TK
```

FUSION GENE PRODUCT

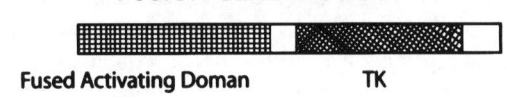

Fused Activating Doman   TK

Rearrangement	Fused Activating Gene	Function	Chromosome
RET/PTC1	H4	Unknown	10q21
RET/PTC2	RI α	Regulatory subunit of cAMP-dependent protein Kinase A	17q23-24
RET/PTC3 RET/PTC4	ELE1 (ARA 70)	Androgen receptor-associated protein (co-transcription factor)	10q11.2
RET/PTC5	GOLGA5 (RFG5)	Gogli integral membrane protein	14q
RET/PTC6	hTIF1 α	Transcription intermediary factor	7q32-34
RET/PTC7	hTIF1 γ (RFG7)	Transcription intermediary factor	1p13
RET/PTC8	Kinectin	Vesicle membrane anchored protein	14q22.1
RET/PTC9	RFG9	Putative intracellular transport protein	18q21-22
RET/PCM1	PCM1	Centrosomal protein	8p22-21.3
ELKS/RET	ELKS	Unknown	12p13

Fig. 4. Patterns of *RET* oncogene rearrangement found in papillary carcinomas.

The fused activating domain derived from the H4 protein is predicted to contain a leucine zipper motif that mediates dimerization and activation of the tyrosine kinase function. The *RET/PTC2* rearrangement features a fusion between the tyrosine kinase domain of *RET* and a portion of the *RI-α* gene (encoding the regulatory subunit of cAMP-dependent PKA) from chromosome 17. This rearrangement is believed to result from a reciprocal translocation between chromosomes 10 and 17. The *RET/PTC3* rearrangement also arises from an inversion and features a fusion between the tyrosine kinase domain of *RET* and a segment of the *ELE1* (*ARA 70*) gene (also located on the long arm of chromosome 10). Following the Chernobyl accident, rare types of *RET/PTC* rearrangements were described. These include a variant of *RET/PTC1 (110)*, *RET/PTC4 (111)*, and other variants of *RET/PTC3 (112,113)*, *RET/PTC5 (114)*, *RET/PTC6 (115)*, *RET/PTC7 (115)*, *RET/PTC8 (116)*, and *RET/PTC9 (117)*. Three other rearrangements—*RET/PCM1 (118)*, *ELKS/RET (119)*, and *RET/PTC1L* (another variant of *RET/PTC1*) *(120)*—were recently described.

RET rearrangements are traditionally thought to be highly specific for papillary thyroid cancer *(96,121)* and are rarely found in tumors of other tissues or in other types of thyroid neoplasms. However, the *RET/PTC* oncogene is frequently activated in Hurthle cell adenomas and carcinomas *(122)* and occasionally in poorly differentiated thyroid tumors, particularly those coexisting or evolving from well-differentiated papillary carcinomas *(123)*. *RET* is typically activated in about 5–35% of sporadic papillary thyroid cancers in different series, but the rate is lower in some geographic areas *(125)* and notably higher (up to 85%) in others *(138–140)*. The reasons for the differences are likely multifactorial and may include geographic and environmental factors, genetic background, patient selection, and technical factors. The prevalence of *RET/PTC* rearrangements in sporadic papillary carcinomas in pediatric populations ranges from 30% to 71% *(101,134, 141,142)*. Occult papillary microcarcinomas frequently harbor *RET/PTC* rearrangements, suggesting a role in early stage pathogenesis *(133)*. *RET* rearrangements may be induced as a result of radiation exposure *(108,109)*, and *RET* activation has been documented in Chernobyl-related papillary cancers in children *(97–107,* see also Chapters 4 and 7*)*. Among the papillary thyroid carcinomas surgically removed up to 10 years following the Chernobyl accident, *RET/PTC3* is the predominant rearrangement *(98–101)*. Pisarchik and colleagues *(102–104)* reported that the spectrum of *RET/PTC* rearrangements appears to be changing as a function of time since the accident. The proportion of *RET/PTC3* rearrangements has declined, whereas the proportion of *RET/PTC1* rearrangements has increased in papillary thyroid cancers surgically removed 10 yr or more after the accident. This finding was independently confirmed by Smida and colleagues *(105)*, as well as by Rabes and coworkers *(106,107)*.

Cell Surface Receptors: G Protein-Coupled Receptors

TSH Receptor

Activating mutations of the TSH receptor have been described in toxic (hyperfunctioning) adenomas *(31)*. It is well known that these adenomas rarely exhibit malignant behavior, which holds to the idea that activation of the adenylate cyclase pathway (Fig. 2) maintains the differentiated thyrocyte phenotype. However, the first report of a TSH receptor mutation in three differentiated thyroid carcinomas was presented *(154)*. The mutation was discovered in the third intracellular loop of the receptor in a region critical for signal transduction. This mutation would be expected to cause constitutive activation of the cAMP pathway. As predicted, the affected cancers had increased basal levels of cAMP. Activating mutations in the TSH receptor are quite rare in differentiated and poorly differentiated thyroid carcinomas; only several cases have been reported *(155–161)*.

Signal Transduction Proteins

RAS Proteins

RAS proteins are activated in various thyroid cancers *(79,93,94,143–146,162–196)*. Single-base activating substitution mutations in codons 12, 13, or 61 have been described in all three *RAS* oncogenes. In addition, activation of *RAS* by gene amplification has also been described in thyroid cancer *(168)*. As previously described, *RAS* mutations are expected to constitutively activate the MAPK cascade (Fig. 1) and will stimulate proliferation, loss of the differentiated phenotype, and genomic instability. Table 2 illustrates data pooled from 21 studies that employed DNA sequencing to confirm the presence of activating *RAS* mutations in codons 12, 13, or 61 of *H-RAS*, *K-RAS*, or *N-RAS*. Whenever possible, data for follicular variant papillary thyroid carcinomas were tabulated separately from data for conventional papillary carcinomas. Furthermore, data regarding Hurthle cell adenomas and Hurthle cell carcinomas were considered separately from other follicular neoplasms whenever available. Carcinomas with evidence of poor differentiation, including those with insular elements, were classified as poorly differentiated carcinomas in this analysis.

As demonstrated in Table 2, activating *RAS* point mutations occur most frequently in poorly differentiated and undifferentiated (anaplastic) carcinomas (40%), suggesting that *RAS* mutations may be a marker for aggressive cancer behavior (189). Additionally, activating *RAS* mutations are more prevalent in follicular (31%) than in conventional papillary thyroid carcinomas (~6%), but follicular variant papillary thyroid carcinomas display a high prevalence of *RAS* mutations (33%), similar to that of follicular carcinomas. These data imply that activating *RAS* mutations are important in the pathogenesis of follicular carcinomas and propose that nearly all papillary cancers with a *RAS* mutation display a follicular growth pattern *(144,187)*. In contrast, activating *RAS* mutations do not appear to have a significant role in the pathogenesis of traditional papillary thyroid carcinomas. The 6% prevalence for traditional papillary carcinomas should be considered an estimate because it was not possible to separate the contribution of follicular variant cases (if any) in every report in Table 2. Interestingly, activating *RAS* mutations are commonly found in both follicular adenomas (18%) and follicular carcinomas (31%), suggesting that *RAS* mutations occur early in the pathogenesis of follicular cancers. For example, the *RAS* mutation may occur before or during the follicular adenoma stage, which might (in certain cases) progress to the follicular carcinoma stage. Particularly, it has been reported that *N-RAS* codon 61 mutations are common in atypical adenomas and follicular carcinomas, which supports the hypothesis that some atypical adenomas are precursors of follicular carcinomas *(190)*. Finally, several studies indicate that mutations in *N-RAS* are more often found in aggressive follicular, papillary, and poorly differentiated thyroid cancers *(172, 175,177,195)*.

Data on Hurthle cell adenomas and carcinomas are limited but signify that *RAS* mutations are not frequently found

Table 2
Prevalence of Activating Point Mutations in Codons 12, 13, or 61 of all Three RAS Genes in Thyroid Neoplasms

Source	PC	PC-FV	FA	HA	FC	HC	PDC/UC
Sugg (79)	2/17	NT	NT	NT	NT	NT	0/3
Park (143)	0/37	NT	1/8	NT	1/3	NT	0/2
Zhu (144)	0/46	11/27	NT	NT	NT	NT	2/3
Soares (145)	2/27	NT	5/34	NT	4/12	NT	NT
Kimura (146)	11/67	NT	NT	NT	NT	NT	NT
Yoshimoto (176)	0/26	NT	5/24	NT	NT	NT	0/2
Manenti (179)	0/31	NT	0/17	0/2	5/21	NT	4/16
Horie (181)	1/22	NT	1/7	NT	NT	NT	NT
Esapa (183)	0/12	1/1	7/38	0/3	4/9	NT	1/1
Naito (184)	6/34	NT	NT	NT	NT	NT	NT
Ezzat (185)	2/16	NT	1/7	NT	1/4	NT	NT
Bouras (186)	5/62	1/4	8/35	NT	1/6	6/11	0/10
De Micco (187)	0/29	4/20	NT	NT	NT	NT	NT
Salvatore (188)	1/15	NT	NT	NT	0/5	NT	1/6
Garcia-Rostan (189)	2/30	NT	NT	NT	2/19	NT	31/58
Vasko (190)	NT	NT	9/46	NT	7/34	NT	NT
Nikiforova (191)	NT	NT	11/23	1/13	17/33	2/19	NT
Pilotti (192)	NT	NT	NT	NT	5/8	NT	5/8
Krohn (193)	NT	NT	0/27	NT	NT	NT	NT
Tallini (194)	NT	NT	NT	0/7	NT	1/4	NT
Fukushima (196)	0/76	NT	NT	NT	4/8	NT	2/7
Totals	32/547 [6%]	17/52 [33%]	48/266 [18%]	1/25 [4%]	51/162 [31%]	9/34 [26%]	46/116 [40%]

Data confirmed by DNA sequence analysis. PC, papillary carcinoma; PC-FV, papillary carcinoma, follicular variant; FA, follicular adenoma; HA, Hurthle cell adenoma; FC, follicular carcinoma; HC, Hurthle cell carcinoma; PDC/UC, poorly differentiated carcinoma/undifferentiated carcinoma (anaplastic); NT, not tested.

in Hurthle cell adenomas but may be more prevalent in Hurthle cell carcinomas. Additional studies on this hypothesis are required owing to the small number of cases reported.

G Proteins

The oncogene *gsp*, which encodes the Gsα subunit, is commonly mutated in hyperfunctioning adenomas (31). Activating *gsp* mutations have been occasionally described in thyroid cancers (175,180,181,197); however, this is not a common feature of malignant thyroid tumors (143, 158,159,161,198). This fact suggests that cAMP is a relevant growth signal that can contribute to oncogenesis in certain circumstances. It is likely that *gsp* must be activated in concert with another oncogene to promote cancer formation.

BRAF

Activation of *BRAF* by single-base substitution has been described in a variety of human tumors, notably melanoma, with a specific substitution in the kinase domain (V600E, formerly called V599E), accounting for the majority of cases (199). *BRAF* mutations at codon 600 (V600E) have been described in 29–69% of papillary thyroid carcinomas in different series (145,146,196,200–203). *BRAF*-activating mutations at codon 600 have also been reported in a subset of poorly differentiated and undifferentiated thyroid cancers (196,200,202) but not in follicular adenomas or carcinomas (145,146,196,200–203). Because both *RAS* and *BRAF* mutations activate the MAPK pathway, it is interesting to note that *BRAF* mutations appear to be a marker for papillary thyroid carcinomas, whereas *RAS* mutations are more often found in follicular carcinomas and follicular variant papillary carcinomas. This evidence suggests that the RAS and BRAF oncoproteins can activate distinct sets of downstream effectors. *BRAF* and *RAS* mutations also appear to be mutually exclusive in papillary carcinomas (145,146,196). Similarly, *BRAF* mutations and *RET/PTC* rearrangements are mutually exclusive in papillary carcinomas (145,146).

Nuclear Transcription Factors

Nuclear transcription factors, such as c-fos and c-myc, are overexpressed at the mRNA level in some thyroid cancers (204,205), but this appears to be a secondary consequence of increased proliferation. No structural rearrangements have been identified in these genes in thyroid cancers.

Nuclear Proteins That Control Genomic Integrity

p53

Data have established that inactivation of the p53 tumor suppressor protein by gene mutation is frequently implicated in the pathogenesis of poorly differentiated and anaplastic (undifferentiated) thyroid carcinomas *(206–215)*. However, most authors have not found *p53* gene mutations in well-differentiated papillary thyroid carcinomas *(206–211,213,216)*. Zou and colleagues *(212)* reported finding *p53* gene mutations in seven well-differentiated papillary carcinomas and three papillary carcinomas with evidence of regional dedifferentiation (solid foci) in a group of 40 papillary carcinomas. Three of the reported mutations did not result in an amino acid change. Salvatore and colleagues *(188)* identified a *p53* mutation in 1 of 30 papillary carcinomas. Similarly, Park and coworkers *(143)* identified a *p53* point mutation in one of 31 papillary thyroid carcinomas. Ho and colleagues *(217)* documented two *p53* point mutations in 41 papillary thyroid carcinomas. Alterations involving *p53* have also been detected in some radiation-related papillary carcinomas (see Chapters 3 and 7). Fagin and associates *(211)* found a *p53* mutation in one of 11 follicular carcinomas, and Zou and colleagues *(212)* identified a mutation in one of four follicular carcinomas.

Some anaplastic carcinomas are thought to arise from pre-existing foci of differentiated thyroid cancer. Strong evidence shows that mutational inactivation of *p53* is involved in the transition from differentiated to undifferentiated (anaplastic) thyroid cancer. Donghi and associates *(210)* studied an anaplastic carcinoma that contained a differentiated region and the undifferentiated portion. A *p53* mutation was present in cells from the undifferentiated area, as well as from a lymph node metastasis, but it was not from cells derived from the more differentiated region. Similar observations were reported by Ito and coworkers *(207)* and Asakawa and Kobayashi *(208)*, which suggest that *p53* mutations arise relatively late in the evolution of anaplastic cancer and support the concept of multistep progression of thyroid carcinogenesis.

MDM2

Zou and colleagues *(218)* found twofold overexpression of MDM2 mRNA in 19% (3/16) of papillary carcinomas and threefold overexpression in a single follicular carcinoma. Jennings and colleagues *(219)* observed nuclear MDM2 protein accumulation in 33% (8/24) of papillary carcinomas. Horie and coworkers *(220)* also documented MDM2 overexpression in 33% (26/78) of papillary carcinomas. These findings imply that p53 might be inactivated in a subset of well-differentiated thyroid carcinomas resulting from the overexpression of MDM2 protein.

Nuclear Proteins That Control the Cell Cycle

Cyclin D1

Overexpression of cyclin D1 has been documented in papillary and follicular thyroid carcinomas *(80,221–228)*, as well as poorly differentiated and anaplastic thyroid carcinomas *(229)*. Overexpression of cyclin D1 in a series of 125 patients with papillary thyroid cancer was shown to be an independent predictor of lymph node metastasis *(222)*. Gene amplification has not been identified as a cause of cyclin D1 overexpression *(223,224,227)*; therefore, upregulation of transcription or a posttranscriptional mechanism is likely.

Nuclear Receptors

PAX8-PPARγ

The peroxisome proliferator-activated receptor-γ (PPARγ) is a critical regulator of adipocyte differentiation *(230)*. PPARγ forms a complex with the retinoid X receptor, and the complex binds to specific sites on DNA where it regulates transcription in response to ligand binding. Abrogation of normal PPARγ function is thought to be important in several types of human cancer, including liposarcomas, colon cancers, and breast cancers *(230)*. Recently, a chromosomal translocation, t(2;3)(q13;p25), resulting in the fusion of the *PPARγ* gene to the thyroid transcription factor *PAX8* gene, has been identified in follicular thyroid carcinomas *(191, 231–233)* and infrequently in follicular adenomas *(232,233, 233a)*. *PAX8-PPARγ* rearrangements have not been identified in papillary carcinomas, including follicular variant papillary carcinomas *(144,231–233)*. Follicular carcinomas may arise via two distinct molecular pathways that involve either *RAS* activation or *PAX8-PPARγ* rearrangement *(191)*.

Cell Surface Adhesion Molecules

CD44

CD44 is a polymorphic family of integral membrane proteoglycans and glycoproteins implicated in diverse processes (e.g., cell–cell adhesion, cell–matrix adhesion, cell migration, and tumor metastasis; *234,235*). CD44 is a major receptor for hyaluronate *(236)*. The heterogeneity of CD44 results from posttranslational modifications and "alternative mRNA splicing" of up to 10 variant exons that encode parts of the extracellular domain. The process of alternative mRNA splicing allows different combinations of the variant exons to be incorporated into CD44 mRNA transcripts, resulting in the generation of multiple different CD44 protein isoforms. In rodent models, some CD44 isoforms can confer metastatic behavior to tumor cells *(237,238)*. Recent data demonstrate that variant CD44 molecules are expressed widely throughout the human body on epithelial cells in a tissue-specific pattern *(239,240)*, signifying that the process of alternative splicing is normally tightly regulated. Significant levels of CD44 protein are expressed on the

Molecular Pathogenesis

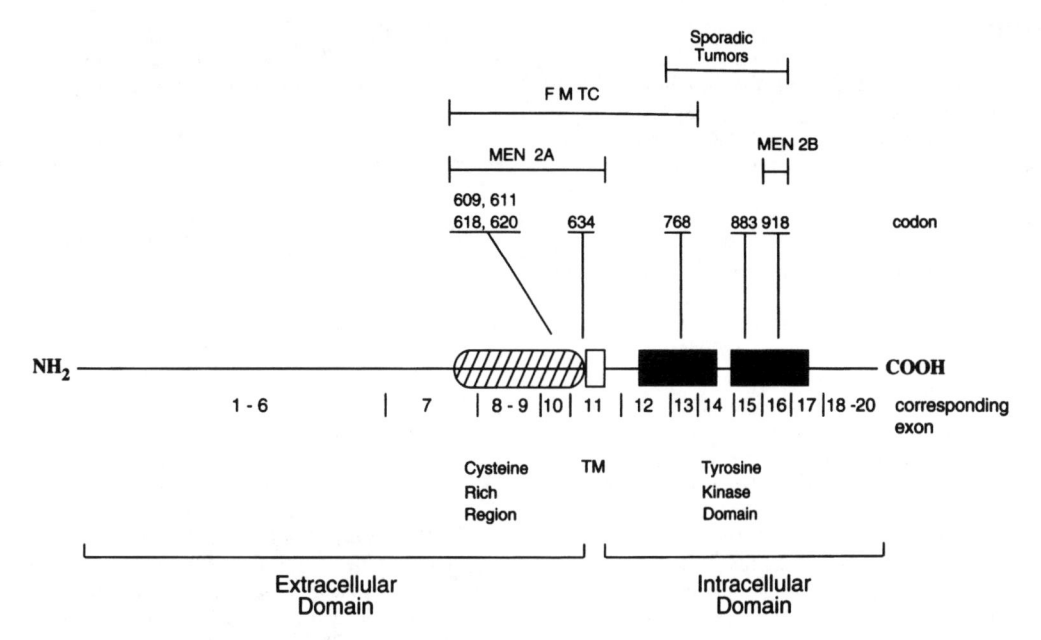

Fig. 5. Map of inherited *RET* mutations predisposing to medullary carcinoma in MEN 2A, MEN 2B, and familial non-MEN medullary carcinoma. Some sporadic medullary carcinomas harbor *RET* mutations in the tumor DNA but not the germline DNA.

plasma membranes of papillary thyroid cancer cells *(241)*. Ermak and coworkers *(242,243)* reported that alternative splicing of CD44 is deregulated in various thyroid lesions (goiters, adenomas, and papillary carcinomas). Papillary carcinomas exhibit specific patterns of aberrant CD44 mRNA splicing *(243)*. These aberrations are postulated to affect the function of CD44 protein molecules on the cell surface and might (at least in part) regulate papillary thyroid cancer growth patterns and metastatic potential.

E-Cadherin

E-cadherin—a calcium-dependent cell adhesion molecule required for normal epithelial differentiation *(244)* and function—is thought to impact tumor invasion. Data from several models suggest that E-cadherin is a suppressor of tumor spreading and invasion *(245,246)*. E-cadherin mRNA levels and protein immunoreactivity are equally high in normal thyroid tissue and benign thyroid disorders but are both markedly reduced in anaplastic thyroid carcinomas *(247)*. In papillary carcinomas, E-cadherin mRNA levels and immunoreactivity are variable, ranging from normal to markedly reduced. The E-cadherin mRNA levels in follicular carcinomas are high, but immunoreactivity varies considerably. A good correlation was found between the level of E-cadherin and steady-state TSH receptor mRNA, suggesting that E-cadherin is a marker of differentiation in thyroid malignancies *(247)*. The loss of E-cadherin expression in anaplastic carcinomas may somewhat explain the aggressive behavior of these cancers at the molecular level.

Genetic Syndromes Associated With Thyroid Cancer

The prevalence of thyroid cancer is increased in certain genetic syndromes *(248–252)*, such as Gardner syndrome, adenomatous polyposis coli, and Cowden's disease. There are also families with a clustering of papillary thyroid carcinomas (familial papillary thyroid cancer syndromes), potentially representing the existence of hereditary non-medullary thyroid carcinoma *(252)*.

MEDULLARY THYROID CARCINOMA

Medullary thyroid carcinomas arise from the C cells of the thyroid and may be sporadic (80%) or familial (20%). The genetic predisposition to develop a familial medullary carcinoma is conferred by a point mutation in the germline DNA that encodes the *RET* oncogene *(253)*. Figure 5 summarizes the current data regarding the status of inherited *RET* mutations in three inherited medullary carcinoma syndromes: MEN2A, MEN2B, and familial non-MEN medullary carcinoma. These mutations serve to constitutively activate the tyrosine kinase function of the *RET* gene product and predispose to the development of neoplasia. Lesions conferring susceptibility to MEN2A map to exons 10 and 11, encoding part of a cysteine-rich region in the extracellular domain of the receptor. MEN2B maps most often to codon 918 in exon 16, which codes for part of the tyrosine kinase domain. Some sporadic tumors also have mutations (in the tumor DNA but not germline DNA) that map to the tyrosine kinase domain.

REFERENCES

1. Lewinski A, Pawlikowski M, Cardinali DP. Thyroid growth-stimulating and growth-inhibiting factors. Biol Signals 1993; 2:313–351.
2. Roger P, Taton M, Van Sande J, Dumont JE. Mitogenic effects of thyrotropin and adenosine 3′,5′-monophosphate in differentiated normal human thyroid cells in vitro. J Clin Endocrinol Metab 1988; 66: 1158–1165.
3. Hershman JM, Lee HY, Sugawara M, Mirell CJ, Pang XP, Yanagisawa M, Pekary AE. Human chorionic gonadotropin stimulates iodide uptake, adenylate cyclase, and deoxyribo-nucleic acid synthesis in cultured rat thyroid cells. J Clin Endocrinol Metab 1988; 67:74–79.
4. Tramontano D, Gushing GW, Moses AC, Ingbar SH. Insulin-like growth factor-I stimulates the growth of rat thyroid cells in culture and synergizes the stimulation of DNA synthesis induced by TSH and Graves'-IgG. Endocrinology 1986; 119:940–942.
5. Roger PP, Dumont JE. Epidermal growth factor controls the proliferation and the expression of differentiation in canine thyroid cells in primary culture. FEBS Lett 1982; 144:209–212.
6. Grubeck-Loebenstein B, Buchan G, Sadeghi R, Kissonerghis M, Londei M, Turner M, et al. Transforming growth factor beta regulates thyroid growth: role in the pathogenesis of nontoxic goiter. J Clin Invest 1989; 83:764–770.
7. Eggo MC, Hopkins JM, Franklyn JA, Johnson GD, Sanders DS, Sheppard MC. Expression of fibroblast growth factors in thyroid cancer. J Clin Endocrinol Metab 1995; 80:1006–1011.
8. Eccles N, Ivan M, Wynford-Thomas D. Mitogenic stimulation of normal and oncogene-transformed human thyroid epithelial cells by hepatocyte growth factor. Mol Cell Endocrinol 1996; 117: 247–251.
9. Lupulescu A. Goiter formation following prostaglandin administration in rats. Am J Pathol 1976; 85:21–35.
10. Pawlikowski M, Kunert-Radek J, Lewinski A. Effect of prostaglandins on the mitotic activity of rat thyroid in organ culture. Endokrynol Pol 1982; 33:129–134.
11. Mine M, Tramontano D, Chin WW, Ingbar SH. Interleukin-1 stimulates thyroid cell growth and increases the concentration of the c-myc proto-oncogene mRNA in thyroid follicular cells in culture. Endocrinology 1987; 120:1212–1214.
12. Raspe E, Laurent E, Andry G, Dumont JE. ATP, bradykinin, TRH and TSH activate the Ca^{2+}-phosphatidylinositol cascade of human thyrocytes in primay culture. Mol Cell Endocrinol 1991; 81:175–183.
13. Sho K, Okajima F, Majid MA, Kondo Y. Reciprocal modulation of thyrotropin actions by Pl-purinergic agonists in FRTL-5 thyroid cells. J Biol Chem 1991; 266:12,180–12,184.
14. Raspe E, Laurent E, Corvilain B, Verjans B, Erneux C, Dumont JE. Control of the intracellular Ca^{2+} concentration and inositol phosphate accumulation in dog thyrocyte primary culture: evidence for different kinetics of Ca^{2+}-phosphatidylinositol cascade activation and for involvement in the regulation of H_2O_2 production. J Cell Physiol 1991; 146:242–250.
15. Ando T, Latif R, Pritsker A, Moran T, Nagayama Y, Davies TF. A monoclonal thyroid-stimulating antibody. J Clin Invest 2002; 110: 1667–1674.
16. Chang F, Steelman LS, Shelton JG, Lee JT, Navolanic PM, Blalock WL, et al. Regulation of cell cycle progression and apoptosis by the Ras/Raf/MEK/ERK pathway. Int J Oncol 2003; 22:469–480.
17. Lemoine NR, Hughes CM, Gullick WJ, Brown CL, Wynford-Thomas D. Abnormalities of the EGF receptor system in human thyroid neoplasia. Int J Cancer 1991; 49:558–561.
18. Egan SE, Giddings BW, Brooks MW, Buday L, Sizeland AM, Weinberg RA. Association of Sos RAS exchange protein with Grb2 is implicated in tyrosine kinase signal transduction and transformation. Nature 1993; 363:45–51.
19. Scheffzek K, Ahmadian MR, Kabsch W, Wiesmuller L, Lautwein A, Schmitz F, Wittinghofer A. The ras-rasGAP complex: structural basis for GTPase activation and its loss in oncogenic ras mutants. Science 1997; 277:333–338.
20. Rochefort P, Caillou B, Michiels FM, Ledent C, Talbot M, Schlumberger M, et al. Thyroid pathologies in transgenic mice expressing a human activated RAS gene driven by a thyroglobulin promoter. Oncogene 1996; 12:111–118.
21. Peyssonnaux C, Eychene A. The Raf/MEK/ERK pathway: new concepts of activation. Biol Cell 2001; 93:53–62.
22. Roberts TM. A signal chain of events. Nature 1992; 360:534–535.
23. Frodin M, Gammeltoft S. Role and regulation of 90 kDa ribosomal S6 kinase (RSK) in signal transduction. Mol Cell Endocrinol 1999; 151:65–77.
24. Figge J, Wright C, Collins CJ, Roberts TM, Livingston DM. Stringent regulation of stably integrated chloramphenicol acetyl transferase genes by E. coli lac represser in monkey cells. Cell 1988; 52:713–722.
25. Liu HS, Scrable H, Villaret DB, Lieberman MA, Stambrook PJ. Control of Ha-RAS-mediated mammalian cell transformation by Escherichia coli regulatory elements. Cancer Res 1992; 52:983–989.
26. Denko NC, Giaccia AJ, Stringer JR, Stambrook PJ. The human Ha-RAS oncogene induces genomic instability in murine fibroblasts within one cell cycle. Proc Nati Acad Sci USA 1994; 91:5124–5128.
27. Finney RE, Bishop JM. Predisposition to neoplastic transformation caused by gene replacement of H-RAS1. Science 1993; 260:1524–1527.
28. Gossen M, Freundlieb S, Bender G, Muller G, Hillen W, Bujard H. Transcriptional activation by tetracyclines in mammalian cells. Science 1995; 268:1766–1769.
29. Saavedra HI, Knauf JA, Shirokawa JM, Wang J, Ouyang B, Elisei R, et al. The RAS oncogene induces genomic instability in thyroid PCCL3 cells via the MAPK pathway. Oncogene 2000; 19:3948–3954.
30. Dremier S, Coulonval K, Perpete S, Vandeput F, Fortemaison N, Van Keymeulen A, et al. The role of cyclic AMP and its effect on protein kinase A in the mitogenic action of thyrotropin on the thyroid cell. Ann NY Acad Sci 2002; 968:106–121.
31. Russo D, Arturi F, Wicker R, Chazenbalk GD, Schlumberger M, DuVillard JA, et al. Genetic alterations in thyroid hyperfunctioning adenomas. J Clin Endocrinol Metab 1995; 80:1347–1351.
32. Ermak G, Davies KJ. Calcium and oxidative stress: from cell signaling to cell death. Mol Immunol 2002; 38:713–721.
33. Harris CC, Hollstein M. Clinical Implications of the p53 tumor-suppressor gene. N Engl J Med 1993; 329:1318–1327.
34. Fields S, Jang SK. Presence of a potent transcription activating sequence in the p53 protein. Science 1990; 249:1046–1049.
35. Vogelstein B, Kinzler KW. p53 function and dysfunction. Cell 1992; 70:523–526.
36. Namba H, Hara T, Tukazaki T, Migita K, Ishikawa N, Ito K, et al. Radiation-induced G1 arrest is selectively mediated by the p53-WAF1/Cip1 pathway in human thyroid cells. Cancer Res 1995; 55:2075–2080.
37. Hartwell L. Defects in a cell cycle checkpoint may be responsible for the genomic instability of cancer cells. Cell 1992; 71:543–546.
38. Clarke AR, Purdie CA, Harrison DJ, Morris RG, Bird CC, Hooper ML, Wyllie AH. Thymocyte apoptosis induced by p53-dependent and independent pathways. Nature 1993; 362:849–852.
39. Livingstone LR, White A, Sprouse J, Livanos E, Jacks T, Tlsty TD. Altered cell cycle arrest and gene amplification potential accompany loss of wild-type p53. Cell 1992; 70:923–935.
40. Srivastava S, Zou ZQ, Pirollo K, Blattner W, Chang EH. Germ-line transmission of a mutated p53 gene in a cancer-prone family with Li-Fraumeni syndrome. Nature 1990; 348:747–749.
41. Hollstein M, Sidransky D, Vogelstein B, Harris CC. p53 mutations in human cancers. Science 1991; 253:49–53.
42. Cho Y, Gorina S, Jeffrey PD, Pavletich NP. Crystal structure of a p53 tumor suppressor-DNA complex: understanding tumorigenic mutations. Science 1994; 265:346–355.

43. Powell Jr DJ, Russell JP, Li G, Kuo BA, Fidanza V, Huebner K, Rothstein JL. Altered gene expression in immunogenic poorly differentiated thyroid carcinomas from RET/PTCp53-/- mice. Oncogene 2001; 20:3235–3246.
44. Oliner JD, Kinzler KW, Meltzer PS, George DL, Vogelstein B. Amplification of a gene encoding a p53-associated protein in human sarcomas. Nature 1992; 358:80–83.
45. Momand J, Zambetti GP, Olson DC, George DL, Levine AJ. The mdm-2 oncogene product forms a complex with the p53 protein and inhibits p53-mediated transactivation. Cell 1992; 69:1237–1245.
46. Oliner J, Pietenpol J, Thiagalingam S, Gyuris J, Kinzler K, Vogelstein B. Oncoprotein MDM2 conceals the activation domain of tumor suppressor p53. Nature 1993; 362:857–860.
47. Kussie PH, Gorina S, Marechal V, Elenbaas B, Moreau J, Levine AJ, Pavletich NP. Structure of the MDM2 oncoprotein bound to the p53 tumor suppressor transactivation domain. Science. 1996; 274:948–953.
48. Barak Y, Juven T, Haffner R, Oren M. mdm2 expression is induced by wild type p53 activity. EMBO J 1993; 12:461–468.
49. Wu X, Bayle JH, Olson D, Levine AJ. The p53-mdm2 autoregulatory feedback loop. Genes Dev 1993; 7:1126–1132.
50. Sher CJ. Cancer cell cycles. Science 1996; 274:1672–1677.
51. Figge J, Breese K, Vajda S, Zhu QL, Eisele L, Andersen TT, et al. The binding domain structure of retinoblastoma-binding proteins. Protein Sci 1993; 2:155–164.
52. DeCaprio JA, Ludlow JW, Figge J, Shew JY, Huang CM, Lee WH, et al. SV40 large tumor antigen forms a specific complex with the product of the retinoblastoma susceptibility gene. Cell 1988; 54: 275–283.
53. Whyte P, Buchkovich KJ, Horowitz JM, Friend SH, Raybuck M, Weinberg RA, Harlow E. Association between an oncogene and an anti-oncogene: the adenovirus E1A proteins bind to the retinoblastoma gene product. Nature 1988; 334:124–129.
54. Ledent C, Dumont J, Vassart G, Parmentier M. Thyroid adenocarcinomas secondary to tissue-specific expression of simian virus-40 large T-antigen in transgenic mice. Endocrinology 1991; 129:1391–1401.
55. Reynolds RK, Hoekzema GS, Vogel J, Hinrichs SH, Jay G. Multiple endocrine neoplasia induced by the promiscuous expression of a viral oncogene. Proc Natl Acad Sci USA 1988; 85:3135–3139.
56. Ledent C, Marcotte A, Dumont JE, Vassart G, Parmentier M. Differentiated carcinomas develop as a consequence of the thyroid specific expression of a thyroglobulin-human papillomavirus type 16 E7 transgene. Oncogene 1995; 10:1789–1797.
57. Hahn WC, Weinberg RA. Rules for making human tumor cells. N Engl J Med 2002; 347:1593–1603.
58. Cahill DP, Kinzler KW, Vogelstein B, Lengauer C. Genetic instability and Darwinian selection in tumours. Trends Cell Biol 1999; 9: M57–M60.
59. Namba H, Matsuo K, Fagin JA. Clonal composition of benign and malignant human thyroid tumors. J Clin Invest 1990; 86:120–125.
60. Thomas GA, Williams D, Williams ED. The clonal origin of thyroid nodules and adenomas. Am J Pathol 1989; 134:141–147.
61. Gerber H, Burgi U, Peter HJ. Etiology and pathogenesis of thyroid nodules. Exp Clin Endocrinol 1993; 101:97–101.
62. Matsuo K, Tang SH, Zeki K, Gutman RA, Fagin JA. Aberrant DNA methylation in human thyroid tumors. J Clin Endocrinol Metab 1993; 77:991–995.
63. Laird PW, Jaenisch R. The role of DNA methylation in cancer genetic and epigenetics. Annu Rev Genet 1996; 30:441–464.
64. Aasland R, Akslen LA, Varhaug JE, Lillehaug JR. Co-expression of the genes encoding transforming growth factor-alpha and its receptor in papillary carcinomas of the thyroid. Int J Cancer 1990; 46:382–387.
65. Mizukami Y, Nonomura A, Hashimoto T, Michigishi T, Noguchi M, Matsubara F, Yanaihara N. Immunohistochemical demonstration of epidermal growth factor and c-myc oncogene product in normal, benign and malignant thyroid tissues. Histopathology 1991; 18:11–18.
66. Williams DW, Williams ED, Wynford-Thomas D. Evidence for autocrine production of IGF-1 in human thyroid adenomas. Mol Cell Endocrinol 1989; 61:139–143.
67. Minuto F, Barreca A, Del Monte P, Cariola G, Torre GC, Giordano G. Immunoreactive insulin-like growth factor I (IGF-I) and IGF-I-binding protein content in human thyroid tissue. J Clin Endocrinol Metab 1989; 68:621–626.
68. Tode B, Serio M, Rotella CM, Galli G, Franceschelli F, Tanini A, Toccafondi R. Insulin-like growth factor I: autocrine secretion by human thyroid follicular cells in primary culture. J Clin Endocrinol Metab 1989; 69:639–647.
69. Boelaert K, McCabe CJ, Tannahill LA, Gittoes NJ, Holder RL, Watkinson JC, et al. Pituitary tumor transforming gene and fibroblast growth factor-2 expression: potential prognostic indicators in differentiated thyroid cancer. J Clin Endocrinol Metab 2003; 88: 2341–2347.
70. Bunone G, Vigneri P, Mariani L, Buto S, Collini P, Pilotti S, et al. Expression of angiogenesis stimulators and inhibitors in human thyroid tumors and correlation with clinical pathological features. Am J Pathol 1999; 155:1967–1976.
71. Poulaki V, Mitsiades CS, McMullan C, Sykoutri D, Fanourakis G, Kotoula V, et al. Regulation of vascular endothelial growth factor expression by insulin-like growth factor I in thyroid carcinomas. J Clin Endocrinol Metab 2003; 88:5392–5398.
72. Viglietto G, Maglione D, Rambaldi M, Cerutti J, Romano A, Trapasso F, et al. Upregulation of vascular endothelial growth factor (VEGF) and downregulation of placenta growth factor (PlGF) associated with malignancy in human thyroid tumors and cell lines. Oncogene 1995; 11:1569–1579.
73. Soh EY, Duh QY, Sobhi SA, Young DM, Epstein HD, Wong MG, et al. Vascular endothelial growth factor expression is higher in differentiated thyroid cancer than in normal or benign thyroid. J Clin Endocrinol Metab 1997; 82:3741–3747.
74. Bauer AJ, Terrell R, Doniparthi NK, Patel A, Tuttle RM, Saji M, et al. Vascular endothelial growth factor monoclonal antibody inhibits growth of anaplastic thyroid cancer xenografts in nude mice. Thyroid 2002; 12:953–961.
75. Bauer AJ, Patel A, Terrell R, Doniparthi K, Saji M, Ringel M, et al. Systemic administration of vascular endothelial growth factor monoclonal antibody reduces the growth of papillary thyroid carcinoma in a nude mouse model. Ann Clin Lab Sci 2003; 33:192–199.
76. Fenton C, Patel A, Dinauer C, Robie DK, Tuttle RM, Francis GL. The expression of vascular endothelial growth factor and the type 1 vascular endothelial growth factor receptor correlate with the size of papillary thyroid carcinoma in children and young adults. Thyroid 2000; 10:349–357.
77. Olayioye MA, Neve RM, Lane HA, Hynes NE. The ErbB signaling network: receptor heterodimerization in development and cancer. EMBO J 2000; 19:3159–3167.
78. Aasland R, Lillehaug JR, Male R, Josendal O, Varhaug JE, Kleppe K. Expression of oncogenes in thyroid tumors: coexpression of c-erbB2/neu and c-erbB. Br J Cancer 1988; 57:358–363.
79. Sugg SL, Ezzat S, Zheng L, Freeman JL, Rosen IB, Asa SL. Oncogene profile of papillary thyroid carcinoma. Surgery 1999; 125:46–52.
80. Bieche I, Franc B, Vidaud D, Vidaud M, Lidereau R. Analyses of MYC, ERBB2, and CCND1 genes in benign and malignant thyroid follicular cell tumors by real-time polymerase chain reaction. Thyroid 2001; 11:147–152.
81. Di Carlo A, Mariano A, Pisano G, Parmeggiani U, Beguinot L, Macchia V. Epidermal growth factor receptor and thyrotropin response in human thyroid tissues. J Endocrinol Invest 1990; 13: 293–299.
82. Bergstrom JD, Westermark B, Heldin NE. Epidermal growth factor receptor signaling activates met in human anaplastic thyroid carcinoma cells. Exp Cell Res 2000; 259:293–299.

83. Heldin NE, Gustavsson B, Claesson-Welsh L, Hammacher A, Mark J, Heldin CH, Westermark B. Aberrant expression of receptors for platelet-derived growth factor in an anaplastic thyroid carcinoma cell line. Proc Natl Acad Sci USA 1988; 85:9302–9306.
84. Di Renzo MF, Narsimhan RP, Olivero M, Bretti S, Giordano S, Medico E, et al. Expression of the met/HGF receptor in normal and neoplastic human tissues. Oncogene 1991; 6:1997–2003.
85. Di Renzo MF, Olivero M, Ferro S, Prat M, Bongarzone I, Pilotti S, et al. Overexpression of the c-MET/HGF receptor gene in human thyroid carcinomas. Oncogene 1992; 7:2549–2553.
86. Ruco LP, Ranalli T, Marzullo A, Bianco P, Prat M, Comoglio PM, Baroni CD. Expression of Met protein in thyroid tumours. J Pathol 1996; 180:266–270.
87. Ivan M, Bond JA, Prat M, Comoglio PM, Wynford-Thomas D. Activated ras and RET oncogenes induce over-expression of c-met (hepatocyte growth factor receptor) in human thyroid epithelial cells. Oncogene 1997; 14:2417–2423.
88. Brinkmann V, Foroutan H, Sachs M, Weidner KM, Birchmeier W. Hepatocyte growth factor/scatter factor induces a variety of tissue-specific morphogenic programs in epithelial cells. J Cell Biol 1995; 131:1573–1586.
89. Scarpino S, Stoppacciaro A, Colarossi C, Cancellario F, Marzullo A, Marchesi M, et al. Hepatocyte growth factor (HGF) stimulates tumour invasiveness in papillary carcinoma of the thyroid. J Pathol 1999; 189:570–575.
90. de Luca A, Arena N, Sena LM, Medico E. Met overexpression confers HGF-dependent invasive phenotype to human thyroid carcinoma cells in vitro. J Cell Physiol 1999; 180:365–371.
91. Ruco LP, Stoppacciaro A, Ballarini F, Prat M, Scarpino S. Met protein and hepatocyte growth factor (HGF) in papillary carcinoma of the thyroid: evidence for a pathogenetic role in tumourigenesis. J Pathol 2001; 194:4–8.
92. Belfiore A, Gangemi P, Costantino A, Russo G, Santonocito GM, Ippolito O, et al. Negative/low expression of the Met/hepatocyte growth factor receptor identifies papillary thyroid carcinomas with high risk of distant metastases. J Clin Endocrinol Metab 1997; 82:2322–2328.
93. Fusco A, Grieco M, Santoro M, Berlingieri MT, Pilotti S, Pierotti MA, et al. A new oncogene in human thyroid papillary carcinomas and their lymph-nodal metastases. Nature 1987; 328:170–172.
94. Bongarzone I, Pierotti MA, Monzini N, Mondellini P, Manenti G, Donghi R, et al. High frequency of activation of tyrosine kinase oncogenes in human papillary thyroid carcinoma. Oncogene 1989; 4:1457–1462.
95. Grieco M, Santoro M, Berlingieri MT, Melillo RM, Donghi R, Bongarzone I, et al. PTC is a novel rearranged form of the RET proto-oncogene and is frequently detected in vivo in human thyroid papillary carcinomas. Cell 1990; 60:557–563.
96. Santoro M, Carlomagno F, Hay ID, Herrmann MA, Grieco M, Melillo R, et al. *Ret* oncogene activation in human thyroid neoplasms is restricted to the papillary cancer subtype. J Clin Invest 1992; 89:1517–1522.
97. Ito T, Seyama T, Iwamoto KS, Mizuno T, Tronko ND, Komissarenko IV, et al. Activated *RET* oncogene in thyroid cancers of children from areas contaminated by Chernobyl accident. Lancet 1994; 344:259.
98. Klugbauer S, Lengfelder E, Demidchik EP, Rabes HM. High prevalence of *RET* rearrangement in thyroid tumors of children from Belarus after the Chernobyl reactor accident. Oncogene 1995; 11:2459–2467.
99. Fugazzola L, Pilotti S, Pinchera A, Vorontsova TV, Mondellini P, Bongarzone I, Greco A, et al. Oncogenic rearrangements of the *RET* proto-oncogene in papillary thyroid carcinomas from children exposed to the Chernobyl nuclear accident. Cancer Res 1995; 55:5617–5620.
100. Rabes HM, Klugbauer S. Radiation-induced thyroid carcinomas in children: high prevalence of RET rearrangement. Verh Dtsch Ges Pathol 1997; 81:139–144.
101. Nikiforov YE, Rowland JM, Bove KE, Monforte-Munoz H, Fagin JA. Distinct pattern of ret oncogene rearrangements in morphological variants of radiation-induced and sporadic thyroid papillary carcinomas in children. Cancer Res 1997; 57:1690–1694.
102. Pisarchik AV, Ermak G, Fomicheva V, Kartel NA, Figge J. The ret/PTC1 rearrangement is a common feature of Chernobyl-associated papillary thyroid carcinomas from Belarus. Thyroid 1998; 8:133–139.
103. Pisarchik AV, Ermak G, Demidchik EP, Mikhalevich LS, Kartel NA, Figge J. Low prevalence of the ret/PTC3r1 rearrangement in a series of papillary thyroid carcinomas presenting in Belarus ten years post-Chernobyl. Thyroid 1998; 8:1003–1008.
104. Pisarchik AV, Yarmolinskii DG, Demidchik YE, Ermak GZ, Kartel NA, Figge J. ret/PTC1 and ret/PTC3r1 rearrangement in thyroid cancer cells, arising in residents of Belarus in the period after the accident at the Chernobyl nuclear power plant. Genetika 2000; 36:959–964.
105. Smida J, Salassidis K, Hieber L, Zitzelsberger H, Kellerer AM, Demidchik EP, et al. Distinct frequency of ret rearrangements in papillary thyroid carcinomas of children and adults from Belarus. Int J Cancer 1999; 80:32–38.
106. Rabes HM, Demidchik EP, Sidorow JD, Lengfelder E, Beimfohr C, Hoelzel D, Klugbauer S. Pattern of radiation-induced RET and NTRK1 rearrangements in 191 post-chernobyl papillary thyroid carcinomas: biological, phenotypic, and clinical implications. Clin Cancer Res 2000; 6:1093–1103.
107. Rabes HM. Gene rearrangements in radiation-induced thyroid carcinogenesis. Med Pediatr Oncol 2001; 36:574–582.
108. Ito T, Seyama T, Iwamoto KS, Hayashi T, Mizuno T, Tsuyama N, et al. In vitro irradiation is able to cause *RET* oncogene rearrangement. Cancer Res 1993; 53:2940–2943.
109. Bounacer A, Wicker R, Caillou B, Cailleux AF, Sarasin A, Schlumberger M, Suarez HG. High prevalence of activating ret proto-oncogene rearrangements, in thyroid tumors from patients who had received external radiation. Oncogene 1997; 15:1263–1273.
110. Elisei R, Romei C, Soldatenko PP, Cosci B, Vorontsova T, Vivaldi A, et al. New breakpoints in both the H4 and RET genes create a variant of PTC-1 in a post-Chernobyl papillary thyroid carcinoma. Clin Endocrinol 2000; 53:131–136.
111. Fugazzola L, Pierotti MA, Vigano E, Pacini F, Vorontsova TV, Bongarzone I. Molecular and biochemical analysis of RET/PTC4, a novel oncogenic rearrangement between RET and ELE1 genes, in a post-Chernobyl papillary thyroid cancer. Oncogene 1996; 13:1093–1097.
112. Klugbauer S, Lengfelder E, Demidchik EP, Rabes HM. A new form of RET rearrangement in thyroid carcinomas of children after the Chernobyl reactor accident. Oncogene 1996; 13:1099–1102.
113. Klugbauer S, Demidchik EP, Lengfelder E, Rabes HM. Molecular analysis of new subtypes of ELE/RET rearrangements, their reciprocal transcripts and breakpoints in papillary thyroid carcinomas of children after Chernobyl. Oncogene 1998; 16:671–675.
114. Klugbauer S, Demidchik EP, Lengfelder E, Rabes HM. Detection of a novel type of RET rearrangement (PTC5) in thyroid carcinomas after Chernobyl and analysis of the involved RET-fused gene RFG5. Cancer Res 1998; 58:198–203.
115. Klugbauer S, Rabes HM. The transcription coactivator HTIF1 and a related protein are fused to the RET receptor tyrosine kinase in childhood papillary thyroid carcinomas. Oncogene 1999; 18:4388–4393.
116. Salassidis K, Bruch J, Zitzelsberger H, Lengfelder E, Kellerer AM, Bauchinger M. Translocation t(10;14)(q11.2:q22.1) fusing the kinectin to the RET gene creates a novel rearranged form (PTC8) of the RET proto-oncogene in radiation-induced childhood papillary thyroid carcinoma. Cancer Res 2000; 60:2786–2789.

117. Klugbauer S, Jauch A, Lengfelder E, Demidchik E, Rabes HM. A novel type of RET rearrangement (PTC8) in childhood papillary thyroid carcinomas and characterization of the involved gene (RFG8). Cancer Res 2000; 60:7028–7032.
118. Corvi R, Berger N, Balczon R, Romeo G. RET/PCM-1: a novel fusion gene in papillary thyroid carcinoma. Oncogene 2000; 19:4236–4242.
119. Nakata T, Kitamura Y, Shimizu K, Tanaka S, Fujimori M, Yokoyama S, Ito K, Emi M. Fusion of a novel gene, ELKS, to RET due to translocation t(10;12)(q11;p13) in a papillary thyroid carcinoma. Genes Chromosomes Cancer 1999; 25:97–103.
120. Giannini R, Salvatore G, Monaco C, Sferratore F, Pollina L, Pacini F, et al. Identification of a novel subtype of H4-RET rearrangement in a thyroid papillary carcinoma and lymph node metastasis. Int J Oncol 2000; 16:485–489.
121. Santero M, Sabino N, Ishizaka Y, Ushijima T, Carlomagno F, Cerrato A, et al. Involvement of *RET* oncogene in human tumours: specificity of RET activation to thyroid tumours. Br J Cancer 1993; 68:460–464.
122. Chiappetta G, Toti P, Cetta F, Giuliano A, Pentimalli F, Amendola I, et al. The RET/PTC oncogene is frequently activated in oncocytic thyroid tumors (Hurthle cell adenomas and carcinomas), but not in oncocytic hyperplastic lesions. J Clin Endocrinol Metab 2002; 87:364–369.
123. Santoro M, Papotti M, Chiappetta G, Garcia-Rostan G, Volante M, Johnson C, et al. RET activation and clinicopathologic features in poorly differentiated thyroid tumors. J Clin Endocrinol Metab 2002; 87:370–379.
124. Donghi R, Sozzi G, Pierotti MA, Biunno I, Miozzo M, Fusco A, et al. The oncogene associated with human papillary thyroid carcinoma (PTC) is assigned to chromosome 10 q11-q12 in the same region as multiple endocrine neoplasia type 2a (MEN2A). Oncogene 1989; 4: 521–523.
125. Zou M, Shi Y, Farid NR. Low rate of RET proto-oncogene activation (PTC/RET^{TPC}) in papillary thyroid carcinomas from Saudi Arabia. Cancer 1994; 73:176–180.
126. Sugg SL, Zheng L, Rosen IB, Freeman JL, Ezzat S, Asa SL. ret/PTC-1, -2, and -3 oncogene rearrangements in human thyroid carcinomas: implications for metastatic potential? J Clin Endocrinol Metab 1996; 81:3360–3365.
127. Said S, Schlumberger M, Suarez HG. Oncogenes and anti-oncogenes in human epithelial thyroid tumors. J Endocrinol Invest 1994; 17:371–379.
128. Delvincourt C, Patey M, Flament JB, Suarez HG, Larbre H, Jardillier JC, Delisle MJ. Ret and trk proto-oncogene activation in thyroid papillary carcinomas in French patients from the Champagne-Ardenne region. Clin Biochem 1996; 29:267–271.
129. Santoro M, Dathan NA, Berlingieri MT, Bongarzone I, Paulin C, Grieco M, et al. Molecular characterization of RET/PTC3; a novel rearranged version of the RET proto-oncogene in a human thyroid papillary carcinoma. Oncogene 1994; 9:509–516.
130. Bongarzone I, Butti MG, Coronelli S, Borrello MG, Santoro M, Mondellini P, et al. Frequent activation of ret protooncogene by fusion with a new activating gene in papillary thyroid carcinomas. Cancer Res 1994; 54:2979–2985.
131. Ishizaka Y, Kobayashi S, Ushijima T, Hirohashi S, Sugimura T, Nagao M. Detection of retTPC/PTC transcripts in thyroid adenomas and adenomatous goiter by an RT-PCR method. Oncogene 1991; 6:1667–1672.
132. Wajjwalku W, Nakamura S, Hasegawa Y, Miyazaki K, Satoh Y, Funahashi H, et al. Low frequency of rearrangements of the ret and trk proto-oncogenes in Japanese thyroid papillary carcinomas. Jpn J Cancer Res 1992; 83:671–675.
133. Sugg SL, Ezzat S, Rosen IB, Freeman JL, Asa SL. Distinct multiple RET/PTC gene rearrangements in multifocal papillary thyroid neoplasia. J Clin Endocrinol Metab 1998; 83:4116–4122.
134. Motomura T, Nikiforov YE, Namba H, Ashizawa K, Nagataki S, Yamashita S, Fagin JA. ret rearrangements in Japanese pediatric and adult papillary thyroid cancers. Thyroid 1998; 8:485–489.
135. Chung JH, Hahm JR, Min YK, Lee MS, Lee MK, Kim KW, et al. Detection of RET/PTC oncogene rearrangements in Korean papillary thyroid carcinomas. Thyroid 1999; 9:1237–1243.
136. Kjellman P, Learoyd DL, Messina M, Weber G, Hoog A, Wallin G, et al. Expression of the RET proto-oncogene in papillary thyroid carcinoma and its correlation with clinical outcome. Br J Surg 2001; 88: 557–563.
137. Mayr B, Potter E, Goretzki P, Ruschoff J, Dietmaier W, Hoang-Vu C, et al. Expression of Ret/PTC1, -2, -3, -delta3 and -4 in German papillary thyroid carcinoma. Br J Cancer 1998; 77:903–906.
138. Lee CH, Hsu LS, Chi CW, Chen GD, Yang AH, Chen JY. High frequency of rearrangement of the RET protooncogene (RET/PTC) in Chinese papillary thyroid carcinomas. J Clin Endocrinol Metab 1998; 83:1629–1632.
139. Chua EL, Wu WM, Tran KT, McCarthy SW, Lauer CS, Dubourdieu D, et al. Prevalence and distribution of ret/ptc 1, 2, and 3 in papillary thyroid carcinoma in New Caledonia and Australia. J Clin Endocrinol Metab 2000; 85:2733–2739.
140. Finn SP, Smyth P, O'Leary J, Sweeney EC, Sheils O. Ret/PTC chimeric transcripts in an Irish cohort of sporadic papillary thyroid carcinoma. J Clin Endocrinol Metab 2003; 88:938–941.
141. Fenton CL, Lukes Y, Nicholson D, Dinauer CA, Francis GL, Tuttle RM. The ret/PTC mutations are common in sporadic papillary thyroid carcinoma of children and young adults. J Clin Endocrinol Metab 2000; 85:1170–1175.
142. Bongarzone I, Fugazzola L, Vigneri P, Mariani L, Mondellini P, Pacini F, et al. Age-related activation of the tyrosine kinase receptor protooncogenes RET and NTRK1 in papillary thyroid carcinoma. J Clin Endocrinol Metab 1996; 81:2006–2009.
143. Park KY, Koh JM, Kim YI, Park HJ, Gong G, Hong SJ, Ahn IM. Prevalences of Gs alpha, ras, p53 mutations and RET/PTC rearrangement in differentiated thyroid tumours in a Korean population. Clin Endocrinol 1998; 49:317–323.
144. Zhu Z, Gandhi M, Nikiforova MN, Fischer AH, Nikiforov YE. Molecular profile and clinical-pathologic features of the follicular variant of papillary thyroid carcinoma. An unusually high prevalence of ras mutations. Am J Clin Pathol 2003; 120:71–77.
145. Soares P, Trovisco V, Rocha AS, Lima J, Castro P, Preto A, et al. BRAF mutations and RET/PTC rearrangements are alternative events in the etiopathogenesis of PTC. Oncogene 2003; 22:4578–4580.
146. Kimura ET, Nikiforova MN, Zhu Z, Knauf JA, Nikiforov YE, Fagin JA. High prevalence of BRAF mutations in thyroid cancer: genetic evidence for constitutive activation of the RET/PTC-RAS-BRAF signaling pathway in papillary thyroid carcinoma. Cancer Res 2003; 63: 1454–1457.
147. Jhiang SM, Caruso DR, Gilmore E, Ishizaka Y, Tahira T, Nagao M, et al. Detection of the PTC/RETTPC oncogene in human thyroid cancers. Oncogene 1992; 7:1331–1337.
148. Jhiang SM, Sagartz JE, Tong Q, Parker-Thornburg J, Capen CC, Cho JY, et al. Targeted expression of the RET/PTC1 oncogene induces papillary thyroid carcinomas. Endocrinology 1996; 137:375–378.
149. Santoro M, Chiappetta G, Cerrato A, et al. Development of thyroid papillary carcinomas secondary to tissue-specific expression of the RET/PTC1 oncogene in transgenic mice. Oncogene 1996; 12: 1821–1826.
150. Russell JP, Powell DJ, Cunnane M, Greco A, Portella G, Santoro M, et al. The TRK-T1 fusion protein induces neoplastic transformation of thyroid epithelium. Oncogene 2000; 19:5729–5735.
151. Greco A, Pierotti MA, Bongarzone I, Pagliardini S, Lanzi C, Delia Porta G. TRK-T1 is a novel oncogene formed by the fusion of TPR and TRK genes in human papillary thyroid carcinomas. Oncogene 1992; 7:237–242.
152. Alberti L, Carniti C, Miranda C, Roccato E, Pierotti MA. RET and NTRK1 proto-oncogenes in human diseases. J Cell Physiol 2003; 195: 168–186.

153. Pierotti MA. Chromosomal rearrangements in thyroid carcinomas: a recombination or death dilemma. Cancer Lett 2001; 166:1–7.
154. Russo D, Arturi F, Schlumberger M, Caillou B, Monier R, Filetti S, Suarez HG. Activating mutations of the TSH receptor in differentiated thyroid carcinomas. Oncogene 1995; 11:1907–1911.
155. Camacho P, Gordon D, Chiefari E, Yong S, DeJong S, Pitale S, Russo D, Filetti S. A Phe 486 thyrotropin receptor mutation in an autonomously functioning follicular carcinoma that was causing hyperthyroidism. Thyroid 2000; 10:1009–1012.
156. Fuhrer D, Tannapfel A, Sabri O, Lamesch P, Paschke R. Two somatic TSH receptor mutations in a patient with toxic metastasising follicular thyroid carcinoma and non-functional lung metastases. Endocr Relat Cancer 2003; 10:591–600.
157. Russo D, Wong MG, Costante G, Chiefari E, Treseler PA, Arturi F, et al. A Val 677 activating mutation of the thyrotropin receptor in a Hurthle cell thyroid carcinoma associated with thyrotoxicosis. Thyroid 1999; 9:13–17.
158. Spambalg D, Sharifi N, Elisei R, Gross JL, Medeiros-Neto G, Fagin JA. Structural studies of the thyrotropin receptor and Gs alpha in human thyroid cancers: low prevalence of mutations predicts infrequent involvement in malignant transformation. J Clin Endocrinol Metab 1996; 81:3898–3901.
159. Esapa C, Foster S, Johnson S, Jameson JL, Kendall-Taylor P, Harris PE. G protein and thyrotropin receptor mutations in thyroid neoplasia. J Clin Endocrinol Metab 1997; 82:493–496.
160. Russo D, Tumino S, Arturi F, Vigneri P, Grasso G, Pontecorvi A, et al. Detection of an activating mutation of the thyrotropin receptor in a case of an autonomously hyperfunctioning thyroid insular carcinoma. J Clin Endocrinol Metab 1997; 82:735–738.
161. Matsuo K, Friedman E, Gejman PV, Fagin JA. The thyrotropin receptor (TSH-R) is not an oncogene for thyroid tumors: structural studies of the TSH-R and the alpha-subunit of Gs in human thyroid neoplasms. J Clin Endocrinol Metab 1993; 76:1446–1451.
162. Lemoine NR, Mayall ES, Wyllie FS, et al. Activated RAS oncogenes in human thyroid cancers. Cancer Res 1988; 48:4459–4463.
163. Suarez HG, DuVillard JA, Caillou B, Schlumberger M, Tubiana M, Parmentier C, Monier R. Detection of activated RAS oncogenes in human thyroid carcinomas. Oncogene 1988; 2:403–406.
164. Lemoine NR, Mayall ES, Wyllie FS, Williams ED, Goyns M, Stringer B, Wynford-Thomas D. High frequency of *RAS* oncogene activation in 11 stages of human thyroid tumorigenesis. Oncogene 1989; 4:159–164.
165. Stringer BM, Rowson JM, Parker MH, Seid JM, Hearn PR, Wynford-Thomas D, et al. Detection of the H-*RAS* oncogene in human thyroid anaplastic carcinomas. Experientia 1989; 45:372–376.
166. Wright PA, Lemoine NR, Mayall ES, Wyllie FS, Hughes D, Williams ED, Wynford-Thomas D. Papillary and follicular thyroid carcinomas show a different pattern of RAS oncogene mutation. Br J Cancer 1989; 60:576–577.
167. Dockhorn-Dworniczak B, Caspari S, Schroder S, Bocker W, Dworniczak B. Demonstration of activated oncogenes of the RAS family in human thyroid tumors using the polymerase chain reaction. Verhandl Dtsch Ges Pathol 1990; 74:415–418.
168. Namba H, Gutman RA, Matsuo K, Alvarez A, Fagin JA. H-*RAS* protooncogene mutations in human thyroid neoplasms. J Clin Endocrinol Metab 1990; 71:223–229.
169. Namba H, Rubin SA, Fagin JA. Point mutations of RAS oncogenes are an early event in thyroid tumorigenesis. Mol Endocrinol 1990; 4:1474–1479.
170. Schark C, Fulton N, Jacoby RF, Westbrook CA, Straus FH, Kaplan EL. *N-RAS* 61 oncogene mutations in Hürthle cell tumors. Surgery 1990; 108:994–999.
171. Suarez HG, du Villard JA, Severino M, Caillou B, Schlumberger M, Tubiana M, et al. Presence of mutations in all three RAS genes in human thyroid tumors. Oncogene 1990; 5:565–570.
172. Karga H, Lee JK, Vickery AL, Thor A, Gaz RD, Jameson JL. *RAS* oncogene mutations in benign and malignant thyroid neoplasms. J Clin Endocrinol Metab 1991; 73:832–836.
173. Shi Y, Zou M, Schmidt H, Juhasz F, Stensky V, Robb D, Farid NR. High rates of *RAS* codon 61 mutation in thyroid tumors in an iodide-deficient area. Cancer Res 1991; 51:2690–2693.
174. Wright PA, Williams ED, Lemoine NR, Wynford-Thomas D. Radiation-associated and "spontaneous" human thyroid carcinomas show a different pattern of *RAS* oncogene mutation. Oncogene 1991; 6:471–473.
175. Goretzki PE, Lyons J, Stacy-Phipps S, Rosenau W, Demeure M, Clark OH, et al. Mutational activation of *RAS* and *gsp* oncogenes in differentiated thyroid cancer and their biological implications. World J Surg 1992; 16:576–581.
176. Yoshimoto K, Iwahana H, Fukuda A, Sano T, Katsuragi K, Kinoshita M, et al. RAS mutations in endocrine tumors: mutation detection by polymerase chain reaction-single strand conformation polymorphism. Jpn J Cancer Res 1992; 83:1057–1062.
177. Hara H, Fulton N, Yashiro T, Ito K, DeGroot LJ, Kaplan EL. N-RAS mutation: an independent prognostic factor for aggressiveness of papillary thyroid carcinoma. Surgery 1994; 116:1010–1016.
178. Kaihara M, Taniyama M, Tadatomo J, Tobe T, Tomita M, Ito K, et al. Specific PCR amplification for N-RAS mutations in neoplastic thyroid diseases. Endocr J 1994; 41:301–308.
179. Manenti G, Pilotti S, Re FC, Della Porta G, Pierotti MA. Selective activation of RAS oncogenes in follicular and undifferentiated thyroid carcinomas. Eur J Cancer 1994; 30A:987–993.
180. Challeton C, BounacerA, Du Villard JA, Caillou B, De Vathaire F, Monier R, et al. Pattern of RAS and gsp oncogene mutations in radiation-associated human thyroid tumors. Oncogene 1995; 11:601–603.
181. Horie H, Yokogoshi Y, Tsuyuguchi M, Saito S. Point mutations of RAS and Gsα subunit genes in thyroid tumors. Jpn J Cancer Res 1995; 86:737–742.
182. Oyama T, Suzuki T, Hara F, Iino Y, Ishida T, Sakamoto A, Nakajima T. N-RAS mutation of thyroid tumor with special reference to the follicular type. Pathol Int 1995; 45:45–50.
183. Esapa CT, Johnson SJ, Kendall-Taylor P, Lennard TW, Harris PE. Prevalence of Ras mutations in thyroid neoplasia. Clin Endocrinol 1999; 50:529–535.
184. Naito H, Pairojkul C, Kitahori Y, Yane K, Miyahara H, Konishi N, et al. Different ras gene mutational frequencies in thyroid papillary carcinomas in Japan and Thailand. Cancer Lett 1998; 131:171–175.
185. Ezzat S, Zheng L, Kolenda J, Safarian A, Freeman JL, Asa SL. Prevalence of activating ras mutations in morphologically characterized thyroid nodules. Thyroid 1996; 6:409–416.
186. Bouras M, Bertholon J, Dutrieux-Berger N, Parvaz P, Paulin C, Revol A. Variability of Ha-ras (codon 12) proto-oncogene mutations in diverse thyroid cancers. Eur J Endocrinol 1998; 139:209–216.
187. De Micco C. ras mutations in follicular variant of papillary thyroid carcinoma. Am J Clin Pathol 2003; 120:803.
188. Salvatore D, Celetti A, Fabien N, Paulin C, Martelli ML, Battaglia C, et al. Low frequency of p53 mutations in human thyroid tumours; p53 and Ras mutation in two out of fifty-six thyroid tumours. Eur J Endocrinol 1996; 134:177–183.
189. Garcia-Rostan G, Zhao H, Camp RL, Pollan M, Herrero A, Pardo J, et al. ras mutations are associated with aggressive tumor phenotypes and poor prognosis in thyroid cancer. J Clin Oncol 2003; 21:3226–3235.
190. Vasko V, Ferrand M, Di Cristofaro J, Carayon P, Henry JF, de Micco C. Specific pattern of RAS oncogene mutations in follicular thyroid tumors. J Clin Endocrinol Metab 2003; 88:2745–2752.
191. Nikiforova MN, Lynch RA, Biddinger PW, Alexander EK, Dorn GW II, Tallini G, et al. RAS point mutations and PAX8-PPAR gamma rearrangement in thyroid tumors: evidence for distinct molecular

pathways in thyroid follicular carcinoma. J Clin Endocrinol Metab 2003; 88:2318–2326.
192. Pilotti S, Collini P, Mariani L, Placucci M, Bongarzone I, Vigneri P, et al. Insular carcinoma: a distinct de novo entity among follicular carcinomas of the thyroid gland. Am J Surg Pathol 1997; 21:1466–1473.
193. Krohn K, Reske A, Ackermann F, Muller A, Paschke R. Ras mutations are rare in solitary cold and toxic thyroid nodules. Clin Endocrinol 2001; 55:241–248.
194. Tallini G, Hsueh A, Liu S, Garcia-Rostan G, Speicher MR, Ward DC. Frequent chromosomal DNA unbalance in thyroid oncocytic (Hurthle cell) neoplasms detected by comparative genomic hybridization. Lab Invest 1999; 79:547–555.
195. Basolo F, Pisaturo F, Pollina LE, Fontanini G, Elisei R, Molinaro E, et al. N-ras mutation in poorly differentiated thyroid carcinomas: correlation with bone metastases and inverse correlation to thyroglobulin expression. Thyroid 2000; 10:19–23.
196. Fukushima T, Suzuki S, Mashiko M, Ohtake T, Endo Y, Takebayashi Y, et al. BRAF mutations in papillary carcinomas of the thyroid. Oncogene 2003; 22:6455–6457.
197. Suarez HG, du Villard JA, Caillou B, Schlumberger M, Parmentier C, Monier R. gsp mutations in human thyroid tumors. Oncogene 1991; 6:677–679.
198. O'Sullivan C, Barton CM, Staddon SL, Brown CL, Lemoine NR. Activating point mutations of the gsp oncogene in human thyroid adenomas. Mol Carcinog 1991; 4:345–349.
199. Davies H, Bignell GR, Cox C, Stephens P, Edkins S, Clegg S, et al. Mutations of the BRAF gene in human cancer. Nature 2002 Jun 27; 417:949–954.
200. Namba H, Nakashima M, Hayashi T, Hayashida N, Maeda S, Rogounovitch TI, et al. Clinical implication of hot spot BRAF mutation, V599E, in papillary thyroid cancers. J Clin Endocrinol Metab 2003; 88:4393–4397.
201. Xu X, Quiros RM, Gattuso P, Ain KB, Prinz RA. High prevalence of BRAF gene mutation in papillary thyroid carcinomas and thyroid tumor cell lines. Cancer Res 2003; 63:4561–4567.
202. Nikiforova MN, Kimura ET, Gandhi M, Biddinger PW, Knauf JA, Basolo F, et al. BRAF mutations in thyroid tumors are restricted to papillary carcinomas and anaplastic or poorly differentiated carcinomas arising from papillary carcinomas. J Clin Endocrinol Metab 2003; 88:5399–5404.
203. Cohen Y, Xing M, Mambo E, Guo Z, Wu G, Trink B, et al. BRAF mutation in papillary thyroid carcinoma. J Natl Cancer Inst 2003; 95:625–627.
204. Terrier P, Sheng ZM, Schlumberger M, Tubiana M, Caillou B, Travagli JP, et al. Structure and expression of c-myc and c-fos proto-oncogenes in thyroid carcinomas. Br J Cancer 1988; 57:43–47.
205. Cerutti J, Trapasso F, Battaglia C, Zhang L, Martelli ML, Visconti R, et al. Block of c-myc expression by antisense oligonucleotides inhibits proliferation of human thyroid carcinoma cell lines. Clin Cancer Res 1996; 2:119–126.
206. Ito T, Seyama T, Mizuno T, Tsuyama N, Hayashi T, Hayashi Y, et al. Unique association of p53 mutations with undifferentiated but not with differentiated carcinomas of the thyroid gland. Cancer Res 1992; 52:1369–1371.
207. Ito T, Seyama T, Mizuno T, Tsuyama N, Hayashi Y, Dohi K, et al. Genetic alterations in thyroid tumor progression: association with p53 gene mutations. Jpn J Cancer Res 1993; 84:526–531.
208. Asakawa H, Kobayashi T. Multistep carcinogenesis in anaplastic thyroid carcinoma: a case report. Pathology 2002; 34:94–97.
209. Nakamura T, Yana I, Kobayashi T, Shin E, Karakawa K, Fujita S, et al. p53 gene mutations associated with anaplastic transformation of human thyroid carcinomas. Jpn J Cancer Res 1992; 83:1293–1298.
210. Donghi R, Longoni A, Pilotti S, Michieli P, Delia Porta G, Pierotti MA. Gene p53 mutations are restricted to poorly differentiated and undifferentiated carcinomas of the thyroid gland. J Clin Invest 1993; 91:1753–1760.
211. Fagin JA, Matsuo K, Karmakar A, Chen DL, Tang SH, Koeffler HP. High prevalence of mutations of the p53 gene in poorly differentiated human thyroid carcinomas. J Clin Invest 1993; 91:179–184.
212. Zou M, Shi Y, Farid NR. P53 mutations in all stages of thyroid carcinomas. J Clin Endocrinol Metab 1993; 77:1054–1058.
213. Dobashi Y, Sugimura H, Sakamoto A, Mernyei M, Mori M, Oyama T, Machinami R. Stepwise participation of p53 gene mutation during dedifferentiation of human thyroid carcinomas. Diagn Mol Pathol 1994; 3:9–14.
214. Takeuchi Y, Daa T, Kashima K, Yokoyama S, Nakayama I, Noguchi S. Mutations of p53 in thyroid carcinoma with an insular component. Thyroid 1999; 9:377–381.
215. Shahedian B, Shi Y, Zou M, Farid NR. Thyroid carcinoma is characterized by genomic instability: evidence from p53 mutations. Mol Genet Metab 2001; 72:155–163.
216. Gerasimov G, Bronstein M, Troshina K, Alexandrova G, Dedov I, Jennings T, et al. Nuclear p53 immunoreactivity in papillary thyroid cancers is associated with two established indicators of poor prognosis. Exp Mol Pathol 1995; 62:52–62.
217. Ho YS, Tseng SC, Chin TY, Hsieh LL, Lin JD. p53 gene mutation in thyroid carcinoma. Cancer Lett 1996; 103:57–63.
218. Zou M, Shi Y, Al-Sedairy S, Hussain SS, Farid NR. The expression of the MDM2 gene, a p53 binding protein, in thyroid carcinogenesis. Cancer 1995; 76:314–318.
219. Jennings T, Bratslavsky G, Gerasimov G, Troshina K, Bronstein M, Dedov I, et al. Nuclear accumulation of MDM2 protein in well-differentiated papillary thyroid carcinomas. Exp Mol Pathol 1995; 62: 199–206.
220. Horie S, Maeta H, Endo K, Ueta T, Takashima K, Terada T. Overexpression of p53 protein and MDM2 in papillary carcinomas of the thyroid: Correlations with clinicopathologic features. Pathol Int 2001; 51:11–15.
221. Basolo F, Caligo MA, Pinchera A, Fedeli F, Baldanzi A, Miccoli P, et al. Cyclin D1 overexpression in thyroid carcinomas: relation with clinico-pathological parameters, retinoblastoma gene product, and Ki67 labeling index. Thyroid 2000; 10:741–746.
222. Khoo ML, Beasley NJ, Ezzat S, Freeman JL, Asa SL. Overexpression of cyclin D1 and underexpression of p27 predict lymph node metastases in papillary thyroid carcinoma. J Clin Endocrinol Metab 2002; 87:1814–1818.
223. Khoo ML, Ezzat S, Freeman JL, Asa SL. Cyclin D1 protein expression predicts metastatic behavior in thyroid papillary microcarcinomas but is not associated with gene amplification. J Clin Endocrinol Metab 2002; 87:1810–1813.
224. Lazzereschi D, Sambuco L, Carnovale Scalzo C, Ranieri A, Mincione G, Nardi F, Colletta G. Cyclin D1 and Cyclin E expression in malignant thyroid cells and in human thyroid carcinomas. Int J Cancer 1998; 76:806–811.
225. Goto A, Sakamoto A, Machinami R. An immunohistochemical analysis of cyclin D1, p53, and p21waf1/cip1 proteins in tumors originating from the follicular epithelium of the thyroid gland. Pathol Res Pract 2001; 197:217–222.
226. Muro-Cacho CA, Holt T, Klotch D, Mora L, Livingston S, Futran N. Cyclin D1 expression as a prognostic parameter in papillary carcinoma of the thyroid. Otolaryngol Head Neck Surg 1999; 120: 200–207.
227. Zou M, Shi Y, Farid NR, Al-Sedairy ST. Inverse association between cyclin D1 overexpression and retinoblastoma gene mutation in thyroid carcinomas. Endocrine 1998; 8:61–64.
228. Wang S, Wuu J, Savas L, Patwardhan N, Khan A. The role of cell cycle regulatory proteins, cyclin D1, cyclin E, and p27 in thyroid carcinogenesis. Hum Pathol 1998; 29:1304–1309.
229. Wang S, Lloyd RV, Hutzler MJ, Safran MS, Patwardhan NA, Khan A. The role of cell cycle regulatory protein, cyclin D1, in the progression of thyroid cancer. Mod Pathol 2000; 13:882–887.

230. Demetri GD, Fletcher CD, Mueller E, Sarraf P, Naujoks R, Campbell N, et al. Induction of solid tumor differentiation by the peroxisome proliferator-activated receptor-gamma ligand troglitazone in patients with liposarcoma. Proc Natl Acad Sci USA 1999; 96:3951–3956.
231. Kroll TG, Sarraf P, Pecciarini L, Chen CJ, Mueller E, Spiegelman BM, Fletcher JA. PAX8-PPARgamma1 fusion oncogene in human thyroid carcinoma. Science 2000; 289:1357–1360.
232. Nikiforova MN, Biddinger PW, Caudill CM, Kroll TG, Nikiforov YE. PAX8-PPARgamma rearrangement in thyroid tumors: RT-PCR and immunohistochemical analyses. Am J Surg Pathol 2002; 26:1016–1023.
233. Marques AR, Espadinha C, Catarino AL, Moniz S, Pereira T, Sobrinho LG, Leite V. Expression of PAX8-PPAR gamma 1 rearrangements in both follicular thyroid carcinomas and adenomas. J Clin Endocrinol Metab 2002; 87:3947–3952.
233a. Dwight T, Thoppe SR, Foukakis T, et al. Involvement of the PAX8/peroxisome proliferator-activated receptor gamma rearrangement in follicular thyroid tumors. J Clin Endocrinol Metab 2003; 88:4440–4445.
234. Gunthert U. CD44: a multitude of isoforms with diverse functions. Curr Top Microbiol Immunol 1993; 184:47–63.
235. Lesley J, Hyman R, Kincade PW. CD44 and its interaction with extracellular matrix. Adv Immunol 1993; 54:271–335.
236. Aruffo A, Stamenkovic I, Melnick M, Underhill CB, Seed B. CD44 is the principal cell surface receptor for hyaluronate. Cell 1990; 61:1303–1313.
237. Hofmann M, Rudy W, Zoller M, Tolg C, Ponta H, Herrlich P, Gunthert U. CD44 splice variants confer metastatic behavior in rats: homologous sequences are expressed in human tumor lines. Cancer Res 1991; 51:5292–5297.
238. Rudy W, Hofmann M, Schwartz-Albiez R, Zoller M, Heider KH, Ponta H, Herrlich P. Two major CD44 proteins expressed on a metastatic rat tumor cell line are derived from different splice variants: each one individually suffices to confer metastatic behavior. Cancer Res 1993; 53:1262–1268.
239. Fox SB, Fawcett J, Jackson DG, Collins I, Gatter KC, Harris AL, et al. Normal human tissues, in addition to some tumors, express multiple different CD44 isoforms. Cancer Res 1994; 54:4539–4546.
240. Mackay CR, Terpe HJ, Stauder R, Marston WL, Stark H, Gunthert U. Expression and modulation of CD44 variant isoforms in humans. J Cell Biol 1994; 124:71–82.
241. Figge J, del Rosario AD, Gerasimov G, Dedov I, Bronstein M, Troshina K, et al. Preferential expression of the cell adhesion molecule CD44 in papillary thyroid carcinoma. Exp Mol Pathol 1994; 61:203–211.
242. Ermak G, Gerasimov G, Troshina K, Jennings T, Robinson L, Ross JS, Figge J. Deregulated alternative splicing of CD44 messenger RNA transcripts in neoplastic and nonneoplastic lesions of the human thyroid. Cancer Res 1995; 55:4594–4598.
243. Ermak G, Jennings T, Robinson L, Ross JS, Figge J. Restricted patterns of CD44 variant exon expression in human papillary thyroid carcinoma. Cancer Res 1996; 56:1037–1042.
244. Fagman H, Grande M, Edsbagge J, Semb H, Nilsson M. Expression of classical cadherins in thyroid development: maintenance of an epithelial phenotype throughout organogenesis. Endocrinology 2003; 144:3618–3624.
245. Chen W, Obrink B. Cell-cell contacts mediated by E-cadherin (uvomorulin) restrict invasive behavior of L-cells. J Cell Biol 1991; 114:319–327.
246. Vleminckx K, Vakaet L, Mareel M, Fiers W, Van Roy F. Genetic manipulation of E-cadherin expression by epithelial tumor cells reveals an invasion suppressor role. Cell 1991; 66:107–119.
247. Brabant G, Hoang-Vu C, Cetin Y, Dralle H, Scheumann G, Molne J, et al. E-cadherin: a differentiation marker in thyroid malignancies. Cancer Res 1993; 53:4987–4993.
248. Plail RO, Bussey HJ, Glazer G, Thompson JP. Adenomatous polyposis: an association with carcinoma of the thyroid. Br J Surg 1987; 74:377–380.
249. Lote K, Andersen K, Nordal E, Brennhovd IO. Familial occurrence of papillary thyroid carcinoma. Cancer 1980; 46:1291–1297.
250. Liaw D, Marsh DJ, Li J, Dahia PL, Wang SI, Zheng Z, et al. Germline mutations of the PTEN gene in Cowden disease, an inherited breast and thyroid cancer syndrome. Nat Genet 1997; 16:64–67.
251. Garniel MR, Mule JE, Alexander LL, Beninghoff DL. Association of thyroid carcioma with Gardner's syndrome in siblings. N Engl J Med 1968; 278:1056–1058.
252. Malchoff CD, Malchoff DM. The genetics of hereditary nonmedullary thyroid carcinoma. J Clin Endocrinol Metab 2002; 87:2455–2459.
253. Mulligan LM, Ponder BAJ. Genetic basis of endocrine disease: multiple endocrine neoplasia type 2. J Clin Endocrinol Metab 1995; 80:1989–1995.

4
Molecular Aspects of Thyroid Cancer in Children

Gary L. Francis

Children with thyroid cancer generally have a more favorable prognosis than adults. This chapter reviews the data that suggest the pattern of ret/PTC, BRAF, and RAS mutations might differ in papillary thyroid carcinoma (PTC) from children and adults. Expression of the insulin-like growth factors (IGFs) and IGF receptors may also differ, as well as the intensity or nature of the immune response. Additional study is warranted to better define the impact of each of these factors on the clinical behavior of thyroid cancers in children.

INTRODUCTION

PTC and follicular thyroid carcinoma (FTC) share important features in children and adults. The majority of tumors are classic PTC, and about one third are multifocal in both age groups (1). Such variants as tall-cell PTC and less well-differentiated PTC are found in adults, but their frequency and prognosis are not well described in children (2). Not as much is known about FTC because it occurs with lesser frequency in both age groups, and it is even less common in children (1).

Despite these similarities, dramatic differences exist in the clinical behavior of thyroid cancers in children, which imply these malignancies might arise through different mechanisms. First, most children present with more widespread disease than adults. At diagnosis, 70% of childhood PTC has already invaded beyond the thyroid capsule or into the regional lymph nodes, and 10–28% already have pulmonary metastases (1–9). The second major difference is that although they present more often with disseminated disease, children are much less likely to die from PTC than adults are (1,2,10). In all published series of childhood PTC, mortality is under 12%, and in many, less than 1% (2,9,11–18). Although this evidence could be biased by relatively short follow-up (averaging 5–10 yr), a few studies have followed children with thyroid cancer for 30 yr or more and still indicate over 90% survival (12,13). This finding is in marked contrast to all other solid tumors in children for which lymphatic spread and pulmonary metastasis are associated with a high mortality rate (12,13). Additionally, following treatment, about half of the children with pulmonary metastases persist with stable disease (12,13). These are remarkable differences when compared to adults with PTC and pulmonary metastases for whom the 10-yr mortality rate may approach as high as 75% (19).

Fewer data exist comparing FTC in children and adults; only one study has compared disease-free survival for children with PTC and FTC (1). Disease-free survival was similar in children with either variant but is usually shorter in adults with FTC vs PTC (1). However, these observations should be interpreted cautiously because the follow-up was somewhat short and number of children was comparatively small.

Finally, dedifferentiated and anaplastic thyroid cancers rarely, if ever, occur in children (2). This could be a function of time in that most anaplastic thyroid cancers in adults are thought to arise through dedifferentiation of PTC or FTC over many years (20). Certainly, the paucity of dedifferentiated thyroid cancers in children improves the overall prognosis, but the prognosis is more favorable for children than adults, even when comparing similar histology and extent of disease at diagnosis (1).

INHERITED CANCER SYNDROMES

Fortunately, thyroid carcinomas are uncommon in children, but this has made elucidation of their molecular origins and a molecular explanation for these differences in clinical behavior much more difficult. Nevertheless, a few inherited forms of PTC occur during childhood and provide insight into

---

*The opinions and assertions contained herein are the private views of the authors and are not to be construed as official or as reflecting the opinions of the Uniformed Services University of the Health Sciences, the Department of the Army, or the Department of Defense.

at least some genetic alterations that might be important. Approximately 5% of PTC is inherited through a dominant mode of transmission (21). These alterations can present as one feature in a variety of inherited tumor syndromes, including Gardner's and Cowden's syndromes. Gardner's syndrome has been linked to mutations in the *APC* gene at chromosome 5q21 (21,22). Affected patients develop various intestinal and dermoid tumors, lipomas, and epidermoid cysts that begin as hamartomas around 10–20 yr of age and progress to carcinoma (21,22). Cowden's syndrome is caused by mutations in the *PTEN* tumor suppressor gene located on chromosome 10q22-q23 that result in overactivation of protein kinase B (Akt; 23). Clinical findings include multiple hamartomas, breast cancer, colon cancer, and nodular goiter. The Carney Complex (spotty skin pigmentation, myxomas, schwannomas, and endocrine overactivity) is caused by a defect in the protein kinase A regulatory subunit type I α gene located on chromosome 17q22-24 and can also be associated, albeit rarely (3.8%), with inherited forms of thyroid cancer (24,25). Although uncommon causes of thyroid cancer, these syndromes should be considered in any patient with a pedigree that suggests dominant transmission. They also provide evidence for the potential importance of mutations on chromosomes 5 and 10 in thyroid cancers of all ages.

RADIATION-INDUCED THYROID CANCERS

However, the vast majority of differentiated thyroid cancers in children are not inherited and probably arise through different mechanisms. Their incidence is dramatically increased following exposure to ionizing radiation, especially at a young age (26). This fact must be considered when comparing the genetic alterations reported in childhood thyroid cancers with those reported in adults, as many studies have included only children exposed to radioactivity after the Chernobyl nuclear accident. In the exposed children, thyroid malignancies appeared as early as 5 yr after the accident, and they developed in patients who were younger than those with "spontaneous" thyroid cancers (27,28). Generally, radiation-induced thyroid cancers appear to be more aggressive and are frequently multifocal (29,30). They commonly exhibit mutations in the *ret* proto-oncogene and express higher levels of vascular endothelial growth factor (VEGF) than any other form of childhood thyroid cancer (31–36). How, or even if, these molecular changes contribute to the more aggressive clinical course of radiation-induced thyroid cancer is not yet known.

Radiation-induced PTC in children have been shown most frequently to harbor chromosomal rearrangements between the *ret* proto-oncogene and regulatory elements of ordinarily unrelated genes (36–39). In radiation-induced PTC of children, this most often generates a specific recombinant gene known as *ret/PTC-3*. Nikiforov et al. found an important spatial geometry that allows ELE-1 and *ret* to recombine following chromosomal breaks that arise from a single radiation track, facilitating the formation of *ret/PTC-3* (40). Consequently, the thyroid is particularly vulnerable to radiation-induced cancer, a possibility that is borne out by all studies of children with radiation-induced thyroid cancer in which *ret/PTC-3* mutations are the most common (41).

RET/PTC MUTATIONS

Even when they are not radiation-induced, about half of childhood PTC contain recombination events between the tyrosine kinase domain of the ret proto-oncogene and regulatory elements of other genes (42). These rearrangements occur in a multitude of upstream regulators, resulting in overexpression of the *ret/PTC* chimeric gene and unregulated ret tyrosine kinase activity (43). The *ret/PTC* mutations are directly transforming in experimental models and are more commonly found from PTC in children than in adults (44). This is true for children with radiation-induced PTC and with spontaneous PTC, but the type of *ret/PTC* rearrangements appears to differ (42,45). The most common mutation in spontaneous childhood thyroid cancer appears to be *ret/PTC-1* (42); it is also the most common *ret/PTC* rearrangement in adults (46). Few studies have correlated the presence or absence of specific *ret/PTC* mutations with the clinical behavior of PTC in children. A single report failed to find any evidence that *ret/PTC* mutations are associated with a more or less favorable outcome in children (42). In contrast, adult PTC harboring a *ret/PTC* mutation may follow a more aggressive clinical course (47,48).

BRAF MUTATIONS

Another group of mutations particularly important in the control of cell proliferation includes those in the small guanosine triphosphate (GTP)-binding proteins (49–51). These mutations affect the signal transduction pathways significant for various key growth factors. Growth factors usually transmit their signals by binding and activating specific membrane-bound cell surface receptors (Fig. 1). Following activation, the receptors associate with docking proteins and small GTP-binding proteins, such as *ras*. BRAF is a serine/threonine kinase that receives a mitogenic signal from *ras* and transmits it to the mitogen-activated protein kinase (MAPK) pathway (52). MAPK activation then leads to more rapid cell division and a distinct survival advantage. Constitutive activation of any one of the effectors along the *ret/PTC-ras-*BRAF-MAPK pathway is sufficient to increase proliferation and, possibly in concert with other events, induce the malignant phenotype (52).

Recent studies of adults with PTC have detected a high incidence of B-RAF mutations (52–54). In fact, B-RAF mutations now appear to be the most frequently reported

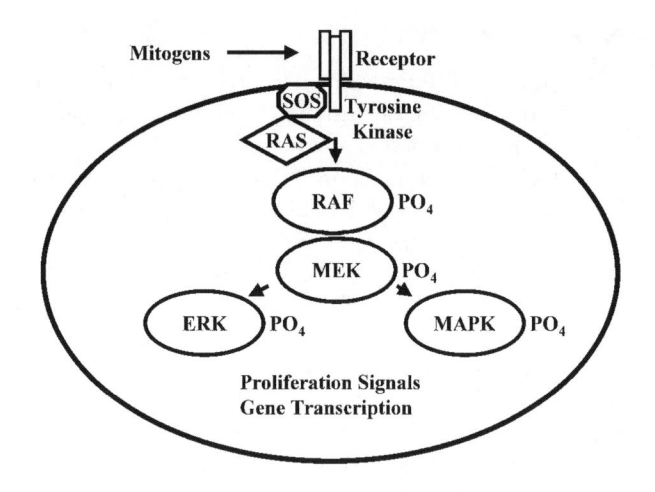

Fig. 1. Membrane-bound receptor signal transduction. Once activated, cell-surface growth factor receptors dock with SOS (SOS1 guanine nucleotide exchange factor) and activate the RAS, RAF, and MAPK pathways that lead to cell division.

genetic alterations in adult PTC *(52–54)*. As of this date, there are no published reports of B-RAF mutations in childhood thyroid cancer, but unpublished observations from the author's own laboratory failed to identify BRAF mutations in a group of 10 well-differentiated PTC from children. Additional studies of BRAF mutations in childhood PTC are soon to be published. Even if the preliminary data in these 10 children with PTC are compared with that of adults, the lack of BRAF mutations in our 10 children with PTC is significantly different from that of published adult series (97 PTC had the B-RAF 1796 T → A transversion/232 analyzed, 42% incidence; $p < 0.01$).

RAS AND OTHER MUTATIONS

Mutations of the *ras* oncogene have been reported with high frequency in benign adenomas and carcinomas from adults but appear to be less frequent in childhood thyroid tumors *(50,54–56)*. Similarly, activating mutations of the α subunit of GTP-binding proteins (Gsα) are rarely found in childhood tumors but are typical in adult thyroid cancers *(57)*.

As mentioned previously, dedifferentiated or anaplastic thyroid cancers occur in adults but almost never during childhood *(2)*. Such poorly differentiated tumors are often found to have mutations in the *p53* tumor suppressor gene *(55,58)*. Owing to the lack of anaplastic cancers, *p53* mutations are expected to be rare in childhood thyroid cancers, and such appears to be the case *(59)*.

It is highly likely that the reduced incidence of *p53* mutations and poorly differentiated thyroid cancers in children contribute to the overall favorable prognosis. However, given their rarity and restriction to poorly differentiated thyroid cancers, *p53* mutations are not likely to explain the more positive prognosis in children in comparison to adults with similar histology and extent of disease. Whether the near-complete lack of B-RAF, *ras*, and Gsα mutations is sufficient to explain these differences remains to be seen, but the near absence of these mutations could be potentially important in promoting the favorable prognosis for children with PTC.

GROWTH FACTORS

Although not transforming in and of themselves, several growth factors and cell cycle regulatory proteins have been implicated during the transformation of the normal thyroid into thyroid cancer and have been investigated independently in children and adults. Generally, expression appears to be a common feature to both age groups, but there are a few important and additional minor quantitative differences.

One major difference involves the expression of IGFs and their receptors. IGF-1 has been detected in 90% of adult PTC and was shown to stimulate the growth of PTC in culture *(60,61)*. However, there was no relationship between IGF-1 expression and the prognosis for adults *(60,61)*. The IGF-1 receptor was also expressed by the majority of adult PTC and significantly correlated with tumor size *(62)*. Vella et al. found that the IGF-1 receptor was expressed only by differentiated thyroid cancers, whereas insulin receptors (IRs) and hybrid receptors formed between the IGF-1 receptor and IR were expressed by poorly differentiated thyroid cancers *(63–65)*. Ordinarily, these hybrid receptors are only expressed during fetal life and confer the ability to bind IGF-2 *(65)*. Adult thyroid cancers with increased expression of hybrid IGF-1 recptors/IRs are most often poorly differentiated and have a poor prognosis *(63–65)*.

To the author's knowledge, such studies have not been fully replicated regarding thyroid cancers in children. However, one study did investigate the expression of IGF-1 and its receptor in a small number of PTC and FTC in children *(66)*. The IGF-1 and IGF-1 receptor were detected in somewhat fewer tumors than in adults (45% and 43%, respectively). Importantly, IGF-1 receptor expression was more intense in invasive, metastatic, recurrent, or persistent tumors. These data support a role for the IGFs, particularly the IGF-1 receptor, in the clinical behavior of childhood thyroid carcinoma. It remains to be determined if the expression of hybrid IGF-1 receptors/IRs arises from or contributes to dedifferentiation.

Another significant protein in thyroid cancer is telomerase. During normal cell division, the terminal ends of the DNA or telomeres are lost, leading to programmed senescence *(67)*. Telomerase is a specific enzyme that replaces telomeric DNA, conferring cellular immortality *(68)*. In adult thyroid cancers, telomerase activity was increased and associated with a high probability of metastasis *(69,70)*. Recent studies also found increased telomerase expression in malignant thyroid tumors in children, suggesting that telomerase expression could allow thyroid cells in either age group to become immortal and accumulate the additional mutations necessary for the full malignant phenotype *(71)*.

Several other factors are produced by thyroid carcinoma and appear important in promoting growth, metastasis, and recurrence. The potent angiogenic stimulus, VEGF, and the VEGF receptor (Flt-1) are expressed by childhood thyroid carcinoma, increased in the largest tumors, and most intense in tumors destined to recur *(72–74)*. In addition, VEGF expression is greater in PTC in children than in adults and even greater in radiation-induced PTC *(75)*. The importance of VEGF in sustaining thyroid carcinoma has been further demonstrated by abrogating the growth of thyroid cancer xenografts with VEGF monoclonal antibodies *(76,77)*.

Nitric oxide (NO) is another potent stimulus for blood flow and angiogenesis. NO is produced by several isoforms of nitric oxide synthase (NOS); of which, endothelial (eNOS) and inducible (iNOS) are potentially important in the thyroid. Both iNOS and eNOS have been detected in adult thyroid neoplasms, but there appeared to be no difference between benign and malignant lesions *(78,79)*. But Kitano et al. detected iNOS only in adult PTC, not in normal thyroid *(79)*. They also showed that most iNOS-containing cells were thyroid follicular cells *(78,79)*. In a recent study of NOS in childhood thyroid cancers, both iNOS and eNOS were detected and increased in benign and malignant thyroid tumors in children *(80)*.

Other key growth factors are the hepatocyte growth factor/scatter factor (HGF/SF) and HGF/SF receptor (cMET). The overexpression of both components of this autocrine/paracrine loop has been reported in childhood tumors with a higher probability of recurrence *(81)*.

IMMUNE CONSIDERATIONS

The host immune response could also be valuable in determining the prognosis for individual patients with thyroid cancer *(82,83)*. Although this occurs in both adults and children with PTC, the immune response might be more robust in children *(82,83)*. Adults with autoimmune thyroiditis and PTC generally have improved disease-free survival, and lymphocytic infiltration of adult PTC is associated with lower stage disease at diagnosis and reduced recurrence risk *(83,84)*. PTC in children and adolescents contain more lymphocytes than PTC in adults, and PTC with the most proliferating lymphocytes have the best prognosis *(82)*. In a recent study of childhood PTC, tumors that contained either CD8+ cells or a combination of CD4+, CD8+, and CD19+ lymphocytes contained more proliferating lymphocytes and were less likely to recur than PTC that contained any other combination of immune cell infiltrates *(85)*. Taken together, these data suggest a complex interplay between host and tumor that could be essential in establishing the clinical outcome for individual patients with thyroid carcinoma.

NIS EXPRESSION

The level of differentiation of individual tumors also has an important role in determining the clinical course. One indicator of differentiated thyroid function is the expression of the sodium-iodide symporter (NIS). NIS is also essential for successful therapy with radioactive iodine. Using either immunostaining or reverse transcriptase polymerase chain reaction, the majority of studies have detected NIS expression in adult thyroid cancers *(86–89)*. A smaller study of childhood PTC not only documented NIS expression in 35% of PTC and 44% of FTC but also found that recurrence developed exclusively from PTC and FTC with undetectable NIS *(90)*. In addition, the dose of ^{131}Iodine required to achieve remission was greater in patients with PTC that had undetectable NIS when compared to patients of similar age and with similar extent of disease for whom NIS expression was unknown *(90)*. Whether this is a direct reflection of the differentiation level or the ability to concentrate radioactive iodine is not clear from these studies, but the presence of NIS expression may be crucial to promote the favorable long-term survival of children with PTC.

SUMMARY

In conclusion, children with thyroid cancer generally have a more positive prognosis than adults do with similar disease status. Although data are limited, there are suggestions that the pattern of mutations in PTC from children differ when compared to those from adults. The ret/PTC rearrangements might be more typical in childhood PTC than adult PTC, with ret/PTC-3 being the most common in radiation-induced tumors and ret/PTC-1 the most common in spontaneous childhood PTC. In contrast, adult thyroid cancers appear to harbor more frequent mutations in BRAF or *ras* oncogenes. Additional growth factors and growth factor receptors are expressed by thyroid cancers in both ages but may differ, especially in the expression of the IGFs and IGF receptors. Lastly, the immune response against thyroid cancers, although evident in both ages, may also be more robust in children. Further study is warranted to better define the impact of each of these factors on the clinical behavior of thyroid cancers in children.

REFERENCES

1. Welch Dinauer CA, Tuttle RM, Robie DK, et al. Clinical features associated with metastasis and recurrence of differentiated thyroid cancer in children, adolescents and young adults. Clin Endocrinol 1998; 49:619–628.
2. McClellan DR, Francis GL. Thyroid cancer in children, pregnant women, and patients with Graves' disease. Endocrinol Metab Clin North Am 1996; 25:27–48.
3. Harness JK, Thompson NW, McLeod MK, Pasieka JL, Fukuuchi A. Differentiated thyroid carcinoma in children and adolescents. World J Surg 1992; 16:547–554.
4. Fassina AS, Rupolo M, Pelizzo MR, Casara D. Thyroid cancer in children and adolescents. Tumori 1994; 80:257–262.

5. Samuel AM, Sharma SM. Differentiated thyroid carcinomas in children and adolescents. Cancer 1991; 67:2186–2190.
6. Samuel AM, Rajashekharrao B, Shah DH. Pulmonary metastases in children and adolescents with well-differentiated thyroid cancer. J Nucl Med 1998; 39:1531–1536.
7. Maxon HR. The role of radioiodine in the treatment of childhood thyroid cancer—a dosimetric approach. In Jacob Robbins M, editor. Treatment of Thyroid Cancer in Childhood. Bethesda, MD: NIDDK, National Institutes of Health, 1992:109–126.
8. Yeh SD, La Quaglia MP. 131I therapy for pediatric thyroid cancer. Semin Pediatr Surg 1997; 6:128–133.
9. Feinmesser R, Lubin E, Segal K, Noyek A. Carcinoma of the thyroid in children—a review. J Pediatr Endocrinol Metab 1997; 10:561–568.
10. Gorlin JB, Sallan SE. Thyroid cancer in childhood. Endocrinol Metab Clin North Am 1990; 19:649–662.
11. Geiger JD, Thompson NW. Thyroid tumors in children. Otolaryngol Clin North Am 1996; 29:711–719.
12. LaQuaglia MP, Telander R. Differentiated and medullary thyroid cancer in children and adolescence. Semin Pediatr Surg 1997; 6: 42–49.
13. LaQuaglia M, Black T, Holcomb G, et al. Differentiated thyroid cancer: clinical characteristics, treatment, and outcome in patients under 21 years of age who present with distant metastases. A report from the Surgical Discipline Committee of the Children's Cancer Group. J Pediatr Surg 2000; 35:955–959.
14. Landau D, Vini L, A'Hern R, Harmer C. Thyroid cancer in children: the Royal Marsden Hospital experience. Eur J Cancer 2000; 36: 214–220.
15. Newman KD, Black T, Heller G, et al. Differentiated thyroid cancer: determinants of disease progression in patients <21 years of age at diagnosis: a report from the Surgical Discipline Committee of the Children's Cancer Group. Ann Surg 1998; 227:533–541.
16. Poth M. Thyroid cancer in children and adolescents. In Wartofsky L, editor. Thyroid Cancer: A Comprehensive Guide to Clinical Management. Totowa, NJ: Humana Press; 2000:121–128.
17. Skinner MA. Cancer of the thyroid gland in infants and children. Semin Pediatr Surg 2001; 10:119–126.
18. Tronko MD, Bogdanova TI, Komissarenko IV, et al. Thyroid carcinoma in children and adolescents in Ukraine after the Chernobyl nuclear accident: statistical data and clinicomorphologic characteristics. Cancer 1999; 86:149–156.
19. Shoup M, Stojadinovic A, Nissan A, et al. Prognostic indicators of outcomes in patients with distant metastases from differentiated thyroid carcinoma. J Am Coll Surg 2003; 197:191–197.
20. Lo CY, Lam KY, Wan KY. Anaplastic carcinoma of the thyroid. Am J Surg 1999; 177:337–339.
21. Ozaki O, Ito K, Kobayashi K, Suzuki A, Manabe Y, Hosoda Y. Familial occurrence of differentiated, nonmedullary thyroid carcinoma. World J Surg 1988; 12:565–571.
22. Camiel MR, Mule JE, Alexander LL, Benninghoff DL. Association of thyroid carcinoma with Gardner's syndrome in siblings. N Engl J Med 1968; 278:1056–1058.
23. Ringel MD, Hayre N, Saito J, et al. Overexpression and overactivation of Akt in thyroid carcinoma. Cancer Res 2001; 61:6105–6111.
24. Bertherat J, Groussin L, Sandrini F, et al. Molecular and functional analysis of PRKAR1A and its locus (17q22-24) in sporadic adrenocortical tumors: 17q losses, somatic mutations, and protein kinase A expression and activity. Cancer Res 2003; 63:5308–5319.
25. Stratakis CA, Kirschner LS, Carney JA. Clinical and molecular features of the Carney complex: diagnostic criteria and recommendations for patient evaluation. J Clin Endocrinol Metab 2001; 86:4041–4046.
26. Thompson DE, Mabuchi K, Ron E, et al. Cancer incidence in atomic bomb survivors. Part II: Solid tumors, 1958-1987 [published erratum appears in Radiat Res 1994; 139:129]. Radiat Res 1994; 137(2 Suppl): S17–S67.
27. Astakhova LN, Anspaugh LR, Beebe GW, et al. Chernobyl-related thyroid cancer in children of Belarus: a case-control study. Radiat Res 1998; 150:349–356.
28. Pacini F, Vorontsova T, Demidchik EP, et al. Post-Chernobyl thyroid carcinoma in Belarus children and adolescents: comparison with naturally occurring thyroid carcinoma in Italy and France. J Clin Endocrinol Metab 1997; 82:3563–3569.
29. Nikiforov Y, Gnepp DR. Pediatric thyroid cancer after the Chernobyl disaster. Pathomorphologic study of 84 cases (1991-1992) from the Republic of Belarus. Cancer 1994; 74:748–766.
30. Antonelli A, Miccoli P, Derzhitski VE, Panasiuk G, Solovieva N, Baschieri L. Epidemiologic and clinical evaluation of thyroid cancer in children from the Gomel region (Belarus). World J Surg 1996; 20: 867–871.
31. Becker DV, Robbins J, Beebe GW, Bouville AC, Wachholz BW. Childhood thyroid cancer following the Chernobyl accident: a status report [published erratum appears in Endocrinol Metab Clin North Am 1996; 25:xi]. Endocrinol Metab Clin North Am 1996; 25:197–211.
32. Bongarzone I, Butti MG, Fugazzola L, et al. Comparison of the breakpoint regions of ELE1 and RET genes involved in the generation of RET/PTC3 oncogene in sporadic and in radiation-associated papillary thyroid carcinomas. Genomics 1997; 42:252–259.
33. Bounacer A, Wicker R, Schlumberger M, Sarasin A, Suarez HG. Oncogenic rearrangements of the ret proto-oncogene in thyroid tumors induced after exposure to ionizing radiation. Biochimie 1997; 79:619–623.
34. Bounacer A, Wicker R, Caillou B, et al. High prevalence of activating ret proto-oncogene rearrangements, in thyroid tumors from patients who had received external radiation. Oncogene 1997; 15:1263–1273.
35. Dobson C, Gupta S, Patel A, et al. Papillary thyroid carcinoma from Russian children exposed to radiation following the Chernobyl nuclear accident are more likely to contain proliferating non-lymphocytic cells. Montreal, Canada: Lawson Wilkins Pediatric Endocrine Society Meeting, 2001.
36. Rabes HM, Klugbauer S. Molecular genetics of childhood papillary thyroid carcinomas after irradiation: high prevalence of RET rearrangement. Recent Results Cancer Res 1998; 154:248–264.
37. Rabes HM, Klugbauer S. Radiation-induced thyroid carcinomas in children: high prevalence of RET rearrangement. Verh Dtsch Ges Pathol 1997; 81:139–144.
38. Beimforh C, Klugbauer S, Demidchik EP, Lengfelder E, Rabes HM. NTRK1 rearrangement in papillary thyroid carcinomas of children after the Chernobyl reactor accident. Int J Cancer 1999; 80:842–847.
39. Klugbauer S, Rabes HM. The transcription coactivator HTIF1 and a related protein are fused to the RET receptor tyrosine kinase in childhood papillary thyroid carcinomas. Oncogene 1999; 18:4388–4393.
40. Nikiforov YE, Koshoffer A, Nikiforova M, Stringer J, Fagin JA. Chromosomal breakpoint positions suggest a direct role for radiation in inducing illegitimate recombination between the ELE1 and RET genes in radiation-induced thyroid carcinomas. Oncogene 1999; 18: 6330–6334.
41. Nikiforov Y. Spatial positioning of RET and H4 following radiation exposure leads to tumor development. Scientific World J 2001; 1: 186–187.
42. Fenton CL, Lukes Y, Nicholson D, Dinauer CA, Francis GL, Tuttle RM. The ret/PTC mutations are common in sporadic papillary thyroid carcinoma of children and young adults. J Clin Endocrinol Metab 2000; 85:1170–1175.
43. Sarasin A, Bounacer A, Lepage F, Schlumberger M, Suarez HG. Mechanisms of mutagenesis in mammalian cells. Application to human thyroid tumours. C R Acad Sci III 1999; 322:143–149.
44. Jhiang SM, Cho JY, Furminger TL, et al. Thyroid carcinomas in RET/PTC transgenic mice. Recent Results Cancer Res 1998; 154:265–270.
45. Tuttle RM, Fenton C, Lukes Y, et al. Activation of the ret/PTC oncogene in papillary thyroid cancer from Russian children exposed to

radiation following the Chernobyl accident. Kyoto, Japan: 12th International Thyroid Congress, 2000.
46. Smida J, Salassidis K, Hieber L, et al. Distinct frequency of ret rearrangements in papillary thyroid carcinomas of children and adults from Belarus. Int J Cancer 1999; 80:32–38.
47. Sugg SL, Zheng L, Rosen IB, Freeman JL, Ezzat S, Asa SL. ret/PTC-1, -2, and -3 oncogene rearrangements in human thyroid carcinomas: implications for metastatic potential? J Clin Endocrinol Metab 1996; 81:3360–3365.
48. Kjellman P, Learoyd DL, Messina M, et al. Expression of the RET proto-oncogene in papillary thyroid carcinoma and its correlation with clinical outcome. Br J Surg 2001; 88:557–563.
49. Farid NR, Zou M, Shi Y. Genetics of follicular thyroid cancer. Endocrinol Metab Clin North Am 1995; 24:865–883.
50. Fenton C, Anderson J, Lukes Y, Dinauer CA, Tuttle RM, Francis GL. Ras mutations are uncommon in sporadic thyroid cancer in children and young adults. J Endocrinol Invest 1999; 22:781–789.
51. Nikiforov YE, Nikiforova MN, Gnepp DR, Fagin JA. Prevalence of mutations of ras and p53 in benign and malignant thyroid tumors from children exposed to radiation after the Chernobyl nuclear accident. Oncogene 1996; 13:687–693.
52. Nikiforova MN, Kimura ET, Gandhi M, et al. BRAF mutations in thyroid tumors are restricted to papillary carcinomas and anaplastic or poorly differentiated carcinomas arising from papillary carcinomas. J Clin Endocrinol Metab 2003; 88:5399–5404.
53. Kimura ET, Nikiforova MN, Zhu Z, Knauf JA, Nikiforov YE, Fagin JA. High prevalence of BRAF mutations in thyroid cancer. Cancer Res 2003; 63:1454–1457.
54. Moretti F, Nanni S, Pontecorvi A. Molecular pathogenesis of thyroid nodules and cancer. Baillieres Best Pract Res Clin Endocrinol Metab 2000; 14:517–539.
55. Suchy B, Waldmann V, Klugbauer S, Rabes HM. Absence of RAS and p53 mutations in thyroid carcinomas of children after Chernobyl in contrast to adult thyroid tumours. Br J Cancer 1998; 77:952–955.
56. Hara H, Fulton N, Yashiro T, Ito K, DeGroot LJ, Kaplan EL. N-ras mutation: an independent prognostic factor for aggressiveness of papillary thyroid carcinoma. Surgery 1994; 116:1010–1016.
57. Waldmann V, Rabes HM. Absence of G(s)alpha gene mutations in childhood thyroid tumors after Chernobyl in contrast to sporadic adult thyroid neoplasia. Cancer Res 1997; 57:2358–2361.
58. Fagin JA, Matsuo K, Karmakar A, Chen DL, Tang SH, Koeffler HP. High prevalence of mutations of the p53 gene in poorly differentiated human thyroid carcinomas. J Clin Invest 1993; 91:179–184.
59. Fenton CL, Patel A, Tuttle RM, Francis GL. Autoantibodies to p53 in sera of patients with autoimmune thyroid disease. Ann Clin Lab Sci 2000; 30:179–183.
60. Silva Filho GB, Maciel RM, Takahashi MH, et al. Study of immunohistochemical expression of insulin-like growth factor I and proliferating cell nuclear antigen in thyroid gland papillary carcinoma and its metastasis. Head Neck 1999; 21:723–727.
61. Yashiro T, Ohba Y, Murakami H, et al. Expression of insulin-like growth factor receptors in primary human thyroid neoplasms. Acta Endocrinol (Copenh) 1989; 121:112–120.
62. Maiorano E, Ciampolillo A, Viale G, et al. Insulin-like growth factor 1 expression in thyroid tumors. Appl Immunohistochem Molecul Morphol 2000; 8:110–119.
63. Belfiore A, Pandini G, Vella V, Squatrito S, Vigneri R. Insulin/IGF-I hybrid receptors play a major role in IGF-I signaling in thyroid cancer. Biochimie 1999; 81:403–407.
64. Vella V, Sciacca L, Pandini G, et al. The IGF system in thyroid cancer: new concepts. Mol Pathol 2001; 54:121–124.
65. Vella V, Pandini G, Sciacca L, et al. A novel autocrine loop involving IGF-II and the insulin receptor isoform-A stimulates growth of thyroid cancer. J Clin Endocrinol Metab 2002; 87:245–254.
66. Gydee H, O'Neill JT, Patel A, Bauer AJ, Tuttle RM, Francis GL. Differentiated thyroid carcinomas from children and adolescents express insulin-like growth factor-1 (IGF-1) and the IGF-1 receptor (IGF-1-R). Cancers with the most intense IGF-1-R expression may be more aggressive. Pediatr Res 2004; 55:1–7.
67. Allsopp RC, Chang E, Kashefi-Aazam M, et al. Telomere shortening is associated with cell division in vitro and in vivo. Exp Cell Res 1995; 220:194–200.
68. Blackburn EH, Greider CW, Henderson E, Lee MS, Shampay J, Shippen-Lentz D. Recognition and elongation of telomeres by telomerase. Genome 1989; 31:553–560.
69. Lo CY, Lam KY, Chan KT, Luk JM. Telomerase activity in thyroid malignancy. Thyroid 1999; 9:1215–1220.
70. Okayasu I, Osakabe T, Fujiwara M, Fukuda H, Kato M, Oshimura M. Significant correlation of telomerase activity in thyroid papillary carcinomas with cell differentiation, proliferation and extrathyroidal extension. Jpn J Cancer Res 1997; 88:965–970.
71. Straight A, Patel A, Fenton C, Dinauer C, Tuttle RM, Francis G. Thyroid carcinomas that express telomerase follow a more aggressive clinical course for children and adolescents. J Endocrinol Invest 2002; 25:302–308.
72. Fenton C, Patel A, Dinauer C, Robie DK, Tuttle RM, Francis GL. The expression of vascular endothelial growth factor and the type 1 vascular endothelial growth factor receptor correlate with the size of papillary thyroid carcinoma in children and young adults. Thyroid 2000; 10:349–357.
73. Huang SM, Lee JC, Wu TJ, Chow NH. Clinical relevance of vascular endothelial growth factor for thyroid neoplasms. World J Surg 2001; 25:302–306.
74. Lennard CM, Patel A, Wilson J, et al. Intensity of vascular endothelial growth factor expression is associated with increased risk of recurrence and decreased disease-free survival in papillary thyroid cancer. Surgery 2001; 129:552–558.
75. Tuttle RM, Patel A, Francis G, et al. Vascular endothelial growth factor (VEGF) and Type 1 VEGF receptor (Flt-1) are highly expressed in Russian papillary thyroid carcinomas. Kyoto, Japan: 12th International Thyroid Congress, 2000.
76. Bauer AJ, Terrell R, Doniparthi NK, et al. Vascular endothelial growth factor monoclonal antibody inhibits growth of anaplastic thyroid cancer xenografts in nude mice. Thyroid 2002; 12:953–961.
77. Bauer AJ, Patel A, Terrell R, et al. Vascular endothelial growth factor monoclonal antibody (VEGF-MAb) inhibits growth of papillary thyroid cancer xenografts. Ann Clin Lab Sci 2003; 33:192–199.
78. Kayser L, Francis D, Broholm H. Immunohistochemical localization of inducible and endothelial constitutive nitric oxide synthase in neoplastic and autoimmune thyroid disorders. Apmis 2000; 108:785–791.
79. Kitano H, Kitanishi T, Nakanishi Y, et al. Expression of inducible nitric oxide synthase in human thyroid papillary carcinomas. Thyroid 1999; 9:113–117.
80. Patel A, Fenton C, Terrell R, et al. Nitrotyrosine, inducible nitric oxide synthase (iNOS), and endothelial nitric oxide synthase (eNOS) are increased in thyroid tumors from children and adolescents. J Endocrinol Invest 2002; 25:675–683.
81. Ramirez R, Hsu D, Patel A, et al. Over-expression of hepatocyte growth factor/scatter factor (HGF/SF) and the HGF/SF receptor (cMET) are associated with a high risk of metastasis and recurrence for children and young adults with papillary thyroid carcinoma. Clin Endocrinol 2000; 53:635–644.
82. Gupta S, Patel A, Folstad A, et al. Infiltration of differentiated thyroid carcinoma by proliferating lymphocytes is associated with improved disease-free survival for children and young adults. J Clin Endocrinol Metab 2001; 86:1346–1354.

83. Loh KC, Greenspan FS, Dong F, Miller TR, Yeo PP. Influence of lymphocytic thyroiditis on the prognostic outcome of patients with papillary thyroid carcinoma. J Clin Endocrinol Metab 1999; 84:458–463.
84. Ozaki O, Ito K, Mimura T, Sugino K, Hosoda Y. Papillary carcinoma of the thyroid. Tall-cell variant with extensive lymphocyte infiltration. Am J Surg Pathol 1996; 20:695–698.
85. Modi J, Patel A, Terrell R, et al. Papillary Thyroid Carcinoma from Children and Adolescents Contain a Mixture of Lymphocytes. J Clin Endocrinol Metab 2003; 88:4418–4425.
86. Jhiang SM, Cho JY, Ryu KY, et al. An immunohistochemical study of Na+/I- symporter in human thyroid tissues and salivary gland tissues. Endocrinology 1998; 139:4416–4419.
87. Caillou B, Troalen F, Baudin E, et al. Na+/I- symporter distribution in human thyroid tissues: an immunohistochemical study. J Clin Endocrinol Metab 1998; 83:4102–4106.
88. Ringel MD, Anderson J, Souza SL, et al. Expression of the sodium iodide symporter and thyroglobulin genes are reduced in papillary thyroid cancer. Mod Pathol 2001; 14:289–296.
89. Saito T, Endo T, Kawaguchi A, et al. Increased expression of the sodium/iodide symporter in papillary thyroid carcinomas. J Clin Invest 1998; 101:1296–1300.
90. Patel A, Jhiang S, Dogra S, et al. Differentiated thyroid carcinoma that express sodium-iodide symporter have a lower risk of recurrence for children and adolescents. Pediatr Res 2002; 52:737–744.

5
Oncogenes in Thyroid Cancer

Katherine B. Weber and Michael T. McDermott

INTRODUCTION

At the time of conception, the human organism is a single cell zygote. During the course of development into an adult, this cell expands into a complex mass of approximately 100 trillion cells, with an enormous variety of shapes, sizes, and functions. Normal tissue growth and development require prolific cell division, exquisitely regulated cell differentiation, and appropriately timed cell death or apoptosis. Neoplastic transformation of tissue generally occurs when abnormal regulatory mechanisms promote excessive cell division, impaired cell differentiation, and/or failure of apoptosis. In most tumor types, this aberrant control originates at the genetic level.

Intensive study of these regulatory mechanisms has led to significant progress in our ability to diagnose, predict biological behavior, and understand the basic molecular pathophysiology of thyroid neoplasms. The upcoming sections explore the major advances in the study of thyroid oncogenes and tumor suppressor genes. As this discussion relies on the knowledge of some basic concepts, the essential elements of the cell cycle and gene function are first briefly reviewed.

THE CELL CYCLE

The life cycle of a cell can be viewed as consisting of two alternating stages: interphase and mitosis (Fig. 1). Interphase—the longer stage—is composed of three substages or phases: gap 1 (G1), DNA synthesis (S), and gap 2 (G2). During the G1 stage, cells use DNA as a template to transcribe mRNA then to translate mRNA, into proteins. In the S phase, DNA is replicated, which doubles the cellular DNA content. During the G2 phase, DNA repair corrects any mutations that occurred during the S phase as the cell makes final preparations for entry into mitosis (1).

Mitosis is a much shorter stage when cell division occurs, comprised of four sequential phases. In prophase, sister chromatids pair by attaching at their centromeres; the nuclear membrane disappears and cytoplasmic spindle fibers begin to form. During metaphase, the chromosomes condense and line up along the equator of the cell attached to the spindles. The anaphase is characterized by the separation of sister chromatids and migration of individual chromatids along the spindles to opposite ends of the cell. In telophase, two new nuclear membranes form and cytoplasmic division (cytokinesis) occurs. The end result is two daughter cells, each with a complete set of 23 chromosome pairs (1).

Meiosis is a more complicated type of cell division that takes place only in germ cells. This process consists of two consecutive cell divisions; however, the second division is not preceded by DNA replication. In contrast to mitosis, meiosis produces four daughter cells, each with only 23 single chromosomes (1).

GENES

The basic blueprints of life are contained within our genes. A gene is a segment of DNA that carries the information necessary for a cell to produce a specific protein. There are approximately 50,000–100,000 genes in every human cell. To be successful, a gene must perform essential functions, such as expression, replication, and repair.

Gene expression (Fig. 2) takes place predominantly during the G1 period of interphase. Genes have two general regions—termed the regulatory and structural (coding) regions. Nuclear proteins (known as transcription factors) bind to the regulatory regions and govern the rate at which the structural region is transcribed into mRNA. mRNA molecules then travel to the cytoplasm where they are translated into the proteins characteristic of that particular cell phenotype. These proteins carry out the functional activities of the cell (1).

Gene replication (Fig. 3) occurs during the S phase. At this time, enzymes known as helicases unwind the DNA double helix, leaving two single strands of unpaired DNA. Using these as templates, DNA polymerases then promote

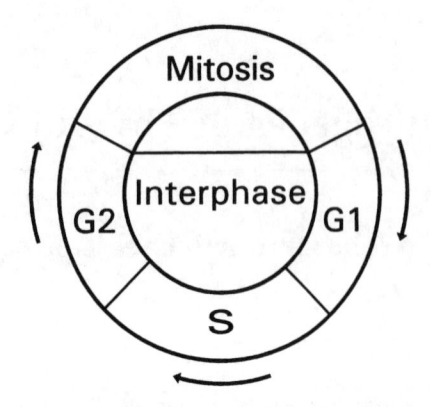

Fig. 1. The cell cycle. The cell cycle consists of two recurring stages: interphase and mitosis. The first substage or phase of interphase is G1, the period during which most gene expression occurs. Then follows the S phase, when DNA replicates, resulting in the number of chromosomes doubling. During G2, DNA repair occurs, and the cell prepares to divide. The cell then enters into the mitosis (or cell division) stage when the cell splits to form two daughter cells.

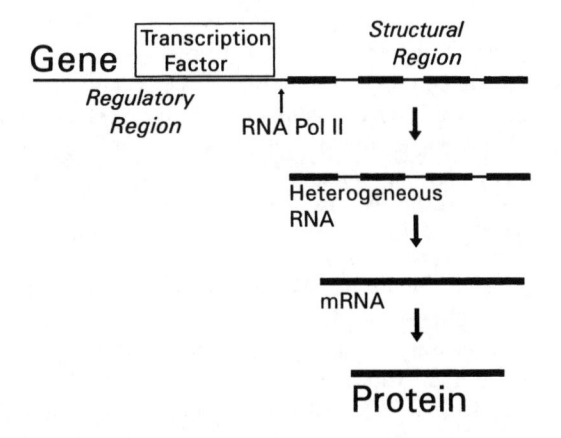

Fig. 2. Gene expression. Genes have both regulatory and structural (coding) regions. Gene expression begins when nuclear transcription factors bind to regulatory regions of target genes. These proteins modulate the rate at which an enzyme, RNA polymerase II (RNA Pol II), transcribes the structural region into heterogeneous RNA. Introns are then removed, leaving mature mRNA that exits the nucleus and attaches to ribosomes where the nucleotide sequence is translated into proteins.

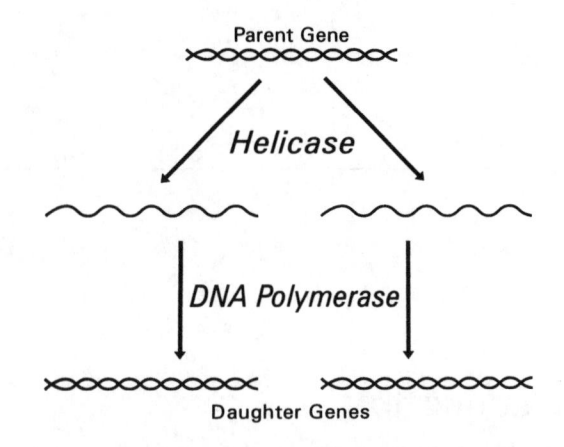

Fig. 3. Gene replication. During the S phase, enzymes known as helicases unwind the DNA double helix, separating it into two single strands. DNA polymerases then utilize the single-strand templates to assemble free nucleotide bases into complementary strands that anneal to these templates, producing two identical molecules of double-stranded DNA that subsequently reacquire their helical structures.

the assembly of free nucleotide bases into two new complementary chains that bind to each of these single strands, which leads to the formation of two new identical DNA double helices *(1)*.

Gene repair, occurring during G2, utilizes a complex set of enzymes collectively referred to as the DNA repair system. Contained within each cell, the human genome consists of approximately three billion nucleotide pairs that are replicated with each cell division. It is estimated that spontaneous mutations occur at a rate of about two per million base pairs during each S phase; thus, as many as 6000 mutations may appear each time a cell divides. The proteins of the DNA repair system rapidly and efficiently scan along the chromosomes to detect and repair most or all of these mutations before the cell proceeds into mitosis *(1)*.

ONCOGENES AND TUMOR SUPPRESSOR GENES

Throughout their lifespan, somatic cells can be thought of as progressing through three overlapping transitional stages (Fig. 4). Stem cells initially proliferate by undergoing repetitive cell division, causing a rapid expansion of immature tissue mass. Subsequently, these cells differentiate into mature cells that deliver the functions characteristic of their particular phenotype. Later, they grow senescent and undergo programmed cell death or apoptosis. Tumor development (or neoplasia) results from stimuli that augment cellular proliferation or impair cell differentiation and/or apoptosis. A diverse set of signaling and effector proteins is involved in the precise regulation of this enormously complex series of events. Mutations in the genes encoding these proteins have been found to underlie the majority of human malignancies *(2)*.

Genes that encode the proteins promoting normal cell proliferation are called *proto-oncogenes*. Proto-oncogenes sometimes develop activating or gain-of-function mutations that result in the production of proteins that are qualitatively

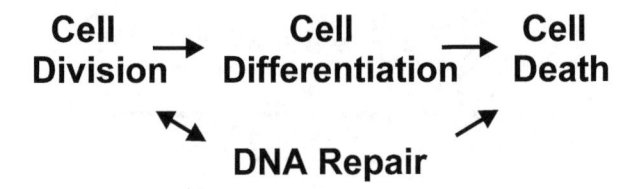

Fig. 4. The three transitional stages in the life of a cell. Stem cells initially proliferate rapidly, greatly expanding their cell numbers. Later, they differentiate into mature cells that perform the functions characteristic of their phenotype. Eventually, they grow senescent and undergo programmed cell death or apoptosis. DNA that is damaged during cell division is repaired by the DNA repair system and returns to the cycle or, if the damage is irreparable, the cell soon dies.

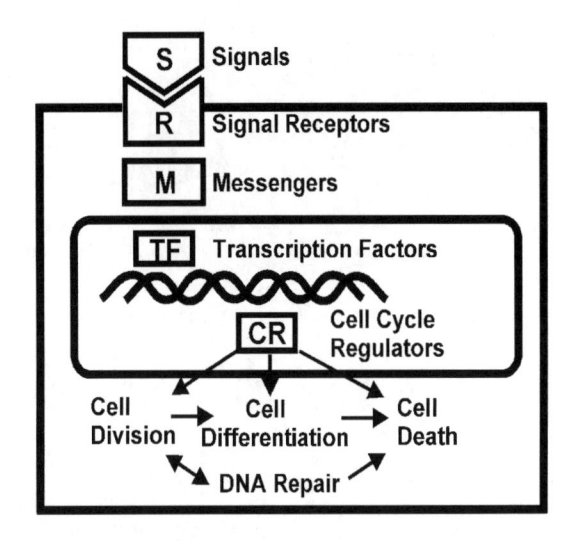

Fig. 5. A model for growth signal transduction. An extracellular signal molecule binds to a cell membrane receptor, resulting in the generation of intracellular messengers that relay the signal to the nucleus by activating transcription factors. Active transcription factors bind to targeted genes to modulate their production of the cell cycle regulatory proteins that ultimately direct the cell to proliferate, differentiate, or die.

overactive or quantitatively excessive and thereby promote over-robust cellular proliferation. These mutated protooncogenes are known as *oncogenes (2–8)*. Oncogene mutations tend to be dominantly expressed and thus become clinically apparent in the heterozygous state. Other genes, termed *tumor suppressor genes (8–12)*, encode the proteins that serve to restrain excessive cellular proliferation or promote cell differentiation and/or apoptosis. Inactivating or loss-of-function mutations of these tumor suppressor genes can also lead to neoplasia; these tend to be recessive and therefore are clinically consequential only when present in the homozygous state. Cells undergoing unregulated proliferation because of an activated oncogene or inactivated tumor suppressor gene are believed to be *transformed*.

Cancer-causing mutations may be either somatic or germline. *Somatic mutations* are those that usually develop in a single cell at any time in life after fertilization. Through some survival advantage conferred by the mutation, the transformed cell expands monoclonally into a solitary tumor mass that may eventually invade or metastasize. In contrast, *germline mutations* originate in a parent and are passed to offspring through a germ cell. Affected offspring have the mutation present diffusely and may thus be susceptible to the development of multiple tumors within a given organ or susceptible to tumors in multiple organs throughout the body. Most known inherited cancer syndromes result from germline mutations in tumor suppressor genes. Accordingly, individuals are born heterozygous at a critical locus but are initially unaffected because of the normal gene at the homologous locus. However, if a somatic mutation later in life inactivates the normal homologous locus, the individual is rendered unable to make any normal suppressor protein and begins to develop cancer.

The complex system that regulates cellular proliferation, differentiation, and apoptosis has many checks and balances. Although a single genetic mutation may initially transform a cell permitting the monoclonal expansion of its progeny, it is unlikely that a single mutation alone could result in the development of highly malignant tumor behavior. Yet, it appears that the unregulated proliferation of a transformed cell predisposes it to develop additional mutations. These, in turn, provide further selective survival advantages by promoting ever-accelerating cell proliferation, tissue invasion, and distant metastases. Indeed, experimental evidence indicates that multiple activated oncogenes and inactivated tumor suppressor genes are often found in highly malignant and metastatic tumors *(13,14)*.

A general model of cellular growth signal transduction is now examined and this model is applied to thyroid growth and function and current concepts of thyroid oncogenesis.

NORMAL GROWTH SIGNAL TRANSDUCTION: A MODEL

Although the precise mechanisms of signal transduction vary considerably among the different bodily tissues, a simple and general model is proposed in Fig. 5. Accordingly, in response to a need for cellular change, an extracellular molecular signal is generated and binds to a specific cell membrane receptor. Consequently, the generation of intracellular messengers relay the message to the nucleus by activating appropriate nuclear transcription factors. These proteins bind to the promoter regions of specific genes to modulate production of the cell cycle regulatory proteins that direct cells to proliferate, differentiate, or undergo apoptosis *(2,12)*.

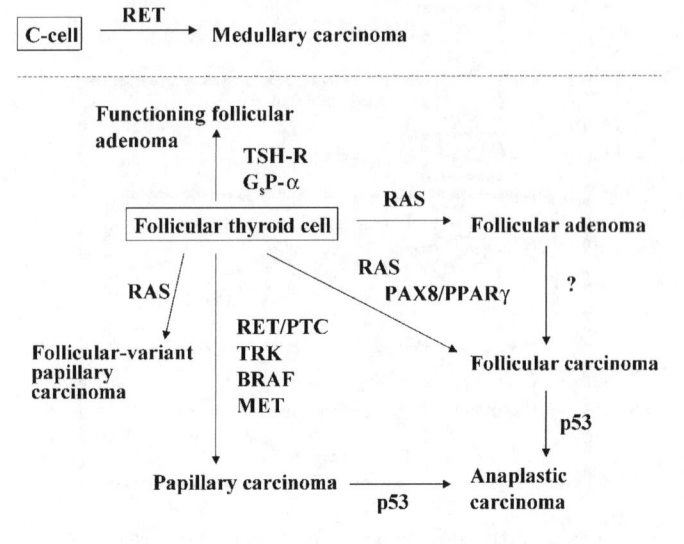

Fig. 6. Pathways to thyroid neoplasia. There appear to be specific pathways of oncogene mutations that lead to each type of thyroid tumor; these pathways are exclusive of each other. Activating mutations of the TSH receptor (TSH-R) and GsP-α genes predispose to the development of autonomously functioning follicular adenomas with a low potential for malignant degeneration. Ras mutations can lead to either follicular adenomas, follicular carcinomas, or follicular variant papillary carcinomas, whereas mutations in PAX8/PPARγ commit the neoplasm to become a follicular carcinoma. Papillary carcinomas can arise from mutations in several different oncogenes, including Ret/PTC, BRAF, MET, and TRK. In contrast, MTC arises from mutations in the Ret protooncogene. Inactivating mutations of the p53 tumor suppressor gene are a final common pathway to anaplastic carcinoma.

COMMON TYPES OF ONCOGENES IN THYROID NEOPLASIA

Oncogenic transformation can affect any element of the normal pathway of signal transduction, leading to constitutive activation of signaling and excess growth and proliferation. One common mutation site in thyroid cancer is at the level of the signal receptor. Particularly in papillary thyroid carcinoma, alterations in receptor tyrosine kinase activity are frequent, including the Ret, Ret/PTC, TRK, and MET oncogenes. Other sites of oncogenic activation include intracellular signaling molecules, such as Ras and BRAF, as well as transcription factors like PAX8/PPARγ and p53.

Two common general mechanisms for oncogene activation in thyroid neoplasia are point mutations and chromosomal translocations or gene rearrangements. Most point mutations are activating mutations of the gene, causing increased production of the gene product. Examples of this in thyroid cancer are Ret, Ras, and BRAF; an example of an inactivating point mutation is *p53*—a tumor suppressor gene that becomes less functional after the mutation. Chromosomal translocations or gene rearrangements are uncommon in most epithelial tumors. However, this mechanism has an important role in thyroid neoplasia. In a gene rearrangement, parts of two different chromosomes are combined, leading to the production of a novel fusion protein (e.g., in thyroid cancer, Ret/PTC, TRK, and PAX8/PPARγ).

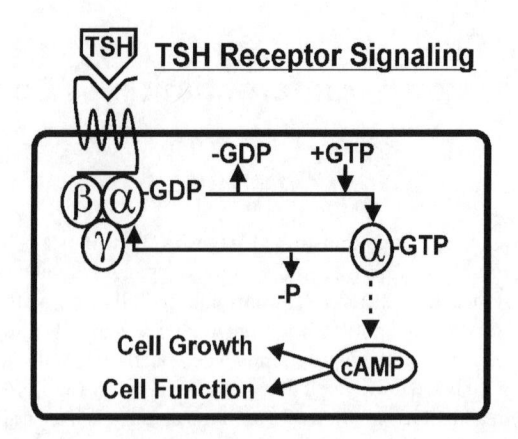

Fig. 7. TSH signal transduction in thyroid cells. TSH binds to the extracellular domain of the TSH receptor, causing dissociation of GsP into its α, β, and γ subunits and release of an α-bound GDP molecule. Then α attaches to a GTP molecule, forming an active dimer that stimulates cAMP production. The α subunit then utilizes intrinsic GTPase activity to deactivate itself by converting the GTP back to GDP. This pathway promotes both thyroid cellular proliferation and thyroid hormone production.

GENERAL MODEL FOR THYROID TUMORIGENESIS

In recent years, there have been many important advances in the study of thyroid oncogenes, bringing forth a greatly enhanced understanding of the different pathways that lead to various types of thyroid tumors. Evidence is mounting that the development of the two most common cancers arising from thyroid follicular cells—papillary and follicular thyroid carcinoma—proceeds along mutually exclusive pathways, suggesting that the initiating event in tumorigenesis commits the neoplasm to one or the other lineage. A proposed model for thyroid tumor development is shown in Fig. 6, and each pathway shown is covered in detail in the following sections.

THE PATHWAY TO FUNCTIONING FOLLICULAR ADENOMAS: THYROTROPIN RECEPTOR AND GsP-α MUTATIONS

The thyrotropin (TSH) receptor is a protein composed of a large extracellular domain, a transmembrane domain with seven-membrane spanning segments, and a short intracellular domain (Fig. 7). It is coupled to a guanine nucleotide-binding stimulatory protein (GsP) that is composed of α, β, and γ subunits and an α-bound guanosine diphosphate

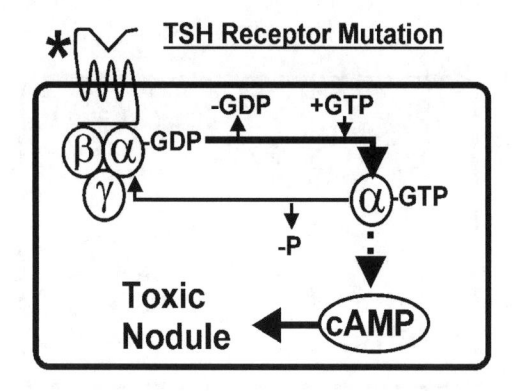

Fig. 8. Activating TSH receptor mutations. Some TSH receptor gene mutations produce a TSH receptor that is constitutively active without a need for TSH binding. Somatic mutations of this type may lead to the development of an autonomously functioning follicular adenoma.

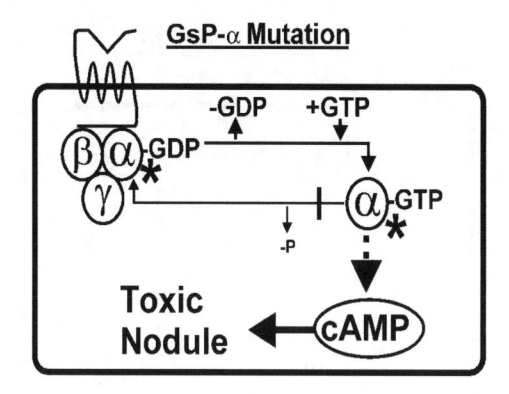

Fig. 9. Activating GsP-α subunit mutations. Mutations in the gene encoding the GsP-α subunit produce an α protein that retains the ability to bind GTP but has deficient intrinsic GTPase activity. Once activated by GTP binding, it is unable to deactivate itself by degrading GTP to GDP. The persistently active α-GTP dimer generates a continuous excess of cAMP that promotes thyroid cell proliferation and function, leading to the development of an autonomously functioning follicular adenoma.

(GDP) molecule. The α subunit has several significant properties: it is inactive when bound to GDP; it is active when bound to guanosine triphosphate (GTP); and it possesses intrinsic GTPase activity that converts GTP to GDP. TSH binding to the TSH receptor extracellular domain stimulates the transmembrane and intracellular domains to initiate an intracellular messenger cascade that begins with the release of GDP and dissociation of GsP into its subunits. Once liberated, the free α subunit attaches to GTP, forming an active dimer that stimulates adenylate cyclase to generate cyclic adenosine monophosphate (cAMP). Utilizing its intrinsic GTPase activity, the α subunit then converts the bound GTP back to GDP, thereby deactivating the α-GTP dimer. The burst of cAMP stimulates protein kinase A, which enlists additional proteins into a messenger cascade that ultimately stimulates thyroid cells to proliferate and produce thyroid hormone (15).

Autonomously functioning follicular adenomas are benign thyroid neoplasms that grow and produce thyroid hormone without any apparent requirement for TSH stimulation. Most of these tumors have been found in some (16–21), but not other (22–24), geographic locations to harbor activating point mutations in the TSH receptor gene, resulting in TSH receptors that are constitutively overactive in the presence or absence of TSH binding. Because the TSH receptor is normally involved in stimulating both thyroid growth and function, these constitutively active TSH receptors promote the neoplastic expansion of a clone of hormone producing thyroid cells (Fig. 8).

Activating mutations of the gene encoding the GsP-α subunit have also been detected in up to 25% of autonomously functioning follicular adenomas (23–26). The mutations described produce an α subunit that has normal GTP-binding ability but lacks intrinsic GTPase activity (Fig. 9). These abnormal α proteins form active α-GTP dimers that generate cAMP continuously and excessively because they have no intrinsic GTPase to deactivate themselves. As GsP-α is a downstream component of the TSH receptor signaling pathway, these activating GsP-α mutations also predispose to the development of benign neoplasms that autonomously proliferate and secrete thyroid hormone. However, neither the TSH receptor nor GsP-α mutations appear to have a significant impact in the development of malignant thyroid neoplasms (23,24,27).

THE PATHWAY TO FOLLICULAR ADENOMAS AND FOLLICULAR CARCINOMAS: RAS AND PAX/PPARγ MUTATIONS

Ras

Ras proteins are an important part of the signaling pathway for thyroid cell proliferation. Three distinct Ras genes are known: *H-RAS*, *K-RAS*, and *N-RAS*. Each codes for a 21-kDa protein that is critical in conveying signals from membrane receptors to the mitogen-activated protein kinase (MAPK) pathway, with the end result being activation of specific gene transcription. (Fig. 10) Like the GsP-α subunit, Ras proteins are inactive when bound to GDP, are active when bound to GTP, and possess intrinsic GTPase activity. In the basal state, Ras is tethered to the cell membrane, bound in an inactive dimeric complex with GDP. The binding of an extracellular ligand to a membrane receptor causes receptor dimerization and phosphorylation of tyrosine residues on the receptor's intracellular domain. The activated receptor then engages two proteins, Grb-2 and Sos, which cooperate to dissociate Ras from GDP. Ras immediately attaches to GTP, forming an active Ras-GTP dimer

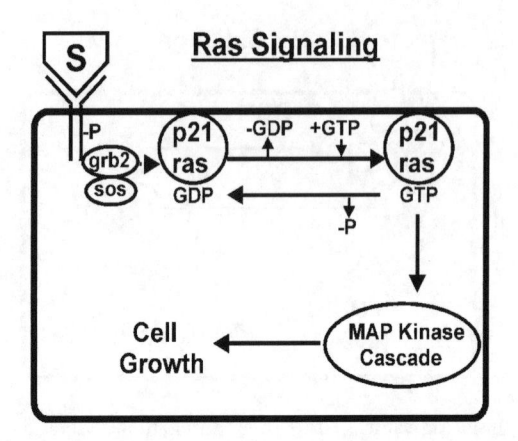

Fig. 10. The Ras-signaling proteins. Ras proteins are bound to GDP molecules as inactive dimers attached to the inner aspect of the cell membrane. When a ligand binds to a Ras-associated receptor, the intracellular portion of the receptor becomes phosphorylated and engages two proteins, Grb-2 and Sos, into a complex that dissociates Ras from GDP. Ras then binds to GTP, forming an active dimer that initiates a protein phosphorylation cascade. Ras then uses its intrinsic GTPase activity to deactivate itself by converting GTP back to GDP. This pathway primarily promotes thyroid cell proliferation.

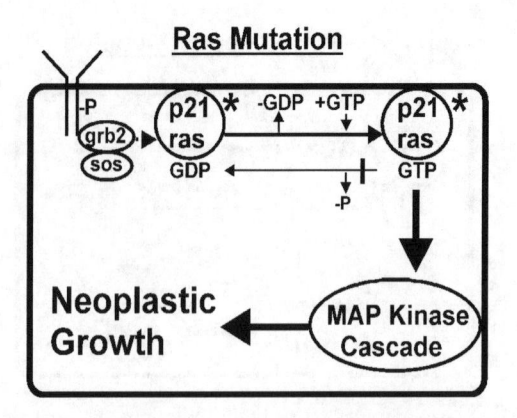

Fig. 11. Activating Ras mutations. Mutations in Ras genes result in the production of Ras proteins that can bind to GTP but that lack intrinsic GTPase activity. The persistently active Ras-GTP dimer excessively stimulates a cascade of protein phosporylations that mostly promote thyroid cell proliferation. This predisposes to the development of nonfunctioning follicular neoplasms.

that initiates a multistep protein phosphorylation cascade. Subsequently, Ras utilizes its intrinsic GTPase activity to disable itself by converting the bound GTP back to GDP. This Ras-associated pathway eventually activates nuclear proteins that primarily promote thyroid cellular proliferation but have little or no known effects on thyroid function.

In thyroid cancer, point mutations have been found in amino acids 12, 13, and 61, leading to the constitutive activation of Ras (28). In a situation analogous to GsP-α, these mutated Ras proteins can bind to GTP but lack the GTPase activity necessary to deactivate the Ras-GTP dimer (Fig. 11). In contrast to GsP-α, however, *Ras* mutations result in overstimulation of a signaling cascade that encourages the growth of nonfunctioning thyroid tumors.

Ras mutations have been found in 40–50% of both follicular adenomas and follicular carcinomas (28–34). Because of their presence in both benign and malignant thyroid lesions, it has been suggested that *Ras* mutations alone may not be sufficient for malignant transformation of thyroid cells but may be an early event in thyroid tumorigenesis that could predispose a cell to further mutations that subsequently lead to malignancy (31).

Interestingly, observed in up to 20% of cases in various series (30,34–36), *Ras* mutations are much less common in papillary thyroid carcinomas. Several intriguing studies have demonstrated *Ras* mutations in 20–43% of follicular variant papillary thyroid carcinomas but not in any cases of classic papillary thyroid carcinoma, suggesting that *Ras* may only be operative in a distinct subset of papillary carcinomas (35).

PAX8/PPARγ

Another oncogene identified as important in the development of follicular thyroid carcinoma is the PAX8/PPARγ fusion gene (Fig. 12). PAX8 is a thyroid-specific nuclear transcription factor that is known to be necessary for the genesis of thyroid follicular cells and the regulation of thyroid-specific gene expression (28,37). Peroxisome-proliferator–activated receptor γ (PPARγ) is a more general nuclear transcription factor that has a role in lipid metabolism, inflammation, differentiation, and tumorigenesis (38). The oncogene is created by a t(2;3)(q13;p25) chromosomal translocation, leading to the fusion of the DNA-binding domains of PAX8 to domains A–F of the PPARγ nuclear receptor (37). Experiments have shown that PAX8/PPARγ exerts a dominant negative effect on wild-type PPARγ transactivation (37). Given that PPARγ ligands can inhibit growth and promote differentiation of thyroid cancer cell lines, the inhibition of normal PPARγ activity by the oncogene may be an important mechanism of thyroid follicular tumorigenesis (37).

PAX8/PPARγ translocations have been identified in 26–63% of follicular carcinomas (31,37,39–41). However, unlike *Ras*, PAX8/PPARγ is rarely seen in follicular adenomas, with the prevalence ranging 0–13% in several series (31,37,39–41). This pattern has led to speculation that PAX8/PPARγ may confer invasive potential at an early stage (31).

One intriguing study showed that in a group of 49 follicular thyroid carcinomas, only one (3%) had both the PAX8/PPARγ rearrangement and *Ras* mutation, whereas 49% had *Ras* mutations alone, and 36% had the PAX8/PPARγ rearrangement alone (31). This would suggest two important conclusions about follicular thyroid tumorigenesis: 85% of

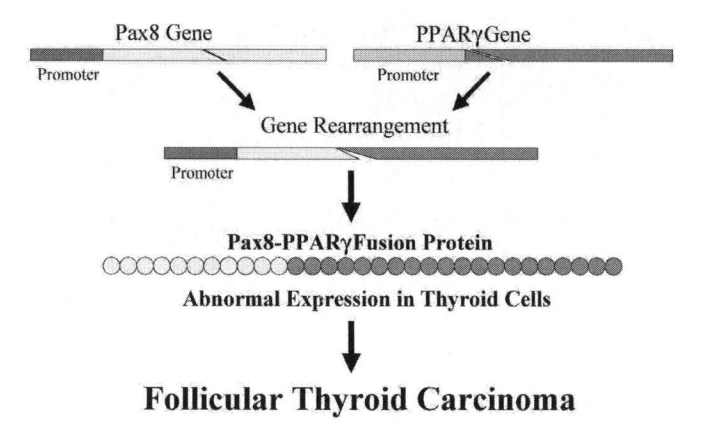

Fig. 12. PAX8/PPARγ fusion gene mutations. The PAX8/PPARγ oncogene is a fusion of the DNA-binding domains of PAX8, a thyroid-specific transcription factor, and the nuclear receptor domains of PPARγ, a more general nuclear transcription factor. The resulting fusion protein exerts a dominant negative effect on PPARγ transactivation, which may allow for promotion of growth in thyroid follicular cells. PAX8/PPARγ is found exclusively in follicular carcinomas. (Color illustration is printed in insert following p. 198.)

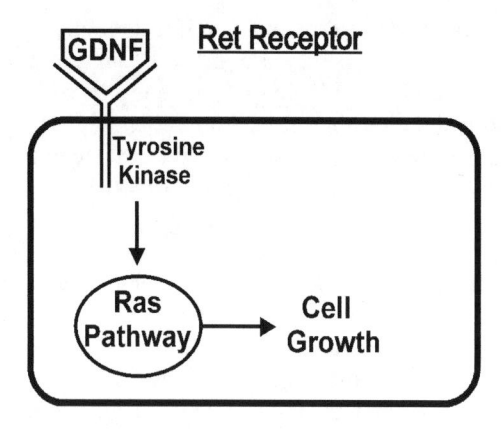

Fig. 13. The Ret receptor. Binding of the GDNF ligand to the extracellular domain of the Ret receptor enhances the intrinsic tyrosine kinase activity of the intracellular domain, resulting in the phosphorylation of downstream proteins that participate in a pathway that promotes cell proliferation. Ret receptors are normally present in thyroid parafollicular C cells but not in the more abundant follicular cells.

follicular thyroid carcinomas are caused by changes in either Ras or PAX8/PPARγ; and these two oncogenes represent two distinct and mutually exclusive pathways to the development of follicular thyroid cancer and could have significant implications for prognosis and therapy.

THE PATHWAY TO MEDULLARY THYROID CARCINOMA: RET MUTATIONS

The Ret receptor is a component of a different signaling cascade that appears to be primarily involved in cell proliferation of neural crest origin (Fig. 13). Ret is a proto-oncogene normally expressed in the calcitonin-producing parafollicular C cells but not in the thyroid hormone–producing follicular cells. Ret has an extracellular ligand-binding domain, a single transmembrane segment, and an intracellular portion that possesses low-level intrinsic tyrosine kinase activity. The ligands that bind to the Ret receptor are members of the glial-cell–derived neurotrophic factor (GDNF) family, including GDNF, neurturin, artemin, and persephin *(42,43)*. GDNF binding results in dimerization of the Ret receptor and significant enhancement of the receptor's tyrosine kinase activity. This results in the activation of various downstream signaling pathways, including Ras, PI3K, MAPK, and JNK that relay the message to the nucleus to promote cell division *(44)*.

Medullary thyroid carcinoma (MTC) is a malignancy of the parafollicular C cells. Approximately 10% are familial, whereas the remainder appears to be sporadic. Familial MTC is an autosomal dominant disorder that occurs in three recognized forms: familial isolated MTC, MTC associated with

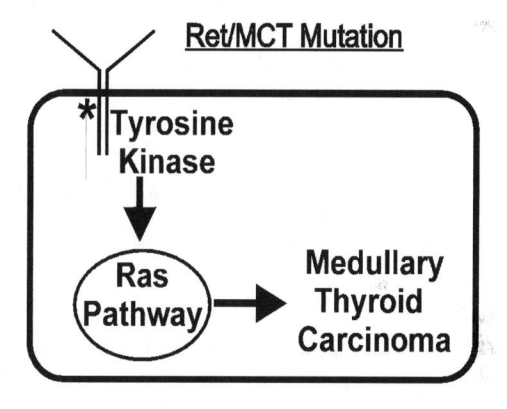

Fig. 14. Activating Ret receptor mutations (Ret/MTC) in the medullary thyroid carcinoma. Germline point mutations in the gene regions that code for the intracellular domain of the Ret receptor produce receptors with enhanced basal tyrosine kinase activity. This leads to excessive activation of downstream proteins that promote C-cell proliferation, predisposing to C-cell hyperplasia and multifocal medullary carcinoma.

the multiple endocrine neoplasia type IIA (MEN IIA) syndrome, and MTC associated with the MEN IIB syndrome. Familial MTC of all three types has been found in over 90% of cases to harbor activating point mutations in the Ret gene *(45–55)*. These lead to constitutively active Ret receptors with a high level of basal tyrosine kinase activity that sets in motion downstream growth signaling cascades, eventually leading to diffuse C cell hyperplasia and multifocal MTC (Fig. 14). The Ret/MTC oncogene has also been detected in some sporadic MTCs *(45,48–51)*. This suggests that sporadic MTC, generally a unifocal tumor, may sometimes arise from a somatic Ret mutation in a single cell; in contrast, familial MTC almost always results from a germline Ret mutation that affects all cells. Not surprisingly, the Ret/MTC oncogene has also been detected in pheochromocytomas from patients with MEN IIA and MEN IIB syndromes *(45–47,50,52)*.

The specific *Ret* mutations causing MEN IIA and MEN IIB have been identified and demonstrate different mechanisms of oncogenic activation. Of MEN IIA mutations, 98% are found in the extracellular domain and change a cysteine residue to a noncysteine residue. These cysteine residues normally form intramolecular disulfide bonds. But when one is mutated, another is left unpaired to form an intermolecular bond with another mutant Ret receptor, causing constitutive dimerization and activation of the receptor *(42,43,56–58)*. Alternatively, in MEN IIB, 95–98% of patients demonstrate a point mutation in the kinase domain of *Ret* that changes a methionine to a threonine. This mutation activates the tyrosine kinase activity, but the ligand is still required for full activation of the receptor *(42–44,59)*. These differing mechanisms to activate the *Ret* oncogene may explain some phenotypic variations between MEN IIA and IIB, perhaps by causing the phosphorylation of different tyrosine residues and the susequent activation of different downstream signaling pathways.

THE PATHWAY TO PAPILLARY THYROID CARCINOMA: RET/PTC, TRK, MET, AND BRAF MUTATIONS

Ret/PTC, TRK, and MET

Papillary thyroid carcinomas commonly arise from mutations in tyrosine kinases, including Ret/PTC, TRK, and MET. The Ret/PTC mutation is a gene rearrangement between the 3′ tyrosine kinase domain of the *Ret* proto-oncogene and the 5′ domain of another gene, which is constitutively expressed in thyroid follicular cells *(28,38)*. This explains how the *Ret* gene, normally only expressed in parafollicular C cells, can be involved in the genesis of papillary thyroid carcinoma. These mutations involve a gene truncation/rearrangement that deletes the coding region for the receptor's extracellular domain and interposes a promoter sequence adjacent to the coding region for the intracellular domain. This leads to the expression and constitutive activation of the intracellular portion of the Ret receptor in thyroid follicular cells (Fig. 15), generating a continuous excess of tyrosine kinase activity that stimulates downstream growth signals to promote thyroid follicular cell neoplasia.

Currently, 10 different Ret/PTC mutations are known: Ret/PTC 1–9 and ELKS/Ret *(28,42,44)*. Seen in more than 90% of papillary thyroid carcinomas, the most typical varieties are Ret/PTC-1 and Ret/PTC-3. Ret/PTC-1 involves the fusion of the Ret tyrosine kinase to a gene called H4, the func-

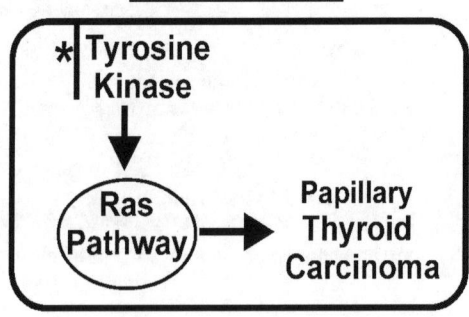

Fig. 15. Activating Ret receptor mutations (Ret/PTC) in papillary thyroid carcinoma. Somatic deletion/rearrangement mutations of the Ret receptor gene in thyroid follicular cells produce a truncated receptor with enhanced basal tyrosine kinase activity. This causes excessive activation of a pathway that promotes thyroid follicular cell proliferation and leads to the development of papillary thyroid carcinoma.

tion of which is unknown. It is the most common mutation in sporadic adult papillary thyroid carcinoma. Ret/PTC-3 involves the fusion of the Ret tyrosine kinase to a gene known as ELE-1, whose function is also currently unclear. This mutation has been associated with more aggressive subtypes of papillary thyroid carcinoma, such as solid and tall-cell variants, and is also seen in children who had a short latency period in developing thyroid cancer after radiation exposure at Chernobyl *(38,42,43,60–62)*.

The Ret/PTC mutation is seen in approx 20–50% of papillary thyroid carcinomas *(63–67)*. Radiation appears to significantly increase the prevalence of this mutation, with Ret/PTC rearrangements seen in 49–87% of thyroid cancers after the Chernobyl incident and in 84% of those developing after therapeutic neck radiation *(38,60,68–70)*.

The TRK proto-oncogene codes for a transmembrane tyrosine kinase receptor whose natural ligand is the neural growth factor. Like Ret/PTC, the oncogene product is a fusion protein that results from a chromosomal rearrangement of the 3′ tyrosine kinase domain of TRK with the 5′ end of one of several ubiquitously expressed foreign genes, causing constitutive tyrosine kinase activation. Demonstrated in up to 10% of papillary thyroid carcinomas *(38,66,71–73)*, this rearrangement is less common than Ret/PTC.

MET is another tyrosine kinase receptor with activity in papillary thyroid carcinoma. Its natural ligand is the hepatic growth factor/scatter factor, a cytokine that stimulates epithelial cell proliferation, motility, and invasion *(74–81)*. Unlike Ret/PTC and TRK, in papillary thyroid carcinoma, MET is activated through overexpression rather than gene rearrangement *(38,82)*. Although it is generally observed in around 50% of papillary thyroid carcinomas, some series have suggested a prevalence as high as 100%, and it is only rarely seen in other varieties of thyroid cancer *(38,82)*.

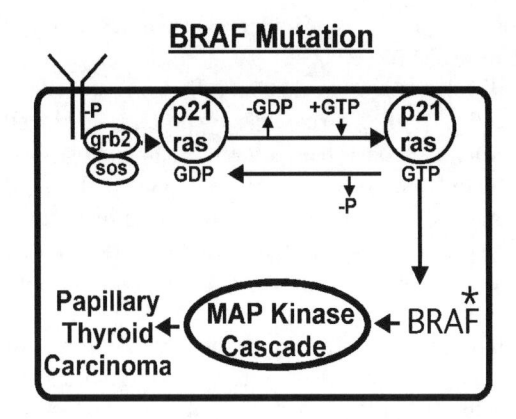

Fig. 16. Activating BRAF mutations. BRAF codes for a cytoplasmic serine-threonine kinase, which is regulated upstream by Ras and causes downstream signaling through the MAPK pathway. A point mutation at codon 599 causes constitutive activation of the kinase, causing continuous downstream signaling and promotion of uncontrolled cell division.

BRAF

BRAF is a proto-oncogene coding for a cytoplasmic serine-threonine kinase (Fig. 16). Ras regulates it upstream, causing downstream signaling through the MAPK pathway. Several studies in papillary thyroid carcinoma have shown a point mutation at codon 599, causing a change from a valine to a glutamine residue. This mutation mimics phosphorylation in the activation segment of the kinase, resulting in continuous signaling down the MAPK pathway and the promotion of uncontrolled cell division *(83)*. The prevalence of the BRAF mutation is estimated at 36–69% of all papillary thyroid carcinomas *(83–88)*. Interestingly, like Ret/PTC, the BRAF mutation has been shown to be unique to papillary thyroid carcinoma *(84,85)*. Also, no overlap is observed between those cancers demonstrating Ret/PTC rearrangements and BRAF mutations *(84,87)*. These observations point to the central importance of the Ret/PTC-Ras-BRAF-MAPK pathway in the development of papillary thyroid carcinoma.

THE PATHWAY TO ANAPLASTIC THYROID CARCINOMA: P53 MUTATIONS

The p53 protein is a multifunctional antiproliferative transcription factor or a tumor suppressor gene product (Fig. 17) that augments the production of regulatory proteins that inhibit cell division and other proteins that promote DNA repair and apoptosis *(89,90)*. Inactivating mutations of the *p53* gene result in the production of nonfunctional p53 proteins that predispose to malignant transformation and progression by multiple mechanisms (Fig. 18). Because abnormal p53 proteins are often catabolized more slowly than normal p53, their presence is frequently discovered by finding increased tissue levels of total p53 protein. Detected

Fig. 17. Normal p53 protein function. The normal p53 protein enters the nucleus and binds to targeted genes where it modulates the production of the cell cycle regulatory proteins that inhibit cell proliferation and promote cell differentiation, DNA repair, and age-appropriate apoptosis.

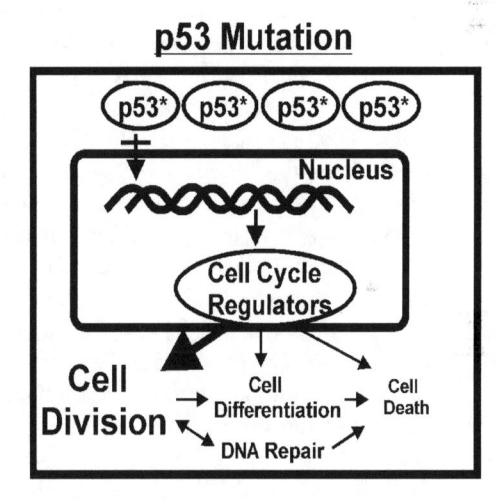

Fig. 18. Inactivating *p53* mutations. Inactivating mutations of the *p53* gene produce a nonfunctional p53 protein that leads to progressive malignant tumor growth by failing to restrain excessive proliferation or failing to induce differentiation, DNA repair, or apoptosis in thyroid cells that have been previously transformed by a primary genetic mutation.

in up to 50% of all malignant tumors, *p53* gene mutations are among the most common genetic abnormalities in human cancer *(91–93)*. They are rarely found in differentiated thyroid carcinomas but have been detected in 20–100% of poorly differentiated and anaplastic thyroid cancers *(94–101)*. This data indicate that most *p53* gene mutations are not primary but instead develop in cells transformed by a prior genetic abnormality and also indicates that they portend progression to a more aggressive tumor phenotype.

CELL CYCLE REGULATORY PROTEINS

Cell cycle regulatory proteins are the end products or effectors of the growth-signaling cascades (Fig. 5; *2, 102,103*). Mutations of the genes encoding these proteins also predispose to neoplasia by a variety of mechanisms (*2,104,105*). The best known protein in this category is pRB—a master regulator that normally serves to halt the cell cycle by preventing cells from progressing past the G1 phase. Initially described in childhood retinoblastomas, inactivating pRB gene mutations have now been detected in multiple tumor types (*106*) and may be involved in the development of thyroid carcinomas (*107*). Cyclins are a separate class of regulatory proteins that promote the passage of cells through the cell cycle. Cyclin D, for example, binds to a cyclin-dependent kinase, forming a complex that inactivates pRB, thereby allowing the cell to progress into the S phase (*2*). Activating mutations of the cyclin genes have been reported in various tumors (*104,105*) but have yet to be demonstrated in thyroid cancers (*107*).

Telomerase is a unique type of regulatory protein normally present only in germ cells. Telomeres are the chromosomal caps that function to prevent chromosomes from sticking together or forming otherwise unstable configurations. Human telomeres consist of approx 2000 repeats of the nucleotide sequence TTGGGG. Each time a cell divides, it loses some of its telomeric sequences. Once telomeres are reduced to a critical length, the cell stops dividing and eventually undergoes apoptosis. Germ cells, however, avoid this fate by producing telomerase, an enzyme that rebuilds telomeres after each cell cycle, allowing germ cells to proliferate continuously throughout the life of the host. Interestingly, telomerase has been detected in nearly 90% of human cancers from various sites (*108,109*); it has been theorized that it may influence the immortalization of malignant cells. Telomerase has also been shown in over 60% of papillary thyroid carcinomas (*110*) but is uncommon in other thyroid tumor types. Clarification of the significance of these findings, and the mechanism by which the normally silent telomerase gene becomes activated into an oncogene in human neoplasms, awaits further investigation.

MAINTENANCE PROTEINS

Angiogenesis factors are proteins produced by growing tissues to stimulate the development of vascular networks to ensure an adequate supply of oxygen and nutrients. Because tumors frequently require a robust vascular supply, and many become hypervascular, it is likely that overexpression of one or more angiogenesis factors has a key supportive role at some point in tumor development (*111*). Basic fibroblast growth factor (FGF) is one angiogenic factor present in normal thyroid tissue and has been shown to increase in several thyroid tumors (*112,113*). The contribution of FGF and other vascular growth factors to the development of thyroid tumors is not yet fully understood but certainly warrants further research (*113*).

Cell adhesion molecules fall into two general categories: cell–cell and cell–matrix adhesion proteins. Cell–cell adhesion proteins, such as the cadherins, maintain tissue integrity by causing the cells of a given organ to stick together. Cell–matrix adhesion proteins, known as integrins, anchor cells to the extracellular matrix; not only does this provide structural integrity, but these cell–matrix links serve as a scaffolding that is required by some cell types for continued cell division (anchorage dependence). Benign neoplasms that remain localized to their tissue of origin probably retain these adhesive proteins, whereas they may be lost or altered in tumors that invade adjacent tissues or metastasize to distant sites (*113–116*). In support of this hypothesis, the expression of E-cadherin, a cell–cell adhesion protein, is significantly reduced in malignant compared to benign thyroid neoplasms, and its absence is associated with an increased risk of metastatic spread (*117*).

CLINICAL APPLICATIONS

The study of oncogenes and tumor suppressor genes has provided scientists and physicians with extremely valuable insights into the pathophysiology of thyroid cancer development and progression. Many of these discoveries have or will soon have important clinical applications in the areas of diagnosis, prognosis, and treatment.

Diagnosis

As specific oncogenes and tumor suppressor genes are characteristic of certain tumor types (Fig. 6), tissue obtained by fine-needle aspiration, at surgery, or from archived samples might soon be screened with an oncogene panel to facilitate an accurate diagnosis. This could be particularly helpful in the preoperative distinction between follicular adenomas and follicular carcinomas. For example, the presence of the PAX8/PPARγ rearrangement would strongly suggest a follicular carcinoma, whereas evidence of Ras would not differentiate between a follicular adenoma and carcinoma (*31*).

Preclinical screening for familial MTC is an area where oncogene testing has already had dramatic impacts on clinical practice. Because this disorder is autosomal-dominant and will be transmitted, on average, to 50% of an affected individual's offspring, family members of an MTC patient must be screened for the disease. Traditionally, family screening includes the measurement of basal and stimulated serum or plasma calcitonin levels to detect members with early involvement. However, these tests do not become positive until either C-cell hyperplasia or frank MTC is present and therefore may not detect disease early enough to effect a cure. Furthermore, when negative, they must be repeated annually until around age 35. In contrast, Ret/MTC genetic testing can be performed on a sample of peripheral blood mononuclear cells, has a sensitivity of over 99%, can detect the disorder at birth, and has to be done only once in each family member *(47,55)*. This oncogene test has all but eliminated the need for calcitonin testing when screening family members for the presence of preclinical or subclinical MTC.

Prognosis

The capability of accurately forecasting the probable future behavior of a tumor is particularly important in the management of thyroid cancer. Most thyroid malignancies are indolent and do not substantially affect life expectancy or lifestyle, but a significant minority recur or metastasize, resulting in morbidity and premature mortality. Prognosis estimates are currently based on clinical features, such as patient age, tumor size, histologic grade, and the presence of local tissue invasion or distant metastases. Oncogene screening of tissue from the primary tumor or recurrent lesions may soon allow more accurate prognostic estimation based on the types or numbers of genetic mutations detected. One example of how oncogenes are currently used for prognosis is in medullary carcinoma, where discovery of the specific *Ret* mutation present in an individual can guide the timing of therapeutic interventions (e.g., total thyroidectomy). Because mutations at certain codons have been shown to be more aggressive than others, patients with high-risk mutations are advised to receive thyroidectomies earlier than those patients with less aggressive genotypes *(42–44)*.

Treatment

Thyroid cancers are usually treated with a combination of surgery, radioactive iodine administration, and L-thyroxine suppression. In the near future, oncogene screening may significantly affect therapeutic decision-making. Awareness of the oncogene profile could help physicians decide, based on prognosis, whether an individual patient should receive a more aggressive or more conservative course of treatment. In this regard, such knowledge could serve as a guide to decisions, such as the optimal extent of surgery, the dose of radioactive iodine, and the degree of L-thyroxine suppression. Furthermore, by more fully illuminating the molecular factors underlying tumor behavior, oncogene screening may lead to the development and use of chemotherapeutic and/or immunologic agents that specifically retard thyroid cell proliferation, promote differentiation into more mature cell types, restore the normal mechanisms of DNA repair and/or apoptosis, and impair tumor angiogenesis or maintain cell–cell and cell–matrix adhesiveness *(118–120)*. Such advances could bring forth a new era of safer and more effective treatment for thyroid cancer.

REFERENCES

1. Jorde LB, Carey JC, White RL. Basic cell biology: structure and function of genes and chromosomes. In Medical Genetics. St. Louis: Mosby-Yearbook, 1995:7–29.
2. Weinberg RA. How cancer arises. Scientific American 1996; 275:62–70.
3. Cline MJ, Slamom DJ, Lipsick JS. Oncogenes: implications for the diagnosis and treatment of cancer. Ann Intern Med 1984; 101:223–233.
4. Gordon H. Oncogenes. Mayo Clin Proc 1985; 60:697–713.
5. Druker BJ, Mamon HJ, Roberts TM. Oncogenes, growth factors, and signal transduction. N Engl J Med 1989; 321:1383–1391.
6. Krontiris TG. Molecular medicine: oncogenes. N Engl J Med 1995; 333:303–306.
7. Latchman DS. Transcription-factor mutations and disease. N Engl J Med 1995; 334:28–33.
8. Friend SH, Dryja TP, Weinberg RA. Oncogenes and tumor-suppressing genes. N Engl J Med 1988; 318:618–622.
9. Weinberg RA. Tumor suppressor genes. Science 1991; 254: 1138–1145.
10. Marshall CF. Tumor suppressor genes. Cell 1991; 64:313–326.
11. Knudson AG. Antioncogenes and human cancer. Proc Natl Acad Sci USA 1993; 90:10914–10921.
12. Hartwell LH, Kastan MB. Cell cycle control and cancer. Science 1994; 266:1821–1828.
13. Vogelstein B, Kinzler KW. The multistep nature of cancer. Trends Genet 1993; 9:138–141.
14. Bishop JM. Cancer: the rise of the genetic paradigm. Genes Dev 1995; 9:1309–1315.
15. Vassart G, Dumont JE. The thyrotropin receptor and the regulation of thyrocyte function and growth. Endocrine Rev 1992; 13:596–611.
16. Paschke R, Tonacchera M, Van Sande J, et al. Identification and functional characterization of two new somatic mutations causing constitutive activation of the thyrotropin receptor in hyperfunctioning autonomous adenomas of the thyroid. J Clin Endocrinol Metab 1994; 79:1785–1789.
17. Porcellini A, Ciullo I, Laviola L, et al. Novel mutations of thyrotropin receptor gene in thyroid hyperfunctioning adenomas. Rapid identification by fine needle aspiration biopsy. J Clin Endocrinol Metab 1994; 79:657–661.
18. Russo D, Arturi F, Wicker R, et al. Genetic alterations in thyroid hyperfunctioning adenomas. J Clin Endocrinol Metab 1995; 80: 1347–1351.
19. Ohno M, Endo T, Ohta K, et al. Point mutations in the thyrotropin receptor in human thyroid tumors. Thyroid 1995; 5:97–100.
20. Parma J, Duprez L, Van Sande J, et al. Constitutively active receptors as a disease-causing mechanism. Mol Cell Endocrinology 1994; 100: 159–162.
21. Van Sande J, Parma J, Tonacchera M, et al. Somatic and germline mutations of the TSH receptor gene in thyroid diseases. J Clin Endocrinol Metab 1995; 80:2577–2585.
22. Takeshita A, Nagayama Y, Yokoyama N, et al. Rarity of oncogenic mutations in the thyrotropin receptor of autonomously functioning thyroid nodules in Japan. J Clin Endocrinol Metab 1995; 80: 2607–2611.
23. Matsuo K, Friedan E, Gejman PV, Fagin JA: The thyrotropin receptor (TSH-R) is not an oncogene for thyroid tumors: structural studies of the TSH-R and the alpha subunit of Gs in human thyroid neoplasms. J Clin Endocrinol Metab 1993; 76:1446–1451.
24. Esapa C, Foster S, Johnson S, et al: G protein and thyrotropin receptor mutations in thyroid neoplasia. J Clin Endocrinol Metab 1997; 82: 493–496.
25. Lyons J, Landis CA, Harsh G, et al. Two G protein oncogenes in human endocrine tumors. Science 1990; 249:655–658.
26. Dumont JE. Thyroid adenoma, Gsa expression and the cyclic adenosine monophosphate mitogenic cascade: A complex relationship. J Clin Endocrinol Metab 1995; 80:1518–1520.
27. Spalmberg D, Sharifi N, Elisei R, et al: Structural studies of the thyrotropin receptor and Gsa in human thyroid cancers: low prevalence of mutations predicts infrequent involvement in malignant transformation. J Clin Endocrinol Metab 1996; 81:3898–3901.

28. Moretti F, Nanni S, Pontecorvi A. Molecular pathogenesis of thyroid nodules and cancer. Ballieres Best Prac Res Clin Endocrinol Metab 2000; 14:517–539.
29. Bos JL. Ras oncogenes in human cancer: a review. Cancer Res 1989; 49:4682–4689.
30. Karga H, Lee JK, Vickery AL, et al: Ras oncogene mutations in benign and malignant thyroid neoplasms. J Endocrinol Metab 1991; 73:832–836.
31. Nikiforova MN, Lynch RA, Biddinger PW, et al. Ras point mutations and PAX8-PPARγ rearrangement in thyroid tumors: evidence for distinct molecular pathways in thyroid follicular carcinoma. J Clin Endocrinol Metab 2003; 88:2318–2326.
32. Lemoine NR, Mayall ES, Wyllie FS, et al. High frequency of ras oncogene activation in all stages of human thyroid tumorigenesis. Oncogene 1989; 4:159–164.
33. Esapa CT, Johnson SJ, Kendall-Taylor P, et al. Prevalence of Ras mutations in thyroid neoplasia. Clin Endocrinol 1999; 50:529–535.
34. Lemoine NR, Mayall ES, Wyllie FS, et al. Activated ras oncogenes in human thyroid cancers. Cancer Res 1988; 48:4459–4463.
35. Zhu Z, Gandhi M, Nikiforova MN, et al. Molecular profile and clinical-pathologic features of the follicular variant of papillary thyroid carcinoma: an unusually high prevalence of ras mutations. Am J Clin Pathol 2003; 120:71–77.
36. Manenti G, Pilotti S, Re FC, et al. Selective activation of Ras oncogenes in follicular and undifferentiated thyroid carcinomas. Eur J Cancer 1994; 30A:987–993.
37. Kroll TG, Sarraf P, Pecciarini L, et al. PAX8/PPARγ1 fusion oncogene in human thyroid carcinoma. Science 2000; 289:1357–1360.
38. Schlumberger M, Pacini F. Oncogenes and tumor suppressor genes. In Thyroid Tumors. Paris: Editions Nucleon, 2003:63–83.
39. Nikiforova MN, Biddinger PW, Caudill CM, et al. PAX8-PPARgamma rearrangement in thyroid tumors: RT-PCR and immunohistochemical analyses. Am J Surg Path 2002; 26:1016–1023.
40. Marques AR, Espadinha C, Catarino AL, et al. Expression of PAX8-PPARγ1 rearrangements in both follicular thyroid carcinomas and adenomas. J Clin Endocrinol Metab 2002; 87:3947–3952.
41. Dwight T, Thoppe SR, Foukakis T, et al. Involvement of the PAX/Peroxisome proliferator-activated receptor γ rearrangement in follicular thyroid tumors. J Clin Endocrinol Metab 2003; 88:4440–4445.
42. Jhiang SM. The RET proto-oncogene in human cancers. Oncogene 2000; 19:5590–5597.
43. Alberti L, Carniti C, Miranda C, et al. RET and NTRK1 protooncogenes in human diseases. J Cell Phys 2003; 195:168–186.
44. Ichihara M, Murakumo Y, Takahashi M. RET and neuroendocrine tumors. Cancer Lett 2004; 204:197–211.
45. Hofstra RMW, Landsvater RM, Ceccherini I, et al. A mutation in the RET protooncogene associated with multiple endocrine neoplasia type 2B and sporadic medullary thyroid carcinoma. Nature 1994; 367:375–376.
46. Smith DP, Eng C, Ponder BAJ. Mutations of the RET proto-oncogene in the multiple endocrine neoplasia type 2 syndromes and Hirschsprung disease. J Cell Science 1994; Suppl18:43–49.
47. Lips CJM, Landsvater RM, Hoppener JWM, et al. Clinical screening as compared with DNA analysis in families with multiple endocrine neoplasia type 2A. N Engl J Med 1994; 31:828–835.
48. Zedenius J, Larsson C, Bergholm U, et al. Mutations of codon 918 in the RET proto-oncogene correlate to poor prognosis in sporadic medullary thyroid carcinomas. J Clin Endo Metabol 1995; 80:3088–3090.
49. Romei C, Elisei R, Pinchera A, et al. Somatic mutations of the ret protooncogene in sporadic medullary thyroid carcinoma are not restricted to exon 16 and are associated with tumor recurrence. J Clin Endocrinol Metab 1996; 81:1619–1622.
50. Jhiang SM, Fithian L, Weghorst CM, et al. RET mutation screening in MEN2 patients and discovery of a novel mutation in a sporadic medullary thyroid carcinoma. Thyroid 1996; 6:115–121.
51. Wohllk N, Cote G, Bugalho MMJ, et al. Relevance of ret protooncogene mutations in sporadic medullary thyroid carcinoma. J Clin Endocrinol Metab 1996; 81:3740–3745.
52. Frank-Raue K, Hoppner W, Frilling A, et al. and the German Medullary Thyroid Cancer Study Group. Mutations of the ret protooncogene in German multiple endocrine neoplasia families: relation between genotype and phenotype. J Clin Endocrinol Metab 1996; 81:1780–1783.
53. Quadro L, Panariello L, Salvatore D, et al. Frequent RET protooncogene mutations in multiple endocrine neoplasia type 2A. J Clin Endocrinol Metab 1994; 79:590–594.
54. Mulligan LM, Ponder BAJ. Genetic basis of endocrine disease: multiple endocrine neoplasia type 2. J Clin Endocrinol Metab 1995; 80:1989–1995.
55. Eng C. The ret proto-oncogene in multiple endocrine neoplasia type 2 and Hirschsprung's disease. N Engl J Med 1996; 335:943–951.
56. Asai N, Iwashita T, Matsuyama M, Takahashi M. Mechanism of activation of the ret proto-oncogene by multiple endocrine neoplasia 2A mutations. Mol Cell Biol 1995; 15:1613–1619.
57. Borrello MG, Smith DP, Pasini B, et al. RET activation by germline MEN2A and MEN2B mutations. Oncogene 1995; 11:2419–2427.
58. Santoro M, Carlomagno F, Romano A, et al. Activation of RET as a dominant transforming gene by germline mutations of MEN2A and MEN2B. Science 1995; 267:381–383.
59. Bongarzone I, Vigano E, Alberti L, et al. Full activation of MEN2B mutant RET by an additional MEN2A mutation or by ligand (GDNF) stimulation. Oncogene 1998; 16:2295–2301.
60. Nikiforov YE. RET/PTC rearrangement in thyroid tumors. Endocr Pathol 2002; 13:3–16.
61. Basolo F, Giannini R, Monaco C, et al. Potent mitogenicity of the RET/PTC3 oncogene correlates with its prevalence in tall-cell variant of papillary thyroid carcinoma. Am J Pathol 2002; 160:247–254.
62. Thomas GA, Bunnell H, Cook HA, et al. High prevalence of RET/PTC rearrangements in Ukrainian and Belarussian post-Chernobyl thyroid papillary carcinomas: A strong correlation between RET/PTC3 and the solid-follicular variant. J Clin Endocrinol Metab 1999; 84:4232–4238.
63. Santoro M, Carlomagno F, Hay ID, et al. Ret oncogene activation in human thyroid neoplasms is restricted to the papillary cancer subtype. J Clin Invest 1992; 89:1517–1522.
64. Jhiang SM, Mazzaferri EL. The ret/PTC oncogene in papillary thyroid carcinoma. J Lab Clin Med 1994; 123:331–337.
65. Grieco M, Santoro M, Berlingieri MT, et al. PTC is a novel rearranged form of the ret proto-oncogene and is frequently detected in vivo in human thyroid papillary carcinomas. Cell 1990; 60:557–563.
66. Bongarzone I, Fugazzola L, Vigneri P, et al. Age-related activation of the tyrosine kinase receptor protooncogenes ret and ntrk1 in papillary thyroid carcinoma. J Clin Endocrinol Metab 1996; 81:2006–2009.
67. Sugg S, Zheng L, Rosen IB, et al. ret/PTC-1, -2, and -3 oncogene rearrangements in human thyroid carcinomas: implications for metastatic potential? J Clin Endocrinol Metab 1996; 81:3360–3365.
68. Lam KY, Lo CY, Leung PS. High prevalence of RET proto-oncogene activation (RET/PTC) in papillary thyroid carcinoma. Eur J Endocrinol 2002; 147:741–745.
69. Bounacer A, Wicker R, Caillou B, et al. High prevalence of activationg ret proto-oncogene rearrangements in thyroid tumors from patients who had received external radiation. Oncogene 1997; 15:1263–1273.
70. Elisei R, Romei C, Vorontsova T, et al. RET/PTC rearrangements in thyroid nodules: studies in irradiated and not irradiated, malignant and benign thyroid lesions in children and adults. J Clin Endocrinol Metab 2001; 86:3211–3216.
71. Bounacer A, Schlumberger M, Wicker R, et al. Search for NTRK1 proto-oncogene rearrangements in human thyroid tumours originated after therapeutic radiation. Br J Cancer 2000; 82:308–314.
72. Greco A, Pierotti MA, Bongarzone I, et al. Trk-T1 is a novel oncogene formed by the fusion of tpr and trk genes in human papillary thyroid carcinomas. Oncogene 1992; 7:237–242.

73. Pierotti MA, Bongarzone I, Borrello MG, et al. Cytogenetics and molecular genetics of carcinomas arising from thyroid epithelial follicular cells. Genes Chromosomes Cancer 1996; 16:1–14.
74. Di Renzo MF, Olivero M, Ferro S. Overexpression of the c-MET/HGF receptor gene in human thyroid carcinomas. Oncogene 1992; 7: 2549–2553.
75. Belfiori A, Gamgemi P, Santomocito MG. Prognostic value of c-MET expression in papillary thyroid carcinoma. Thyroid 1995; 5:5–13.
76. Ruco LP, Ranalli T, Marzullo A, et al. Expression of Met protein in thyroid tumours. J Pathol 1996; 180:266–270.
77. Belfiori A, Gangemi P, Costantino A, et al. Negative/low expression of the Met/hepatocyte growth factor receptor identifies papillary thyroid carcinomas with high risk of distant metastases. J Clin Endocrinol Metab 1997; 82:2322–2328.
78. Trovato M, Villari D, Bartolone L, et al. Expression of the hepatocyte growth factor and c-met in normal thyroid, non-neoplastic, and neoplastic nodules. Thyroid 1998; 8:125–131.
79. Oyama T, Ichimura E, Sano T, et al. c-Met expression of thyroid tissue with special reference to papillary carcinoma. Pathol Int 1998; 48:763–768.
80. Zanetti A, Stoppacciaro A, Marzullo A, et al. Expression of Met protein and urokinase-type plasminogen activator receptor (uPA-R) in papillary carcinoma of the thyroid. J Pathol 1998; 186:287–291.
81. de Luca A, Arena N, Sena LM, Medico E. Met overexpression confers HGF-dependent invasive phenotype to human thyroid carcinoma cells in vitro. J Cell Physiol 1999; 180:365–371.
82. Ramirez R, Hsu D, Patel A, et al. Over-expression of hepatocyte growth factor/scatter factor (HGF/SF) and the HGF/SF receptor (cMET) are associated with a high risk of metastasis and recurrence for children and young adults with papillary thyroid carcinoma. Clin Endocrinol 2000; 53:635–644.
83. Nikiforova MN, Kimura ET, Gandhi M, et al. BRAF mutations in thyroid tumors are restricted to papillary carcinomas and anaplastic or poorly differentiated carcinomas arising from papillary carcinomas. J Clin Endocrinol Metab 2003; 88:5399–5404.
84. Kimura ET, Nikiforova MN, Zhu A, et al. High prevalence of BRAF mutations in thyroid cancer: genetic evidence for constitutive activation of the RET/PTC-RAS-BRAF signaling pathway in papillary thyroid carcinoma. Cancer Res 2003; 63:1454–1457.
85. Cohen Y, Xing M, Mambo E, et al. BRAF mutation in papillary thyroid carcinoma. J Natl Cancer Inst 2003; 95:625–627.
86. Xu X, Quiros RM, Gattuso P, et al. High prevalence of BRAF gene mutation in papillary thyroid carcinomas and thyroid tumor cell lines. Cancer Res 2003; 63:4561–4567.
87. Soares P, Trovisco V, Rocha AS, et al. BRAF mutations and RET/PTC rearrangements are alternative events in the etiopathogenesis of PTC. Oncogene 2003; 22:4578–4580.
88. Fukushima T, Suzuki S, Mashiko M, et al. BRAF mutations in papillary carcinomas of the thyroid. Oncogene 2003; 22:6455–6457.
89. Lane DP: p53, guardian of the genome. Nature 1992; 358:15-16.
90. Marx J. How p53 suppresses cell growth. Science 1993; 262: 1644–1645.
91. Frebourg T. Cancer risks from germline p53 mutations. J Clin Invest 1992; 90:1637–1641.
92. Harris CC. Medical progress: clinical implications of the p53 tumor suppressor gene. N Engl J Med 1993; 329:1318–1327.
93. Greenblat MS, Bennet WP, Hollstein M, et al. Mutations in the p53 tumor suppressor gene: Clues to cancer aetiology and molecular pathogenesis. Cancer Res 1994; 54:4855–4878.
94. Dobashi Y, Sakamoto A, Sugimura H, et al. Overexpression of p53 as a possible prognostic factor in human thyroid carcinoma. Am J Surg Pathol 1993; 17:375–381.
95. Dobashi Y, Sugimura H, Sakamoto A, et al. Stepwise participation of p53 gene mutation during dedifferentiation of human thyroid carcinomas. Diagn Mol Pathol 1994; 3:9–14.
96. Nakamura T, Yana I, Kobayashi T, et al. p53 gene mutations associated with anaplastic transformation of human thyroid carcinomas. Jpn J Cancer Res 1992; 83:1293–1298.
97. Ito T, Seyma T, Mizuno T, et al. Unique association of p53 mutations with undifferentiated but not with differentiated carcinoma of the thyroid. Cancer Res 1992; 52:1369–1371.
98. Fagin JA, Matsuo K, Karmakar A, et al. High prevalence of mutations of the p53 gene in poorly differentiated human thyroid carcinomas. J Clin Invest 1993; 91:179–184.
99. Donghi R, Longoni A, Pilotti S, et al. Gene p53 mutations are restricted to poorly differentiated and undifferentiated carcinomas of the thyroid gland. J Clin Invest 1993; 91:1753–1760.
100. Zedenius J, Larsson C, Wallin G, et al. Alterations of p53 and expression of WAF1/p21 in human thyroid tumors. Thyroid 1996; 6:1–9.
101. Zou M, Shi Y, Farid NR. p53 mutations in all stages of thyroid carcinomas. J Clin Endocrinol Metab 1993; 77:1054–1058.
102. Doree M, Galas S. The cyclin-dependent protein kinases and the control of cell division. FASEB J 1994; 8:1114–1121.
103. Morgan DO. Principles of CDK regulation. Nature 1995; 374: 131–134.
104. Hartwell L. Defects in the cell cycle checkpoint may be responsible for genomic instability of cancer cells. Cell 1992; 71:543–546.
105. Kamb A, Gravis S, Weaver-Feldheus J, et al. A cell cycle regulator potentially involved in genesis of many tumor types. Science 1994; 264:436–440.
106. Cyrns VL, Thor A, Xu H-J, et al. Loss of the retinoblastoma tumor-suppressor gene in parathyroid carcinoma. N Engl J Med 1994; 330: 757–761.
107. Farid NR, Zou M, Shi Y. Genetics of follicular thyroid cancer. Endocrinol Metab Clin NA 1995; 24:865–883.
108. Haber DA. Telomeres, cancer and immortality. N Engl J Med 1995; 332:955–956.
109. Greider CW, Blackburn EH. Telomeres, telomerase and cancer. Sci Am 1996; 274:92–97.
110. Haugen BR, Nawaz S, Markham et al. Telomerase activity in benign and malignant thyroid tumors. San Diego, CA: The 69th Annual Meeting of the American Thyroid Association 1996, Nov 14–17.
111. Folkman J. Fighting cancer by attacking its blood supply. Sci Am 1996; 275:150–154.
112. Cuevas P, Gonzalez A-M, Carceller F, Baird A. Vascular response to basic fibroblast growth factor when infused onto normal adventitia or into the injured media of the rat carotid artery. Circ Res 1991; 69:360–369.
113. Bernstein LR, Liotta LA. Molecular mediators of interactions with extracellular matrix components in metastasis and angiogenesis. Cur Opin Oncol 1994; 6:106–113.
114. Ruoslahti E, Reed JC. Anchorage dependence, integrins and apoptosis. Cell 1994; 77:477–478.
115. Akiyama SK, Olden K, Yamada KM. Fibronectin and integrins in invasion and metastasis. Cancer Metastasis Rev 1996; 14:173–189.
116. Ruoslahti E. How Cancer Spreads. Sci Am 1996; 275:72–77.
117. Scheumann GFW, Hoang-Vu C, Cetin Y, et al. Clinical significance of E-cadherin as a prognostic marker in thyroid carcinomas. J Clin Endocrinol Metab 1995; 80:2168–2172.
118. Oliff A, Gibbs JB, McCormick F: New molecular targets for cancer therapy. Sci Am 1996; 275:144–149.
119. Old LJ. Immunotherapy for cancer. Sci Am 1996; 275:136–143.
120. Bassi V, Vitale M, Feliciello A, et al. Retinoic acid induces intercellular adhesion molecule-1 hyperexpression in human thyroid carcinoma cell lines. J Clin Endocrinol Metab 1995; 80:1129–1135.

6
Apoptosis in Thyroid Cancer

Su He Wang and James R. Baker, Jr.

INTRODUCTION

Apoptosis has emerged as an important process in both carcinogenesis and as the response to anticancer treatments for thyroid tumors. Thyroid cancer has been associated with alterations in an increasing number of apoptotic molecules. Our knowledge of apoptosis offers hope for better diagnosis, therapy, and staging thyroid cancer. This chapter discusses data from recent publications and our laboratory work on apoptosis in thyroid cancer. Three main aspects are addressed: apoptotic pathways in cancer; how apoptosis is linked to the development of thyroid cancer; and the possible therapeutic implications of the molecular regulation of apoptosis.

As outlined in other chapters, thyroid cancer is the most common endocrine malignancy. Thyroid cancer can be divided into four types: papillary thyroid carcinoma (PTC) and follicular thyroid carcinoma (FTC), both of which may be classified as differentiated thyroid carcinoma; anaplastic thyroid carcinoma (ATC), also called undifferentiated thyroid carcinoma; and medullary thyroid carcinoma (MTC). Except for MTC derived from parafollicular C cells, all other thyroid cancers originate from follicular epithelial cells. Based on the data obtained over a 10-yr period from 53,856 patients with thyroid cancer in the United States, percentages of the four types of thyroid cancer are: 78% PTC, 13% FTC, 4% MTC, and 2% ATC *(1)*.

The etiology of thyroid cancer is not yet fully known. However, it is believed that its development is a multifactor and multistep process. Several issues are thought to predispose people to thyroid cancer, including radiation, nutrition, sex hormones, environment, and genetics. It is possible that all these factors relate to apoptotic mechanisms. Radiation is probably one of the most well-studied predisposing factors. The source of radiation is usually traceable, such as from the therapeutic or diagnostic use of radiation and from environmental disasters. The effects are dose-dependent and show strong age dependence, with exposure in childhood and adolescence showing almost an order of magnitude higher in the incidence of cancer *(2)*. Both iodine deficiency and excess iodine can contribute to the development of thyroid cancer *(3,4)*.

There are also reports describing other nutritional factors, e.g., goitrogens as an etiologic factor for thyroid cancer *(5)*. Apparently, anything leading to compensatory increases in thyrotropin will increase the risk of thyroid tumors. One specific feature of thyroid carcinoma is its predilection for women of reproductive age relative to men, suggesting a role of sex hormones in the formation of thyroid cancer. The incidence of thyroid carcinoma is three times more frequent in women than in men *(6)*. An elevated risk has also been documented in women who use estrogens for gynecological reasons but not in postmenopausal women on low-dose estrogens *(7)*. Environmental pollution by hexachlorobenzene and tetrachlorodibenzo-*p*-dioxin may cause an increased incidence of thyroid cancer *(8)*. Living near volcanic lava has also been reported as a risk factor for thyroid cancer *(9)*. Although a responsible gene is not identified for thyroid cancer, its occurrence has been reported in several familial syndromes *(10)*. Women under 35 yr of age with familial adenomatous polyposis—a disease associated with altered apoptosis—have been estimated to have a 160-fold higher risk of thyroid cancer than the general population *(11)*.

Apoptosis or programmed cell death is an active process in which a cell dies for the benefit of the whole organism; this mode of cell death is critical in the development and maintenance of multicellular organisms. Apoptosis is characterized by specific morphological features. The process starts with chromatin aggregation along the inner walls of the nuclear envelope and is followed by cytoplasmic shrinkage, membrane blebbing, extensive DNA degradation, and nuclear pyknosis. Finally, the cell condenses into membrane-bound fragments that are eliminated by surrounding macrophages without an inflammatory reaction. Most aforementioned factors are involved in cell proliferation and growth; they can be directly or indirectly linked with apoptosis.

From: *Thyroid Cancer: A Comprehensive Guide to Clinical Management, 2/e*
Edited by: L. Wartofsky and D. Van Nostrand © Humana Press Inc., Totowa, NJ

Although radiation has been reported in the induction of apoptosis in thyrocytes *(12)*, its carcinogenesis may be more related to its ability to damage DNA and cause mutation in tumor-suppressive genes, including *p53 (13)*. It is reported that high iodine concentrations increase the rate of Fas-induced apoptosis in thyrocytes, but low concentrations of iodine are able to inhibit apoptosis *(14)*. Iodine may reduce the sensitivity of PTC cells to apoptotic stimulation via increasing the activity of heme oxygenase and *p21 (15)*. The growth stimulatory effect of estrogen has been intensively studied in various estrogen receptor (ER)-expressing cells. Estrogen protects neuronal cells and cardiac myocytes from apoptosis by regulating Bcl-2 family protein expression *(16)*. It has been demonstrated that estrogen stimulates cell proliferation of breast and ovary cancer cells by upregulating the expression of Bcl-2 *(17,18)*. Estrogen also has a growth stimulatory role in thyroid cancer cells similar to its effect on other ER-expressing cells *(19)*. Environmental pollution, including tetrachlorodibenzo-*p*-dioxin, may suppress apoptosis by stimulating transforming growth factor-α (TGF-α) production *(20,21)*. A connection between proliferation and apoptosis was observed in familial adenomatous polyposis, and the process of tumorigenesis is characterized by a stepwise increase in resistance to apoptosis, followed by an increase in cycling cells *(22,23)*.

APOPTOSIS AND CANCER

The deregulation of apoptosis has been implicated in various clinical disorders, including cancer. Two fundamental lesions are believed to be the underlying pathogenesis of cancer. The first is mutations that give rise to excessive proliferation; the second is a disruption of apoptotic signaling that allows mutated cells to continue to proliferate and to live beyond their normal life span, perpetuating cycles of mutation and oncogenesis. This cycle of mutational activity results in the accumulation of active oncogenes and defective tumor suppressor genes within cells, which makes apoptosis unable to restrict cellular proliferation, and the balance between proliferation and apoptosis is shifted in favor of the former *(24)*.

Apoptosis has an essential role in the elimination of mutated or transformed cells from the body. During the development of cancer, cancer cells and their precursors must develop highly efficient (and usually multiple) mechanisms to avoid apoptosis. In fact, aborting apoptosis is regarded as one of the hallmarks of cancer cells *(25)*. A frequent, apparently paradoxical finding in tumors and their precursor lesions is an increased rate of apoptosis, while at the same time, there is an increased resistance to apoptosis as well. The increased apoptosis reflects the enormous pressure of these abnormal cells to undergo programmed cell death, whereas the increased resistance represents defense mechanisms developed by the mutated cell in an effort to survive. Without the development of apoptotic resistance early during tumorigenesis, the preneoplastic cells would not survive long enough to become invasive cancers. Because apoptosis involves a complex network of interacting checks and balances utilizing several hundreds of genes, cancer cells must develop resistance to apoptosis at multiple levels.

Apoptotic cell death is now known to be mediated through the activation of caspases—a family of cysteine proteases that act as common death effector molecules in various forms of cell death *(26,27)*. Caspases are synthesized as inactive zymogens, which can be proteolytically cleaved at two (or three in some cases) aspartate residues to generate the active mature enzyme. These cleavage events remove an NH2-terminal peptide and separate the small and large subunits of the proenzyme to generate a mature heterotetrameric caspase that comprises two large and two small subunits. The generation of active caspases forms a cascade in which initiator caspases interact with specific adapter molecules to facilitate their own autoprocessing. The activated initiator caspases then cleave and activate the downstream executioner caspases, which finally target cells to dismantle. To date, two major pathways for caspase activation have been described *(28,29)* and are headed by caspase-8 (death receptor-mediated apoptosis) and caspase-9 (mitochondria-mediated apoptosis), respectively (Fig. 1).

The death receptor-mediated apoptotic pathway can be achieved by one of several death receptors when bound by the appropriate ligands, including tumor necrosis factor (TNF), FasL, and TNF-related apoptosis-inducing ligand (TRAIL). Currently, the most clearly understood aspect of the receptor pathway is the interaction between the Fas receptor and its ligand, FasL, and the activation of the TNF-R1 by TNF. The interaction between the death receptor and its ligand results in receptor aggregation and recruitment of the adaptor molecule Fas-associated death domain and caspase-8. Upon recruitment, caspase-8 becomes activated and initiates apoptosis by direct cleavage of downstream effector caspases. Ultraviolet irradiation, growth factor deprivation, and increased reactive oxygen species cause apoptosis through the mitochondria-mediated apoptotic pathway, which is initiated by the release of apoptogenic factors (e.g., cytochrome c). Cytochrome c forms a multiprotein complex with the adaptor molecule Apaf-1 and procaspase-9. Procaspase-9 is activated upon recruitment to this complex, then activates the effector caspases. The receptor and mitochondria pathways can be interconnected at different levels *(30,31)*. Following death receptor stimulation, caspase-8 activation may result in cleavage of Bid—a BH3 domain containing protein of the Bcl-2 family—to a truncated form of Bid (tBid). tBid may stimulate cytochrome c release and subsequently initiate a mitochondrial amplification loop. In addition, mitochondria-triggered caspase-6 cleavage may feed back to the receptor pathway by cleaving caspase-8 *(32)*.

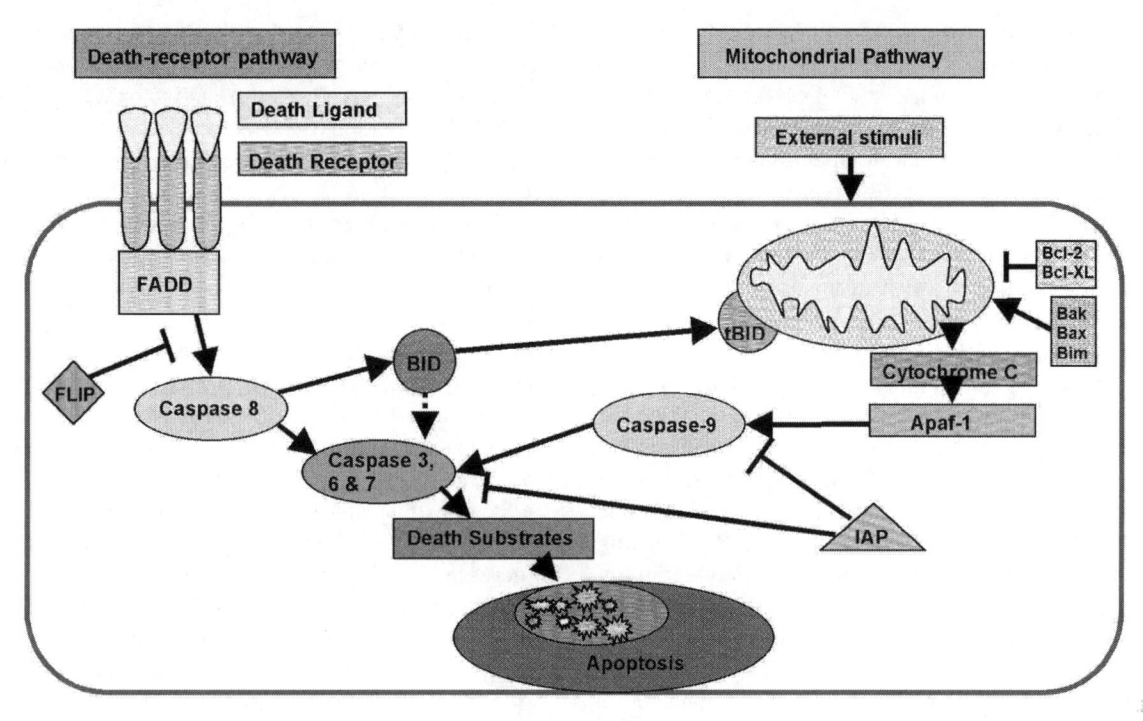

Fig. 1. Death receptor–mediated and mitochondria-mediated pathways lead to apoptotic cell death. (Color illustration is printed in insert following p. 198.)

APOPTOSIS IN THYROID CARCINOGENESIS

Increasing evidence suggests that apoptosis plays a significant role in the development of thyroid cancer. An early study of PTC showed that the apoptotic index calculated by the result of terminal dUTP nick-end labeling (TUNEL) was directly related to the p53 protein but inversely correlated with the antiapoptotic molecule Bcl-2 (33). Resistance to apoptosis and the ability to proliferate appear to be different among different types of thyroid cancer cells. But they increase with tumor aggressiveness, from PTC to poorly differentiated and undifferentiated thyroid cancers. Among various apoptotic molecules, the Fas/FasL system has been extensively investigated in thyroid cancer. Fas-mediated apoptosis is considered a key mechanism of T cell-mediated cytotoxicity against neoplastic cells. Thyroid cancer cells express a significant level of Fas. Upon anti-Fas antibody stimulation in vitro in the presence of interferon γ and cycloheximide, the cancer cells can undergo apoptosis, suggesting that the Fas on the thyroid cancer cells is functional when there are certain cytokines and protein inhibitors available (34). Although Fas is functional in thyroid cancer cells, it may not be able to induce apoptosis, and resistance to Fas is found in thyroid cancer cells (35–37). The mechanism responsible for the resistance is not yet known, but it may be related to reduced numbers of Fas receptors available on the cell surface or to a change in the thyroid cytokine microenvironment. Fas expression has been documented to be lower in thyroid nodules (38). Studies have indicated the existence of regulators that block apoptosis in thyroid cancer cells; thus, proinflammatory cytokines may induce apoptosis in noncancer thyroid cells but not in thyroid cancer cells (36,39). The levels of Fas and FasL in different thyroid cancer cells may substantially differ, and the expression of Fas has been found to be negatively associated with the advanced stage of thyroid cancer (40). Furthermore, the Fas level is significantly higher in well-differentiated PTC and FTC than in poorly differentiated or undifferentiated PTC and FTC. These observations are consistent with the finding that there is an increasing resistance to apoptosis when thyroid cancer becomes more aggressive (33).

As mentioned above, cancer cells usually develop resistance to apoptosis at multiple levels. One proven example applies to thyroid cancer cells. Thyroid cancer cells cannot only escape apoptosis by either reducing Fas expression on their cell membrane and/or displaying blockers that inhibit the Fas/FasL system (35–38) but can also utilize the Fas/FasL system to downregulate the ability of immune surveillance to kill tumor cells by inducing apoptosis of infiltrating lymphocytes and other immune effector cells (36,41). Therefore, FasL expression may correlate with more aggressive types of thyroid cancer (36). Thyroid cancer cells are not killed by their own FasL because of their inherent resistance to Fas-mediated apoptosis *(35–37,39)*. Such FasL-mediated suppression of immune surveillance is called "Fas counterattack" or the "tumor immune privilege" *(42,43)*.

In addition to the involvement of Fas/FasL death receptor-mediated apoptosis in the development of thyroid cancer, mitochondria-mediated apoptosis—represented by the alternation of Bcl-2 family members—may also have a role in the promotion of thyroid cancer cell growth. High levels of Bcl-2 and Bcl-xL, both of which are antiapoptotic, are found in malignant epithelial cells from PTC, FTC, and ATC *(44)*. Furthermore, the level of proapoptotic Bax is reduced in thyroid cancer *(45)*. The aberrant expression of Bcl-2, Bcl-xL, and Bax is thought to result from a change in the cytokine microenvironment of the thyroid, especially interleukin (IL)-4 and IL-10 *(44,45)*. Obviously, the changes in Bcl-2 family members disturb the balance between proapoptotic Bax and antiapoptotic Bcl-2 and Bcl-xL, thereby reducing the sensitivity of thyroid cancer cells to apoptotic stimuli. This assumption is in line with the observation that Bcl-2 expression is inversely correlated with the apoptotic index in thyroid cancer cells *(33)*.

The function of Bcl-2 and its other family members is closely associated with *p53*. For example, *p53* is able to upregulate proapoptotic Bax and Bak in a variety of cell types *(46,47)*. Unfortunately, evidence linking *p53* and Bcl-2 family members in thyroid cancer is lacking thus far. However, it has been confirmed that *p53* has a role in the development of thyroid cancer. Immortalized thyroid cancer cells demonstrated homozygous *p53* abrogation in three of four lines studied *(48,49)*. Mutations of tumor suppressor genes, e.g., *p53* and *p16*, are thought to be important events in thyroid tumor progression once the early stages of oncogene-driven cell transformation have been established *(50)*. Poorly differentiated thyroid cancer cells via the overexpression of *p53* can show reduced proliferation and exhibit malignant behavior *(51)*, suggesting that thyroid cancer cells lacking *p53* activity are more likely to grow fast and are less sensitive to apoptosis. A recent study showed that the *p73* protein—a member of the *p53* family—is also dysfunctional in thyroid cancer *(52)*. Thyroid cancer cells with the functional impairment of *p73* are unresponsive to DNA-damaging agents, failing to elicit cell-cycle arrest and apoptosis.

Peroxisome-proliferator–activated receptor γ (*PPARγ*) is another molecule that has recently gained much attention for its role in apoptosis and tumor development. *PPARγ* activation is capable of inducing apoptosis, thus inhibiting tumor growth *(53,54)*. This activation may counteract the uncontrolled proliferation and malignant cell growth through induction of apoptosis or promotion of cellular terminal differentiation. In fact, *PPARγ* is expressed differently in different types of thyroid cancer cells. A study shows that *PPARγ* mRNA and protein are found in about half of FTC but not in PTC and multinodular hyperplasias *(55)*. In another study in a mouse model of FTC, pathways mediated by *PPARγ* are repressed, whereas other antiapoptotic molecules, such as TGF-β and nuclear factor κB, are upregulated *(56)*. The alteration of *PPARγ* may serve not only as a tumor marker for diagnostic purposes but also as a promising target for cancer therapy.

Several other apoptotic molecules have been studied in thyroid cancer. A study by Miyakawa et al. shows that the proapoptotic molecule, phosphorylated Akt, is increased in PTC, and the increased Akt is accompanied by an elevated phosphorylated Bad *(57)*. Activation of Akt and Bad may contribute to the progression of PTC by stimulating cell proliferation and/or preventing apoptosis. Sunde et al. discovered a novel thyroid-specific gene: thyroid cancer 1 (TC-1; *58*). The role of TC-1 in the development of thyroid cancer is demonstrated by the overexpression of TC-1 in normal thyroid cells. The normal thyroid cells with TC-1 display increased proliferation rates and anchorage-independent growth in soft agar, whereas apoptosis rates are decreased. Ito et al. revealed that survivin, an inhibitor of apoptosis, frequently expresses in FTC, PTC, and ATC, and its expression is significantly increased in advanced stages of thyroid cancers *(59)*. Chung et al. showed that the expression of Gadd45 γ—a protein involved in DNA replication, cell cycle control, and apoptosis—is reduced in ATC. Furthermore, its reexpression can result in apoptosis and significant inhibition of cell proliferation *(60)*. The pathway of these relatively new molecules is not quite clear; further studies need to confirm the alterations found.

POTENTIAL APOPTOTIC INTERVENTION FOR THYROID CANCER

Therapies designed to stimulate apoptosis in target cells increasingly have a central role in the prevention and treatment of human cancer, including thyroid cancer. For several decades, the classical view of an anticancer drug mechanism has relied on the specific interaction of a drug with its target; such an interaction can lead to tumor cell death via its direct and injurious effect on the proliferating tumor cells. However, emerging data based on an increasing understanding of the cell cycle control and apoptosis process indicate that, rather than being intrinsically toxic, many anticancer drugs merely stimulate tumor cells to self-destruction via apoptosis. Studies have demonstrated that most, if not all, of currently available anticancer drugs (including those that target DNA replication, DNA integrity, and cytokines) induce apoptosis in thyroid cancer cells. For example, paclitaxel and manumycin are now known to induce apoptosis in ATC via stimulating *p21* expression *(61)*. Lovastin induces apoptosis of ATC by inhibiting protein geranylation of the Rho family *(62)*. UCN-01, a selective protein kinase inhibitor, can significantly induce apoptosis of various types of thyroid cancer cells, probably by inhibiting the expression of Bcl-2, as the overexpression of Bcl-2 can block the UNC-01–activated cell death pathway *(63)*. Some extracts from traditional Chinese herb medicines have also shown a strong antiproliferative effect via provoking apoptosis in MTC *(64)*. Some attempts to target apoptotic genes have also been made using the antisense approach. In an in vitro experiment, Kim et al. demonstrated that antisense Bcl-2 can significantly enhance chemotherapeutic efficacy in undifferentiated thyroid cancer cells *(65)*. However, this antisense approach may not be feasible in vivo without further modification of the oligonucleotides because they are difficult to deliver.

With the tremendous amount of knowledge gained about apoptosis, the challenge is how this information can be applied to kill tumor cells selectively while sparing normal cells. In this regard, some promising therapies for certain types of thyroid cancer cells have emerged, e.g., the application of TRAIL in the treatment of thyroid cancer. TRAIL can selectively kill thyroid tumor cells without affecting normal thyroid cells *(66)*; further study reveals that interferon γ can sensitize TRAIL-mediated apoptosis in thyroid cancer cells via upregulation of Bak *(39)*. *PPAR*γ ligands also appear to be an effective class of therapeutic agents for thyroid cancer. Various *PPAR*γ ligands, including troglitazone, 15-deoxy-12,14-prostaglandin J2, and BRL 49653, have been tested for successful inhibition of thyroid cancer cells by inducing apoptosis *(67–70)*. It seems that normal thyroid cells will not be significantly targeted by *PPAR*γ because much more is expressed in thyroid cancer cells than in their adjacent normal thyroid cells *(67)*.

CONCLUSIONS

A number of molecules determine whether a cell will die or arrest its growth. As discussed above, apoptosis in thyroid cancer is a multifactor and multistep process. Although the role of Fas/FasL, Bcl-2 family members, *p53*, and some other apoptotic molecules have been demonstrated in thyroid cancer, our understanding of the interaction between these molecules is still very limited. The crosstalk that occurs between many upstream signals and downstream effectors presents a considerable challenge to the ongoing study of apoptosis in thyroid cancer. However, these complexities should also provide many opportunities for rewarding molecule exposure and the discovery of novel therapeutic agents.

REFERENCES

1. Hundahl SA, Fleming ID, Fremgen AM, Menck HR. A National Cancer Data Base report on 53,856 cases of thyroid carcinoma treated in the U.S., 1985-1995. Cancer 1998; 83:2638–2648.
2. Ron E, Lubin JH, Shore RE, et al. Thyroid cancer after exposure to external radiation: a pooled analysis of seven studies. Rad Res 1995; 141:259–277.
3. Frich L, Akslen LA, Glattre E. Increased risk of thyroid cancer among Norwegian women married to fishery workers—a retrospective cohort study. Br J Cancer 1997; 76:385–389.
4. Kanno J, Onodera H, Furuta K, Maekawa A, Kasuga T, Hayashi Y. Tumor-promoting effects of both iodine deficiency and iodine excess in the rat thyroid. Toxicol Pathol 1992; 20:226–235.
5. Kanno J, Matsuoka C, Furuta K, Onodera H, Miyajima H, Maekawa A, Hayashi Y. Tumor promoting effect of goitrogens on the rat thyroid. Toxicol Pathol 1990; 18:239–246.
6. Correa P, Chen VW. Endocrine gland cancer. Cancer 1995; 75(Suppl 1): 338–352.
7. Ron E, Kleinerman RA, Boice JD, et al. A population-based case-control study of thyroid cancer. J Natl Cancer Inst 1987; 79:1–12.
8. Nishimura N, Yonemoto J, Miyabara Y, Sato M, Tohyama C. Rat thyroid hyperplasia induced by gestational and lactational exposure to 2,3,7,8-tetrachlorodibenzo-p-dioxin. Endocrinology 2003; 144: 2075–2083.
9. Kung TM, Ng WL, Gibson JB. Volcanoes and carcinoma of the thyroid: a possible association. Arch Environ Health. 1981; 36:265–267.
10. Gorson D Familial papillary carcinoma of the thyroid. Thyroid 1992; 2:131–132.
11. Plail RO, Bussey HJ, Glazer G, Thomson JP. Adenomatous polyposis: an association with carcinoma of the thyroid. Br J Surg 1987; 74: 377–380.
12. Del Terra E, Francesconi A, Meli A, Ambesi-Impiombato FS. Radiation-dependent apoptosis on cultured thyroid cells. Physica Medica 2001; 17(Suppl 1):261–263.
13. Weihrauch M, Bader M, Lehnert G, Wittekind C, Tannapfel A, Wrbitzky R. Carcinogen-specific mutation pattern in the p53 tumour suppressor gene in UV radiation-induced basal cell carcinoma. Intl Arch Occup Environ Health 2002; 75:272–276.
14. Feldkamp J, Pascher E, Perniok A, Scherbaum WA. Fas-mediated apoptosis is inhibited by TSH and iodine in moderate concentrations in primary human thyrocytes in vitro. Horm Metab Res 1999; 31: 355–358.
15. Chen GG, Liu ZM, Vlantis AC, Tse GM, Leung BC, van Hasselt CA. Heme oxygenase-1 protects against apoptosis induced by tumor necrosis factor-alpha and cycloheximide in papillary thyroid carcinoma cells. J Cell Biochem 2004; 92:1246–1256.
16. Christoph H, Marion L, Alexandra B., et al. Differential mechanisms of neuroprotection by 17 beta-estradiol in apoptotic versus necrotic neurodegeneration. J Neurosci 2001; 21:2600–2609.
17. Wang TTY, Phang JM. Effects of estrogen on apoptotic pathways in human breast cancer cell line MCF-7. Cancer Res 1995; 55:2487–2489.
18. Bu SZ, Yin DL, Ren HX, et al. Progesterone induces apoptosis and up-regulation of p53 expression in human ovarian carcinoma cell lines. Cancer 1997; 79:1944–1950.
19. Manole D, Schildknecht B, Gosnell B, et al. Estrogen promotes growth of human thyroid tumor cells by different molecular mechanisms. J Clin Endocrinol Metab 2001; 86:1072–1077.
20. Davis JW II, Lauer FT, Burdick AD, Hudson LG, Burchiel SW. Prevention of apoptosis by 2,3,7,8-tetrachlorodibenzo-p-dioxin (TCDD) in the MCF-10A cell line: correlation with increased transforming growth factor alpha production. Cancer Res 2001; 61: 3314–3320.
21. Schrenk D, Schmitz HJ, Bohnenberger S, Wagner B, Worner W. Tumor promoters as inhibitors of apoptosis in rat hepatocytes. Toxicol Lett 2004; 149:43–50.
22. Weiss H, Jacobasch KH, Haensch W, Streller B, Hieke B. Significance of apoptosis in the process of tumorigenesis in colorectal mucosa and adenomas in FAP patients. Anal Cell Pathol 1997; 14:61–73.
23. Strater J, Koretz K, Gunthert AR, Moller P. In situ detection of enterocytic apoptosis in normal colonic mucosa and in familial adenomatous polyposis. Gut 1995; 37:819–825.
24. Evan GI, Vousden KH. Proliferation, cell cycle and apoptosis in cancer. Nature 2001; 411:342–348.
25. Hanahan D, Weinberg RA. The hallmarks of cancer. Cell 2000; 100: 57–70.

26. Shi Y. Mechanisms of caspase activation and inhibition during apoptosis. Molecular Cell 2002; 9:459–470.
27. Bratton SB, MacFarlane M, Cain K, Cohen GM. Protein complexes activate distinct caspase cascades in death receptor and stress-induced apoptosis. Exp Cell Res 2000; 256:27–33.
28. Gupta S. Molecular signaling in death receptor and mitochondrial pathways of apoptosis. Intl J Oncol 2003; 22:15–20.
29. Schultz DR, Harrington WJ Jr. Apoptosis: programmed cell death at a molecular level. Sem Arthritis Rheum 2003; 32:345–369.
30. Sprick MR, Walczak H. The interplay between the Bcl-2 family and death receptor-mediated apoptosis. Biochim Biophys Acta 2004; 1644:125–132.
31. Roy S, Nicholson DW. Cross-talk in cell death signaling. J Exp Med 2000; 192:F21–F25.
32. Slee EA, Adrain C, Martin SJ. Serial killers: ordering caspase activation events in apoptosis. Cell Death Differ 1999; 6:1067–1074.
33. Basolo F, Pollina L, Fontanini G, Fiore L, Pacini F, Baldanzi A. Apoptosis and proliferation in thyroid carcinoma: correlation with bcl-2 and p53 protein expression. Br J Cancer 1997; 75:537–541.
34. Arscott PL, Stokes T, Myc A, Giordano TJ, Thompson NW, Baker JR Jr. Fas (CD95) expression is up-regulated on papillary thyroid carcinoma. J Clin Endocrinol Metab 1999; 84:4246–4252.
35. Mitsiades N, Poulaki V, Tseleni-Balafouta S, Koutras DA, Stamenkovic I. Thyroid carcinoma cells are resistant to FAS-mediated apoptosis but sensitive tumor necrosis factor-related apoptosis-inducing ligand. Cancer Res 2000; 60:4122–4129.
36. Mitsiades N, Poulaki V, Mastorakos G, et al. Fas ligand expression in thyroid carcinomas: a potential mechanism of immune evasion. J Clin Endocrinol Metab 1999; 84:2924–2932.
37. Mezosi E, Yamazaki H, Bretz JD, et al. Aberrant apoptosis in thyroid epithelial cells from goiter nodules. J Clin Endocrinol Metab 2002; 87:4264–4272.
38. Andrikoula M, Vartholomatos G, Tsangaris GT, Bafa M, Tzortzatou-Stathopoulou F, Tsatsoulis A. Fas and Bcl-2 protein expression in thyrocytes of patients with nodular goiter. Eur J Endocrinol 2001; 145:403–407.
39. Wang SH, Mezosi E, Wolf JM, et al. IFNgamma sensitization to TRAIL-induced apoptosis in human thyroid carcinoma cells by upregulating Bak expression. Oncogene 2004; 23:928–935.
40. Basolo F, Fiore L, Baldanzi A, et al. Suppression of Fas expression and down-regulation of Fas ligand in highly aggressive human thyroid carcinoma. Lab Investig 2000; 80:1413–1419.
41. Matiba B, Mariani SM, Krammer PH. The CD95 system and the death of a lymphocyte. Sem Immunol 1997; 9:59–68.
42. Walker PR, Saas P, Dietrich PY. Role of Fas ligand (CD95L) in immune escape: the tumor cell strikes back. J Immunol 1997; 158:4521–4524.
43. Hahne M, Rimoldi D, Schroter M, Romero P, Schreier M, French LE, et al. Melanoma cell expression of Fas(Apo-1/CD95) ligand: implications for tumor immune escape. Science 1996; 274: 1363–1366.
44. Stassi G, Todaro M, Zerilli M, et al. Thyroid cancer resistance to chemotherapeutic drugs via autocrine production of interleukin-4 and interleukin-10. Cancer Res 2003; 63:6784–6790.
45. Vella V, Mineo R, Frasca F, Mazzon E, Pandini G, Vigneri R, Belfiore A. Interleukin-4 stimulates papillary thyroid cancer cell survival: implications in patients with thyroid cancer and concomitant Graves' disease. J Clin Endocrinol Metab 2004; 89:2880–2889.
46. Pearson AS, Spitz FR, Swisher SG, Kataoka M, Sarkiss MG, Meyn RE, et al. Up-regulation of the proapoptotic mediators Bax and Bak after adenovirus-mediated p53 gene transfer in lung cancer cells. Clin Cancer Res 2000; 6:887–890.
47. Pohl U, Wagenknecht B, Naumann U, Weller M. p53 enhances BAK and CD95 expression in human malignant glioma cells but does not enhance CD95L-induced apoptosis. Cell Physiol Biochem 1999; 9:29–37.
48. Fagin JA, Matsuo K, Karmakar A, Chen DL, Tang SH, Koeffler HP. High prevalence of mutations of the p53 gene in poorly differentiated human thyroid carcinomas. J Clin Investig 1993; 91:179–184.
49. Wright PA, Lemoine NR, Goretzki PE, Wyllie FS, Bond J, Hughes C, et al. Mutation of the p53 gene in a differentiated human thyroid carcinoma cell line, but not in primary thyroid tumours. Oncogene 1991; 6:1693–1697.
50. Fagin JA. Minireview: branded from the start-distinct oncogenic initiating events may determine tumor fate in the thyroid. Mol Endocrinol 2002; 16:903–911.
51. Moretti F, Farsetti A, Soddu S, et al. p53 re-expression inhibits proliferation and restores differentiation of human thyroid anaplastic carcinoma cells. Oncogene 1997; 14:729–740.
52. Frasca F, Vella V, Aloisi A, Mandarino A, Mazzon E, Vigneri R, Vigneri P. p73 tumor-suppressor activity is impaired in human thyroid cancer. Cancer Res 2003; 63:5829–5837.
53. Jiang M, Shappell SB, Hayward SW. Approaches to understanding the importance and clinical implications of peroxisome proliferator-activated receptor gamma (PPARgamma) signaling in prostate cancer. J Cell Biochem 2004; 91:513–527.
54. Chen GG, Lee JF, Wang SH, Chan UP. Ip PC, Lau WY. Apoptosis induced by activation of peroxisome-proliferator activated receptor-gamma is associated with Bcl-2 and NF-kappaB in human colon cancer. Life Sci 2002; 70:2631–2646.
55. Kroll TG, Sarraf P, Pecciarini L, et al. PAX8-PPARgamma-1 fusion oncogene in human thyroid carcinoma. Science 2000; 289:1357–1360.
56. Ying H, Suzuki H, Furumoto H, et al. Alterations in genomic profiles during tumor progression in a mouse model of follicular thyroid carcinoma. Carcinogenesis 2003; 24:1467–1479.
57. Miyakawa M, Tsushima T, Murakami H, Wakai K, Isozaki O, Takano K. Increased expression of phosphorylated p70S6 kinase and Akt in papillary thyroid cancer tissues. Endocrine J 2003; 50: 77–83.
58. Sunde M, McGrath KC, Young L, Matthews JM, Chua EL, Mackay JP. Death AK. TC-1 is a novel tumorigenic and natively disordered protein associated with thyroid cancer. Cancer Res 2004; 64: 2766–2773.
59. Ito Y, Yoshida H, Uruno T, et al. Expression is significantly linked to the dedifferentiation of thyroid carcinoma. Oncol Rep 2003; 10:1337–1340.
60. Chung HK, Yi YW, Jung NC, et al. Gadd45gamma expression is reduced in anaplastic thyroid cancer and its reexpression results in apoptosis. J. Clin Endocrinol Metab 2003; 88:3913–3920.
61. Yang HL, Pan JX, Sun L, Yeung SC. p21 Waf-1 (Cip-1) enhances apoptosis induced by manumycin and paclitaxel in anaplastic thyroid cancer cells. J Clin Endocrinol Metab 2003; 88:763–772.
62. Wang SH, Phelps E, Utsugi S, Baker JR Jr. Susceptibility of thyroid cancer cells to 7-hydroxystaurosporine-induced apoptosis correlates with Bcl-2 protein level. Thyroid 2001; 11:725–731.
63. Rinner B, Siegl V, Purstner P, et al. Activity of novel plant extracts against medullary thyroid carcinoma cells. Anticancer Res 2004; 24:495–500.
64. Poulaki V, Mitsiades CS, Kotoula V, et al. Regulation of Apo2L/tumor necrosis factor-related apoptosis-inducing ligand-induced apoptosis in thyroid carcinoma cells. Am J Pathol 2002; 161:643–654.
65. Kim R, Tanabe K, Uchida Y, Emi M, Toge T. Effect of Bcl-2 antisense oligonucleotide on drug-sensitivity in association with apoptosis in undifferentiated thyroid carcinoma. Intl J Mol Med 2003; 11: 799–804.
66. Ahmad M, Shi Y. TRAIL-induced apoptosis of thyroid cancer cells: potential for therapeutic intervention. Oncogene 2000; 19: 3363–3371.
67. Martelli ML, Iuliano R, Le Pera I, Sama I, Monaco C, Cammarota S, et al. Inhibitory effects of peroxisome poliferator-activated receptor gamma on thyroid carcinoma cell growth. J. Clin Endocrinol Metab 2002; 87:4728–4735.

68. Hayashi N, Nakamori S, Hiraoka N, Tsujie M, Xundi X, Takano T, et al. Antitumor effects of peroxisome proliferator activate receptor gamma ligands on anaplastic thyroid carcinoma. Intl J Oncol 2004; 24:89–95.
69. Chen SY, Lu FJ, Gau RJ, Yang ML, Huang TS. 15-Deoxy-delta12,14-prostaglandin J2 induces apoptosis of a thyroid papillary cancer cell line (CG3 cells) through increasing intracellular iron and oxidative stress. Anticancer Drugs 2002; 13:759–765.
70. Ohta K, Endo T, Haraguchi K, Hershman JM, Onaya T. Ligands for peroxisome proliferator-activated receptor gamma inhibit growth and induce apoptosis of human papillary thyroid carcinoma cells. J. Clin Endocrinol Metab 2001; 86:2170–2177.

7
Radiation-Induced Thyroid Cancer

James J. Figge, Timothy Jennings, Gregory Gerasimov, Nikolai Kartel, Dima Yarmolinsky, and Gennady Ermak

Radiation is one of the few accepted risk factors for thyroid cancer. Numerous studies have confirmed that the thyroid gland is one of the most radiation-sensitive human organs and that thyroid cancer is one of the most common radiogenic malignancies. Analysis of these studies is problematic, however, owing to difficulties in dose assessment, long-term follow-up of thousands of exposed subjects, definition and confirmation of pathological diagnoses, and differences in exposure modalities.

The first part of this chapter briefly outlines the nature and methods of the most significant studies to date and analyzes the data available to define the characteristics of the risks of radiation to the thyroid on subsequent development of thyroid cancer. The second part of the chapter presents an update on thyroid cancer in children exposed to fallout from the Chernobyl accident. Terminology used throughout the chapter is defined in Table 1.

PATHOLOGY

Knowledge of the pathology of radiation injury to the thyroid is essential to understanding the data from previous long-term follow-up studies. Thyroid glands exposed to external beam or ^{131}I radiation show a variety of histological abnormalities, most often multinodularity, distorting fibrosis, oncocytic change, and chronic inflammation (1–3). At higher (>1.5 Gy) doses, hyperplastic nodules may show cytologic atypia, which requires careful scrutiny to distinguish from malignancy (4). The incidence of benign adenomas in patients who received thyroid irradiation is also greatly increased over nonirradiated individuals, as demonstrated by virtually every study of such populations. Many studies failed to distinguish between benign nodules and carcinoma and are therefore excluded from this discussion.

As early as 1949, Quimby and Werner (5) suggested the possibility of a relationship between radiation and the subsequent development of thyroid carcinoma. Winship and Rosvoll (6) began collecting data on children with thyroid cancer in 1948, and their final report on 878 cases worldwide represents the largest to date. They found a history of radiation in 76% of 476 children with available records. Most received radiation for enlarged thymus or tonsils and adenoids, with an average thyroid dose of 0.512 Gy and an average interval to diagnosis of 8.5 yr; 72% of the cancers were of papillary type, and 18% were follicular. Cervical lymph node metastases were present in 74% of cases, with bilateral neck disease in 32%. Nearly 20% had pulmonary involvement, generally at presentation. The authors noted a sharp rise in thyroid cancer incidence in 1945, with the greatest number of cases presenting between 1946 and 1959. They attributed the subsequent decline to the curtailment of the practice of head and neck irradiation in children.

A number of additional studies (7,8) have confirmed that the majority of radiation-induced thyroid carcinomas are well-differentiated papillary adenocarcinomas that more frequently present with extrathyroidal spread and bilateral thyroid lobe involvement but with similar recurrence and mortality rates to tumors in nonirradiated patients. The patients are also younger at diagnosis, usually less than 35 yr of age, with an average interval to clinical presentation of 25–30 yr. The incidence of radiation-induced thyroid carcinoma appeared to increase from 1940 to at least 1970, but since the discontinuation of widespread use of X-ray therapy in infancy, this trend has decreased (9,10).

Clinically occult papillary microcarcinomas are generally not included in analysis of these data, but they are often detected by pathologists examining thyroids removed for larger benign nodules. Autopsy studies have demonstrated prevalence rates of papillary microcarcinoma (≤1 cm diameter) of up to 33.7% in general populations, and ethnic and/or geographic differences exist (11,12) (see Chapter 2). The prevalence of carcinoma is also dependent on the extent of surgery, the amount of resected thyroid tissue processed for histological assessment, and the absolute number of sections

From: *Thyroid Cancer: A Comprehensive Guide to Clinical Management*, 2/e
Edited by: L. Wartofsky and D. Van Nostrand © Humana Press Inc., Totowa, NJ

Table 1
Definition of Terminology

Term	Definition, Conversion Factors
Gray (Gy)	The Gy is the unit of absorbed dose, the amount of energy imparted by ionizing radiation to a unit mass of tissue; 1 Gy corresponds to 1 joule per kg. 1 Gy = 100 rad
Sievert (Sv)	The sievert is the unit of effective dose. When exposure is to mixed radiation (e.g., α and γ), their contribution is weighted to give an equivalent dose. A further weighting is made to account for different susceptibilities of various tissues. 1 Sv = 100 rem
Becquerel (Bq)	The Bq is the unit of activity, the number of radioactive transformations taking place per second. 1 curie = 3.7×10^{10} Bq
Relative risk (RR)	The risk of developing cancer in a radiation-exposed subject compared to the risk in an unexposed individual.
Excess relative risk (ERR)	RR = ERR + 1. The ERR is usually specified per Gy. For example, if the ERR is 2.0 per Gy, then the RR would be 3.0 for a 1-Gy exposure, and 5.0 for a 2-Gy exposure.
Excess absolute risk (EAR)	Usually expressed per 10,000 person-years per Gy. Defines the increase in the absolute risk of developing cancer as a result of radiation exposure.

examined by the pathologist *(13)*. Care is required in evaluating studies with regard to these issues.

Although radiation exposure has a role in the development of clinical papillary carcinoma, the extent of such risk in a given population cannot always be ascertained, as the number of people at risk may be unknown. Currently, it is estimated that 9% of thyroid cancers may be attributable to radiation *(14)*. Because radiation-induced thyroid carcinomas rarely include the more aggressive anaplastic and medullary types, its fatality rate is between 3% and 9% *(15)*.

A small but significant number of patients with anaplastic thyroid carcinoma have had a history of prior exposure to external irradiation or ^{131}I. Such therapy for differentiated thyroid cancer might theoretically induce transformation to an anaplastic carcinoma, but because most cases of anaplastic carcinoma show areas of differentiated tumor, this phenomenon may be an aspect of the natural history of these tumors and may therefore not be a consequence of radiation *(16)*.

PRIOR STUDIES

External Radiation

Introduction

From 1920 to 1960, γ radiation was commonly used to treat a variety of benign conditions, including several head, neck, and upper thoracic sites, which resulted in thyroid gland exposure. In 1950, Duffy and Fitzgerald *(17)* found that 9 of 28 children with thyroid cancer had received prior irradiation of the thymus as infants. Subsequent reports *(18,19)* confirmed that the risk of thyroid cancer in children exposed to high-dose radiation and the use of radiation to treat benign disease slowly diminished. Also, the risk of radiation has been analyzed in patients treated for malignant disease, in occupational settings, and in situations of inadvertent exposure.

Atomic Bomb Survivors

A fixed cohort of nearly 80,000 survivors of the atomic bomb exposures in Hiroshima and Nagasaki, Japan, has been followed since 1958 by the Atomic Bomb Casualty Commission and its successor, the Radiation Effects Research Foundation. In a comprehensive report *(20)* on the incidence and risk estimates for solid tumors diagnosed between 1958 and 1987, the thyroid had one of the highest solid tumor risk estimates in the Life Span Study cohort, with occult tumors excluded. The mean estimated thyroid dose was 0.264 Sv, and a strong linear dose-response was demonstrated. Persons exposed when younger than age 10 yr had an excess relative risk (ERR) of 9.46, over three times greater than those in their second decade (see Table 2). Although earlier studies *(21)* suggested otherwise, this report *(20)* showed that those individuals over the age of 20 yr at the time of the blast had no excess of thyroid cancer. Mortality data from the Life Span Study contributed little support for an increased risk of thyroid cancer, because the disease causes so few deaths *(22)*.

Cervical Tuberculous Adenitis

Tisell and colleagues *(23)* evaluated 444 patients treated with X-rays for cervical tuberculous lymphadenitis between 1913 and 1951 in Goteborg, Sweden. The mean age at irradiation was 19 yr, with almost 50% of patients between 15 and 24 yr of age. The calculated absorbed dose to the thyroid ranged from 0.40 to 50.90 Gy (median: 5.2 Gy; mean: 7.2 Gy); 25 thyroid cancers were found, all but one palpable, with a mean observation time of 43 yr. The mean and median latency periods were 40 yr to diagnosis. A positive correlation was shown between absorbed dose and the probability of developing carcinoma, even after doses of more than 20 Gy. No significant correlation between age at irradiation and the risk of developing cancer was detected.

Table 2
Major Cohort Studies of External Radiation in Childhood

Study (Ref.)	No. Exposed	Age at Exposure	Thyroid Dose	Follow-up	ERR/Gy 95% CI
Atomic bomb (20)	79,972	17.6 yr	0.264 Sv	1,950,567 PY	1.15/Sv (0.5–2.1)
Age < 10					9.46/Sv (4.1–19)
Hemangioma (25)	14,351	6 mo	0.26 Gy	406,355 PY	4.92/Gy
Hemangioma (26)	11,807	5 mo	0.12 Gy	370,517 PY	7.5/Gy (0.4–18)
Tonsils and adenoids (27)	4,296	4.4 yr	0.59 Gy	33 yr	3.0/Gy (1–40)
Thymus (33)	2,657	5 wk	1.36 Gy	37.1 yr	9.0/Gy (4.2–22)
Tinea (34)	10,834	7.4 yr	0.09 Gy	30.2 yr	30/Gy

ERR/Gy, excess relative risk per gray; CI, confidence interval; PY, person-years.

Cutaneous Hemangioma

Furst and coworkers (24) conducted follow-up with 18,030 patients with skin hemangioma who were treated with external beam radiation between 1920 and 1959 at the Karolinska Hospital. At the time of therapy, 82% were less than 1 yr of age (median age: 6 mo). Treatment methods varied, but the relative risk (RR) of thyroid cancer was only slightly increased (1.18) in the group treated with radium-226 or orthovoltage X-rays. In patients receiving contact X-rays or no radiation, no increased risk was noted. An estimation of absorbed thyroid doses was not made.

A similar analysis (25) of a cohort of 14,351 infants less than 18 mo of age (mean: 6 mo) irradiated for hemangioma during the period of 1920–1959 in Stockholm covered 406,355 person-years at risk, with a mean follow-up of 39 yr. The mean absorbed thyroid dose was 0.26 Gy. The Swedish Cancer Registry documented 17 thyroid cancers. Excess cancers began 19 yr after radiation and persisted for at least 40 yr following radiation therapy (see Table 2).

Another study (26) involved 11,807 infants treated with radium-226 between 1930 and 1965 in Goteborg, Sweden at a median age of 5 mo. The mean absorbed thyroid dose was 0.12 Gy. Follow-up through the Swedish Cancer Registry yielded 15 thyroid cancers (ERR = 7.5/Gy; see Table 2).

Tonsils/Adenoids

Extensive data has been reported by Schneider and colleagues (27–30) from long-term follow-up studies of more than 5300 subjects who received external radiation for various benign head and neck abnormalities, principally for enlarged tonsils and adenoids, during 1939–1962. In analyzing 4296 of these individuals with an average age at first exposure of 4.4 yr and an average thyroid dose of 0.59 Gy, they found that ERR was 3/Gy for thyroid cancer (see Table 2). With a mean follow-up of 33 yr, the majority of cases occurred in the interval between 20 and 40 yr after radiation therapy, peaking at 25–29 yr, with a significant decline in risk with increasing age at exposure (27). Additional data from this source includes information on the effect of screening, as well as characteristics of the secondary thyroid cancers. The authors documented recurrent malignancy in 13.5% of the 296 patients with thyroid cancer, nearly all within 10 yr after primary tumor resection. Significant risk factors for recurrence were the size of the primary lesion, number of lobes involved, histological type, vessel invasion, and lymph node metastasis (28). Longer-term follow-up of 118 cases occurring before intensive screening showed recurrences in 23.7% of this total; 39% of cancers in children recurred vs 15.6% in adults. This established an inverse relationship between the frequency of recurrence and the patient's age at surgery (also between the frequency of recurrence and latency period between radiation and surgery). Age at radiation and treatment dose were not related to recurrences (29). Another aspect explored in this group was the possibility of a radiation sensitivity within the population at risk. Patients with secondary salivary gland and/or neural tumors of the head and neck region had a significantly increased frequency of thyroid cancer compared to patients with neither of these tumors, suggesting that additional factors, such as radiation sensitivity, may account for this increased risk (30).

Acne

Paloyan and Lawrence (31) found that 20 of 224 patients referred for thyroidectomy for solitary nodules had received antecedent radiation for the treatment of acne vulgaris. Of the 20 patients, 12 had thyroid cancer 9–41 yr after radiation therapy. Complete records were unavailable, and no statistical analysis was reported. To date, no comprehensive survey of such patients has been performed.

Thymus

Analysis of radiotherapy's effect for thymic enlargement in infancy on subsequent neoplastic disease was initiated by Hempelmann and colleagues in Rochester, New York in the 1950s. They established that the risk of cancer was proportional to the thyroid dose and raised concern that persons of Jewish ancestry might be at greater risk (32). Extended

37-yr average follow-up (33) of 2657 of these exposed infants and 4833 of their siblings via mail surveys through 1986 confirmed a linear dose–response relationship, with an ERR of 9/Gy (see Table 2). The median age at radiation therapy was 5 wk, and 95% were under 34 wk of age. Estimated thyroid doses ranged from 0.03 to over 10 Gy, with a mean of 1.36 and median of only 0.3 Gy. None of the dose fractionation variables examined (dose per fraction, number of fractions, and interval between fractions) was significant in modifying risk.

Tinea Capitis

A major long-term study (34) of 10,834 subjects who received X-ray therapy for tinea capitis between 1948 and 1960 in Israel were compared with the effects with a similar number of nonirradiated individuals and 5392 nonirradiated siblings. All irradiated subjects were under 16 yr old at the time of treatment, with a mean age of 7.4 yr. The mean thyroid dose was 0.093 Gy, with the dose highly inversely correlated with age at exposure owing to the proximity of the thyroid to the X-ray fields in smaller children. The Israel Cancer Registry documented 98 thyroid cancers, showing a mean interval of 17.1 yr from radiation therapy to diagnosis. A much higher excess risk of thyroid cancer was found than in other studies (Table 2), possibly relating to the underestimation of thyroid doses as a result of patient movement. An increased risk in Jewish patients may also have been a factor.

A similar study of 2215 children irradiated for tinea capitis in New York found no thyroid cancers through a mailed questionnaire after an average 20.5-yr follow-up (35). However, there were less than 300 females, and the expected number of thyroid cancers would have been only 2.9 (36). The mean age at treatment was 7.9 yr; the estimated thyroid dose was 0.06 Gy (35).

Previous Malignancy

Tucker and colleagues (37) reported on the experience of the Late Effects Study Group, which followed a roster of 9170 patients surviving any type of malignancy in childhood for over 2 yr. The period of risk extended to death, the last follow-up, or the date of developing any form of second malignancy, whether of the thyroid or not. The mean age at initial tumor diagnosis was 7 yr, and 45% of all patients were less than 5 yr old. The duration of follow-up beginning 2 yr after initial diagnosis was 2–48 yr (mean: 5.5 yr), with an aggregate follow-up of 50,609 person-years. The radiation dose to the thyroid ranged from 0 to 76 Gy (mean: 12.5; median: 3.6 Gy). The authors documented 23 secondary thyroid cancers through their 13 centers, yielding a 53-fold increased risk over matched controls, and a significantly increased RR was shown among those with early age at initial cancer diagnosis. All the thyroid cancer patients had received at least 1 Gy to the thyroid.

A study of 1787 patients treated for Hodgkin's disease (38) at Stanford University between 1961 and 1989 included 1677 patients who had thyroid radiation, most receiving 44 Gy. The mean age at time of treatment was 28 yr (range: 2–82 yr). After an average follow-up of 9.9 yr, they found six thyroid cancers 9–19 (median: 13) yr after therapy began for a RR of 15.6 times expected. The age of these six patients ranged from 5 to 32 yr at the time of exposure.

Additional studies (39–43) have assessed the risk of radiation therapy for malignancies on the subsequent occurrence of thyroid and other second cancers. These include investigations of large populations of women treated for uterine cervical cancer and males with testicular malignancy; no increased risk of secondary thyroid cancer has been demonstrated, but one such study in women found a slight insignificant excess (RR =1.1; 39). In this study, as well as the others, the thyroid gland was outside the field of direct radiation, and the estimated average thyroid dose was 0.15 Gy.

Occupational Exposure

Occupational exposure to low-dose radiation has been analyzed in large studies of workers in the nuclear industry. In a report on mortality among radiation workers in the United Kingdom, thyroid cancer was the only malignancy for which the standardized mortality ratio was raised, but the ERR was low (1.05/Sv; 44). A similar study of employees of the UK Atomic Energy Authority demonstrated a slight, but not significant, increase in mortality from thyroid cancer (45). Additional mortality studies in the United States (46–48) failed to demonstrate excess thyroid cancer deaths among nuclear materials workers. To date, no analysis of cancer incidence has been performed in such a cohort.

A study of cancer incidence among medical diagnostic X-ray workers in China (49) found 7 thyroid cancers in 27,011 individuals employed between 1950 and 1980, with nearly 700,000 person-years of observation. Thyroid cancers were increased among workers employed for 10 yr or more and among those who began such work before 1960. No dosimetry measurements were obtained. A study of more than 143,000 members of the American Registry of Radiologic Technologists (50) from 1926 to 1982, who were evaluated through questionnaires, revealed a total of 220 self-reported thyroid cancers vs an expected number of approx 100 cases. However, these data are preliminary however, and do not include confirmation of the diagnoses, nor are thyroid dose estimates yet available.

Mortality analysis by review of death certificates of British radiologists who died between 1897 and 1976 failed to demonstrate an excess of thyroid cancers (51). Similar mortality data from North American radiologists did not demonstrate any excess deaths from thyroid cancer compared to other specialty physicians during 1920–1969 (52).

Prenatal Exposure

The cancer risk of prenatal irradiation has been analyzed in atomic bomb survivors and from diagnostic imaging. Although some studies have found evidence of an increased incidence of childhood cancer following prenatal abdominal X-ray exposure, thyroid cancer rates have never been shown to increase. Many of these reports have been based on mortality data *(53,54)*, which would not be expected to show an increase for thyroid cancer, but several have utilized incidence data as well *(55–57)*. Yet, these studies are confounded by a number of factors, including difficulties in dose estimation and maternal issues that may affect the risk of subsequent malignancy, such as prenatal care, maternal age, sibship position, and prior miscarriage. Follow-up by death records and tumor registries of 1630 of the 2802 individuals surviving *in utero* exposure from the Japanese atomic bombs disclosed only one thyroid cancer until 1984 *(58)*.

Internal Irradiation

Introduction

Human exposure to ^{131}I has been analyzed in patients treated for hyperthyroidism and at smaller doses (<1 mCi) for diagnostic thyroid scans. Radioactive fallout containing ^{131}I and short-lived radioiodines has also resulted in human thyroid irradiation. Although it is believed that ^{131}I is considerably less effective in producing thyroid abnormalities than X-radiation, one of the best controlled animal studies suggests that the carcinogenic effects are similar *(59)*. Shorter-lived radioisotopes of iodine are more destructive because of the greater penetration of their β rays and faster dose rate, but their ability to produce thyroid cancer relative to X-rays is uncertain.

Populations Near Nuclear Facilities

Research from the United States and United Kingdom *(60,61)* have investigated the mortality from cancer among people residing near nuclear power plants. Although such analyses are problematic owing to relocation of potentially exposed people, case ascertainment in different areas, information on individual radiation exposures, and various social issues, an increase in thyroid cancer deaths has not yet been reported. The Chernobyl accident is considered separately below.

HANFORD NUCLEAR SITE

In 1986, it was revealed that the Hanford Atomic Products Operations in Richland, Washington had released ^{131}I into the environment over a period of years, the greatest during 1944–1947. The Hanford Thyroid Disease Study *(62)* reported that the thyroid glands of 3441 people born in the vicinity of the Hanford plant between 1940 and 1946 had been thoroughly examined and thyroid dose reconstruction calculations had been performed. The final Hanford report *(62)*, released in 2002, failed to demonstrate an increased risk of thyroid cancer from exposure to Hanford's ^{131}I atmospheric releases. A review of the study by the National Research Council of the National Academy of Sciences *(63)* concluded that the imprecision of dose estimates weakened the statistical power of the study. Therefore, although the study did not detect a dose–response relationship, the data are not strong enough to determine whether there is a small incremental risk associated with ^{131}I exposure.

Diagnostic ^{131}I

In a multicenter cohort *(64)* study of 35,074 patients, 50 thyroid cancers were observed through the Swedish Cancer Registry vs an expected number of 39.4 in the general population. This incidence was not significantly greater than expected and may have been influenced by the prevalence of underlying thyroid disease in this selected population. The mean age at first ^{131}I examination was about 44 yr, with a mean total dose of 52 μCi and absorbed dose of 0.5 Gy. The mean follow-up was 20 yr, with 527,056 person-years at risk, excluding the first 5 yr after examination.

Therapeutic ^{131}I

Several studies of the effect of ^{131}I therapy for hyperthyroidism on subsequent malignancy have been performed. The largest of these *(65)* from the Cooperative Thyrotoxicosis Therapy Follow-up Study evaluated 35,593 patients, including 23,020 treated with ^{131}I. An elevated risk of thyroid cancer mortality following ^{131}I treatment was documented *(65)*; however, in absolute terms, the excess number of thyroid cancer deaths was small.

In a group of 4557 patients who received ^{131}I therapy for hyperthyroidism between 1951 and 1975 in Sweden, Holm *(66)* found no increased risk of thyroid cancer at doses estimated at 60–100 Gy. The mean age at treatment in this study was 56 yr and an average follow-up time of only 9.5 yr. An excess of thyroid cancer was found by Hoffman and associates *(67)* in a study of 1005 women treated with ^{131}I at the Mayo Clinic, but this excess was not statistically significant. In the study with the longest follow-up period (mean of 15 yr for 85% of recipient patients surviving), Holm and coworkers *(68)* found no increased risk of thyroid cancer in 3000 subjects treated for hyperthyroidism or cardiac disease, based on Swedish Cancer Registry data. Further mortality studies *(69,70)* in women receiving ^{131}I therapy for hyperthyroidism have shown no excess thyroid cancer deaths.

At the Cleveland Clinic *(71)*, 87 children and adolescents less than 18 yr of age when they received ^{131}I treatment for hyperthyroidism were evaluated. The mean ^{131}I dose was 9.75 mCi. No thyroid cancers were detected in these patients or their offspring; the mean follow-up period was 12.3 yr. Although ^{131}I in therapeutic doses may affect substantial cell killing and thereby mitigate any tumorigenic impact on the thyroid, long-term follow-up of exposed populations is needed to establish the effect of ^{131}I on subsequent thyroid cancer risk.

Fallout

SOUTHWESTERN UNITED STATES

People living in Nevada and Utah near the nuclear test site were exposed to radioactive fallout in the 1950s. At least 87 of the atmospheric tests between 1951 and 1958 resulted in offsite contamination (72). Thyroid dose estimates range from 0.46 (73) to 25 Gy or more (72) with added uncertainty regarding the amount of consumption of contaminated milk. It is not known whether short-lived isotopes of iodine were involved. Thyroid examination 12–18 yr later of 5179 children from the area of greatest exposure failed to disclose any increase in abnormalities (73). However, an interview survey of a 1951 cohort of 4125 Mormons in this area disclosed an excess incidence of thyroid cancers from 1958 to 1980 (72). This report was challenged by a subsequent mortality study of this region, which found no excess thyroid cancer deaths (74). Owing to the lack of accurate dose information in this setting, no definite conclusions regarding the risk of fallout exposure are possible.

CONTINENTAL UNITED STATES

The National Cancer Institute published estimates of ^{131}I thyroid doses in the Continental United States from fallout exposure related to the Nevada tests of the 1950s (75). An ecologic study of thyroid cancer death rates across the continental United States suggested an association with the thyroid dose received by children under 1 yr of age but failed to demonstrate increased risk from doses received at ages 1–15 yr (76). This result may relate to biases inherent in an ecologic study design, especially limitations introduced by studying a mobile population. Based on the National Cancer Institute data, a committee of the US National Academy of Sciences Institute of Medicine and National Research Council (77) estimated that an excess of 11,300 thyroid cancer cases could be attributed to exposure from the Nevada atomic bomb testing. It was further calculated that 45% of these cases had already occurred at the time of the report (1999).

MARSHALL ISLANDS

In 1954, after detonation of a 15-megaton nuclear device at Bikini, an unanticipated windshift caused exposure to fallout of at least 300 people on at least three of the atolls of the Marshall Islands (78–80). Late effects of this exposure have been predominantly thyroid abnormalities from absorbed radioiodines (^{131}I, ^{132}I, ^{133}I, and ^{135}I), as well as penetrating whole-body γ radiation. Significant uncertainty exists regarding thyroid doses; rough estimates average 3.12 Gy in all exposed children. Although a significant increase in nodular thyroid disease and hypothyroidism has been shown throughout the northern atolls, few cancers have been documented, and the estimated risk only 1.9 times greater than unexposed Marshallese. The risk of thyroid cancer was lower in children under 10 yr old at irradiation than in older populations, suggesting that dose estimates might be too low and that significant cell killing occurred in the younger group, which is reflected by their higher incidence of hypothyroidism. No thyroid cancer has been detected in the 10 individuals exposed *in utero*, but two developed benign nodules.

OTHER INCIDENCES

Wiklund and colleagues (81) studied a cohort of 2034 reindeer-breeding Lapps who had ingested large amounts of radioactive fallout products from nuclear weapons tests in the USSR. Exposure was through the lichen-reindeer-man food chain. From 1961 to 1984, an abundance in thyroid cancer incidence was not detected through the Swedish Cancer Registry.

^{131}I Risk in Children and Adolescents

Data in the literature regarding ^{131}I exposures in individuals under age 20 are sparse (82). Exposed populations were small, and only small numbers of thyroid cancer (23 cases) have been reported. Because of these factors, and the fact that some subjects were being investigated for thyroid diseases and others were administered ^{131}I doses in the cell-sterilization range, there is insufficient scientific information to make conclusions about the risk posed by ^{131}I in children and adolescents.

ANALYSIS OF RISK ASSESSMENT

Introduction

The association between radiation exposure and subsequent thyroid cancer has been conclusively demonstrated in epidemiological studies of children receiving head and neck irradiation and in survivors of the atomic bomb exposures in Japan. These studies indicate that radiation to the thyroid at high doses (>1 Gy) is highly linked with the subsequent development of cancer; the effect at lower doses is difficult to assess. Previous studies to assess doses of less than 0.10 Gy have produced no conclusive evidence of significant risk, but the requisite sample of greater than 100,000 exposed individuals and a similar control population have not been identified and analyzed.

Modifying Factors

Type and Duration of Exposure

External radiation is roughly four to five times as effective in causing thyroid cancer as is ^{131}I for each unit of absorbed dose (83), with other isotopes of iodine probably having an effect between that of ^{131}I and external radiation. Fractionation appears to provide an approx 30% reduction in the tumorigenic effect on the thyroid (84). However, X-ray technicians may have an increased risk over the general population (49,50).

Age at Irradiation

The thyroid is more radiosensitive in children than in adolescents and similarly more so in adolescents than in adults. Tucker and colleagues (37) found that individuals treated at an early age and also after lower doses of radiation appeared to have a higher RR of thyroid cancer, suggesting some increased sensitivity to radiation. Shore *(83)* estimated that the geometric mean ERR of thyroid cancer following irradiation in adulthood was about 10% of that in children. In the atomic bomb survivors, thyroid cancer in children had one of the highest ERR estimates among solid malignancies, whereas there was virtually no ERR for thyroid cancer in adults *(20)*. Large studies of women treated with radiation therapy for cervical cancer *(39,40)* are among the few in adults that have demonstrated an excess risk for thyroid cancer, but the confidence intervals were very wide in each study.

Sex

The absolute risk in females is two to four times that of males, but the ERR/Gy is about the same in both sexes. In a study by Lundell and associates *(25)*, most thyroid cancers occurred in females, but because of their higher background incidence rate, the sex-specific RR estimates were similar. Ron and associates *(34)* and Shore and coworkers *(85)* reported a greater excess number of cancers among females compared to males but no significant difference in the RR estimates. According to the report of the BEIR V Committee *(86)*, females are about three times as susceptible to radiogenic and nonradiogenic thyroid cancer as males.

Race

The risk appears to be greater in individuals of Jewish ancestry. Thyroid cancer risks varied among different Jewish subgroups in the Israeli Tinea study, with those born in Israel having one third the risk of those born in the Middle East or North Africa. Because the fathers of those born in Israel were themselves born in the Middle East or North Africa, environmental, rather than genetic, issues seem to be operative *(86)*.

Iodine Deficiency

Iodine deficiency is a possible promoting factor, as decreased thyroid hormone results in increased stimulation of the thyroid epithelium by thyrotropin (TSH). However, at least two human studies indicate the opposite effect, and thyroid cancer is associated with a high dietary iodine intake *(83)*. To date, only a few reports exist on iodine deficiency's influence on the risk of radiation-induced thyroid cancer *(87,88)*.

Parity

The observation that thyroid cancer among the exposed Marshall Island population occurred exclusively in multiparous women implied that parity might increase the chance of radiation-induced thyroid cancer. Shore and colleagues *(33)* demonstrated that older age at first childbirth significantly increased the risk of radiation-induced thyroid cancer in patients irradiated for thymic enlargement in infancy. A similar effect was found with older age at menarche. Other studies reveal that a history of miscarriage increased this risk, especially for younger women *(83)*.

Latency Period

The interval between initial exposure to radiation and detection of thyroid cancer varies widely among human clinical studies, from 5 to 50 yr after irradiation, largely reflecting the study's follow-up interval. The latency period may also increase with the individual's age at irradiation.

Effect of Screening

Based on an intensive screening program that started in 1974 in Chicago, Ron and colleagues *(89)* reported that adjusted incidence rates of secondary thyroid cancer were seven times greater during the screening period (1974–1979) than before.

Temporal Pattern

The temporal pattern of risk remains uncertain owing to the limited long-term follow-up data available. Schneider and colleagues *(27)* estimated that the increased risk of radiation-induced thyroid cancer probably lasts throughout life. Similarly, Thompson and colleagues *(20)* found no evidence for decreased risk with time after exposure. Ron and coworkers *(34)* reported a continued increase in risk over their entire study period of up to 38 yr. Shore and collaborators *(33)* indicated that the risk ratio declined over time but remained highly elevated at least 45 yr after irradiation. Excess risk began 5 yr after exposure.

Shore and coworkers *(33)* found that the ERR decreased during the entire study period, but that there was no significant change over time in excess absolute risk (EAR). Conversely, Ron and coworkers *(34)* demonstrated no significant change in ERR but a continuing increase in EAR during the entire study period (mean follow-up: 30 yr). These somewhat contradictory results highlight the need for even longer follow-up periods to clarify the temporal pattern.

Dose–Response Relationship

A strong dose–response relationship between radiation and incidence of thyroid cancer has been documented in Japanese atomic bomb survivors *(20)* and in studies of children and adolescents *(25,27,34,85)*. A pooled analysis *(84)* of seven major studies over a wide range of doses demonstrated an ERR of 7.7 per Gy (95% confidence limits: 2.1–28.7). For those exposed to radiation before age 15 yr, linearity best described the dose–response relationship, even at 0.10 Gy. Although risk estimates are generally those of the linear no-threshold model, at very high doses, these estimates might not be valid because of cell killing *(15)*. Regardless of possible threshold effects at high doses owing to cell killing, the greatest need is for an understanding of carcinogenic effects of low-dose radiation.

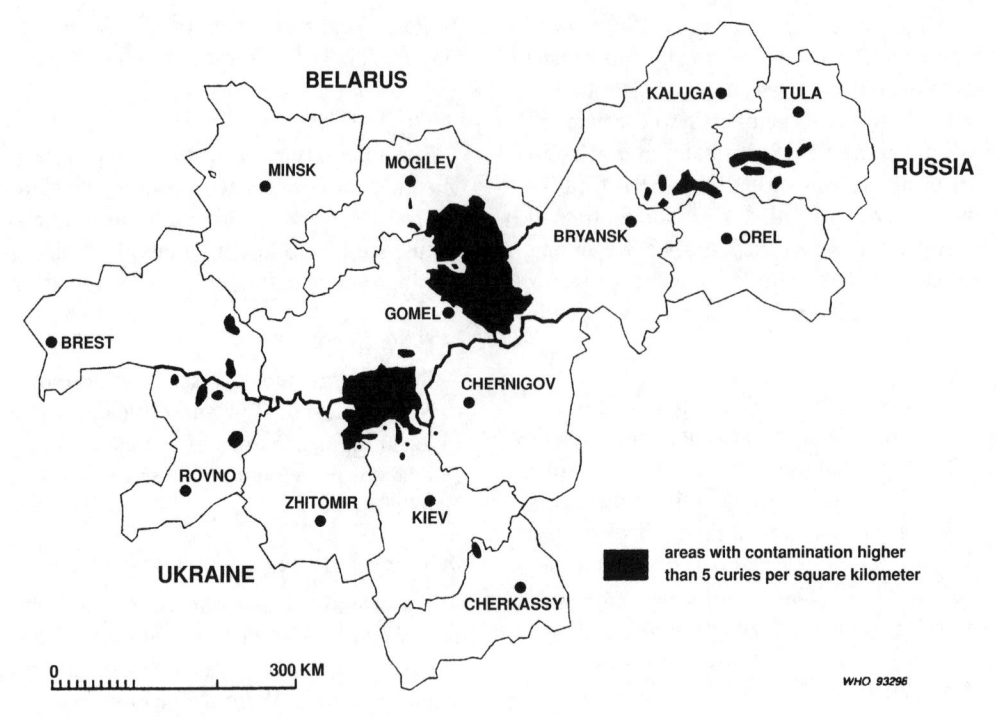

Fig. 1. Map showing the distribution of ^{137}Cs in Belarus, Ukraine, and Russia. (From ref. *100*, courtesy of the World Health Organization.)

THE CHERNOBYL ACCIDENT AND THYROID CANCER

Radioactivity Release

Without question, the Chernobyl accident was the worst technological disaster in the history of nuclear power generation. On April 26, 1986 at 1:23 AM, two explosions occurred (from steam and hydrogen) in reactor 4 of the Chernobyl nuclear power station, ejecting large amounts of radioactive material into the atmosphere. Subsequently, the graphite within the reactor ignited, and fuel elements in the core of the reactor melted, resulting in the release of volatile radioactive products over a 10-d period. The immediate cause of the accident was operator error, but the reactor design (which lacked a concrete containment vessel) has been implicated in the serious consequences of the accident. Initial estimates from officials in Moscow *(90)* indicated that approx 4% of the total activity of the core escaped into the atmosphere, resulting in the release of some 50 million Ci (2×10^{18} Bq). However, other researchers concluded that the release was much greater *(91,92)*. After 18 mo of study at the reactor site, Sich *(93,94)* estimated that the total release was actually in the range of 120–150 million Ci. Over 80 different isotopes were released *(95)*; the most abundant volatile isotopes were those of iodine (^{131}I, ^{132}I, ^{133}I, and ^{135}I), tellurium (^{132}Te), and cesium (^{134}Cs and ^{137}Cs). Some radioactive isotopes released during the accident naturally decayed to isotopes of iodine, e.g., ^{132}Te has a 3-d half-life and decays to ^{132}I.

Geographic Distribution of Volatile Radioactive Isotopes

The distribution of volatile radioactive isotopes to different geographic regions was governed by the prevailing meteorologic conditions *(96–99)*. The initial plume of volatile isotopes drifted over northern Ukraine and the Gomel oblast (region) of southern Belarus (Fig. 1). Contaminated air masses moved west and then northwest, sweeping across the Brest and Grodno oblasts of Belarus, causing the deposition of isotopes in Sweden on April 27. The wind direction changed to the northeast and to the east on April 29, and a large cloud of radioactivity drifted over southern Belarus and the southwestern corner of the Russian Federation. A substantial deposit of radioactivity in the Gomel and Mogilev oblasts of Belarus and the Bryansk oblast of Russia resulted from rainfall during April 28–30, which washed fallout from the cloud onto the ground. Another substantial deposit about 500 km from Chernobyl was formed when the same cloud drifted over the Kaluga-Tula-Orel oblasts of Russia. Rain during April 28–30 washed fallout to the ground in these regions. Winds changed to the south, then shifted to the southwest during the last few days of the accident, contaminating the Balkans and Alps. The World Health Organization (WHO) estimated that 4.9 million people lived in areas where ground surface contamination exceeded 1 Ci/km^2 *(100)*. About 2.3 million children lived in locations that were significantly contaminated at the time of the accident *(101)*.

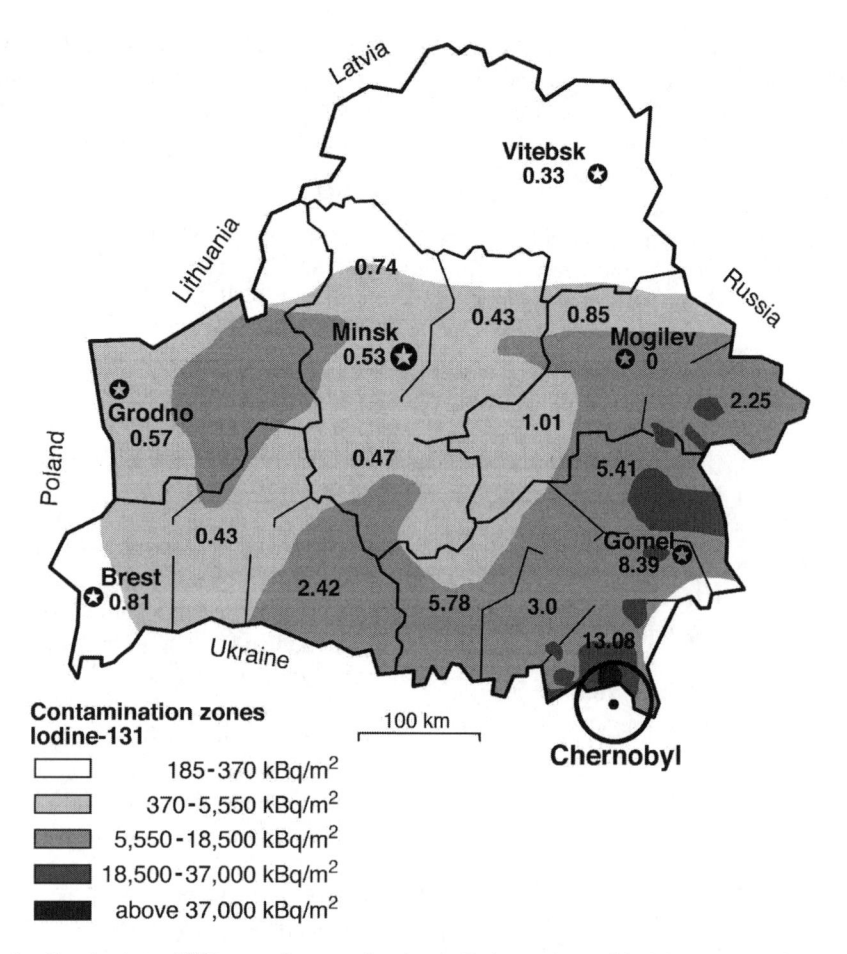

Fig. 2. Map showing the distribution of ^{131}I ground contamination in Belarus. Annual incidence rates of thyroid cancer in children in different geographic districts are shown per 100,000 children (based on data in ref. *135*). (From ref. *103* with permission of the American Association for the Advancement of Science.) (Color illustration is printed in insert following p. 198.)

Cesium-137 Release

Approximately 2 million Ci (8×10^{16} Bq) of ^{137}Cs was released, causing widespread soil contamination *(96,102)*. The distribution of ^{137}Cs, which has a half-life of approx 30 yr, has been carefully mapped *(89)* and was deposited in the following manner: Belarus, 33.5%; Russia, 24%; Ukraine, 20%; Sweden, 4.4%; and Finland, 4.3%. The areas with the highest ^{137}Cs contamination are shown in Fig. 1.

Radioiodine Release

The heaviest initial exposure to the population resulted from isotopes of iodine. According to recent studies, the release of ^{131}I (half-life: 8.05 d) was 40–50 million Ci (approx 1.7×10^{18} Bq), representing about 50–60% of the core inventory *(102–105)*. By comparison, the Three Mile Island accident released only 15–20 Ci of ^{131}I in the United States in 1979. During the first month following the Chernobyl accident, the major source of internal radiation exposure was ^{131}I, which was acquired by inhalation and ingestion of contaminated food. Deposits of ^{131}I on pasturelands and gardens in the rural agricultural areas surrounding the reactor introduced this radioisotope into the food chain. Ingestion of contaminated milk was the most important source of internal ^{131}I exposure in children *(97)*. Consumption of contaminated leafy vegetables was a secondary source of internal ^{131}I exposure.

Short-lived isotopes of iodine, such as ^{132}I (half-life: 2.3 h) and ^{133}I (half-life: 21 h) were also released from Chernobyl-4. Very few direct measurements of radioiodines were made in the initial days following the explosion. Therefore, data regarding ^{132}I and ^{133}I, which were important primarily in the first days after the accident, are scarce. Measurements made on April 28, 1986 in Warsaw, Poland, revealed that 28% of the radioactivity in the air was from short-lived iodine isotopes *(106)*. Thus, populations near the reactor location were exposed to ^{132}I and ^{133}I via inhalation for at least 1 or 2 d.

Following the accident, a limited number of measurements of the ground deposition density of ^{131}I were conducted in Belarus by the Belarus Institute of Nuclear Physics (Minsk; *107*). A map (Fig. 2) of the ^{131}I deposition in Belarus *(103)* shows some obvious differences in the distribution of

^{131}I compared with the pattern of ^{137}Cs ground contamination (Fig. 1). Particularly, the Gomel and Mogilev oblasts were both heavily contaminated with ^{137}Cs, with relatively less contamination in the Brest oblast. In contrast, the ^{131}I contamination was highest in the Gomel oblast, and lower but significant levels of deposition were seen in both the Mogilev and Brest oblasts. The contamination in the Brest oblast arose from the initial plume of radioactivity that passed over this area during the first day of the accident.

Reconstruction of Thyroid Doses

Ideally, to support careful epidemiological studies, accurate thyroid dose reconstructions are needed that separate out the contribution of (1) external radiation, (2) internal radiation owing to ^{131}I (from both inhalation and ingestion) and (3) internal radiation from the short-lived iodine isotopes (^{132}I and ^{133}I), because these three components may have differing potential to cause thyroid cancer. For example, ^{132}I and ^{133}I, which decay more rapidly than ^{131}I, deliver their radiation dose over a shorter time interval and could theoretically have a carcinogenic effect on thyroid tissue similar to that of X-rays (108). It has been suggested (101) that the majority of thyroid exposure (85%) was from internally concentrated ^{131}I derived from ingestion. Approximately 15% was estimated to have been derived from inhalation of short-lived iodine isotopes.

Following the accident, direct measurements of thyroid radioactive iodine content were made in Belarus, Russia, and the Ukraine. From these, the exposure to ^{131}I can be extrapolated, but the measurements were made too late to provide useful information on ^{132}I and ^{133}I. Furthermore, the direct measurements were made on only a small proportion of the affected population. Thyroid dose reconstruction is required to determine the exposure for the rest of the population. Many factors may account for the variability in thyroid doses received by different individuals in the same geographic area. For example, many families grew their own vegetables and obtained milk from their own cows. Many individuals were outdoors most of the day at the time of the accident and slept with the windows open at night, thereby maximizing their exposure to ^{131}I by inhalation. The thyroid dose is known to be inversely related to thyroid mass. Thus, for a given uptake of ^{131}I, children achieve a higher thyroid dose than adults. The iodine level in the diet also influences the efficiency of uptake of ^{131}I. Southern Belarus suffers from mild iodine deficiency, with some relatively isolated pockets of severe iodine deficiency (109,110). Iodine supplementation measures had lapsed by 1985. The subsequent implications are that individuals living in iodine-deficient areas would have a greater thyroid uptake of radioiodine than those living in iodine-replete areas. An effective prophylaxis program utilizing potassium iodide, as was administered in Poland (99), could have limited radioiodine exposure. As exposed inhabitants were not immediately informed of the accident, and there was no immediate effort to systematically prophylax the population, potassium iodide was not administered early enough (if at all) in Belarus, Ukraine, and Russia to be effective.

Belarus

Direct measurements of thyroid ^{131}I content were made during May and June of 1986 in approx 300,000 individuals living in the contaminated areas of Belarus. About 200,000 records were verified and form the basis of a database for the calculation of individual thyroid doses of Belarussian residents (111–117). Roughly 150,000 individuals in the database were interviewed regarding lifestyle and diet. Thyroid dose estimates have been completed for 130,000 residents of the Gomel and Mogilev oblasts and Minsk City who had direct thyroid measurements completed before June 6. Estimates were based on the direct measurements and information on lifestyle and diet (e.g., level of milk consumption). Calculations assumed ^{131}I intake by inhalation and ingestion of fresh milk after a single deposition of fallout on pasture grass (111). Average thyroid doses have also been estimated for individuals living in 800 rural settlements without direct thyroid measurements. These reconstructions are calculated using the aforementioned database, considering the level of consumption of fresh cows' milk. A dose reconstruction study involving two cities and 2122 settlements in Belarus, as well as one city and 607 settlements in the Bryansk district of the Russian Federation, estimated an ERR of 23 per Gy (112).

Reported average thyroid doses of ^{131}I in Belarussian children living in different contaminated raions (administrative districts) of the Gomel and Mogilev oblasts ranged from 0.15 to 4.7 Gy (111–117). Young children (age ≤7) in these districts generally received thyroid doses that were 3–5 fold higher than those recorded in adults living in the same district. Several hundred children in Belarus received doses of 10 Gy or more to the thyroid; the highest thyroid dose did not exceed 60 Gy.

Russian Federation

In addition to the 130,000 direct measurements in Belarus, 28,000 measurements were made in the Kaluga oblast, and 2000 measurements were made in the Bryansk oblast of Russia (118–120). These oblasts also suffered from mild-to-moderate iodine deficiency (110). The mean thyroid dose owing to iodine radionuclides in children in Bryansk was 0.5 Gy, but it was 2.2 Gy in the more heavily contaminated zones. In the Kaluga oblast the mean dose in children was 0.25 Gy. In the more heavily contaminated areas, the mean dose was 0.5 Gy, and individual doses were as high as 10 Gy.

Ukraine

Direct measurements of thyroid ^{131}I content were made in 150,000 people in the Ukraine in May to June of 1986,

Table 3
Incidence of Thyroid Cancer in Children (Under Age 15 at Diagnosis)

Location	Rate		
	1981–1985	1986–1990	1991–1994
Belarus	0.3	4.0	30.6
Gomel oblast	0.5	10.5	96.4
Ukraine	0.5	1.1	3.4
Kiev, Chernigov, Cherkassy, Rovno, and Zhitomir oblasts	0.1	2.0	11.5
Russia			
Bryansk and Kaluga oblasts	0	1.2	10.0

Annual incidence rates per million children under age 15 are given. Data from ref. *101*.

including 108,000 children and adolescents age 0–18 yr *(121–125)*. The measurements were conducted in four of the northern oblasts: Chernigov, Kiev, Zhitomir, and Vinnytsia. Large-scale thyroid dose reconstructions were carried out using the direct measurements in combination with environmental data and information on personal behavior and intake of milk and leafy vegetables. Empirical relations were developed between parameters of ^{131}I intake and the level of ^{137}Cs soil contamination and the distance and direction from the nuclear plant. These relations allowed estimation of thyroid ^{131}I content in territories without direct measurements, such as the Cherkassy and Rovno oblasts. In different administrative regions of northern Ukraine, average thyroid doses from ^{131}I in children and adolescents ranged from 0.03 to 1.6 Gy.

Thyroid Cancer Incidence in Children

Following the Chernobyl accident, Prisyazhiuk and colleagues *(126)* reported a small increase in thyroid cancer cases in children from three districts in the northern Ukraine within 80 km of the nuclear plant. Another report from the Ukraine followed *(127)*. Local physicians had simultaneously detected a marked increase in the rate of childhood thyroid cancer in Belarus, starting in 1990 and primarily affecting the Gomel oblast *(99,128–131)*. Whereas only one or two cases of thyroid cancer were seen annually in the Gomel oblast during 1986–1989, there were 14 cases in 1990 and 38 cases in 1991. Most cases from Belarus (128/131) were diagnosed as papillary carcinomas. The initial reports were met with some skepticism by the international scientific community. Therefore, a team of international scientists under the auspices of the WHO and Swiss government visited Belarus in July of 1992 to verify the accuracy of the histologic diagnoses of thyroid cancer. The international team studied the histologic specimens from 104 children diagnosed with thyroid cancer since 1989 and agreed with the diagnosis in 102 cases *(132)*. The team also reported a marked increase in the incidence of childhood cancer (age ≤14) in Gomel from 1990 onward, with 80 cancers per million children each year by 1992, compared with the usual background rate of around one case of cancer per million children each year.

Subsequent data *(101)* have shown a continued increase in thyroid cancer incidence in children from Belarus, northern Ukraine (Kiev, Chernigov, Cherkassy, Rovno, and Zhitomir oblasts), and southwestern Russia (Bryansk and Kaluga oblasts) since the accident (Table 3). As shown, rates are expressed as cases of pediatric (age ≤14) thyroid cancer per million children each year.

Belarus

The annual pediatric (age ≤14) thyroid cancer incidence rate in Belarus increased from 0.3 per million in 1981–1985 to 30.6 per million in 1991–1994, a 100-fold increase. A total of 333 cases of pediatric thyroid cancer were diagnosed in Belarus from 1986 to 1994 *(101,133,134)*. During 1995, 91 additional cases were diagnosed (57 in the first 7 mo of the year). Yet, there were only seven pediatric cases in Belarus for 9 yr preceding the accident (1977–1985). In the Gomel oblast, the incidence rate increased nearly 200-fold up to 96.4 per million.

Of the 390 pediatric cases reported in Belarus through mid-1995, 54.3% were from the Gomel oblast, and 21.8% were from the Brest oblast. Only 1.8% of cases were from the Vitebsk oblast, which was not contaminated following the Chernobyl accident. Annual childhood thyroid cancer incidence rates for different geographic zones in Belarus are shown in Fig. 2 (in cases per 100,000 children/year for 1990–1991). There is a strong correlation between these incidence rates and soil ^{131}I contamination levels (Fig. 2), as documented by the study of Abelin and colleagues *(135–137)*. As noted by those authors, the higher incidence rates occurred along the two paths taken by the initial clouds of volatile radioisotopes: one pathway to the west and the other to the northeast. The highest annual incidence rate (130.8/million) was found in the southern part of the Gomel oblast, adjacent to Chernobyl, where the ^{131}I contamination level was highest. The association between childhood thyroid

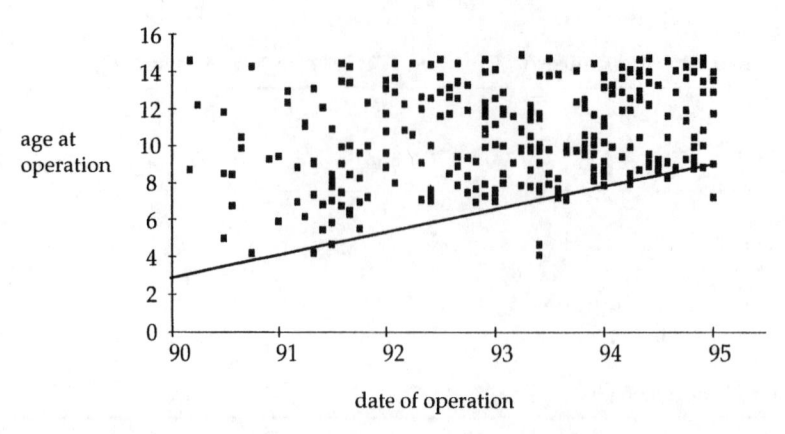

Fig. 3. Graph showing the age of Belarussian children at the time of thyroid surgery vs the date of surgery. The bold line corresponds to the age of a child born on November 26, 1986. Note that very few cases fall below the bold line. (From ref. *138*, courtesy of the European Commission.)

cancer incidence and ^{131}I deposition suggests that radioactive isotopes of iodine had an etiological role in the pathogenesis of the thyroid cancers.

The ratio of affected girls to boys in Belarus was 1.5 : 1.0. Most affected children (386/390) were born either before the accident or near the time of the accident; only four of the children were born after 1986. The rate of thyroid cancer in children born after 1986 is low and approximates baseline levels before the accident. Figure 3 shows data from 298 children diagnosed with thyroid cancer at the Pathology Institute in Minsk from 1990 to 1994 *(138)*. Note that there is a sharp cutoff age (Fig. 3, bold line) below which few young children have presented with thyroid cancer, and the cutoff age increases with time. The bold line in Fig. 3 represents children who were born on November 26, 1986. Children born on this date would have been approx 10-wk gestational age at the time of the Chernobyl accident. Because the fetal thyroid gland can concentrate iodine by 12 wk, these children could have theoretically sustained significant thyroid exposure to ^{131}I *in utero* during the first month following the accident. These data strongly suggest that intrathyroidal accumulation of radioactive iodine isotopes—either *in utero* or after birth—was an important factor in the pathogenesis of the pediatric thyroid cancers in Belarus.

An analysis of thyroid cancer cases in Belarus by cohorts, defined according to the patient's date of birth, is shown in Fig. 4 *(136,139)*. Clearly, increasing numbers of cases have occurred in each cohort at least until 1993. The largest number of new thyroid cancer cases has occurred in individuals who were age 4 and younger at the time of the accident (birth date: 1982–1986), followed by those who were age 5–9 (birth date: 1977–1981); however, individuals as old as 19 at the time of the accident were still at risk. These data suggest that younger children are most susceptible to the carcinogenic effects of radioactive iodine isotopes.

The peak incidence of childhood papillary thyroid carcinoma (in patients up to age 14) occurred in Belarus in 1995 at 40 cases per million. Subsequently, a gradually decreasing frequency of papillary carcinoma has been observed in this age group. There were 84 cases observed in 1996, 66 cases in 1997, 54 cases in 1998, 49 cases in 1999, and 31 cases in 2000 *(140)*. This represents a total of 708 childhood cases presenting in Belarus from 1986 until 2000. After the latter half of 2001, only sporadic thyroid cancers were found in Belarussian children. The decrease is readily explained because over time, exposed individuals will reach age 15 or older and will no longer be reported in the data for children (up to age 14). In keeping with this analysis, since 1997, the incidence of thyroid cancer has increased in Belarussian adolescents age 15–18 yr old at the time of diagnosis or surgery. In 2001, the incidence was 112 per million in this patient cohort *(141)*.

Russian Federation

In the contaminated oblasts of the Russian Federation, an increased incidence of thyroid cancer in children and adolescents has been registered *(101,119,142,143)*. The annual prevalence in children (age ≤14) in the Bryansk and Kaluga oblasts has increased from background to 10 per million. The major increase occurred in the Bryansk oblast, with 21 cases reported between 1986 and 1994.

Ukraine

Between 1986 and 1994, 211 children (age ≤14) underwent surgery for thyroid cancer in the Ukraine *(101, 121,122,144,145)*. The incidence in children increased from 0.4 to 0.6 per million pre-Chernobyl to 4 per million by 1992–1994. The ratio of girls to boys was 1.4 : 1.0. In the five most northern oblasts (Kiev, Chernigov, Zhitomir, Cherkassy, and Rovno) that were heavily contaminated by the Chernobyl accident, the incidence was much higher: 11.5 per million children. About 60% of the cases in the Ukraine originated from these five oblasts out of 25 oblasts in the country. Only two children presenting with thyroid cancer were born after 1986, equivalent to an incidence of

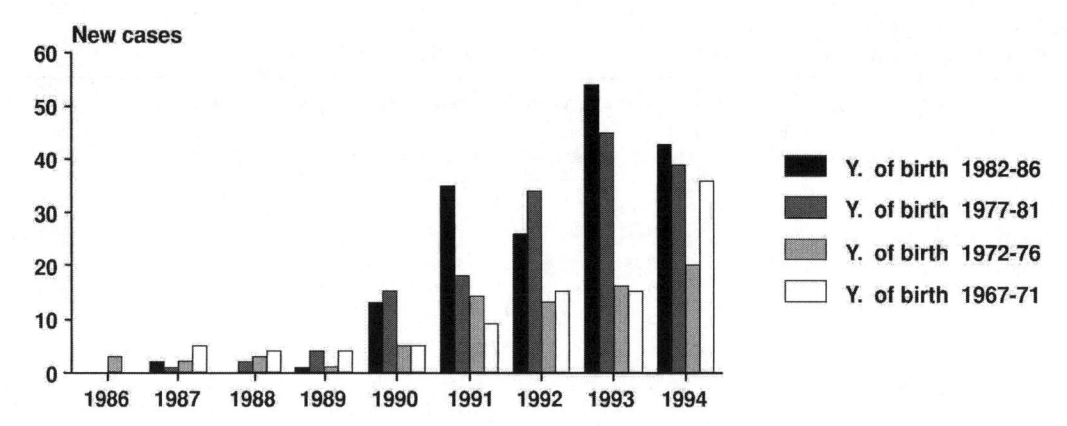

Fig. 4. Graph showing the number of new thyroid cancer cases during each year from 1986 to 1994 in cohorts of Belarussian children defined by year of birth. (From ref. *139*, courtesy of the European Commission.)

less than 1 per million each year in children born after 1986. In Pripyat, located 3.5 km from the Chernobyl plant, the incidence in children and adolescents who were age 0–18 yr old at the time of the accident was 137 per million by 1990–1992. Throughout the Ukraine, there was a 30-fold gradient in thyroid cancer incidence rates in individuals age 0–18 at the time of the accident, directly corresponding to the gradient in thyroid doses from ^{131}I exposure *(122)*. This relationship between cancer incidence and thyroid ^{131}I dose strongly supports a role for radioactive iodine isotopes in the pathogenesis of the cancers.

Pathologic and Biologic Features of the Pediatric Thyroid Cancers

The pathologic features of the thyroid cancers presenting after the Chernobyl accident in children from Belarus, the Ukraine, and Russia have been well characterized *(146–155)*. With few exceptions, all the cases have been papillary carcinomas. Several histological subtypes have been noted *(146–149)*: classical papillary architecture, often with mixed papillary/follicular elements (approx 11%); a mixture of solid and follicular structures (73%); and the diffuse sclerosing type (8%). Primary tumors were 1 cm or larger in diameter in the vast majority of cases (79–88.5% in three series; *133,150,151*).

Thyroid tumors that arise in children are typically more aggressive than those that arise in adults *(156–161)*. This phenomenon was also true in the Chernobyl-related cases. The tumors were often widely invasive within the thyroid gland (33% in one series *[151]*; 59% of cases in another series *[146]*). There was direct invasion of extrathyroidal tissue (T4 stage) in a high proportion of cases (48–63%; *133,134,144, 146,150,154*). Lymphatic invasion was present in 77% of cases and blood vessel invasion in 15–32% *(146,150,151)*. Regional lymph node metastases (N1 stage) were present in 59–88% of cases *(133,144,150,151,154)*. Distant metastases (M1 stage, usually to lung) were present in 5–9% of cases *(133,150,154)*.

Only a few cases showed features of "occult" or microcarcinoma. Taken together, these pathological and biological features argue strongly against the cancers being incidental findings *(162–164)*. In nearly all cases, the cancers represented clinically significant disease; only 9% of the children in one series from Belarus were staged at T1 N0 M0 *(150)*.

MOLECULAR CHARACTERIZATION OF CHERNOBYL-ASSOCIATED PAPILLARY THYROID CARCINOMAS

Ret *Oncogene*

Activation of the *ret* oncogene (see Chapters 3 and 5) by chromosomal rearrangement was initially reported in four of seven Chernobyl-associated pediatric cases by Ito and coworkers *(165)* and is the most characteristic type of molecular alteration in post-Chernobyl papillary thyroid carcinomas *(165–186)*. An analysis of pooled data regarding *ret* rearrangements from eight published studies *(166–168, 177–182)* is presented in Table 4. For purposes of this analysis, those cases diagnosed or undergoing surgery on or before April 26, 1996 are reported in part A; those presenting after April 26, 1996 are reported in part B. The original published case series have been segregated into two groups according to this criterion. For example, the first 37 cases of Smida et al. *(182)* underwent surgery from April 21, 1993 to April 16, 1996 and are recorded in part A. The remaining 14 from this series underwent surgery from May 3, 1996 to February 14, 1997 and are recorded in part B. The 191 cases of Rabes et al. *(177,178)* were divided into groups of 61 and 130 by the original authors using the same criterion. Case numbers 3, 4, 5, and 6 as published by Pisarchik et al. *(179, 180)* underwent surgery in February, 1996 and are included in part A. Cases numbered 7–39 underwent surgery from October 2, 1996 to December 27, 1996 and are reported in part B. All individuals reported in this analysis were under age 20 at the moment of the accident (April 26, 1986).

Table 4
Studies of *Ret* Rearrangements in Post-Chernobyl Papillary Thyroid Cancers

A. Latency Period* ≤10 yr (April 26, 1986 through April 26, 1996)

Authors (ref.)	N	Dates of Diagnosis	Ret/PTC1	Ret/PTC2	Ret/PTC3
Fugazzola et al. *(166)*	6	1991–1992	0 (0%)	1 (17%)	3 (50%)
Nikiforov et al. *(167)*	38	1991–1992	6 (16%)	1 (3%)	22 (58%)
Klugbauer et al. *(168)*	12	1993–1995	2 (17%)	0 (0%)	6 (50%)
Smida et al. *(182)*	37	1993–4/16/1996	8 (22%)	0 (0%)	11 (29%)
Rabes et al. *(177,178)*	61	1993–4/26/1996	9 (15%)	0 (0%)	24 (39%)
Pisarchik et al. *(179)*	4	2/1996	1 (25%)	NT	NT
Pisarchik et al. *(180)*	3	2/1996	NT	NT	1 (33%)
Pooled Data			26 (16%)	2 (1.3%)	67 (43%)

B. Latency Period >10 yr (after April 26, 1996)

Authors (ref.)	N	Dates of Diagnosis	Ret/PTC1	Ret/PTC2	Ret/PTC3
Pisarchik et al. *(179)*	27	10/1996–12/1996	8 (30%)	NT	NT
Pisarchik et al. *(180)*	12	10/1996–12/1996	NT	NT	0 (0%)
Pisarchik et al. *(181)*	37	1998	8 (22%)	NT	5 (14%)
Smida et al. *(182)*	14	5/1996–1997	4 (29%)	0 (0%)	2 (14%)
Rabes et al. *(177,178)*	130	5/1996–1998	39 (30%)	0 (0%)	14 (11%)
Pooled Data			59 (28%)	0 (0%)	21 (11%)

*Interval between exposure and diagnosis/surgery. NT, not tested.

As demonstrated in Table 4, part A, *ret*/PTC3 is the most prevalent form of *ret* rearrangement in post-Chernobyl papillary carcinomas diagnosed during the first decade following the accident (until April 26, 1996). The overall prevalence of *ret*/PTC3 in these cases is 43%, whereas the prevalence of *ret*/PTC1 is 16% and that of *ret*/PTC2 is only 1.3%.

In contrast with the earlier case series, Pisarchik and colleagues *(179)* found a higher prevalence of *ret*/PTC1 rearrangements (29%) in 31 post-Chernobyl papillary thyroid carcinomas presenting in 1996. However, the prevalence of *ret*/PTC3 was found to be quite low (7%) in a subset of these cases *(180)*. Pisarchik and colleagues *(180)* suggested that there was a switch in the ratio of *ret*/PTC3 to *ret*/PTC1 rearrangements in late (1996) vs early (1991–1992) post-Chernobyl papillary thyroid cancers. Smida and colleagues *(182)* independently arrived at a similar conclusion after studying 51 Chernobyl-related cases. These authors *(182)* suggested that *ret*/PTC3 may be typical for radiation-associated childhood papillary thyroid carcinomas with a short latency period, whereas *ret*/PTC1 may be a marker for carcinomas appearing after a longer latency period. These observations are confirmed by the pooled analysis in Table 4, part B. The overall prevalence of *ret*/PTC3 in these later cases is significantly lower at 11%, whereas the prevalence of *ret*/PTC1 is higher at 28%.

In addition to influencing the latency period, the type of *ret* rearrangement correlates strongly with morphological variants of papillary thyroid carcinoma. Nikiforov and colleagues *(167)* first reported that post-Chernobyl papillary thyroid carcinomas with a solid differentiation pattern are associated with *ret*/PTC3, and the classic papillary differentiation pattern is related to the *ret*/PTC1 rearrangement. This finding has been confirmed by Rabes and colleagues *(177,178)*, as well as Thomas and colleagues *(183–185)*, and similar results have been obtained in transgenic mice *(187–189)*.

The results regarding *ret* rearrangements are particularly interesting in view of the recent demonstration that X-irradiation (50–100 Gy) in vitro can induce *ret* oncogene rearrangements in undifferentiated human thyroid carcinoma cells *(190)*. Furthermore, Bounacer and colleagues *(191)* reported a high frequency of *ret* rearrangements (primarily *ret*/PTC1) in papillary thyroid carcinomas originating from patients with a history of external radiation. Similar results using immunohistochemistry were reported by Collins and colleagues *(192)*. Taken together, they suggest that *ret* rearrangements are important in the pathogenesis of radiation-induced papillary thyroid carcinomas, and the specific type of molecular rearrangement (*ret*/PTC1 vs *ret*/PTC3) may influence the biology of the cancer (e.g., the latency period and morphological variant).

Other Genetic Loci

Other genetic loci have been investigated *(138, 146,193–200)* including *NTRK1*, *p53*, the TSH receptor, and the three *ras* genes (*H-RAS*, *K-RAS*, and *N-RAS*). Chromosomal rearrangements associated with the *NTRK1* gene *(193)* have been identified infrequently in post-Chernobyl papillary thyroid carcinomas *(177,178,194)*. Nikiforov and colleagues *(195)* used single-strand conformation polymorphism analysis and found a *p53* missense mutation in 1 of 33 Chernobyl-associated papillary thyroid carcinomas (3%) involving codon 160. Hillebrandt and coworkers *(196,197)* used temperature gradient gel electrophoresis (TGGE) and identified only one *p53* missence mutation (involving codon 258) out of 70 post-Chernobyl papillary thyroid carcinomas. Smida and colleagues *(198)* found five cases of a silent mutation in *p53* codon 213 out of 24 Chernobyl-related papillary carcinomas. Suchy and colleagues *(199)* studied 34 cases of post-Chernobyl papillary carcinomas but found no mutations in *p53*. Santoro et al. *(184)* analyzed 35 cases with TGGE and found no *p53* mutations. Pisarchik and colleagues *(200)* used polymerase chain reaction with direct sequencing and identified *p53* mutations in 5 of 24 cases. One alteration involving codon 167 (CAG→CAT) in all five cases resulted in the substitution of HIS for GLN. The second alteration involving codon 183 (TCA→TGA) in all five cases led to a premature termination codon. Alterations of the TSH-receptor and *RAS* genes are very rare, suggesting that mutations in these genes do not have a significant role in the pathogenesis of Chernobyl-associated thyroid cancers.

EPIDEMIOLOGICAL CONSIDERATIONS

Following the initial reports of thyroid cancer cases in the regions surrounding Chernobyl, there were many questions about whether the cases were related to the accident or simply represented increased ascertainment *(89,201,202)*. The data reviewed in this chapter support the contention that nearly all the cancer cases were correctly diagnosed, and the majority represented clinically important disease, not incidental cases found by screening. Some oblasts that received little radiation (Vitebsk) were subjected to intensive screening but yielded very few cases. Thus, increased ascertainment cannot explain the dramatic and sustained increase in incidence that has been documented. The large number of cases and latency period support an association with the accident *(108)*. In addition, data reviewed previously suggest that radioiodine isotopes are implicated in the pathogenesis of the cancers. A small case-control epidemiological study has provided some further evidence for this point by demonstrating a dose–response relationship at the level of the individual thyroid dose *(203,204)*. A study by Jacob et al. *(205)* showed a linear dose–response relationship between the thyroid dose, resulting from internal ^{131}I exposure and the risk of thyroid cancer. A recent analysis by Shibata et al. *(206)* further supports the concept that direct external or internal exposure to ^{131}I and short-lived radioiodine isotopes was a causative factor in the pediatric thyroid cancers. An analysis of children who lived within a 150-km radius from Chernobyl revealed that cancer frequently developed in children born in 1983–1986; however, no cases were seen in children born in 1987–1989. This is most likely explained by natural degradation of ^{131}I and short-lived radioiodine isotopes, as well as erosion of these isotopes from the contaminated territory by wind and rain. More large-scale epidemiological studies are in progress *(207)*. Other questions to be addressed are the exact contributions of ^{131}I vs short-lived radioiodines. The contribution of tellurium also needs to be established. The possible contribution of other environmental factors (industrial pollution and iodine deficiency), and host factors (e.g., increased genetic predisposition to increased sensitivity to radiation effects) should also be considered *(208)*.

Studies in the Tula Oblast of Russia

Gerasimov (The Russian Endocrinology Research Center) and Figge have conducted field surveys between 1991 and 1995 in the Arsenyevo district of the Tula Oblast in Russia, an area contaminated with ^{137}Cs at a density of 5–15 Ci/km^2, and in the Yasnagorsk district, a noncontaminated area. Both regions had mild iodine deficiency with urinary iodine levels of 7–9 µg/dL. The distribution of benign thyroid lesions from both regions was similar. A papillary thyroid cancer was diagnosed in 1991 in one female from Arsenyevo who was 12 yr old in 1986. As pointed out by Williams *(164)*, it is not known why areas contaminated with fairly high levels of fallout in southwest Russia appear to have fewer thyroid cancer cases than in Belarus. An answer to this question will be important to understand the factors involved in thyroid cancer pathogenesis.

REFERENCES

1. Hanson GA, Komorowski RA, Cerletty JM, Wilson SD. Thyroid gland morphology in young adults: normal subjects versus those with prior low-dose neck irradiation in childhood. Surgery 1983; 94:984–988.
2. Spitalnik PF, Straus FH. Patterns of human thyroid parenchymal reaction following low-dose childhood irradiation. Cancer 1978; 41:1098–1105.
3. Freedberg AS, Kurland GS, Blumgart HL. The pathologic effects of I-131 on the normal thyroid gland of man. J Clin Endocrinol 1952; 12:1315–1348.
4. Carr RF, LiVolsi VA. Morphologic changes in the thyroid after irradiation for Hodgkin's and non-Hodgkin's lymphoma. Cancer 1989; 64:825–829.
5. Quimby EH, Werner SC. Late radiation effects in roentgen therapy for hyperthyroidism. JAMA 1949; 140:1046–1047.
6. Winship T, Rosvoll RV. Thyroid carcinoma in childhood: final report on a 20 year study. Clinical Proceedings of the Children's Hospital of Washington, DC 1970; 26:327–349.
7. Roudebush CP, Asteris GT, DeGroot LJ. Natural history of radiation-associated thyroid cancer. Arch Intern Med 1978; 138:1631–1634.
8. Samaan NA, Schultz PN, Ordonez NG, Hickey RC, Johnston DA. A comparison of thyroid carcinoma in those who have and have not had head and neck irradiation in childhood. J Clin Endocrinol Metab 1987; 64:219–223.
9. Mehta MP, Goetowski PG, Kinsella TJ. Radiation induced thyroid neoplasms 1920 to 1987: a vanishing problem? Int J Radial Oncol Biol Phys 1989; 16:1471–1475.

10. Akslen LA, Haldorsen T, Thoresen SO, Glattre E. Incidence pattern of thyroid cancer in Norway: influence of birth cohort and time period. Int J Cancer 1993; 53:183–187.
11. Harach HR, Franssila KO, Wasenius V-M. Occult papillary carcinoma of the thyroid: a "normal" finding in Finland—a systematic autopsy study. Cancer 1985; 56:531–538.
12. Sampson RJ, Woolner LB, Bahn RC, Kurland LT. Occult thyroid carcinoma in Olmsted County, Minnesota: prevalence at autopsy compared with that in Hiroshima and Nagasaki, Japan. Cancer 1974; 34:2072–2076.
13. Wilson SD, Komorowski R, Cerletty J, Majewski JT, Hooper M. Radiation-associated thyroid tumors: extent of operation and pathology technique influence the apparent incidence of carcinoma. Surgery 1983; 94:663–667.
14. Robbins J. Thyroid cancer: a lethal endocrine neoplasm—NIH conference. Ann Intern Med 1991; 115:133–147.
15. Mettler FA, Upton AC. Carcinogenesis at specific sites. In Medical Effects of Ionizing Radiation. Philadelphia, PA: WB Saunders, 1995:130–139.
16. Aldinger KA, Samaan NA, Ibanez M, Hill CS. Anaplastic carcinoma of the thyroid: a review of 84 cases of spindle and giant cell carcinoma of the thyroid. Cancer 1978; 41:2267–2275.
17. Duffy BJ, Fitzgerald PJ. Cancer of the thyroid in children: a report of 28 cases. J Clin Endocrinol Metab 1950; 10:1296–1308.
18. Simpson CL, Hempelmann LH. The association of tumors and roentgen-ray treatment of the thorax in infancy. Cancer 1957; 10:42–56.
19. Saenger EL, Silverman FN, Sterling TD, Turner ME. Neoplasia following therapeutic irradiation for benign conditions in childhood. Radiology 1960; 74:889–904.
20. Thompson DE, Mabuchi K, Ron E, Soda M, Tokunaga M, Ochikubo S, et al. Cancer incidence in atomic bomb survivors. Part II: Solid tumors, 1958-1987. Radiat Res 1994; 137:817–867.
21. Parker LN, Belsky JL, Yamamoto T, Kawamoto S, Keehn RJ. Thyroid carcinoma after exposure to atomic radiation: a continuing survey of a fixed population, Hiroshima and Nagasaki, 1958-1971. Ann Intern Med 1974; 80:600–604.
22. Schull WJ. Atomic bomb survivors: patterns of cancer risk. Prog Cancer Res Ther 1984; 26:21–36.
23. Fjalling M, Tisell L-E, Carlsson S, Hansson G, Lundberg L-M, Oden A. Benign and malignant thyroid nodules after neck irradiation. Cancer 1986; 58:1219–1224.
24. Furst CJ, Lundell M, Holm LE, Silfversward C. Cancer incidence after radiotherapy for skin hemangioma: a retrospective cohort study in Sweden. J Natl Cancer Inst 1988; 80:1387–1392.
25. Lundell M, Hakulinen T, Holm L-E. Thyroid cancer after radiotherapy for skin hemangioma in infancy. Radiat Res 1994; 140:334–339.
26. Lindberg S, Karlsson P, Arvidsson B, Holmberg E, Lundberg LM, Wallgren A. Cancer incidence after radiotherapy for skin haemangioma during infancy. Acia Oncol 1995; 34:735–740.
27. Schneider AB, Ron E, Lubin J, Slovall M, Gierlowski TC. Dose-response relationships for radiation-induced thyroid cancer and nodules: evidence for the prolonged effects of radiation on the thyroid. J Clin Endocrinol Metab 1993; 77:362–369.
28. Schneider AB, Recant W, Pinsky SM, Ryo UY, Bekerman C, Shore-Freedman E. Radiation-induced thyroid carcinoma: clinical course and results of therapy in 296 patients. Ann Intern Med 1986; 105:405–412.
29. Viswanathan K, Gierlowski TC, Schneider AB. Childhood thyroid cancer: characteristics and long-term outcome in children irradiated for benign conditions of the head and neck. Arch Pediatr Adolesc Med 1994; 148:260–265.
30. Schneider AB, Shore-Freedman E, Weinstein RA. Radiation-induced thyroid and other head and neck tumors: occurrence of multiple tumors and analysis of risk factors. J Clin Endocrinol Metab 1986; 63:107–112.
31. Paloyan E, Lawrence AM. Thyroid neoplasms after radiation therapy for adolescent acne vulgaris. Arch Dermatol 1978; 114:53–55.
32. Hempelmann LH, Hall WJ, Phillips M, Cooper RA, Ames WR. Neoplasms in persons treated with x-rays in infancy: fourth survey in 20 years. J Natl Cancer Inst 1975; 55:519–530.
33. Shore RE, Hildreth N, Dvoretsky P, Andresen E, Moseson M, Pasternack B. Thyroid cancer among persons given x-ray treatment in infancy for an enlarged thymus gland. Am J Epidemiol 1993; 137:1068–1080.
34. Ron E, Modan B, Preston D, Alfandary E, Stovall M, Boice JD. Thyroid neoplasia following low-dose radiation in childhood. Radiat Res 1989; 120:516–531.
35. Shore RE, Albert RE, Pasternack BS. Follow-up study of patients treated by x-ray epilation for tinea capitis: resurvey of post-treatment illness and mortality experience. Arch Environ Health 1976; 31:17–24.
36. Ron E, Modan B. Thyroid and other neoplasms following childhood scalp irradiation. Prog Cancer Res Ther 1984; 26:139–151.
37. Tucker MA, Morris Jones PH, Boice JD, Robison LL, Stone BJ, Stovall M, et al. Therapeutic radiation at a young age is linked to secondary thyroid cancer. Cancer Res 1991; 51:2885–2888.
38. Hancock SL, Cox RS, McDougall IR. Thyroid diseases after treatment of Hodgkin's disease. N Engl J Med 1991; 325:599–605.
39. Boice JD, Day NE, Andersen A, Brinton LA, Brown R, Choi NW, et al. Second cancers following radiation treatment for cervical cancer: an international collaboration among cancer registries. J Natl Cancer Inst 1985; 74:955–975.
40. Boice JD, Engholm G, Klienerman RA, Blettner M, Stovall M, Lisco H, et al. Radiation dose and second cancer risk in patients treated for cancer of the cervix. Radiat Res 1988; 116:3–55.
41. Arai T, Nakano T, Fukuhisa K, Kasamatsu T, Tsunematsu R, Masubuchi K, et al. Second cancer after radiation therapy for cancer of the uterine cervix. Cancer 1991; 67:398–405.
42. Hay JH, Duncan W, Kerr GR. Subsequent malignancies in patients irradiated for testicular tumours. Br J Radiol 1984; 57:597–602.
43. Fossa SD, Langmark F, Aass N, Andersen A, Lothe R, Borrasen AL. Second non-germ cell malignancies after radiotherapy of testicular cancer with or without chemotherapy. Br J Cancer 1990; 61:639–643.
44. Kendall GM, Muirhead CR, MacGibbon BH, O'Hagan JA, Conquest AJ, Goodill AA, et al. Mortality and occupational exposure to radiation: first analysis of the National Registry for Radiation Workers. BMJ 1992; 304:220–225.
45. Beral V, Inskip H, Fraser P, Booth M, Coleman D, Rose G. Mortality of employees of the United Kingdom Atomic Energy Authority, 1946-1979. BMJ 1985; 291:440–447.
46. Wilkinson GS, Tietjen GL, Wiggs LD, Galke WA, Acquavella JF, Reyes M, et al. Mortality among plutonium and other radiation workers at a plutonium weapons facility. Am J Epidemiol 1987; 125:231–250.
47. Checkoway H, Pearce N, Crawford-Brown DJ, Cragle DL. Radiation doses and cause-specific mortality among workers at a nuclear materials fabrication plant. Am J Epidemiol 1988; 127:255–266.
48. Wing S, Shy CM, Wood JL, Wolf S, Cragle DL, Frame EL. Mortality among workers at Oak Ridge Nationaal Laboratory: evidence of radiation effects in follow-up through 1984. JAMA 1991; 265:1397–1402.
49. Wang J-X, Boice JD, Li B-X, Zhang J-Y, Fraumeni JF. Cancer among medical diagnostic x-ray workers in China. J Natl Cancer Inst 1988; 80:344–350.
50. Boice JD, Mandel JS, Doody MM, Yoder RC, McGowan R. A health survey of radiologic technologists. Cancer 1992; 69:586–598.
51. Smith PG, Doll R. Mortality from cancer and all causes among British radiologists. Br J Radiol 1981; 54:187–194.
52. Mátanosla GM, Seltser R, Sartwell PE, Diamond EL, Elliott EA. The current mortality rates of radiologists and other physician specialists: specific causes of death. Am J Epidemiol 1975; 101:199–210.

53. Stewart A, Kneale GW. Radiation dose effects in relation to obstetric x-rays and childhood cancers. Lancet 1970; 1:1185–1188.
54. Mole RH. Childhood cancer after prenatal exposure to diagnostic x-ray examinations in Britain. Br J Cancer 1990; 62:152–168.
55. Oppenheim BE, Griem ML, Meier P. Effects of low-dose prenatal irradiation in humans: analysis of Chicago Lying-in data and comparison with other studies. Radiat Res 1974; 57:508–544.
56. Harvey EB, Boice JD, Honeyman M, Flannery JT. Prenatal x-ray exposure and childhood cancer in twins. N Engl J Med 1985; 312:541–545.
57. Rodvall Y, Pershagen G, Hrubec Z, Ahlbom A, Pedersen NL, Boice JD. Prenatal x-ray exposure and childhood cancer in Swedish twins. Int J Cancer 1990; 46:362–365.
58. Yoshimoto Y, Kato H, Schull WJ. Risk of cancer among children exposed in útero to A-bomb radiations, 1950-1984. Lancet 1988; 2:665–669.
59. Lee W, Chiacchierini RP, Shleien B, Telles NC. Thyroid tumors following I-131 or localized X irradiation to the thyroid and pituitary glands in rats. Radiat Res 1982; 92:307–319.
60. Forman D, Cook-Mozaffari P, Darby S, Davey G, Sratton I, Doll R, Pike M. Cancer near nuclear installations. Nature 1987; 329:499–505.
61. Jablon S, Urubec Z, Boice JD. Cancer in populations living near nuclear facilities: a survey of mortality nationwide and incidence in two states. JAMA 1991; 265:1403–1408.
62. Davis S, Kopecky KJ, Hamilton T. Hanford Thyroid Disease Final Report. Seattle, WA: Fred Hutchinson Cancer Research Center, 2002.
63. Committee on an Assessment of Centers for Disease Control and Prevention Radiation Studies from DOE Contractor Sites: Subcommittee to Review the Hanford Thyroid Disease Study Final Results and Report, National Academy of Sciences. Review of the Hanford Thyroid Disease Study Draft Final Report. Washington, DC: National Academies Press, 2000.
64. Holm L-E, Wiklund KE, Lundell GE, Bergman NA, Bjelkengren G, Cederquist ES, et al. Thyroid cancer after diagnostic doses of iodine-131: a retrospective cohort study. J Natl Cancer Inst 1988; 80:1132–1138.
65. Ron E, Doody MM, Becker DV, Brill AB, Curtis RE, Goldman MB, et al. Cancer mortality following treatment for adult hyperthyroidism. JAMA 1998; 280:347–355.
66. Holm L-E. Malignant disease following iodine-131 therapy in Sweden. Prog Cancer Res Ther 1984; 26:263–271.
67. Hoffman DA, McConahey WM, Fraumeni JF, Kurland LT. Cancer incidence following treatment of hyperthyroidism. Int J Epidemiol 1982; 11:218–224.
68. Holm L-E, Dahlqvist I, Israelsson A, Lundell G. Malignant thyroid tumors after iodine-131 therapy: a retrospective cohort study. N Engl J Med 1980; 303:188–191.
69. Hoffman DA, McConahey WM, Diamond EL, Kurland LT. Mortality in women treated for hyperthyroidism. Am J Epidemiol 1982; 115:243–254.
70. Goldman MB, Maloof F, Monson RR, Aschengrau A, Cooper DS, Ridgway EC. Radioactive iodine therapy and breast cancer: a follow-up study of hyperthyroid women. Am J Epidemiol 1988; 127:969–980.
71. Safa AM, Schumacher OP, Rodriguez-Antunez A. Long-term follow-up results in children and adolescents treated with radioactive iodine (I-131) for hyperthyroidism. N Engl J Med 1975; 292:167–171.
72. Johnson CJ. Cancer incidence in an area of radioactive fallout downwind from the Nevada test site. JAMA 1984; 251:230–236.
73. Rallison ML, Dobyns BM, Keating PR, Rail JE, Tyler FH. Thyroid disease in children: a survey of subjects potentially exposed to fallout radiation. Am J Med 1974; 56:457–463.
74. Machado SG, Land CE, McKay FW. Cancer mortality and radioactive fallout in southwestern Utah. Am J Epidemiol 1987; 125:44–61.
75. National Cancer Institute. Estimated Exposures and Thyroid Doses Received by the American People from Iodine-131 in Fallout Following Nevada Atmospheric Nuclear Bomb Tests: a Report from the National Cancer Institute. U.S. Department of Health and Human Services, 1997.
76. Gilbert ES, Tarone R, Bouville A, Ron E. Thyroid cancer rates and 131-I doses from Nevada atmospheric nuclear bomb tests. J Natl Cancer Inst 1998; 90:1654–1660.
77. Committee on Thyroid Screening Related to I-131 Exposure, Institute of Medicine, and Committee on Exposure of the American People to I-131 from the Nevada Atomic Bomb Tests, National Research Council. Exposure of the American People to Iodine-131 from Nevada Nuclear-Bomb Tests: Review of the National Cancer Institute Report and Public Health Implications. Washington, DC: National Academies Press, 1999.
78. Conard RA, Paglia DE, Larsen PR, Sutow WW, Dobyns BM, Robbins J, et al. Review of medical findings in a Marshallese population twenty-six years after accidental exposure to radioactive fallout. Brookhaven National Laboratory Report 1980; BNL 51261.
79. Conard RA. Late radiation effects in Marshall Islanders exposed to fallout 28 years ago. Prog Cancer Res Ther 1984; 26:57–71.
80. Hamilton TE, van Belle G, LoGerfo JP. Thyroid neoplasia in Marshall Islanders exposed to nuclear fallout. JAMA 1987; 258:629–636.
81. Wiklund K, Holm L-E, Eklund G. Cancer risks in Swedish Lapps who breed reindeer. Am J Epidemiol 1990; 132:1078–1082.
82. Shore RE. Human thyroid cancer induction by ionizing radiation: summary of studies based on external irradiation and radioactive iodines. In Karaoglou A, Desmet G, Kelly GN, Menzel HG, editors. The Radiological Consequences of the Chernobyl Accident. Brussels: European Commission, 1996:669–675.
83. Shore RE. Issues and epidemiological evidence regarding radiation-induced thyroid cancer. Radiat Res 1992; 131:98–111.
84. Ron E, Lubin JH, Shore RE, Mabuchi K, Modan B, Pottern LM, et al. Thyroid cancer after exposure to external radiation: a pooled analysis of seven studies. Radiat Res 1995; 141:259–277.
85. Shore RE, Woodard E, Hildreth N, Dvoretsky P, Hempelmann L, Pasternack B. Thyroid tumors following thymus irradiation. J Natl Cancer Inst 1985; 74:1177–1184.
86. National Academy of Sciences. Committee on the Biological Effects of Ionizing Radiations: Health Effects of Exposure to Low Level of Ionizing Radiation (BEIR V). Washington, DC: National Academy Press, 1990.
87. Shakhtarin VV, Tsyb AF, Stepanenko VF, Orlov MY, Kopecky KJ, Davis S. Iodine deficiency, radiation dose, and the risk of thyroid cancer among children and adolescents in the Bryansk region of Russia following the Chernobyl power station accident. Int J Epidemiol 2003; 32:584–591.
88. Niedziela M, Korman E, Breborowicz D, et al. A prospective study of thyroid nodular disease in children and adolescents in western Poland from 1996 to 2000 and the incidence of thyroid carcinoma relative to iodine deficiency and the Chernobyl disaster. Pediatr Blood Cancer 2004; 42:84–92.
89. Ron E, Lubin J, Schneider AB. Thyroid cancer incidence. Nature 1992; 360:113.
90. USSR State Committee on the Utilization of Atomic Energy. The Accident at the Chernobyl Nuclear Power Plant and Its Consequences. Information compiled for the International Atomic Energy Agency Experts Meeting, August 25-29, 1986, Vienna. Moscow: USSR State Committee on the Utilization of Atomic Energy, 1986.
91. Travis J. Chernobyl explosion. Inside look confirms more radiation. Science 1994; 263:750.
92. Warman EA. Paper presented at the New York Chapter Health Physics Society symposium on the effects of the nuclear reactor accident at Chernobyl. Upton, NY: Brookhaven National Laboratory, April 3, 1987.
93. Sich AR. Chernobyl thesis. Science 1994; 266:1627–1628.

94. Stone R. The explosions that shook the world. Science 1996; 272:352–354.
95. Sobotovich E, Bondarenko G, Petriaev E. Geochemistry of Chernobyl radionuclides. In Karaoglou A, Desmet G, Kelly GN, Menzel HG, editors. The Radiological Consequences of the Chernobyl Accident. Brussels: European Commission, 1996:477–483.
96. Izrael YA, De Cort M, Jones AR, et al. The atlas of caesium-137 contamination of Europe after the Chernobyl accident. In Karaoglou A, Desmet G, Kelly GN, Menzel HG, editors. The Radiological Consequences of the Chernobyl Accident. Brussels: European Commission, 1996:1–10.
97. Balonov M, Jacob P, Likhtarev I, Minenko V. Pathways, levels and trends of population exposure after the Chernobyl accident. In Karaoglou A, Desmet G, Kelly GN, Menzel HG, editors. The Radiological Consequences of the Chernobyl Accident. Brussels: European Commission, 1996:235–249.
98. Tsaturov YS, De Cort M, Dubois G, Izrael YA, Stukin ED, Fridman SD, et al. The need for standardization in the analysis, sampling and measurement of deposited radionuclides. In Karaoglou A, Desmet G, Kelly GN, Menzel HG, editors. The Radiological Consequences of the Chernobyl Accident. Brussels: European Commission, 1996: 425–433.
99. Kazakov VS, Demidchik EP, Astakhova LN. Thyroid cancer after Chernobyl. Nature 1992; 359:21.
100. World Health Organization. International programme on the health effects of the Chernobyl accident. Geneva: World Health Organization, 1993.
101. Stsjazhko VA, Tsyb AF, Tronko ND, Souchkevitch G, Baverstock KF. Childhood thyroid cancer since accident at Chernobyl. BMJ 1995; 310:801.
102. Williams N, Balter M. Chernobyl research becomes international growth industry. Science 1996; 272:355–356.
103. Balter M. Children become the first victims of fallout. Science 1996; 272:357–360.
104. Goldman M, Catlin R, Anspaugh L. Health and Environmental Consequences of the Chernobyl Nuclear Power Plant Accident. Washington, DC: U.S. Department of Energy Report DOE/ER 0332, 1987.
105. Lange R, Dickerson MH, Gudiksen PH. Dose estimates from the Chernobyl accident. Nucl Technol 1988; 82:311–323.
106. Nauman J, Wolff J. Iodine prophylaxis in Poland after the Chernobyl reactor accident: benefits and risks. Am J Med 1993; 94:524–532.
107. Dubina YV, Schekin YK, Guskina LN. Systematisation and verification of the spectrometrical analysis data of soil, grass, milk and milk products samples with results of 131-iodine measurements. (In Russian) Minsk, Belarus, 1990.
108. Becker DV, Robbins J, Beebe GW, Bouville AC, Wachholz BW. Childhood thyroid cancer following the Chernobyl accident. Endocrinol Metab Clin North Am 1996; 25:197–211.
109. Mityukova T, Astakhova L, Asenchyk L, Orlov M, Van Middlesworth L. Urinary iodine excretion in Belarus children. Eur J Endocrinol 1995; 133:216–217.
110. Gerasimov G, Alexandrova G, Arbuzova M, Butrova S, Kenzhibaeva M, Kotova G, et al. Iodine defficiency disorders (IDD) in regions of Russia affected by Chernobyl. In Karaoglou A, Desmet G, Kelly GN, Menzel HG, editors. The Radiological Consequences of the Chernobyl Accident. Brussels: European Commission, 1996: 813–815.
111. Gavrilin Y, Khrouch V, Shinkarev S, Drozdovitch V, Minenko V, Shemyakina E, et al. Estimation of thyroid doses received by the population of Belarus as a result of the Chernobyl accident. In Karaoglou A, Desmet G, Kelly GN, Menzel HG, editors. The Radiological Consequences of the Chernobyl Accident. Brussels: European Commission, 1996:1011–1020.
112. Jacob P, Kenigsberg Y, Zvonova I, Goulko G, Buglova E, Heidenreich WF, et al. Childhood exposure due to the Chernobyl accident and thyroid cancer risk in contaminated areas of Belarus and Russia. Br J Cancer 1999; 80:1461–1469.
113. Gavrilin YI, Gordeev KI, Ivanov VK, Ilyin LA, Kondrusev AI, Margulis UY, et al. The process and results of the reconstruction of internal thyroid doses for the population of contaminated areas of the Republic of Belarus. (In Russian) Vestn Acad Med Sci 1992; 2:35–43.
114. Ilyin LA, Balonov MI, Buldakov LA, et al. Radiocontamination patterns and possible health consequences of the accident at the Chernobyl nuclear power station. J Radiol Prot 1990; 10:13–29.
115. Gavrilin YI, Gordeev KI, Ilyin LA, et al. Results of thyroid dose assessment for contaminated territories of Belarussia. (In Russian) Bull Acad Med Sci USSR 1991; 8:35.
116. Gavrilin YI, Khrouch VT, Shinkarev SM. Internal thyroid exposure of the residents in several contaminated areas of Belarus. (In Russian) J Med Radiol 1993; 6:15–20.
117. Khrouch VT, Gavrilin YI, Shinkarev SM, et al. Generalization of results of individual thyroid dose reconstruction: determination of connections between parameters of contamination of people residences and levels of irradiation on thyroid glands. (In Russian) Minsk, Belarus, Moscow: Final Report of Institute of Biophysics, Moscow Contract N 7-17/93 with the Ministry of Public Health, 1994.
118. Stepanenko V, Gavrilin Y, Khrousch V, et al. The reconstruction of thyroid dose following Chernobyl. In Karaoglou A, Desmet G, Kelly GN, Menzel HG, editors. The Radiological Consequences of the Chernobyl Accident. Brussels: European Commission, 1996: 937–948.
119. Tsyb AF, Parshkov EM, Shakhtarin VV, Stepanenko VF, Skvortsov VF, Chebotareva IV. Thyroid cancer in children and adolescents of Bryansk and Kaluga regions. In Karaoglou A, Desmet G, Kelly GN, Menzel HG, editors. The Radiological Consequences of the Chernobyl Accident. Brussels: European Commission, 1996: 691–697.
120. Zvonova I, Balonov MI. Radioiodine dosimetry and prediction of thyroid effects on inhabitants of Russia following the Chernobyl accident. In Merwin SE, Balonov MI, editors. The Chernobyl Papers, vol. I: Doses to the Soviet Population and Early Health Effects Studies. Richland, WA: Research Enterprises, 1993:71–126.
121. Sobolev B, Likhtarev I, Kairo I, Tronko N, Oleynik V, Bogdanova T. Radiation risk assessment of the thyroid cancer in Ukrainian children exposed due to Chernobyl. In Karaoglou A, Desmet G, Kelly GN, Menzel HG, editors. The Radiological Consequences of the Chernobyl Accident. Brussels: European Commission, 1996: 741–748.
122. Likhtarev IA, Sobolev BG, Kairo IA, Tronko ND, Bogdanova TI, Oleinic VA, et al. Thyroid cancer in the Ukraine. Nature 1995; 375: 365.
123. Likhtarev IA, Shandala NK, Gulko GM, Kairo IA, Chepurny NI. Ukrainian thyroid doses after the Chernobyl accident. Health Phys 1993; 64:594–599.
124. Likhtarev I, Sobolev B, Kairo I, et al. Results of large scale thyroid dose reconstruction in Ukraine. In Karaoglou A, Desmet G, Kelly GN, Menzel HG, editors. The Radiological Consequences of the Chernobyl Accident. Brussels: European Commission, 1996: 1021–1034.
125. Likhtarev IA, Gulko GM, Sobolev BG, et al. Thyroid dose assessment for the Cherginov region (Ukraine): estimation based on 131I thyroid measurements and extrapolation of the results to districts without monitoring. Radiat Environ Biophys 1994; 33:149–166.
126. Prisyazhiuk A, Pjatak OA, Buzanov VA, Reeves GK, Beral V. Cancer in the Ukraine, post-Chernobyl. Lancet 1991; 338:1334–1335.
127. Oleynic VA, Cheban AK. Thyroid cancer in children of Ukraine from 1981 to 1992. In Robbins J, editor. Treatment of Thyroid Cancer in Childhood. Proceedings of a workshop on September 10-11, 1992, at the National Institutes of Health. Publication No. DOE/EH-0406 1992; 35.

128. Astakhova LN. Condition of the thyroid system and peculiarity of forming its pathology in the BSSR population under influence of the iodine-radionuclides in connection with Chernobyl nuclear accident. (In Russian) Zdravoohranenie Belorussi 1990; 6:11–15.
129. Astakhova LN, Demidchuk EP, Davydova EV, et al. Health status of Byelorussian children and adolescents exposed to radiation as consequence of the Chernobyl atomic energy station accident. (In Russian) Vestn Akad Med Nauk USSR 1991; 11:25–27.
130. Okeanov AE, Averkin YI. Analysis of malignant neoplasms in population of the Republic of Belarus before and after the Chernobyl accident. In Matyukhin VA, Astakhova LN, Konigsberg YE, Nalivko SN, editors. Catastrophe at the Chernobyl Atomic Energy Station and Estimation of Health State of Population of the Republic of Belarus. Minsk: Research Institute of Radiation Medicine, 1991:25–33.
131. Astakhova LN, Vorontsova TV, Drozd VM. Thyroid nodule pathology in children of Belarus following the Chernobyl accident. In Robbins J, editor. Treatment of Thyroid Cancer in Childhood. Proceedings of a workshop on September 10-11, 1992, at the National Institutes of Health. Publication No. DOE/EH-0406 1992; 35.
132. Baverstock K, Egloff B, Finchera A, Ruchti C, Williams D. Thyroid cancer after Chernobyl. Nature 1992; 359:21–22.
133. Demidchik EP, Kazakov VS, Astakhova LN, et al. Thyroid cancer in children after the Chernobyl accident: clinical and epidemiological evaluation of 251 cases in the Republic of Belarus. In Nagataki S, editor. Nagasaki Symposium on Chernobyl: Update and Future. Amsterdam: Elsevier, 1994:21.
134. Demidchik EP, Drobyshevskaya IM, Cherstvoy ED, et al. Thyroid cancer in children in Belarus. In Karaoglou A, Desmet G, Kelly GN, Menzel HG, editors. The Radiological Consequences of the Chernobyl Accident. Brussels: European Commission, 1996:677–682.
135. Abelin T, Averkin JI, Egger M, et al. Thyroid cancer in Belarus post-Chernobyl: improved detection or increased incidence? Soz Praventivmed 1994; 39:189–197.
136. Averkin JI, Abelin T, Bleuer JP. Thyroid cancer in children in Belarus: ascertainment bias? Lancet 1995; 346:1223–1224.
137. Abelin T, Egger M, Ruchti C. Belarus increase was probably caused by Chernobyl. BMJ 1994; 309:1298.
138. Williams ED, Cherstvoy E, Egloff B, et al. Interaction of pathology and molecular characterization of thyroid cancers. In Karaoglou A, Desmet G, Kelly GN, Menzel HG, editors. The Radiological Consequences of the Chernobyl Accident. Brussels: European Commission, 1996:699–714.
139. Abelin T, Averkin JI, Okeanov AE, Bleuer JP. Thyroid cancer in Belarus: the epidemiologic situation. In Karaoglou A, Desmet G, Kelly GN, Menzel HG, editors. The Radiological Consequences of the Chernobyl Accident. Brussels: European Commission, 1996:727–730.
140. Malko M. Chernobyl radiation induced thyroid cancers in Belarus. Joint Institute of Power and Nuclear Research, National Academy of Science of Belarus, pp. 240–255. Available on: www-j.rri.kyoto-u.ac.jp/NSRG/reports/ kr79/kr79pdf/Malko2.pdf.
141. Demidchik YE, Demidchik EP. Thyroid carcinomas in Belarus 16 years after the Chernobyl disaster. In Proceedings of Symposium of Chernobyl-Related Health Effects. Tokyo, Japan: Radiation Effects Association, 2002.
142. Tsyb AF, Parshkov EM, Ivanov VK, Stepanenko VF, Matveenko EG, Skoropad YD. Disease indices of thyroid and their dose dependence in children and adolescents affected as a result of the Chernobyl accident. In Nagataki S, editor. Amsterdam: Elsevier Science, 1994:9–19.
143. Remennik LV, Starinsky VV, Mokina VD, et al. Malignant neoplasms on the territories of Russia damaged owing to the Chernobyl accident. In Karaoglou A, Desmet G, Kelly GN, Menzel HG, editors. The Radiological Consequences of the Chernobyl Accident. Brussels: European Commission, 1996:825–828.
144. Tronko N, Bogdanova T, Komissarenko I, et al. Thyroid cancer in children and adolescents in Ukraine after the Chernobyl accident. In Karaoglou A, Desmet G, Kelly GN, Menzel HG, editors. The Radiological Consequences of the Chernobyl Accident. Brussels: European Commission, 1996: 683–690.
145. Tronko N, Epstein Y, Oleinik V, et al. Thyroid gland in children after the Chernobyl accident (yesterday and today). In Nagataki S, editor. Nagasaki symposium on Chernobyl: update and future. Amsterdam: Elsevier, 1994:31–46.
146. Williams ED, Tronko ND. Molecular, Cellular, Biological Characterization of Childhood Thyroid Cancer. Brussels: European Commission, 1996.
147. Cherstvoy E, Pozcharskaya V, Harach HR, Thomas GA, Williams ED. The pathology of childhood thyroid carcinoma in Belarus. In Karaoglou A, Desmet G, Kelly GN, Menzel HG, editors. The Radiological Consequences of the Chernobyl Accident. Brussels: European Commission, 1996:779–784.
148. Bogdanova T, Bragarnik M, Tronko ND, Harach HR, Thomas GA, William ED. The pathology of thyroid cancer in Ukraine post Chernobyl. In Karaoglou A, Desmet G, Kelly GN, Menzel HG, editors. The Radiological Consequences of the Chernobyl Accident. Brussels: European Commission, 1996:785–789.
149. Abrosimov AY, Lushnikov EF, Tsyb AF, Harach HR, Thomas GA, Williams ED. The pathology of childhood thyroid tumours in the Russian Federation after Chernobyl. In Karaoglou A, Desmet G, Kelly GN, Menzel HG, editors. The Radiological Consequences of the Chernobyl Accident. Brussels: European Commission, 1996:791–793.
150. Furmanchuk AW, Averkin JI, Egloff B, et al. Pathomorphological findings in thyroid cancers of children from the Republic of Belarus: a study of 86 cases occurring between 1986 ("post-Chernobyl") and 1991. Histopathology 1992; 21:401–408.
151. Nikiforov Y, Gnepp DR. Pediatric thyroid cancer after the Chernobyl disaster. Cancer 1994; 74:748–766.
152. Williams ED. Thyroid cancer in United Kingdom children and in children exposed to fallout from Chernobyl. In Nagataki S, editor. Nagasaki symposium on Chernobyl: update and future. Tokyo, Japan: Elsevier, 1994.
153. Nikiforov Y, Gnepp DR, Fagin JA. Thyroid lesions in children and adolescents after the Chernobyl disaster: implications for the study of radiation tumorigenesis. J Clin Endocrinol Metab 1996; 81:9–14.
154. Pacini F, Vorontsova T, Demidchik EP, et al. Diagnosis, surgical treatment and follow-up of thyroid cancers. In Karaoglou A, Desmet G, Kelly GN, Menzel HG, editors. The Radiological Consequences of the Chernobyl Accident. Brussels: European Commission, 1996: 755–763.
155. Nikiforov YE, Heffess CS, Korzenko AV, Fagin JA, Gnepp DR. Characteristics of follicular tumors and nonneoplastic thyroid lesions in children and adolescents exposed to radiation as a result of the Chernobyl disaster. Cancer 1995; 76:900–909.
156. Sierk AE, Askin FB, Reddick RL, Thomas CG. Pediatric thyroid cancer. Pediatr Pathol 1990; 10:877–893.
157. Harness JK, Thompson NW, Nishiyama RH. Childhood thyroid carcinoma. Arch Surg 1971; 102:278–284.
158. Richardson JE, Beaugie JM, Brown CL, Doniach I. Thyroid cancer in young patients in Great Britain. Br J Surg 1974; 61:85–89.
159. Tallroth E, Backdahl M, Einhorn J, Lundell G, Lowhagen T, Silfversward C. Thyroid carcinoma in children and adolescents. Cancer 1986; 58:2329–2332.
160. Mizukami Y, Michigishi T, Nonomura A, et al. Carcinoma of the thyroid at young age: a review of 23 patients. Histopathology 1992; 20:63–66.
161. Robbins J. Characteristics of spontaneous and radiation induced thyroid cancers in children. In Nagataki S, editor. Nagasaki Symposium on Chernobyl: Update and Future. Amsterdam: Elsevier, 1994:81.
162. Williams ED. Radiation-induced thyroid cancer. Histopathology 1993; 23:387–389.
163. Willams ED. Chernobyl, eight years on. Nature 1994; 371:556.

164. Williams D. Thyroid cancer and the Chernobyl accident. J Clin Endocrinol Metab 1996; 81:6–8.
165. Ito T, Seyama T, Iwamoto KS, Mizuno T, Tronko ND, Komissarenko IV, et al. Activated RET oncogene in thyroid cancers of children from areas contaminated by Chernobyl accident. Lancet 1994; 344:259.
166. Fugazzola L, Pilotti S, Pinchera A, et al. Oncogenic rearrangements of the RET proto-oncogene in papillary thyroid carcinomas from children exposed to the Chernobyl nuclear accident. Cancer Res 1995; 55:5617–5620.
167. Nikiforov YE, Rowland JM, Bove KE, Monforte-Munoz H, Fagin JA. Distinct pattern of ret oncogene rearrangements in morphological variants of radiation-induced and sporadic thyroid papillary carcinomas in children. Cancer Res 1997; 57:1690–1694.
168. Klugbauer S, Lengfelder E, Demidchik EP, Rabes HM. High prevalence of RET rearrangement in thyroid tumors of children from Belarus after the Chernobyl reactor accident. Oncogene 1995; 11:2459–2467.
169. Rabes HM, Klugbauer S. Radiation-induced thyroid carcinomas in children: high prevalence of RET rearrangement. (German) Verh Dtsch Ges Pathol 1997; 81:139–144.
170. Klugbauer S, Lengfelder E, Demidchik EP, Rabes HM. A new form of RET rearrangement in thyroid carcinomas of children after the Chernobyl reactor accident. Oncogene 1996; 13:1099–1102.
171. Klugbauer S, Demidchik EP, Lengfelder E, Rabes HM. Molecular analysis of new subtypes of ELE/RET rearrangements, their reciprocal transcripts and breakpoints in papillary thyroid carcinomas of children after Chernobyl. Oncogene 1998; 16:671–675.
172. Fugazzola L, Pierotti M, Vigano E, Pacini F, Verontsova T, Bongarzone I. Molecular and biochemical analysis of RET/PTC4, a novel oncogeneic rearrangement between RET and ELE1 genes, in a post-Chernobyl papillary thyroid cancer. Oncogene 1996; 13:1093–1097.
173. Klugbauer S, Demidchik EP, Lengfelder E, Rabes HM. Detection of a novel type of RET rearrangement (PTC5) in thyroid carcinomas after Chernobyl and analysis of the involved RET-fused gene RFG5. Cancer Res 1998; 58:198–203.
174. Klugbauer S, Rabes HM. The transcription coactivator HTIF1 and a related protein are fused to the RET receptor tyrosine kinase in childhood papillary thyroid carcinomas. Oncogene 1999; 18:4388–93.
175. Salassidis K, Bruch J, Zitzelsberger H, Lengfelder E, Kellerer AM, Bauchinger M. Translocation t(10;14)(q11.2:q22.1) fusing the kinectin to the RET gene creates a novel rearranged form (PTC8) of the RET proto-oncogene in radiation-induced childhood papillary thyroid carcinoma. Cancer Res 2000; 60:2786–2789.
176. Klugbauer S, Jauch A, Lengfelder E, Demidchik E, Rabes HM. A novel type of RET rearrangement (PTC8) in childhood papillary thyroid carcinomas and characterization of the involved gene (RFG8). Cancer Res 2000; 60:7028–7032.
177. Rabes HM, Demidchik EP, Sidorow JD, et al. Pattern of radiation-induced RET and NTRK1 rearrangements in 191 post-Chernobyl papillary thyroid carcinomas: biological, phenotypic, and clinical implications. Clin Cancer Res 2000; 6:1093–1103.
178. Rabes HM. Gene rearrangements in radiation-induced thyroid carcinogenesis. Med Pediatr Oncol 2001; 36:574–582.
179. Pisarchik AV, Ermak G, Fomicheva V, Kartel NA, Figge J. The ret/PTC1 rearrangement is a common feature of Chernobyl-associated papillary thyroid carcinomas from Belarus. Thyroid 1998; 8:133–139.
180. Pisarchik AV, Ermak G, Demidchik EP, Mikhalevich LS, Kartel NA, Figge J. Low prevalence of the ret/PTC3r1 rearrangement in a series of papillary thyroid carcinomas presenting in Belarus ten year post-Chernobyl. Thyroid 1998; 8:1003–1008.
181. Pisarchik AV, Yarmolinskii DG, Demidchik YE, Ermak GZ, Kartel NA, Figge J. ret/PTC1 and ret/PTC3r1 rearrangement in thyroid cancer cells, arising in residents of Belarus in the period after the accident at the Chernobyl nuclear power plant. (In Russian) Genetika 2000; 36:959–964.
182. Smida J, Salassidis K, Hieber L, et al. Distinct frequency of ret rearrangements in papillary thyroid carcinomas of children and adults from Belarus. Int J Cancer 1999; 80:32–38.
183. Thomas GA, Bunnell H, Cook HA, et al. High prevalence of RET/PTC rearrangements in Ukrainian and Belarussian post-Chernobyl thyroid papillary carcinomas: a strong correlation between RET/PTC3 and the solid-follicular variant. J Clin Endocrinol Metab 1999; 84:4232–4238.
184. Santoro M, Thomas GA, Vecchio G, et al. Gene rearrangement and Chernobyl related thyroid cancers. Br J Cancer. 2000; 82:315–322.
185. Williams ED, Abrosimov A, Bogdanova T, et al. Thyroid carcinoma after Chernobyl latent period, morphology and aggressiveness. Br J Cancer 2004; 90:2219–2224.
186. Elisei R, Romei C, Vorontsova T, et al. RET/PTC rearrangements in thyroid nodules: studies in irradiated and not irradiated, malignant and benign thyroid lesions in children and adults. J Clin Endocrinol Metab 2001; 86:3211–3216.
187. Jhiang SM, Sagartz JE, Tong Q, et al. Targeted expression of the RET/PTC1 oncogene induces papillary thyroid carcinomas. Endocrinology 1996; 137:375–378.
188. Santoro M, Chiappetta G, Cerrato A, et al. Development of thyroid papillary carcinomas secondary to tissue-specific expression of the RET/PTC1 oncogene in transgenic mice. Oncogene 1996; 12:1821–1826.
189. Powell DJ Jr, Russell J, Nibu K, et al. The RET/PTC3 oncogene: metastatic solid-type papillary carcinomas in murine thyroids. Cancer Res 1998; 58:5523–5528.
190. Ito T, Seyama T, Iwamoto KS, et al. In vitro irradiation is able to cause RET oncogene rearrangement. Cancer Res 1993; 53:2940–2943.
191. Bounacer A, Wicker R, Caillou B, et al. High prevalence of activating ret proto-oncogene rearrangements, in thyroid tumors from patients who had received external radiation. Oncogene 1997; 15:1263–1273.
192. Collins BJ, Chiappetta G, Schneider AB, et al. RET expression in papillary thyroid cancer from patients irradiated in childhood for benign conditions. J Clin Endocrinol Metab 2002; 87:3941–3946.
193. Butti MG, Bongarzone I, Ferraresi G, Mondellini P, Borrello MG, Pierotti MA. A sequence analysis of the genomic regions involved in the rearrangements between TPM3 and NTRK1 genes producing TRK oncogenes in papillary thyroid carcinomas. Genomics 1995; 28:15–24.
194. Beimfohr C, Klugbauer S, Demidchik EP, Lengfelder E, Rabes HM. NTRK1 re-arrangement in papillary thyroid carcinomas of children after the Chernobyl reactor accident. Int J Cancer. 1999; 80:842–847.
195. Nikiforov YE, Nikiforova MN, Gnepp DR, Fagin JA. Prevalence of mutations of ras and p53 in benign and malignant thyroid tumors from children exposed to radiation after the Chernobyl nuclear accident. Oncogene 1996; 13:687–693.
196. Hillebrandt S, Streffer C, Reiners C, Demidchik E. Mutations in the p53 tumor suppressor gene in thyroid tumors of children from areas contaminated by the Chernobyl accident. Int J Radial Biol 1996; 69:39–45.
197. Hillebrandt S, Streffer C, Demidchik EP, Biko J, Reiners C. Polymorphisms in the p53 gene in thyroid tumors and blood samples of children from areas in Belarus. Mutat Res 1997; 381:201–207.
198. Smida J, Zitzelsberger H, Kellerer AM, et al. P53 mutations in childhood thyroid tumors from Belarus and in thyroid tumors without radiation history. Int J Cancer 1997; 73:802–807.
199. Suchy B, Waldmann V, Klugbauer S, Rabes HM. Absence of RAS and p53 mutations in thyroid carcinomas of children after Chernobyl in contrast to adult thyroid tumors. Br J Cancer 1998; 77:952–955.
200. Pisarchik AV, Ermak G, Kartel NA, Figge J. Molecular alterations involving p53 codons 167 and 183 in papillary thyroid carcinomas

from Chernobyl-contaminated regions of Belarus. Thyroid 2000; 10:25–30.
201. Beral V, Reeves G. Childhood thyroid cancer in Belarus. Nature 1992; 359:680–681.
202. Shigematsu I, Thiessen JW. Childhood thyroid cancer in Belarus. Nature 1992; 359:681.
203. Beebe GW. Epidemiologic studies of thyroid cancer in the CIS. In Karaoglou A, Desmet G, Kelly GN, Menzel HG, editors. The Radiological Consequences of the Chernobyl Accident. Brussels: European Commission, 1996:731–740.
204. Astakhova LN, Anspaugh LR, Beebe GW, Bouville A, Drozdovitch VV, Garber V, et al. Chernobyl-related thyroid cancer in children of Belarus: a case-control study. Radiat Res 1998; 150:349–356.
205. Jacob P, Goulko G, Heidenreich WF, et al. Thyroid cancer risk to children calculated. Nature 1998; 392:31–32.
206. Shibata Y, Yamashita S, Masyakin VB, Panasyuk GD, Nagataki S. 15 years after Chernobyl: new evidence of thyroid cancer. Lancet 2001; 358:1965–1966.
207. Robbins J, Dunn JT, Bouville A, et al. Iodine nutrition and the risk from radioactive iodine: a workshop report in the Chernobyl long-term follow-up study. Thyroid 2001; 11:487–491.
208. Cardis E, Okeanov AE. What is feasible and desirable in the epidemiologic follow-up of Chernobyl. In Karaoglou A, Desmet G, Kelly GN, Menzel HG, editors. The Radiological Consequences of the Chernobyl Accident. Brussels: European Commission, 1996: 835–850.

8
Classification of Thyroid Malignancies

Yolanda C. Oertel

We follow the World Health Organization (WHO) Histological Classification of Thyroid Tumors (1) and that of the AFIP Atlas of Tumor Pathology (2). See Table 1.

Many thyroid cancers arise in essentially normal thyroid tissue. Most grow slowly and are amenable to appropriate treatment. The majority are papillary cancers, especially in those areas of the world in which adequate iodides are present in the diet and environment.

Proper handling of the tissues is crucial to produce good histological sections for accurate diagnosis. Incomplete fixation of any thyroid tissue may produce loss of cellular details and pale nuclei in the sections (thus, a superficial resemblance to the nuclei of papillary carcinoma).

The pathologist must provide the following: weight of the specimen; exact size of the neoplasm; its relation to the borders of the thyroid gland; if there is a capsule present around the tumor; whether the neoplastic cells extend directly beyond the border of the thyroid (and if so, which tissues are involved); histological diagnosis of the tumor (including the histologic patterns and mitotic activity); and whether any lymph nodes in the specimen contain metastatic tumor. Brief descriptions are also needed of the nonneoplastic thyroid parenchyma and any other thyroid tumors present, and if so, their histological diagnoses. The results of special procedures (e.g., immunoperoxidase stains, analysis of nuclear ploidy, *in situ* hybridization of nucleic acids) should be provided if these are available at reasonable cost.

Critical assessment of any special laboratory procedures is important if they are significant in the pathologic interpretation. The reagents must be of high quality, the technical assistance should be skillful, and all the personnel involved must be experienced.

SPECIAL STUDIES

Evaluation of nuclear DNA content by flow cytometry or imaging photometry suggests that aneuploidy in the differentiated carcinomas may have adverse effects on survival in patients who do not have metastases at the time of initial diagnosis (3–5). Apparently, aneuploidy does not have diag-

Table 1
Classification of Thyroid Tumors

Primary Malignant Tumors
  Malignant tumors of follicular cells
    Follicular carcinoma
    Papillary carcinoma
    Poorly differentiated carcinoma
    Undifferentiated (anaplastic) carcinoma
  Malignant tumors of C cells
    Medullary carcinoma
  Malignant tumors of mixed follicular and C cells
  Miscellaneous epithelial tumors
    Squamous cell carcinoma, adenosquamous carcinoma, mucin-producing carcinoma
    Hyalinizing trabecular neoplasms (predominantly adenomas)
    Neoplasms associated with familial intestinal adenomatous polyposis
    Mucoepidermoid carcinoma
    Thymic and related neoplasms
    Teratomas
  Malignant nonepithelial tumors
    Malignant lymphoma
    Sarcomas
Secondary Tumors
  Metastatic melanoma
  Metastatic renal cell carcinoma
  Metastatic mammary carcinoma
  Metastatic pulmonary carcinoma

nostic significance. Studies of H-*ras*, K-*ras*, and N-*ras* proto-oncogenes demonstrate mutations in some follicular carcinomas as opposed to adenomas (6). The N-*ras* mutation in papillary carcinoma increases the chance of death (7). The p53 protein is a tumor suppressor protein with a rapid turnover. If it is inactivated or present in a mutant form, it accumulates in the nuclei. Detecting this protein indicates a loss of differentiation and is associated with unfavorable prognosis factors. It has been found in numerous examples of poorly differentiated and undifferentiated carcinomas, contrasting its absence or infrequent occurrence in differentiated carcinomas

(8–10). Conversely, *bcl-2* expression is rare in undifferentiated carcinoma but is common in well-differentiated carcinoma and poorly differentiated carcinoma *(11)*. More recently, emphasis is being placed on the molecular profile of thyroidal neoplasms instead of their morphological appearance to differentiate between benign and malignant tumors *(12)*.

REFERENCES

1. Hedinger C, Williams ED, Sobin LH. Histological typing of thyroid tumours. World Health Organization International Histological Classification of Tumours, 2nd ed. Berlin: Springer-Verlag, 1988.
2. Rosai J, Carcangiu ML, DeLellis RA. Tumors of the thyroid gland. In Rosai J, Sobin H, editors. Atlas of Tumor Pathology, 3rd Series, Fasc 5. Washington, DC: A. F. I. P, 1992.
3. Hay ID. Papillary thyroid carcinoma. Endocrinol Metab Clin North Am 1990; 19:545–576.
4. Pasieka L, Zedenius J, Auer G, et al. Addition of nuclear DNA content to the AMES risk-group classification for papillary thyroid cancer. Surgery 1992; 112:1154–1160.
5. Nishida T, Nakao K, Hamaji M, Nakahara M, Tsujimoto M. Overexpression of p53 protein and DNA content are important biologic prognostic factors for thyroid cancer. 1996; 119:568–575.
6. Sciacchitano S, Paliotta DS, Nardi F, Sacchi A, Andreoli M, Pontecorvi A. PCR amplification and analysis of RAS oncogenes from thyroid cytologic smears. Diagn Mol Pathol 1994; 3:114–121.
7. Hara H, Fulton N, Yashiro T, Ito K, DeGroot LJ, Kaplan EL. N-Ras mutation: an independent prognostic factor for aggressiveness of papillary thyroid carcinoma. Surgery 1994; 116:1010–1016.
8. Fagin JA, Matsuo K, Karmaker A, Chen DL, Tang S-H, Koeffler HP. High prevalence of mutations of the p53 gene in poorly differentiated human thyroid carcinomas. J Clin Invest 1993; 91:179–184.
9. Donghi R, Longoni A, Pilotti S, Michieli P, Delia Porta G, Pierotti MA. Gene p53 mutations are restricted to poorly differentiated and undifferentiated carcinomas of the thyroid gland. J Clin Invest 1993; 91:1753–1760.
10. Soares P, Cameselle-Teijeiro J, Sobrinho-Simoes M. Immunohistochemical detection of p53 in differentiated, poorly differentiated and undifferentiated carcinomas of the thyroid. Histopathology 1994; 24:205–210.
11. Pilotti S, Collini P, Del Bo R, Cattoretti G, Pierotti MA, Rilke F. A novel panel of antibodies that segregates immunocytochemically poorly differentiated carcinoma from undifferentiated carcinoma of the thyroid gland. Am J Surg Pathol 1994; 18:1054–1064.
12. Mazzanti C, Zeiger MA, Costourous N, Umbricht C, Westra WH, Smith D, et al. Using gene expression profiling to differentiate benign versus malignant thyroid tumors. Cancer Res 2004; 64:2898–2903.

9
Staging of Thyroid Cancer

Leonard Wartofsky

DEFINITION AND UTILITY OF STAGING

In general, the "stage" of a cancer refers to a phase in the course of the tumor when it has reached some defined level of extent. The extent of the tumor is a measure of its size and whether it has spread elsewhere. As thyroid cancers grow, they are first confined to the thyroid gland, then may extend in variable degrees to the subcutaneous tissues and lymph nodes of the neck, and finally, potentially to distant sites of the body. Staging a tumor allows a more accurate description of the extent of disease in a given patient in objective and standardized terms. Staging permits communication between patients and physicians about their prognosis. This is facilitated by the fact that clinical investigators analyze and report their experience with various therapeutic approaches and express their results based on the staging of their patient population. Then therapeutic approaches may be selected for the patient based on these published studies on treatment results in comparably staged patients. A standardized staging vocabulary also allows more precise communication among physicians about the degree of disease present.

Thus, examining the thyroid cancer literature enables a better perspective of the potential outcome for our patients according to the results seen in hundreds or thousands of other patients at the same stage of disease. Prediction of outcome relates to prognosis of the various thyroid cancers and is discussed by Burch in several chapters below related to specific tumors. Prognosis may be expressed as life expectancy or the likelihood of achieving a full cure, remission, possible residual, but nonlife-threatening, persistent disease, or in the worst case scenario, death. Tumors classified as stage 1 or 2 are typically considered to be "low risk" tumors with excellent-to-good prognosis, whereas stage 3 or 4 tumors are often described as being "high risk," implying a greater chance of residual disease after initial treatment, recurrence, or death. The overwhelming majority of thyroid cancer patients will fall into stages 1 and 2 and have excellent prognosis with little risk for recurrence or death

from their disease. In one large Mayo Clinic review of over 1400 patients with papillary thyroid cancer (PTC) (1), there was a remarkable 25-yr survival of 97% in patients who had complete surgical resection of their apparent disease. Thirty-year survival rates of 75–85% are not unusual for such patients with low death rates. Stage 2 and 3 patients may have recurrences that require additional therapy but may still be at relatively low risk of death. A worse prognosis is associated with extensive local invasion at presentation and even more so with distant metastases, especially those to bone.

Outcome in patients with papillary cancer may vary widely because some of these tumors may be very small (<1.0 cm) or so-called "microcarcinomas," and these tumors show little evidence of invasion and usually have an excellent outcome. Alternatively, other PTCs may grow rapidly, invade tissues aggressively, metastasize widely, and ultimately cause death. Staging of PTC is based on the patient characteristics that have been shown to impact prognosis. Many clinical and pathologic characteristics have been evaluated as predictors of tumor behavior and ultimate patient prognosis. For example, both the extent of disease and age of the patient at presentation are important determinants of outcome (2,3). The extent of disease could refer to invasion of the tumor into extrathyroidal soft tissues of the neck, spread to regional lymph nodes, or metastases to more distant sites. The extent of disease may be determined by clinical, radiological, and pathological examinations to include biopsy of suspicious lymph nodes. Awareness of distant metastases may be suggested by the finding of high levels of serum thyroglobulin postoperatively but may not be confirmed until a total-body radioisotopic survey scan is performed (4).

STAGING SCORING SYSTEMS
AMES System

A large number of staging systems currently exist that have been developed at various medical centers over the

Table 1
TNM Staging System

Tumor Size
TX	Primary tumor cannot be assessed
T0	No evidence of primary tumor
T1	Tumor ≤2 cm in greatest dimension limited to thyroid
T2	Tumor >2 cm but <4 cm in greatest dimension and limited to the thyroid
T3	Tumor >4 cm in greatest dimension limited to the thyroid, or tumor of any size with minimal extrathyroid extension (e.g., to sternothyroid muscle or perithyroid soft tissues)
T4a	Tumor of any size extending beyond the thyroid capsule and invading local soft tissues, larynx, trachea, esophagus, or recurrent laryngeal nerve
T4b	Tumor invading prevertebral fascia, mediastinal vessels, or encasing carotid artery in the neck

Nodes
NX	Regional nodes cannot be assessed
N0	No metastases to regional nodes
N1	Metastases to regional nodes are present
N1A	To level 6 (pretracheal, paratracheal, prelaryngeal, and Delphian lymph nodes)
N1B	In other unilateral, bilateral, or contralateal cervical or mediastinal lymph nodes

Metastases
MX	Presence of distant metastases cannot be assessed
M0	No distant metastases
M1	Distant metastases are present

past several decades. Most systems include the key prognostic factors of patient age, tumor size, and extent of disease but may add other characteristics thought to lend greater specificity to the staging. According to preference, bias, or experience, different staging systems may be favored by various endocrinologists or may be more popular at certain specific medical centers. One such system, known as the AMES system, where the AMES letters refer to age (A), metastases (M), extent of tumor (E), and tumor size (S). This system classifies patients as either low or high risk (5). Low-risk patients would include: tumor size less than 5 cm, papillary cancer without evidence of extrathyroidal invasion, follicular carcinoma without major vascular or capsular invasion, and tumors in men less than 40 yr old or women under 50 yr old without evidence of metastatic disease. Any tumor that does not meet these criteria would be classified as high risk. Cady and Rossi (5) reported 89% of 310 patients were low-risk patients seen to have a recurrence rate of 5%, whereas the remaining high-risk patients had a recurrence rate of 55%. The same group reported the 20-yr survival statistics on a subsequent larger series of 1019 patients, of whom the low-risk patients had a recurrence rate of 5% and a survival of 98% compared to 50% in the high-risk group (6). Moreover, recurrence in the high-risk patients was associated with a 75% mortality. They concluded that the AMES criteria were valid predictors of risk.

TNM System

Some differences pertain to staging systems used by clinicians compared to those used by pathologists. One of the most popular staging systems is called the "TNM" classification system, developed by the American Joint Commission on Cancer (AJCC), and it is used by pathologists for most malignancies as well as for thyroid cancer. TNM refers to tumor size (T), involvement of lymph nodes (N), and the presence of distant metastases (M). Based on the tumor characteristics, the disease stage is described by assigning a numerical score to each of the characteristics reflecting the extent of disease present. The AJCC system was developed in 1959, derived from an earlier European system initiated by the International Union Against Cancer or Union Internationale Contre le Cancer (UICC; 7). Updated versions of the AJCC manual for staging are published every few years; the most recent is the sixth edition published in 2002 (3).

Tumor Size

For tumor size, designations of T-0 to T-4 reflect a range of tumor sizes and whether local invasion was seen. For example, a small tumor of less than 2 cm confined to the thyroid is classified as T1; a very large tumor or one invading local tissues would be a T4, with intermediate levels designated as T2 or T3. Tumor size refers to the original single malignant nodule or the largest nodule in a gland with multifocal lesions. As can be seen in Table 2, it is only in patients over age 45 that tumor size influences the "T" score in the TNM system and ultimately the designated stage of disease. This is so because virtually all patients underage 45 fall into the category of low risk (stages 1 or 2) and by definition, there are no young patients classified as stage 3 or stage 4. The impact of tumor size on prognosis can be recognized by examining outcomes in a large series of patients with PTC seen at the Mayo Clinic *(8)*. Cancer-specific mortality was directly related to increasing tumor size with a 20-yr mortality of 0.8% for patients with tumors less than 2.0-cm diameter; 6% for tumors 2.0–3.9 cm; 16% for tumors 4.0–6.9 cm; and 50% for tumors greater than 7 cm. When the tumor was confined to the thyroid, the death rate was 1.9%, whereas those patients whose tumor extended through the thyroid capsule into the surrounding tissues of the neck had a 20-yr mortality of 28%. Outcomes were the most poor in those patients with distant metastases at presentation who experienced a 10-yr mortality rate of 69%, compared to 3% in patients with tumors confined to the neck.

Multifocality

In the majority (~70%) of patients with thyroid cancer, the tumor is confined to one lobe or one side of the thyroid gland; in about 20–40% of patients, the tumor is found in the contralatreral lobe as well. Some studies have suggested that multifocal tumors may have a worse prognosis *(9)*, but this notion is controversial. Multifocality of cancer may relate to "seeding" of the tumor throughout the gland via intrathyroidal lymphatics or direct extension, but molecular typing also has demonstrated that many arise *de novo*. Multifocal tumors are also seen when there is a history of some carcinogenic environmental factor, such as exposure to external or internal radiation as seen after the Chernobyl nuclear plant accident in the Soviet Union in April 1986. Multifocal tumors are more likely to have regional lymph node involvement *(10)*.

Lymph Node Involvement

The "N" designation describes the extent of lymph nodes involved. Regional lymph nodes are defined as bilateral cervical and upper mediastinal nodes. Several staging systems include subcategories designated "A" or "B" to describe whether the involved lymph nodes were on the side of the neck of the original cancer or on the opposite side. About 35–40% of patients presenting with papillary thyroid cancer have involvement of either cervical or mediastinal lymph nodes, or both. When a papillary cancer is more aggressive, as evident by widespread involvement throughout the thyroid gland, the likelihood of lymph node metastases approaches 75% *(9)*. In addition to the staging of lymph node involvement based on the surgical findings, the extent of lymph node involvement can be determined by ultrasound examinations of the neck or by computed tomography (CT) or magnetic resonance imaging (MRI) scans of the neck and mediastinum. The significance of lymph node metastases in the neck on prognosis and ultimate outcome has been debated. Different perspectives from different authors or medical centers may be owing to application of varying staging criteria to thyroid cancers of different pathologic type and grade. Two large series of patients from the Mayo Clinic *(8)* and Memorial Sloan Kettering *(10)* concluded that the presence of tumor in lymph nodes had no adverse impact on either recurrence or survival. However, another series of patients reported by Mazzaferri and Jiang *(9)*, that differed from the latter two series by the inclusion of the effect of routine radioiodine ablation on outcome, did demonstrate that lymph node metastases in the neck were an important independent predictive factor for both recurrence and survival. Most workers in the field of thyroid cancer now accept the importance of neck node metastases, and this is reflected in the various staging systems described in this chapter.

Beasley et al. *(11)* reviewed their experience with 347 patients with stage 1 disease and another 118 patients with stage 2 disease. Patients with multifocal intrathyroidal disease were more likely to have neck node metastases, and those patients with positive neck nodes had higher rates of recurrence and lower rates of disease-free survival, as well as reduced overall survival. Those patients who presented with disease in lymph nodes outside of the central compartment of the neck (e.g., in the lateral compartments of the neck or in the mediastinum) were seen to have a greater than six-fold relative risk of recurrence. Because of this greater risk, it may be argued that larger ablative doses of radioiodine should be employed in such patients, and a more frequent or greater degree of tumor surveillance should be exercised.

Distant Metastases

Distant metastases are scored as either present (M1) or absent (M0). Loh and coworkers *(2)* found the TNM system of staging to be a useful method in regard to correlation with observed outcomes based on a retrospective analysis of 700 patients over a 25-yr period. A CT or MRI may be useful to determine if there are distant metastases as well. Because of their propensity to invade blood vessels, follicular carcinomas are more likely to spread to distant sites in the lung or bone. The presence of distant metastases to the lung or bone is typically discovered on the first postoperative and postradioiodine therapy nuclear scan. For bone, radioactive iodine is generally more useful to detect metastases than technetium pyrophosphate.

Impact of Age on Staging

In the AJCC system, two patients ages 25 and 47, with comparable tumor size and distant metastases, could be quite differently staged. The first could have stage 2, and the older patient could have stage 4 because the AJCC system puts a great deal of weight on patient age (see Table 2). Indeed, age of diagnosis appears to be the most important factor in terms of having an impact on prognosis, with clearly more aggressive tumor behavior likely after age 40–45. In one large retrospective review of 15,698 cases of thyroid cancer, age was a stronger predictor of survival for patients with follicular carcinoma than for papillary carcinoma *(12)*.

Table 2
Impact of Age on TNM Staging

	Less Than 45 yr of Age	45 yr or Older
Stage 1	any T, any N, M0	T1, N0, M0
Stage 2	any T, any N, M1	T2, N0, M0
Stage 3	N/A	T3, N0, M0 or T1–T3, N1A, M0
Stage 4A	N/A	T1–T3, N1B, M0
		T4a, N0–N1, M0
4B		T4b, Nx, M0
4C		Tx, Nx, M1

The staging for PTC is designated as stage 1, 2, 3, or 4 based on the TNM status and age of patient. N/A

The impact of age on prognosis also can be seen in the outcomes of a large series of patients with PTC seen at the Mayo Clinic over a 40-yr period (8). Cancer-specific mortality rates at 20 yr were 0.8% for patients below 50 yr of age; 7% for patients 50–59 yr of age; 20% for patients 60–69 yr of age; and 47% for patients ages 70 or older. Although not as important as age, the size of the original tumor is also important; tumors less than 1.5 cm have the best prognosis, and those more than 4 cm have the worst prognosis. Finally, a worse prognosis is also associated with extensive local invasion and even more so with distant metastases, especially those to bone. Some investigators have also incorporated the histological grade of the tumor into the prognostic score (1,13).

Histologic Variants of Papillary Cancer

Most patients with stage 1 or 2 PTC present with disease that is readily amenable to treatment, i.e., low-risk tumor. Not infrequently, pathologists see many follicular elements interspersed within the usual papillary cancer, and these tumors are designated as "follicular" variants of PTC. However, in their biological and clinical course, these tumors tend to behave like papillary cancers, rather than like follicular cancers. However, some subtypes of PTC typically behave somewhat more aggressively and, consequently, tend to have a worse prognosis than the common forms of papillary thyroid cancer. These subtypes are known by the pathologic terms used to describe the microscopic appearance of the cells and include tumors designated as the "tall-cell" variant, the "columnar" variant, and "insular" papillary thyroid cancer (14). Because these variant tumors are relatively more rare, inferences regarding prognosis from small published series may not be accurate. Sywak et al. (15) collated all the cases in the published literature and analyzed 209 cases of the tall-cell variant, concluding that it was a more aggressive tumor that was associated with distant metastases in 22% of patients and had a tumor-related mortality of 16%. Similar outcomes with the tall-cell variant were observed by Prindiville et al. (16). When encapsulated, the columnar cell variant had an excellent prognosis but was associated with an even higher mortality rate of 32% when not encapsulated (41 reported cases). The insular variant (213 cases) was also shown as more aggressive, with a 64% likelihood of recurrence or distant metastases and a 32% mortality rate. Although these variants may behave more aggressively and may be associated with higher risk, the staging is not done differently from that of typical papillary carcinoma.

TNM Updates

Periodic updated versions of the AJCC or UICC staging systems may revise assigned scoring, thereby impacting comparisons of outcomes to those reported in the literature according to earlier and different criteria. In this regard, Dobert et al. (17) examined the influence of the differences between the recent UICC fifth and sixth editions by retrospectively applying the two scoring systems to a group of 169 patients. Comparing the two versions indicated that 32% of the patients would have been stage 1 by the fifth edition, whereas the sixth edition placed 49% as stage 1. As a result, fifth edition–scored T1 tumors had a 1-yr relapse-free interval of 100% compared to 96.8% of T1 tumors scored by the sixth edition. Although the latter difference constitutes a slightly worse prognostic determination, Dobert et al. concluded that the differences did not appear to be sufficient enough to alter management strategies. In a comparison and evaluation of six different staging systems, Brierley et al. (18) concluded that no system provided any advantage over the TNM system and advocated its universal use to facilitate communication between medical centers worldwide.

Ohio State Scoring System

Although it has not been applied widely, Mazzaferri and colleagues proposed a variant on staging that is referred to as the Ohio State University Staging system (9). Their system was based on a retrospective multivariate analysis of 1355 patients. Stage 1 patients had tumors less than 1.5 cm

Table 3
The Ohio State University Experience

Stage	% of Patients	Disease-Specific Mortality (%)
1	13	0
2	70	6
3	15	14
4	2	65

in size; stage 2 patients had tumors between greater than 1.5 but less than 4.5 cm or lymph node metastases or greater than 3 multifocal tumors; patients were considered as stage 3 if their tumors were greater than 4.5 cm or if they had extrathyroidal extension of tumor; and patients with distant metastases were classified as stage 4. As seen in Table 3, there was a clear correlation between mortality and stage of disease.

AGES System

Physicians at the Mayo Clinic described and applied a staging system known as AGES (A, age; G, histologic grade; E, extent; and S, tumor size; *19*). Low-risk stage 1 patients were seen to have an excellent prognosis with a 1% 20-yr disease-specific death rate compared to 20%, 67%, and 87% mortality for stages 2, 3, and 4, respectively. The AGES schema likely never became popular because it requires knowledge of tumor grade that is rarely reported by pathologists. Members of the same Mayo Clinic group subsequently modified AGES by devising the MACIS grading system, which eliminates the need to know tumor grade *(19)*. The Mayo group incorporated all the other factors into their MACIS scoring system (see below), which can reliably predict outcome based on data at initial presentation.

MACIS System

The MACIS scoring system is defined as metastases (M), age (A), completeness of resection (C), invasion (I), and tumor size (S) *(20)*. Hay *(1)* and others identified three varieties of presentation that reflected a different prognostic category regarding tumor recurrence. The three most important factors were the presence of postoperative local metastatic nodes, postoperative distant metastases, and local recurrence in the thyroid bed or adjacent tissue other than lymph nodes. They believe this scoring system can more reliably predict outcome based on data at initial presentation than the TNM system, which is limited to fewer characteristics. Using the MACIS system, they described 20-yr disease-specific mortality rates that directly correlated with the magnitude of scores (see Tables 4 and 5).

NTCTCS System

The most recently developed staging system was proposed by Sherman et al. *(21)* from the empirical develop-

Table 4
The MACIS Scoring System

Metastases	Absent	0
	Present	3
Patient age	<40	3.1
	>40	0.08 × age
Resection	Complete	0
	Incomplete	1
Invasion	Absent	0
	Present	1
Tumor size		0.3 × size in cm

Table 5
Correlation of MACIS Score with Mortality

Score	Stage	Mortality Rates (%)
<6	1	1
6–6.99	2	11
7–7.99	3	44
>8	4	76

ment of a classification that considered patient data in a registry derived from 14 different medical centers, known as the National Thyroid Cancer Treatment Cooperative Study (NTCTCS). Prospective information on 1607 patients was analyzed and validated on the basis of initial follow-up. A comparison of the NTCTCS system to the other systems was performed for prediction of the disease-free state. The NTCTCS system provided somewhat better correlation than the AMES or Ohio State systems but did not appear to provide any advantage over the TNM system. The system was criticized as unnecessary and potentially flawed by Cady *(22)* and Sherman countered with a lively rebuttal *(23)*.

FOLLICULAR THYROID CANCER

Staging for follicular thyroid cancer (FTC) is done exactly the same as for PTC. Stage 1 follicular tumors, like papillary tumors, tend to have an excellent prognosis. The key underlying difference between these two cancer types is that the follicular cancers tend to be more invasive, invading blood vessels in the thyroid gland that can then lead to hematogenous metastases to bone and lung. Several studies have attempted to determine which features or characteristics of a follicular tumor might be associated with a more negative prognosis. In one analysis *(21)*, age at diagnosis, tumor size, poor differentiation, and extracervical metastases were the most important staging factors. These more "negative" features appear to be similar to those for papillary tumors and include age greater than 45 yr, tumor size more than 4 cm, invasion of tumor into blood vessels or the capsule of the thyroid, extension of the cancer beyond the thyroid gland, and metastases to distant sites (e.g., bones and lungs). In a retrospective review of 504 patients with FTC, Simpson et al. (24) identified age at diagnosis, extrathyroidal invasion, primary tumor size, distant metastases, nodal involvement, and postoperative status as independently important prognostic factors. In another retrospective review of 214 patients with FTC (25), recurrence rates were less in those patients given radioiodine ablation, and no deaths occurred during a mean follow-up of 8.8 yr, except in those with distant metastases at the time of presentation. Brennan et al. reported a retrospective analysis of 100 patients with FTC followed for up to 32 yr (mean 17 yr) who had an overall cancer-related mortality of 19% (26). Multivariate analysis suggested a "multiplier" effect with patients illustrating several negative prognostic features doing more poorly than those with only one negative indicator. High-risk patients with two or more negative risk predictors had a 5-yr survival rate of 47% and a 20-yr survival rate of 8%.

MEDULLARY THYROID CANCER

Management and outcomes for medullary thyroid cancer (MTC) differ greatly from those for follicular cell–derived thyroid cancers (27). As may be seen in all of the various staging systems described below for MTC, patient age is not considered. Because the etiology and natural history of MTC differs broadly from that of follicular cell cancers, there may be some rationale for the development and use of a more specific analysis of staging and prognosis based on distinctions between familial and sporadic MTC and for the various described somatic and germline ret mutations.

ANAPLASTIC CARCINOMA OF THE THYROID

Because papillary thyroid cancer and FTC together account for about 95% of thyroid cancers, this chapter generally relates to these well-differentiated cancers. Prognostic issues related to anaplastic thyroid cancer and MTC are discussed in Chapters 67 and 83. With very few exceptions, anaplastic cancer always has a poor prognosis and is automatically staged as stage 4, regardless of tumor size, patient age, or the presence of distant metastases (29,30) The current practice in staging anaplastic tumors is only to break the category down into stage 4A (surgically removable), 4B (not surgically removable), or 4C (with distant metastases).

RELATION OF STAGING TO PROGNOSIS

Prognosis of the different types of thyroid cancer is discussed by Burch in specific chapters, and the topic is only briefly addressed here for well-differentiated follicular cancer in the context of staging. When analyzing reports or retrospective analyses of outcomes based on stage from different centers, it is important to note whether the patients' routine initial management (e.g., total thyroidectomy and radioiodine ablation) were comparable. Following thyroidectomy for papillary lesions more than 1.5 cm, most workers employ radioiodine in doses of 30–150 mCi to ablate residual tissue and facilitate follow-up monitoring (4) as discussed in Chapters 26 and 27. Early patient series have indicated that ^{131}I ablation of thyroid remnants was followed by a significantly lower recurrence rate (8,31,32), but the conviction that such management is absolutely necessary in all patients and actually improves prognosis has been disputed by some experts (1,33). For example, Hay et al. retrospectively reviewed 2444 PTC patients at the Mayo Clinic over a 60-yr period and compared outcomes in the low-risk patients treated in the early decades without radioiodine ablation to those treated in the later decades with ablation (34). They observed no difference in the rates of tumor recurrence or mortality rates from thyroid cancer, thereby implying that ablation did not improve outcomes and was not necessary in low-risk tumors. Alternatively, Simpson and coworkers (24) in a series of 321 patients, found that fewer recurrences occurred in those patients who underwent ablation, and 20-yr survival was greater (90% vs 40%). Similarly, another retrospective analysis of 700 patients suggested that patients not treated with radioiodine ablation had a 2.1-fold greater risk of recurrence of their malignancy ($p = .0001$) but no difference in death rates (2). A careful meta-analysis of the

NTCCTS Clinical Staging of MTC

Stage	Description
Stage 1	C-cell hyperplasia
Stage 2	Tumor less than 1 cm confined to thyroid with negative lymph nodes
Stage 3	Tumors 1 cm or more or tumor of any size with positive nodes
Stage 4	Tumors of any size with metastases outside the neck or with extrathyroidal extension

AJCC Staging of MTC

Stage	Description	4-yr Mortality (28)
Stage 1	Tumor less than 1 cm confined to the thyroid gland	0
Stage 2	Tumor more than 1 cm or with extrathyroidal extension and negative lymph nodes	13%
Stage 3	Tumors of any size with positive nodes	56%
Stage 4	Tumors of any size with distant metastases	100%

DeGroot Staging of MTC

Stage	Description
Stage 1	Tumor confined to the thyroid gland
Stage 2	Tumor limited to the thyroid and cervical lymph nodes
Stage 3	Tumor extending beyond the thyroid or lymph nodes
Stage 4	Tumor with distant metastases

literature concluded that ablation would reduce recurrence rates and improve outcome in high-risk patients, but definitive proof of necessity for ablation of low-risk tumors remains marginally convincing (35). The reasons are not clear for the different outcomes in those studies supporting ablative therapy vs those that do not, and the issue for low-risk tumors remains controversial. Several authors cite the need for a randomized, controlled clinical trial to address this question (36,37).

Finally, the importance of age should be emphasized as a prognostic factor and can be appreciated by noting that all patients less than 45 yr old without distant metastases are classified as stage 1, and those with distant metastases are not classified any higher than stage 2. The overwhelming majority of patients will fall into stages 1 and 2, with excellent prognosis and little risk for recurrence or death from their disease. There was a remarkable 25-yr survival (97%) in 1408 patients reviewed by Hay (1) who had complete surgical resection of their apparent disease. For such patients, 30-yr survival rates of 75–85% are not unusual. Stages 2 and 3 patients may have recurrences that require additional therapy but remain at relatively low risk for death (1,9,31,34). Numerous other factors have been assessed relating to prognosis, such as thyroglobulin levels (38,39) and large lymph node metastases (40). Most analyses tend to conclude that the most important staging factors influencing prognosis are patient age at diagnosis and the presence of distant metastases. A significant negative subsequent factor is a persistently elevated thyroglobulin (Tg) at 1-yr postoperation (41).

Blood vessel invasiveness has been cited by some authors as a correlate of tumor aggressiveness and prognosis. In a review of 358 patients with differentiated thyroid cancer, Furlan et al. (42) concluded that this was not necessarily the case regarding outcome for the short term of PTC and long term of FTC. Employing either the MACIS, TNM, or AMES criteria, angioinvasive PTC did have a worse prognosis, but the latter tumors were larger than nonangioinvasive tumors, raising the question of whether tumor size is the relevant parameter.

In the final analysis, it may not make a great difference which staging system is used; virtually all consider the most important factors, but it would obviously be optimal if we all used the same system to facilitate communication. In one comparison analysis (43), the TNM, AMES, AGES, and MACIS systems all provided comparably useful information correlating with prognosis. In another study (44) comparing MACIS, TNM, and AMES, the TNM system fared better in predicting disease-related mortality likely because it was the only system to include nodal metastases.

Although staging does allow more accuracy in predicting outcomes, true prognosis will be better defined as the course of the disease is observed over months to years. This is because clinical staging typically is done early in the course of the disease, i.e., before any definitive treatment and on the basis of physical examination, imaging studies, and biopsy. Pathologic staging can be done shortly after thyroidectomy with the examination of the surgical specimen for precise tumor size and presence of involved lymph nodes or after the first administration of radioiodine. Data derived from correlations of stage and prognosis from large series of patients are, of course, average data. The stage designation may not accurately predict the outcome in a single given patient who may do better or worse than predicted. Those who have a worse outcome do because their tumors may become more aggressive with time than the average anticipated for a given stage of tumor. One major clinical difficulty for both patients and their physicians is dealing with the indolent nature of these tumors. Thyroid cancer cells are usually slow-growing; while this is favorable for recurrence and death rates, it also implies the absolute necessity for long-term meticulous follow-up because there can be recurrences in patients believed to be disease-free as late as 15–20 yr after their original presentation.

STAGING IN CHILDREN

Thyroid cancer in children and adolescents is generally managed like that in adults (45,46), with the same approaches: near total thyroidectomy, radioiodine ablation, radioiodine therapy for recurrence, and long-term monitoring with serum thyroglobulin measurements. Staging is done in a similar manner. The MACIS system has been used in the pediatric age group with excellent negative predictive value for persistent disease (47). Because of the importance of age as a prognostic factor and the obvious fact that these patients are young by definition, the prognosis tends to be excellent in children even with extensive local spread of disease. Indeed, in contrast to adults, the majority of children with thyroid cancer will already have local tumor spread in the neck to the lymph nodes at the time of initial diagnosis. Moreover, as many as 10–20% of children and adolescents will have distant metastases at diagnosis, such as tumor in the lung, compared to only 5% in adults (48). Despite this apparently more aggressive appearance of these tumors in children, the prognosis for cure remains good with therapy, with less than 10% of children dying from their disease—a prognosis that is significantly better than mortality rates seen in adults. An exception to this general experience occurs in young children under 8 yr of age, who may have more aggressive disease for unknown reasons. However, because of the usual excellent results with therapy, some physicians question whether aggressive approaches to therapy with large-dose radioiodine are necessary in children as it may be in adults, given the long-term radiation side effects that may ensue for these children. No clearcut studies answer this question yet, but some physicians treating children with thyroid cancer will reserve aggressive radioiodine therapy for those with disease that has spread to the outside of the thyroid gland. Thus, as with adults, a reasonable approach is to individualize therapy rather than adopt an arbitrary standard approach, and long term follow-up and monitoring is essential owing to the slow-growing nature of thyroid cancer (49).

REFERENCES

1. Hay ID. Papillary thyroid carcinoma. Endocrinol Metab Clin North Am 1990; 19:545–576.
2. Loh K-C, Greenspan FS, Gee L, et al. Pathological tumor-node-metastasis (pTNM) staging for papillary and follicular thyroid carcinomas: a retrospective analysis of 700 patients. J Clin Endocrinol Metab 1997; 82:3553–3562.
3. American Joint Committee on Cancer. The thyroid gland. In AJCC Cancer Staging Manual, 6th ed. New York, NY: Springer, 2002; 77–87.
4. Sweeney DC, Johnston GS. Radioiodine therapy for thyroid cancer. Endocr Metab Clin N Amer 1995; 24:803–840.
5. Cady B, Rossi R. An expanded view of risk-group definition in differentiated thyroid carcinoma. Surgery 1988; 104:947–953.
6. Sanders LE, Cady B. Differentiated thyroid cancer: reexamination of risk groups and outcome of treatment. Archives Surg 1998; 133:419–425.
7. UICC 2002. Sobin LH, Wittekind C, editors. TNM Classification of Malignant Tumors, 6th ed. New York: Wiley-Liss, 2002; 52–56.
8. McConahey Wm, Hay ID, Woolner LB, et al. Papillary thyroid cancer treated at the Mayo Clinic, 1946 through 1970: initial manifestations, pathologic findings, therapy, and outcome. Mayo Clin Proc 1986; 61: 978–996.
9. Mazzaferri EL, Jhiang SM. Long-term impact of initial surgical and medical therapy on papillary and follicular thyroid cancer. Am J Med 1994; 97:418–428.
10. Shah JP, Loree TR, Dharker D, et al. Prognostic factors in differentiated carcinoma of the thyroid gland. Am J Surg 1992; 164:658–661.
11. Beasley NJP, Lee J, Eski S, et al. Impact of nodal metastases on prognosis in patients with well-differentiated thyroid cancer. Arch Otolaryngol Head Neck Surg 2002; 128:825–828.
12. Gilliland FD, Hunt WC, Morris DM, Key CR. Prognostic factors for thyroid carcinoma: a population based study of 15698 cases from the surveillance, epidemiology and end results (SEER) program 1973-1991. Cancer 1997; 79:564–573.
13. Samaan NA, Schultz PN, Hickey RC, et al. Well differentiated thyroid carcinoma and the results of various modalities of treatment: a retrospective review of 1599 cases. J Clin Endocrinol Metab 1992; 75: 714–720.
14. Burman KD, Ringel MD, Wartofsky L. Unusual types of thyroid neoplasms. Endocrin Metab Clin N Amer 1996; 25:49–68.
15. Sywak M, Pasieka JL, Ogilvie T. A review of thyroid cancer with intermediate differentiation. J Surg Oncol 2004; 86:44–54.
16. Prendiville S, Burman KD, Ringel MD, et al. Tall cell variant: an aggressive form of papillary thyroid carcinoma. Otolaryngol Head Neck Surg 2000; 122:352–357.
17. Dobert N, Menzel C, Oeschger S, Grunwald F. Differentiated thyroid carcinoma: The new UICC 6th edition TNM cassification system in a retrospective analysis of 169 patients. Thyroid 2004; 14:65–70.
18. Brierley JD, Panzarella T, Tsang RW, et al. A comparison of different staging systems predictability of patient outcome. Thyroid carcinoma as an example. Cancer 1997; 79:2414–2423.
19. Hay ID, Grant CS, van Heerden JA, et al. Papillary thyroid microcarcinoma: A study of 535 cases observed in a 50-year period. Surgery 1987; 102:1088–1095.
20. Hay ID, Bergstralh EJ, Goellner JR, et al. Predicting outcome in papillary thyroid carcinoma: development of a reliable prognostic scoring system in a cohort of 1779 patients surgically treated in one institution during 1940 through 1989. Surgery 1993; 114:1050–1058.
21. Sherman SI, Brierley JD, SperlingM, et al. Prospective multicenter study of thyroid carcinoma treatment: initial analysis of staging and outcome. National Thyroid Cancer Treatment Cooperative Study Registry Group. Cancer 1998; 83:1012–1021.
22. Cady B. Staging in thyroid carcinoma. Cancer 1998; 83:844–847.
23. Sherman SI. Staging of thyroid carcinoma—reply. Cancer 1998; 83:848–850.
24. Simpson WJ, McKinney SE, Carruthers JS, et al. Papillary and follicular thyroid cancer: Prognostic factors in 1,578 patients. Am J Med 1987; 83:479–488.
25. Young RL, Mazzaferri EL, Rahe AJ, Dorfman SG. Pure follicular thyrid carcinoma: impact of therapy in 214 patients. J Nucl Med 1980; 21:733–737.
26. Brennan MD, Bergstralh EJ, van Heerden JA, McConahey WM. Follicular thyroid cancer treated at the Mayo Clinic, 1946 through 1970: initial manifestations, pathologic findings, therapy, and outcome. Mayo Clin Proc 1991; 66:11–22.
27. Massoll N, Mazzaferri El. Diagnosis and management of medullary thyroid carcinoma. Clin Lab Med 2004; 24:49–83.
28. Dottorini ME, Assi A, Sironi M, et al. Multivariate analysis of patients with medullary thyroid carcinoma. Prognostic significance and impact on treatment of clinical and pathologic variables. Cancer 1996; 77:1556–1565.
29. McIver B, Hay ID, Giuffrida DF, et al. Anaplastic thyroid carcinoma: a 50-year experience at a single institution. Surgery 2001; 130:1028–1034.
30. Pasieka JL. Anaplastic thyroid cancer. Curr Opinion Oncol 2003; 15:78–83.
31. Mazzaferri EL, Young RL, Oertel JE, et al. Papillary thyroid carcinoma: the impact of therapy in 576 patients. Medicine 1977; 56:171–196.
32. Mazzaferri EL, Young RL. Papillary thyroid carcinoma: A 10 year follow-up report of the impact of therapy in 576 patients. Am J Med 1981; 70:511–518.
33. Schlumberger M, Hay ID. Use of radioactive iodine in patients with papillary and follicular thyroid cancer: towards a selective approach. J Clin Endocrinol Metab 1998; 83:4201–4203.
34. DeGroot LJ, Kaplan EL, McCormick M, Straus FH. Natural history, treatment, and course of papillary thyroid carcinoma. J Clin Endocrinol Metab 1990; 71:414–424.
35. Sawka AM, Thephamongkhol K, Brouwers, et al. J Clin Endocrinol Metab 2004; 89:3668–3676.
36. Haugen BR. Editorial: Patients with differentiated thyroid carcinoma benefit from radioiodine remnant ablation. J Clin Endocrinol Metab 2004; 89:3665–3667.
37. Mazzaferri EL. Editorial: A randomized trial of remnant ablation—In search of an impossible dream? J Clin Endocrinol Metab 2004; 89:3662–3664.
38. Tubeau M, Touzery C, Arveux P, et al. Predictive value for disease progression of serum thyroglobulin levels measured in the postoperative period and after (131)I ablation therapy in patients with differentiated thyroid cancer. J Nucl Med 2004; 45:988–994.
39. Torre EM, Carballo MTL, Erdozan RMR, et al. Prognostic value of thyroglobulin serum levels and 131-I whole-body scan after initial treatment of low-risk differentiated thyroid cancer. Thyroid 2004; 14:301–306.
40. Sugitani I, Kasai N, Fujimoto Y, Yanagisawa A. A novel classification system for patients with PTC : Addition of the new variables of large (3 cm or greater) nodal metastases and reclassification during the follow-up period. Surgery 2004; 135:139–148.
41. Eichhorn W, Tabler H, Lippold R, et al. Prognostic factors determining long-term survival in well-differentiated thyroid cancer: an analysis of 484 patients undergoing therapy and aftercare at the same institution. Thyroid 2003; 13:949–958.
42. Furlan JC, Bedard YC, Rosen IB. Clinicopathologic significance of histologic vascular invasion in papillary and follicular thyroid carcinomas. J Amer Coll Surg 2004; 198:341–348.
43. D'Avanzo A, Ituarte P, Treseler P, et al. Prognostic scoring systems in patients with follicular thyroid cancer: A comparison of different

staging systems in predicting the patient outcome. Thyroid 2004; 14:453–458.

44. Voutilainen PE, Siironen P, Franssila KO, et al. AMES, MACIS, and TNM prognostic classifications in papillary thyroid carcinoma. Anticancer Res 2003; 23:4283–4288.

45. Chow S, Law S, Mendenhall W, et al. Differentiated thyroid carcinoma in childhood and adolescence—clinical course and role of radioiodine. Pediatr Blood Cancer 2004; 42:176–183.

46. Hung W, Sarlis NJ. Current controversies in the management of pediatric patients with well-differentiated nonmedullary thyroid cancer: a review. Thyroid 2002; 12:683–702.

47. Powers PA, Dinauer CA, Tuttle RM, Francis GL. The MACIS score predicts the clinical course of papillary thyroid carcinoma in children and adolescents. J Pediatr Endocrinol 2004; 17:339–343.

48. LaQuaglia M, Black T, Holcomb G, et al. Differentiated thyroid cancer: clinical characteristics, treatment, and outcome in patients under 21 years of age who present with distant metastases. A report from the Surgical Discipline Committee of the Children's Cancer Group. J Pediatr Surg 2000; 35:955–959.

49. Powers PA, Dinauer CA, Tuttle RM, Francis GL. Treatment of recurrent papillary thyroid carcinoma in children and adolescents. J Pediatr Endocrinol 2003; 16:1033–1040.

10
Thyroid Cancer in Children and Adolescents*

Merrily Poth

INTRODUCTION

Thyroid cancer is the most common endocrine tumor in children. It comprises 0.5–1.5% of childhood tumors and is the most common malignant tumor of the head and neck in young people *(1,2)*. Although it is more common in adults than in children, approx 10% of all cases are diagnosed before age 21 *(3)*. The histology of the disease in childhood is like it is in adults, but the disease's presentation and behavior is significantly different when it occurs in children and adolescents. For example, even though thyroid cancer is relatively uncommon in children and adolescents, a mass identified in the thyroid before age 21 is much more likely to be malignant than when the same finding occurs in an older patient *(4)*. The disease is more often advanced at diagnosis with local and even distant metastasis, and it subsequently continues to behave more aggressively with more frequent recurrence *(5,6)*. In adults, especially older patients, this aggressive behavior would be accompanied by a poor long-term prognosis. However, in general, despite its aggressive behavior, thyroid cancer in children usually has an excellent prognosis when appropriately treated. It is important for caregivers to have adequate understanding of its presentation so that valuable time is not lost before evaluation can occur and treatment can begin.

In a recent excellent review, Hung and Sarlis *(7)* suggested that children and adolescents with differentiated thyroid cancer (DTC) should be treated as two separate disease populations. They felt that the disease in older children and adolescents presents and behaves much as it does in adults, and data from adult studies could be applied after mid-puberty. It was their opinion that the disease behaved differently only in children younger than age 10 yr, and it was only then that different parameters needed to be applied. Although there is some rationale to this proposal, in our experience, the age division is not so clear. We have treated a small number of young patients with rapidly growing tumors, overwhelming metastatic behavior, and resistance to cure. However, most younger patients have tumors that behave much like those in adolescents, with both local and distant spread early but an excellent response to therapy and good long-term response to treatment. We have not seen a break point in age where the tumor appears to behave differently. Certainly, the same considerations of potential negative effects of therapy vs long-term prognosis apply to all children and adolescents. For those reasons, we believe that DTC in children and adolescents is worthy of consideration separately from the adult disease.

EPIDEMIOLOGY AND GENERAL RISK FACTORS

The incidence of thyroid cancer varies from 1 to 6 per 100,000 individuals under the age of 21 *(8,9)*. While in some reported series, this incidence appears to be increasing over time *(10,11,11a)*, in other studies, it is found to be relatively constant, aside from episodic increases in specific geographic areas, usually associated with exposure to radiation *(9,12,13)*.

There are no careful and comprehensive epidemiological studies of the potential factors influencing the incidence of thyroid cancer in children. The sparse available data examining the incidence in racial groups appear to show a greater incidence of papillary cancer in whites compared to blacks and with an equal or increased incidence of follicular tumors in blacks *(14)*. The role of gender in regard to the incidence of thyroid cancer is similar to the adult population, with a greater incidence in older female children and adolescents than in males; ratios reported range from 2.5–6.0 to 1 *(14,15)*. However, this relatively greater prevalence is not seen in the very young, in whom the ratio may be unity or even reversed.

---

*The opinions and assertions contained herein are the private view of the author and are not to be construed as official or as reflecting the opinions of the Uniformed University of the Health Sciences or the Department of Defense.

From: *Thyroid Cancer: A Comprehensive Guide to Clinical Management, 2/e*
Edited by: L. Wartofsky and D. Van Nostrand © Humana Press Inc., Totowa, NJ

The interaction of other risk factors, particularly radiation, with gender is not clear. One investigator reported an extremely increased risk in male children treated with radiation for Hodgkin's disease (16), whereas others have not found such a difference in the relative risk after radiation between male and female children (13,17,18). Generally, there is a relatively constant and low incidence of thyroid cancer in young children and steady increased incidence beginning in early puberty (19,20).

Analysis of the effect of iodine dietary content on thyroid cancer has shown an increased incidence of papillary cancer in areas where iodine intake is high and follicular lesions where iodine intake is low (21). However, these data have not been separately analyzed for children. The recent experience with radiation exposure at Belarus (see Chapter 7) has illuminated an important interaction between iodine deficiency and increased vulnerability to thyroid cancer in children after radiation exposure (22).

The possible interaction of other thyroid diseases, particularly Hashimoto's thyroiditis, on the prevalence of thyroid cancer is somewhat controversial. Some studies imply that malignancy in the presence of thyroiditis is increased (23,24), whereas other authors refute such an association. The topic is complicated by the general failure of the literature on the potential association to exhibit clearly defined criteria for the diagnosis of Hashimoto's thyroiditis (25). Recent studies examining pathological specimens of thyroid cancer for the presence of lymphocytic infiltration, and correlations with prognosis (26), add to the uncertainty around this issue. While autoimmune thyroid disease is common in children and adolescents, no separate reports analyze either the effect of lymphocytes in tumor specimens from children or the incidence of cancer in children with and without autoimmune thyroid disease.

There are several situations where thyroid cancer appears to be genetic. The syndrome of familial adenomatous polyposis or Gardner syndrome is associated with an increased risk of papillary thyroid cancer, which typically presents in adolescence (27). Thyroid cancer is also associated with other specific syndromes, including Cowden's and the Carney complex, while other families appear to have an isolated propensity for papillary cancer (28–31). The vast majority of these patients are diagnosed in young adulthood. It would seem logical to institute increased surveillance during adolescence for potential at-risk individuals based on family history.

Radiation as a Risk Factor

The most important risk factor for the development of thyroid cancer is exposure to ionizing radiation. As a matter of policy, all children with a history of significant exposure to radiation, including radiation therapy for malignancy, should be prospectively monitored for thyroid dysfunction and the occurrence of thyroid nodules and cancer. Although radiation exposure is clearly a risk factor for the development of thyroid cancer in adults and children, the effects are markedly exaggerated when the exposure occurs in childhood. Children show an increased sensitivity to radiation effects and increased occurrence of thyroid cancer even after relatively small doses of radiation. Thay also have a pronounced decrease in latency in the time between radiation exposure and occurrence of thyroid neoplasm (32,33).

Many studies have confirmed the strong relationship between radiation exposure and thyroid cancer. The first of such studies in children was by Duffy and Fitzgerald in 1950, who reported on 28 children with thyroid cancer, 10 of whom had received radiation treatment for an enlarged thymus (34). In a 1961 review of findings on 562 cases of thyroid cancer in children, Winship and Rosvoll found that almost 80% reported previous irradiation for enlarged thymus, hypertrophied tonsils and adenoids, nevi, or angiomas (35).

Further analysis of the effects of radiation therapy for benign conditions continues to be published by investigators, and all reports validated the association. A study reviewing therapeutic radiation for ringworm of the scalp compared 10,834 irradiated persons, designating 5392 siblings as controls (36). They found a relative risk for thyroid cancer of 4.0 and an excess risk of 1.2/10,000 persons per year and reported a linear dose–response curve with an average absolute excess risk of 12.5 person-years per cGy. In addition, their study also supported the relative increased sensitivity of younger children to radiation exposure, reporting an increased risk for children irradiated before age 5 compared to children irradiated at older ages. Two other studies have reported similarly increased relative risk of 7.5–10 per Gy for infants and children irradiated for a variety of benign medical conditions (37,38).

A comprehensive paper by Ron and colleagues in 1995 summarized the data, adding a study of atomic bomb exposure, a childhood cancer study, and two different studies of children irradiated for enlarged tonsils and adenoids to the studies of tinea capitis and thymus irradiation that are described above (39). Their summary noted excess relative risks, which varied from 1.1 to 32.5 per Gy with excess absolute risks of 2.6–7.6. They confirmed the reported linear relationship between radiation dose and risk, with increased risk even with doses as low as 0.1 Gy. They also emphasized that the increased risk continues for up to 40 yr after irradiation. Recent papers, following these and other radiation-exposed children, have reconfirmed the risk and relationship between dose and ultimate risk (18,32,40,40a,40b).

Children no longer receive radiation therapy for treatment of benign disease; however, treatment for childhood cancer often includes radiation therapy. As patient survival with childhood cancer continues to improve, a large population of surviving patients have sustained significant incidental radiation exposure to the thyroid. Based on the previous experience with thyroid cancer after radiation for benign conditions, these patients would be expected also to be at risk for thyroid cancer. This question is discussed briefly by Ron et al. *(39)*, and numerous other studies involving patients given radiation therapy for malignant conditions have validated this relationship. One study that included a group of patients with a variety of childhood tumors reported a 4.6% incidence of thyroid cancer after a mean follow-up period of only 11 yr *(41)*. Another report of 9170 patients who survived childhood cancer for at least 2 yr found that the risk of thyroid cancer increased by a factor of 53 over the general population *(42)*. This study found the risk highest in patients treated for neuroblastoma and Wilms tumors; the authors attributed this to the fact that these were the patients who were the youngest when they received their radiation therapy. A study of patients who received radiation therapy for Hodgkin's disease *(43)* found, in addition to thyroid nodules and cancers, a high incidence of autoimmune thyroid disease and hypothyroidism. This report also indicated hypothyroidism frequently occurs after a dose of 30 Gy to the gland. Thus, it seems appropriate to follow such patients prospectively, with yearly thyrotropin (TSH) assays and careful monitoring for nodules. Thyroid hormone therapy should be instituted as soon as an increase in TSH is seen.

Another group reporting on patients with Hodgkin's lymphoma after radiation therapy have recommended annual ultrasound evaluation to aid the earliest identification of nodules and malignancy *(44)*. The frequency and even necessity of serial ultrasounds is currently debated; those in favor of this approach suggest that serial ultrasound would provide improved surveillance in a group of patients with a high risk of nodular disease and cancer. Others argue that this approach would lead to increased stress, anxiety, and the potential need for fine-needle aspiration biopsy and/or surgery. The question remains unsettled because the chance of malignancy is real, and earlier diagnosis would significantly benefit the patient. Although using ultrasound to follow these patients has not been established as standard of care, it would be reasonable to conduct an ultrasound study at baseline, along with a careful thyroid exam. At minimum, annual thyroid exams and serum TSH levels should be followed, and ultrasound examinations should be used to evaluate any minor or questionable abnormality during physical examination.

In an interesting study, Mazonakis used anthropomorphic phantoms to quantify thyroid exposure after radiation treatment of brain tumors. Whereas an adult treated with radiation would have an increased thyroid cancer risk of 1.1 or less, the excess relative risk for a treated child would range between 0.6 and 14.9 *(45)*.

All these data relative to radiation and thyroid cancer in children pale when considered in the context of the vast numbers of thyroid cancer cases that followed the 1986 tragic accident in Chernobyl, where an unprecedented 40–50 million Ci of ^{131}I was released into the atmosphere *(46;* see Chapter 7). The resulting radioactive material was widely dispersed and entered into the food chain. While the radiation was inhaled and ingested by both children and adults, the exposure per body mass was undoubtedly greater in the children. The subsequent increase in childhood thyroid cancer has been widely reported. Early attempts to attribute even part of this "epidemic" to increased surveillance have been effectively rebutted *(47,48)*. The occurrence of cancer correlated with the distance from the event (49,50) and showed an unexpectedly short latency of 3 yr. Risk of thyroid cancer was much higher in younger children, and the largest proportion of affected children were those less than 1 yr of age at the time of their exposure *(49,50)*. Overall, more than 55% of the thyroid cancers were reported in children less than 4 yr of age at exposure *(49,50)*.

Essentially, all the thyroid tumors in this population were papillary carcinomas, and the female-to-male ratio of affected children reported was 1.15:1. The behavior of the tumors has been similar to thyroid cancer in children without a history of radiation exposure, where a high percentage of tumors show capsular invasion at the time of diagnosis, and most tumors present with lymph node metastases *(50)*. Clearly, the full magnitude of this event has not been realized, and continued surveillance is likely to lead to the discovery of more lesions *(50a)*.

These patients offer insights into the causality of thyroid cancer in children, particularly in relation to the impact of exposure to large doses of varying radioiodine isotopes. For many years, there has been concern over exposure to ^{131}I used for diagnostic studies of thyroid function and for treatment of hyperthyroidism. Although there are no published studies of large groups of children followed for the subsequent development of thyroid cancer after extensive doses of radiation from diagnostic studies, case reports of thyroid cancer are developing in such children, suggesting a possible relationship *(51)*. With these data in mind, it is appropriate and logical that surveillance of these patients should continue. However, to date, studies of ^{131}I used for diagnostic studies or treatment of thyroid disease have failed to show an increase in malignancy after this exposure *(52,53)*.

The search for genetic markers in tumors of patients developing thyroid cancer after radiation exposure has been fruitful. A 1996 analysis reported *p53* gene mutations in 4 of 22 patients with a history of radiation exposure compared to no mutations in 18 thyroid cancer patients without radiation exposure *(54)*. Recent attempts to look for such markers in thyroid cancers following the Chernobyl accident are ongoing. To date, activating RET/PTC proto-oncogene rearrangements, particularly RET/PTC-3 rearrangements, appear to be quite common *(55–57)*. This data seems quite convincing, but many of these studies did not include a control group of thyroid cancers from patients without radiation exposure. As a consequence, the data may overrepresent the incidence of genetic changes found in children without a history of radiation exposure. The analysis in a recent study did not detect presence of a specific genetic "signature" in post Chernobyl tumors (57a). Thus, although the importance of genetic mutations in thyroid cancers occurring after radiation exposure appears fairly well established, it remains to be seen to what degree these molecular mechanisms differ from those in spontaneous pediatric thyroid cancer. (See Chapter 4 by Gary Francis in which this issue is explored in detail.)

CLINICAL PRESENTATION

Both the presentation and behavior of thyroid cancer in children differs somewhat from that of adults. The extent of disease at diagnosis is often greater than in adults, and the disease more often persists or recurs after initial treatment. Despite this aggressive behavior, the long-term prognosis for eventual cure is excellent, and mortality from disease is low with appropriate follow-up and treatment.

In children, the incidence of local invasion of tumor or spread to lymph nodes approaches 90%, and distant metastases to lung are present at diagnosis in up to 20%. More than half of the cases of papillary thyroid cancer present as a neck mass, with or without a palpable thyroid lesion (58–63). The importance of considering thyroid cancer in the diagnosis of neck mass in children cannot be overemphasized.

The discovery of a neck mass or solitary thyroid nodule most often occurs during a routine physical examination for school or participation in a sports program, but it is not uncommon for the patient or a family member to detect a mass and request an evaluation. Other symptoms, such as dysphagia, hoarseness, or pain, are less common in children with thyroid cancer at presentation.

Because the disease is relatively rare, there are no systematic prospective studies of the effects of specific approaches to treatment regarding disease morbidity or mortality. However, several long-term retrospective studies are underway using a large clinical database and molecular biology techniques to develop better ways to predict the relative aggressiveness of individual tumors and examine the outcomes of therapy in a more systematic way (64). Current methods to therapy, along with data regarding both long- and short-term issues of each therapeutic approach, are discussed in Chapter 41.

PATHOLOGIC DIAGNOSES

The distribution of pathologic types of thyroid cancer in children does not differ markedly from that in younger adults. The most common form seen is papillary, which composes 70–90% of all thyroid cancers in this age group, with follicular cancers comprising most of the rest (59–66). The larger numbers of tumors characterized as papillary in more recent series are a result of the change in classification to include all of the former "follicular variant of papillary" tumors as papillary. Upon analysis, all the tumors with some papillary characteristics are felt to behave as papillary cancers, leading to the newer classification system. Cancers that develop in children after radiation exposure have an even larger proportion of papillary tumors (67,68), with essentially all such tumors exhibiting histologic characteristics of papillary disease. Anaplastic cancer is extremely rare in children, less than 1% of the total in all reported series. When it occurs, it appears to have the same poor prognosis as it does in older patients. Medullary thyroid cancer occurs in children, as in adults, in association with multiple endocrine neoplasia; this disease is considered in great detail in other sections of this book (see Chapters 67–73).

REFERENCES

1. Clark RM, Rosen IB, Laperriere NJ. Malignant tumors of the head and neck in a young population. Am J Surg 1982; 144:459–462.
2. Bernstein L, Gurney JG. Carcinomas and other malignant epithelial neoplasms. ICCC XI. 2001. Pediatric monograph, NCI SEER. Available at: seer.cancer.gov/publications/childhood.
3. Buckwalter JA, Gurll NJ, Thomas Jr. CG. Cancer of the thyroid in youth. World J Surg 1981; 5:15–25.
4. Newman KD. The current management of thyroid tumors in childhood. Semin Pediatr Surg 1993; 2:69–74.
5. Zohar Y, Strauss M, Laudan N. Adolescent versus adult thyroid carcinoma. Laryngoscope 1986; 96:555–559.
6. McClellan DR, Francis GL. Thyroid cancer in children, pregnant women, and patients with Graves' disease. Endocrinol Metab Clin North Am 1996; 25:27–48.
7. Hung W, Sarlis NJ. Current controversies in the management of pediatric patients with well-differentiated nonmedulllary thyroid cancer: A review. Thyroid 2002; 12:683–702.
8. Zimmerman D, Hay I, Bergstralh E. Papillary thyroid carcinoma in children. Treatment of Thyroid Cancer in Childhood. Bethesda, MD: National Institutes of Health, 1992; 3–10.
9. Harach HR, Williams ED. Childhood thyroid cancer in England and Wales. Br J Cancer 1995; 72:777–783.
10. Sala E, Olsen JH. Thyroid cancer in the age group 0-19: time trends and temporal changes in radioactive fallout. Eur J Cancer 1993; 29A: 1443–1445.
11. Zheng T, Holford TR, Chen Y, Ma JZ, Flannery J, Liu W. Time trend and age-period-cohort effect on incidence of thyroid cancer in Connecticut, 1935-1992. Int J Cancer 1996; 67:504–509.
11a. Hodgson NC, Button J, Solorzano CC. Thyroid cancer: is the incidence still increasing? Ann Surg Oncol 2004; 11:1093–1097.
12. Thoresen S, Akslen LA, Glattre E, Haldorsen T. Thyroid cancer in children in Norway 1953-1987. Eur J Cancer 1993; 29A:365–366.
13. Mangano JJ. A post-Chernobyl rise in thyroid cancer in Connecticut, USA. Eur J Cancer Prevent 1996; 5:75–81.
14. Correa P, Chen VW. Endocrine gland cancer. Cancer 1995; 75:338–352.
15. dos Santos Silva I, Swerdlow AJ. Sex differences in the risks of hormone-dependent cancers. Am J Epidemiol 1993; 138:10–28.
16. Sankila R, Garwicz S, Oslen JH, et al. Risk of subsequent malignant neoplasms among 1,641 Hodgkin's disease patients diagnosed in childhood and adolescence: a population based cohort study in five Nordic countries. J Clin Oncol 1996; 14:1442–1446.
17. Thompson DE, Mabuchi K, Ron E, et al. Cancer incidence in atomic bomb survivors. Part II; Solid tumors, 1958-1987. Radial Res 1994; 137:817–867.
18. Acharya S, Sarafoglou K, LaQuaglia M, et al. Thyroid neoplasms after therapeutic radiation for malignancies during childhood and adolescence. Cancer 2003; 97:2397–2403.
19. Ceccarelli C, Pacini F, Lippi F, et al. Thyroid cancer in children and adolescents. Surgery 1988; 104:1143–1148.

20. Zimmerman D, Jay ID, Gough IR, et al. Papillary thyroid carcinoma in children and adults: long-term follow-up of 1039 patients conservatively treated at one institution during three decades. Surgery 1988; 104:1157–1166.
21. Belfiore A, Giuffrida D, LaRosa GL, et al. High frequency of cancer in cold thyroid nodules occurring at young age. Acta Endocrinol 1989; 121:197–202.
22. Shakhtarin VV, Tsyb AF, Stepanenko VF, Orlov MY, Kopecky KJ, Davis S. Iodine deficiency, radiation dose, and the risk of thyroid cancer among children and adolescents in the Bryansk region of Russia following the Chernobyl power station accident. Int J Epidemiol 2003; 32:584–591.
23. Ott RA, Calandra DB, McCall A, Shah KH, Lawrence AM, Paloyan E. The incidence of thyroid carcinoma in patients with Hashimoto's thyroiditis and solitary cold nodules. Surgery 1985;1202–1206.
24. Okayasu I, Fujiwara M, Hara Y, Tanaka Y, Rose NR. Association of chronic lymphocytic thyroiditis and thyroid papillary carcinoma: a study of surgical cases among Japanese, and white and African Americans. Cancer 1995; 76:2312–2318.
25. Kamma H, Fujii K, Ogata T. Lymphocytic infiltration in juvenile thyroid carcinoma. Cancer 1988; 62:1988–1993.
26. Matsubayashi S, Kawai K, Matsumoto Y, et al. The correlation between papillary thyroid carcinoma and lymphocytic infiltration in the thyroid gland. J Clin Endocrinol Metab 1995; 80:3421–3424.
27. Bell B, Mazzaferri EL. Familial adenomatous polyposis (Gardner's syndrome) and thyroid carcinoma. Digest Dis Sci 1993; 38:185–189.
28. Kwok CG, McDougall IR. Familial differentiated carcinoma of the thyroid: report of five pairs of siblings. Thyroid 1995; 5:295–297.
29. Lote K, Andersen K, Nordal E, Brennhovd IO. Familial occurrence of papillary thyroid carcinoma. Cancer 1980; 46:1291–1297.
30. Eng C. Editorial: Familial papillary thyroid cancer—many syndromes, too many genes? J Clin Endocrinol Metab 2000; 85:1755–1756.
31. Sandrini F, Matyakhina L, Sarlis NJ, et al. Regulatory subunit type 1-α of protein kinase A (*PRKAR1A*): A tumor suppressor gene for sporadic thyroid cancer. Genes Chromosomes Cancer 2002; 35:182–192.
32. Bhatia S, Yasui Y, Robison LL, et al. High risk of subsequent neoplasms continues with extended follow-up for the late effects study group. J Clin Oncol 2003; 21:4386–4394.
33. Farahati J, Demidchik EP, Biko J, Reiners C. Inverse association between age at the time of radiation exposure and extent of disease in cases of radiation-induced thyroid carcinoma in Belarus. Cancer 2000; 88:1470–1476.
34. Duffy BJ Jr, Fitzgerald PJ. Thyroid cancer in childhood and adolescence; report on 28 cases. J Clin Endocrinol 1950; 10:1296–1308.
35. Winship T and Rosvoll RV. Childhood thyroid carcinoma. Cancer 1961; 14:734–743.
36. Ron E, Madon B, Preston D, Alfandary E, Stovall M, Boice JD. Thyroid neoplasia following low-dose radiation in childhood. Radiat Res 1989; 120:516–531.
37. Lindberg S, Karlsson P, Arvidsson B, Holmberg E, Lindber LM, Wallgren A. Cancer incidence after radiotherapy for skin haemangioma during infancy. Acta Oncol 1995; 34:735–740.
38. Shore RE, Hildreth N, Dvoretsky P, Andresen E, Moseson M, Pasternack B. Thyroid cancer among persons given X-ray treatment in infancy for an enlarged thymus gland. Am J Epidemiol 1993; 137:1068–1080.
39. Ron E, Lubin JH, Shore RE, et al. Thyroid cancer after exposure to external radiation: a pooled analysis of seven studies. Radiat Res 1995; 141:259–277.
40. Niedziela M, Korman E, Breborowicz D, et al. A prospective study of thyroid nodular disease in children and adolescents in western Poland from 1996 to 2000 and the incidence of thyroid carcinoma relative to iodine deficiency and the Chernobyl disaster. Pediatr Blood Cancer 2004; 42:84–92.
40a. Gow KW, Lensing S, Hill DA, et al. Thyroid carcinoma presenting in childhood or after treatment of childhood malignancies: An institutional experience and review of the literature. J Pediatr Surg 2003; 38:1574–1580.
40b. Acharya S, Sarafoglou K, Laquaglia M, et al. Thyroid neoplasms after therapeutic radiation for malignancies during childhood and adolescence. Cancer 2003; 97:2397–2403.
41. Vane D, King DR, Boles ET Jr. Secondary thyroid neoplasms in pediatric cancer patients: increased risk with improved survival. J Pediatr Surg 1984; 109:855–860.
42. Tucker MA, Morris Jones PH, et al. Therapeutic radiation at a young age is linked to secondary thyroid cancer. Cancer Res 1991; 51:2885–2888.
43. Hancock SL, Cox RS, McDougall IR. Thyroid disease after treatment of Hodgkin's disease. N Engl J Med 1991; 325:599–605.
44. Healy JC, Shafford EA, Reznek RH, et al. Sonographic abnormalities of the thyroid gland following radiotherapy in survivors of childhood Hodgkin's disease. Br J Radiol 1996; 69:617–623.
45. Mazonakis M, Damilakis J, Varveris H, Fasoulaki M, Gourtsoyiannis N. Risk estimation of radiation-induced thyroid cancer from treatment of brain tumors in adults and children. Int J Oncol 2003; 22:221–225.
46. Becker DV, Robbins J, Beebe GW, Bouville AC, Wachholz BW. Childhood thyroid cancer following the Chernobyl accident. Thyroid Cancer II 1996; 25:197–211.
47. Abelin T, Averkin JI, Egger M, et al. Thyroid cancer in Belarus post-Chernobyl: improved detection or increased incidence? Soz Praventiv Med 1994; 39:189–197.
48. Baverstock KF. Thyroid cancer in children in Belarus after Chernobyl. World Health Stat Q 1993; 46:204–208.
49. Nikiforov YE, Gnepp DR, Fagin JA. Thyroid lesions in children and adolescents after the Chernobyl disaster: implications for the study of radiation tumorigenesis. J Clin Endocrinol Metab 1996; 81:9–14.
50. Nikiforov YE, Gnepp DR. Pediatric thyroid cancer after the Chernobyl disaster: pathomorphologic study of 84 cases (1991-1992) from the Republic of Belarus. Cancer 1994; 74:748–766.
50a. Mahoney MC, Lawvere S, Falkner KL, et al. Thyroid cancer incidence trends in Belarus: Examining the impact of Chernobyl. Int J Epidemiol 2004; 33:1025–1033.
51. Pillay R, Graham-Pole J, Miraldi F, Yulish B, Newman A, Liebman J. Diagnostic x-irradiation as a possible etiologic agent in thyroid neoplasms of childhood. J Pediatr 1982; 101:566–568.
52. Holm LE, Wiklund KE, Lundell GE, et al. Thyroid cancer after diagnostic doses of iodine-131: a retrospective cohort study. J Natl Cancer Inst 1988; 80:1132–1138.
53. Shore RE. Issues and epidemiological evidence regarding radiation-induced thyroid cancer. Radiat Res 1992; 131:98–111.
54. Fogelfield L, Bauer TK, Schneider AB, Swartz JE, Zitman R. p53 gene mutation in radiation-induced thyroid cancer. J Clin Endocrinol Metab 1996; 81:3039–3044.
55. Ito T, Seyama T, Iwamoto KS, et al. Activated RET oncogene in thyroid cancers of children from areas contaminated by Chernobyl accident. Lancet 1994; 344:259.
56. Fugazzola L, Pilotti S, Pinchera A, et al. Oncogenic rearrangements of the RET protooncogene in papillary thyroid carcinomas from children exposed to the Chernobyl nuclear accident. Cancer Res 1995; 55: 5617–5620.
57. Elisel R, Romel C, Soldatenko PP, et al. New breakpoints in both the H4 and RET genes create a variant of PTC-1 in a post-Chernobyl papillary thyroid carcinoma. Clin Endocrinol 2000; 53:131–136.
57a. Detours V, Wattel S, Venet D, et al. Absence of a specific radiation signature in post-Chernobyl thyroid cancers. Brit J Cancer 2005; 92:1545–52.
58. Jocham A, Joppich I, Hecker W, Knorr D, Schwarz HP. Thyroid carcinoma in childhood: management and follow-up of 11 cases. Eur J Pediatr 1994; 153:17–22.
59. Samuel AM, Sharma SM. Differentiated thyroid carcinomas in children and adolescents. Cancer 1991; 67:2186–2190.

60. Ceccarelli C, Pacini F, Lippi F, et al. Thyroid cancer in children and adolescents. Surgery 1988; 104:1143–1148.
61. Viswanathan K, Gierlowski TC, Schneider AB. Childhood thyroid cancer: characteristics and long-term outcome in children irradiated for benign conditions of the head and neck. Arch Pediatr Adolesc Med 1994; 148:260–263.
62. Harness JK, Thompson NW, McLeod MK, Pasieka JL, Fukuuchi A. Differentiated thyroid carcinoma in children and adolescents. World J Surg 1992; 16:47–54.
63. Schlumberger M, De Vathaire F, Travagli JP, et al. Differentiated thyroid carcinoma in childhood: long term follow-up of 72 patients. J Clin Endocrinol Metab 1987; 65:1088–1094.
64. Welch-Dinauer CA, Tuttle RM, Robie DK, et al. Clinical features associated with metastasis and recurrence of differentiated thyroid cancer in children, adolescents and young adults. Clin Endocrinol 1998; 49:619–628.
65. Fassina AS, Rupolo M, Pelizzo MR, Casara D. Thyroid cancer in children and adolescents. Tumori 1994; 80:257–262.
66. Lamberg BA, Karkinen-Jaaskelainen M, Franssila KO. Differentiated follicle-derived thyroid carcinoma in children. Acta Pediatr Scand 1989; 78:419–425.
67. Nikiforov YE, Gnepp DR. Pathomorphology of thyroid gland lesions associated with radiation exposure: the Chernobyl experience and review of the literature. Adv Anat Pathol 1999; 6:78–91.
68. Nikiforov YE, Rowland JM, Bove KE, Monforte-Munoz H, Fagin JA. Distinct pattern of ret oncogene rearrangements in morphological variants of radiation-induced and sporadic thyroid papillary carcinomas in children. Cancer Res 1997; 57:1690–1694.

11
Recombinant Human Thyrotropin

Matthew D. Ringel and Stephen J. Burgun

INTRODUCTION

Initial management of patients with thyroid cancer generally includes surgical thyroidectomy, eradication of iodine-avid tissue (benign or malignant) with radioactive iodine, and long-term treatment with L-thyroxine at doses sufficient for suppression of pituitary production of thyrotropin (TSH; *1,2*). Thyroid cancer recurs in 20–40% of patients, requiring long-term monitoring for tumor recurrence or progression *(3)*. Similar to most other malignancies, monitoring is done by physical examination, measurement of tissue or tumor-specific serum markers, and radiographic and sonographic imaging. Measurements of serum thyroglobulin concentrations and radioiodine whole-body imaging are used most frequently to monitor thyroid cancer patients *(1,4)*. Both of these modalities measure relatively thyroid-specific functions. However, the sensitivities of iodine scanning and thyroglobulin measurement are limited by the small, relative amount of thyroid tissue present in patients treated by thyroidectomy and dedifferentiation of tumor cells compared to normal thyrocytes. Therefore, for optimal sensitivity, both radioiodine imaging and serum thyroglobulin measurement require stimulation of thyroid tissue by elevated TSH levels. Moreover, elevated serum concentrations of TSH are also required for radioiodine therapy.

To attain the elevated serum TSH concentrations needed for accurate monitoring, protocols have been designed to stimulate endogenous pituitary TSH production and secretion. Most commonly, L-thyroxine is withdrawn 4–6 wk before radioiodine scanning and serum thyroglobulin measurement. To limit the duration of symptomatic hypothyroidism, patients are frequently treated with triiodothyronine (T_3), an agent with a shorter circulating half-life than L-thyroxine, for 2–3 wk following discontinuation of thyroxine. Most patients attain an adequate serum TSH concentration (>30 mU/L) 2–3 wk after discontinuation of T_3, allowing for scanning and thyroglobulin measurement *(1)*. Several days after scanning and/or therapy, one or both types of thyroid hormone are restarted. Using this paradigm, patients are clinically hypothyroid for approx 4–8 wk, which results in substantial morbidity, including lethargy, depression, irritability, and limited ability to work *(5–7)*. Moreover, elevated TSH levels for extended periods of time have been associated with rapid growth of metastatic tumor tissue, resulting in clinical compromise, particularly among patients with central nervous system metastases *(8,9)*. For these reasons, effective alternative methods for thyroid cell stimulation that require limited thyroid hormone withdrawal *(10,11)* or do not require thyroid hormone withdrawal at all have been sought for many decades *(12)*. This chapter reviews the history of alternative forms of thyroid cell stimulation using exogenous thyroid-stimulating agents, with particular emphasis on the recent development of recombinant human TSH (rhTSH).

EXOGENOUS THYROTROPIN-RELEASING HORMONE

Initial attempts to stimulate endogenous production of pituitary TSH production without thyroxine stimulation were performed using exogenous thyrotropin-releasing hormone (TRH), administered as intramuscular (IM) or intravenous (IV) injections or as an oral preparation. When administered IV, TRH is rapidly inactivated and has a half-life of 4–5 min. TSH peaks approx 20–30 min following TRH administration in normal individuals, but this response is blunted in patients with hyperthyroidism or those on thyroxine suppression *(13–15)*. Repeated doses and infusions have been shown to enhance the TSH response to TRH, but this agent has proven to be too cumbersome for clinical use *(16)*.

Several groups subsequently evaluated oral TRH as an adjunct to standard thyroxine withdrawal or as a method to elevate the serum TSH concentration while patients remain on their L-thyroxine suppression *(16–18)*. Longer periods of TSH elevation were observed with oral TRH when compared to IV or IM TRH administration, particularly when used to augment the TSH rise of thyroxine withdrawal. However, TRH administration alone was less effective in stimulating iodine uptake than standard thyroid hormone withdrawal, despite similar rises in serum TSH concentrations (17). When used in combination with thyroxine withdrawal and lithium carbonate, oral TRH administration did not enhance the iodine uptake vs withdrawal only (19).

More recent data suggest that the glycosylated forms of TSH secreted after acute stimulation with IV TRH may differ from the usual circulating forms of TSH (20). Human TSH contains three asparagine-linked oligosaccharide chains that when fully processed, terminate either with sialic acid linked to galactose or with sulfate attached to N-acetylgalactosamine. Two of these oligosaccharide chains are attached to the α-subunit, and one chain is attached to the β-subunit. The biological importance of these glycosylated forms remains to be completely determined; however, different forms exert different cellular effects in vitro, with unique metabolism and serum half-lives, as well as specific affinities for association with the α-subunit (21–27). Therefore, it is possible that the forms of TSH released following TRH stimulation may not have equivalent biological activity to those present with a more gradual development of hypothyroidism or in the absence of T_3. This may explain the apparent dissociation between iodine uptake and serum TSH concentration after TRH administration. Studies evaluating the importance of the glycosylation pattern on in vivo and in vitro function of rhTSH are detailed below.

BOVINE THYROTROPIN

Seidlin and colleagues (28) and Stanley and Astwood (29) first reported administration of bovine TSH to stimulate radioiodine uptake in humans. Benua and colleagues (30) subsequently reported their 18-yr experience with bovine TSH to augment iodine uptake in patients already hypothyroid following thyroidectomy and ablation using a 2-d dosing regimen. There were 20 patients studied, and only a minimal increase in iodine uptake was seen; however, these patients were already hypothyroid at the time of the bovine TSH administration.

The administration of bovine TSH during thyroxine therapy as an alternative to thyroid hormone withdrawal in preparation for radioiodine scanning was first reported in 1953 by Sturgeon et al. (31); and then revisited by Catz et al. in 1959 (32,33). These reports suggested that bovine TSH administration may be an acceptable alternative to thyroid hormone withdrawal in selected cases. In addition, a cellular rationale for use of bovine TSH in patients was obtained when similar binding and activity was seen for human and bovine TSH in the chick bioassay (34). Schneider and coworkers (35) subsequently showed similar enhancement of thyroid iodine uptake in normal subjects following injection of either bovine or human pituitary TSH.

The similar activities of bovine and human TSH provided a basis for clinical studies designed to evaluate the efficacy of bovine TSH-stimulated radioiodine scanning and treatment in patients with thyroid cancer during thyroid hormone therapy and after a period of thyroxine withdrawal. Pharmacokinetic studies showed a peak serum TSH concentration 4 h after IM administration of bovine TSH; by 10 h, serum concentrations had decreased by 50% (36). Initial results in thyroid cancer patients suggested that administration of bovine TSH was effective, but it did not stimulate iodine uptake as well as thyroid hormone withdrawal (36,37).

Local and systemic adverse events were associated with bovine TSH administration, including local induration, nausea, vomiting, urticaria, and anaphylaxis (38,39). These were specifically evident in patients treated multiple times (37). Because of these allergic reactions and the diminished efficacy of the agent with repeated doses, patients were studied for the development of neutralizing antibodies to bovine TSH. Detectable circulating, neutralizing antibodies developed in the majority of patients who received multiple doses of bovine TSH (40–42). These antibovine TSH antibodies also interfered with measurement of endogenous TSH, hindering the ability to monitor patients for efficacy of thyroid hormone suppression therapy (43–47). With the development of specific immunoassays against human TSH, it was determined that these antibodies were either directed against bovine TSH alone or cross-reacted with bovine and human TSH (42,44). Therefore, there was concern that these antibodies may modulate the bioactivity of endogenous TSH and bovine TSH, limiting subsequent use of radioiodine therapy with either method of stimulation.

A series of in vitro bioassay studies confirmed that the antibodies generated by bovine TSH were partially neutralizing to both bovine and human TSH (40,42). However, the effect on bovine TSH bioactivity was more pronounced. Owing to the combination of relative ineffectiveness with multiple dosing and the development of antibodies, the popularity of bovine TSH use subsequently diminished, and this agent is currently not available in the United States for clinical use.

HUMAN THYROTROPIN

Human Pituitary TSH

Human pituitary TSH was proposed as useful in preparing patients for radioiodine scanning. Studies reporting kinetics in humans show effective stimulation of thyroid hormone production and iodine uptake (48–51). Yet, enthusiasm for the potential use of human pituitary TSH waned when in the early 1980s, several cases of Creutzfeld-Jakob syndrome were reported in patients treated with human pituitary growth hormone (52). In addition, the purity of the human TSH preparation was questioned. Although useful in the laboratory as a standard, clinical use of human pituitary TSH became unlikely because of the unacceptable potential risk of slow-virus transmission.

Recombinant Human TSH

In Vitro Studies

The cloning of the gene encoding the human TSH-β subunit *(53,54)* brought forth the possibility of producing rhTSH using molecular techniques. After several years, bioactive rhTSH was successfully manufactured by several groups by cotransfecting mammalian cells with complementary DNAs that encode both the common human α-subunit and human TSH-β subunit *(21,23,55–58)*. As noted above, the human TSH protein is glycosylated at three sites: two on the α-subunit and one on the β-subunit. The glycosylated forms of TSH found in the pituitary are heterogeneous and may differ from the predominant circulating forms. Because bacterial cells do not possess the enzymes necessary for protein glycosylation, the use of more labor-intensive mammalian gene expression systems was required. This chapter discusses rhTSH derived from transfected Chinese hamster ovary (CHO) cells, as it has been manufactured commercially in large amounts and has been used in clinical studies.

The recombinant protein was isolated from the cotransfected CHO cells and purified by several methods *(55–58)*. In vitro activity and the chemical structure of rhTSH were compared to the international human pituitary TSH standards utilized in clinical assays. Binding studies revealed that rhTSH had high affinity for human TSH receptors expressed endogenously on human fetal thyroid cells *(59)* and for human TSH receptors expressed on CHO cells transfected with TSH receptor cDNA *(25,26,55–58)*. Furthermore, rhTSH binding was not species-specific, displaying relatively high affinities for both endogenous rat TSH receptors expressed on Fisher rat thyroid cells (FRTL-5) and mouse TSH receptors *(25,26,62)*. rhTSH was also functionally active in all TSH receptor–expressing cell types analyzed both in vitro and in vivo *(25,26,55–62)*.

These in vitro studies led to several in vivo animal studies in mice and rats *(60–62)* and primates *(63)* that revealed enhanced serum TSH concentrations and radioiodine uptake following administration of rhTSH. Careful analysis of the differences in activity between the batches of rhTSH both in vitro and in vivo was then performed. In those studies, it became apparent that there was a poor correlation between in vitro and in vivo activity, and differences in the glycosylation patterns of the batches were responsible.

As noted above, three oligosaccharide chains are attached to the endogenous α- and β-subunits of TSH that terminate either with a sialic acid bound to a galactose residue or a sulfate bound to N-acetylgalactosamine. Because the sulfotransferases and GalNAc transferases are found only in pituitary cells, rhTSH produced in cells lacking these enzymes (e.g., CHO cells) contains only the sialylated form. Both human pituitary TSH and rhTSH contain a heterogeneous mixture of glycosylated forms. The difference in bioactivity between the different batches of rhTSH appeared to vary with the pH of the reaction conditions in the bioreactor used for protein manufacturing *(61)*. Specifically, the in vitro bioactivity was higher for the more basic sulfated forms of rhTSH compared to the more acidic sialylated forms. However, the in vivo bioactivity of the sialylated form was greater than that of the sulfated form, presumably related to its longer serum half-life. The sulfated form is excreted in the kidneys and has a relatively short half-life, whereas the sialylated form is metabolized in the liver, resulting in a longer serum half-life *(22–26,61)*. In addition, Magner and colleagues *(20)* identified sialylated TSH as the predominant circulating TSH glycoprotein. Therefore, along with its greater in vivo activity, sialylated rhTSH may be more similar to circulating endogenous TSH than either sulfated rhTSH or human pituitary extract.

Clinical Studies

"NORMAL" SUBJECTS

Although several studies of rhTSH were performed in euthyroid animals, only one published study has been reported in "normal" human subjects. Ramirez et al. *(64)* evaluated six euthyroid subjects with no prior history of thyroid disease, normal thyroid physical examinations, and no biochemical evidence of thyroid disease. The subjects received 0.6 U of rhTSH IM on 3 consecutive days. Serum TSH, T_4, T_3, free thyroxine index, and thyroglobulin were monitored every 4 h for the first 12 h, at 24, 72, and 96 h, and 7 d after dose administration. The development of antibodies against human TSH following the injections was also assessed. Serum TSH rose from a baseline of 1.3 mU/L to a mean of 40 mU/L in 4 h, peaked after 24 h, and then decreased to below baseline 7 d after the injection. Serum T_3 and T_4 concentrations showed similar patterns, except that the peak occurred after 48 h with continued elevation (still within the normal range) after 1 wk. Serum thyroglobulin also rose following recombinant TSH administration, but the maximal rise did not occur until 48–72 h after the dose. The rhTSH was well tolerated, and no patients developed anti-TSH antibodies. Radioiodine uptake was not measured in this study.

PATIENTS WITH THYROID CANCER

Several studies and case reports of use of rhTSH in patients with thyroid cancer have been published in the literature *(9,65–67)*. The focus of this section is on the phases I, II, and III clinical trials that address rhTSH administration for diagnostic scans and measurements of serum thyroglobulin. In these studies, because of ethical considerations, patients were prepared first by rhTSH during thyroid hormone therapy, then by thyroid hormone withdrawal. Randomization of scan order would have subjected some patients to a second period of hypothyroidism in preparation for radioiodine therapy. Therefore, the possibility of reduced sensitivity of the withdrawal scan secondary to "stunning" by the first scanning dose must be considered as a potential confounding factor. However, several studies, and clinical experience, suggest that the incidence of "stunning" is low, particularly when using low (2–5 mCi)-scanning doses; thus, the effects of this bias are likely to be minimal *(1,7)*.

In 1994, Meier and coworkers *(67)* performed a phase I/II clinical trial designed to compare the efficacy and pharmacokinetics of various dosing regimens of rhTSH administration on iodine uptake and serum thyroglobulin concentrations in patients with thyroid cancer. In addition, they also compared the efficacy of the various rhTSH preparation regimens with standard thyroid hormone withdrawal. They evaluated 19 patients with differentiated thyroid cancer. All patients were treated with triiodothyronine (T_3) for an average of 37 d before receiving rhTSH. Suppressed serum TSH concentrations were documented in these patients, and they were randomized to receive a single IM injection of recombinant TSH (10, 20, 30, or 40 U) or multiple doses (2 or 3) of 10 U or two doses of 20 U at 24-h intervals while they remained on T_3. Laboratory evaluation included serum concentrations of TSH, thyroglobulin, free T_4, total T_3, and antithyroglobulin antibodies. Diagnostic whole-body radioiodine scans using 1–2 mCi of ^{131}I were performed 48 h after the last rhTSH injection. After the ^{131}I scan, patients were withdrawn from T_3 for an average of 29 d until the serum TSH concentration was above 30 mU/L. Patients then received a second diagnostic whole-body ^{131}I scan. Patients were treated as clinically indicated based on the results of the scans and serum thyroglobulin concentrations. Diagnostic scans using the two preparations were compared by independent, blinded nuclear medicine physicians and then compared later as paired samples, in which the reviewers were blinded to the order and dates of the two scans.

The pharmacokinetic study revealed that serum TSH concentrations were maximally elevated with higher doses of rhTSH. Yet, the lower 10-U dose resulted in mean serum TSH concentrations similar to withdrawal (127 mU/L vs 77 mU/L, respectively) after one dose, with a greater peak after the second dose (mean value: 220 mU/L). The TSH elevation was maintained for a longer period of time with a multiple-injection schedule. In the blinded review of scans, radioiodine scans were read as equivalent in 17/19 (89%) patients. In two patients, the withdrawal scans were considered superior. In the paired evaluation, scans were of equivalent quality in 12/19 cases; in four cases, the rhTSH scan was superior, and in three cases, the withdrawal scan was superior.

The iodine uptake was lower in the rhTSH scans than in withdrawal preparation in 72% of patients, regardless of dosing regimen. The uptake was similar in the group prepared with one or two doses of 10 U and one dose of 20 U. There was no correlation between the degree of TSH elevation and percentage uptake between the rhTSH groups. Retention of the ^{131}I dose in the neck was measured in seven patients. A twofold greater dose retention was demonstrated after thyroid hormone withdrawal than after rhTSH administration. This difference was corrected by controlling for whole-body retention. Thus, the likely cause of the longer retention time in the thyroid hormone withdrawal scans was thought to be reduced metabolism and renal clearance of iodine in the hypothyroid subjects.

Serum thyroglobulin concentrations also increased in response to the rhTSH. Similar to the response in normal euthyroid subjects, maximal serum concentrations in the thyroid cancer patients occurred 48 and 72 h postadministration. Serum thyroglobulin concentration increased more than twofold in 79% of patients after thyroid hormone withdrawal, compared to 58% of patients after rhTSH. No data are provided about the frequency of lesser thyroglobulin elevations or the correlation between withdrawal and rhTSH-induced elevations; 4 of 19 patients with circulating antithyroglobulin antibodies were included in the study.

None of the patients in the study showed detectable levels of circulating antibodies against human TSH. Quality-of-life assessment using both the Billewicz Scale *(6)*, to assess hypothyroid symptoms, and the Profile of Mood State Comparison (68), to assess changes in mood and other psychological symptoms, revealed more frequent abnormal scores during thyroid hormone withdrawal.

Thus, this phase I/II study showed that in most patients, rhTSH preparation for diagnostic whole-body scans was as efficacious as withdrawal scanning. However, lower neck radioiodine uptake and retention of isotope, along with lower rises in serum thyroglobulin, were seen following rhTSH preparation. Patients tolerated the medication well and had far fewer symptoms compared to withdrawal preparation. The two-injection 10-U regimen produced similar rises in TSH to higher dose regimens and was well tolerated.

Based on the results of this phase I/II trial, a phase III trial was initiated to further compare the diagnostic utility of rhTSH with standard withdrawal scanning. Ladenson and colleagues *(7)* reported the results of a similarly designed study of 152 patients with thyroid cancer who received rhTSH (0.9 mg IM) on 2 consecutive days during thyroid hormone suppression therapy with either L-T_4 or T_3, followed by a thyroid hormone withdrawal scan 4–6 wk later (Fig. 1). Thyroxine suppression was confirmed by serum TSH concentrations. Patients received 2–4 mCi doses of radioiodine 1 d after the second dose of rhTSH and were scanned 2 d later. Serum concentrations of TSH and urinary iodine were measured. In 35 patients, serum thyroglobulin and antithyroglobulin antibodies were also measured. Whole-body radioiodine scans were interpreted by three independent reviewers in a blinded manner, and the results were compared. Hypothyroid symptoms and mood alterations were measured by the Billewicz Scale *(6)* and the Profiles of Mood States Comparison (68), respectively. Of the initial 152 patients enrolled, 127 were included in the

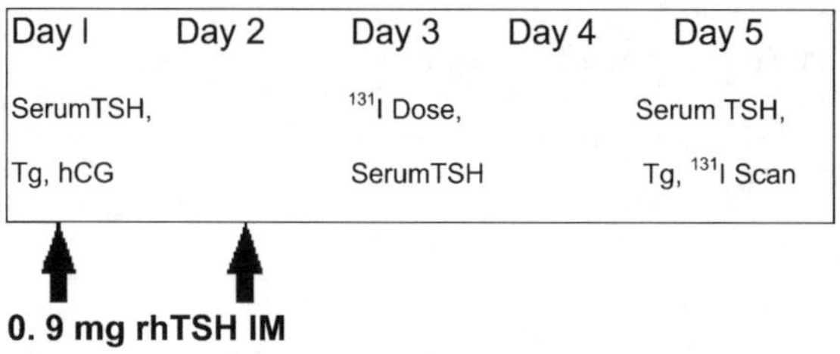

Day 1	Day 2	Day 3	Day 4	Day 5
SerumTSH, Tg, hCG		^{131}I Dose, SerumTSH		Serum TSH, Tg, ^{131}I Scan

↑ ↑
0.9 mg rhTSH IM

Fig. 1. Recommended dosing regimen for rhTSH: 0.9 mg of rhTSH (bioequivalence is 10 U/mg protein, Second World Health Organization International Reference Preparation, Thyrotropin, Human, for Bioassay) is administered on 2 consecutive days. Based on prior studies, the maximal rise in serum TSH occurs 24 and 48 h after the last dose of rhTSH, and the maximal rise in serum thyroglobulin (Tg) concentrations occurs 72 h after the last dose. Pregnancy tests (serum human chorionic gonadotropin [hCG]) should be obtained in all women of childbearing age before rhTSH administration.

study evaluation. The majority of patients not included in the analysis were excluded for undefined protocol violations.

Mean serum TSH concentrations were 132 mU/L 24 h after the second rhTSH dose and 101 mU/L following thyroid hormone withdrawal. In 51% of patients, scans revealed no uptake in both the withdrawal and rhTSH prepared scans. Among the 62 patients with uptake identified on one or both scans, 45 had thyroid bed uptake, 10 had cervical metastases, and 7 had distant metastases. Scans were considered discordant if additional areas of uptake were seen on one scan compared to the other, even if no change in tumor stage occurred. RhTSH and withdrawal scans were concordant in 66% of the patients with positive scans. The rhTSH scan was superior in 5%; the withdrawal scan was superior in 29%. Tumor stage was altered by the scan discordance in 6 or 17 patients with metastases. Including the concordant negative scans, the overall concordance rate for the 127 patients was 83%. rhTSH scans were dominant in 3% of cases, and withdrawal scans were superior in 14% of cases.

Similar to the phase I/II study, local neck radioiodine uptake was lower after rhTSH preparation, but when normalized for the differences in whole-body retention of ^{131}I, no difference was noted. Symptoms of hypothyroidism were significantly less common at the time of the rhTSH administration than after thyroid hormone withdrawal. Serum cholesterol, triglyceride, uric acid, and creatinine concentrations were also lower at the time of rhTSH stimulation than following withdrawal of thyroid hormone.

Serum thyroglobulin concentrations were measured in 35 of the patients. After rhTSH administration, thyroglobulin values were highest at 72–96 h after the first dose. Thyroglobulin rose to a value greater than 5 ng/mL in 13 patients after rhTSH and in 14 patients after withdrawal. No patients developed anti-TSH antibodies, including seven patients who previously received rhTSH in the phase I/II study. Adverse events were noted in 48 of 152 subjects. The most frequent adverse effect was nausea, which occurred in 25 patients and was generally mild and self-limited.

This phase III trial using a two-dose regimen demonstrated that among patients with recurrent or residual thyroid tissue, rhTSH preparation of patients for radioiodine scanning resulted in inferior scans in 29% of cases. This frequency of inferior scans was concerning, and several of these patients were treated differently according to the discordant scan. However, many may have also been identified as requiring ^{131}I treatment based on their rhTSH-stimulated serum thyroglobulin concentrations. Measurement of an rhTSH-stimulated thyroglobulin appeared to be quite sensitive and concordant with thyroid hormone withdrawal–stimulated thyroglobulin. Unfortunately, this laboratory test was obtained from only 35 of the 127 patients in this study. Most patients tolerated the rhTSH well, and symptoms of hypothyroidism were dramatically reduced with the use of rhTSH.

Several reasons could account for the greater sensitivity of withdrawal scans compared to rhTSH scans. Among these reasons: (1) reduced renal clearance of the ^{131}I in hypothyroidism present after withdrawal results in a higher bioavailability for the iodine-avid tissue; (2) the longer duration of the elevated TSH levels after withdrawal may be important for maximally stimulating iodine uptake; and (3) the potentially higher total-body iodine stores owing to continuing L-thyroxine therapy *(11)*.

To further define a potential role for rhTSH as a monitoring agent and to reevaluate the dosing regimen, a second phase III clinical trial compared the two-injection regimen to a three-injection regimen in 226 patients *(69)*. This study was also intended to better evaluate the sensitivity of rhTSH-stimulated thyroglobulin concentrations. The protocol was designed in a similar manner to the study of Ladenson and coworkers *(7)*, but patients were randomized to receive either two or three 0.9-mg IM doses of rhTSH. Patients received ^{131}I 24 h after the last dose of rhTSH, were scanned using 2–4 mCi ^{131}I 2 d later, and serum thyroglobulin concentrations were measured 48 and 72 h after the last dose of rhTSH. Following this scan, patients were withdrawn from thyroid hormone for diagnostic scans, serum thyroglobulin measurements, and treatment as needed.

In this study, scan discordance was defined as uptake on one scan that altered the stage of disease. Using this definition, the overall concordance rate between rhTSH and withdrawal ^{131}I whole-body scans was 89%. Of the discordant studies, whole-body scans after withdrawal were interpreted as dominant in 8% of cases, and rhTSH-stimulated scans were superior in 4% of cases. No statistically significant difference between the accuracy of rhTSH-stimulated scans and withdrawal scans was identified. Moreover, no statistically significant differences were seen between the two rhTSH preparation regimens. Combined data from the two

Table 1
Diagnostic Accuracy of rhTSH Monitoring and Thyroid Hormone Withdrawal vs Thyroid Hormone Withdrawal

Scans	Two Injections (%)	Three Injections (%)
A. Concordance Between rhTSH-Stimulated Scans[a]		
Thyroid whole-body scans	N = 240	N = 107
Concordance	207 (86)	94 (88)
Discordance	33 (14)	13 (12)
Positive whole-body scans	N = 110	N = 60
Concordance	77 (70)	47 (78)
Discordance	33 (30)	13 (22)
rhTSH scan superior	6 (5)	5 (8)
Withdrawal scan superior (% of positive scans)	27 (24)	8 (13)
B. Combined rhTSH Scans and Tg Concentrations vs a "Gold Standard" of Positive Withdrawal Scan and/or an Elevated Withdrawal Thyroglobulin Concentration		
Withdrawal scan and/or Tg > 10 ng/mL[b]	N = 77	N = 86
rhTSH scan + or Tg > 10 ng/mL		
Sensitivity (%)	94	97
Specificity (%)	93	81
Metastases on withdrawal scan	N = 9	N = 23
rhTSH scan + or Tg ≥ 3 ng/mL N (%)	9 (100)	23 (100)

[a]Hormone withdrawal scans are compared. Data for the two-injection regimen are combined from the two phase III trials. Overall concordance rates and concordance rates for those patients in whom at least one scan displayed uptake are shown. The definition of discordance differed in the two phase III studies (see text).

[b]Data are from the second phase III study only. Analysis of all subjects using 5 ng/mL as a positive rhTSH value yielded similar results to the 10 ng/mL value. Using the presence of uptake on rhTSH scanning or a rhTSH-stimulated thyroglobulin greater than 3 ng/mL identified recurrence in all of 32 patients with cervical and/or extracervical metastases.

Tg, thyroglobulin.

phase III trials comparing the utility of the two- and three-injection regimens for radioiodine scanning vs withdrawal scanning are summarized in Table 1A.

Serum thyroglobulin measurements were measured 48 and 72 h after the last dose of rhTSH and following thyroid hormone withdrawal using a highly sensitive radioimmunoassay. Serial samples from individual patients were measured on the same assay. Analysis using different thyroglobulin values to identify disease presence (detectable iodine-avid tissue on diagnostic and/or posttherapy scan) was performed for both basal and stimulated values. The lowest concentration that provided the greatest accuracy for stimulated thyroglobulin concentrations using rhTSH or thyroid hormone withdrawal was established as 3 ng/mL. At values of 3 ng/mL or more, the sensitivity and specificity were 72% and 95% for rhTSH-stimulated thyroglobulin and 71% and 100% for the withdrawal-stimulated thyroglobulin measurements, respectively. Patients with circulating antithyroglobulin antibodies were excluded from this analysis. In general, serum thyroglobulin rose to similar levels after rhTSH stimulation and thyroid hormone withdrawal. The interpretation of these thyroglobulin data is dependent on the reproducibility of the thyroglobulin assay at lower values—a factor that varies greatly between different commercial laboratories. This is particularly critical when interpreting values in the 2–10-ng/mL range. Using a TSH-stimulated value of 5 or 10 ng/mL as a "positive value," the combination of rhTSH-stimulated thyroglobulin and scan was 94% sensitive and 93% specific in predicting iodine-avid tissue on subsequent withdrawal and/or posttherapy scan. When a stimulated thyroglobulin value 3 ng/mL or greater was used in combination with scanning, rhTSH stimulation identified all 32 patients with cervical or distant metastases. Data from the second phase III study that evaluated the accuracy of combining the rhTSH scan and thyroglobulin measurement to identify metastases are summarized in Table 1B.

Recent literature has advocated the use of rhTSH-stimulated thyroglobulin alone, without the use of a diagnostic whole-body ^{131}I scan for patients at low risk of metastasis. Several investigators noted a discordance between L-thyroxine withdrawal, TSH-stimulated thyroglobulin results and whole-body scanning, indicating optimal sensitivity and less false-negative results with the TSH-stimulated thyroglobulin than whole-body scintigraphy (70–72). At 6–12 mo postoperative therapy with 100 mCi, Callieux and associates detected at least 1.0 ng/mL of thyroglobulin after L-thyroxine withdrawal in 46 of 256 patients (70). Diagnostic ^{131}I scintigraphy showed no uptake in 236 patients (92%). Iodine uptake did not correlate with the thyroglobulin level. Of the 210 with hypothyroid thyroglobulin concentration less than 1.0 ng/mL, only two had recurrent disease in 3 yr follow-up. Of 15 patients with hypothyroid thyroglobulin concentrations of 10 ng/mL or more, three had detectable thyroid bed uptake on scintigraphy, but five demonstrated persistent disease. The 37 patients from this cohort with hypothyroid concentrations greater than 1.0 ng/mL were followed further, and nine had evidence of disease between 3 and 117 mo after intitial surgery. Of these recurrences, only one was detected by pulmonary uptake on diagnostic ^{131}I scintigraphy. The diagnostic scans were negative in the other eight cases (71).

These studies were corroborated by both retrospective and prospective studies of rhTSH-stimulated thyroglobulin alone as the method of surveillance after thyroidectomy and thyroid remnant ablation. A retrospective review of 107 patients with differentiated thyroid cancer, without thyroglobulin antibodies, compared the results of rhTSH-stimulated thyroglobulin and 4-mCi (3.8–5.1 mCi) ^{131}I diagnostic whole-body scintigraphy (73). Persistent disease was found in 11 patients. At an rhTSH-stimulated thyroglobulin concentration of 2.0 ng/mL or more, there was 100% sensitivity and 100% negative predictive value. The diagnostic scan did not identify the site of disease in any case and had a 73% false-negative rate.

The use of rhTSH-stimulated thyroglobulin alone was studied prospectively in a multicenter trial of 300 patients with differentiated thyroid cancer and negative thyroglobulin antibody testing (74). Serum thyroglobulin increased by at least 2 ng/mL in 53 patients (18%) after rhTSH. Of 267 patients with baseline thyroxine-suppressed thyroglobulin less than 1 ng/mL, 26 (10%) had at least 2 ng/mL of stimulated thyroglobulin. Of the 53 patients with net increases of at least 2 ng/mL of thyroglobulin, 33 (62%) had a history of negative ^{131}I whole-body scans.

These findings culminated in an expert summary in 2003, advocating the use of rhTSH-stimulated thyroglobulin as the preferred method of surveillance for patients with differentiated thyroid cancer at low risk for metastasis (75). This consensus was limited to patients at clinically low risk for persistent or recurrent disease, or cancer death, and without thyroglobulin antibodies. The use of sensitive immunometric thyroglobulin assays was advocated, along with a sensitive immunoassay for the thyroglobulin antibody. An rhTSH-stimulated thyroglobulin concentration of 2.0 ng/mL was set as the threshold for further intervention. Although hypothyroid and euthyroid rhTSH-stimulated thyroglobulin measurements were considered comparable for disease detection, the authors opined that rhTSH was preferable to L-thyroxine withdrawal because of the likelihood of hypothyroid symptoms and potential loss of productivity after withdrawal.

SUMMARY OF RHTSH IN THYROID CANCER

Based on the three controlled clinical studies performed in a limited number of patients, it appears that rhTSH is a safe alternative to thyroid hormone withdrawal in the detection of recurrent or residual thyroid cancer. There also appears to be no significant advantage of the three-injection regimen when compared to the two-injection regimen. RhTSH preparation for ^{131}I scanning appears to be less sensitive than thyroid hormone withdrawal; however, the combined use of scanning and measurements of serum thyroglobulin improves the sensitivity of rhTSH monitoring. RhTSH preparation avoids the severe transient hypothyroidism that occurs with thyroid hormone withdrawal.

The advantages must be balanced against the risk of recurrence in each individual patient, and it is important to realize that rhTSH has been studied only in diagnostic testing, not for radioiodine therapy. Therefore, patients with high-risk tumors, or patients being prepared for post-thyroidectomy ablation, may not be appropriate for rhTSH screening. In addition, reliance on serum thyroglobulin measurements depends on the absence of antithyroglobulin antibodies and the sensitivity and reproducibility of the particular thyroglobulin immunoassay—factors that vary greatly between different laboratories.

In many patients, performance of rhTSH-stimulated thyroglobulin testing without diagnostic whole-body ^{131}I scanning may be appropriate for surveillance after thyroidectomy and radioiodine ablation, in addition to clinical and ultrasound examination. This strategy is limited to patients with a history of differentiated thyroid cancer at low risk for recurrence or cancer death and without interfering thyroglobulin antibodies. For this population, the rhTSH-stimulated ^{131}I whole-body scan has been less sensitive for detection of persistent disease and may not add any diagnostic information beyond the rhTSH-stimulated thyroglobulin measurement.

Larger clinical studies are needed to adequately address several questions regarding the clinical use of rhTSH. First, what is the sensitivity of rhTSH in patients with poorly differentiated tumors; second, is there a role for rhTSH stimulation for ^{131}I treatment in selected individuals? A critical issue is standardization of thyroglobulin assays, because the most effective use of rhTSH relies heavily on an assay with high reproducibility in the lower range. A suggested algorithm for use of rhTSH as a diagnostic agent, while monitoring patients for recurrence of thyroid cancer based on the current data, is depicted in Fig. 2. Similar algorithms were recently published (76,77), and determination of the optimal

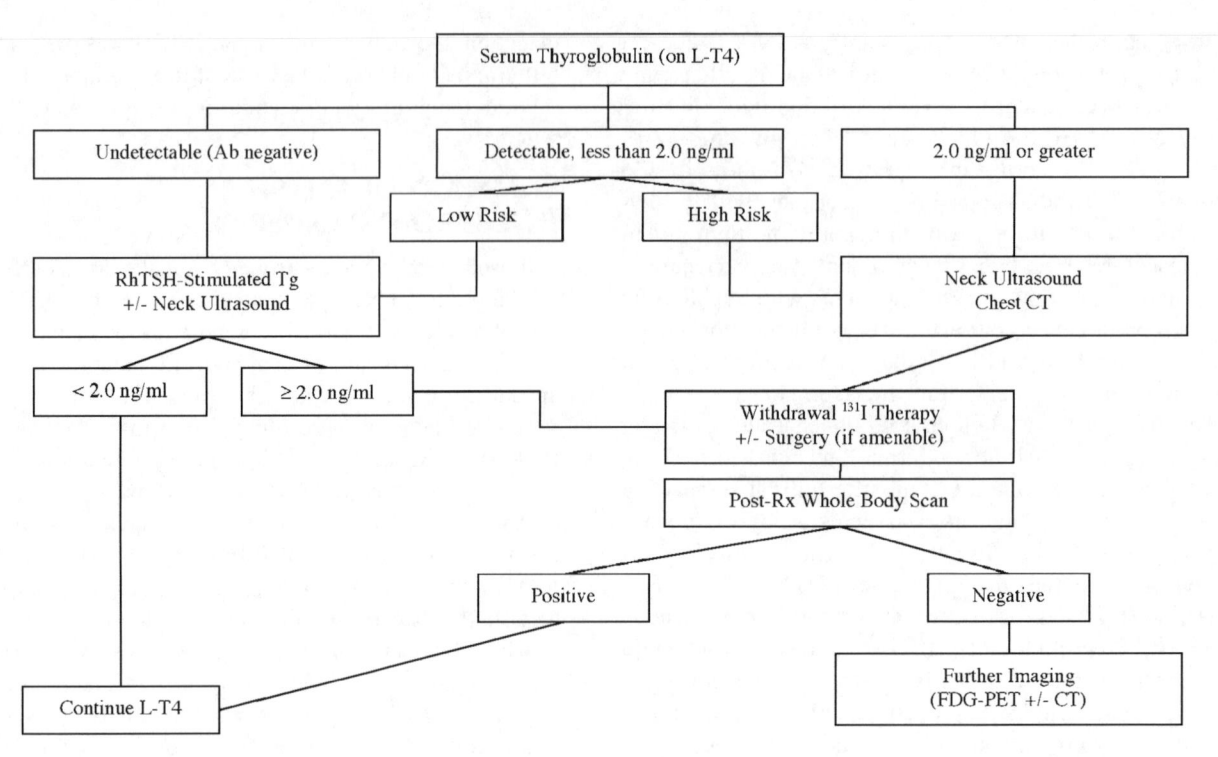

Fig. 2. Algorithm for monitoring thyroid cancer recurrence. This algorithm applies to patients already treated with thyroidectomy and remnant ablation with ^{131}I and is highly dependent on an accurate thyroglobulin (Tg) assay, with absence of the Tg antibody. Patients with elevated serum Tg levels (>2 ng/mL) on TSH-suppression therapy, or those with high-risk tumors and more modest elevations (0.5–2.0 ng/mL), have a high likelihood of recurrence and are likely to require radioiodine therapy or surgery, depending on the extent of prior therapy. These patients should have radiographic imaging to search for surgically amenable recurrence (e.g., neck lymph nodes) and, if negative, opt for thyroid hormone withdrawal scan and/or treatment. Patients with low-risk tumors and small elevations of Tg on suppression (0.5–2.0 ng/mL) should be evaluated by rhTSH-stimulated Tg with or without a scan and neck sonogram. Patients with low-risk tumors and undetectable serum Tg on suppression should have a rhTSH-stimulated Tg with or without a scan and neck ultrasound to monitor for recurrence. The frequency of evaluation depends on the years since diagnosis and other factors. If the Tg concentration rises, thyroid hormone withdrawal for therapy and other radiographic imaging should be anticipated to identify surgically amenable recurrences. The value of 2 ng/mL used as a threshold value for stimulated Tg is based on published data using highly accurate assays in the absence of antithyroglobulin antibodies. The incremental rise of serum thyroglobulin concentration following rhTSH administration, particularly the thyroglobulin assay, and other clinical factors may warrant radiographic evaluations for rhTSH-stimulated concentrations different than 2 ng/mL. If rhTSH scans are obtained, uptake outside of the thyroid bed may also dictate the need for surgical excision or ^{131}I therapy, depending on the site of uptake.

use of rhTSH in thyroid cancer requires further study and more extensive clinical use.

rhTSH in Other Conditions

No clinical trials have been reported using rhTSH to facilitate therapy for thyroid diseases other than thyroid cancer. Clinical trials using rhTSH as preparation for radioiodine therapy of toxic and nontoxic, large goiters are ongoing. RhTSH may be particularly useful if the overall iodine uptake of the goiter is low. In addition, it may prove to be a useful adjunct to ^{123}I scanning in patients with poor-quality scans possibly related to iodine exposure. In the determination of serum TSH concentrations, rhTSH may be a more standardized and easily replenishable source of concentration controls than human pituitary TSH (78,79).

FUTURE DIRECTIONS

More clinical experience and clinical trials are needed for a full assessment of the utility of rhTSH in monitoring patients with thyroid cancer. Recent reports by Skudlinski and colleagues (80), as well as Grossman and colleagues (81), raise the possibility of developing TSH receptor superagonists with enhanced effects on iodide uptake. Grossman et al. inserted four mutations in the common α subunit and three mutations in the TSH-β subunit in locations, according to the crystallographic structure of human chorionic gonadotropin and its homology with TSH. This mutated TSH protein displays a 1000-fold greater affinity for the TSH receptor and a 100-fold greater in vivo activity than wild-type TSH. Although this agent has not been tested in humans, similar superagonists of the TSH receptor may improve the sensitivity of rhTSH preparation for diagnostic testing in thyroid cancer and other disorders *(82)*.

SUMMARY

The development of rhTSH as an adjunct for diagnostic testing in patients with thyroid cancer may enable physicians to limit the morbidity associated with monitoring techniques. Although there are some concerns regarding sensitivity of the agent, screening for recurrence by rhTSH-stimulated thyroglobulin with or without ^{131}I scanning may be appropriate for many patients with low-risk tumors. Mutated forms of TSH with enhanced bioactivity may improve the sensitivity of monitoring techniques that do not require thyroid hormone withdrawal. Further studies and more extensive clinical experience are needed to fully delineate the role for this exciting new agent in the detection and treatment of thyroid cancer and other thyroid conditions.

REFERENCES

1. Singer PA, Cooper DS, Daniels GH, et al. Treatment guidelines for patients with thyroid nodules and well-differentiated thyroid cancer. Arch Intern Med 1996; 156:2165–2172.
2. Solomon BL, Wartofsky L, Burman KD. Current trends in the management of well differentiated papillary thyroid carcinoma. J Clin Endocrinol Metab 1996; 81:333–339.
3. Mazzaferri EL, Jiang SM. Long-term impact of initial surgical and medical therapy on papillary and follicular cancer. Am J Med 1994; 89:418–428.
4. Ozata M, Suzuki S, Miyamoto T, et al. Serum thyroglobulin in the follow-up of patients with treated differentiated thyroid cancer. J Clin Endocrinol Metab 1994; 778:188–196.
5. Dow KH, Ferrell BR, Annelo C. Quality of life changes in patients with thyroid cancer after withdrawal of thyroid hormone therapy. Thyroid 1997; 7:613–619.
6. Billewicz WZ, Chapman RS, Crooks J, et al. Statistical methods applied to the diagnosis of hypothyroidism. Q J Med 1969; 38: 255–266.
7. Ladenson PW, Braverman LE, Mazzaferri EL, et al. Comparison of administration of recombinant human thyrotropin with withdrawal of thyroid hormone for radioactive iodine scanning in patients with thyroid carcinoma. N Engl J Med 1997; 337:888–896.
8. Stakianakis GN, Stillman TG, George JM. Thyroxine withdrawal in thyroid cancer. Ohio State Med J 1975; 71:79–82.
9. Goldberg LD, Ditchek NT. Thyroid carcinoma with spinal cord compression. JAMA 1981; 245:953–954.
10. Guimaraes V, Degroot LJ. Moderate hypothyroidism in preparation for whole body 131I scintiscans and thyroglobulin testing. Thyroid 1996; 6:69–73.
11. Maxon HR. Recombinant human thyrotropin symposium: Detection of residual and recurrent thyroid cancer by radionuclide imaging. Thyroid 1999; 9:443–446.
12. Robbins J. Recombinant human thyrotropin seminar: Pharmacology of bovine and human thyrotropin: an historical perspective. Thyroid 1999; 9:451–453.
13. Wide L, Dahlberg PA. Quality requirements of basal S-TSH assays in predicting an S-TSH response to TRH. Scand J Clin Lab Invest 1981; 40:101.
14. Sawin CT, Hershman JM. The TSH response to thyrotropin-releasing hormone (TRH) in young adult men: intra-individual variation and relation to basal serum TSH and thyroid hormones. J Clin Endocrinol Metab 1976; 42:809–816.
15. Spencer CA, Schwarzbein D, Guttler RB, et al. Thyrotropin (TSH)-releasing hormone stimulation test responses employing third and fourth generation TSH assays. J Clin Endocrinol Metab 1993; 76: 494–498.
16. Fairclough PD, Cryer RJ, McAllister J, et al. Serum TSH responses to intravenously and orally administered TRH in man after thyroidectomy for carcinoma of the thyroid. Clin Endocrinol 1973; 2:351–359.
17. Wenzel KW, Meinhold H, Bogner U, et al. Serum TSH levels in thyroidectomized patients after withdrawal of thyroid hormone therapy or oral administration of TRH. Acta Endocrinol 1973; 173(Suppl):15.
18. Eissner D, Hahn K, Grimm W. Oral TRH stimulation in patients with thyroid carcinoma. ROFO 1983; 138:95–100.
19. Ang ES, Teh HS, Sundram FX, Lee KO. Effect of lithium and oral thyrotrophin-releasing hormone (TRH) on serum thyrotropin (TSH) and radioiodine uptake in patients with well differentiated thyroid carcinoma. Singapore Med J 1995; 36:606–608.
20. Magner JA, Kane J, Chou ET. Intravenous thyrotropin (TSH)-releasing hormone releases human TSH that is structurally different from basal TSH. J Clin Endocrinol Metab 1992; 74:1306–1311.
21. Schaaf L, Leiprecht A, Saji M, et al. Glycosylation variants of human TSH selectively activate signal transduction pathways. Mol Cell Endocrinol 1997; 132:185–194.
22. Szkudinski MW, Thokatura NR, Weintraub BD. Subunit-specific functions of N-linked oligosaccharides in human thyrotropin: role of terminal residues of alpha and beta subunit oligosaccharides in clearance and bioactivity. Proc Natl Acad Sci USA 1995; 92:9062–9066.
23. Cannone C, Papandreou MJ, Medri G, et al. Biological and immunochemical characterization of recombinant human thyrotrophin. Glycobiology 1995; 5:473–481.
24. Szkudlinski MW, Thokatura NR, Bucci I, et al. Purification and characterization of recombinant human thyrotropin (TSH) isoforms produced by Chinese hamster ovary cells: the role of sialylation and sulfation in TSH bioactivity. Endocrinology 1993; 133:1490–1503.
25. Thokatura NR, Desai RK, Bates LG, et al. Biological activity and metabolic clearance of a recombinant human thyrotropin produces in Chinese hamster ovary cells. Endocrinology 1991; 128:341–348.
26. Thokatura NR, Szkudlinski MW, Weintraub BD. Structure-function studies of oligosaccharides of recombinant human thyrotropin by sequential deglycosylation and resialylation. Glycobiology 1994; 4: 525–533.
27. Matzuk MM, Kornmeier CM, Whitfield GK, et al. The glycoprotein α-subunit is critical for secretion and stability of the human thyrotropin β-subunit. Mol Endocrinol 1988; 2:95–100.
28. Seidlin SM, Oshry E, Yalow AA. Spontaneous and experimentally induced uptake of radioactive iodine in metastases from thyroid carcinoma: a preliminary report. J Clin Endocrinol 1948; 8:423–432.
29. Stanley MM, Astwood EB. The response of the thyroid gland in normal human subjects to the administration of thyrotropin, as shown by studies with I-131. Endocrinology 1949; 44:49–60.
30. Benua RS, Sonenberg M, Leeper RD, Rawson RW. An 18 year study of the use of beef thyrotropin to increase I-131 uptake in metastatic thyroid cancer. J Nucl Med 1964; 5:796–801.
31. Sturgeon CT, Davis FE, Catz B, et al. Treatment of thyroid cancer metastases with TSH and I-131 during thyroid hormone medication. J Clin Endocrinol Metab 1953; 13:1391–1407.
32. Catz B, Petit D, Starr P. The diagnostic and therapeutic value of thyrotropic hormone and heavy dosage scintigrams for the demonstration of thyroid cancer metastases. Am J Med Sci 1959; 237:158–164.
33. Catz B, Petit DW, Schwartz M, et al. Treatment of cancer of the thyroid postoperatively with suppressive thyroid medication, radioiodine, and thyroid-stimulating hormone. Cancer 1959; 12:371–383.
34. Reichert LE Jr. On the relationship between human thyrotropin research standard A, the United States Pharmacopeia thyrotrophin

34. standard (bovine) and the International Standard for thyrotrophin (bovine). J Clin Endocrinol 1970; 31:331–333.
35. Schneider PB, Robbins J, Condliffe PG. Thyroid response to human thyrotropin in man. J Clin Endocrinol Metab 1965; 25:514–517.
36. Hershman JM, Edwards CL. Serum thyrotropin (TSH) levels after thyroid ablation compared with TSH levels after exogenous bovine TSH: implications for ^{131}I treatment of thyroid carcinoma. J Clin Endocrinol 1972; 34:814–818.
37. Hays MT, Solomon DH, Werner SC. The effect of purified bovine thyroid-stimulating hormone in man. II. Loss of effectiveness with prolonged administration. J Clin Endocrinol Metab 1961; 21:1475–1482.
38. Krishnamurthy GT. Human reactive to bovine TSH: concise communication. J Nucl Med 1978; 19:284–286.
39. Sherman WB, Werner SC. Generalized allergic reaction to bovine thyrotropin. JAMA 1964; 190:244–245.
40. Hays MT, Solomon DH, Pierce JG, Carsten ME. The effect of purified bovine thyroid-stimulating hormone in man. I. Dose-response characteristics studies with I132. J Clin Endocrinol Metab 1961; 21:1469–1474.
41. Melmed S, Harada A, Hershman JM, Krishnamurthy GT, Bland WH. Neutralizing antibodies to bovine thyrotropin in immunized patients with thyroid cancer. J Clin Endocrinol Metab 1980; 51:358–363.
42. Hays MT, Solomon DH, Beall GN. Suppression of human thyroid function by antibodies to bovine thyrotropin. J Clin Endocrinol Metab 1967; 27:1540–1549.
43. Greenspan FS, Lowenstein JM, West MN, Okerlund MD. Immunoreactive material to bovine TSH in plasma from patients with thyroid cancer. J Clin Endocrinol Metab 1972; 35:795–798.
44. Frohman LA, Baron MA, Schneider AB. Plasma immunoreactive TSH: spurious elevation due to antibodies to bovine TSH which cross-react with human TSH. Metabolism 1982; 31:834–840.
45. Greenspan FS, Lew W, Okerlund MD, et al. Falsely positive bovine TSH radioimmunoassay responses in sera from patients with thyroid cancer. J Clin Endocrinol Metab 1974; 38:1121–1122.
46. Sain A, Sham R, Singh A, et al. Erroneous thyroid-stimulating hormone radioimmunoassay results due to interfering anti-bovine thyroid-stimulating hormone antibodies. Am J Clin Pathol 1979; 71:540–542.
47. Chaussain JL, Binet E, Job JC. Antibodies to human thyrotropin in the serum of certain hypopituitary dwarfs. Rev Eur Etudes Clin Biol 1972; 17:95–99.
48. Uller RP, van Herle AJ, Chopra IJ. Comparison of alterations in circulating thyroglobulin, triiodothyronine and thyroxine in response to exogenous (bovine) and endogenous (human) thyrotropin. J Clin Endocrinol Metab 1973; 37:741–745.
49. Kuku SF, Harsoulle P, Kjed M, Fraser TR. Human thyrotrophic hormone kinetics and effects in euthyroid males. Horm Metab Res 1975; 7:54–59.
50. Law A, Jack GW, Tellez M, Edmonds CJ. In vivo studies of a human thyrotrophin preparation. J Clin Endocrinol 1986; 110:375–378.
51. Ridgway EC, Weintraub BD, Maloof F. Metabolic clearance and production rates of human thyrotropin. J Clin Invest 1974; 53:8895–8903.
52. Brown P, Gadjusek DC, Gibbs Jr CJ, Asher DM. Potential epidemic of Creutzfeld-Jakob disease from human growth hormone therapy. N Engl J Med 1985; 110:375–378.
53. Hayashizaki Y, Miyai K, Kato K, Matsubara K. Molecular cloning of the human thyrotropin beta-subunit gene. FEBS Lett 1985; 188:394–400.
54. Wondisford FE, Radovick S, Moates JM, et al. Isolation and characterization of the human thyrotropin-beta subunit gene. J Biol Chem 1988; 263:12,538–12,542.
55. Watanabe S, Hayashizaki Y, Endo Y, et al. Production of human thyroid stimulating hormone in Chinese hamster ovary cells. Biochem Biophys Res Commun 1987; 149:1149–1155.
56. Hussain A, Zimmerman CA, Boose JA, et al. Large scale synthesis of recombinant human thyrotropin using methotrexate amplification: chromatographic, immunological, and biological characterization. J Clin Endocrinol Metab 1996; 81:1184–1188.
57. Cole ES, Lee K, Lauziere K, et al. Recombinant human thyroid-stimulating hormone: development of a biotechnology product for detection of metastatic lesions of thyroid carcinoma. Biotechnology 1993; 11:1014–1024.
58. Wondisford FE, Usala SJ, DeCherney GS, et al. Cloning of the human thyrotropin β-subunit gene and transient expression of biologically active human thyrotropin after gene transfection. Mol Endocrinol 1988; 2:32–39.
59. Huber GK, Fong P, Concepción ES, Davies TF. Recombinant human thyroid-stimulating hormone: initial bioactivity assessment using human fetal thyroid cells. J Clin Endocrinol Metab 1991; 72:1328–1331.
60. Leitolf H, Szkudlinski MW, Thotakura NR, et al. Effects of continuous and pulsatile administration of pituitary rat thyrotropin and recombinant human thyrotropin in a chronically cannulated rat. Horm Metab Res 1995; 27:173–178.
61. East-Palmer J, Szkudlinski MW, Lee J, et al. A novel nonradio-active in vivo bioassay of thyrotropin (TSH). Thyroid 1995; 5:55–59.
62. Colzani RM, Alex S, Fang S-L, et al. The effect of recombinant human thyrotropin (rhTSH) on thyroid function in mice and rats. Thyroid 1998; 8:797–801.
63. Braverman LE, Pratt BM, Ebner S, Longcope C. Recombinant human thyrotropin stimulated thyroid function and radioactive iodine uptake in the rhesus monkey. J Clin Endocrinol Metab 1992; 74:1135–1139.
64. Ramirez L, Braverman LE, White B, Emerson CE. Recombinant human thyrotropin is a potent stimulator of thyroid function in normal subjects. J Clin Endocrinol Metab 1997; 82:2836–2839.
65. Ringel MD, Ladenson PW. Diagnostic accuracy of ^{131}I scanning with recombinant human thyrotropin versus thyroid hormone withdrawal in a patient with metastatic thyroid carcinoma and hypopituitarism. J Clin Endocrinol Metab 1996; 81:1724–1725.
66. Rudavsky AZ, Freeman LM. Treatment of scan-negative, thyroglobulin-positive metastatic thyroid cancer using radioiodine 131I and recombinant human thyroid stimulating hormone. J Clin Endocrinol Metab 1997; 82:9–10.
67. Meier CA, Braverman LE, Ebner SA, et al. Diagnostic use of recombinant human thyrotropin in patients with thyroid carcinoma (phase I/II study). J Clin Endocrinol Metab 1994; 78:188–196.
68. Albrecht RR, Ewing SJ. Standardizing administration of the Profile of Moods States (POMS): development of alternative word lists. J Personal Assess 1989; 53:31–39.
69. Haugen BR, Pacini F, Reiners C, et al. A comparison of recombinant human thyrotropin and thyroid hormone withdrawal for the detection of thyroid remnant or cancer. J Clin Endocrinol Metab 1999; 84:3877–3885.
70. Cailleux AF, Baudin E, Travagli JP, et al. Is diagnostic iodine-131 scanning useful after total thyroid ablation for differentiated thyroid cancer? J Clin Endocrinol Metab 2000; 85:175–178.
71. Baudin E, Do Cao C, Cailleux AF, et al. Positive predictive value of serum thyroglobulin levels, measured during the first year of follow-up after thyroid hormone withdrawal, in thyroid cancer patients. J Clin Endocrinol Metab 2003; 88:1107–1111.
72. Robbins RJ, Chon JT, Fleisher M, et al. Is the serum thyroglobulin response to recombinant human thyrotropin sufficient, by itself, to monitor for residual thyroid carcinoma? J Clin Endocrinol Metab 2002; 87:3242–3247.
73. Mazzaferri EL, Kloos RT. Is diagnostic iodine-131 scanning with recombinant human TSH useful in the follow-up of differentiated thyroid cancer after thyroid ablation? J Clin Endocrinol Metab 2002; 87:1490–1498.

74. Wartofsky L, et al. Management of low-risk well-differentiated thyroid cancer based only on thyroglobulin measurement after recombinant human thyrotropin. Thyroid 2002; 12:583–590.
75. Mazzaferri EL, Robbins RJ, Spencer CA, et al. A consensus report of the role of serum thyroglobulin as a monitoring method for low-risk patients with papillary thyroid carcinoma. J Clin Endocrinol Metab 2003; 88:1433–1441.
76. Ladenson PW. Recombinant human thyrotropin symposium: Strategies for thyrotropin use to monitor patients with treated thyroid carcinoma. Thyroid 1999; 9:429–433.
77. Mazzaferri EL. Recombinant human thyrotropin symposium: An overview of the management of papillary and follicular thyroid carcinoma. Thyroid 1999; 9:421–427.
78. Ribela MT, Bianco AC, Bartolini P. The use of recombinant human thyrotropin produced by Chinese hamster ovary cells for the preparation of immunoassay reagents. J Clin Endocrinol Metab 1996; 81:249–256.
79. Morgenthaler NG, Pampel I, Aust G, et al. Application of a bioassay with CHO cells for the routine detection of stimulating and blocking autoantibodies to the TSH-receptor. Horm Metab Res 1998; 30:162–168.
80. Szkudlinski MW, Teh NG, Grossman M, et al. Engineering human glycoprotein hormone superactive analogues. Nature Biotechnol 1996; 14:1257–1263.
81. Grossmann M, Leitolf H, Weintraub BD, et al. A novel strategy for rational design of protein hormone superagonists. Nature Biotechnol 1998; 16:871–875.
82. Weintraub BD, Szkudlinski MW. Recombinant human thyrotropin symposium: development and in vitro characterization of human recombinant thyrotropin. Thyroid 1999; 9:447–450.

Part II
General Considerations II
Nuclear Medicine

12
History of the Role of Nuclear Medicine in the Thyroid Gland and its Diseases
A Personal Perspective

Henry N. Wagner, Jr.

INTRODUCTION

No organ of the body has been more important in the development of nuclear medicine than the thyroid gland. The use of nuclear medicine in the care of patients with thyroid disease illustrates most of the general principles upon which the field is based. After I finished my internal medicine residency at Johns Hopkins and two subsequent years as a Clinical Associate at the National Institutes of Health (NIH), I had 1 yr before I had to return to Johns Hopkins as Chief Resident on the Osler Medical Service. Because endocrinology was the most exciting area of medicine at that time (the late 1950s), I decided to spend a year as a postdoctoral fellow at Hammersmith Hospital in London, working in the department of Dr. Russell Fraser. That year opened my eyes to the use of radioactive tracers in medicine.

My exposure to the use of iodine-132 in patients with thyroid disease at Hammersmith Hospital in 1957 led me into the field that was to become "nuclear medicine." For the first time, I saw the types of information that radioactive isotopes could provide that were so helpful in the care of my patients. The methods were sensitive, specific, and could be used to examine the chemistry within the body via radiation detectors outside of the body. The information was dynamic, rather than static, with space and time joining to quantitatively document the chemistry of the living human body. We now had the tools to examine and quantitatively characterize the dynamic state of the processes that are the basis of life.

One of my responsibilities was to separate the short-lived iodine-132 from its parent radionuclide tellurium-132 through the process of distillation. The iodine-132 had a 2.5-h half-life. The physicist at Hammersmith Hospital, Dr. John Mallard, advised me to visit Drs. Stang and Richards at the Brookhaven National Laboratory (BNL) after I returned to the United States. They had developed a method that separated short-lived "daughter" radionuclides from their longer-lived "parent" radionuclides. Iodine-132 with a half-life of 3 h could be eluted from a column containing the longer-lived tellurium-132. This type of "radionuclide generator," often called a "cow," would have a major effect on nuclear medicine, particularly in making the radionuclide technetium-99m, available from its parent molybdenum-132.

For example, in a patient with a nodule within the thyroid, I used a Geiger counter to measure the radiation from the injection of iodine-132 into the patient. A plastic grid was used to delineate points 1 cm apart across the patient's neck. "Isocount" lines were then drawn to provide a crude image of the radioactivity distribution from the thyroid. If the radioactivity from the region of the nodule was less than in the surrounding thyroid, the nodule was "cold" and was much more likely to be thyroid cancer than if it accumulated radioiodine (i.e., was "hot"). We learned that one of the functions malignant thyroid cells lose is the ability to accumulate radioiodine.

It also became possible to take advantage of the fact that the thyroid accumulates technetium-99m pertechnetate in the same manner as radioiodine. Paul Harper, from the University of Chicago, was the first to recognize that the ready availability, short half-life, type of radioactive decay by isomeric transition, and 150 keV photons emitted in the process of radioactive decay of technetium-99m made this radionuclide ideal for external imaging of the human body with the recent invented Anger camera. The BNL molybdenum/technetium generator was advertized from 1951 to 1953, 3 yr before Harper recognized it to have such great potential (Fig. 1).

Various disorders of the thyroid gland may be found when a patient or the examining physician initially detects an enlargement of the gland or nodules in the neck, or the patient begins to develop symptoms of nervousness and weight loss from the increased secretion of thyroid hormones, known as hyperthyroidism. Radioactive iodine or its analog, technetium-99m pertechnetate, makes it possible to examine the biochemical processes within the thyroid gland itself and quantify the increased or decreased incorporation of iodine

From: *Thyroid Cancer: A Comprehensive Guide to Clinical Management, 2/e*
Edited by: L. Wartofsky and D. Van Nostrand © Humana Press Inc., Totowa, NJ

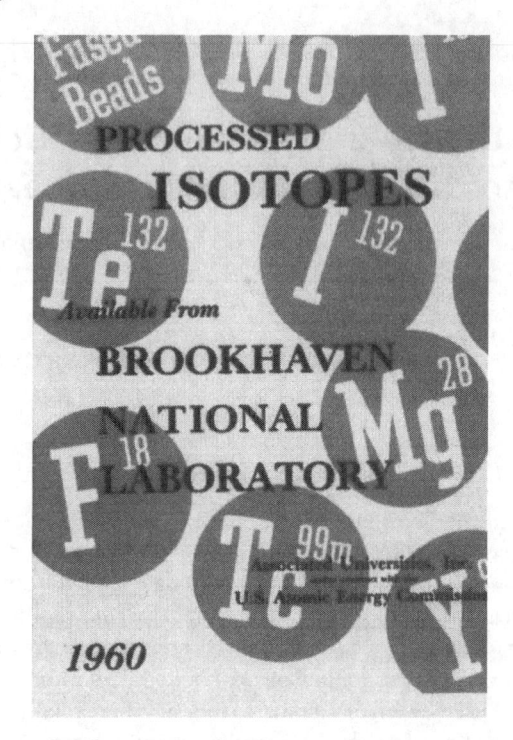

Fig. 1. Catalogue of the BNL in 1961, offering for sale a tellurium-132/iodine-132 generator, as well as a molybdenum-99/technetium-99m generator. This was 3 years before technetium-99m was used in patients.

into the gland or release of synthesized hormone secreted by the gland. Imaging procedures, including radionuclide imaging, ultrasound, and magnetic resonance imaging, can provide structural details (e.g., delineation of nodules or enlargement of the gland). Examining the structure, function, and biochemistry of the thyroid not only provides the diagnosis but also a way to plan and monitor the effect of surgery or drug treatment.

BERNARD AND THE BIRTH OF PHYSIOLOGY

In the late 19th century, Claude Bernard, a French physician, paved the way for scientific medicine as we know it today. The driving interest of his life was "to search for an understanding, in terms of physics and chemistry, of those processes by which we live, by which we become ill, by which we are healed, and by which we die." He showed how medicine could move beyond the use of anatomy in defining disease, the approach that had begun with Vesalius in 1543.

During the last several decades, development has moved into the "molecular" era of medicine, but most diseases are still defined on the basis of abnormalities in gross pathology, histopathology, microbiology, and biochemistry of body fluids. What is now termed "molecular imaging" began with the use of radioactive iodine to examine the thyroid in patients with decreased or increased thyroidal function. The characterization of regional molecular abnormalities which began with the use of radioactive iodine, provides a way to identify disease at the molecular level, progressing from the level of the whole body, organ, tissue, or cellular level. Molecular imaging can provide quantitative parameters of a specific regional molecular process, e.g., the incorporation of radioiodine into the thyroid and synthesis of thyroid hormones. These "molecular phenotypes" may help define a person's state of health and disease. Medicine has gone beyond the physician's challenge to locate the patient's problem in a specific organ. Claude Bernard was the first to point out how difficult it was to deduce the function of an organ from its structure. Functional paradigms, so many of which were developed in endocrinology, lay ahead. The focus on the cells of the body led to a cellular theory of disease, i.e., histopathology, which even today retains a dominant position in the process of medical diagnosis but is being extended by "quantitative molecular imaging," the essence of nuclear medicine.

MOLECULAR IMAGING

At the end of the 19th century, the French physicist Henri Becquerel was exploring the consequences of Roentgen's discovery of X-rays when he accidentally discovered what became known as radioactivity. He placed a phosphorescent uranium salt in a lightproof envelope that contained an unexposed photographic plate and set it in the sunlight. He reasoned that if the plate showed black spots where the salt was, this would be from X-rays excited by the sun, and the black spots apparently confirmed his theory. However, then there was a period of cloudy weather, and by usual habit, he developed some photographic plates that had been lying in a dark drawer with bits of uranium salt on them without any exposure to the sun. To his astonishment, the darkened areas were again observed where the uranium salt had been. As has often been said, discovery depends on a "prepared mind." Becquerel concluded that the uranium salts were giving off penetrating X-rays, even when in their natural unstimulated state. Radioactivity had been discovered.

Using a radiation detector invented by her husband, Pierre, Marie Curie (who suggested the term "radioactivity") began to isolate the active fraction of pitchblende, a result that was so interesting that Pierre dropped the pursuit of his own research and joined his wife in her efforts. Their first discovery was that another source of radioactivity existed in pitchblende, in addition to uranium. This source was thorium. Even more intriguing, the radiation did not have the low energy of X-rays but emitted far more energetic and penetrating rays.

Hevesy and Paneth invented the most important principle of nuclear medicine—the tracer principle—in Vienna in 1913 (Fig. 2). They monitored the movement of lead from the soil into plants, then back into the soil when the plants died. In this way, the dynamic processes that characterize life could be monitored. Early instruments to make these mea-

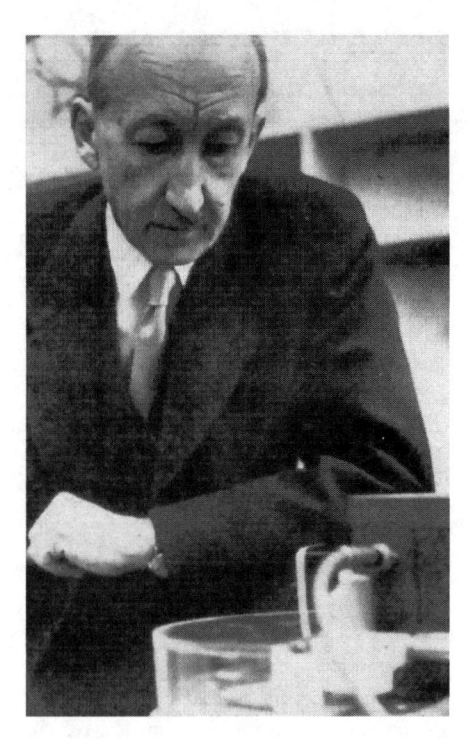

Fig. 2. George Hevesy, inventor of the tracer principle—the most fundamental in nuclear medicine.

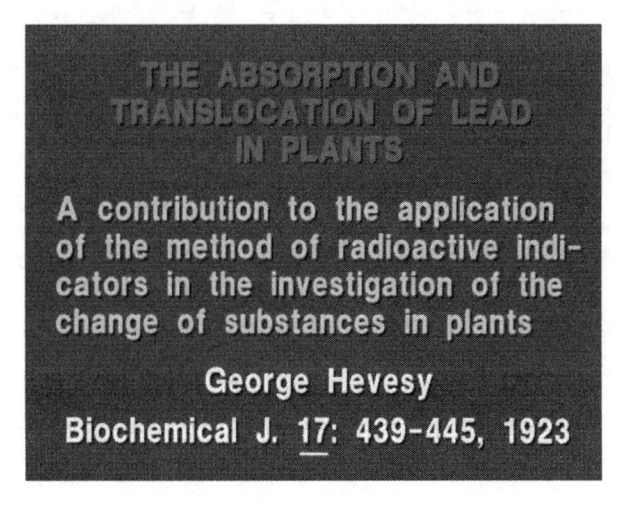

Fig. 3. Hevesy's first article describing the tracer principle.

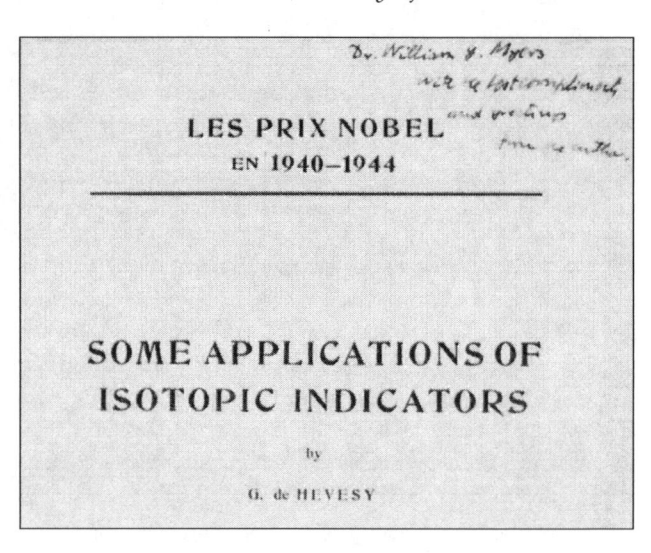

Fig. 4. The title page of Hevesy's Nobel Prize lecture in 1943.

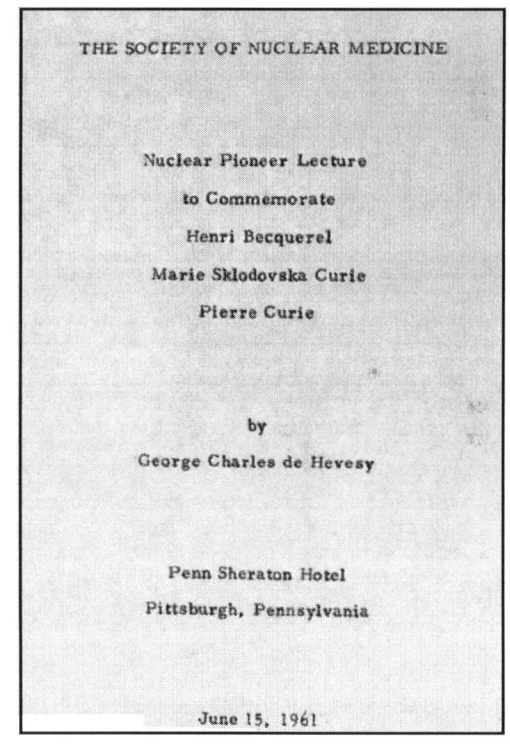

Fig. 5. The Nuclear Pioneer lecture that was delivered by Hevesy at the meeting of the Society of Nuclear Medicine.

surements included the piezoelectric device used by the Curies, photographic plates used by Rutherford and others, the cloud chamber that was invented by the Scottish physicist Wilson in 1895, the gold leaf electroscope, and the Geiger counter, perfected in 1928. Hevesy and Paneth relied on the gold leaf electroscope.

The most fundamental principle of molecular imaging is that the radioactive tracer has no biological effects on the biochemical processes within the organism being studied. This principle, first defined by Hevesy (Figs. 3–5), entails that these "indicators," as they were called by Hevesy, could be used as representatives of the same element as they moved through the biological system. If larger amounts of the radioactive tracer were given, the biological process under study could be suppressed, which made radionuclide therapy possible.

In the 1940s, the initial reports of using radioactive iodine to treat diseases of the thyroid, and radioactive phosphorus to treat leukemia, were greeted with great enthusiasm by the

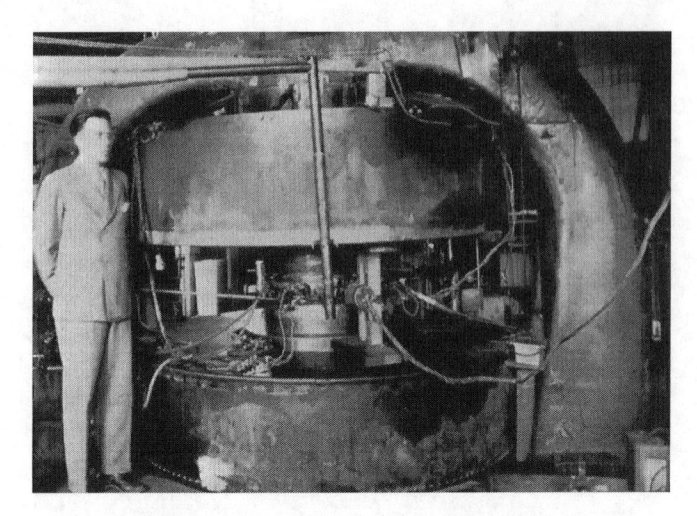

Fig. 6. Ernest Lawrence, inventor of the cyclotron.

"The medical cyclotron of the
Crocker Radiation Laboratory"
Ernest O. Lawrence
Science 90: 407-408, 1939

Fig. 7. Publication of a description of the first "medical" cyclotron.

PROMISING NUCLIDES OF THE FUTURE

Cyclotron: ^{11}C, ^{13}N, ^{15}O, ^{18}F, ^{123}I, ^{52}Fe ^{199m}Hg, ^{49}Cr, ^{61}Cu, ^{62}Zn, ^{73}Se, ^{111m}Cd, and ^{117}Sb

Reactor: ^{87m}Sr, ^{131}Cs, ^{77}Ge, ^{104}Pd, ^{159}Gd ^{175}Yb, and ^{193}Os

Fig. 8. Radionuclides that can be generated by a cyclotron.

medical profession and public. It was envisioned that these forerunners would be followed by a whole series of similar radioactive "magic bullets" that would seek out and destroy diseased tissues within the human body.

In 1931, at the University of California in Berkeley, Ernest Lawrence invented the cyclotron (Figs. 6–8), which was the first major source of radioactive elements. In 1942, Enrico Fermi (Fig. 9) invented the nuclear reactor that could provide an even wider source of radioactive elements and compounds. The invention of the nuclear reactor, a product of the Manhattan District Project of World War II, made

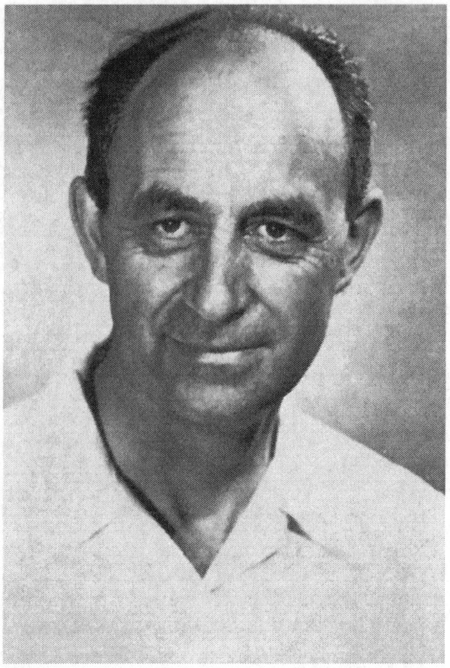

Fig. 9. Enrico Fermi, inventor of the nuclear reactor, in 1942.

large quantities of useful radioactive elements available to scientists and physicians throughout the world. In 1934, Frederick Joliot and Irene Curie (Fig. 10) had made the startling discovery that practically every chemical element could be made radioactive by particle bombardment. Bombardment with high-energy particles, such as protons, was possible in a cyclotron, as progressively high voltages of electricity could be produced conveniently. This made it possible to produce hundreds of isotopes of different elements, including carbon, nitrogen, and oxygen, which are enormously important in living systems. Indeed, carbon defines organic chemistry—the chemistry of life. Lawrence and his colleagues immediately recognized the great biomedical potential of the cyclotron.

At the end of the war in October 1945, President Truman appointed a commission to establish control of the production and use of atomic power in the United States, which led to the creation of a civilian Atomic Energy Commission (AEC). The AEC would direct all atomic energy programs, ranging from bomb production to nuclear power, as well as medical and research uses of radioactive materials. Its mission was stated as follows:

". . . It is hereby declared to be the policy of the people of the United States, that, subject at all times to the paramount objective of assuring the common defense and security, the development and utilization of atomic energy shall, as far as practicable, be directed toward improving the public welfare, increasing the standard of living, strengthening free competition in private enterprise, and promoting world peace."

History of Nuclear Medicine

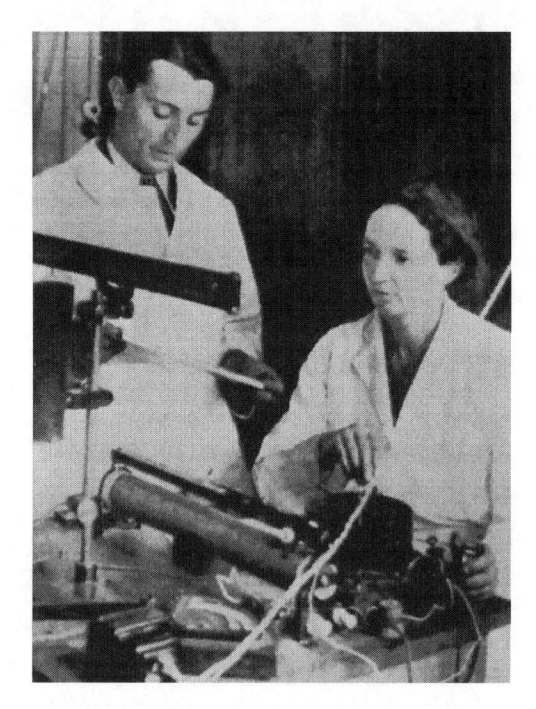

Fig. 10. Frederick Joliot and Irene Curie, who discovered artificial radioactivity in 1932.

A major debate at that time was whether atomic energy should be kept secret and totally held within the government, as the military wished. Others believed that secrecy was a hopeless task; thus, the path should be "control" after worldwide release of nuclear energy and other "peaceful uses of atomic energy." The explosion of a Soviet atomic bomb on September 23, 1949 catalyzed the belief that atomic energy could not be kept secret.

On December 8, 1953, President Eisenhower delivered his famous "Atoms For Peace" speech before the United Nations General Assembly in New York. The President said:

> "It is not enough to take this weapon out of the hands of soldiers. It must be put in the hands of those who know how . . . to adapt it to the arts of peace . . . This greatest of destructive forces can be developed into a great boon for the benefit of all mankind . . . if the entire body of the world's scientists and engineers had adequate amounts of fissionable material with which to test and develop their ideas, that this capability would be rapidly transformed into universal, efficient, and economic usage."

His proposals resulted in the establishment of the International Atomic Energy Agency, which came into being in 1959.

It took until 1954, 1 yr after Eisenhower's speech, for the Atomic Energy Act to be amended to allow private ownership of nuclear reactors and other uses of fissionable materials, rights previously limited to the AEC. In collaboration with industry, the AEC initiated a 5-yr Reactor Development Program. By 1956, this program had received $15 billion in federal funds.

The longer half-lives of single photon–emitting radionuclides, such as iodine-131, iodine-123, and technetium-99m, greatly simplified their availability, use, and cost in comparison to cyclotron-produced radionuclides. The physical characteristics of technetium-99m—its half-life, type of decay, and energy of its photon emissions—made it ideal for radiation detection from outside of the body. The invention of generators enables short-lived radionuclides to be available away from their production site.

THE DISCOVERY OF THYROID DISEASE

Since ancient times, an enlargement of the neck was often recognized as a manifestation of disease, rather than just a sign of beauty in certain women. In the first century AD, Pliny the Elder wrote: "Only men and swine are subject to swellings in the throat, which are mostly caused by the noxious quality of the water they drink." In the 12th century, the ashes of sponges and seaweed were used for the treatment of goiter. In the painting entitled "The Flagellation of Christ," painted in 1515, one of the persons gazing at Christ has clear evidence of a multinodular goiter. In 1527, Paracelsus lectured to his students that drinking water was a cause of goiter and he postulated that the offending substance was iron oxide. It was not until centuries later that iodine was identified as the substance in seaweed and other marine products that could prevent goiter.

In 1809, the discovery of the element iodine is an example of the frequent scientific advances made by wartime research *(1–3)*. A saltpeter manufacturer named Courtois discovered gaseous iodine but did not realize that it was an element. Sir Humphrey Davy reported that iodine was an element in 1813. A description of Coindet's discovery was reported in 1824 in the *Edinburgh Medical and Surgical Journal*: "We learn from the first memoir of Dr. J. C. Coindet that in the year 1813 . . . he introduced iodine into medical treatment" *(4)*. Chatin, a Professor of Pharmacy in Paris, published an extensive series of papers on the geographic distribution of iodine and recommended iodination of the water supply in 1852 *(5)*. His recommendations were ignored by the French Academy of Sciences. Over 50 yr elapsed before further studies focused on the use of iodine in the prevention of endemic goiter. Renewed interest arose in 1896 with the work of Baumann, who showed that the human thyroid contained large amounts of iodine *(6)*. In 1915, E. C. Kendall crystallized thyroxine from thyroid tissue, and in 1926, C. R. Harington determined its chemical structure. In 1954 Gross and Pitt-Rivers identified a related molecule with only three, not four, iodine atoms. The compound triiodothyronine (T3) was physiologically more active than thyroxine (T4) and was thought to be a product of thyroxine. The latter is the major molecule secreted by

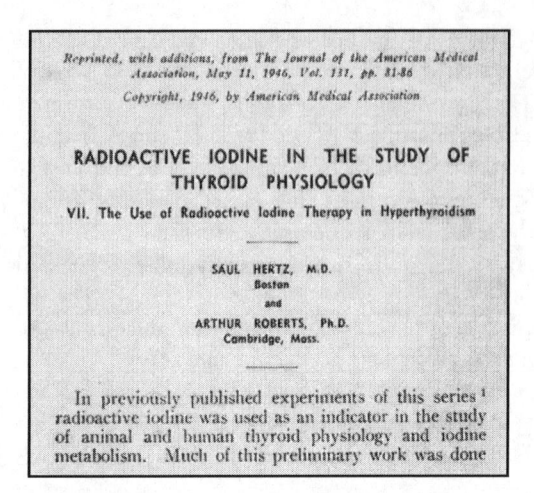

Fig. 11. First publication on accumulation of radioiodine by the thyroid.

the thyroid, which we subsequently learned was converted to T3 in other tissues via the process of deiodination.

The clinical manifestations of overactivity of the thyroid (hyperthyroidism) were first described by C. H. Parry in 1825. It is often called "Graves' disease," because of Robert Graves' report in 1835 that described the manifestations of enlargement of the thyroid, palpitations, and exophthalmos (7). He most clearly attributed the manifestations to disease of the thyroid.

Paracelsus described cretinism in 1603, but it was not until William Gull in 1874 (8) and W. M. Ord in 1878 (9) that descriptions were introduced of the clinical manifestations of decreased thyroid function, called "myxedema." The relationship between the thyroid and iodine has been known for a long time. The ancient Chinese recognized the existence of goiter and its reduction in size or even disappearance by eating burnt sponge and the seaweed Sargassum. The use of seaweed to treat goiter is described in Chinese literature dating back to 2700 BC. Burnt sponge was used as therapy in 1600 BC. Eating animal thyroid to decrease swelling in the neck dates back to 500 AD. Iodine was first discovered in seaweed by Courtois (1811), in sea sponges by Fyfe (1819), and in the thyroid by Baumann (1895). As long ago as 1816 and 1820, Proust and Coindet recommended iodine for the treatment of goiter. Thyroxine was crystallized in pure form by Kendall in 1914, and chemical synthesis of the hormone was accomplished 12 yr later by Harington.

Goiters have been pictured in paintings for many centuries and were often noted in areas around the world where the soils were deficient in iodine (10). In addition to its important role to prevent iodide deficiency goiter and hypothyroidism, iodine was also first used to treat hyperthyroidism by Plummer in 1923 (11). Characterization of various dietary and environmental goitrogens led to the observation that members of the thiocarbamide class of chemicals effectively perturb the synthesis of thyroxine and triiodothyronine. This

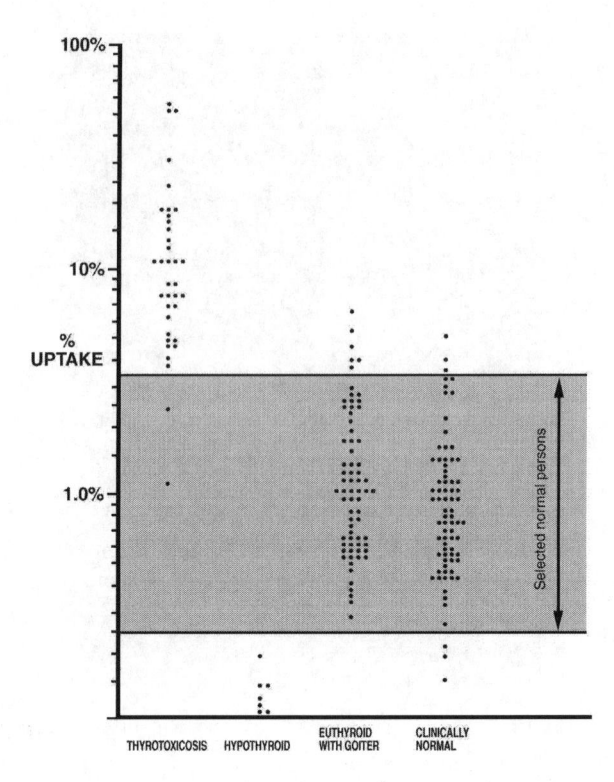

Fig. 12. Differentiation of hyperthyroidism from normal persons in the accumulation of radioiodine.

group includes derivatives of thioacetamide, thiourea, mercaptoimidazole (imidazolethione), and thiouracil. Several of these compounds proved useful in probing the biosynthetic pathway for thyroxine: thiocyanate, propylthiouracil, N-methyl-2-mercaptoimidazole, and thiourea. Toxicities of these drugs and their various metabolites have limited the therapeutic value of these agents. Consequently, early research on the thyroid has diverged in two directions of study: hormonal regulation of the thyroid gland and intrathyroidal production of thyroxine.

Beginning in 1907, David Marine in Michigan began a series of observations and experiments in dogs that led him to conclude in 1924 that hyperplasia of the thyroid was a response to iodine deficiency. He also found that goiter was an exaggeration of this normal physiological process, an excellent example of the relationship between nutrition and disease, as well as a homeostatic process in disarray (12,13).

The use of radioiodine to help diagnose disease of the thyroid gland began in 1940 (Figs. 11–13). Seaborg and Livingston produced iodine-131 in Ernest Lawrence's laboratory in Berkeley. For his discoveries of the transuranic elements and his determination of their chemistry, Seaborg was awarded the 1951 Nobel Prize in chemistry.

Measuring the rate of accumulation of the iodine-131 tracer with an external radiation detector directed at the patient's neck made it possible to differentiate between decreased, normal, and increased function of the thyroid

History of Nuclear Medicine

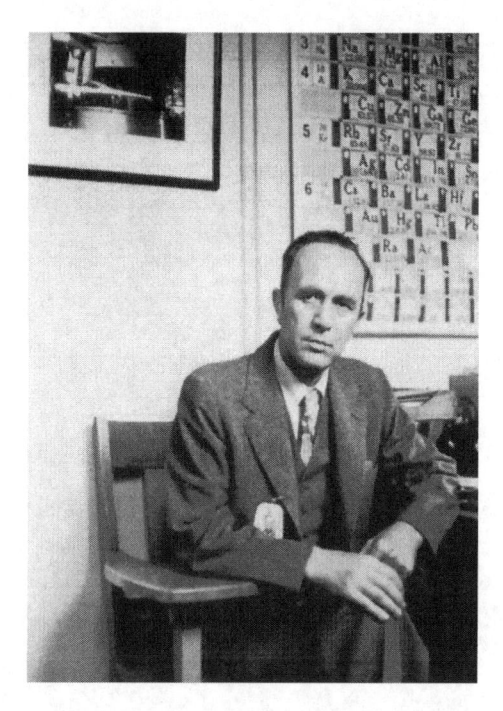

Fig. 13. Joseph Hamilton, at the Lawrence Berkeley Laboratory, who described the accumulation of radioiodine by the thyroid.

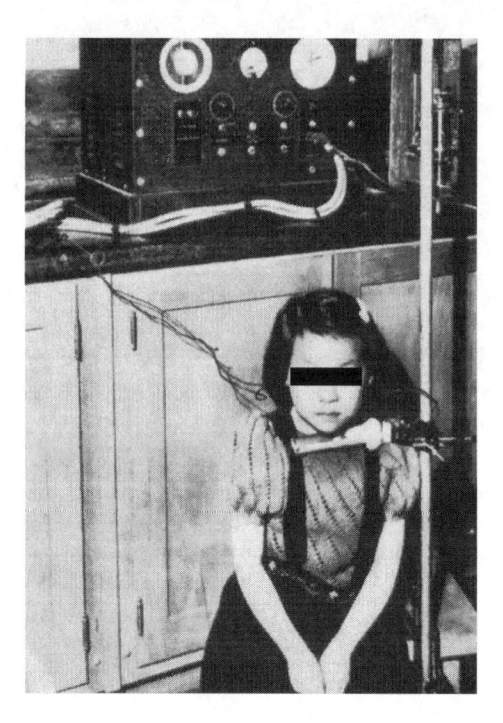

Fig. 14. Early measurement of radioiodine uptake by the thyroid using a Geiger counter.

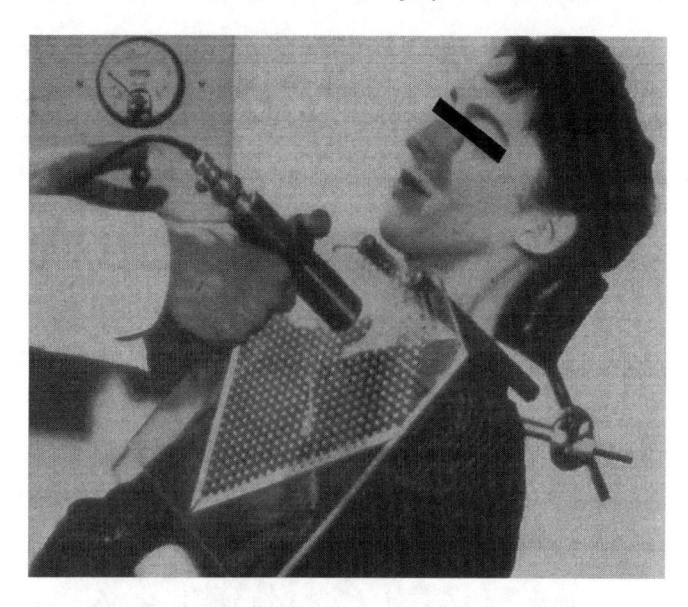

Fig. 15. My task at Hammersmith Hospital, London (1957), measuring the accumulation of iodine-132 in a patient with a thyroid nodule.

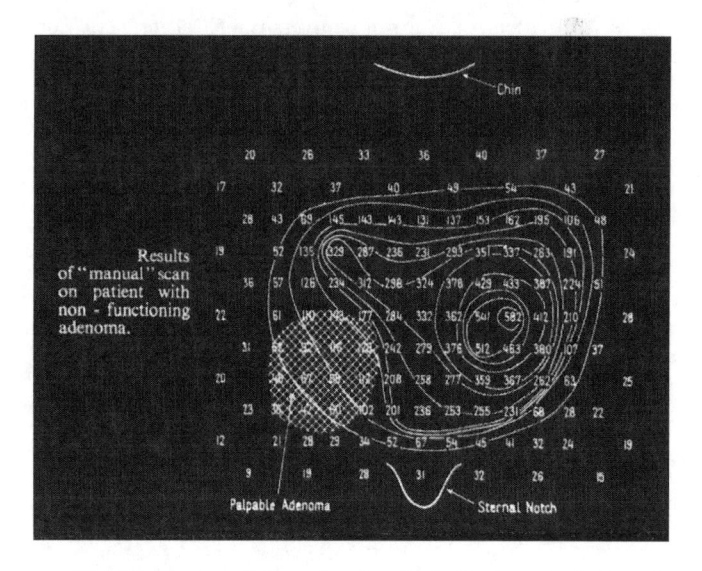

Fig. 16. "Isocount" lines showing the lack of accumulation of iodine-132 in a "cold" nodule of the thyroid.

(Figs. 12, 14). Radioisotope scanning was invented by Benedict Cassen in 1950 and was used to examine patients with thyroid disease, especially goiter (Figs. 17–20). Scintillation detectors with focused collimators to localize the source of radioactivity were connected to mechanical styluses. These styluses would print out the spatial distribution of radioactive iodine in the neck of the patient and detect single and multiple nodules of the thyroid. Hal Anger improved the imaging procedure by replacing the mechanical stylus with a flashing light that activated the photographic emulsion on X-ray film.

An early clinical example of its efficacy was the demonstration that an avid accumulation of iodine-131 in a mass beneath the sternum proved to be a substernal goiter. One of the most important contributions to the field of nuclear medicine was made by Anger, in view of the millions of patients all over the world, whose diagnosis and treatment depended on the use of the "Anger camera." In 1951, Anger learned

123

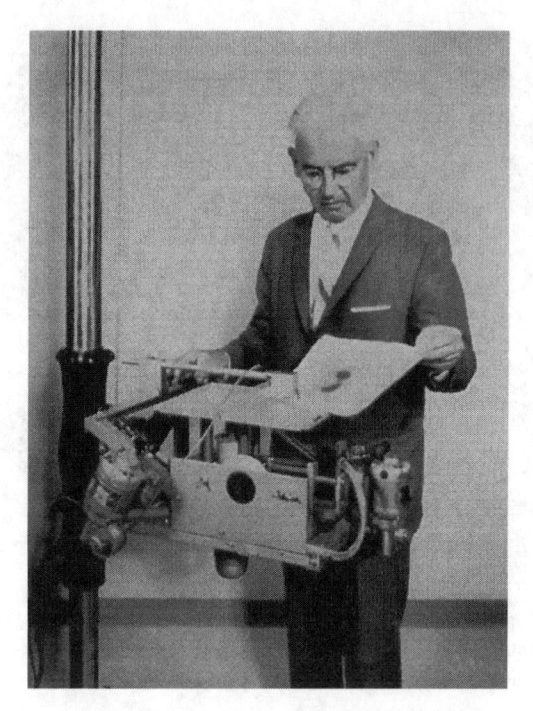

Fig. 17. Benedict Cassen (University of California at Los Angeles), who invented the first automatic "rectilinear" scanner in 1951.

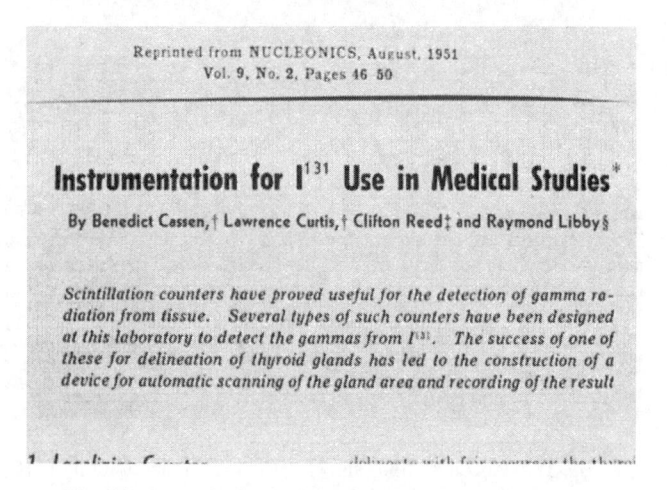

Fig. 18. Cassen's first publication describing the scanner.

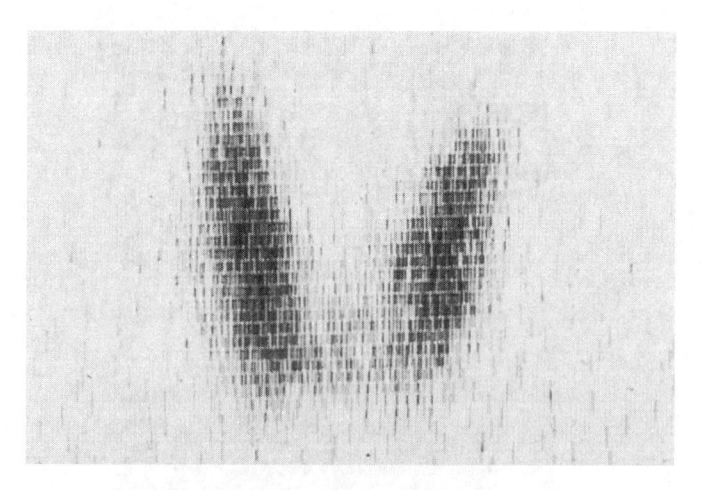

Fig. 19. Early image of radioiodine in the thyroid made with the Cassen scanner.

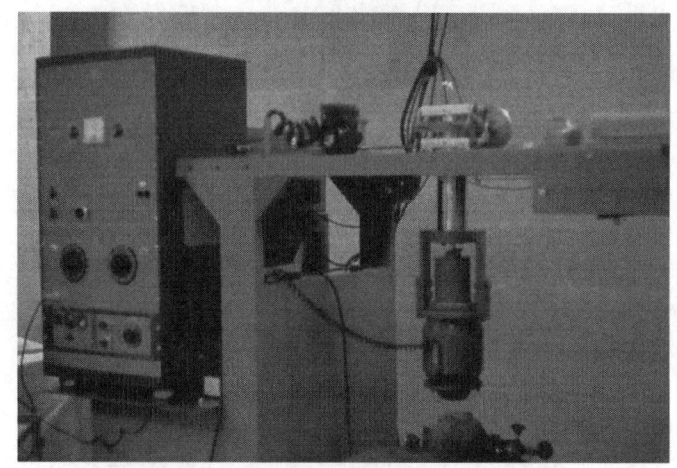

Fig. 20. First rectilinear scanner at Johns Hopkins in 1958.

about the invention of the rectilinear scanner by Cassen at University of California at Los Angeles. He recognized that the mechanical movement of the crystal radiation detector over the patient's body was a serious limitation and set out to develop a γ ray camera that would simultaneously record the photons coming from the patient's body.

In 1948, Anger worked at the Donner Laboratory, which was part of the Lawrence Radiation Laboratory, named for Ernest Lawrence, inventor of the cyclotron in the early 1930s. John Lawrence, brother of Ernest, was head of the Donner Laboratory. Among the first projects to which Anger was assigned was the modification of the 184-in. cyclotron to be used for irradiation of pituitary tumors with high-energy deuterons. During World War II, the 184-in. cyclotron had been converted to a large-scale spectrograph, or "calutron," and was used to produce the uranium-235 for the first atomic bomb.

The first γ camera report by Anger was on the use of a pinhole camera for in vivo studies (*14*; Figs. 21–24). γ photons from iodine-131 in a patient with metastatic cancer near the skin were used to produce images with a pinhole collimator in front of a 2- × 4-in. thallium-activated sodium iodide crystal 5/6 in. thick. Another key publication was entitled, *The Gamma-pinhole Camera and Image Amplifier*.

The first scintillation camera was described in an article entitled "A New Instrument for Mapping Gamma-Ray Emitters" in *Biology and Medicine Quarterly Report*. The instrument was exhibited at the 1958 annual meeting of the Society of Medicine and later that year at the meeting of the American Medical Association. As expected, the new invention was warmly received, and the next step was its commercial development.

History of Nuclear Medicine

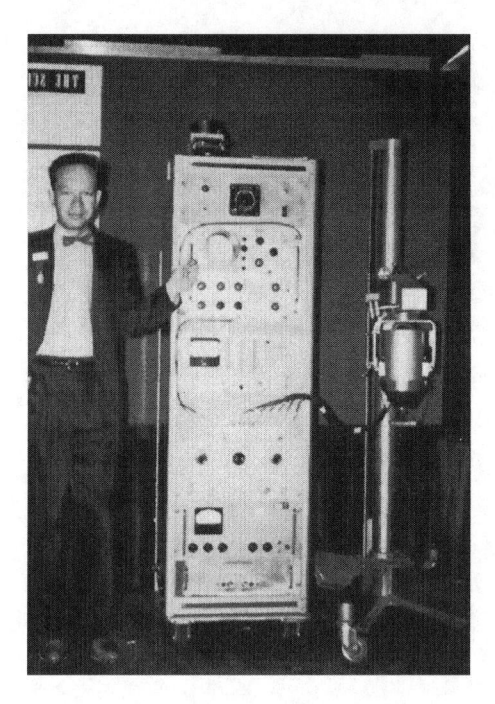

Fig. 21. Hal Anger and the first scintillation camera at an exhibit at the 1958 annual meeting of the Society of Nuclear Medicine.

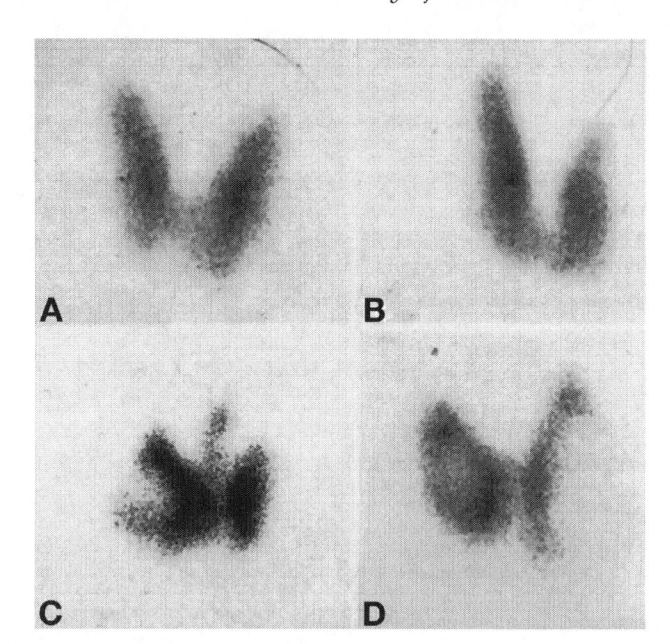

Fig. 22. Images of technetium-99m in the thyroid made with the Anger camera and a pinhole collimator.

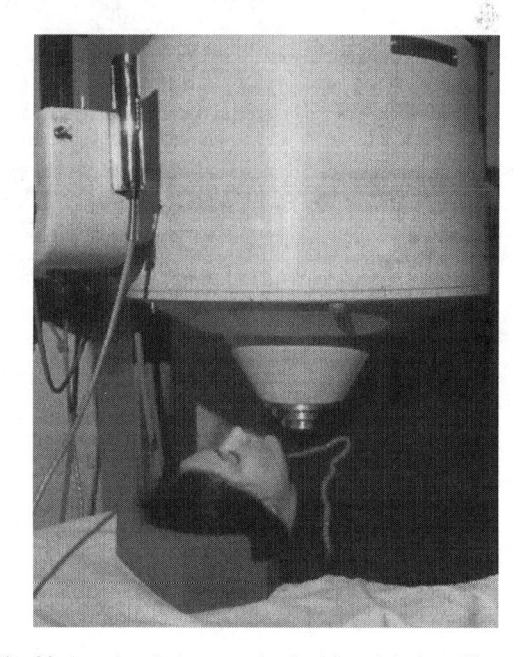

Fig. 23. A patient being examined with a pinhole collimator and the Anger camera.

One property that makes radioactive isotopes, such as iodine-123 or iodine-131 (or technetium-99m), valuable is that they can be accurately and specifically measured when present in exceedingly small concentrations. The γ rays that are emitted by the specific isotopes can be accurately counted at the body's surface by the external radiation detectors. The most fundamental property is their use as tracers to solve problems that could not otherwise be addressed. The radioactive tracers have the biochemical properties that are identical to the molecules being traced.

An avid or excessive accumulation of radioiodine by the thyroid gland is a manifestation of hyperthyroidism but may also be observed in patients with iodine-avid nontoxic goiter. In such patients, the thyroid can be accumulating abnormally high amounts of iodine but producing inadequate amounts of thyroxine. An abnormally low rate of radioiodine accumulation by the thyroid may be caused by abnormally high serum iodine levels, as well as from decreased function owing to the disease, hypothyroidism. Inflammation of the thyroid (thyroiditis) is often manifested by an abnormally low accumulation of radioiodine.

The benefit of imaging the sites and rates of radioiodine by the thyroid is reflected in the:

1. Identification of the nature of masses beneath the sternum.
2. Identification of thyroidal tissue beneath the tongue or in other unusual places (Fig. 25).
3. Detection of residual thyroidal tissue after an attempt to totally remove the thyroid surgically.
4. Detection of multinodular goiter when only one nodule can be felt by physical examination.
5. Differentiation of functional ("hot") from nonfunctioning ("cold") nodules to help determine the probability of thyroid cancer.
6. Detection of metastatic thyroid cancer in the lungs, skeleton, or elsewhere in the body.

Ionizing radiation serves two purposes in medicine: to provide information in low doses and to kill hyperactive or cancerous cells in high doses. In the case of thyroid cancer, radioiodine scans are used to detect residual thyroid tissue

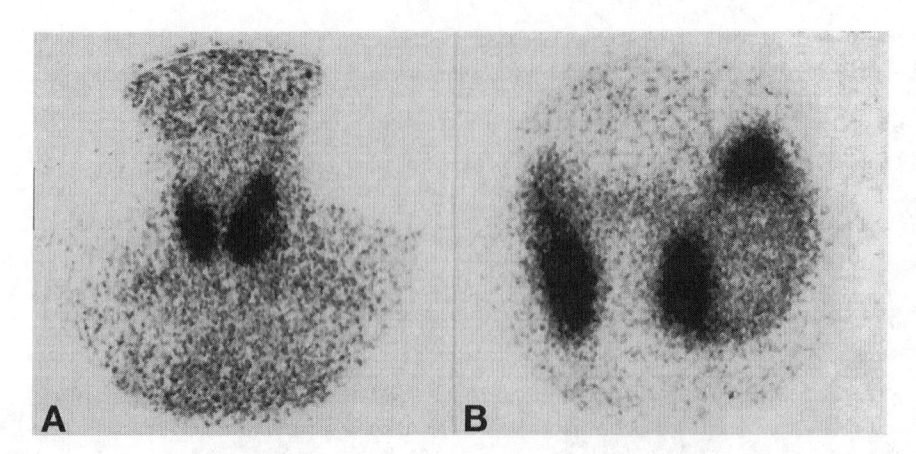

Fig. 24. An example of the improved spatial resolution with the pinhole collimator and the Anger camera.

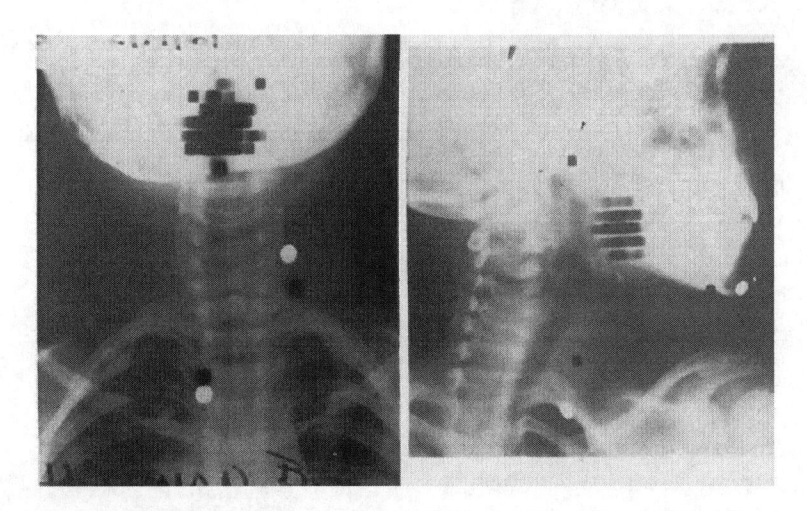

Fig. 25. Superimposed ("fused") image of radioiodine accumulation in a sublingual mass on a simultaneously obtained X-ray in 1961. Fiducial markers were used to make the correct superimposition.

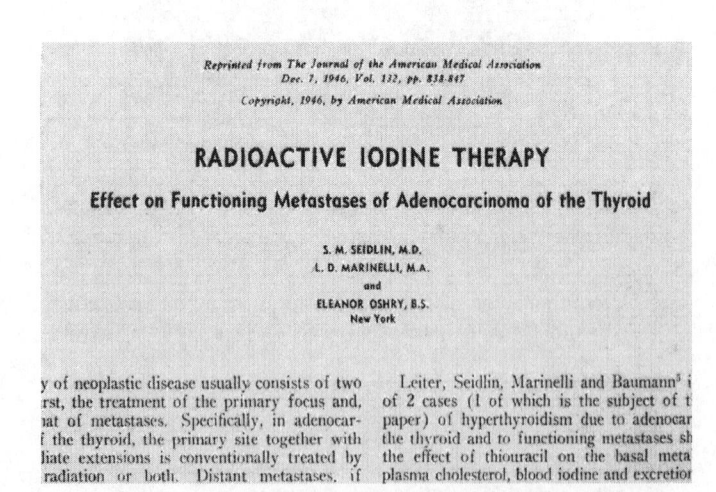

Fig. 26. First description of radioiodine in the treatment of thyroid disease.

or identify distant metastatic disease if the metastatic lesions accumulate radioiodine. Most cancers of the thyroid consist of differentiated cells that accumulate radioiodine; as a result, radioiodine is used in high doses to kill cancerous cells (Fig. 26). The radiotracer F-18 fluorodeoxyglucose can detect metastases that do not accumulate radioiodine because the cancerous cells are primitive and undifferentiated, without the ability to accumulate radioiodine (Figs. 27 and 28). Details of F-18 fluorodeoxyglucose scanning are discussed in Chapters 34, 61, 71, 76, 80).

Nuclear medicine now has a great effect on medical practice and biomedical research and is likely to increase its role in the future. The greatest impact will be on treatment. Not all patients confirm to either a "one operation fits all," or "one dose fits all" in the case of drug therapy. We now know that the doses of isotopes, as well as drugs, require adjustment in the individual patient. Efficacy, side effects, and

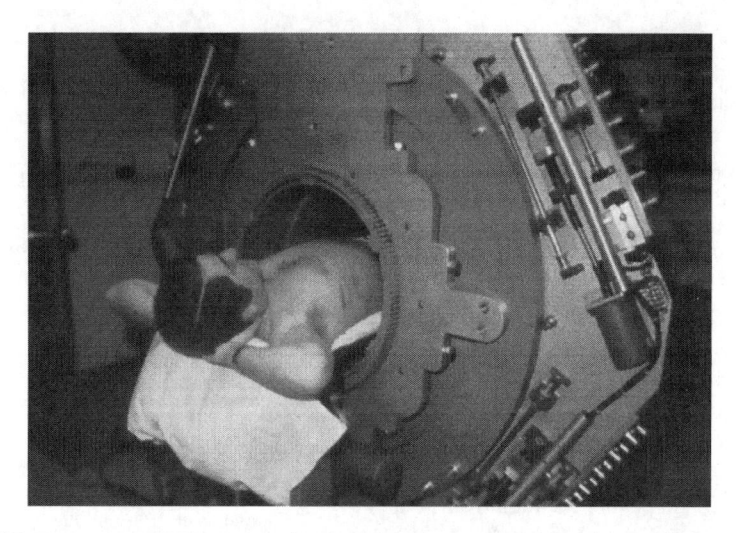

Fig. 27. The author (HNW) being examined in a positron emission tomography scanner.

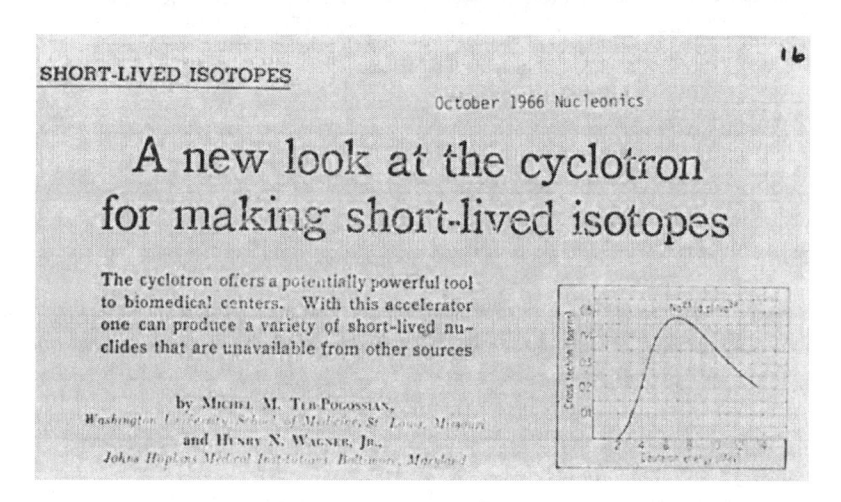

Fig. 28. A 1966 publication describing the value of positron emission tomography scanning of positron-emitting radionuclides.

duration of treatment must all be assessed periodically in every patient for maximum safety and effectiveness.

Mainstream medical instrumentation companies are becoming increasingly involved in the development of what were originally called "novel imaging" devices. Their increased capital investment and competitive activities are clearly benefiting physicians but, even more importantly, benefitting patients and the health care system. Industry is collaborating with academic and private research programs and cooperating with large pharmaceutical companies in the application of molecular imaging to drug design and development. The president and CEO of General Electric Medical, Joseph M. Hogan, stated recently: "In the years to come, we envision a health care system that uses molecular medicine to diagnose and treat patients before symptoms appear and treatments that are tailored to an individual based on his or her genetic makeup." In the "NIH Roadmap for Medical Research in the 21st Century," Dr. Elias Zerhouni, the first radiologist to head the NIH, included "molecular imaging" as a major initiative, directed toward the presymptomatic detection of disease, personalized medicine based on molecular targets, and phenotypic characterization of genetic abnormalities.

ATOMS FOR PEACE AFTER HALF A CENTURY

In the official government report on the development of the atomic bomb during 1940–1945, in a book by Henry D. Smyth, he states:

"The possible uses of nuclear energy are not all destructive, and the second direction in which technical development can be expected is along the path of peace . . . there is no immediate prospect for running cars with nuclear power or lighting houses with radioactive lamps, although there is a good probability that nuclear power for special purposes could be developed within 10 years and that plentiful supplies of radioactive materials can have a profound effect on scientific research and perhaps on the treatment of certain diseases in a similar period."

Would we be where we are today, in benefiting from the results of using radiation in biomedical research and health care, if our government had applied the same regulations concerning biomedical radiation that they have been applied to other uses of radiation, such as nuclear energy? In a report last year on radiation standards, the General Accounting Office of the US government, the investigative arm of Congress, said: "The standards administered by EPA and NRC to protect the public from low-level radiation exposure do not have a conclusive scientific basis, despite decades of research."

The EPA advocates a standard for all radiation exposure from a single source or site at 15 mrem per year, with no more than 4 mrem coming from ground water. In comparison, a standard chest X-ray gives about 10 mrem to the chest, which is equivalent to 1 or 2 mrem to the whole body. The NRC sets its acceptable level of radiation exposure from any one source at 25 mrem a year. In contrast, the natural level of background radiation in the United States averages about 350 mrem per year, and in some areas of the country, it is many times higher than that. Yet, there is no evidence that the effects of environmental radiation in such areas as Colorado are greater than elsewhere in the United States.

People absorb about 100 mrem of radiation each year from cosmic rays alone, and in Denver, exposure from cosmic rays averages 200 mrem per year. According to the *New York Times*, the quandary over how to set radiation levels does not result from a lack of research or analysis.

SUMMARY

In summary, the thyroid and its associated diseases have been important in the development of nuclear medicine, which has had a major impact on the diagnosis, treatment, and understanding of thyroid disease. With the anticipated increased use of iodine-124 and use of other upcoming radiopharmaceuticals, the relationship of the thyroid and radiotracer molecular imaging continues and is certain to further expand.

REFERENCES

1. Chattway FD. The discovery of iodine. Chem News 1909; 99:193.
2. Sharp G. The history of iodine, the iodides, and iodoform. Pharm J 1913; 91:98.
3. Boussingault JB. Ann Chim Phys 1831; 45:41, and 1833; 54:163.
4. Chatin A. Series of papers. Compt Rend Acad Sci 1850–1876.
5. Coindet JC. Decouverte d'un nouveau remede contre goiter. Bibl Britannique 1820; 14:190.
6. Baumann E. Hoppe-Seyl 1896; 2:21, 319.
7. Graves RJ. Clinical lectures. Lond Med Surg J (Part II) 1835; 7:516.
8. Gull WW. On a cretinoid state supervening in adult life in women. Trans Clin Soc (Lond) 1874; 7:180.
9. Ord WM. On myxoedema, a term proposed to be applied to an essential condition in the "cretinoid" affection occasionally observed in middle-aged women. Medico-chirurgical Transactions 1878; 61:57–78.
10. Kimball OP. History of the prevention of endemic goiter. Bull World Health Organ 1958; 9:241.
11. Plummer HS. Results of administering iodine to patients having exophthalmic goiter. JAMA 1923; 80:1953.
12. Marine D. Etiology and prevention of simple goiter. Medicine 1924; 3:453.
13. Marine D. Endemic goiter: a problem in preventive medicine. Ann Intern Med 1954; 41:875–876.
14. Anger H. Use of a gamma-ray pinhole camera for in vivo studies. Nature 1952; 170:200–201.

13
Prophylaxis Against Radiation Exposure from Radioiodine

Jacob Robbins and Arthur B. Schneider

INTRODUCTION

The major cause of accidental exposure to radioactive iodine that would endanger a sizable population is its release from the core of a functioning nuclear power-generating facility. Because the half-lives of the iodine radionuclides of interest are 8 d or less, an accident at a reactor that has been inactive for a relatively brief period would not create a risk. For similar reasons, it is unlikely that a terrorist act involving a "dirty bomb," or reactor waste products, would require prophylactic measures to protect the thyroid gland. This discussion applies primarily to large populations exposed to volatile radioiodines, rather than individuals who might be exposed in the setting of a scientific laboratory.

Protection against a nuclear accident includes sheltering from fallout, avoiding ingestion of contaminated food, and evacuation from the contaminated area. Milk is especially important because grazing animals harvest fallout from large areas, and iodine is concentrated by the mammary glands into milk. However, these measures may be insufficient or too slow to provide complete thyroid protection, whereas blockade of thyroid iodine uptake by a sufficiently high blood level of stable iodide can be achieved quickly, even in advance of exposure. Potassium iodide (KI), of course, will only protect the thyroid gland and only against internal radiation from radioactive iodine.

The accident in 1986 at Chernobyl in the USSR (now Chornobyl in the Ukraine) has provided answers to several questions: whether a nuclear power accident can indeed result in thyroid cancer, what the minimal amount of internal thyroid radiation is that might be responsible, and whether high doses of KI can be safely administered to a large population. Fallout of radioiodine in regions as far as 150 miles from the plant, depending on wind and weather conditions, was sufficient to cause a major increase in the occurrence of thyroid nodules and thyroid cancer in children (1). Initial dose estimates, still undergoing analysis, indicate that the minimal thyroid dose might be as low as 0.6 cGy (2). Side effects after administration of KI to millions of children and adults in Poland were uncommon, mild, and reversible (3).

Furthermore, as much as 30% of thyroid radiation received by children who were evacuated from Pripyat, the closest village, and in other children as far away as Poland, has been attributed to inhalation (3,4). A portion of the inhaled radionuclides can be radioiodines with half-lives measured in hours and with possibly higher oncogenic potential than the major component, ^{131}I (5).

PHARMACOLOGY OF KI

The major blocking effect of excess iodine on thyroid iodine accumulation occurs at the basal membrane of the thyroid follicular cell (6). The active transport of the small physiological concentration of iodide by the Na/I symporter is overwhelmed by the much higher concentration derived from the recommended doses of KI (see below). The 100 mg of iodine in a 130-mg tablet of KI exceeds the normal dietary iodine intake (approx 200 µg) by nearly three orders of magnitude. In addition, excess iodine near the apical cell membrane interferes with the organification of thyroglobulin and thyroid hormone formation, and any iodide that enters the cell is rapidly excreted (7). A third effect of excess iodine interferes with thyroid hormone release from the gland, but this does not effectively compromise the major beneficial effect on iodine accumulation.

Iodide is rapidly absorbed from the intestinal tract and quickly excreted in the urine (8). As shown in Table 1, the greatest protection is provided when KI is given 1 h before exposure but is still substantial if it is given within 8 h after exposure (9,10). A high level of protection persists for 1 or 2 d after KI is ingested; thus, daily administration is adequate if needed for continued protection.

KI is currently available as 130- and 65-mg tablets without a prescription in individually sealed, light-proof wrapping (11). Provided that the tablets are not placed in extreme conditions, it is likely that the shelf-life has no practical limit. For infants (see Side Effects section), smaller doses must be prepared, either by dissolving the tablet or using an available iodide solution. Detailed information for home preparation of solutions from 130- or 65-mg tablets have

Table 1
KI Protection Against a Single ^{131}I Exposure

Hours between KI and ^{131}I ingestion	−96	−48	−1	0	2	3	8
Percent protection	Very little	≈80	Highest	98	80	60	40

Data at 0 and 3 h are experimental (see ref. 9). Other data are derived from models (see ref. 10).

Table 2
WHO and FDA Guidelines for KI Use in a Radiation Emergency

	Exposure Threshold (cGy)^a		KI Dose (mg)	
	WHO 1999	FDA 2001	WHO 1999	FDA 2001
Adults >40 yr	500	500	130	130
18–40 yr	10	10	130	130
Pregnant or lactating	1	5	130	130
Adolescents	1	5	130	65–130^b
Children 3–12 yr	1	5	65	65
>1 mo–3 yr	1	5	32	32
<1 mo	1	5	16	16

^{a}1 cGy or 10 mGy is equivalent to 1 rad.
^{b}Dose can vary with age or body size.

been provided on the Food and Drug Administration (FDA) website (12).

SIDE EFFECTS

Potential side effects of KI are thyroid-related (hypothyroidism, hyperthyroidism, and neonatal goiter), gastrointestinal (nausea, vomiting, diarrhea, and pain), allergy-related (angioedema, arthralgia, eosinophilia, and urticaria), and skin rashes.

Nonthyroidal side effects were mild and infrequent among 12,040 children living in Poland at the time of the Chernobyl accident. Most children received a single dose of KI (15 mg for newborn infants; 50 mg for children under 5 yr; 70 mg for others), but some had multiple doses, and a few had been given tincture of iodine (3). The most common were vomiting (2.38%) and skin rashes (1.07%). Of 5061 adults, most receiving one dose of 70-mg KI, vomiting was reported in 0.85% and skin rashes in 1.24%. It was estimated that only about 0.2% of the population administered KI had medically significant adverse reactions. Two adults with chronic obstructive lung disease and known sensitivity to iodides were hospitalized for acute respiratory distress.

In evaluating the occurrence of thyroid-related side effects in follow-up studies in Poland (3), no significant change in the prevalence of thyroid disease or abnormal thyroid function was detected, aside from the case of newborn infants. In 3214 infants given KI during the first days of life and tested during the third to fifth days, 12 (0.37%) had elevated thyrotropin (TSH). Although TSH returned to normal by days 16–20 of life, and follow-up in the second to third year of life detected no abnormality, the possibility of a subtle effect on cognitive development was not excluded.

RADIATION GUIDELINES

As a result of the Chernobyl experience, the World Health Organization (WHO) in 1999 (13), and the US FDA in 2001 (14), revised their published guidelines for iodine prophylaxis in radiation emergencies. Their recommendations are summarized in Table 2. Both organizations provide considerable background information and justification for their recommendations as part of their guidelines. There are only two differences: the estimated thyroid radiation dose that triggers KI administration to children and the KI dose to use for adolescent children. Both conclude that adults over 40 yr should receive KI only to prevent thyroid gland damage by a high-radiation dose. This is because their risk of radiation-induced thyroid cancer is low, and their risk of KI-induced thyroid-related side effects, especially transient hypo- and hyperthyroidism, is relatively high. In subsequent communications (11,14), the FDA has emphasized that the safety of KI in children and young adults, as well as the expected uncertainty of the extent of radiation exposure in an emergency, permits flexibility in deciding when to administer KI and how much to give. The main exceptions to this are fetuses, infants, and pregnant women. The infant's thyroid, and probably the fetal thyroid after the first few months of gestation, are both particularly susceptible to the carcinogenic effects of radiation along with radiation-induced hypothyroidism. Because of their small size, the relative uptake of radioactive iodine (quantity/unit volume) is high. Therefore, it is especially important to provide protection with KI in these cases, but the lowest effective KI dose should be used. In lactating mothers, the amount of iodide secreted in the milk is too low to protect the infant; therefore, both mother and child should be given KI. The FDA has provided detailed information on the preparation of KI doses for infants using the currently available KI tablets (Table 2; *12*), and has approved a pediatric KI solution.

KI AVAILABILITY AND DISTRIBUTION

For KI prophylaxis to be effective, it must be available within hours of the time of need, the public must be adequately informed in advance, and the appropriate health and radiation agencies must give timely and accurate information to the populace. Strong differences of opinion exist between those who believe that KI should be provided and those who believe it should not. The latter cite the following to support their view:

1. Nuclear reactors in the United States and most other countries are designed better than the reactor at Chernobyl. They are less likely to have an accident, able to mitigate an accident, and strong enough to withstand most foreseeable terroristic acts *(15)*.
2. The provision of KI has serious legal and logistical problems. In fact, some organizations (including schools) have rejected storing KI for these reasons *(16)*.
3. Some people may misunderstand the role of KI and not evacuate contaminated areas.

Alternatively, based on the evidence, many organizations, including the American Thyroid Association, the American Academy of Pediatrics, the Endocrine Society, and the American Association of Clinical Endocrinologists, have endorsed its use. As a result of these differing views, it is not surprising that there is a great disparity between countries and between localities within countries regarding whether or how they have planned for KI use *(16)*.

The US Nuclear Regulatory Commission has long required that KI be made available in and immediately surrounding a nuclear power station for staff and people who cannot be evacuated. The commission now requires that states with population within a 10-mile radius of the station should consider KI in their emergency planning. The federal government provides KI tablets if they are requested, but it is a prerogative of the states to plan for its distribution and/or stockpiling.

As required by a congressional mandate to assess strategies for distribution and administration of KI, a committee of the US National Academy of Sciences recently completed its work and has published a detailed report *(16)*. Although the committee confirmed the safety and efficacy of KI, it concluded that the geographic and logistic diversity among the states was too great to accommodate a uniform national program. Instead, the committee recommended that KI distribution plans be developed by the states with federal support, and it provided detailed suggestions for program development. It also advised that the federal government maintain KI stockpiles sufficient to ensure that an adequate supply of KI tablets is available for the target population and should develop a distribution system to supplement the states' programs. The development of a national program was suggested to evaluate the different KI distribution plans to assess health effects of KI use in the case that KI administration is implemented after an emergency.

SUMMARY

KI provides a safe and effective means to protect the thyroid gland from internal radiation following an accident that releases radioiodines. Despite continuing differences in opinion concerning the need for KI, knowledge derived from the Chernobyl accident has convinced many that provision of KI stockpiles and, in some cases, predistribution, is necessary for the public's safety. The WHO, FDA, and the Nuclear Regulatory Commission, as well as the governments of most of the developed nations, have promulgated guidance and regulations for KI use in radiation emergencies. Assistance with planning for this use has been initiated by a committee of the US National Academy of Sciences.

REFERENCES

1. Becker DV, Robbins J, Beebe GW, et al. Childhood thyroid cancer following the Chernobyl accident. Endocrinol Metab Clin North Am 1996; 25:197–211.
2. Astakhova LN, Anspaugh LR, Beebe GW, et al. Chernobyl-related thyroid cancer in children of Belarus: A case-control study. Radiat Res 1998; 150:349–356.
3. Naumann J, Wolff J. Iodide prophylaxis in Poland after the Chernobyl reactor accident. Benefits and risks. Am J Med 1993; 94:524–532.
4. Balonov M, Kaidanovsky G, Zvonova I, et al. Contributions of short-lived radioiodines to thyroid doses received by evacuees from the Chernobyl area estimated using early in vivo activity measurements. Radiat Prot Dosimetry 2003; 105:593–599.
5. Schneider AB, Robbins J. Ionizing radiation and thyroid cancer. In Fagin JA, editor. Thyroid Cancer. Boston, MA: Kluwer Academic Publishers, 1998:27–47.
6. Verger P, Aurengo A, Geoffroy B, Le Guen B. Iodine kinetics and effectiveness of stable iodine prophylaxis after intake of radioactive iodine: a review. Thyroid 2001; 11:353–360.
7. Wolff J. Iodide prophylaxis for reactor accidents. In Nagataki S, Yamashita S, editors. Nagasaki Symposium Radiation and Human Health. Amsterdam: Elsevier Science B.V., 1996:227–237
8. Takamura N, Hamada A, Yamaguchi N, et al. Urinary iodine kinetics after oral loading of potassium iodine. Endocr J 2003; 50: 589–593.
9. Blum M, Eisenbud M. Reduction of thyroid irradiation from I-131 by potassium iodide. J Am Med Assoc 1967; 200:1036–1040.

10. Zanzonico PB, Becker DV. Effects of time of administration and dietary iodine levels on potassium iodide (KI) blockade of thyroid irradiation by I-131 from radioactive fallout. Health Phys 2000; 78:660–667.
11. Available at: www.fda.gov/cder/drugprepare/KI_Q&A.htm
12. Available at: www.fda.gov/cder/drugprepare/kiprep
13. World Health Organization. Guidelines for Iodine Prophylaxis Following Radiation Accidents: Update 1999. Geneva, 1999.
14. U.S. Food and Drug Administration, Guidance. Potassium Iodide as a Thyroid Blocking Agent in Radiation Emergencies. 2001.
15. Chapin DM, Cohen KP, Davis WK, et al. Nuclear safety. Nuclear power plants and their fuel as terrorist targets. Science 2002; 297:1997–1999. (Comment in: Science 2003; 299:201–203.)
16. Distribution and Administration of Potassium Iodide in the Event of a Nuclear Incident. Washington: The National Academies Press, 2004.

14
Radioiodine Whole Body Imaging*

Frank B. Atkins and Douglas Van Nostrand

INTRODUCTION

Radioiodine imaging is an important diagnostic modality for the evaluation of well-differentiated thyroid carcinoma. A basic understanding of the physics, radioisotopes, equipment, and imaging techniques help the endocrinologist fully comprehend the logistics, interpretation, strengths, and weaknesses of this diagnostic tool. This chapter presents a primer of the subjects noted in Table 1.

OVERVIEW OF ATOMS AND ISOTOPES

An atom is made up of a center (nucleus) and electrons, which circle around the nucleus in nearly the same way as satellites orbit the earth. A particular atom is designated by one or two letters, such as "I" for iodine, and is a distinct chemical element. The nucleus is composed of protons and neutrons. The total number of protons and neutrons equals the mass number, which is labeled as "A." The number of protons is called the "atomic number" and is labeled as "Z." These qualifying labels are usually placed above and below the letter or letters used to designate the chemical element as noted in Fig. 1.

This label is often shortened to include only the mass number, e.g., ^{131}I. In this case, the "I" identifies the element (iodine), and the "131" indicates the total number of protons and neutrons in the atom.

Although a given chemical element must always have the same number of protons, the number of neutrons may vary. In other words, the atomic number (Z) must always be the same, but the mass number (A) will change as the number of neutrons in the nucleus change. When only the number of neutrons differs, those atoms of the same element are called isotopes. ^{131}I, ^{123}I, ^{124}I, and ^{127}I are all isotopes of the same chemical element, iodine, and are different because of the different number of neutrons in the nucleus. While all have 53 protons, ^{131}I has 78 neutrons, ^{123}I has 70 neutrons, ^{124}I has 71 neutrons, and ^{127}I has 74 neutrons. The number of neutrons affects the isotope's physical characteristics, which include the half-life and decay (see below), but the neutrons have no effect on its chemical behavior. Two isotopes—^{131}I and ^{123}I—are used routinely, and a third, namely ^{124}I, has recently become available for the diagnosis and possible treatment of thyroid carcinoma.

An important and distinct characteristic of the various isotopes of radioiodine is how that particular radioiodine releases its energy as it transforms from one iodine to another more stable element. This release of energy is called "decay," but this terminology is misleading. Although decay suggests deterioration, nothing is being destroyed. The element is only changing to another form with the release of energy.

The several types of decay have been discussed in "Radiation and Radioactivity" (see Chapter 44). One method is releasing a wave. These waves are similar to light but cannot be seen by the human eye and can pass through tissue. These "waves of energy" are γ (gamma) *waves* or *rays* and can be seen only by special devices: γ *cameras*. Just as there are different types of light, there are different types of γ waves. The γ cameras used by the nuclear medicine physician or nuclear radiologist not only have the ability to see the γ waves but also have the ability to identify the types of γ wave.

Another way of releasing energy is in the form of a particle, which is similar to those particles that comprise the current that flows to and through a light bulb. The particle could be negatively or positively charged and is referred to as a β particle. The negatively charged β particles are identical to *electrons*, whereas the positively charged particles are called *positrons*. With this form of radioactive decay, energy is released by the nucleus as it "throws off" an electron or positron.

The methods of energy release are shown schematically in Fig. 2 (^{131}I) and Fig. 3 (^{123}I). The decay of ^{124}I is complex and beyond the scope of this chapter; however, a simplified decay scheme is shown in Fig. 4. When ^{123}I decays, it releases

---

*A significant portion of this chapter has been reproduced from Van Nostrand D, Bloom G, Wartofsky L, Thyroid Cancer: A Guide for Patients, with permission from Keystone Press, Inc.

From: *Thyroid Cancer: A Comprehensive Guide to Clinical Management*, 2/e
Edited by: L. Wartofsky and D. Van Nostrand © Humana Press Inc., Totowa, NJ

Table 1

Overview of Atoms and Isotopes
Advantages and Disadvantages of Radioiodine Isotopes
Overview of the γ Camera
Types of Nuclear Medicine Imaging Systems
Types of Whole-Body Scintigraphy
Selection of Radioisotope and Prescribed Activity
Utility of Posttherapy Scans

$$^A I_Z$$

Fig. 1. Notation of an element. "I" represents the element. The superscript "A" represents the atomic weight, which is the total number of protons and neutrons. The subscript "Z" is the atomic number, which is the number of protons and determines the element, iodine. Alternative forms might be written without the superscripts and subscripts, such as 131-I or I-131.

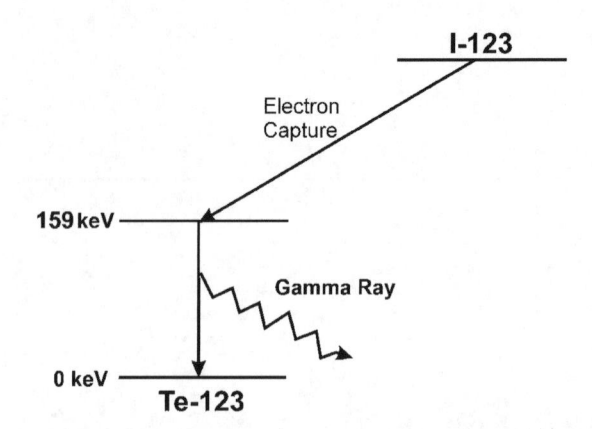

Fig. 3. Electron capture decay for ^{123}I. This is a simplified visual representation of the decay of ^{123}I, which does so by a process known as *electron capture*. In an unstable nucleus that contains too many positively charged particles or protons, electron capture is a mode of radioactive decay in which one of the protons in the nucleus captures one of the atom's orbital electrons. These two particles combine in such a way that the negative charge of the electron and positive charge of the proton effectively cancel each other out to produce a neutral particle, a *neutron*, which remains in the nucleus. Following the capture, the nucleus usually emits a γ ray.

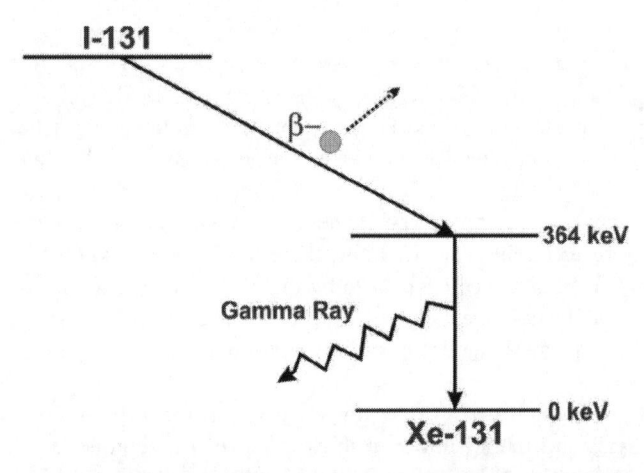

Fig. 2. β− decay for ^{131}I. This is a very simplified visual representation of the decay of ^{131}I, which does so by a process known as β− *emission*. β− emission is a mode of radioactive decay by which an unstable nucleus, one containing too few positively charged particles or protons, can become more stable. In this case, one of the neutral particles in the nucleus, i.e., the neutron, transforms into a proton. As this particle was originally neutral before changing to a positively charged particle, it must then also form a negatively charged particle, so that the two charges cancel each other. The negatively charged particle produced is identical to the electrons that are the constituents of matter. However, because the electron does not belong within the confines of the nucleus, it is forcefully ejected during the transformation process. To identify this particle as having originated from within the nucleus, "β," is used—β particle. Following the emission of the β particle, the nucleus usually emits a γ ray, in this case one which carries 364 keV of energy.

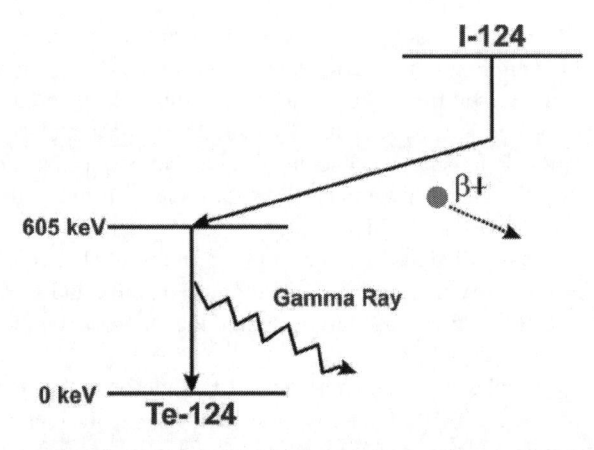

Fig. 4. Positron emission (β+) decay for ^{124}I. This is a simplified visual representation of the decay of ^{124}I, which does so by a process known as *positron emission*. Positron emission, like electron capture, is a mode of radioactive decay for an unstable nucleus that contains too many protons. In this case, to get rid of the excess positive charge, the proton transforms into a neutron and ejects a particle, which has the same mass as an electron except that it is positively charged. This positively charged electron is a positron or a β+ particle. Particles of this type are referred to as antiparticles. The ultimate fate of the positron is that after it loses most of its energy traveling through several millimeters of surrounding matter, the positron will combine with an electron. The two particles will annihilate each other with the subsequent production of two γ rays each with 511 keV of energy that travel in nearly opposite directions from the site of annihilation. It is these annihilation γ rays that are imaged using a PET scanner, which also exploits their simultaneous production and directionality of the two γ rays to form the image.

Table 2
Radioiodines Used for Imaging of Thyroid Diseases

	Decay Mode	Half-Life	Gamma Energy (keV)	Production Method	Typical Prescribed Activity mCi (MBq)
^{123}I	Electron capture	13.6 h	159	Cyclotron methods. One method, referred to as a (p,5n), produces ^{123}I with no ^{124}I contamination and little ^{125}I. The other approach, referred to as (p,2n), has a number of impurities that have high-energy γ's and long half-lives. These contaminations reduce image quality and increase the radiation exposure of the patient.	0.4–4.0 (15–148.8)
^{124}I	Positron emission	4.2 d	511	Cyclotron	2–4 (74–148)
^{125}I	Electron capture	60.2 d	35	Cyclotron. Not used for imaging because the γ energy is too low. Also, the long half-life results in a significant radiation burden to the patient. This has primarily been used for radioimmunoassays and other in vitro laboratory tests.	Not used for imaging owing to long half-life and low energy of γ ray.
^{127}I	Stable	–	–	Naturally occurring	N/A
^{131}I	β-decay	8.02 d	364	Reactor produced either from direct bombardment of a target by neutrons or from the reprocessing of spent fuel rods from a nuclear power plant.	Uptakes: 0.005 (0.185) Imaging: 1–5 (37–185) Treatment: 29–1000 (1.07–37 GBq)

γ waves. When ^{131}I decays, it releases several types of γ waves, as well as a β particle. When ^{124}I decays, it releases energy in many different ways; the diagnostically important method is by the release of a positron. This positron collides with an electron, and both the positron and electron disintegrate or annihilate each other with the conversion of mass into two γ waves of the same energy, which are released 180° apart.

Another important characteristic of any radionuclide is its half-life, which is the time it takes for half of the atoms to decay. The half-life could be seconds, minutes, hours, or days, but it is the same for all atoms of a given isotope. For example, if you had 100 atoms of ^{131}I, it would take 8.06 d for 50 of the atoms to transform into the element, xenon. For ^{123}I, this same process would take 13.3 h for 50 atoms to transform into tellurium, and for ^{124}I, it would take 4.2 d. A summary of the decay mode, half-life, γ energy, production method, and typical prescribed activity are noted in Table 2.

ADVANTAGES AND DISADVANTAGES OF RADIOIODINE ISOTOPES OF ^{123}I, ^{131}I, AND ^{124}I

Some advantages and disadvantages of ^{123}I, ^{131}I, and ^{124}I are summarized in Table 3. The contents of this table are likely to change over time as a result of fluctuations in the cost of these isotopes or as new information becomes available.

OVERVIEW OF THE γ CAMERA

As noted above, the basic instrument used in nuclear medicine to form an image of the radionuclide distribution within the patient is the γ camera. This terminology is derived from the fact that it generates a two-dimensional (2D) image of an object (like a photographic camera) by detecting γ radiation, a particular type of radiation that is emitted from the tracer within the patient. Although there are numerous designs and configurations of γ cameras, most have one important component in common: the type of radiation detector used

Table 3
Comparison of ^{123}I, ^{124}I, and ^{131}I

	^{123}I	^{124}I	^{131}I
Expense	$$	$$$	$
Readily available	Y	Just becoming available	Y
Reimbursed by Insurance	Y	N	Y
Useful in the treatment of differentiated thyroid carcinoma	N	Y[a]	Y
Useful for dosimetry (blood/bone marrow)	Possibly	Y	Y
Useful for dosimetry (lesion)	Limited	Y	Limited
Stunning	No	Possibly	Possibly
Risk to personnel handling patient and radionuclide	Low	Medium	Medium
Necessity of radiation safety precautions for patient and public	N	Y	Y
Image quality	Good	Excellent	Fair
Delayed imaging (>48 h)	N[b]	Y	Y
PET scanner required	N	Y	N
Tomographic images (routinely)	N	Y	N
Image fusion with other modalities	N	Y	N

[a]The energy of the positron and half-life of ^{124}I would make it technically feasible for this radioiodine to be used for the treatment of differentiated thyroid carcinoma. However, even if sufficient quantities could be produced in today's market, the cost would be prohibitive.

[b]Multiple studies have demonstrated the ability to obtain images at 48 h after administration of ^{123}I, and with higher prescribed activity, further delayed imaging may be possible.

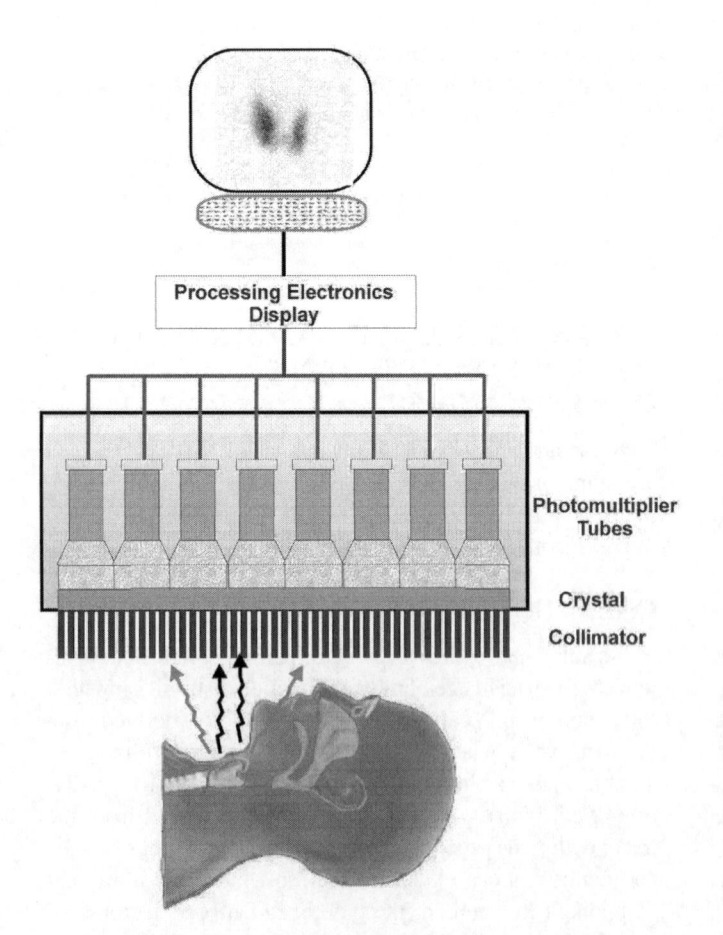

Fig. 5. Components of a γ camera. See text for discussion.

to measure the γ radiation. The kind of device in question is a *scintillation detector*, as it is based on measuring a small burst of light that is produced by the γ radiation as it passes through the detector. For this reason, a γ camera is also frequently referred to as a *scintillation camera*. The technology is not new; in fact, the γ camera has been used in medical imaging since its invention by Hal Anger in the early 1960s. This is discussed further in Chapter 12 entitled the "History of Nuclear Medicine in Thyroid Disease." Since the γ camera was introduced, its design and performance has evolved considerably into the sophisticated device that is in widespread use today. Although there are numerous versions of γ cameras currently available on the market, four components are common to virtually all of them: collimator, scintillation crystal, photomultiplier tubes, and the electronics/computers to process and display the image. These components are shown in the Fig. 5.

Collimator

The γ rays produced by the radioiodine within the patient are emitted randomly in all directions. However, to form an image requires knowledge or information about the direction that the γ ray is traveling. Because it is not possible to determine this directly, a collimator is used instead. The most common design of a γ camera collimator is shown in the Fig. 6. It usually consists of a set of holes or channels (typically several thousand) in a block of lead, each of which is parallel to all the others. Hence, it is referred to as a *parallel-hole* collimator. γ rays that are traveling in a direction that pass through the channel will make it to the

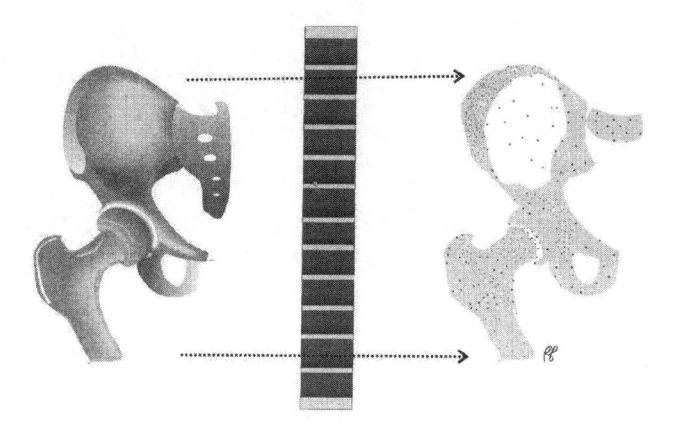

Fig. 6. Parallel-hole collimator. The collimator is an essential component of the γ camera. One type shown in this figure is a parallel-hole collimator because each channel through which the γ rays must pass before they can be recorded in the image is parallel to all of the other channels or holes. See text for more discussion. Reproduced with permission from *Essentials of Nuclear Medicine Physics*, Blackwell Publishers, Inc.

opposite side and enter the detector. Most γ rays that would cross from one channel to another will be absorbed in the lead that separates the holes and will not be recorded in the image. As a result, the γ rays that pass through the collimator form a distribution on its exit side, which is a representation of the radionuclide distribution within the patient.

To form an accurate representation of the distribution of radioiodine within the patient, it is important that as few γ rays as possible that have crossed between channels reach the detector. The γ rays that do are referred to as *penetration radiation*. Because of the nature of the passage of γ rays through material, it is not possible to completely stop all penetration, but it can be minimized through appropriate design and construction.

Several variables could be used to characterize the design of such a collimator and will have an impact on the quality of the image formed. These variables include the diameter of the hole, thickness of the collimator, and spacing between holes. By making the channel or hole wider, more γ rays will pass through the collimator and will be recorded in the image. Therefore, the statistical noise* in the image will be reduced. The importance of counts on the overall image quality is illustrated in Fig. 7.

However, the larger hole is less selective about the direction that the γ ray is traveling; therefore, the uncertainty about where the γ ray originated from within the patient is greater. Thus, larger channels will produce images with less statistical noise but also less sharpness or detail, i.e., greater blurring of images. The thickness of the material that separates one channel from an adjacent channel affects the amount of radiation that "penetrates" the collimator. Increasing this thickness reduces the penetration but also reduces the number of γ rays recorded in the image. Once again, the statistical noise can become a limiting factor. Furthermore, if it is too thick (>1 mm), the pattern of the holes or channels in the collimator can be visualized as it is superimposed on the patient's image. To compensate for this effect, the collimators can be increased in total height to maintain the spacing between channels at acceptable values.

Another important characteristic of γ rays is that the higher the energy of the photon, the more difficult it is to stop or absorb that radiation. This factor has a major impact on collimator design. Consequently, collimators are designed specifically for certain energy ranges. A typical and important rule followed in collimator design is that the number of γ rays that penetrate the collimator septa should be less than approx 2% of the total number that pass through the collimator. Because ^{131}I emits a relatively high-energy γ ray (364 keV), it is important to use a collimator that has been designed for high-energy imaging. Usually, the penetration radiation is spread out diffusely over the entire patient image, but if there is a small intense area of ^{131}I concentration in the patient, it will be manifested as a star-like artifact, with rays projecting outward from the center like the points on a star. The number of points and shape of this artifact depends on the layout of the channels and shape of the hole in the collimator. Basically, the projections are along paths where the material that separates one hole from its neighbor is the thinnest. An example is shown in Fig. 8.

The parallel-hole collimator is the most widely used type in nuclear medicine, but the pinhole collimator is another particularly useful design in imaging small organs like the thyroid gland.

The pinhole collimator is much simpler than the parallel-hole collimator in terms of its design and construction. The bulk of this collimator consists of a large lead conical shell with the tip cut off. The base of the cone will cover a large portion of the γ camera crystal. The purpose of this shell is to shield the detector from the γ rays that do not pass through the collimator itself. As implied by the name, the pinhole collimator itself consists of a single small hole (often

---

Statistical noise is a colloquial term used to describe the amount of variation that is produced in a sample or measurement. Suppose, for example, we have a patio composed of large number of square tiles, and it is raining lightly. After a short time, we count the number of raindrops that have fallen on each tile. Even though we expect each of the tiles to receive the same amount of rain, there will be a variation in the number from one tile to the next. This is due to the random nature of the location of the individual raindrops. The underlying structure of the nuclear medicine image is likewise composed with an arrangement of "tiles," which are picture elements (also called "pixels"). The image displayed on the monitor is simply a visual representation of the number of γ rays (i.e., raindrops) that have struck each small area of the detector and is converted into the relative brightness or darkness of each pixel. The smaller the number of γ rays recorded in each pixel, the greater the relative variation from pixel to pixel and hence, the greater the statistical noise in the image.

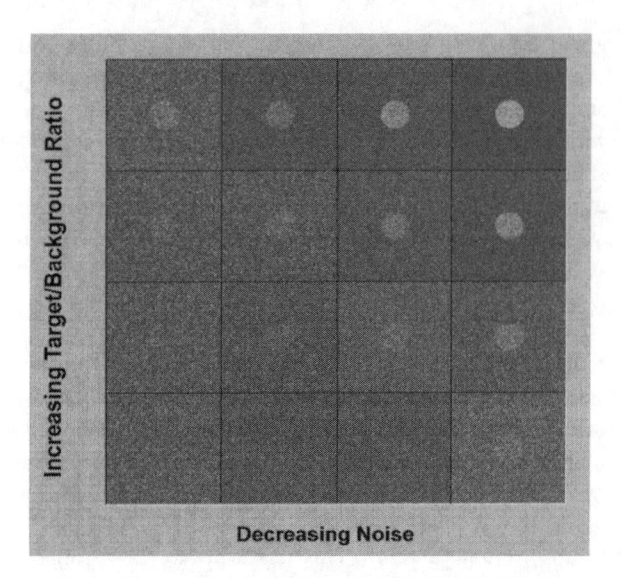

Fig. 7. Relationships of spatial resolution and detected events. This figure illustrates the importance of both counts (the number of γ rays recorded in the image) and the contrast (the relative ability of the tissue to concentrate the radionuclide compared to its surrounding tissues) on the ability to "detect" a lesion. The lesion in this case is a circular area in a uniform background. Along each row of this grid, the contrast is a constant value but increases progressively from the bottom to the top. Likewise, the statistical variations in the image (called "noise") are the same along a given column but decrease progressively from left to right. The box at the lower left has the lowest lesion contrast and the greatest noise level, whereas the box in the upper right corner has the highest lesion contrast and the least noise level. If you examine the bottom row, you will probably only be confident that the lesion is present for the last box. However, the lesion is present in every box; it is just obscured by the noise. For the second row from the bottom, the lesion is probably just detectable in the next to last box. Similarly, for the next row up, the lesion is detectable in the last three boxes. This illustrates that as the contrast increases, the lesion can be detected in the presence of greater noise levels.

The contrast depends on a number of physiological parameters that affect the ability of the metastatic thyroid tissue to concentrate the radioiodine relative to surrounding background tissues. One common way for the nuclear medicine physician to try and increase the lesion contrast is to delay the time of imaging an additional 24 h or longer. This takes advantage of the fact that nonprotein-bound iodine is generally cleared or eliminated from normal tissues faster than it is from functioning thyroid metastasis. As a result, the contrast may increase over time, which would be equivalent to moving to a higher row in this image. What can also be observed in this figure is that even low-contrast lesion can be "seen" if the statistical noise is small enough. Noise can be reduced by recording more γ rays in the image. There are a variety of ways in which the number of detected γ rays can be increased. The simplest is to increase the imaging time. Another option might be to increase the administered prescribed activity. However, in the case of ^{131}I, this might increase the risk of stunning. The patient could be imaged sooner after the administration of the radioiodine while there is more activity in the patient, but this would result in a smaller lesion contrast as noted above.

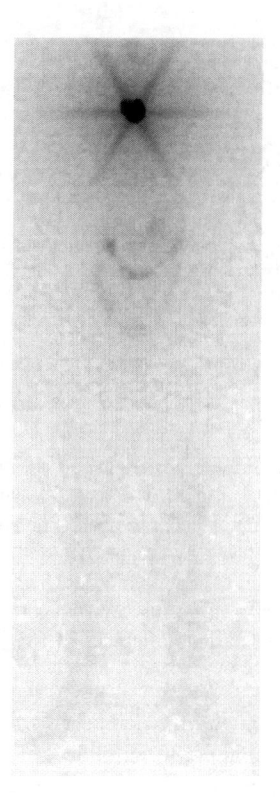

Fig. 8. Star artifact on radioiodine whole-body scan. See text and Chapter 15 for discussion.

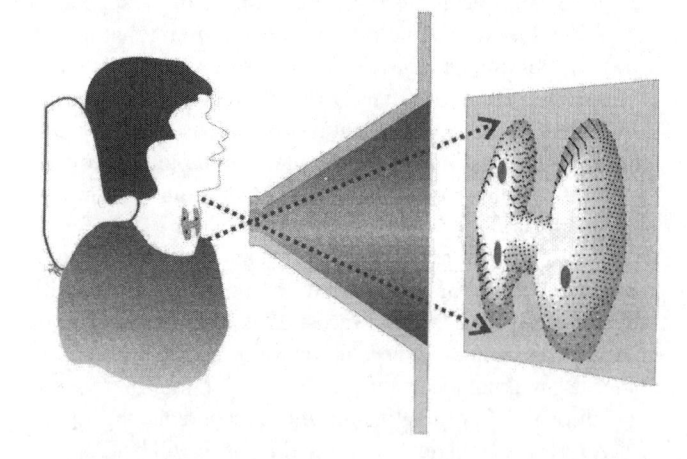

Fig. 9. Pinhole collimator. See text for discussion. Reproduced with permission from *Essentials of Nuclear Medicine Physics*, Blackwell Publishers, Inc.

referred to as an *aperture*) in the truncated tip of the cone. The diameter of this aperture is typically several millimeters. Ideally, the only γ rays that can reach the detector and contribute to the image are those that are emitted from the patient, pass through the pinhole, and strike the crystal. As γ rays travel along a straight line, each point on the crystal would then correspond to a small volume within the patient. This is illustrated in Fig. 9.

How well defined the patient's image is depends partly on how large the pinhole is. If it is too large, then γ rays from a broader region of the organ being imaged can pass through the aperture and strike the same location on the crystal. As a result, the image is not sharp. Alternatively, if the aperture is too small, then very few γ rays will pass through the opening, and the image (although sharp) will be of poor quality because of statistical limitations of low counts. For this reason, pinhole collimators are usually designed so that the aperture is changeable to accommodate different imaging conditions and requirements. A typical set of pinholes might include a diameter range of 2, 4, 6, and 8 mm. Generally, for lower energy γ and higher administered activities (e.g., ^{99m}Tc pertechnetate), the smaller 2–4-mm pinhole is used; for higher energies (e.g., ^{131}I), a larger 6–8-mm pinhole is used.

For parallel-hole collimators, penetration of the collimator by γ waves is also a problem for pinhole collimators. For this reason, the insert assembly is often manufactured using Tungsten, which is a strong metal that can be machined and is about 1.5 times more than the density of lead. Consequently, it is even more effective than lead at reducing the penetration radiation. Another advantage is its strength. Lead is a soft metal and can be easily damaged. For some research applications, an even denser metal has been used, i.e., *depleted uranium*. Naturally occurring uranium consists of a mixture by weight of three radionuclides of uranium: ^{238}U (99.27%), ^{235}U (0.72%), and ^{234}U (0.0054%). The uranium used in nuclear power plants requires an "enriched" form in which the fraction of ^{235}U has been increased from 0.72% to about 1.5–3%. Depleted uranium is the uranium remaining after the enrichment process contains only about 0.2% of the fissionable ^{235}U. This material is even denser than tungsten and is about two times greater than the density of lead.

There are a number of important differences between pinhole and parallel-hole collimators. One is the *field of view* (FOV), how large an area of the patient the γ camera can image. For the parallel-hole collimator, the size of the FOV is essentially the physical size of the detector itself (aside from dead space around the periphery). However, for pinhole collimators, the area of an organ that can be imaged depends on how far the organ is from the pinhole. For objects only about 5 cm from the pinhole, the FOV is about one fourth to one third of the dimensions of the detector. As the object moves closer to the pinhole, the FOV decreases. In addition, as objects move away from the pinhole collimator, the number of γ rays that can pass through the pinhole falls off rapidly. Consequently, pinhole collimators are used to image small organs, such as the thyroid gland and neck bed, which can be positioned close to the collimator.

Scintillation Crystal

Once the γ ray passes through the collimator, it must then be detected. This involves the use of a special type of material that will produce a brief flash of light (*scintillation*) when a γ ray interacts. This flash itself only lasts less than a 1/1,000,000 of a second. Although not all materials possess this capability, many that do are in a physical form, which we refer to as a "crystal," i.e., the atoms are lined up in a regular periodic structure. There are many different scintillation crystals, but the most commonly used for γ cameras is sodium iodide (NaI). The primary reasons for using NaI are the natural abundance of the raw materials and relative ease of growing the large crystals needed for this application. Both of these factors contribute to a relatively low cost for this component of the imaging system. The usual representation of the sodium iodide crystal is NaI(Tl). This indicates that a small amount (~0.1%) of thallium (Tl) has been intentionally included in the growth of this scintillation crystal. A small amount of this impurity has been found to significantly increase the amount of light produced in the crystal by the radiation. When a γ ray interacts in the crystal, two important features help in the imaging process: (1) the light emanates from the point at which the γ interacts, and (2) the intensity of the light is proportional to the energy of the γ ray. The first factor allows an image of the location of the γ ray to be generated (i.e., where it came from in the patient), and the second factor allows the discrimination of γ rays of different energies, which then allows the discrimination of different radionuclides and γ wave scatter within the patient. Most γ cameras use a single, rectangular, large-area scintillation crystal that is capable of imaging a substantial portion of the patient at one time. Typical FOV are 20 in. wide by 15 in. in length.

Photomultiplier Tubes (PMT)

These electronic devices are designed for a single purpose—to detect and measure small amounts of light in a short period of time. The γ camera consists of an array of photomultipliers (see Fig. 10), which cover the surface of the scintillation crystal. Generally 2–3-in. diameter PMTs are used so that 50–100 of these devices are required. Each time a scintillation event occurs in the crystal (a γ ray is detected), some resultant light is detected by the PMT, and an electrical signal is produced. The more light that is "seen" by a PMT, the greater the signal it produces. Although "photomultiplier" implies the multiplication of photos (see Fig. 11), the PMT multiplies the electrical signal.

Processing Electronics and Image Display

The last component in the γ camera imaging chain is associated with the processing of the electrical signals from the PMTs and conversion of this information into an image. The closer a PMT is to the source of the light (i.e., the point in the crystal where the γ ray was absorbed), the more light it sees. Hence, the greater the electrical signal, the closer the PMT is to the scintillation event. By examining the signal distribution from a cluster of PMTs surrounding the interaction site, it is possible to determine the location of the γ interaction in

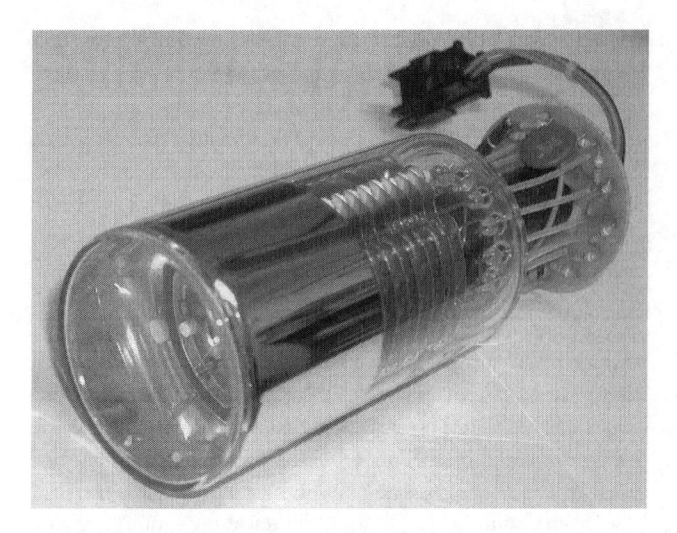

Fig. 10. Photomultiplier tube. The left end of the tube is coupled to the crystal. See text for discussion.

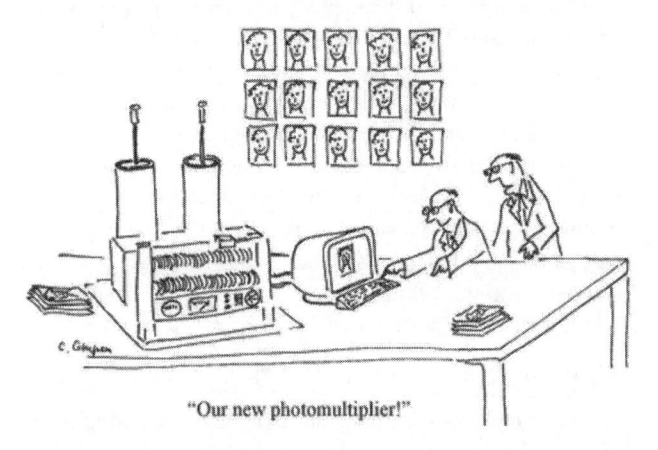

Fig. 11. See text. Photo was reproduced with permission of the Dr. Claus Grupen, the creator.

the crystal itself with some degree of precision. In fact, despite the PMTs fairly large size (typically about 75 mm in diameter), this approach for localization can determine the site with a precision of about ±2.0 mm. Finally, the information from each detected event is stored in a 2D array, and each element of the array (called a pixel for picture element) contains the total number of γ rays that were detected at that location in the crystal during the entire acquisition period. The image displayed on the computer is a representation of the radioactivity distribution in the patient. Usually, the image is displayed in black and white, with the scale or darkness proportional to the number of γ rays that came from that region of the patient.

NUCLEAR MEDICINE IMAGING TECHNIQUES

Several techniques can be used to image thyroid tissue and well-differentiated thyroid cancer using the γ camera.

Static Planar Imaging

The operating principles of the γ camera were described in the previous section. As indicated, this device consists of a large-area crystal to detect the γ rays and a collimator to select the γ rays on the basis of their direction of travel. Usually, the collimator is a parallel-hole design, which means that the γ rays recorded in the image are only those that are traveling (more or less) in a direction that is perpendicular to the crystal. If the detector has a dimension, e.g., of 15 by 20 in., then the area of the patient that would be examined is also approximately the same size. If the area of interest were much smaller than the camera area, such as the thyroid bed, then the detector would not be utilized efficiently. In this case, a different type of collimator might be used instead, i.e., a pinhole collimator. On the contrary, the FOV of the γ camera may not be large enough to cover all the areas of the patient that need to be examined. In this instance, a series of images are acquired with the patient repositioned in front of the γ camera. Each image is often referred to as a "static" image.

Whole-Body Imaging (Metastatic Survey)

The whole-body or metastatic survey is a routinely performed imaging procedure to detect the metastatic spread of well-differentiated thyroid carcinoma. As thyroid cancer can metastasize to regions well outside the thyroid bed, it is necessary to image or *survey* a large portion of the patient's body. Hence, it is often referred to as *whole-body* scanning. In practice, however, the area scanned usually extends from the head to the knee or just below the knee because thyroid cancer rarely metastasizes more distally than this. The radionuclide used for this purpose is one of the radioisotopes of iodine. In the past, this has been generally ^{131}I; but more recently, ^{123}I has had increased usage, and the positron-emitter ^{124}I may have an important role in the not-too-distant future.

For either ^{123}I or ^{131}I, the device used is the γ camera to generate a 2D image of the radionuclide distribution within the patient, who is really a 3D object. Because some radiation is absorbed within the patient's body, the resulting image will be influenced to a greater extent by the radioiodine that is located closer to the patient's surface on the side that the γ camera is positioned. Thus, concentrations of activity (metastases) that are located posteriorly within the patient might not be visualized when viewed anteriorly and vice versa. Images are therefore obtained routinely from both the anterior and posterior projections.

To reduce imaging time, most systems currently employ two γ cameras that are mounted on a gantry, allowing the detectors to be positioned directly opposite each other, with the patient located between them (see Fig. 12). In this case, the anterior and posterior images can be acquired simultaneously. Furthermore, because the FOV along the length of

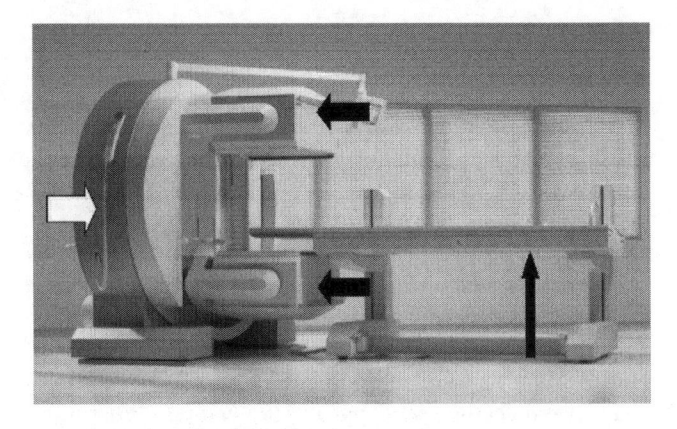

Fig. 12. Dual-head nuclear medicine γ camera. The thick arrows represent the dual γ camera heads. The thin arrow represents the patient table, and the open arrow represents the camera gantry. Photo courtesy of Siemens Medical Solutions USA, Inc.

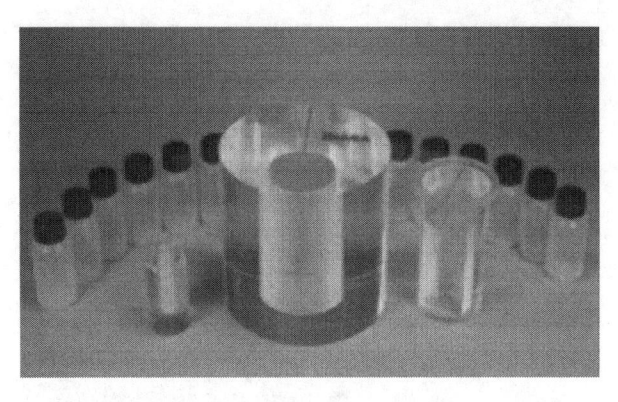

Fig. 13. Thyroid phantom. See text for discussion. Photo courtesy of Biodex Medical Systems, Inc.

the patient is typically only approx 15 in., multiple sets of images need to be acquired to cover or survey the patient's whole body. Although this could be accomplished by imaging each section of the patient individually, with some slight overlap between sections, this is a time-consuming approach for the patient and the technologist. Ultimately, the nuclear medicine physician must deal with assembling these images from all the different sections into the proper presentation. To facilitate the imaging of a substantial length of the patient, most imaging systems also have the capability of continuously scanning over the length of the patient as the data is collected. This scanning can either involve the patient's bed moving between the detectors or the camera gantry traversing along a track. In either case, the imaging system has been designed to incorporate the relative position of the γ cameras and table to generate a single image from each detector over the entire length that was scanned.

Radioiodine Uptake

An important factor often used to help select the prescribed activity for ablation or treatment of well-differentiated thyroid cancer with radioiodine is the *uptake*. Uptake is a measure of the fraction (usually expressed as a percentage) of the administered radioiodine present in some specific tissue at the time of measurement—usually 24 h after dosing. The tissue in question could be the thyroid gland, thyroid remnant left after near-total thyroidectomy, or metastatic thyroid carcinoma. The uptake is a significant parameter because it may directly impact the radiation dose that can be delivered to the tissue targeted for treatment and, hence, the potential effectiveness of the radioiodine therapy. The calculation is simple:

Uptake (%) = radioactivity in tissue × 100 / administered activity

Although the radioactivity in the tissue is measured at a specific time after the administration, the value used in this equation is what it would have been at the time of administration. Thus, this value is corrected for the decay of the radionuclide between the time of administration and measurement. If ^{123}I is being used for this measurement, then this amounts to a factor of about 3.4 for a 24-h period.

At issue is how to determine the activity in the tissue. There are basically two approaches to measure the uptake and use different instrumentation: an uptake probe and a γ camera. As the radiation detectors count γ rays while the patient is given an amount of radioiodine measured in units of *activity*, i.e., millicuries (mCi) or mega-Becquerel (MBq) then some calibration of the counts into radioactivity would be needed. In addition, because the thyroid gland is at some depth, albeit small, within the patient's neck, some loss of γ rays is from their absorption within the patient. Consequently, a separate measurement of a known amount of radioactivity (calibration source) of the radioiodine used for the uptake is also measured using the same device. In this case, the calibration source is (1) placed inside a phantom designed to mimic a typical neck size and tissue depth, and (2) the phantom is positioned in front of the uptake probe in the same manner as the patient would be. The neck phantom has been standardized by the International Atomic Energy Agency and is shown in Fig. 13.

A solid plastic cylinder simulates the neck of a patient approx 5 in. in diameter by 5 in. in height with a cylindrical hole that extends partially through the phantom and is offset toward the "anterior" surface. If capsules containing the standard radioiodine are used, they are placed inside the plastic insert shown just to the left of the neck phantom. This insert is then placed inside the holder to the right of the neck, and the assembly is inserted into the hole in the phantom. If liquids are used instead of capsules, then one of the vials is filled with the radioiodine and placed into the insert. Frequently, the same capsule(s) to be administered to the patient are used for the calibration. The denominator in the

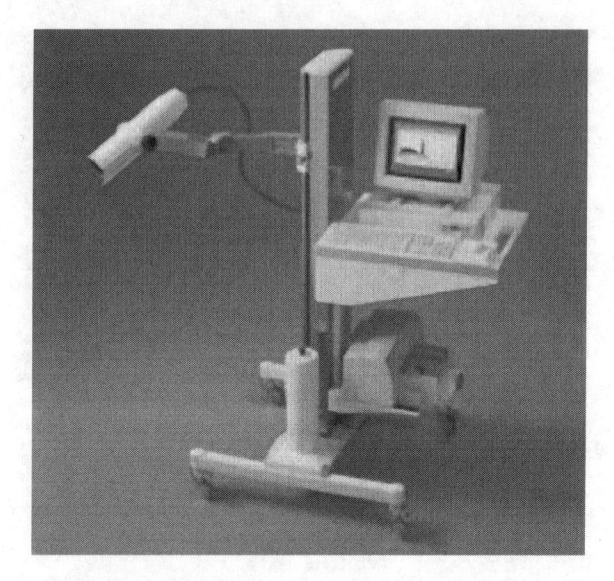

Fig. 14. Thyroid uptake probe. See text for discussion. Photo courtesy of Biodex Medical Systems, Inc.

equation above is simply the counts recorded using this measurement; no additional corrections are required.

Uptake Probe

The uptake probe typically uses a single small NaI (Tl) radiation detector that is mounted onto an articulating arm. The diameter of this detector is generally between 1 and 2 in. A collimator is in front of the detector and is a slightly tapered, cylindrical, lead-based shell of about 5 in. in length that blocks γ rays from striking the detector unless they originate from a reasonably small volume at the end of the collimator. Because γ rays travel along straight lines, the size of the sensitive volume gradually increases with distance from the detector. Systems specifically designed as thyroid uptake probes are commercially available, and an example is shown in Fig. 14.

The arm holding the probe can move vertically along the counterbalanced stand to allow easy positioning over the anterior surface of the thyroid bed of the seated patient. The γ radiation emanating from the patient is then counted for about 5 min. As the number of γ rays that would strike the detector depends strongly on the distance of the source from the probe, there is also a movable device mounted on the side of the probe that allows the patient to be positioned at a consistent and reproducible distance about 3 in. from the collimator.

Acquisition Parameters and Technique

Scintigraphic protocols for imaging well-differentiated thyroid cancer depend on which radioiodine was administered and the mode of operation of the γ camera. To evaluate the patient for metastatic spread of the thyroid cancer, a large portion of the body must be imaged from the head to about the knees. Although this can be accomplished in different ways, the most common technique is a whole-body scan, which was discussed earlier in this chapter. Today, most scintillation cameras are mounted on a gantry that enables either the patient bed to continuously translate the patient through the imaging field or the gantry and camera to "scan" along the length of the patient. In either case, a single image can be produced in which the width is equal to the camera's active width, whereas the height of the image corresponds to the distance that was scanned. Typically, the maximum length that can be scanned is approx 200 cm. Furthermore, many scintillation camera systems currently have two detectors, such that anterior and posterior projections can be acquired simultaneously, thereby reducing the overall imaging time. If the imaging system is not capable of whole-body scanning, then separate overlapping images that span the appropriate length of the patient can be used. The whole-body scan or survey is an indispensable diagnostic tool; nevertheless, the image quality is not quite as good as that obtained from a static or "spot" view of a particular area of the patient.

Table 4 lists typical acquisition parameters that might be used to acquire each image for the different modes of operation (whole-body scanning, static images, and pinhole images) for ^{123}I and ^{131}I. For some parameters, the values listed are guidelines and might differ somewhat between facilities. Additional information is also available from the Society of Nuclear Medicine (1).

Positron Emission Tomography (PET) Scanner

Because ^{124}I is a position-emitting radionuclide, a different device is required to image this radioiodine: the PET scanner, which is discussed further in Chapter 34 entitled "PET Imaging."

TYPES OF WHOLE-BODY SCINTIGRAPHY

Understanding the different types of radioiodine whole-body scanning can be confusing because a whole-body scan can be performed many different ways, and the terminology varies between imaging facilities and also within the same facility. To aid the understanding and communication of the many different types of radioiodine whole-body scans, three factors are typically included in the name (see Table 5).

Time Points of Scanning

Scans are typically performed at four time points during the patient's medical care.

Time Point 1: Preablation Scan

The first scan is performed typically 4–6 wk after the patient's initial thyroid surgery and before the first radioiodine ablation, hence, the terms *preablation scan, first diagnostic scan*, or *postoperative* scan.

Table 4
Typical Acquisition Parameters

		Whole-Body Scanning			
Radionuclide	Collimator	Peak (keV)	Window	Speed	Matrix
^{123}I	Low energy	159	15–20%	4–6 cm/min	512 × 1024
^{131}I	High energy	362	15–20%	4–6 cm/min	512 × 1024
		Static Imaging			
Radionuclide	Collimator	Peak (keV)	Window	Time/View	Matrix
^{123}I	Low energy	159	15–20%	10–20 min	256 × 256
^{131}I	High energy	362	15–20%	10–20 min	256 × 256
		Pinhole Imaging			
Radionuclide	Pinhole Insert	Peak (keV)	Window	Time	Matrix
^{123}I	4 mm	159	15–20%	10–20 min	256 × 256
^{131}I	6 mm	362	15–20%	10–20 min	256 × 256

Table 5
Factors for Describing Radioiodine Whole Body Scan

The point in time during the patient's medical care when the scan is performed.
The type of thyroid stimulation used in preparation for the scan.
The specific radioiodine used.

The objectives of this scan are:

1. To visually assess the extent and distribution of normal thyroid tissue still remaining after the thyroidectomy.
2. To qualitatively demonstrate and quantitatively measure (uptake probe) the amount of radioiodine in the thyroid bed, which could affect the empiric, ablative prescribed activity of radioiodine.
3. To evaluate the presence of metastasis, such as in the cervical lymph nodes, bones, lungs, or brain, which may alter the immediate management of the patient.

Although most facilities perform these preablation scans, a few facilities have eliminated them (2,3). These facilities typically use a single empiric prescribed activity of radioiodine for all initial ablations in adults, regardless of the results from the initial preablation scan. At this time, no conclusive scientific data is present indicating whether one approach is better than the other. Nevertheless, this author believes that these scans are valuable for the reasons noted above and in Table 6. For the minor inconvenience to the patient and a cost equivalent to about one computed tomography (CT) scan, the information obtained is useful and could alter the physician's management of the patient.

Time Point 2: Follow-Up as a Screen for Recurrent Cancer

As part of the follow-up and monitoring for recurrent well-differentiated thyroid cancer in patients who have had a thyroidectomy and radioiodine ablation, a radioiodine whole-body scan may be used, and this is frequently a *surveillance scan*. These scans may be performed as soon as 6 mo or possibly as long as 2 yr after the patient's initial ablation. Most surveillance scans are performed at approx 1 yr after ablation, then periodically at increasing time intervals. However, with the availability of thyroglobulin blood levels that can be used as a tumor marker, many facilities have stopped performing surveillance scans as part of the patient's routine follow-up and monitoring (4–7).

Time Point 3: When Metastasis is Suspected

A scan may also be performed when recurrence of thyroid cancer is already known to be present or is suggested based on an elevated or rising thyroglobulin blood level, positive cytology obtained by fine-needle aspiration of a lymph node, a new mass on physical exam, or findings suggesting recurrence on CT, ultrasound, magnetic resonance (MR), or PET. Although some facilities also refer to this as a surveillance scan, the objective of this scan is no longer for surveillance. Rather, the objective of this scan depends on the patient's clinical situation. For example, if the patient's serum thyroglobulin level is rising, the objective of the scan may be to try to localize the site of the recurrent cancer for possible surgery, to determine whether the thyroid cancer has radioiodine uptake and could benefit from radioiodine treatment, or both. However, if a new mass is

Table 6
Utility of the Preablation Scan[a]

Demonstration of the pattern and percent uptake of iodine in the thyroid bed or neck area that could, in turn, alter the management, therapeutic prescribed activity, or both. Examples include:

1. A single area of significant uptake, such as 5–30%, which suggests considering additional surgery or modifying the empiric prescribed activity of radioiodine.[b]
2. A single area of low uptake such as 1%, which suggests modifying the empiric prescribed activity of radioiodine.[b]
3. A pattern of radioiodine uptake consistent with cervical metastasis that may suggest (1) further evaluation with MR or ultrasound, (2) additional fine-needle aspiration, surgery, or both and/or (3) the use a larger empiric prescribed activity of radioiodine.

Demonstration of distant metastasis that may alter the evaluation and/or the management of the patient prior to radioiodine treatment. Examples include:

1. Focal or diffuse uptake in lung that may warrant further evaluation with CT without contrast, pulmonary function tests, and dosimetry to determine the maximum tolerable prescribed activity without exceeding 48-h retained whole-body or retained lung restrictions. The latter may increase or decrease prescribed activity relative to an empiric prescribed activity and may help minimize the potential for acute radiation pneumonitis and pulmonary fibrosis.
2. Focal area suggesting bone metastasis that may need further evaluation with CT, larger empiric prescribed activity, dosimetry and/or coordination of subsequent external radiotherapy or radiofrequency ablation.
3. Focal uptake in the head that may warrant an MR exam of the brain. If the focal area is a brain metastasis, then the empiric prescribed activity may require a reduction, and/or the pretreatment management of the patient may be altered to include steroids, glycerol, and/or mannitol.

[a]This author believes that a preablation scan has value. In an unpublished retrospective review of 115 patients, the preablation scan modified the patient's evaluation, surgical management, pretreatment radioiodine management, or prescribed activity of radioiodine in 15% of the patients.
[b]Various reports suggest that the prescribed activity for residual thyroid tissue in the thyroid bed be increased or decreased based upon the radioiodine uptake (see Chapter 26, refs. *32–36*).

---

present, and its cytology by fine-needle aspiration is positive, the objective of the scan may be to determine whether it can be potentially treated with radioiodine and if there are other sites of metastasis similar to some of those listed in Table 6 that may alter management.

Time Point 4: Posttherapy Scan

This scan is typically performed between 1 and 12 d after the patient's radioiodine ablation or treatment. Posttherapy scans have a particular advantage over the other scans discussed because of the much higher prescribed activity of radioiodine used for the patient's ablation or treatment. As a result, these scans may demonstrate thyroid tissue or metastases that could not be detected on the postoperative or preablation scans owing to statistical noise. Although the information provided by the posttherapy scan typically does not alter the patient's immediate management, it could have an impact on subsequent follow-up and evaluation. This is discussed in more detail later in this chapter.

Method of Thyroid Stimulation

Patients may be prepared either by withdrawing their thyroid hormone for a sufficiently long period to elevate their endogenous thyrotropin (TSH) level or by administering recombinant TSH. This subject has been discussed in Chapters 27, 46, 48.

Type of Radioiodine

Finally, and as already discussed earlier in this chapter, the whole-body scan is performed with ^{123}I, ^{131}I, or ^{124}I.

Thus, by knowing these previous three factors, the physician has a better understanding of the wide spectrum of terms employed, types of whole-body scans available, and which whole-body scan may have been performed for their patients. Examples of terminology are shown in Table 7.

SELECTION OF RADIOISOTOPE AND PRESCRIBED ACTIVITY

As already noted in the Introduction, radioiodine whole-body scintigraphy is a valuable diagnostic tool in the assessment of patients with thyroid cancer. Two of the most controversial areas of radioiodine whole-body scanning involve the: (1) selection of the radioisotope and (2) prescribed activity to administer. The choices of radioiodine isotopes are ^{131}I, ^{123}I, and ^{124}I, and the physical characteristics

Table 7
Terminology of Radioiodine Whole-Body Scanning

^{123}I postoperative withdrawal scan
^{123}I postoperative rhTSH scan
^{123}I preablation withdrawal scan
^{123}I preablation rhTSH scan
^{123}I first-time withdrawal scan
^{123}I first-time rhTSH scan
^{131}I postoperative withdrawal scan
^{131}I postoperative rhTSH scan
^{131}I preablation withdrawal scan
^{131}I preablation rhTSH scan
^{131}I first-time withdrawal scan
^{131}I first-time rhTSH scan
^{123}I surveillance withdrawal scan
^{123}I surveillance rhTSH scan
^{131}I surveillance withdrawal scan
^{131}I surveillance rhTSH scan
^{131}I withdrawal scan and dosimetry
^{131}I rhTSH scan and dosimetry
Posttherapy scan

Reproduced with permission from Van Nostrand D, Bloom G, Wartofsky L. Thyroid Cancer: A Guide for Patients, Keystone Press, Inc., 2004.

of each have already been discussed earlier in this chapter. This section presents an overview of the choices of ^{131}I, ^{123}I, and ^{124}I, as well the arguments for no preablation or surveillance scans and concludes with this author's recommendations. Further discussion regarding thyroid hormone withdrawal vs recombinant human (rh) TSH injections can be found in Chapters 27, 46, 48. Additional information regarding ^{124}I is also available below (p.146).

^{131}I

The most frequently used radiopharmaceutical to date is ^{131}I (8,9). Its major advantages are its long historical use, availability, reasonable cost, and half-life. ^{131}I has been used for clinical imaging for over 50 yr, is readily available, and is relatively inexpensive for a diagnostic radiopharmaceutical. The half-life is approx 8 d, which allows additional delayed imaging to be performed as long as 3 or 4 d, possibly even longer after administering ^{131}I. The value of delayed scanning is to allow significantly more time for the patient's background radioactivity to clear. Although the radioactivity of the normal or abnormal thyroid tissue may also have clearance over time, this decrease in radioactivity within the thyroid tissue or metastasis is typically less than the clearance of the whole-body background radioactivity. This causes increasing thyroid tissue-to-background ratios of radioactivity, thereby increasing the detection of functioning normal and abnormal thyroid tissue. The long half-life of ^{131}I also allows dosimetry to be performed, including whole-body counting, blood specimens, and urine specimens to be obtained and measured 5 d and even longer after radioiodine administration.

The major disadvantage of ^{131}I is the potential of "stunning." The concept and arguments regarding "stunning" are discussed in Chapter 36. In brief, stunning is the short-term reduction of radioiodine uptake after diagnostic amounts of prescribed activities of ^{131}I, secondary to the radiation dose to the tissue. Again, as discussed elsewhere, this can reduce the therapeutic effect of a radioiodine treatment of ^{131}I administered shortly after a diagnostic study.

^{123}I

As an alternative to ^{131}I, ^{123}I has been used, and its advantages and disadvantages have been previously noted in Table 3. No known stunning has been reported using ^{123}I, and given the relatively small estimated radiation doses from diagnostic amounts of ^{123}I, thyroid stunning of any significant degree is highly unlikely. ^{123}I also has better imaging characteristics than ^{131}I, resulting in high-quality images, and ^{123}I does not require a high- or medium-energy collimator. This allows great flexibility for obtaining images by various γ cameras within a nuclear medicine facility. Although the availability and cost for ^{123}I were previously problematic, ^{123}I is now becoming more widely available in more countries, and the cost of ^{123}I has decreased as its use has increased.

Studies Involving ^{123}I

In evaluating (1) the prescribed activity of ^{123}I, (2) the time of imaging after dosing ^{123}I, and (3) the detection of thyroid tissue and thyroid cancer metastasis with ^{123}I relative to ^{131}I, multiple studies have been reported (10–15,17–22).

Naddaf (10) compared 13 ^{123}I scans in 10 patients with posttherapy ^{131}I scans. The ^{123}I scans were performed 4, 24, and 48 h after the oral administration of 10 mCi (370 MBq) of ^{123}I. Anterior and posterior whole-body images were obtained for 60 min. The posttherapy scans were performed 5–7 d after 75–217 mCi (2.78–8 GBq) of ^{131}I. Of functioning thyroid tissue, 27 cites were identified on the posttherapy ^{131}I scans, and 24 of the 27 sites were identified on the ^{123}I scan. No comment was made regarding the relative utility of imaging ^{123}I at 4, 24, and 48 h.

Mandel et al. (9) evaluated 14 patients in whom the ^{123}I scans were obtained 5 h after administration of 1.3–1.5 mCi (48–56 MBq) ^{123}I. The ^{131}I scans were obtained at 48 h after the administration of 3 mCi (111 MBq) of ^{131}I. These scans were then compared with posttherapy scans performed 7 d after radioiodine therapy. There were 35 foci identified, and ^{123}I images demonstrated that all 35 foci were in the thyroid bed and neck, whereas only 32 of 35 foci (91%) were seen on the pretherapy ^{131}I scan. Mandel et al. concluded that ^{123}I resulted in improved quality of images relative to ^{131}I in patients undergoing thyroid remnant ablation.

Berbano (12) reported that 15 of 16 patients had concordant findings on the ^{123}I scans relative to the ^{131}I scans.

Only one patient had an additional site identified on the ^{131}I scan, which was not identified on the ^{123}I scan, and this was a patient with metastatic disease. The prescribed activity of ^{123}I was 10 mCi (370 MBq). The ^{131}I scans were performed after radioiodine therapy, with prescribed activities ranging from 75 to 200 mCi (2.8–7.4 GBq). Berbano (12) also evaluated ^{123}I scans at 24 and 48 h after dosing. He reported no advantage for imaging at 48 h in comparison to 24 h.

Maxon (13) evaluated 13 administrations of ^{123}I in 11 patients. The average prescribed activity of ^{123}I was 20.1 mCi (743 MBq); the ^{123}I scans were compared with scans performed 2–3 d after ^{131}I therapy. He reported no false-negative ^{123}I scans when those scans were imaged at 18–24 h after administration of ^{123}I. Scans performed 2 h after ^{123}I administration had a false-negative rate of 38% (5/13). Pretherapy scans with ^{131}I were performed with 2 mCi (74 MBq) of ^{131}I, and the results of analyzing the ^{123}I scans with ^{131}I scans were not reported.

Yaakob (14) examined 13 patients with ^{123}I with prescribed activities of 0.8–1.0 mCi (30–37 MBq). Images were obtained 24 h after ^{123}I administration and compared with scans performed 7–10 d after ^{131}I therapy. There were 11 ^{123}I scans that correlated with the posttherapy scan. One patient had an additional area detected on the ^{131}I posttherapy scan that was not detected on ^{123}I scan, and one patient had an additional area detected on the ^{123}I scan that was not seen on the ^{131}I posttherapy scan. The latter was attributed to physiologic esophageal activity.

Shankar (15) compared ^{123}I and ^{131}I scans in 26 patients. The ^{123}I scans were performed 4 h after the administration of 1.5 mCi (55.5 MBq) of ^{123}I, and the ^{131}I scans were performed 48 h after the administration of 3 mCi (111 MBq) of ^{131}I. ^{123}I scans identified 56 foci of activity, whereas the ^{131}I scan demonstrated only 44 of the 56 foci seen on the ^{123}I scan. All 56 foci of activity were seen on the posttherapy ^{131}I scan, and the posttherapy ^{131}I scan showed one additional area not seen on the ^{123}I scan. Of the 56 foci, 54 foci were in the neck and thyroid bed, with one focus each in the mediastinum and lung. In a separate report, Shankar, et al. (16) demonstrated that the imaging with ^{123}I was superior at 24 h relative to 5 h after administration of the ^{123}I.

In a comparison of ^{123}I scans with posttherapy ^{131}I scans, Gerard et al. (17) identified 37 sites on posttherapy scan; 26 were identified with ^{123}I for a sensitivity of 70%. Of the 11 sites missed by ^{123}I, 7 were seen on the posttreatment scan relative to the early scan. A total of 10 patients had 48-h ^{123}I scans, and 8 were of good quality. Lesion detection was improved on the 48-h scans. ^{123}I scans after withdrawal of thyroid hormone were performed with 3–5 mCi (111–185 MBq) ^{123}I at 6, 24, and 48 h.

Alzahrani et al. (18) had 238 pairs of pretherapy ^{123}I scans and posttherapy ^{131}I scans with a concordance rate of 94%.

Siddiqi (19) compared ^{123}I whole-body scans to posttherapy ^{131}I scans in 12 patients who had elevated serum thyroglobulin levels and previous negative ^{131}I whole-body scans. On subsequent evaluations, the ^{123}I dose was 5 mCi (185 MBq), and images were obtained at 2 and 24 h after administration of ^{123}I. The posttherapy scans were performed 4–7 d after the therapy with 150 mCi (5.55 GBq). The ^{123}I scans were concordant with the ^{131}I posttherapy scan in 11 of 12 patients.

Sarkar et al. (20) compared ^{123}I and ^{131}I in 12 patients, and both revealed residual disease in nine patients. ^{131}I detected metastases in five studies of four patients. In four of the five studies, ^{123}I missed metastases shown by ^{131}I in eight body regions including the neck, mediastinum, lungs, and bone, and detected three other sites of metastasis only in retrospect. No lesion was better seen with ^{123}I than ^{131}I. Although ^{123}I is adequate for imaging residual disease, it appears to be less sensitive than ^{131}I for minimal thyroid cancer metastasis.

Khan et al. (21) compared ^{123}I scans with prescribed activity of 1.5–3.0 mCi (5.55–111 MBq) with posttherapy ^{131}I in 183 patients, showing a similar number of lesions in similar locations in 91%, but the time of imaging was not noted. Nine patients (4.5%) had more lesions detected in the ^{123}I scan when compared to the 7-d posttherapy ^{131}I scan. Likewise, nine patients had more lesions detected on the 7-d posttherapy scan. Posttherapy scans were obtained 7 d after 60–200 mCi (2.22–7.4 GBq). It is assumed that some of these lesions were included in earlier reports from the same institution (9,15).

Anderson et al. (22) evaluated 101 consecutive ^{123}I and 101 consecutive ^{131}I scans after preparation with rhTSH injections. There were 96 patients in the ^{131}I group and 98 patients in the ^{123}I group who had received previous ^{131}I ablations or treatments. They used 3 mCi (111 MBq) of ^{123}I and 4 mCi (148 MBq) of ^{131}I, and images were obtained 24 h after ^{123}I and 48 h after ^{131}I. The rhTSH-stimulated ^{123}I scans and thyroglobulin levels were concordant in 90% (91/101) of patients; the results of rhTSH-stimulated ^{131}I scans and thyroglobulin levels were concordant in 84% (85/101) of patients. ^{123}I whole-body scans detected nine foci of disease in six patients, and ^{131}I whole-body scans detected 10 foci of disease in 9 patients. Anderson proposed that rhTSH-stimulated ^{123}I scans might prove to be as sensitive as rhTSH-stimulated ^{131}I scans for the detection of metastatic disease.

^{124}I

^{124}I is a positron-emitting radioisotope and has recently become commercially available. The advantages and disadvantages of ^{124}I have been previously noted in Table 3 and include superior image quality, tomographic images, bone marrow and metastatic lesion dosimetry, and the ability to fuse the tomographic images with CT, MR, or both. The physical half-life of ^{124}I is approx 4 d, which is sufficiently long enough to allow delayed imaging and dosimetry. The dominant disadvantages of ^{124}I are its availability (production sites

Table 8
Factors that Affect Scanning and Radioisotope Selection

Time of the whole-body scintigraphy
    First scan, which is performed after initial diagnosis, thyroidectomy, and prior to radioiodine ablation
    Surveillance scan*
    Pretreatment scan*
Patient preparation
    Thyroid hormone withdrawal
    rhTSH injections
Whether thyroglobulin levels are obtained before or simultaneously with radioiodine scan
Presence or absence of increased thyroglobulin blood levels when suppressed or stimulated prior to whole-body scanning
Physician's belief in the potential for stunning
Physician's approach to the selection of prescribed activities for first-radioiodine ablations (e.g., fixed or variable empiric prescribed activity or dosimetrically determined prescribed activity)
Physician's approach to subsequent selection of prescribed activities for treatment of well-differentiated metastatic thyroid carcinoma (e.g., "blind treatments," and empiric vs dosimetrically determined prescribed activity for treatments)

*Defined in text.

are limited), cost, and requirement for a PET imaging system. Another potential disadvantage of ^{124}I is stunning, as the radiation-absorbed dose is about half that of a comparable prescribed activity of ^{131}I. A few studies have already been reported using ^{124}I, *(23,24)* and further research is needed.

No Scan

An alternative to whole-body scanning is to skip the scan at any or all of the time points. The advantages of not performing a scan are the elimination of: (1) the cost and inconvenience of a scan and (2) the possibility of stunning if ^{131}I or ^{124}I is used. Appreciation of the distribution of residual activity in the thyroid bed, metastases, or both is accomplished by the posttherapy scan, which is superior to postoperative, preablation whole-body scans conducted with low diagnostic prescribed activity (see below). However, this approach requires the administration of an empirically prescribed activity of radioiodine ablation for all adult patients and the philosophy that any information that would be derived from the postoperative preablation scans would not alter the patient's treatment. As noted, Schlumberger et al. *(2)* use this approach and have reported good success.

^{99m}Tc Pertechnetate

No significant clinical study has been reported to this author's knowledge to evaluate the utility of ^{99m}Tc pertechnetate for the postoperative preablation scan. If the objective of the postoperative preablation scans is solely to modify an empiric ablative prescribed activity based on the pattern and quantitative trapping of ^{99m}Tc pertechnetate in the thyroid bed, then ^{99m}Tc pertechnetate imaging and a 20-min trapping may have a role, and this may warrant further study.

Whether or Not to Scan and Which Radioiodine Isotope to Use

So, does one scan or not, and if one scans, what isotope of radioiodine does one use? The choice depends on multiple factors, such as those shown in Table 8, as well as which factor(s) the physician considers the most important. Four of the more common situations are discussed, followed by several recommendations.

Initial Ablation

For those facilities that administer a standard empiric prescribed activity for ablation and would not alter their treatment based on any radioiodine scan findings, a scan is obviously unnecessary and no radioisotope is administered.

For those facilities that believe that a radioiodine scan offers useful information prior to the first ablation, the use of ^{123}I is an excellent choice. Not only does this author believe that preablation scans are useful (as already discussed above and in Table 6), this author also believes that if ^{123}I is available, it is the radioisotope of choice.

^{123}I is a reasonably cost-effective isotope that can demonstrate both the pattern and percent uptake of radioiodine activity in the thyroid bed. Its sensitivity is as good or at least comparative to ^{131}I to show functioning metastasis that would result in altering management of anticipated intial radioiodine ablation or treatment. Although ^{123}I may arguably miss a small focus with low uptake in residual thyroid disease or metastasis, the failure to detect these small or low-uptake foci will be infrequent. In addition, regardless of whether there is significant stunning from ^{131}I, ^{123}I completely eliminates the possibility and consideration of stunning. Regarding ^{124}I, this author does not believe it is warranted for routine postoperative preablation scans

Surveillance Scan

The term, "surveillance scan," has been used in a number of contexts. For this chapter, a surveillance scan is a radioiodine scan performed at some routine interval, which is typically 6 mo to 1–2 yr after ablation or treatment. The objective of this scan is to screen for metastatic functioning of well-differentiated thyroid cancer in patients who are in clinical remission. Clinical remission is defined here as no evidence of disease on physical exam and undetectable serum thyroglobulin levels on thyroid hormone suppression.

As used in this section, surveillance scan should be differentiated from a "pretreatment scan," which is defined again as a radioiodine scan performed in "anticipation" of radioiodine treatment in patients with documented or highly suspicious recurrent local thyroid cancer or metastases.

The objectives of the surveillance scans are to detect and localize. The objectives of the pretreatment scan are to (1) determine whether radioiodine is a therapeutic option (in those facilities that only administer radioiodine when the metastatic diseases takes up iodine); (2) assess patterns of radioiodine uptake that would alter prescribed activity for treatment and/or (3) lesional dosimetry, and/or whole-body dosimetry that would change prescribed activity for treatment.

AFTER THYROID HORMONE WITHDRAWAL OR rhTSH STIMULATION

Although surveillance scans have been frequently performed every 6 mo to 1 or 2 yr after the initial ablation of residual thyroid tissue, the utility and cost of such a surveillance scan in a patient who is in clinical remission (low-risk group) has been questioned. A strong argument can be made that the performance of these scans—regardless of the radioiodine used—is no longer cost-effective (4–7). This fact is especially true when the patient must undergo a prolonged period of hypothyroidism during thyroid hormone withdrawal.

However, if a physician believes a surveillance scan is still valuable for his or her patients, then which isotope should be used? As discussed earlier in this chapter, the initial data is promising, indicating that the sensitivity of ^{123}I is equivalent or nearly equivalent to ^{131}I, but a large portion of this data involved comparisons between ^{123}I and ^{131}I for normal residual thyroid tissue, not metastatic disease. Although the initial reports comparing ^{123}I to ^{131}I for recurrence or metastases are positive, this author believes that if a physician is going to perform a surveillance scan, then ^{131}I should be used until the initial positive reports are confirmed. Perhaps ^{124}I will be an option in the future, but with its high cost and the low reported yield from surveillance scans in these low-risk patients, the use of ^{124}I in this population currently appears unappealing.

Pretreatment Scans

A. BEFORE TREATMENT WITH AN EMPIRIC PRESCRIBED ACTIVITY OF RADIOIODINE

We believe that the preferred radioiodine isotope is ^{123}I if: (1) the patient has known or highly suspected recurrent or metastatic disease; (2) the physician anticipates treating with an empiric prescribed activity; and (3) a prescribed activity will be administered even if the scan is negative (a "blind treatment"). This choice is again based on the objective of the scan, i.e., identification of findings that would potentially alter management. The findings are similar to some already noted in Table 4.

B. BEFORE TREATMENT WITH DOSIMETRICALLY DETERMINED PRESCRIBED ACTIVITY OF RADIOIODINE

We believe that the preferred radioiodine isotope is ^{131}I if: (1) the patient has known or highly suspected recurrent disease or metastatic disease; and (2) the physician anticipates treating with a dosimetrically determined prescribed activity. Although the prescribed activity may vary from 1 to 4 mCi (37–148 MBq), the lowest prescribed activity that still allows the performance of dosimetry should be used to minimize the risk of stunning. In the author's facility, this ranges from 1 to 2 mCi (37–74 MBq). For ^{123}I, high-prescribed activities (up to 20 mCi [740 MBq]) have been used (13), and further study is warranted using high diagnostic prescribed activity of ^{123}I for dosimetry. Initial studies have already demonstrated the potential of ^{124}I for dosimetry (23,24), but additional research is needed regarding its potential for stunning.

In summary, many factors and how each physician weighs those factors affect whether a scan is performed, and if a scan is performed, which iodine isotope is used and the amount of that isotope used. The guidelines that this author presently uses are summarized in Table 9.

UTILITY OF POSTTHERAPY SCANS

Posttherapy scans performed between 1 and 12 d after radioiodine ablation or treatment have been shown to be useful (3,25–30a). Fatourechi et al. (29) reported that 13% of (17/117) posttherapy scans demonstrated an abnormal foci of ^{131}I that was originally undetected on the pretherapy scan. The areas of newly detected abnormal uptake were located in the neck (5), lung (5), mediastinum (4), bone (2), and adrenal (1). The prescribed activity of the pretherapy scan was 3 mCi (111 MBq) of ^{131}I, and posttherapy images were obtained between 1 and 5 d after therapy. The likelihood of detecting new uptake on the posttherapy scans decreases after each successive treatment. Sherman et al. (27) reported 22% (31/143) new lesions detected on the posttherapy scan that were not seen on the pretreatment scan. They used

Table 9
Recommendations for Radioiodine Scanning

First-time preablation scan	^{123}I using 2–4 mCi (74–148 MBq) with imaging at 24–48 h
Surveillance scan* after thyroid hormone withdrawal in low-risk patients in clinical remission*	1. No scan 2. If scan is to be performed, then ^{131}I with 2–4 mCi (74–148 MBq) and imaging at 48–72 h
Surveillance scan* after rhTSH for stimulated thyroglobulin levels in low-risk patients in clinical remission	1. No scan 2. If scan is to be performed along with the scheduled injection of rhTSH, then ^{131}I with 4 mCi (148 MBq) and imaging at 48 h
Pretreatment scan* with the intent to treat with an empiric prescribed activity of radioiodine.	^{123}I using 2–4 mCi (74–148 MBq) with imaging at 24–48 h
Pretreatment scan* with the intent to treat with dosimetrically determined prescribed activity of radioiodine	^{131}I using the lowest prescribed activity possible to perform dosimetry while minimizing potential stunning (typically 1–2 mCi [37–74 MBq])

*Defined in text.

2–5 mCi (74–185 MBq) for the pretherapy scan, and the posttherapy scan was performed between 5 and 12 d after therapy. In regard to the effects of posttherapy scans on management strategies, Fatourechi et al. (29) reported that 9% of scans affected management (e.g., future decisions about plans for diagnostic scanning or ^{131}I therapy) or changed the patient's risk-group category. Posttherapy scans are widely performed and accepted as useful.

SUMMARY

Radioiodine whole-body scans are important diagnostic tools in the evaluation of patients with well-differentiated thyroid carcinoma. With a basic understanding of such factors as radio-elements, scientific notation, decay, physical half-life, γ cameras, and protocols, the endocrinologist will have a better understanding of how the radioiodine whole-body scans are performed, as well as their utility and controversial aspects. The next chapter presents a primer and atlas for the basic interpretation of radioiodine whole-body scans.

REFERENCES

1. Procedure Guideline for Extended Scintigraphy for Differentiated Thyroid Cancer. Society of Nuclear Medicine, 2003; 19–23.
2. Schlumberger M, Tubiana M, De Vathaire F, et al. Long term results of treatment of 283 patients with lung bone and metastases from differentiated thyroid carcinoma. J Clin Endocrinol Metab 1998; 63:960–967.
3. Pacini F, Lippi F, Formica N, et al. Therapeutic doses of iodine-131 reveal undiagnosed metastases in thyroid cancer patients with detectable serum thyroglobulin levels. J Nucl Med 1987; 28: 1888–1891.
4. Cailleux AF, Baudin E, Travagli JP, Schlumberger RM. Is diagnostic iodine-131 scanning useful after total thyroid ablation for differentiated thyroid cancer? J Clin Endocrinol Metab 2000; 85:175–178.
5. Wartofsky L. Clinical utility of rh-TSH-stimulated thyroglobulin testing without scan in the follow-up of differentiated thyroid cancer. Denver, Co: Program of the 83rd Annual Meeting of the Endocrine Society; 2000:P2–P535.
6. Mazzaferri EL, Kloos RT. Is diagnostic iodine-131 scanning with recombinant human TSH useful in the follow-up of differentiated thyroid cancer after thyroid ablation? J Clin Endocrinol Metab 2002; 87: 1490–1498.
7. Wartofsky L. Using baseline and recombinant human TSH-stimulated Tg measurements to manage thyroid cancer without diagnostic I-131 scanning. J Clin Endocrinol Metab 2002; 87:1486–1489.
8. Maxon HR, Smith HR. Radioiodine-131 in the diagnosis and treatment of metastatic well-differentiated thyroid cancer. Endocrinol Metab Clin North Am 1990; 19:685–718.
9. Mandel SJ, Shankar LK, Benard F, et al. Superiority of iodine-123 compared with iodine-131 scanning for thyroid remnants in patients with differentiated thyroid cancer. Clin Nuc Med 2001; 26:6–9.
10. Jeevanram RK, Shah DH, Shama M, et al. Influence of initial large dose on subsequent uptake of therapeutic radioiodine in thyroid cancer patient. Nucl Med Biol 1986; 13:277.
11. Naddaf S, Young I, Rapun R, et al. Comparison between iodine-123 (I-123) and iodine-^{131}I sodium iodide total body scanning in thyroid cancer patients. J Nucl Med 1996; 37:251P.
12. Berbano B, Naddaf S, Echemendia, et al. Use of iodine-123 as a diagnostic tracer for neck and whole body scanning in patients with well-differentiated thyroid cancer. Endocrine Practice 1998; 4:11–16.
13. Maxon JR, Thomas SR, Washburn LC, et al. High-activity ^{123}I for the diagnostic evaluations of patients with thyroid cancer. J Nucl Med 1993; 34:42P.
14. Yaakob W, Gordon L, Spicer KM, Nitke SJ. The usefulness of iodine-123 whole-body scans in evaluating thyroid carcinoma and metastases. J Nucl Med Tech 1999; 27:279–281.

15. Shankar LK, Mandel S, Benard F. The promising role of ^{123}I Scintigraphy in the management of differentiated thyroid cancer. J Nucl Med 2002; 43:526.
16. Shankar LK, Yamamoto AJ, Alavi A, et al. Comparison of I-123 scintigraphy at 5 and 24 hours in patients with differentiated thyroid cancer. J Nucl Med 2002; 43:72–76.
17. Gerard SK, Cavalieri RR. ^{123}I diagnostic thyroid tumor whole-body scanning with imaging at 6, 24, and 48 hours. Clin Nuc Med 2002; 27:1–8.
18. Alzahrani AS, Bakheet S, Mandil MAL, et al. ^{123}I isotope as a diagnostic agent in the follow-up of patients with differentiated thyroid cancer: comparison with post ^{131}I therapy whole body scanning. J Clin Endocrinol Metab 2001; 86:5294–5300.
19. Siddiqi A, Foley RR, Britton KE, et al. The role of ^{123}I diagnostic imaging in the follow-up of patients with differentiated thyroid carcinoma as compared to ^{131}I scanning; avoidance of negative therapeutic uptake due to stunning. Clin Endocrinol 2001; 55: 515–521.
20. Sarkar SD, Kalapparambath TP, Palestro CJ. Comparison of ^{123}I and ^{131}I for whole body imaging in thyroid cancer. J Nucl Med 2002; 43: 632–634.
21. Khan J, Hickeson M, Zhuang HM, et al. Diagnostic scanning by ^{123}I vs ^{131}I in thyroid remnant following surgery for differentiated thyroid cancer. J Nucl Med 2002; 43:129P.
22. Anderson GS, Fish S, Nakhoda K, et al. Comparison of ^{123}I and ^{131}I for whole body imaging after stimulation by recombinant human thyrotropin: a preliminary report. Clin Nucl Med 2003; 28:93–96.
23. Eschmann, SM, Reischl G, Bilger K, et al. Evaluation of dosimetry of radioiodine therapy in benign and malignant thyroid disorders by means of iodine-124 and PET. Euro J Nuclear Med 2002; 29: 760–767.
24. Sgouros G, Kolbert KS, Sheikh A, et al. Patient-specific dosimetry for I-131 thyroid cancer therapy using I-124 PET and 3-dimensional-internal dosimetry (3D-ID) software. J Nucl Med 2004; 45: 1366–1372.
25. Nemec J, Rohling S, Zamarazil V, Pohunkova D. Comparison of the distribution of diagnostic and thyroablative I-131 in the evaluation of differentiated thyroid cancers. J Nucl Med 1997; 20:92–97.
26. Balachandran S, Sayle BA. Value of thyroid carcinoma imaging after therapeutic doses of radioiodine. Clin Nucl Med 1981; 6:162–167.
27. Sherman SI, Tielens ET, Sostre S, et al. Clinical utility of post treatment radioiodine scans in the management of patients with thyroid carcinoma. J Clin Endocrinol Metab 1994; 78:629–634.
28. Spies WG, Wojtowicz CH, Spies SM, et al. Value of post-therapy whole-body I-131 imaging in the evaluation of patients with thyroid carcinoma having undergone high-dose I-131 therapy. Clin Nucl Med 1989; 14:793–800.
29. Fatourechi V, Hay ID, Mullan BP, et al. Are post therapy radioiodine scans informative and do they influence subsequent therapy of patients with differentiated thyroid cancer? Thyroid 2000; 10:573–577.
30. Pineda JD, Lee T, Ain K, et al. Iodine-131 therapy for thyroid cancer patients with elevated thyroglobulin and negative diagnostic scan. J Clin Endocrinol Meta 1995; 80:1488–1492.
30a. Rosario PWSD, Barroso AL, Rezende LL, et al. Post I-131 therapy scanning in patients with thyroid carcinoma metastases; an unnecessary cost or a relevant contribution? Clin Nuc Med 2004; 29:795–798.
31. Dorn R, Kopp J, Vogt H, et al. Dosimetry-guided radioactive iodine treatment in patients with metastatic differentiated thyroid cancer: largest safe dose using a risk-adapted approach. J Nuc Med 2003; 44:451–456.
32. Thomas SR, Maxon HR, Kereiakes JG, Saenger EL. Quantitative external counting techniques enabling improved diagnostic and therapeutic decisions in patients with well differentiated thyroid cancer. Radiology 1997; 122:731–737.
33. Comtois R, Theriault C, Del Vecchio P. Assessment of the efficacy of iodine-131 for thyroid ablation. J Nucl Med 1993; 34:1927–1930.
34. Maxon HR, Englaro EE, Thomas SR, et al. Radioiodine-131 therapy for well differentiated thyroid cancer—a quantitative radiation dosimetric approach: Outcome and validation in 85 patients. J Nucl Med 1992; 33:1132–1136.
35. Maxon HR, Englaro EE, Thomas SR, et al. Radioiodine-131 therapy for well differentiated thyroid cancer—a quantitative radiation dosimetric approach: Outcome and validation in 85 patients. J Nucl Med 1992; 33:1132–1136.
36. Hodgson DC, Brierley JD, Tsang RW, Panzarella T. Prescribing 131-I iodine based on neck uptake produces effective thyroid ablation and reduced hospital stay. Radiother Oncol 1998; 47:325–330.

15
Primer and Atlas for the Interpretation of Radioiodine Whole-Body Scintigraphy

Douglas Van Nostrand, Reetha Bakthula, and Frank B. Atkins

INTRODUCTION

Radioiodine whole-body scintigraphy remains an important diagnostic modality in the evaluation of patients with well-differentiated thyroid carcinoma. The advantages and disadvantages of the various radioiodine isotopes, and how the images are obtained, were discussed in Chapter 14. This chapter presents a primer and atlas for the interpretation of radioiodine whole-body scintigraphy. The objective of the primer is to present a simple, consistent, and reliable approach to the evaluation and interpretation of radioiodine whole-body scans. The objectives of the atlas are to demonstrate (1) a spectrum of residual activity in the thyroid bed; (2) a spectrum of nonthyroidal physiological uptake; (3) various patterns of metastatic disease; (4) examples of false-positives and artifacts; and (5) several techniques to help the interpreter differentiate metastatic disease from physiologic uptake, false-positives, and artifacts. Although all patterns of physiologic uptake, false-positive uptake, and artifacts cannot be presented, a comprehensive review of the literature of thyroidal uptake, nonthyroidal uptake, false-positives, and artifacts of radioiodine uptake is presented in Chapter 16.

Primer

A SYSTEMATIC APPROACH FOR THE EVALUATION AND INTERPRETATION OF RADIOIODINE WHOLE-BODY SCANS

When a medical student or physician in-training sees a radioiodine whole-body scan for the first time, the initial response is frequently either, "it's easy—just look for the hot spots," or "the findings are so nonspecific." However, both responses are incorrect. The interpretation of radioiodine whole-body scans is not easy, and the findings can be very specific.

Like most nuclear medicine scans, the process of interpreting radioiodine whole-body scans can be divided into three simple but important steps: (1) ensuring adequate quality of the imaging technique, (2) observation, and (3) interpretation.

The first step is to review the scan in terms of the quality of the imaging technique. Ensuring that adequate quality of the scan has been achieved is not difficult but is frequently taken for granted. Failure to ensure that the scan is performed according to the facility's procedural guidelines can be without exaggeration—disastrous. The physician must ensure quality by:

1. Interviewing the patient before beginning the scan to ascertain his or her compliance with thyroid hormone withdrawal, thyrotropin injections, and/or low-iodine diet.
2. Reviewing β human choriogonadotropin (hCG) levels when warranted, thyrotropin (TSH) blood levels, images, and the placement of markers; and when necessary
3. Questioning the technologist regarding window settings, exposure intensity, duration of imaging, counts, scanning speed, collimator, and other factors that may affect the acquisition of the images.

This is only a partial list. However, without first ensuring adequate quality of technique, the remaining steps may have reduced or no value.

The second step is simply to observe and describe all areas of increased radioactivity on the whole-body scan or camera views. The physician who states that the radioiodine whole-body scan is easy typically performs only this step.

The third step of interpretation involves the evaluation of each area of increased radioactivity noted on the previous step for etiology. The physician who claims that the radioiodine whole-body scans are nonspecific, albeit at times correct, usually does not use the databases and tools discussed below to markedly improve the specificity of radioiodine uptake. Five databases are noted in Table 1; many of the tools for evaluating radioiodine accumulation are listed in Table 2. Although most of these tools fall into the category of "common sense," they are not commonly considered.

From: *Thyroid Cancer: A Comprehensive Guide to Clinical Management*, 2/e
Edited by: L. Wartofsky and D. Van Nostrand © Humana Press Inc., Totowa, NJ

Table 1
Five Databases

Patient's detailed history for specific scan findings
Normal physiologic distribution and patterns of radioiodine at various times after dosing
Normal variants
Artifacts
Tools to distinguish all of the above from metastasis

Table 2
Tools to Help Distinguish Metastases from Nonthyroidal Physiological Uptake, False-Positives, and Artifacts

Obtain "uptake-specific" history, such as:
   Recent surgery
   Other diseases
   Colostomies
   Prostheses
   Dentures
   Contact lens, artificial eye, and so on
Examine the patient regarding:
   Colostomies
   Ureterostomies, nephrostomies
   Skin lesions
Localize the area of radioiodine accumulation within the patient with:
   Marker images with external radioactive sources placed on the patient to provide anatomical reference points on the scan, e.g., to help establish that the region of uptake corresponds to the submandibular gland or a palpable mass
   Marker image to help localize area of radioactivity on scan or patient, which, in turn, may help facilitate the evaluation of the area on CT, MRI, or ultrasound
   Lateral views to localize the radioiodine as deep or superficial, such as helping to differentiate rib from lung, sternum from mediastinum, gastrointestinal tract from bone, and brain from bone
Improve resolution:
   Pinhole images
Manipulate the radioactivity:
   Decontamination
   Additional views 1 or 2 d later
   Administration of water
   Administration of sialogogues (lemon)
   Administration of laxatives
Compare:
   With previous study
Perform additional diagnostic studies, such as:
   Chest X-ray
   Plain films
   Ultrasound
   CT
   MRI
   PET
   Bone scan
   Renal scan

CT, computed tomography; MR, magnetic resonance imaging; PET, positron emission tomography.

Similarly, despite these tools not guaranteeing a determination of the etiology of all areas of increased radioiodine uptake, their use can help reduce the frequency of false-positive and artifactual findings. They can also increase the value of the radioiodine whole-body scan for the patient. In addition, the physician who follows these guidelines will discover that the radioiodine whole-body scans are neither easy nor nonspecific.

Atlas

ATLAS OF RADIOIODINE WHOLE-BODY SCANS

The atlas is divided into six sections:

1. The spectrum of thyroid tissue uptake (Figs. 1–5).
2. The spectrum of nonthyroidal physiological uptake (Figs. 6–14).
3. Some patterns of metastatic disease (Figs. 15–25).
4. Examples of false-positive uptake and artifacts (Figs. 26–30 and Chapter 16).
5. Several tools to help differentiate metastases from nonthyroidal physiological uptake, false-positives, and artifacts (Figs. 31–34).
6. Miscellaneous (Fig. 35).

For each scan, only the teaching point for the figure is typically noted and discussed in the legend.

Primer and Atlas

PART 1
The Spectrum of Thyroid Tissue Uptake

PREOPERATIVE THYROID SCAN WITH HYPOFUNCTIONING AREA

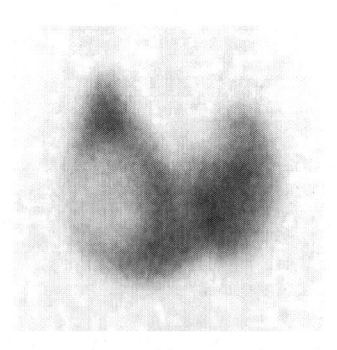

Fig. 1. This is a preoperative pinhole collimator image of the thyroid performed 24 h after the administration of ^{123}I. A large hypofunctioning area is noted in the right lobe, which corresponded to a palpable nodule. The patient subsequently had fine-needle aspiration with cytology that demonstrated well-differentiated papillary thyroid carcinoma. The patient had a near-total thryoidectomy. Reproduced with permission from Keystone Press, Inc. (*1*).

Comment: Although preoperative thyroid scans are not routinely performed as a baseline for future comparison with a postoperative radioiodine whole-body scan, it is possible that the preoperative scan could be valuable. The preoperative scan may help differentiate residual normal thyroid tissue (e.g., functioning thyroid tissue in a pyramidal lobe, the thyroglossal track, or aberrant thyroid tissue) from metastatic disease on a postoperative scan. Metastatic disease typically appears as a hypofunctioning area on a preoperative scan and as a functioning area on a postoperative scan. Despite the presence of the radioactivity on the initial preoperative scan not conclusively proving that the radioactivity is physiologic and not malignant, it would support this.

But why does metastatic disease appear "cold" on thyroid scans and "hot" on radioiodine whole-body scans? The primary site or metastases of well-differentiated thyroid cancer can take up radioiodine, but the degree of this uptake is generally much less than the surrounding normal functioning thyroid tissue and, as a result, appears "cold" on a preoperative thyroid scan. However, after most of the thyroid gland has been surgically removed, and the residual thyroid tissue ablated with radioiodine, metastases will then frequently appear "hot" and functioning relative to background activity.

MINIMAL POSTOPERATIVE RESIDUAL THYROID TISSUE (THYROID REMNANT)

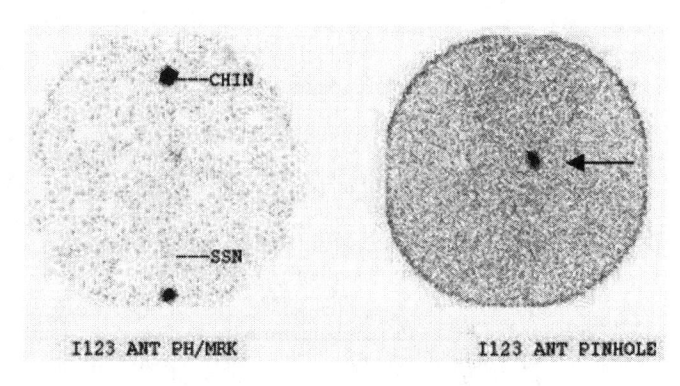

Fig. 2. The pinhole collimator image on the left represents a marker image, in which the chin and suprasternal notch (SSN) are marked by placing radioactive sources on the patient. After the markers are removed and without moving the patient, a second pinhole collimator image is performed for a significantly longer interval of time. The resulting image on the right demonstrates a single well-defined focal area of modest radioiodine uptake in the upper aspect of the thyroid bed. The patient received radioiodine to ablate this minimal residual thyroid tissue. (The label for the SSN is slightly higher than the actual marker.)

Comment: The surgeon typically leaves behind some normal residual thyroid tissue because of the surgeon's objective to avoid injury to the laryngeal nerves and to preserve some parathyroid tissue. However, the volume and the number of individual foci of thyroid tissue left by the surgeon varies not only between surgeons but also among patients operated on by the same surgeon.

A question frequently asked is whether or not this focus of uptake could represent a focus of metastatic thyroid carcinoma. It is possible but not likely. Again, the surgeon seeks to remove any areas of metastatic thyroid carcinoma while leaving normal thyroid tissue to spare the recurrent laryngeal nerve and leave functioning parathyroid tissue. Although it is possible to remove all thyroid tissue while leaving only distant metastatic thyroid carcinoma, it is less likely.

Could thyroid carcinoma still be present in the remaining normal residual thyroid tissue? Yes, and this is one of the objectives of radioiodine ablation, i.e., the destruction of any additional area of thyroid cancer embedded within the remaining remnant of normal thyroid tissue.

MARKED POSTOPERATIVE RESIDUAL THYROID TISSUE

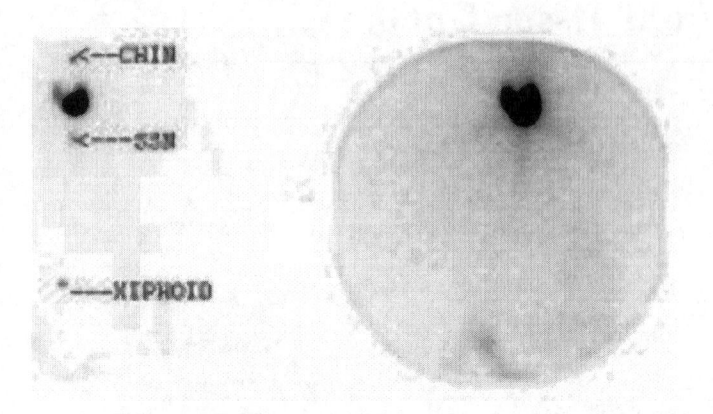

Fig. 3. The parallel collimator image on the left represents a marker image in which the chin, SSN, and xiphoid are all marked. After the markers are removed, and without moving the patient, a second parallel-hole collimator image is performed for a significantly longer time. The resulting image on the right demonstrates a focus of significant increased radioiodine uptake. This figure, together with the previous figure, illustrates the two extremes of residual thyroid activity after a near-total thyroidectomy.

Comment: Because of the significant amount of thyroid tissue remaining in the thyroid bed after the initial surgery, additional surgery may have to be considered. However, whether more surgery is warranted is beyond the scope of this chapter.

If the facility administers a fixed empiric prescribed activity of radioiodine for ablation, regardless of the result of these postoperative scans, then these scans would obviously not need to be performed. However, many facilities use these scans along with uptakes to modify the treatment approach (see Chapter 14 entitled "Radioiodine Whole-Body Scintigraphy").

FUNCTIONING THYROID TISSUE IN THE THYROGLOSSAL TRACT

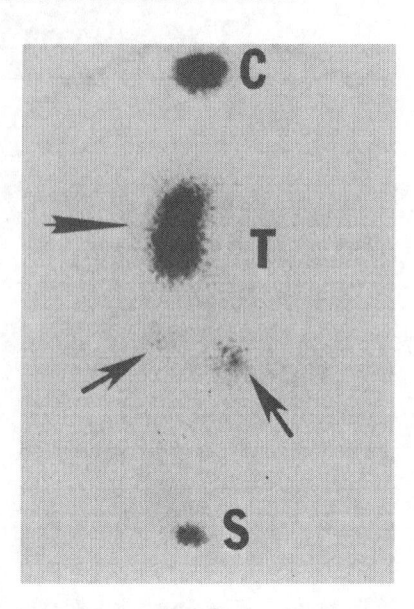

Fig. 4. An ^{131}I image of the neck bed was performed using a pinhole collimator. An elongated area of radioactivity is present in the midline at the level of the thyroid cartilage (T) and is consistent with the functioning thyroid tissue within the thyroglossal duct remnant (arrowhead). Two small foci of residual radioactivity are also noted in the thyroid bed (arrows). The location of the chin (C) and suprasternal notch (S) are marked using cobalt sources. Reproduced with permission from Lippincott, Williams, and Wilkins (2).

Comment: The thyroid gland embryologically develops from the foramen cecum at the junction of the anterior two thirds and posterior one third of the tongue. It then descends and bifurcates in the neck. During thyroid development and migration, various embryologic maldevelopments may occur, including functioning thyroid tissue in the thyroglossal tract (as noted above), lingual thyroid, and aberrant thyroid tissue (see Table 1 in Chapter 16 entitled "False Positives and Artifacts of Radioiodine Imaging").

The diagnosis of thyroglossal duct remnant is suggested by the midline location and the linear-oval distribution of radioactivity. Although one can help exclude esophageal activity with techniques, such as clearing the esophageal activity by drinking water and repeating the scan (see Table 2 and Fig. 9 in this chapter), one may not be able to differentiate thyroglossal duct remnant from local lymph node metastasis. However, based on the combination of the intensity, location, and presence of the radioactivity on the presurgical scan, thyroglossal duct remnant would be most likely.

STRUMA OVARII

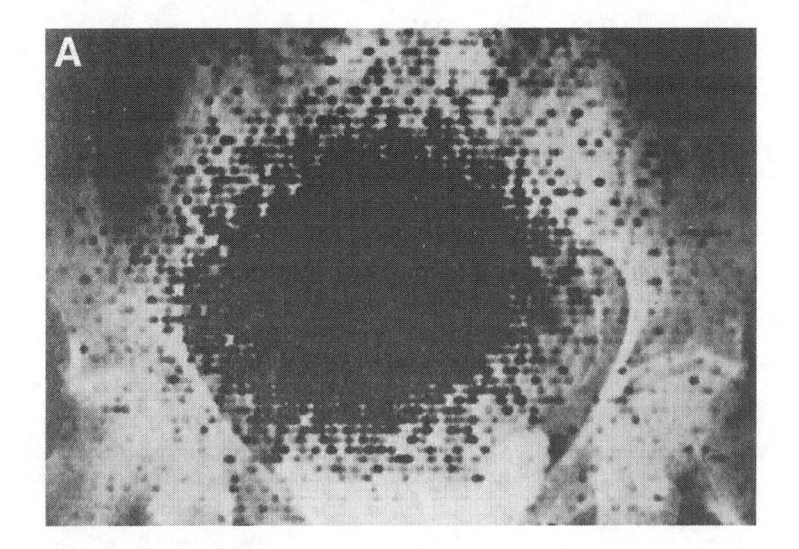

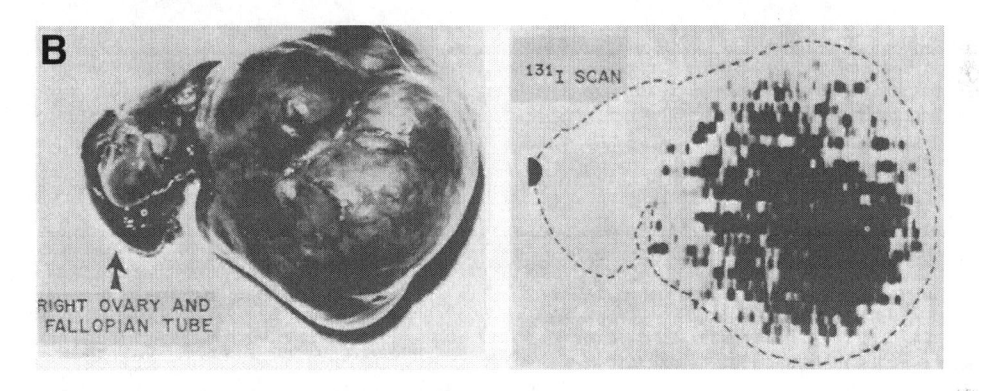

Fig. 5. Part **A** is an overlay of the patient's ^{131}I rectilinear scan onto her pelvic radiograph, and this combined image demonstrates ^{131}I uptake in the pelvic region. This uptake corresponded to a 10-cm pelvic mass, which was an infarcted teratoma composed mostly of active thyroid tissue (struma ovarii). With the bladder catheterized, the 24-h ^{131}I uptake over the mass was 17%. The image on the left in part **B** is the gross surgical specimen; the image on the right is the corresponding in vitro ^{131}I image of the specimen. The ^{131}I had been administered 9 d prior to surgery. Reproduced with permission from the *Journal of Nuclear Medicine (6)*.

Comment: Although struma ovarii itself is very rare, the likelihood of the simultaneous occurrence with thyroid carcinoma is even more remote *(3–5)*. Pelvic or abdominal ^{131}I uptake in struma ovarii could be mistaken for metastatic thyroid carcinoma *(6,7)*.

PART 2
Nonthyroidal Physiologic Uptake

"FACIAL" RADIOACTIVITY

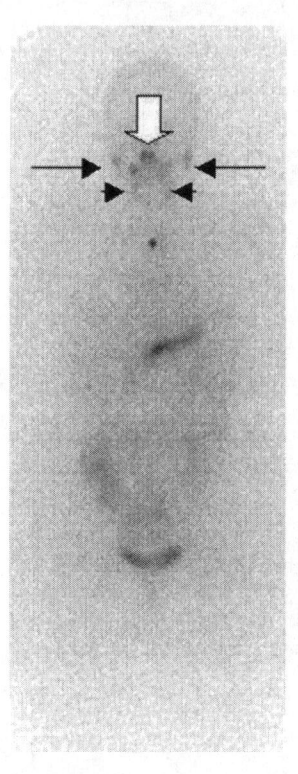

Fig. 6. The above radioiodine whole-body image was performed 48 h after the ^{131}I administration. Physiological uptake is present in the facial area. Modest uptake is found in the parotid glands (long, black, thin arrows), and less intense radioactivity is noted in the submandibular glands (short, black, thin arrows). Slightly more intense activity is indicated in the midline (white arrow), which is most likely nasal uptake (see Figs. 7 and 8), and a small asymmetric area (no arrow) is noted slightly inferior to the nasal area and medial to the right parotid (no arrow), consistent with asymmetric oropharyngeal activity.

Comment: Radioiodine normally concentrates in the salivary glands, including the parotid, submandibular, and sublingual glands, and is secreted into the oral pharynx. Uptake may also be present in the nasal area, which is discussed further below.

"FACIAL" RADIOIODINE ACCUMULATION

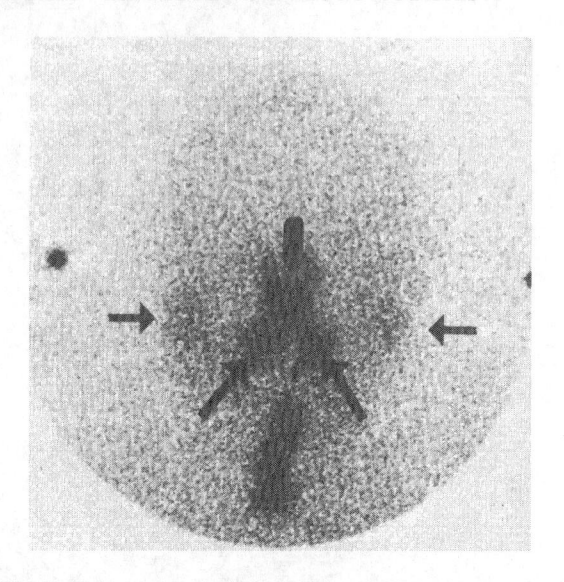

Fig. 7. Using a parallel-hole collimator of the head, face, and neck, this anterior image demonstrates typical areas of facial uptake and the variability of radioactivity in more detail than Fig. 6. Normal radioiodine uptake is noted in the parotid (short arrows), with slightly greater activity in the right parotid relative to the left. More intense radioactivity is found in the mouth and/or sublingual salivary gland area (long arrows). On this anterior image, no definitive radioiodine accumulation is noted in the submandibular glands. The radioactivity in the midline (thick arrow) represents nasal activity. The faint radioactivity that outlines the head is secondary to residual radioactivity in the blood pool. (The radioactivity in the midline below the two long arrows was discussed in the legend to Fig. 4.) Reproduced with permission from Lippincott, Williams, and Wilkins (2).

Comment: Uptake in the facial area can be variable. Although the radioactivity in each group of salivary glands is usually symmetrical, this is not always the case (as noted here). Asymmetric uptake may be caused by disease of the salivary gland, asymmetric development of the salivary glands, previous radioiodine treatment that resulted in asymmetric sialoadenitis, or even a slight rotation of the head during imaging.

Kulkarni et al. (8) has suggested that assessment of salivary gland uptake on the postoperative preablation/therapy scan may help predict sialoadenitis. If this is confirmed, the scan may help identify patients for whom the management should be altered, such as a reduced ablative or therapeutic prescribed activity and/or additional medications administered prophylactically to try to reduce the radiation exposure to the salivary glands from the treatment.

"FACIAL UPTAKE"

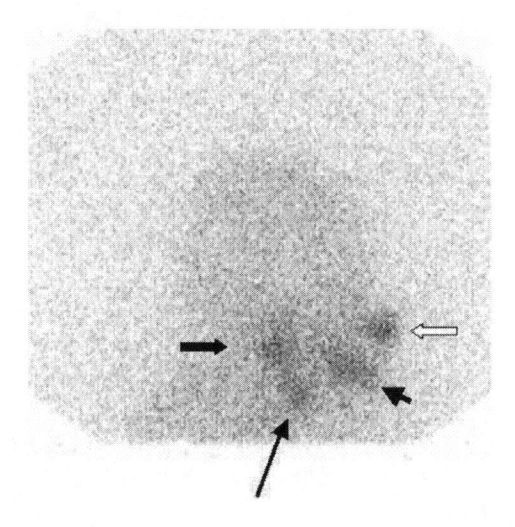

Fig. 8. This right lateral view of the head was obtained approx 72 h after the administration of ^{131}I. It demonstrates radioiodine accumulation in the nose (open arrow), parotid gland (medium-length arrow), submandibular gland (long arrow), and oral pharyngeal area (short arrow).

Comment: Uptake in the nose is a common finding. Norby et al. *(9)* reported that 95% (20/21) of patients had nasal radioactivity greater than background on whole-body scans performed 72 h after the administration of 5 mCi (18.5 MBq) of ^{131}I. The intensity of radioiodine accumulation was 1+ (greater than background but less than parotid gland and/or mouth activity) in 33% (6/20); 2+ (equal to parotid and/or mouth) in 33% (6/20); and 3+ (greater than parotid and/or mouth) in 40% (8/20). The pattern was ovoid in 75% (15/20) of patients but could also be linear.

The mechanism of radioiodine accumulation in the nose is not known. However, mucous glands are present in the tip of the nose and may be responsible. Focal uptake in the tip of the nose should not be considered a bone metastasis. Nasal pain and epistaxis have been reported after large therapeutic prescribed activities (200–400 mCi [7.4–14.8 GBq]) of radioiodine, and they are hypothesized to be the result of significant radiation-absorbed dose to the tip of the nose *(10)*. Assessment of the radioiodine whole-body scan may help identify patients who may be at risk for these nasal side effects and who may warrant a change in management, such as reduced prescribed activity and/or medication(s) to reduce the nasal uptake.

ESOPHAGUS: SWALLOWED RADIOACTIVITY OR ABERRANT THYROID TISSUE?

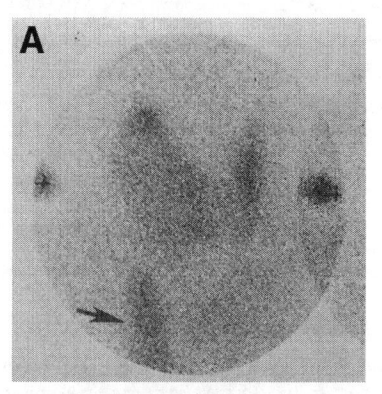

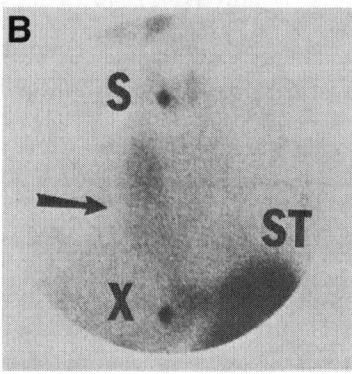

Fig. 9. Although these preoperative thyroid images were performed using ^{99m}TcO$_4$, they illustrate the potential pitfall of esophageal radioactivity. The anterior image of the thyroid performed using a pinhole collimator (**A**) demonstrates a large linear area of radioactivity inferior to the right lobe of the thyroid (arrow). Image (**B**) was obtained with a parallel-hole collimator and shows that the radioactivity extends to the xiphoid region (large arrow). After the patient drank several glasses of water, the radioactivity cleared. The patient had achalasia, and the area of radioactivity most likely represented persistent radioactivity in the dilated esophagus, which had been secreted by the salivary glands and swallowed (X, xiphoid; S, suprasternal notch; ST, stomach). Reproduced with permission from Lippincott, Williams, and Wilkins *(2)*.

Comment: ^{131}I, like ^{99m}TcO$_4$, may end up in the esophagus via several mechanisms. First, the ^{131}I that concentrates in the salivary glands may be secreted into the oropharynx and subsequently swallowed into the esophagus. Second, ^{131}I that is secreted by the gastric mucosa into the stomach may reflux into the esophagus. Third, ectopic gastric mucosa in the esophagus, such as a Barrett's esophagus, may secrete ^{131}I. Although the esophageal radioactivity from any of these mechanisms should clear rapidly, stasis may occur with Zenker's diverticulum or achalasia. To help differentiate physiological radioactivity from metastases, further manipulations may be necessary.

THYMUS

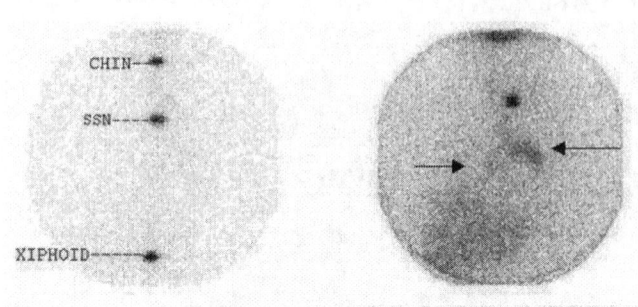

Fig. 10. The parallel-hole collimator image on the left represents a marker image, in which the location of the chin, SSN, and xiphoid are marked. After the markers are removed, and without moving the patient, a second parallel-hole collimator image was performed for a significantly longer time. These images were performed several days after radioiodine ablation. The image on the right demonstrates a bilobed area of radioactivity present in the mediastinum (arrows) secondary to normal thymic uptake. The modest radioactivity noted in the lower corner of the image is in the liver, which is discussed on page 179.

Comment: Radioiodine uptake in thymus has been reported by multiple authors, and the uptake has been observed in both hyperplastic and normal thymic tissue *(11–17)*. Wilson et al. has also reported $^{99m}TcO_4$ uptake in a thymoma *(12)*. The mechanism of radioiodine accumulation in the thymus is not known, but Vermiglio et al. *(13)* have suggested that the radioiodine localizes in cystic Hassall's bodies. Although thymic uptake is more frequently observed in children, it can also be seen in adults *(11)*.

In a group of 175 patients, Davidson *(17a)* reported radioiodine accumulation in thymus in four of 325 diagnostic scans and three of 200 posttreatment scans. Michigishi *(17b)* has suggested that the mediastinal uptake may become more prominent after successive ^{131}I therapies. Uptake in the thymus should not be mistaken for mediastinal metastasis. Computed tomography (CT) without contrast may be helpful in confirming the presence of thymic tissue or confirming an abnormal mass or nodes that suggest metastases.

CARDIAC BLOOD POOL

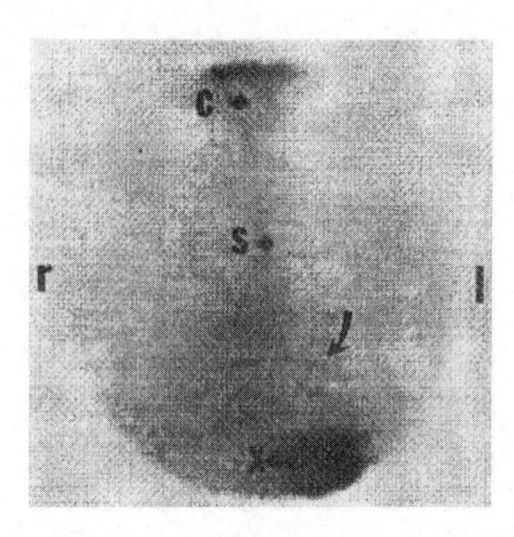

Fig. 11. This anterior neck and chest image was obtained 24 h after the administration of 1.0 mCi (37 MBq) of ^{131}I orally. Increased radioiodine activity is noted in the cardiac region (curved arrow) and represents normal cardiac blood pool activity at this time point. This area cleared on the 72-h image (not shown). The chin (C), suprasternal notch (S), and xiphoid (X) are noted using cobalt markers. The right (r) and left (l) side of the patient are also marked. Reproduced with permission from Lippincott, Williams, and Wilkins *(2)*.

Comment: The physician should be alert for and recognize blood pool activity, which may be more frequent on 24-h images with either ^{131}I or ^{123}I. It is normal and should not be mistaken for diffuse metastasis. Blood pool radioactivity may mask metastasis in both the lower lung and possibly the lower hilar regions. Delayed views on subsequent days may be needed to allow further clearance of the blood pool (background) activity.

DIFFUSE LIVER RADIOACTIVITY

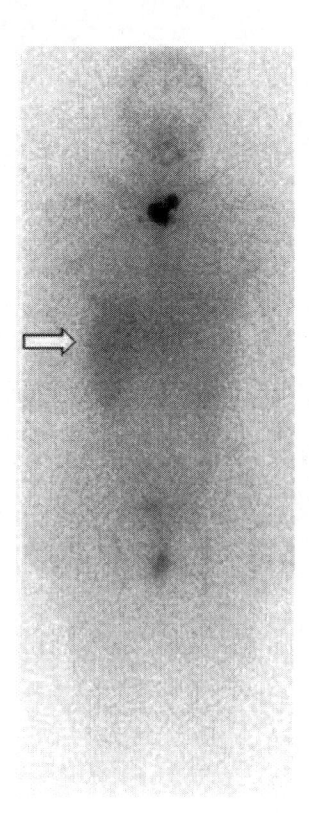

Fig. 12. This posttherapy ^{131}I whole-body scan was performed approx 12 d after ablation with ^{131}I and demonstrates diffuse radioactivity in the liver (arrow). Reproduced with permission from Keystone Press, Inc. *(18)*.

Comment: Ziessman *(14)* reported that liver uptake is commonly seen in 44% (12/27) of patients and 35% (21/60) of scans and can be present on posttherapy scans, as well as on diagnostic scans. Of 19 posttherapy scans performed following 30–200 mCi (1.11–7.4 GBq) of ^{131}I, liver radioactivity was present on a subjective scale of 3+ in six, 2+ in four, 1+ in four, and 0 in five. In contrast, of 41 patients receiving 2–10 mCi (74–370 MBq) of ^{131}I, liver radioactivity was present on the same scale with 3+ in one, 2+ in two, 1+ in six, and 0 in 32. The posttherapy scans were performed 3–7 d after the therapy, and the diagnostic scans were performed 48 h after administration of the diagnostic prescribed activity.

Chung et al. *(15)* reported that 60% of 399 patients and 36% of 1115 radioiodine whole-body scans had diffuse hepatic uptake more than grade 2, which was defined as definite but faint liver activity. In the diagnostic scans, 12% showed uptake in the liver, whereas the frequency of liver uptake on posttherapy scans increased based on the therapy dose. Liver uptake was present in 39% of scans performed after treatment with 30 mCi (1.11 GBq), 62% after 75–100 mCi (2.775–3.7 GBq), and 71.3% after 150–200 mCi (5.55–7.4 GBq). Similarly, as the uptake in residual thyroid tissue increased visually, the liver intensity also increased. However, 15 patients showed diffuse liver uptake without uptake in the thyroid or metastases. Chung et al. *(15)* also showed a relationship of the degree of hepatic uptake to release of ^{131}I-labeled thyroglobulin.

Zeissman *(14)* also reported that the presence of liver uptake correlated with both the administered prescribed activity of ^{131}I and the absolute thyroid uptake (actual number of millicuries of ^{131}I in the thyroid) but not with the percent uptake. With few exceptions, patients with liver visualization had an absolute thyroid uptake of more than 1 mCi (37 MBq), and most without liver visualization had thyroid uptake of less than 1 mCi (37 MBq). He also suggested that the longer the time interval between administration of the radioiodine and the time to imaging, the greater the frequency would be, as well as the degree of increased uptake of liver radioactivity.

Radiolabeled thyroxine localizes in the liver within hours after injection *(16)*, and the liver deiodinates 40% of the whole-body T-4 and 70% of the T-3 production *(17)*.

GASTROINTESTINAL RADIOACTIVITY

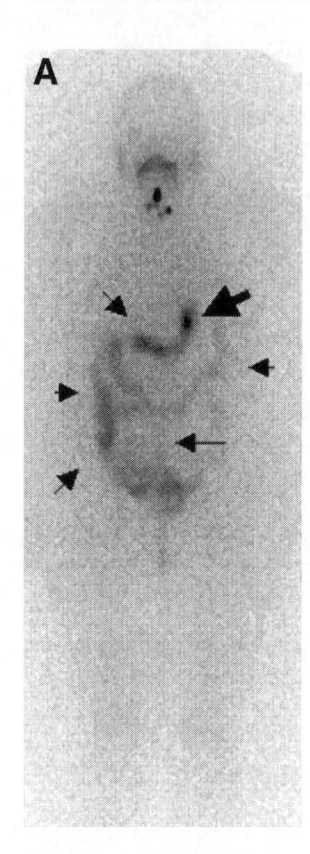

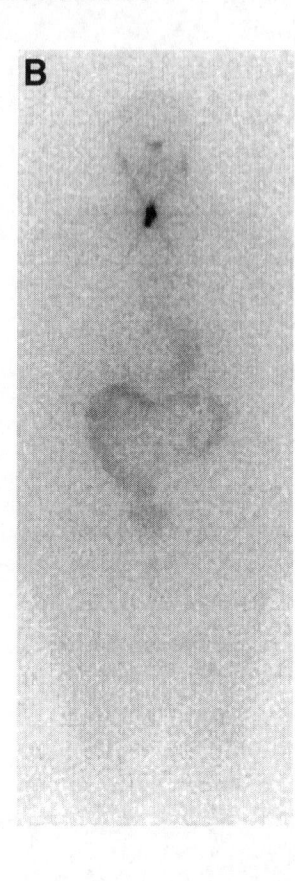

Fig. 13. Part **A** demonstrates normal physiologic radioactivity in the stomach (large arrow) and gastrointestinal system (small arrowheads). The patterns of gastrointestinal radioactivity are variable (part **B**).

Comment: Radioiodine in the stomach and gastrointestinal tract may be secondary to a combination of at least three mechanisms: swallowed radioactive saliva, radioactivity secreted by the gastric mucosa, and deiodinated thyroid hormone in the liver excreted through the biliary tree.

Because it is highly unusual for well-differentiated thyroid carcinoma to metastasize to the gastrointestinal system, differentiating physiological gastrointestinal uptake from a gastrointestinal metastasis is not a diagnostic problem. Rather, the problem is differentiating physiological gastrointestinal uptake from a metastasis in bone. This is usually facilitated by the pattern, localization, and use of multiple tools as listed in Table 2. A radioactive focus with a tubular, not focal pattern, that localizes on lateral views to abdomen, not bone, and that changes configuration on delayed views with or without laxatives is indicative of gastrointestinal radioactivity. Single-photon emission computed tomography (SPECT) [123]I scans or positron emission tomography (PET) [124]I scans fused with SPECT bone scans or CTs are potentially helpful additional options.

In addition to the above, delayed and lateral views may help assess the bones that are obscured by overlying gastrointestinal radioactivity. Identification of significant gastrointestinal radioactivity on a diagnostic scan may encourage the physician to manage more aggressively a patient with stool softeners and/or laxatives after ablation or treatment. This may reduce the amount and residence time of the radioactivity in the intestine, thereby reducing the radiation absorbed dose to the gastrointestinal tract.

URINARY BLADDER

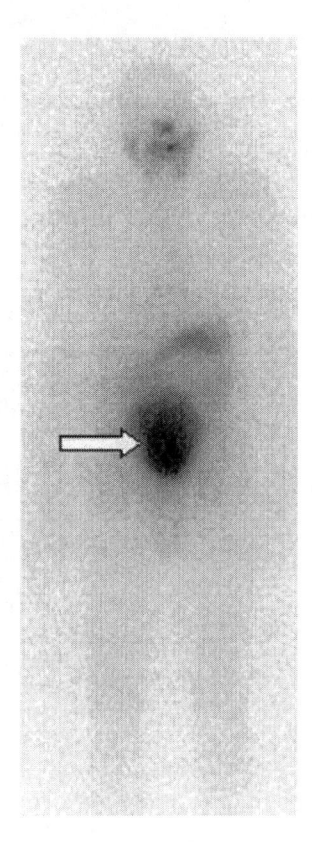

Fig. 14. A large area of radioactivity is noted in the pelvic area, extending into the lower abdomen (white arrow), which is a distended urinary bladder. Gastrointestinal activity is also noted slightly cephalad.

Comment: The kidneys are the principal means by which the radioiodine is cleared from the body; of course, radioiodine will accumulate in the urinary bladder. The importance of urinary bladder radioactivity is that:

1. It is very variable in intensity of configuration.
2. It should not be mistaken for bony metastasis.
3. It can obscure the assessment of the underlying pelvic bones for bony metastases.
4. The patient should be encouraged to void before beginning the scan.
5. Hydration and frequent voiding after radioiodine ablation will help reduce the radiation exposure to the urinary bladder wall, adjacent bowel, colon, ovaries, and so on.
6. Distended bladders, such as this patient's bladder, may need to be catheterized to minimize the radiation exposure to the urinary bladder wall after radioactivity ablation or treatment.

PART 3
Patterns of Metastatic Disease

REGIONAL LYMPH NODE METASTASIS

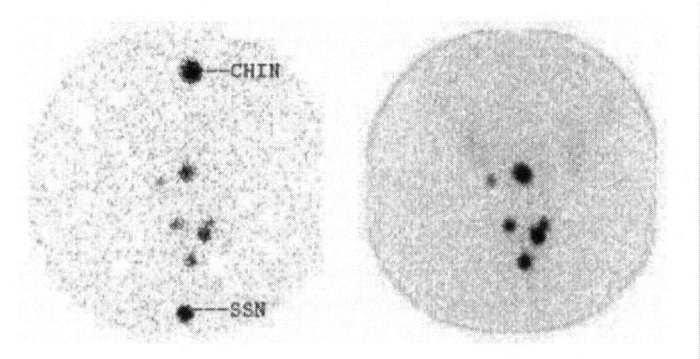

Fig. 15. The pinhole collimator image on the left represents a marker image in which the location of the chin and SSN are marked. After the markers are removed, and without moving the patient, a second pinhole collimator image is performed for a significantly longer time. The resulting image on the right demonstrates six areas of focal radioactivity. Several of these were confirmed as cervical lymph nodes with metastatic disease.

Comment: This author (DVN) proposes that as the number of focal areas of radioactivity increases, the likelihood of lymph node metastases, rather than just residual preoperative tissue, increases; however, the author is unaware of any significant study to confirm this relationship.

If metastatic disease is confirmed in the lymph nodes using fine-needle aspiration, then additional surgery may need to be considered prior to performing radioiodine ablation or treatment.

Although some facilities will give a fixed empiric prescribed activity for ablation or treatment in this patient, other facilities will consider increasing the empiric prescribed activity of radioiodine or will perform lesional dosimetry, as described by Thomas and Maxon *(19,20)*.

MEDIASTINAL METASTASIS

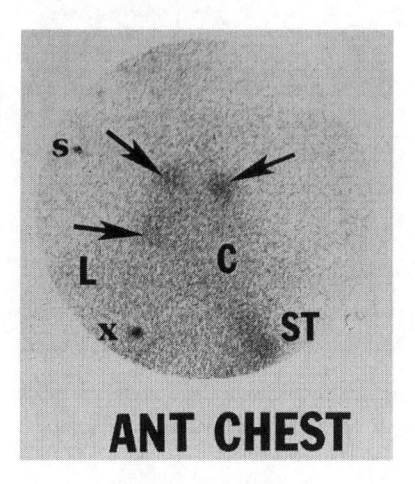

Fig. 16. This parallel-hole collimator image of the chest demonstrates three areas of metastasic thyroid cancer in the mediastinum (black arrows). s represents the level of the SSN, but the marker was placed to the right side of the patient. x designates the xiphoid, but this marker is also placed to the right of the midline. L represents lower lung area, C represents cardiac areas, and ST represents the stomach. Reproduced with permission from Lippincott, Williams, and Wilkins *(2)*.

Comment: This is an example of metastasis to the mediastinal lymph nodes, which is a frequent location of metastasis from well-differentiated thyroid carcinoma. The determination of the prescribed radioactivity to treat this patient is problematic. The prescribed activity could range from an empiric fixed prescribed activity of 100 mCi (3.7 GBq) to 300 mCi (11.1 GBq). Lesional dosimetry, blood (bone marrow) dosimetry, or both have also been performed to help determine an appropriate prescribed radioactivity for treatment.

Pulmonary Metastasis: Patterns

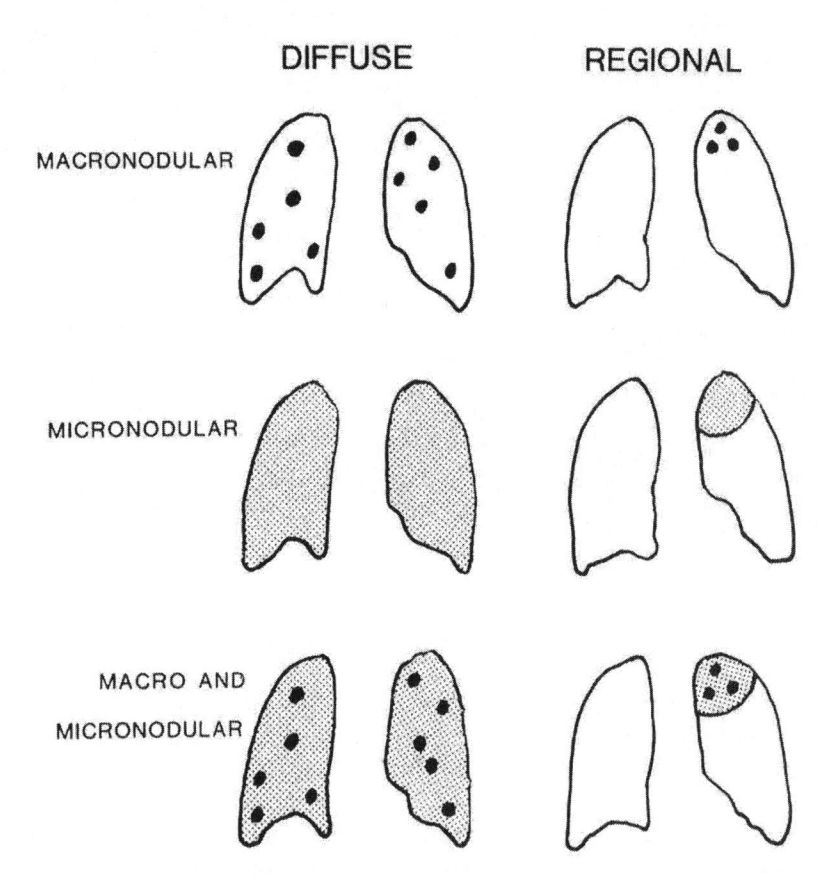

Fig. 17. The above drawings demonstrate three potential patterns of radioactive uptake secondary to metastasic thyroid cancer to the lungs. These patterns are macronodular (upper), micronodular (middle), and mixed (lower) and may also be diffuse or regional. Reproduced with permission from Lippincott, Williams, and Wilkins (2).

Comment: The terms "micronodular" and "macronodular" may be used to describe the pattern of pulmonary metastases on either radioiodine scan or radiographs, albeit most authors use the terms to describe radiograph findings. Although no precise measurement differentiates macronodular from micronodular metastases, 1 cm or greater has been used by Schlumberger as the threshold for macronodular and less than 1 cm as micronodular (21). Casara et al. (36) have used the threshold of more than 5 millimeters as macronodular and less than 5 mm as micronodular. Pulmonary metastasis may present in a wide spectrum of patterns, from a diffuse miliary pattern of micrometastases throughout both lungs with good radioiodine uptake and normal chest X-ray, to a pattern of a single large focal macronodular metastasis on chest X-ray with no radioiodine uptake.

Although the association of the pattern of pulmonary metastasis to either prognosis or the frequency and severity of side effects of radioiodine treatment has not been well characterized (see Chapters 40 and 64 regarding "Prognosis" and Chapter 45 entitled "Radioiodine Treatment"), several potential relationships have been suggested. First, good uptake of radioiodine in a diffuse miliary pattern may be associated with a better prognosis than multiple focal macronodular metastases with poor radioiodine uptake (21–25). In addition, when the chest X-ray/CT is negative for evidence of pulmonary metastasis, Hindié et al. (25a) observed that the prognosis may be even better. Schlumberger et al. (23) observed complete remission in 83% of lesions that were not visible on chest X-ray, in 53% of micronodular (<1 cm), and in only 14% of macronodular (>1 cm) metastases. However, the pattern of diffuse functioning micronodular metastases may be more likely to be associated with diffuse acute radiation pneumonitis, pulmonary fibrosis, or both, rather than the latter pattern (see Chapter 45 entitled "Radioiodine Treatment").

PULMONARY METASTASIS: DIFFUSE MILIARY (MICRONODULAR) METASTASES

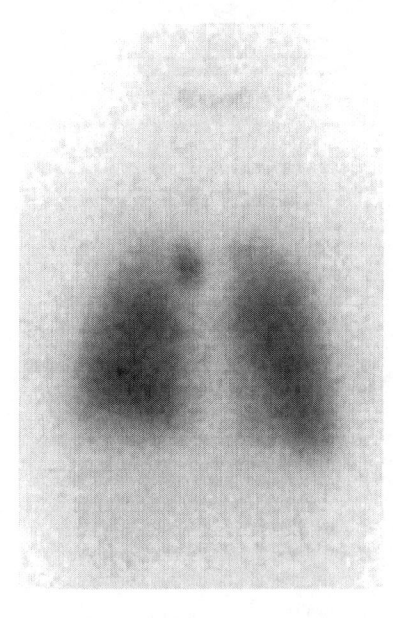

Fig. 18. This is a whole-body anterior image performed 72 h after the administration of ^{131}I. Marked diffuse radioactivity is noted throughout both lung fields, which is typical for a miliary pattern of pulmonary metastasis. The radiograph demonstrates a miliary pattern throughout both lungs. Although the scan suggests a focal area of radioactivity in the upper medial aspect of the right lung, the radiographs showed only a similar miliary pattern. Histopathologic examination confirmed papillary follicular well-differentiated thyroid carcinoma. Owing to the intense uptake in both lungs, the outline of the patient's body is not readily visualized using these brightness and contrast settings. Reproduced with permission from Keystone Press, Inc. *(18)*.

Comment: Several authors have reported that this pattern is associated with a good prognosis. However, this patient may be more susceptible to acute radiation pneumonitis, fibrosis, or both after radioiodine therapy. As previously discussed, the selection of an appropriate prescribed treatment activity for treatment is problematic. In the adult patient, the prescribed activity has ranged between an empiric fixed prescribed activity of 100 mCi (3.7 GBq) to 300 mCi (11.1 GBq). This author suggests that bone marrow (blood) dosimetry, as described by Benua and Leeper, has value in determining the maximum allowable prescribed activity and has a long history of successful usage, with little or no acute radiation pneumonitis and/or pulmonary fibrosis when appropriate restrictions are followed. (See Chapter 47 entitled "Dosimetry" and Chapter 50 entitled "Side Effects of ^{131}I for Ablation and Treatment of Well-Differentiated Thyroid Carcinoma.")

PULMONARY METASTASIS: MACRONODULAR

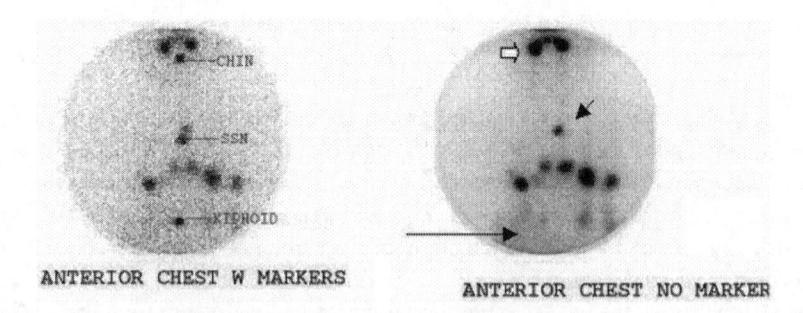

Fig. 19. The parallel-hole collimator image on the left represents a marker image in which the location of the chin, SSN, and xiphoid are marked. After the markers are removed, and without moving the patient, a second parallel-hole collimator image was performed for a significantly longer time. The resulting image on the right demonstrates multifocal macronodular metastases in the lung and possibly mediastinum (short arrow). The activity designated by the long arrow was physiologic liver activity.

Comment: Again, the selection of an appropriate prescribed treatment activity is problematic and discussed above. Unlike the previous figure, this pattern of pulmonary metastases may be associated with a lower likelihood of diffuse acute radiation pneumonitis and/or pulmonary fibrosis. In addition, if either one or both occur, the diffuse acute radiation pneumonitis or fibrosis should be more localized to the area around the macronodules. However, as reported in the external radiation therapy literature, abscopal effects may occur, which are pulmonary changes outside the radiation port *(24–26)*.

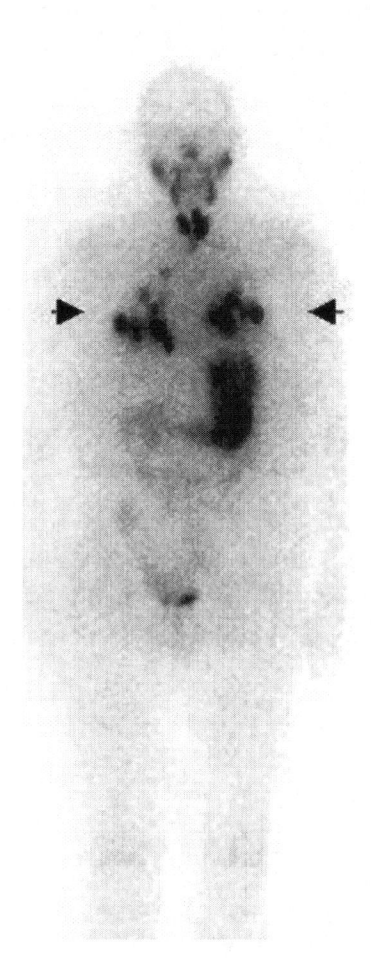

Fig. 20. This whole-body image performed 48 h after radioiodine administration again demonstrates predominantly macronodules more localized to the mid- and lower lung fields (arrow heads).

PULMONARY METASTASIS: MACRO AND MICRONODULAR

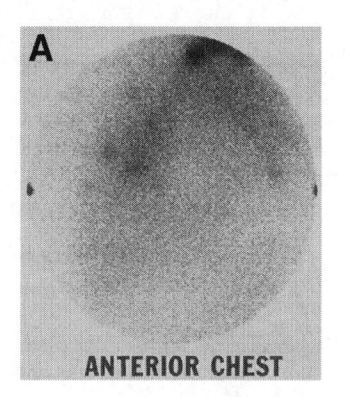

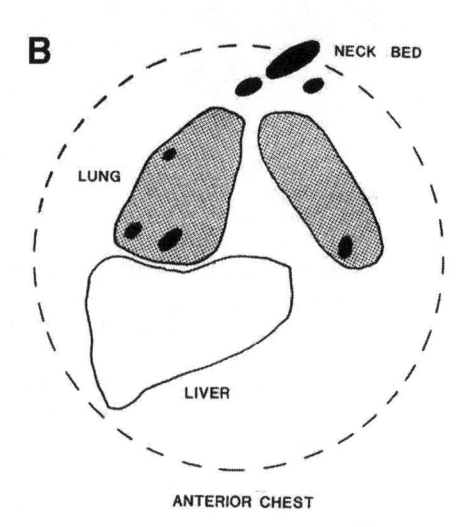

Fig. 21. The patient was shifted slightly to his left for this anterior chest and abdominal image (**A**), and the accompanying diagram (**B**) should aid in identification of the findings. This image demonstrates increased radioiodine in the thyroid bed, diffuse moderately increased radioiodine throughout most of both lungs (which is indicative of micronodular metastases), and faint but definite focal areas of increased radioiodine in the mid- to lower lung fields. The focal areas of radioactivity were attributed to pulmonary macronodular metastases. The CT of the chest confirmed both micronodular and macronodular pattern in the lung without any changes in the bones to account for bony metastasis. Trace amount of radioactivity is noted in the liver and is normal. This case demonstrates that both pulmonary patterns of macronodular and micronodular disease may occur together. Reproduced with permission from Lippincott, Williams, and Wilkins *(2)*.

LIVER METASTASES

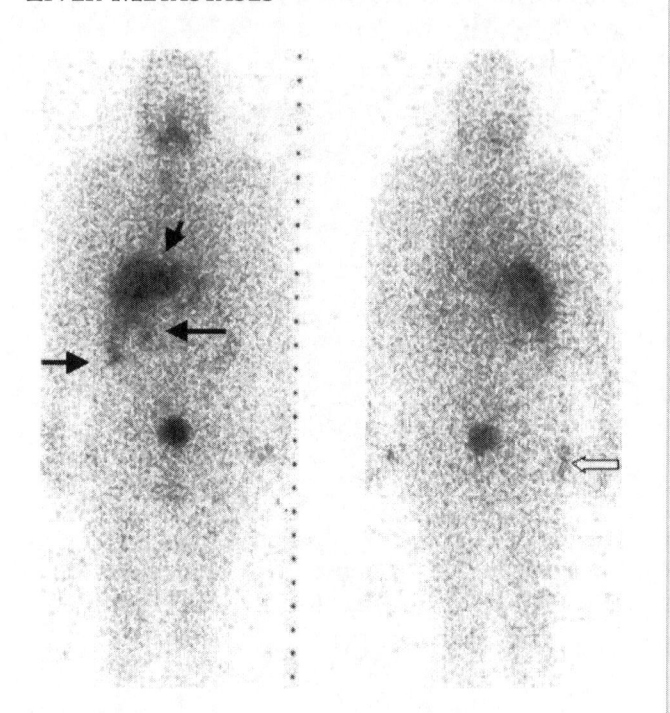

Fig. 22. These whole-body images demonstrate inhomogeneous accumulation of ^{131}I in the liver (black arrows) secondary to confirmed multiple liver metastases. The patient had a total thyroidectomy, and the images were performed prior to ^{131}I treatment. The left and right panels are the anterior and posterior whole-body images, respectively. Metastases to the lung were also present. A radioactivity-contaminated handkerchief (white arrow) is seen in the posterior view in the right pocket. These images were contributed by Milton G. Gross, MD, University of Michigan Medical School, Ann Arbor, MI.

Comment: Metastasis to the liver is rare but does occur. Physiological radioiodine uptake in the liver can be distinguished from metastatic disease by assessment of the pattern of uptake (diffuse vs focal), distribution of uptake (homogeneous versus inhomogeneous), intensity (low vs high), and absolute uptake of radioactivity elsewhere, such as the thyroid bed. Physiological uptake would be typically more diffuse, more homogeneous, have lower intensity, and associated with significant uptake of radioactivity in the thyroid bed or in other functioning metastases *(14)*. (See Fig. 12 of physiological liver uptake above.) Metastases would be more focal, inhomogeneous, and not necessarily associated with significant uptake of radioactivity elsewhere. Of course, further diagnostic imaging, such as with CT, magnetic resonance imaging (MRI), or ultrasound, should be useful.

No significant data are available regarding how the presence of liver metastases would influence the prescribed activity of radioiodine or the side effects of radioiodine in patients with liver metastases. A hyperfunctioning liver metastasis has been reported *(27)*.

BONE METASTASES

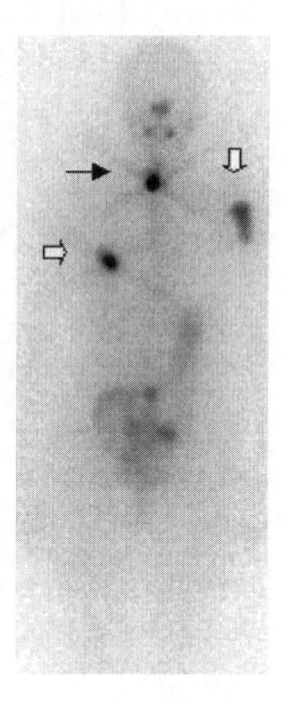

Fig. 23. This pretherapy whole-body scan performed 72 h after administration of ^{131}I demonstrates abnormal radioiodine uptake in the proximal left humerus and one of the anterior right ribs (white arrows). The abnormality in the left humerus was confirmed histopathologically to be metastatic well-differentiated thyroid carcinoma, and a CT of right anterior ribs confirmed changes consistent with bone metastasis.

Significant residual radioactivity is noted in the thyroid bed consistent with postoperative residual thyroid tissue after a near-total thyroidectomy (black arrow). Note the starburst-pattern artifact of radioactivity in the area of uptake in the thyroid bed and possibly the right rib (see Fig. 28).

Comment: Focal uptake that appears to be in the bone on anterior and/or posterior views should be confirmed with lateral or oblique views. Bone uptake should not be taken as prima facie evidence for metastatic bone disease. Plain radiographs, CT without contrast, and/or MRI should be performed to help confirm the presence of metastases or to identify other etiologies for the bony uptake. If a metastasis to the bone is confirmed, consider (1) increasing the empiric prescribed treatment activity; (2) determining the maximal prescribed treatment activity by dosimetry; and/or (3) treating with external-beam radiotherapy. Radiofrequency ablation has also been used with success (see Chapter 54).

BRAIN METASTASIS

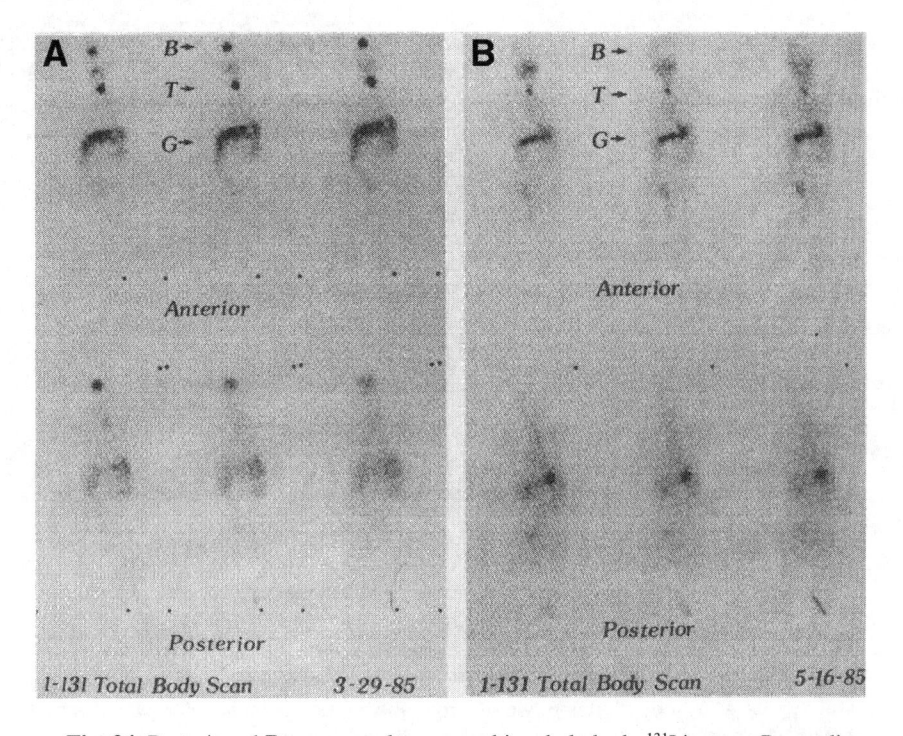

Fig. 24. Parts **A** and **B** are coronal tomographic whole-body ^{131}I images. Proceeding from left to right and top to bottom, the coronal slices progress from anterior to posterior. Part **A** demonstrates abnormal radioiodine accumulation in the head (B), which was confirmed as an intracerebral metastasis. Activity is present in the thyroid bed (T) and gastrointestinal areas (G). After the intracerebral metastasis was resected, repeat images approx 48 d after administration (part **B**) illustrates resolution of the abnormal uptake in the intracerebral metastasis with residual faint background activity. The latter was attributed to postoperative blood pool. Reproduced with permission of the American Medical Association *(29)*.

Comment: Focal uptake that appears to be in the brain on anterior and/or posterior views should be confirmed, if possible, with lateral or oblique views. An MRI is also warranted. Intracerebral metastases are infrequent. Misaki et al. *(28)* report intracerebral metastasis in 5.4% of 167 patients who had lung or bone metastases. In this group, none of the brain lesions had significant uptake of radioiodine despite accumulation in most of the extracerebral metastases.

Management includes surgical resection, stereotactic radiosurgery, external beam irradiation, and/or radioiodine. If radioiodine is to be administered for the treatment of intracerebral metastasis, pretreatment of the patient with steroids, glycerol, or mannitol should be considered.

RENAL METASTASIS

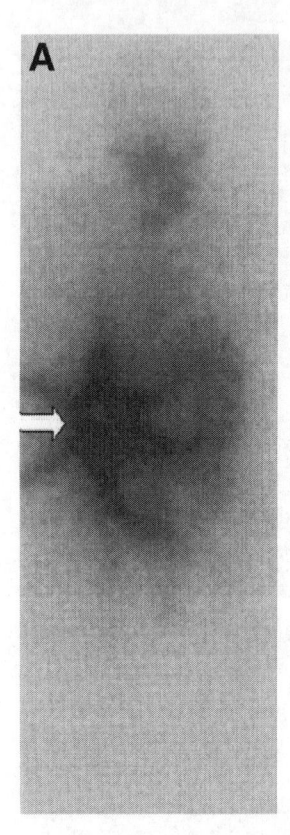

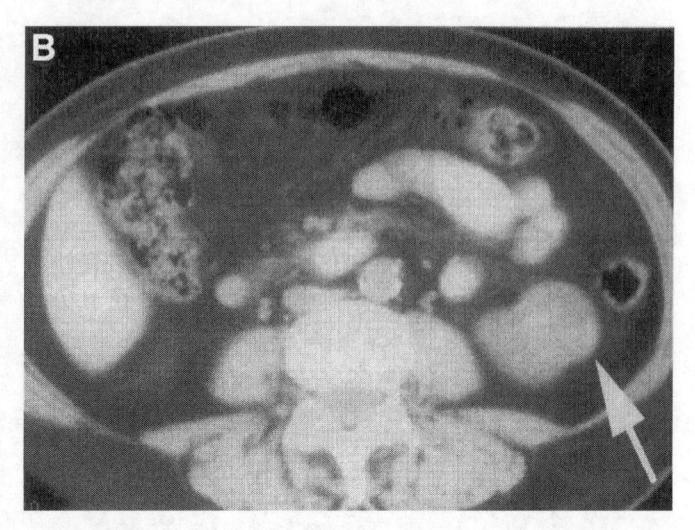

Fig. 25. Part **A** is a posttherapy posterior ^{131}I whole-body scan that demonstrates a prominent "star" artifact (white arrow) in the upper left quadrant of the abdomen, which was secondary to a renal metastasis from well-differentiated thyroid cancer. The "star" artifact is discussed in Fig. 28. Part **B** is the transverse CT image of the abdomen, demonstrating (white arrow) the metastasis in the inferolateral aspect of the kidney. Metastatic well-differentiated thyroid cancer was confirmed in the renal mass by histopathology. Reproduced with permission of Mary Ann Liebert, Inc. *(30)*.

Comment: Renal metastasis from well-differentiated thyroid carcinoma has been reported but is rare *(30,31)*. Radioiodine is excreted by the kidneys, and radioiodine accumulation in the kidney secondary to radioiodine retention in the renal collecting system should not be mistaken for a renal metastasis *(31)*.

PART 4
Examples of False-Positive Uptake and Artifacts

OVARIAN CYSTADENOMA

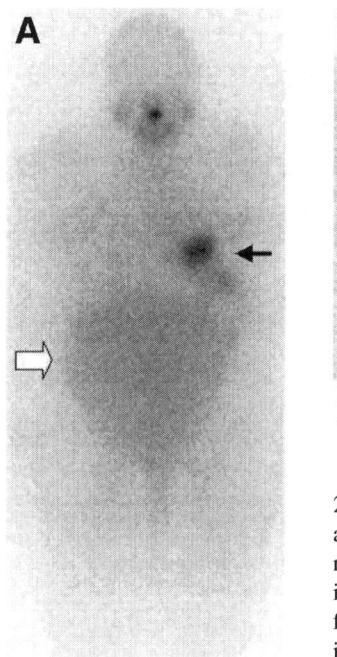

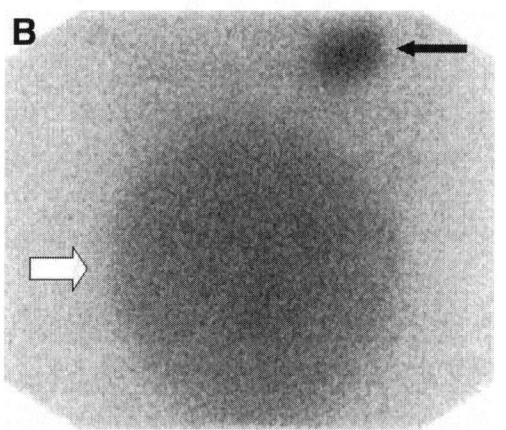

Fig. 26. The whole-body scan (**A**) was performed 24 h after the administration of 1 mCi (37 MBq) of ^{123}I and demonstrates a large circular area of modest radioiodine accumulation (white arrow). **B** is a static image of the abdominal-pelvic area showing the same finding (white arrow). Surgery confirmed a large ovarian cystadenoma. The more intense radioiodine accumulation in the left upper quadrant of the abdomen (black arrows) was attributed to physiological activity in the stomach.

Comment: Radioiodine accumulation in an ovarian cystadenoma has been reported *(32)*. The mechanism of radioiodine accumulation in the ovarian cyst is unknown.

Dentures

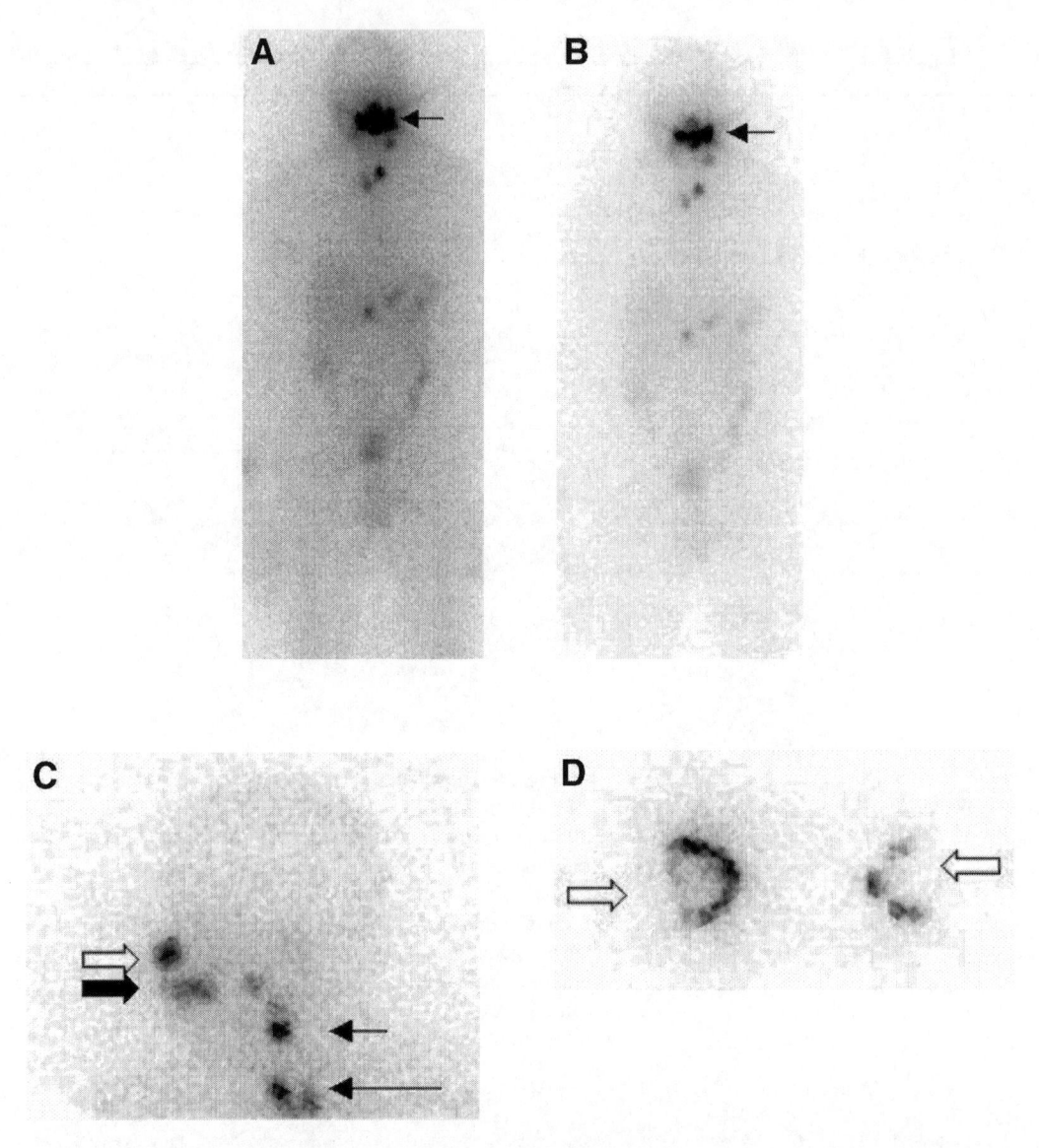

Fig. 27. The whole-body radioiodine image (**A**) demonstrates uptake in the neck and face; however, the radioactivity in the mouth area is more prominent than usual (arrow in high intensity image in **A** and low-intensity image in **B**). Upon further history and after removal of the patient's dentures, the patient was reimaged, and the radioactivity in the mouth region was normal (**C**) (large white arrow nose; large black arrow oral area; thin black arrow salivary gland or metastases; long thin arrow thyroid tissue). Separate images of the upper and lower dentures illustrated the significant radioactivity around the dentures (**D**) (white arrows).

Comment: The etiologies of false-positive areas of radioiodine accumulation are extensive and discussed in detail in Chapter 16. Uptake from poor dental hygiene has been reported *(33)*.

SEPTAL PENETRATION

Fig. 28. This whole-body scan was performed 48 h after the oral administration of 4 mCi (148 MBq) of ^{131}I and demonstrates significant uptake in the thyroid bed, which is not a radioactive marker. Radioactivity is noted, projecting outward in six symmetrical linear "rays" from the intense focal area of radioactivity in the thyroid bed. Owing to the configuration of this pattern, this area has been described as a "star" artifact.

Comment: For a full discussion, see Chapter 14. This is truly an "artifact" because the events being recorded in the image along those projections did not originate at those locations within the patient but instead are malpositioned events that come from the thyroid bed uptake. This phenomenon occurs throughout the image, but it is only apparent around areas of intense radioiodine concentration.

In brief, the γ waves from the ^{131}I have penetrated the thinnest portion of the lead septa of the parallel-hole collimator and are thus visualized. The thinnest portion may depend on the shape and construction of the collimator. In this example, the collimator hole is a hexagon, and the thinnest portion is that portion of the septa between each junction.

This artifact may limit the ability of the scan to show nearby functioning metastases. In addition, because of the intense radioiodine uptake in the thyroid bed, the pattern of radioactivity in that area cannot be demonstrated. As pointed out in the previous figure, this may be important for comparison with subsequent scans. A pinhole collimator does not produce this artifact and will resolve this dilemma.

OFF-PEAK ARTIFACTS

Fig. 29. The above image is a whole-body scan obtained 48-h postadministration of ^{131}I. No identifiable uptake, structure, or outline of the body is noted. The technologist was using an incorrect energy peak for ^{131}I.

Comment: As noted at the beginning of the chapter, the physician must ensure that the images are obtained according to the facility's protocol and are of diagnostic quality. Although the newer cameras help minimize the various set-up and acquisition errors and the nuclear medicine technologist should be able to identify and correct these errors, errors may still occur. The interpreting physician must still have a good working knowledge of technical artifacts to be able to identify and troubleshoot them. This figure is an example of one of the many technical artifacts "off peak."

Low Counts

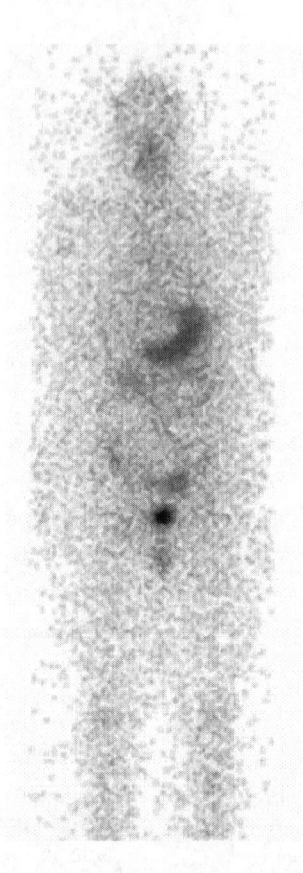

Fig. 30. This whole-body scan was performed 48 h after the administration of ^{131}I. The image appears "grainy" because of low counts.

Comment: Low counts in the image may be the result of such factors as (1) low diagnostic prescribed activity administered, (2) partially infiltrated dose, (3) delayed imaging in a patient with fast clearance, or (4) shortened acquisition time of the study owing to the technologist.

When there are insufficient counts in a whole-body scan, the sensitivity of the scan for the detection of functioning metastases is reduced. The higher the counts are, the more likely that significant accumulation of radioiodine can be differentiated from background and noise.

PART 5
Tools to Help Differentiate Metastases from Nonthyroidal Physiologic Uptake, False-Positives, and Artifact

THE VALUE OF "UPTAKE-SPECIFIC" HISTORY AND PATIENT EXAMINATION

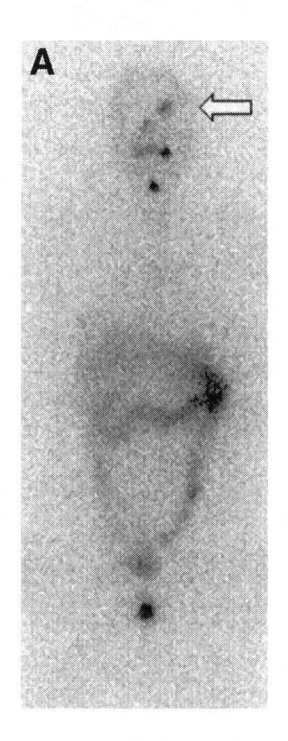

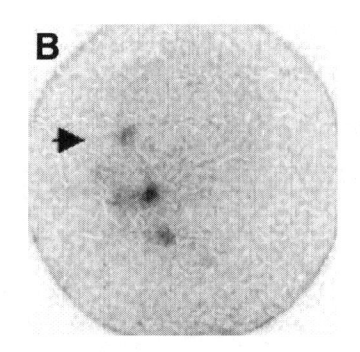

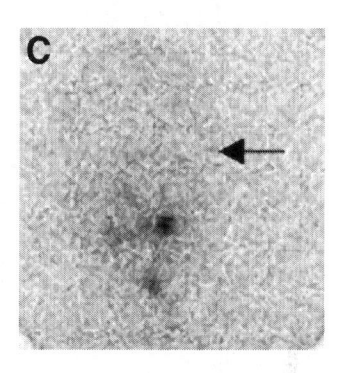

Fig. 31. This whole-body scan (**A**) was performed 24 h after the administration of low prescribed activity of ^{123}I (500 µCi [18.5 MBq]) and demonstrated several asymmetric areas of uptake in the neck and face. The area of interest is the accumulation of radioactivity in the left eye or skull region (arrow). The lateral view (**B**) suggests that the uptake was either in the left eye or adjacent bone, raising the possibility of an unusual bone metastasis (arrow). With additional "uptake-specific" history and examination, it was determined that the patient was found to have an artificial eyeball prosthesis on this side. After removing the artificial eyeball and reimaging the face, the foci of radioactivity disappeared (**C**) (arrow).

Comment: "Uptake-specific" history (i.e., questions directed specifically at areas of suspicious uptake seen on the scan) and examination of the patient can frequently resolve the etiology of an area of radioactivity uptake and improve the specificity of the whole-body radioiodine scan. Although this teaching point should be self-evident, knowledge of an adequate history and a thorough physical examination are not universal. Uptake secondary to an artificial eyeball *(34)* should not be interpreted as bone or brain metastasis.

This is only one example of the wide spectrum of false-positive or artifactual radioiodine accumulation (see Chapter 16).

UTILITY OF PINHOLE COLLIMATOR IMAGES

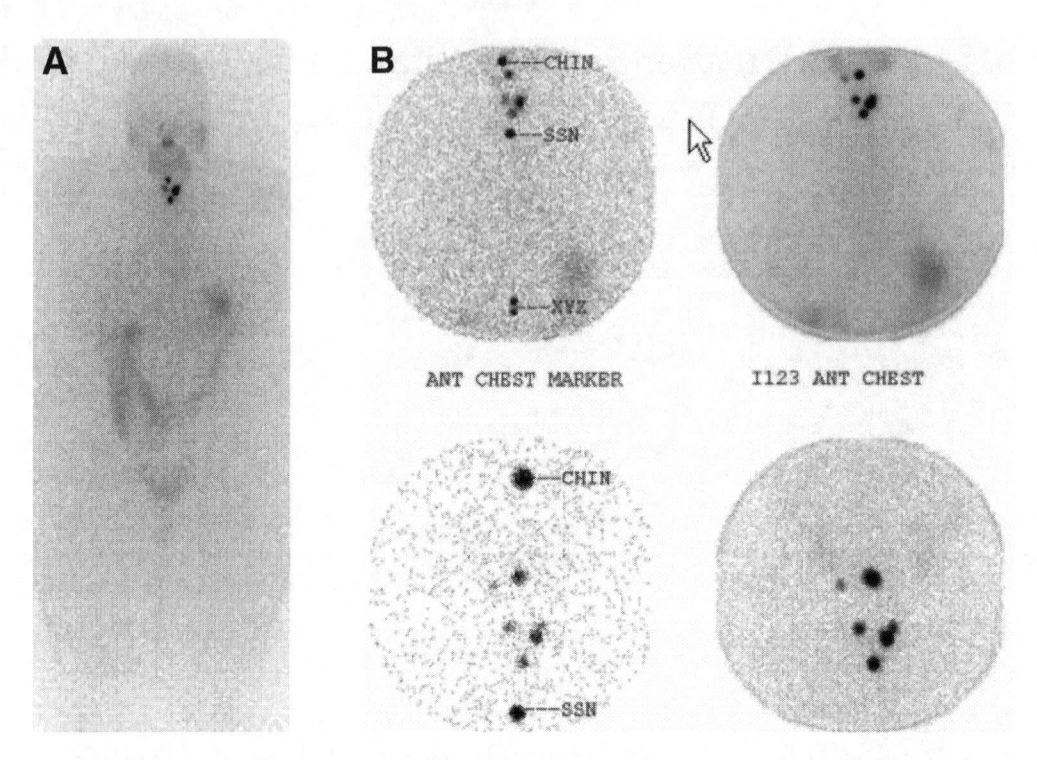

Fig. 32. This figure demonstrates the utility of pinhole collimator images, which are discussed in more detail in Chapter 14. **A** is the whole-body image that shows four distinct areas of uptake in the thyroid bed consistent with normal residual tissue remaining after a near-total thyroidectomy. In **B**, the upper left image was obtained using a parallel-hole collimator, along with external markers placed over the chin, SSN and xiphoid (XYZ) to "mark" these anatomical locations on the image. After the markers are removed, and without moving the patient, a second image was performed for a significantly longer time. The resulting image on the upper right demonstrates five areas of thyroid tissue. The lower set of images of **B** were obtained using a pinhole collimator with the "marker" image on the left. The image on the lower right, which has no markers, illustrates six distinct foci of radioiodine accumulation.

Comment: Pinhole collimator images have higher resolution than "spot-camera" or whole-body camera images performed with a parallel-hole collimator for small targeted areas, e.g., the thyroid bed. In this patient, the differentiation of six, rather than four, foci of radioiodine accumulation suggests a higher likelihood of cervical lymph node metastases.

For those facilities that administer a fixed empiric prescribed activity of radioiodine for ablation without first performing a scan, or regardless of the scan findings, the additional findings seen on the pinhole collimator images would not be of value. However, for those facilities that will either reconsider additional surgery, increase the prescribed activity used for the ablation in the event of cervical metastasis, or both, then pinhole collimator images are valuable.

The pinhole images also provide a superior baseline study for future comparison. If the patient has persistent elevation of serum thyroglobulin levels or develops evidence of some other recurrence, a previous baseline pinhole collimator image helps differentiate whether the radioactivity on a new scan is a new region or one of the previous areas that was not successfully ablated.

Value of Lateral Views

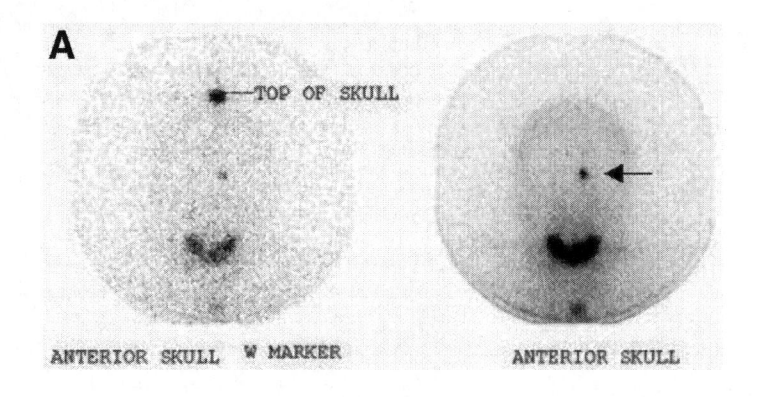

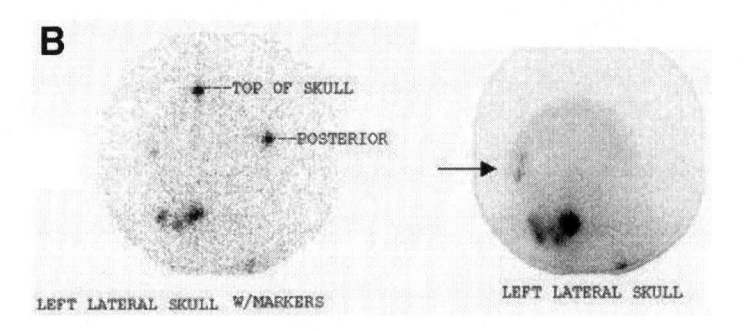

Fig. 33. The image on the upper left of **A** was obtained using a parallel-hole collimator camera, taken of the head in the anterior view with a marker on the top of the calvarium (a "spot-camera" view). The acquisition time was only long enough to allow the marker to be clearly visualized. The marker was then removed, and without moving the patient, an image was performed for a significantly longer duration. This latter image (shown on the upper right) demonstrates a focus of intense radioactivity in the midline (arrow). The radioactivity immediately inferior to this represents physiological oropharyngeal-nasal radioiodine accumulation. The lateral view with markers (left image in **B**) and without markers (right image in **B**) suggests that the radioactivity is in the bone, not the brain, which a noncontrast CT confirmed.

Comment: Lateral views can be useful to further localize radioactivity and are frequently helpful to improve the specificity of radioiodine accumulation. Although the lateral view may not always localize conclusively the radioiodine accumulation, it may still be useful either (1) as a guide for CT and MRI evaluation, or (2) for comparison with future scans.

Further confirmation is always warranted such as with a noncontrast CT or MRI.

VALUE OF PATIENT MARKERS

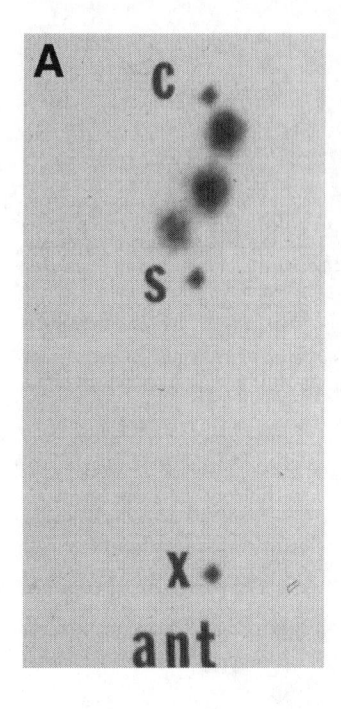

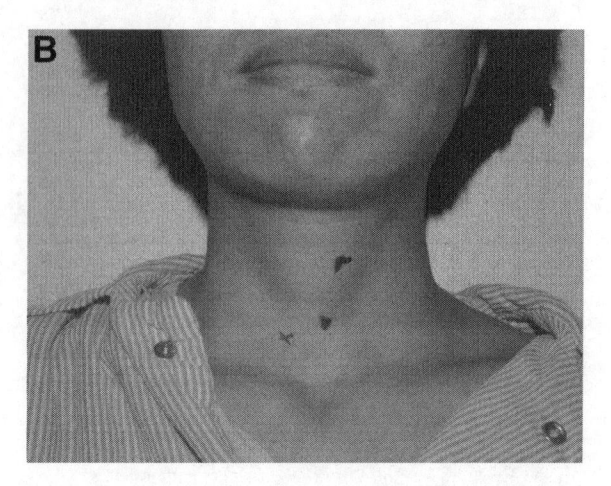

Fig. 34. Part **A** is an anterior (ant) parallel-hole collimator image obtained 48 h after ^{131}I administration. Radioactive markers are placed at the chin (c), suprasternal notch (s), and xiphoid (x). Three focal areas of radioiodine uptake are noted in the thyroid bed. With the use of a radioactive marker, these areas were localized to the patient's skin (**B**).

Comment: As already noted in many earlier figures, radioactive markers can be useful to denote anatomical landmarks and are frequently so indispensable that they are virtually mandatory. Marking the patient's skin can also be valuable by demonstrating that an area of radioiodine accumulation localizes to a palpable mass, lymph node, or salivary gland. Subsequently, these anatomic markers may guide fine-needle aspiration (with or without ultrasound guidance), thereby helping determine the etiology of the radioiodine accumulation. Of note, radioactive markers should not be positioned in such a way that the uptake is obscured under the marker, except when used to localize the region within the patient.

PART 6
MISCELLANEOUS

^{124}I PET

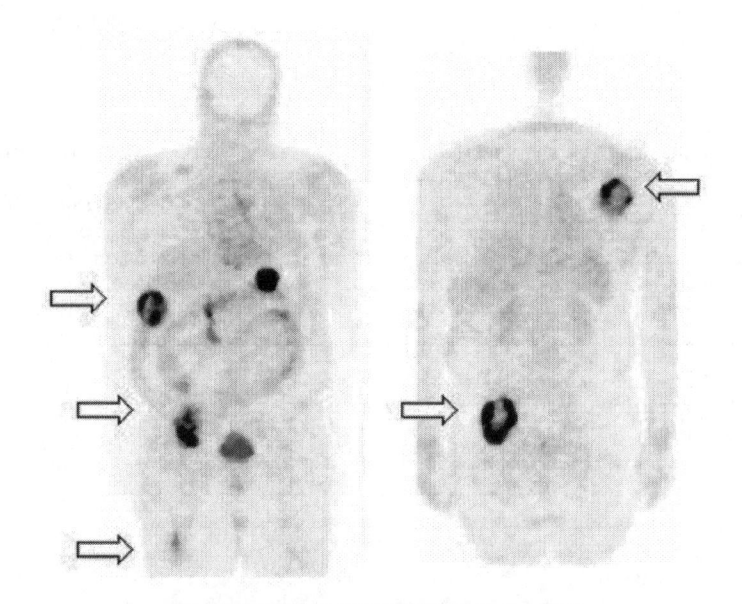

Selected coronal slices

Fig. 35. The above high-quality tomographic whole-body images were obtained after the administration of the positron-emitting radioisotope ^{124}I using a PET-imaging system. The anterior (left) and posterior (right) scans chosen from the complete set of coronal whole-body images demonstrate multiple areas of functioning metastases (white arrows). Image reproduced with permission of the author and the *Journal of Nuclear Medicine (35)*.

Comment: The potential advantages and disadvantages of ^{124}I PET have already been discussed in Chapters 14 and 34. The advantages include:

- Higher resolution
- Tomographic images
- A half-life that permits delayed imaging
- The ability to perform lesional and blood (bone marrow) dosimetry
- The ability to coregister the PET images with CT, MRI, or both for more precise anatomical localization

The present disadvantages are availability, cost, and the potential for stunning.

REFERENCES

1. Wartofsky L. Thyroid nodules. In Van Nostrand D, Bloom G, Wartofsky L, editors. Thyroid Cancer: A Guide for Patients. Baltimore: Keystone Press, Inc., 2004; 15–31.
2. Manier S, Van Nostrand D, Atkins F, Wu SY. I-131 neck and chest scintigraphy. In Van Nostrand D, Baum S, editors. Primers and Atlases of Clinical Nuclear Medicine. Philadelphia: J.B. Lippincott Co., 1988.
3. Makani S, Kim W, Gaba AR. Struma Ovarii with a focus of papillary thyroid cancer: a case report and review of the literature. Gynecol Oncol 2004; 94:835–839.
4. Griffiths AN, Jain B, Vine SJ. Papillary thyroid carcinoma of struma ovarii. J Obstet Gynaecol 2004; 24:92–93.
5. DeSimone CP, Lele SM, Modesitt SC. Malignant struma ovarii: a case report and analysis of cases reported in the literature with focus on survival and I-131 therapy. Gynecol Oncol 2003; 89:543–548.
6. Yeh EI, Mead RC, Ruetz PP. Radionuclide study of struma ovarii. J Nucl Med 1973; 14:118–124.
7. Salvatore M, Rufini V, Daudone MS, et al. Occasional detection of "struma ovarii" in a patient with thyroid cancer. Radiol Med 1991; 744–767.
8. Kulkarni K, Kim SM, Intenzo C. Can salivary gland uptakes on a diagnostic I-131 scan predict acute salivary gland dysfunction in patients receiving radioiodine therapy for thyroid cancer? J Nucl Med 2004; 5S:291P
9. Norby EH, Neutze J, Van Nostrand D, et al. Nasal radioiodine activity; a prospective study of frequency, intensity, and pattern. J Nucl Med 1990; 31:52–54.
10. Van Nostrand D, Neutze J, Atkins F. Side effects of "rational dose" iodine-131 therapy for metastatic well differentiated thyroid carcinoma. J Nucl Med 1986; 27:1519–1527.
11. Jackson GL, Flickinger FW, Graham WP, Kennedy TJ. Thymus accumulation of radioactive iodine. Penn Med 1979; 11:37–38.
12. Wilson RL, Cowan R. Tc-99m pertechnetate uptake in a thymoma: Case report. Clin Nucl Med 1982; 7:149–150.
13. Vermiglio F, Baudin E, Travagli P, et al. Iodine concentration by the thymus in thyroid carcinoma. J Nucl Med 1996; 37:1830–1831.
14. Ziessman HA, Bahar H, Fahey FH, Dubiansky V. Hepatic visualization of iodine-131 whole-body thyroid cancer scans. J Nucl Med 1987; 28:1408–1411.
15. Chung JK, Lee YJ, Jeong YM, et al. Clincal significance of hepatic visualization on iodine-131 whole body scan in patients with thyroid carcinoma. J Nucl Med 1997; 38:1191–1195.
16. Oppenheimer JH. Thyroid hormones in liver. Mayo Clin Proc 1972; 47:854–863.
17. Hillier AP. Deiodination of thyroid hormones by the perfused rat liver. J Physiol 1972; 222:475–485.
17a. Davidson J, McDougall IR. How frequently is the thymus seen on whole-body iodine-131 diagnostic and post-treatment scans? Eur J Nucl Med 2000; 27:425–430.
17b. Michigishi T, Mizukami Y, Shuke N, et al. Visualization of the thymus with therapeutic doses of radioiodine in patients with thyroid cancer. Eur J Nucl Med 1993; 20:75–79.
18. Van Nostrand. Radioiodine whole body scanning: overview and the different types of scans for well-differentiated thyroid cancer. In Van Nostrand D, Bloom G, Wartofsky L, editors. Thyroid Cancer: A Guide for Patients. Baltimore: Keystone Press, Inc., 2004; 111–123.
19. Thomas SR, Maxon HR, Kereiakes JG. In vivo quantitation of lesion radioactivity using external counting methods. Med Phys 1976; 3:253–255.
20. Thomas SR, Maxon HR, Kereiakes JG, Saenger EL. Quantitative external counting techniques enabling improved diagnostic and therapeutic decisions in patients with well-differentiated thyroid cancer. Radiology 1997; 122:731–737.
21. Schlumberge M, Challeton C, De Vathaire F, et al. Radioactive iodine treatment and external radiotherapy for lung and bone metastases from thyroid carcinoma. J Nucl Med 1996; 37:598–605.
22. Nemec J, Zamrazil V, Pohunkova D, Roohling S. Radioiodide treatment of pulmonary metastases of differentiated thyroid cancer. Results and prognostic factors. Nuklearmedizin 1979; 18:86–90.
23. Schlumberger M, Tubiana M, De Vathaire F, et al. Long-term results of treatment of 283 patients with lung and bone metastases from differentiated thyroid cancer. J Clin Endocrinol Metab 1986; 63:960–967.
24. Bennett DE, Million RR, Ackerman IV. Bilateral radiation pneumonitis. A complication of the radiotherapy of bronchogenic carcinoma. Cancer 1969; 23:1001–1018.
25. Fulkerson WJ, McLendon RE, Prosnitz LR. Adult respiratory distress syndrome after limited radiotherapy. Cancer 1986; 57:1941–1946.
25a. Hindié E, Melliere D, Lange F, et al. Functioning pulmonary metastases of thyroid cancer: does radioiodine influence the prognosis? J Nucl Med 2003; 30:974–981.
26. Monson JM, Start P, Reilly JJ, et al. Clinical radiation pneumonitis and radiographic changes after thoracic radiation therapy for lung carcinoma. Cancer 1998; 82:842–850.
27. Guglielmi R, Pacella CM, Dottorini ME, et al. Severe thyrotoxicosis due to hyperfunctioning liver metastasis from follicular carcinoma: treatment with (131)I and interstitial laser ablation. Thyroid 1999; 9:173–177.
28. Misaki T, Iwata M, Kasagi K, Konishi J. Brain metastasis from differentiated thyroid cancer in patients treated with radioiodine for bone and lung lesions. Ann Nucl Med 2000; 14:111–114.
29. Parker LN, Wu SY, Kim DD, et al. Recurrence of papillary thyroid carcinoma presenting as a focal neurologic deficit. Arch Int Med 1986; 146:1985–1987.
30. Smallridge RC, Castro MR, Morris JC, et al. Renal metastases from thyroid papillary carcinoma: study of sodium iodide symporter expression. Thyroid 2001; 11:795–804.
31. Bakheet SM, Hammami MM, Powe J. False-positive radioiodine uptake in the abdomen and the pelvis: radioiodine retention in the kidneys and review of the literature. Clin Nucl Med 1996; 21:932–937.
32. Kim EE, Pjura G, Gobuty A, et al. 131-I uptake in a benign serous cystadenoma of the ovary. Eur J Nucl Med 1984; 9:433–435.
33. Morgan R, Cote M. Abnormal uptake of I-131 mimicking salivary gland uptake in a patient with diffuse dental disease. Clin Nucl Med 2000; 25:314–315.
34. Howarth DM, Forstrom LA, O'Connor MK, et al. Patient-related pitfalls and artifacts in nuclear medicine imaging. Semin Nuc Med 1996; 26:295–307.
35. Sgouros G, Kolbert KS, Sheikh A, et al. Patient-specific dosimetry for 131I thyroid cancer therapy using 124-I PET and 3-dimensional-internal dosimetry (3D-ID) software. J Nucl Med 2004; 45:1366–1372.
36. Casara D, Rubello D, Saladini G, et al. Different features of pulmonary metastases in differentiated thyroid cancer: natural history and multivariate statistical analysis of prognostic variables. J Nucl Med 1993; 34:1626–1631.

16
False-Positive Radioiodine Scans in Thyroid Cancer

Brahm Shapiro, Vittoria Rufini, Ayman Jarwan, Onelio Geatti, Kimberlee J. Kearfott, Lorraine M. Fig, Ian D. Kirkwood, John E. Freitas, and Milton D. Gross

INTRODUCTION

The whole-body radioiodine scan remains an important component in the postoperative treatment of patients with well-differentiated thyroid cancer. Because normal thyroid tissue remnants and residual or metastatic foci of well-differentiated thyroid cancer have the unique ability to concentrate, organify, and store radioiodine, the whole-body scan provides a depiction of those tissues that can be ablated with therapeutic doses of radioiodine. Over time, it has become obvious that the whole-body scan may also reveal foci of radioiodine accumulation from a wide variety of other causes.

This chapter provides an update of an article in the *Seminars of Nuclear Medicine** in 2000 that detailed the pathophysiological classification of artifacts, anatomic and physiological variants, and nonthyroidal diseases that may give rise to false-positive whole body scans in postoperative patients with thyroid cancer. These include ectopic foci of normal thyroid tissue, nonthyroidal physiological sites (e.g., choroid plexus, salivary glands, gastric mucosa, and urinary tract), contamination by physiological secretions, ectopic gastric mucosa, other gastrointestinal abnormalities, urinary tract abnormalities, mammary abnormalities, serious cavities and cysts, inflammation and infection, nonthyroidal neoplasms, and other unexplained causes.

For over four decades, whole-body radioiodine scanning of patients with thyroid cancer after a thyroidectomy has been widely accepted as a central component of the treatment of this disease (1–14). The value of the technique lies in its ability to detect foci of residual normal thyroid tissue, as well as tumor and metastatic spread to remote sites. The modality may depict disease that is otherwise undetectable by any other modality (6,8–10,15). Furthermore, uptake of radioiodine on diagnostic studies permits the selection of patients for whom radioiodine therapy is an appropriate alternative (6,8,9,15).

All of this is based on the unique property of thyroid tissue to concentrate, organify, and retain radioiodine (2,7–9, 11–19). Many thyroid cancers retain this characteristic property; thus, foci of uptake on postthyroidectomy scans are considered highly specific for thyroid tissue, whether it is residual remnant, normal, or malignant in the neck or elsewhere (2,7–9,11–19). This specificity is unfortunately reduced by uptake in other tissues that can concentrate radioiodine but do not retain it in organic form (Fig. 1). These include the choroid plexus, salivary glands, nasopharynx, and stomach; furthermore, excretion via the kidney, liver, and gut may depict these organs and the bladder (2,6–9, 11,16,17,18). The literature is replete with a growing collection of reports of uptake in these organs and tissues and their associated diseases, as well as other pathological processes (1,4,6,8,12–16,21–24).

The accurate interpretation of postthyroidectomy whole-body radioiodine images requires a thorough knowledge and understanding of all these potential confounding phenomena (1,2,4,6–9,15,21,22,24). Imaging after the therapeutic administration of large activities of radioiodine permits verification of the biodistribution of the therapeutic prescribed activity and may represent an otherwise greater extent of disease (6–9). The same problem of interpretation applies in this posttherapeutic situation as in diagnostic imaging. Unfortunately, the literature is widely scattered and consists primarily of isolated case reports and small series, or it is hidden within larger works as anecdotal descriptions (1,3, 4,6,8,12,16,21–24). We have sought to approach this problem via a detailed review with the available data based on the underlying physiological principles governing the biodistribution of radioactive iodine. This method permits a logical classification and pathophysiological interpretation of the

---

*Modified from ref. *214* with permission from Elsevier.

From: *Thyroid Cancer: A Comprehensive Guide to Clinical Management, 2/e*
Edited by: L. Wartofsky and D. Van Nostrand © Humana Press Inc., Totowa, NJ

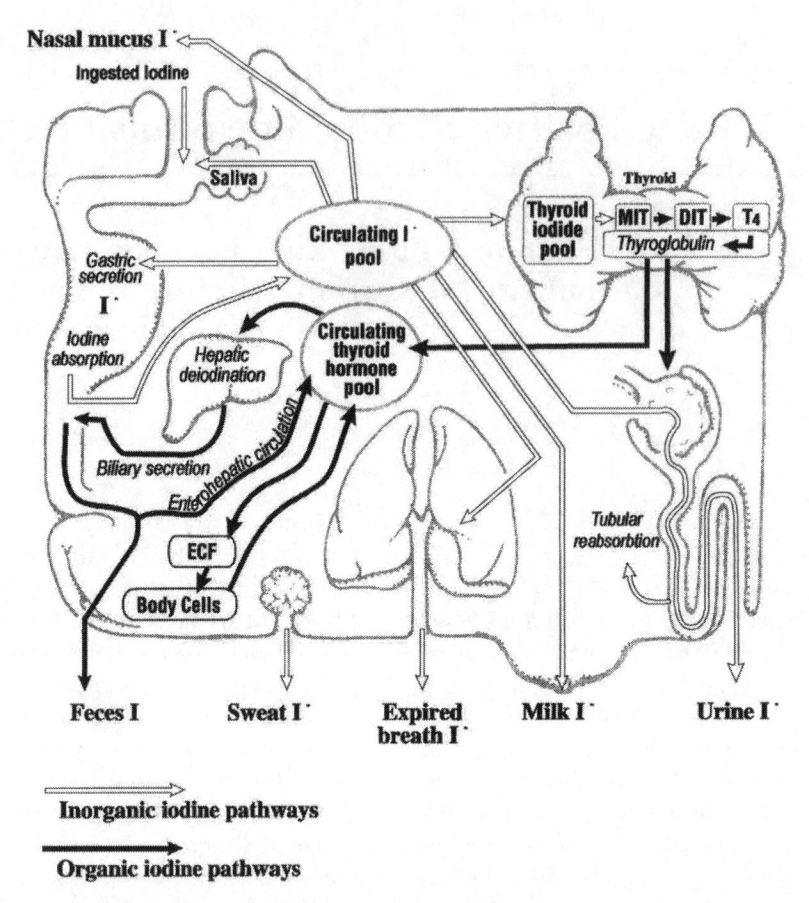

Fig. 1. A schematic representation of iodine metabolism. (From ref. *214* with permission from Elsevier.)

disparate literature concerning artifacts, anatomical and physiological variants, and nonthyroidal diseases responsible for false-positive radioiodine scans in thyroid cancer. The administration of large activities of radioiodine for the treatment of residual or metastatic well-differentiated thyroid cancer is a uniquely effective systemic therapy when applied to appropriate patients *(3,5–9,11)*. Correct interpretation of posttherapy images may prevent misinterpretation and the inappropriate use of radioiodine therapy.

ECTOPIC NORMAL THYROID TISSUE

The embryological origin of the thyroid gland from the foramen cecum, at the junction between the anterior two thirds and posterior one third of the tongue, with its subsequent descent and bifurcation in the neck, leads to a wide variety of abnormalities owing to embryological maldevelopment (Table 1; *4,25–59*). Thus, complete failure to migrate causes a lingual thyroid (Fig. 2), and incomplete migration results in a high cervical thyroid, whereas excessive migration causes a superior mediastinal thyroid or even a paracardiac gland *(4,25–43)*. Foci of functioning tissue may remain anywhere along the embryological thyroglossal duct tract *(4,25–27,31,42–44)*. Abnormal migration results in widely divergent ectopic foci (e.g., esophageal, intratracheal, and intrahepatic; *4,25–27,34,35,45,46,60–62*). The so-called "lateral aberrant thyroid tissue" is highly controversial; many believe that it is, in fact, well-differentiated thyroid cancer metastatic to, and completely replacing, cervical lymph nodes with an occult thyroidal primary *(4,26,27,54,58–60)*. Finally, normally differentiated thyroid tissue may occur in the ovary (struma ovarii), either as the thyroidal component of a teratoma, an isolated finding, or as a malignancy *(4,26,27,47–57)*.

PHYSIOLOGICAL SITES OF NONTHYROIDAL UPTAKE OR BIODISTRIBUTION

Although thyroid tissue is unique in its ability to organify iodide and synthesize thyroid hormones, a variety of glandular tissues share with the thyroid gland the ability to actively transport radioiodine against a chemical gradient from the plasma into the secretory lumen (Table 2; *2,18,63*). Concentration gradients of up to 20:1 can be achieved. Tissues that share this property include gastric mucosa, nasal

Table 1
Ectopic Normal Thyroid Tissue

Ectopic Normal Thyroid Tissue Sites	Mechanism for Radioiodine Uptake	Embryonic Thyroid Migration/Development
Lingual thyroid (4,26–29,43)	Normal thyroid radioiodine uptake/organification	Failure to migrate (descend)
High cervical thyroid (4,15,26,27,30,31,34,43)	Same as above	Incomplete migration
Thoracic superior mediastinal thyroid (4,26,27,36–40)	Same as above	Excessive migration
Paracardiac thyroid (4,26,36,37,40,41)	Same as above	Same as above
Intracardiac (struma cordis)		
Pericardial		
Thyroglossal tract (4,26,27,31,42,43,62)	Same as above	Foci of functioning thyroid tissue along the route of migration, may be stimulated by ↑TSH postthyroidectomy
Esophageal thyroid (4,26,27,35,43,46)	Same as above	Abnormal migration
Intratracheal thyroid (4,26,35,45)	Same as above	Same as above
Ovarian thyroid (struma ovarii) (4,26,27,48–56)	Same as above	Differentiation of thyroid tissue in a benign ovarian teratoma/malignant with metastases
Lateral aberrant thyroid (4,16,26,27,57–59)	Same as above	Many/all are metastases to cervical lymph nodes
Intrahepatic thyroid tissue (4,26,27,34,60,61)	Same as above	Must be distinguished from biliary cyst(s)

Source: From ref. *214* with permission from Elsevier.

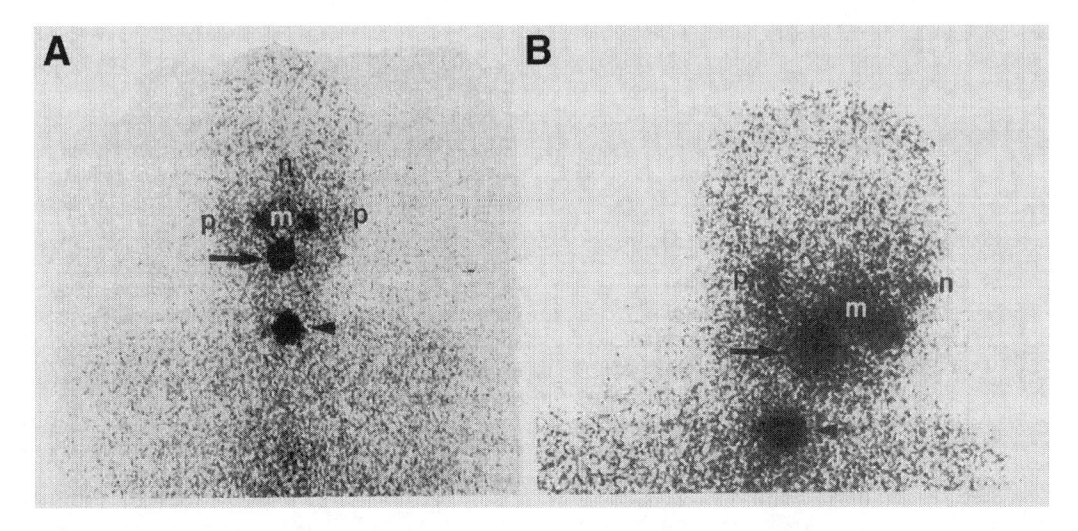

Fig. 2. (**A**) Anterior and (**B**) lateral views of the head, neck, and upper chest 24 h after 2 mCi (74 MBq) of radioiodine following a total thyroidectomy for papillary thyroid cancer. There was a small thyroid bed remnant (arrowhead) and normal uptake of radioiodine in the nose (n), mouth (m), and parotid glands (p). The intense midline focus of uptake below the floor of the mouth was owing to a lingual thyroid remnant in the base of the tongue (arrow). (From ref. *214* with permission from Elsevier.)

Table 2
Physiological Sites of Nonthyroidal Uptake or Biodistribution

Physiological Sites of Nonthyroidal Uptake/Distribution	Mechanism for Radioiodine Uptake	Comments About Normal Biodistribution
Normal cardiac blood pool displaced by pectus excavatum (4,106)	Radioiodine transported from site of absorption via circulation	Activity fades as blood pool clears with time (not to be confused with lung lesions)
Carotid ectasia (4,21,73,107)	Radioiodine transported from site of absorption via circulation	Activity fades as blood pool clears with time (not to be confused with tumor spread to cervical lymph nodes)
Salivary gland uptake (4,6,18,31,63,74)	Site of active radioiodine transport	Knowledge of normal biodistribution required for image interpretation
Gastric mucosal uptake (4,18,72)	Site of active radioiodine transport	Same as above
Nasal mucosal uptake (4,66,72,73,76,77,85)	Site of active radioiodine transport	Same as above
Gut activity (4,72) by gastric mucosa	Translocation of activity secreted	Same as above
Urinary tract excretion (4,24,94,95)	Major route of clearance	Same as above
Choroid plexus uptake (4)	Site of active radioiodine transport	Not to be confused with brain or skull metastases
Persistant uptake in cardiac and great vessel blood pool or dilated veins (2,4,73,96,97,109)	Slow renal clearance in renal disease or absent renal clearance in renal failure and on dialysis	Slow or absent renal clearance from blood pool owing to kidney disease
Nonlactating breast uptake (4,18,70,84,86,87)	Site of active radioiodine transport	Usually faint, but intensity may be quite variable (not to be confused with lung metastases)
Lactating breast uptake (see Fig. 3) (4,15,18,64,67–69,71,72,75,80–82,85,87,93)	Site of active radioiodine transport	Uptake may be intense; breastfeeding must stop before scintigraphy, as significant radioiodine may be transferred to the infant
Liver uptake (4,101,102,104,105,155)	Hepatic uptake of radioiodine-labeled thyroid hormones synthesized by functioning normal or neoplastic thyroid tissue	The uptake by normal residual thyroid tissue or functioning thyroid cancer deposits is usually obvious
Gallbladder uptake (4,94,105,155)	Enterohepatic excretion of radioiodine thyroid hormone and metabolites	Unusual cause for focal uptake in right upper quadrant may be discharged into gut by gallbladder
Swallowed saliva in pharynx and esophagus (4,65,83)	Activity translated from site of secretion in salivary glands	Knowledge of normal biodistribution required for image interpretation, restudy after swallow of water
Lacrimal gland (4,91)	Site of active radioiodine transport	Secretion in tears

Source: From ref. 214 with permission from Elsevier.

mucosa, salivary glands, lacrimal gland, and the lactating or nonlactating breast (Fig. 3; *2,4,15,18,63,94*). Although not a glandular epithelium, the choroid plexus is nevertheless a site of secretory function for the formation of cerebrospinal fluid (CSF) that also shows radioiodine uptake *(4)*.

Being a small ion, iodide is readily cleared by glomerular filtration and subsequently subject to a balance between tubular secretion and reabsorption, such that the urine is the principal route of radioiodine excretion *(2,4,24,94–96)*. Clearance of radioiodine is delayed in patients on dialysis *(96–100)*. Urinary iodide concentration or excretion rates are a good index of the state of iodine nutrition.

Thyroid hormones undergo metabolic degradation and excretion in conjugated form into the gut *(4,72)*. Hence, radioiodine uptake by the liver that exists several days after radioiodine administration is an index of the amount of functioning (hormone-synthesizing) tissue present *(4,72,76,94,101–104)*. The gallbladder may occasionally be depicted when biliary excretion is extensive *(4,101,102,104, 105)*. The majority of the iodine-containing compounds excreted via the liver undergo further metabolism and reabsorption, with reutilization in an enterohepatic circulation *(4,102,104,105)*.

After the prompt and efficient absorption of radioiodine in the upper gastrointestinal tract, the anion is carried to all bodily tissues via circulation, and particularly at earlier imaging time points, radioiodine within the vascular compartment may be visualized *(4,106)*. Examples of artifactual cardiovascular depictions include the heart and great vessels, especially in the presence of pectus excavatum and carotid ectasia *(2,4,21,73,96–98,107)*. In the presence of renal insufficiency, clearance from the vascular compartment will be delayed.

CONTAMINATION BY PHYSIOLOGICAL SECRETIONS

Several potentially misleading artifacts can arise from contamination by physiological or pathological secretions derived from those organs that are capable of uptake and excretion of radioiodine (Table 3). These include urine, saliva, nasal secretions, other respiratory tract secretions, sweat, vomit, and breast milk (Figs. 4 and 5; *1,10,22,64, 67–69,72–74,76,92,110–127)*. Any focus of radioiodine uptake for which there is not an obvious physiological or pathological cause must be suspected as arising from contamination by secretions. The patient should always be imaged in a clean gown; if necessary, this should be replaced after an attempt is made to wash away any unexplained foci of radioiodine *(95,110,117,128–130)*.

Irritants or foreign bodies may exaggerate this phenomenon, such as tracheostomy tubes, bronchitis, nose rings, ocular prostheses, chewing gum or chewing tobacco *(11,92,116,117,122,123)*. Unless sweating is excessive from a fever or high environmental temperature, this route of excretion is seldom prominent but may be increased in cystic fibrosis *(110,112,113,117,124)*.

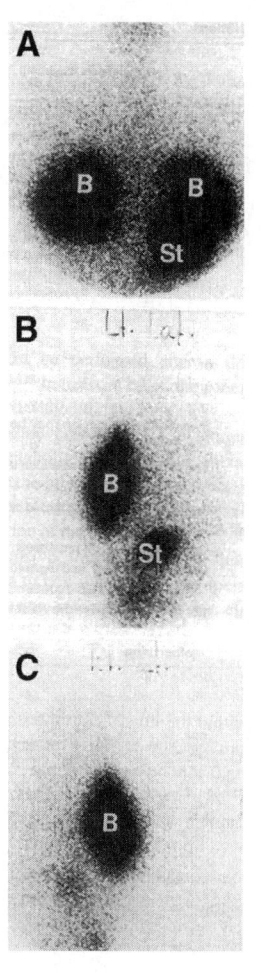

Fig. 3. A diagnostic 2-mCi (74 MBq) radioiodine scan was performed 1 wk after cessation of breastfeeding. The patient has been breastfeeding for 18 mo. Some milk could still be expressed from the breast. (Panel **A**) Anterior, (panel **B**) left lateral, and (panel **C**) right lateral images of the neck and chest, showing (B) intense bilateral breast uptake and normal gastric uptake (S). This clearly demonstrates that a delay of longer than 1 wk after weaning is required for resolution of breast uptake of radioiodine. (From ref. *214* with permission from Elsevier.)

ECTOPIC GASTRIC MUCOSA

The ability of gastric mucosa to concentrate radioiodine is a prominent feature on whole-body radioiodine scintigraphy, and this property is retained by ectopic gastric mucosa (Table 4; *4,18,21,73,89,131–142)*. Ectopic gastric mucosa may arise *de novo* as an abnormality of embryological development in diverticuli (e.g., Meckel's diverticulum) or in duplication cysts almost anywhere along the foregut and mid-gut, or as a component of ovarian or other teratomas

Table 3
Contamination by Physiological Secretions

Sources of Contamination by Physiological Secretions	Mechanism for Radioiodine Uptake*	Comments About Normal Radioiodine Biodistribution
Urine (see Fig. 1) (22,95,108–120)	Major route of radioiodine excretion	Clothing must be changed just before scanning; attempts to wash away unexplained foci should always be made if there is any suspicion of contamination (not to be confused with pathological uptake)
Saliva (see Fig. 1) (63,78,93,116,117,120–122)	Active radioiodine transport into saliva	Typically onto hair, skin, clothing. May be seen on neurosurgical immobilization frame
Nasal secretions (66,73,76,77,93,114,115,117–120)	Active radioiodine transport by mucus glands	Same as above
Nasal secretions on nose ring (115)	Active radioiodine transport by mucus glands and drying on ring	Same as above
Respiratory secretions (especially with tracheostomy) (see Fig. 11) (117,122,123)	Active radioiodine transport by mucus glands	Same as above
Sweat (108,112,113,117,124)	Active radioiodine transport into sweat	Sweat iodide excretion may be greater in cystic fibrosis
Vomit (72,117)	Active radioiodine transport into gastric secretions	Vomiting may occur as a side effect of radioiodine therapy
Breast milk (1,64,67,68,72,75,80,90,92,125–127)	Active radioiodine transport into milk (iodine is an essential micronutrient for the infant)	Activity may be transmitted to infant
Lacrimal on artificial eye (91,93,121)	Active radioiodine transport into tears stimulate salivation with transport of radioiodine saliva	Could be washed off prosthesis
Chewing gum and chewing tobacco (116)		Gum, tobacco quid, and expectorated saliva may cause extensive contamination
External contamination (source unknown) (95,110,117,128–130)	Origin of contamination not always obvious	Contamination above the waist is usually saliva/nasal, below the waist is often urine

*Consequence of normal physiological concentration or route of excretion.
Source: From ref. 214 with permission from Elsevier.

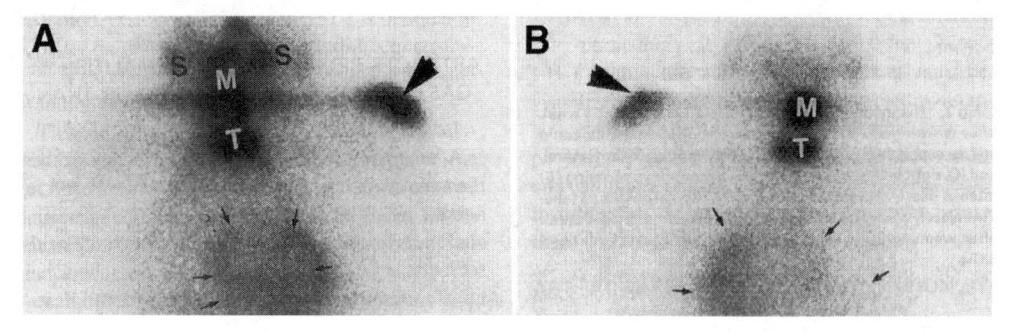

Fig. 4. (A) Anterior and **(B)** posterior views of the neck and chest in a patient 6 wk after a near-total thyroidectomy for papillary thyroid cancer obtained 24 h after a 2-mCi (74 MBq) radioiodine tracer dose shows (s) normal salivary gland uptake and (m) mouth activity. There was extensive salivary contamination of the shirt over the patient's shoulder (arrowhead) and a prominent halo around the heart from a pericardial effusion caused by hypothyroidism (small arrows). (From ref. *214* with permission from Elsevier.)

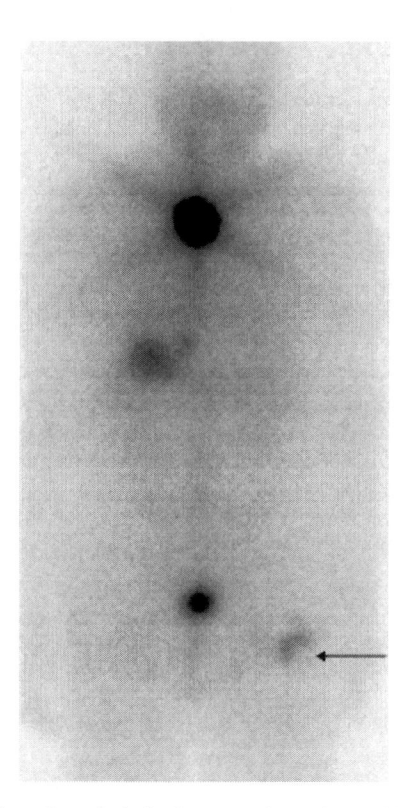

Fig. 5. Anterior whole-body scan of a patient with significant thyroid remnant activity in the neck. A focus of radioiodine in the region of the hip (arrow) is a handkerchief in the patient's left pocket.

(44,89,131,133). Chronic inflammatory changes may cause metaplastic transformation of gastrointestinal epithelium of various types to gastric mucosa [e.g., squamous to gastric mucosa in Barrett's esophagus and gastric metaplasia in chronic colitis *(144)*]. Finally, normal gastric mucosa may be anatomically displaced to abnormal anatomic sites. Mechanisms for this phenomenon include a hiatal hernia (Fig. 6A,B) and surgeries, e.g., gastric pullthrough *(4,18, 21,89,133–137,139–141)*.

ABNORMALITIES OF GASTROINTESTINAL UPTAKE OTHER THAN ECTOPIC GASTRIC MUCOSA

Many pathophysiological processes other than active gastric transport of radioiodine may result in altered radioiodine biodistribution (Table 5). These processes include active concentration by salivary glands, with secretion into saliva and subsequent abnormal transfer of the radioactivity into upper gastrointestinal diverticuli, delay by mechanical esophageal stricture, or dysmotility *(4,16,18,31,65,72,83,89, 117,123,130,144–148)*. When radioiodine is used in capsule form, rather than in solution, poorly dissolved capsules may be retained in the esophagus under these circumstances *(149)*. Asymmetrical depiction of the salivary glands may follow ductal obstruction owing to stone (Fig. 7), stricture, or tumor *(4,6,8,16,18,31,63,72,74,149–154)*. Prior surgery or radiotherapy may reduce salivary gland radioiodine uptake; this may be asymmetrical. Intraluminal radioiodine within the upper gastrointestinal tract is derived from swallowed saliva or active gastric secretion and can be refluxed into the esophagus (Fig. 8; *4,18,65,72,83,89,131,147,150, 151)*. This phenomenon is extremely common, and to distinguish esophageal reflux activity from mediastinal nodal metastases, studies must be performed after a drink of water *(3,4,6,8,16,89,142)*. In resistant cases, the patient may have to be studied while sitting upright.

Prominent depiction of the colon may be the result of radioiodine secreted by the stomach, radioiodine-labeled metabolites of thyroxine metabolism excreted into the bile, and possible direct secretion by colonic mucosa *(1,3, 4,7,8,16,94,101,102,104,105,155,156)*. When extensive, this degrades the quality of images because of possible masking of metastatic sites and decreasing information density elsewhere in the scan, as well as increasing colonic radiation exposure *(156)*. The decreased colonic motility, which almost always accompanies the hypothyroidism required for whole-body radioiodine studies, is a major

Table 4
Uptake by Ectopic Gastric Mucosa

Sites of Uptake by Ectopic Gastric Mucosa	Mechanism for Radioiodine Uptake	Comments About Normal Function of Gastric Mucosa
Meckel's diverticulum *(4,131)*	Owing to normal active radioiodine transport into gastric secretions	Gastric mucosa at abnormal site
Gastric duplication cysts (may occur in esophagus, duodenum, and small bowel) *(4,89,133)*	Same as above	Gastric mucosa at abnormal site
Normal stomach in abnormal locations (hiatal hernia, gastric pull through; see Fig. 6A,B) *(4,18,2189,133–141)*	Same as above	Displacement of stomach from normal site
Barrett's esophagus *(142)*	Same as above	Gastric mucosa present at abnormal site in esophagus

Source: From ref. *214* with permission from Elsevier.

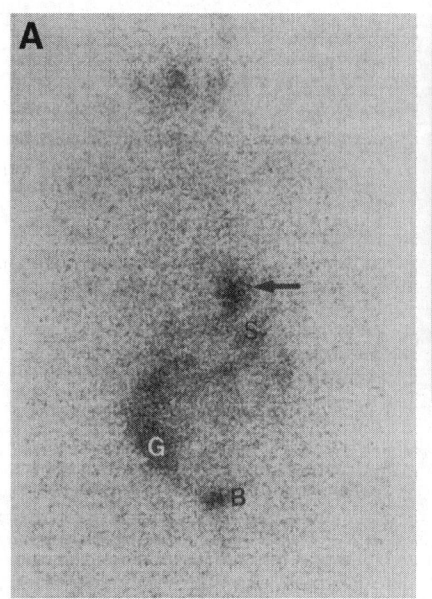

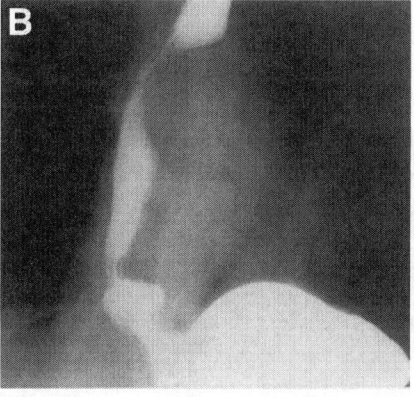

Fig. 6. (Panel **A**) Whole-body anterior image obtained 24 h after a dose of 2 mCi (74 MBq) of radioiodine in a patient with papillary thyroid carcinoma after a total thyroidectomy and radioiodine ablation of thyroid remnants. There is normal uptake of radioiodine in the nasopharynx and salivary glands, stomach (s), and gut (G) and excretion via the bladder (B), as well as a focus above the stomach (arrow) owing to a hiatal hernia. (This was confirmed by a barium study, see Fig. 6B.) (Panel **B**) Barium study showing the presence of a small hiatal hernia. (From ref. *214* with permission from Elsevier.)

contributing factor *(156)*. The appropriate use of laxatives should help remedy this problem *(156)*.

URINARY TRACT ABNORMALITIES

The urinary tract is the principal route of iodide excretion after glomerular filtration of the small anion and is a balance between tubular secretion and reabsorption (Table 6; *2–4,17,19,24,89*). Thus, the urine within the bladder is often the most radioactive site on the whole-body radioiodine scan, particularly at 24- and 48-h postadministration *(2,3, 6–8,16,21,24,89,120)*. Consequently, all dilations, diverticuli, and fistulae of the kidney, ureter, and bladder may show focal radioiodine retention *(3,4,6–8,16,24,27,89,120)*. The same is true of ectopic, horseshoe, and transplanted kidneys *(24)*. Renal cysts may show radioiodine uptake if they communicate with the urinary tract or if the epithelium that lines them has the capacity to concentrate and secrete iodide *(24,157)*. The simultaneous depiction of the urinary tract with a suitable renal tract–imaging agent, such as ^{99m}Tc-DTPA or ^{99m}Tc-MAG3 may be useful in characterizing the nature of these urinary tract abnormalities.

Table 5
Abnormalities of Gastrointestinal Uptake Other Than Ectopic Gastric Mucosa

Sites of Other Abnormalities of Gastrointestinal Uptake	Mechanism for Radioiodine Uptake (Normal Transport into Secretions)	Comments About Abnormal Motility or Structure
Zenker's diverticulum (143,144)	Active radioiodine transport into saliva	Retention of activity in swallowed saliva in diverticulum
Stricture of esophagus (83,145)	Active radioiodine transport into saliva	Retention of saliva above stricture
Achalasia/esophageal dysmotility (31,65,130,146,152,153)	Active radioiodine transport into saliva	Delayed clearance from esophagus
Poorly dissolved radioiodine capsule (149)	Lack of absorption and retention in the esophagus	Often combined with retention of saliva above stricture and delayed clearance from esophagus
Colonic bypass of esophagus (135,141)	Active radioiodine transport into saliva and gastric secretions	Delayed clearance and reflux from stomach
Gastroesophageal reflux (1,16,72,89,139)	Active radioiodine transport into gastric secretions.	Reflux of gastric activity into esophagus is common; always rescan after a drink of water if mediastinal activity is present
Abnormal location of bowel with normal radioiodine content (e.g., diaphragmatic or other hernias) (72,132,137,155)	Active radioiodine secreted into the lumen in patients	Luminal radioiodine activity observed at abnormal location
Constipation (156)	Active radioiodine transport into gastric secretions and translocation by luminal transport to small bowel and colon	Delayed transport of luminal radioiodine activity owing to abnormal colonic motility (may be a result of hypothyroidism)
Parotid gland uptake (154)	Active radioiodine secreted into the lumen in patients with ectasia	Pooling of activity in dilated duct as distinct from diffuse uptake in gland
Asymmetrical salivary glands (150)	Active radioiodine transport into saliva	Obstruction of salivary duct by stone, stricture, or tumor (or absence of normal gland owing to prior surgical removal or injury by radiation therapy)

Source: From ref. 214 with permission from Elsevier.

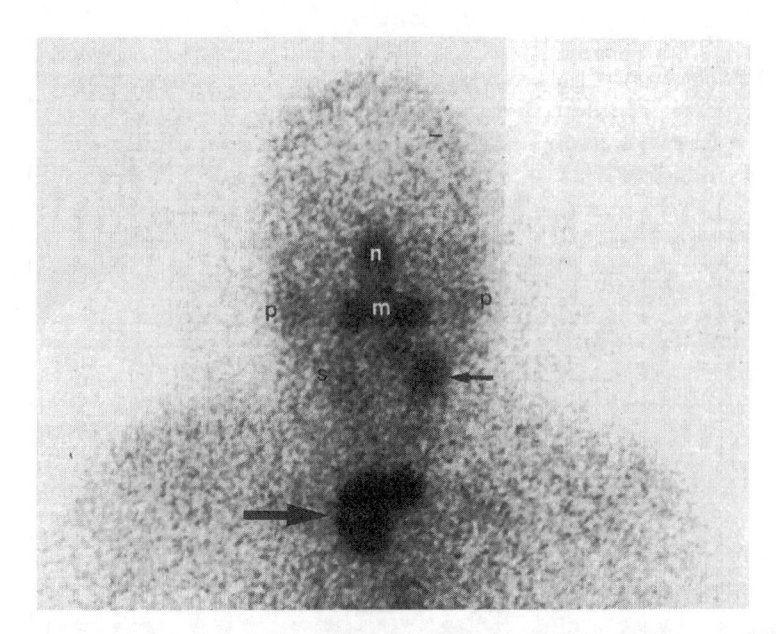

Fig. 7. Anterior scan of head, neck, and chest done 24 h after a 2-mCi (74 MBq) dose of radioiodine in a patient following near-total thyroidectomy for papillary thyroid cancer. There was a large thyroid remnant (large arrow), normal radioiodine uptake in the nose (n), mouth (m), parotid glands (p), and right submandibular gland (s). There was increased radioiodine uptake in the left submandibular gland from an obstructing stone (small arrow). (From ref. *214* with permission from Elsevier.)

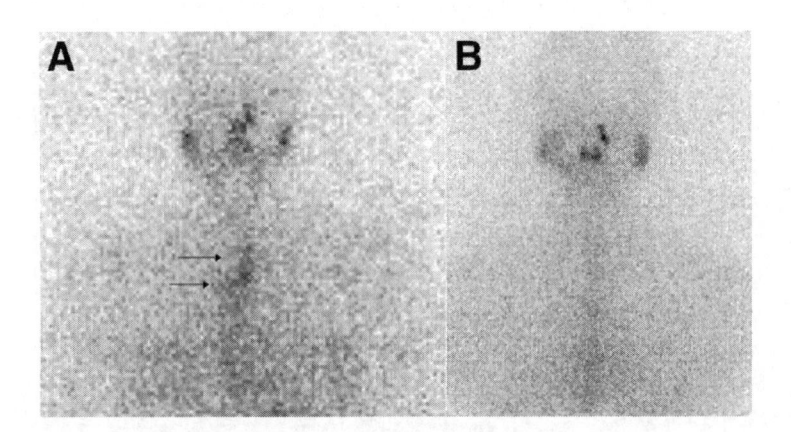

Fig. 8. Early (**A**) and late (**B**) anterior head and chest scans demonstrate radioiodine activity in the neck and chest (arrows) on the 24-h, but not in the 48-h postradioiodine administration image. This is an example of retained esophageal radioiodine that could be mistaken for either residual thyroid tissue, thyroid cancer in the thyroid bed, or metastases.

MAMMARY VARIATIONS AND ABNORMALITES

The glandular epithelium of the breast during lactation is capable of actively transporting the essential micronutrient iodide from plasma into milk with an efficiency of 20 to 1 (Table 7; *17,18,64,67,68,75,82,90,92,95,96,125–127, 162–167*). The lactating breast shows intense radioiodine uptake *(4,15,18,64,67–69,71,72,75,80–82,85,87,93)*. This is under systemic hormonal influence, including priming by estrogens, secretory stimulation by prolactin, and milk ejection by oxytocin, which acts on both breasts. In addition, local reflex secretory stimulation occurs, such that radioiodine uptake is greater in the breast, which is stimulated in asymmetrical or unilateral suckling. The phenomenon of breast uptake persists for weeks or even months after lactation ceases. Faint to moderate radioiodine uptake is also seen in nonlactating breast tissue, presumably from the same epithelial mechanism that operates in lactation *(4,18,70,84,86,87)*. This uptake may be symmetrical or asymmetrical and may

Table 6
Urinary Tract Abnormalities

Sites of Urinary Tract Abnormalities	Mechanism for Radioiodine Uptake	Comments About Slow Clearance From Urinary Tract or Abnormal Structures in Communication With Urinary Tract*
Hydronephrosis, extrarenal pelvis, and calyectasis (3,4,6,8,21,24,27)	Renal clearance of radioiodine into the urine as the major route of excretion	Slow clearance from dilated and/or obstructed renal collecting system
Renal cysts (24,157)	Same as above	Cyst communicates with urinary tract or nephrons
Urinary tract diverticuli (e.g., affecting renal pelvis, ureter, and bladder (4,6,8,21,24,27)	Same as above	Delayed clearance from diverticuli
Urinary tract fistulae (4,6,8,21,24,93)	Same as above	Radioiodine in urine transferred to abnormal locations by fistulous communications
Atonic or dilated bladder (4,6,8,21,24,27)	Same as above	Delayed clearance from bladder owing to obstruction or abnormal motility
Ectopic kidney or transplanted kidney (1,4,8,24,27,93)	Same as above	Normal renal handling of radioiodine at abnormal location

*Simultaneous imaging of urinary tract with suitable radiopharmaceutical (e.g., ^{99m}TC-DTPA or ^{99m}TC-MAG3) may be helpful.
Source: From ref. 214 with permission from Elsevier.

Table 7
Mammary Abnormalities

Sites of Mammary Abnormalities	Mechanism for Radioiodine Uptake*	Comments About Related Abnormalities of Location or Structure
Unilateral mammary hypertrophy (84,86,158,159)	Site of active radioiodine transport	Asymmetrical exaggeration of normal breast uptake
Supernumerary breast (92)	Site of active radioiodine transport	Additional foci of breast tissue may be found from axilla to groin
Asymmetrical lactation (92,158–160)	Site of active radioiodine transport	Asymmetrical suckling may stimulate radioiodine uptake into breast with greatest milk secretion
Lactational duct cyst (161)	Site of active radioiodine transport	Cyst may be lined with epithelium able to transport radioiodine into cyst lumen

*Breast duct epithelium actively transports radioiodine into the lumen.
Source: From ref. 214 with permission from Elsevier.

also be seen in unilateral mammary hypertrophy, supernumery breasts, and lactational duct cysts (Figs. 9 and 10; 84,86,92,158–161).

UPTAKE IN SEROUS CAVITIES AND CYSTS

The epithelial lining pleura, peritoneum, and pericardium are not able to actively transport radioiodine but may be permeable to passive diffusion even in the absence of inflammation (Table 8). This leads to the accumulation of radioiodine in pleural, peritoneal, and pericardial effusions, scrotal hydroceles, and pleuropericardial cysts (22,165–169). Similar processes appear to operate in ovarian cysts and lymphoepithelial cysts (167,168).

UPTAKE IN SITES OF INFLAMMATION OR INFECTION

Inflammation, whether it is sterile (autoimmune, traumatic, or ischemic) or from infection, results in increased blood flow caused by vasodilation, increased capillary

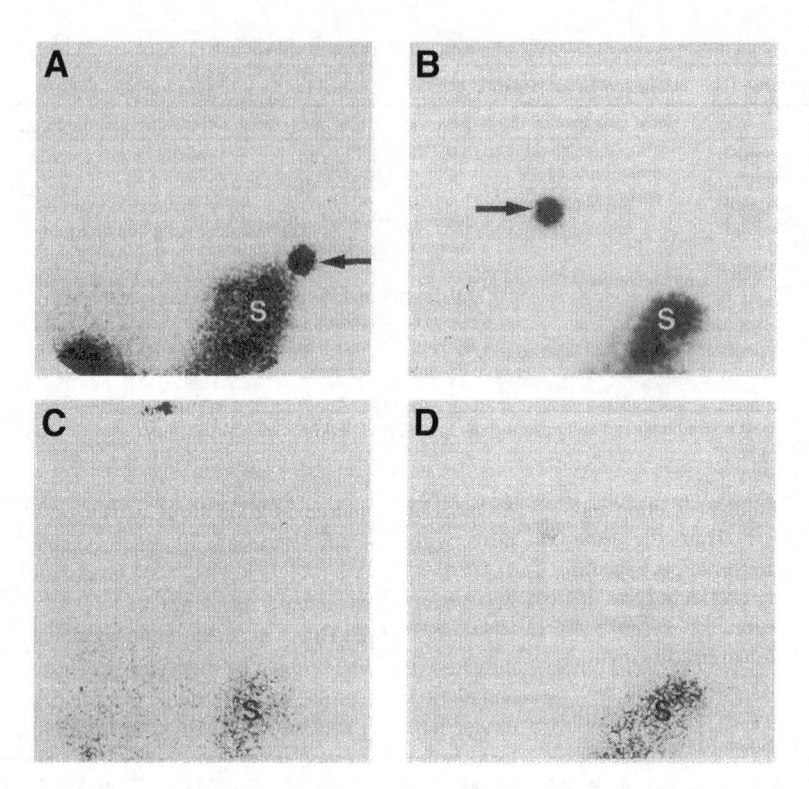

Fig. 9. Diagnostic radioiodine scans of the chest performed 24 h after a 2-mCi (74 MBq) tracer dose in a patient with a previously resected papillary thyroid carcinoma (anterior [**A**], left lateral [**B**]). A small intense focus of activity corresponded to a palpable breast cyst. After aspiration of the cyst fluid contents, the radioiodine uptake disappeared as shown in **C** (anterior) and **D** (left lateral), which are images obtained for lesser total counts. This indicates that the vast majority of the radioiodine activity was in the cyst fluid. Normal gastric uptake (S). (From ref. *214* with permission from Elsevier.)

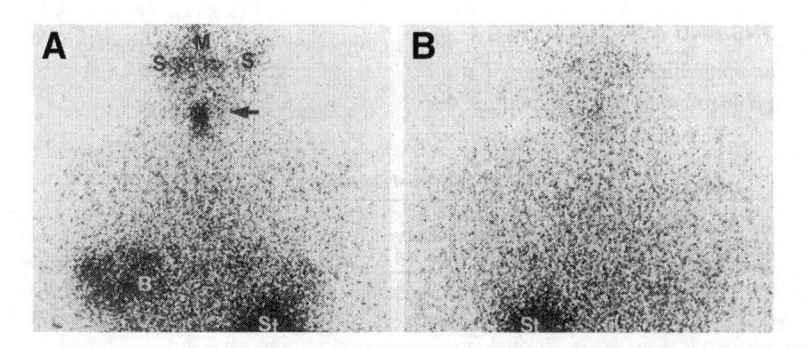

Fig. 10. (Panel **A**) Anterior and (panel **B**) posterior head, neck, and chest views 24 h after administration of 2 mCi (74 MBq) of radioiodine in a patient with papillary thyroid cancer after a prior thyroidectomy. Note thyroid bed radioiodine uptake (arrow) and normal stomach (St), salivary gland (S), and mouth (M) uptake. There is intense radioiodine uptake in the right breast (B; note clear visualization anteriorly but not posteriorly). The patient had ceased breastfeeding just prior to tracer administration but had only been feeding her infant from the right breast for months. Thus, although the hormonal milieu of both breasts was the same (e.g., prolactin levels) the local effect of suckling was important in radioiodine uptake by the lactating breast. (From ref. *214* with permission from Elsevier.)

permeability owing to the complex interplay of inflammatory cells, immune mediators, lymphokines, and other systemic and paracrine mediators (Table 9). This leads to radioiodine accumulation at sites of inflammatory and infectious processes in which increased blood flow delivers increased levels of radioiodine. The radioiodine diffuses through the capillaries that are rendered highly permeable, with accumulation in the increased extracellular water space (edema fluid) (Fig. 11; *1,6,12,22,93,121,151,166,167, 170–186*). These processes seem to be independent of the active iodide transport seen in thyroid, gastric, salivary, and other specialized epithelia *(18)*.

Table 8
Uptake in Serous Cavities and Cysts

Sites of Uptake in Serous Cavities or Cysts	Mechanism for Radioiodine Uptake	Comments About Diverse Locations and Factors That May Be Involved
Pericardial effusion (not associated with inflammation; see also Table 9) (22,165,168)	Cysts are lined by epithelia not able to actively transport	May be associated with hypothyroidism
Scrotal hydrocele (169)	Radioiodine; passive diffusion into cyst fluid with subsequent slow clearance	Must be distinguished from urinary contamination
Lymphoepithelial cysts (169)	Same as above	
Ovarian cysts (168,172)	Same as above	This does not include lesions (teratomas) with ectopic gastric, salivary gland, or thyroid epithelium
Pleuropericardial cysts (171)	Same as above	

Source: From ref. *214* with permission from Elsevier.

Table 9
Uptake in Sites of Inflammation or Infection*

Uptake in Sites of Inflammation/Infection	Mechanism for Radioiodine Uptake	Comments About Diverse Locations Possible*
Pulmonary (e.g., rheumatoid lung, bronchiectasis, fungal infection, or acute respiratory tract infection) (23,93,170–176)	Inflammation results in increased perfusion, vasodilation, and capillary permeability	Increased production of mucus may be an additional factor
Pericarditis (165,166)	Same as above	Frequently autoimmune in cause
Skin burns, superficial abrasions (169,175)	Same as above	Does not need to be infected to show radioiodine uptake
Dental disease/periodontal surgery (12,177,178)	Same as above	May not be clinically evident
Arthritis (e.g., rheumatoid) (179)	Same as above	Usually noninfected inflammatory lesion
Sinusitis and chronic sinusitis (1,93,180,182)	Same as above	Increased production of mucus may be an additional factor
Dacryocystitis (1,96)	Same as above	Increased uptake in gland beyond that owing to concentration in tears
Psoriatic plaques (6)	Same as above	Noninfected inflammatory lesion
Acute or chronic cholecystitis (181)	Same as above	Biliary excretion may also occur
Scalp folliculitis (182,183)	Same as above	Same as above
Sialoadenitis (154)	Same as above	Same as above
Recent myocardial infarct (184)	Increased capillary permeability and inflammation in region of infarcted myocardium implies coronary redistribution	Should not be confused with normal gastric uptake of radioiodine or activity in a hiatal hernia
Infected sebaceous cyst (181,185)	Inflammation results in increased perfusion, vasodilation, and capillary permeability	Sebaceous glands may also concentrate radioiodine
Frontal sinus mucocele (171,180,182)	Sinus mucosa capable of iodide transport	To be distinguished from acute or chronic sinusitis
Site of needle biopsy (186)	Inflammation at site of trauma	Uninfected inflammation

*Inflammatory process need not be of infectious etiology.
Source: From ref. *214* with permission from Elsevier.

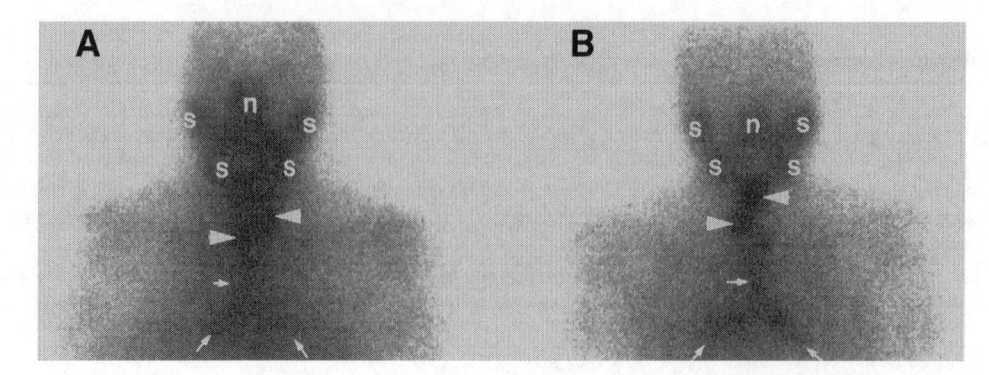

Fig. 11. (A) Anterior and (B) posterior head, neck, and chest views obtained 3 d after a 175-mCi (6.48 GBq) therapy dose of radioiodine 6 wk after a total thyroidectomy and tracheostomy for an invasive papillary carcinoma that had infiltrated the larynx. There was normal uptake of radioiodine in the salivary glands (s) and nasopharynx (n). An intense uptake of radioiodine was in the region of the thyroid bed and tracheostomy (large arrowheads), and faint abnormal uptake of radioiodine throughout the tracheobronchial tree, which had the appearance of an inverted Y (small arrows). This was caused by tracheobronchitis associated with the tracheostomy. (From ref. *214* with permission from Elsevier.)

Table 10
Uptake by Nonthyroidal Neoplasms

Sites of Nonthyroidal Neoplasms	Mechanism for Radioiodine Uptake	Comments Regarding Both Primary and Metastatic Tumors*
Gastric adenocarcinoma *(70,187,188)*	Actively transport of radioiodine	Probably from preservation of normal gastric mucosal active iodide
Meningioma *(189,190)*	Mechanism unclear (highly vascular)	—
Lung cancer (adenocarcinoma, oat cell carcinoma, and squamous cell carcinoma) *(176,189,191–193)*	Bronchial mucus glands actively transport radioiodine	This would explain uptake in adenocarcinoma but not squamous or oat cell cancers
Salivary adenocarcinoma (Warthin's tumor) *(195)*	Salivary glands actively transport radioiodine	Other salivary tumors are less likely to show radioiodine uptake; must be distinguished from uptake owing to ductal obstruction
Ovarian adenocarcinoma and ovarian cystadenoma *(168)*	Mechanism unclear	Mechanism differs from that in ovarian teratomas
Ovarian teratoma (benign/malignant) *(47–53,55,196–199)*	Uptake of radioiodine into salivary gland, gastric mucosa or thyroid gland tissue in tumor	Tissues that normally take up radioiodine may differentiate in such tumors
Teratomas at other sites (benign or malignant) *(200)*	Same as above	Tissues that normally take up radioiodine may differentiate in such tumors
Uterine fibromyoma (see Fig. 12)	Mechanism unclear	May be difficult to separate from bladder and bowel activity
Abdominal neurilemoma *(70,201)*	Same as above	May be difficult to separate from bladder and bowel activity

*Some, but by no means all, of these tumors are derived from tissues that can normally concentrate radioiodine.
Source: From ref. *214* with permission from Elsevier.

UPTAKE BY NONTHYROIDAL NEOPLASMS

Various nonthyroidal neoplasms have been shown to have radioiodine uptake, albeit only in a minority of such lesions (Table 10; *47–53,55,67,70,167,168,187–202*). The mechanisms for this uptake are probably diverse and include (1) the increased vascularity and capillary permeability similar to that seen in inflammation and infection (meningiomas, ovarian adenocarcinoma and cystadenoma, uterine fibroma (Fig. 12), and neurilemoma *(70,168,190,198,201,202)*, and (2) many tumors derived from epithelia that show normal physiological iodide transport *(18)*. Such include gastric

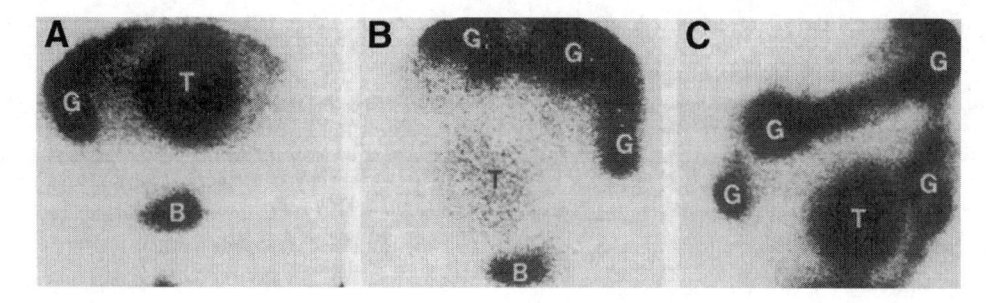

Fig. 12. Diagnostic studies performed 24 h after a dose of 2 mCi (74 MBq) of radioiodine as part of a metastatic survey in a patient after a total thyroidectomy for papillary cancer. There was intense and extensive gut radioactivity (G) owing to the constipation caused by the hypothyroidism required in preparation for the scan. There was normal urinary excretion of radioiodine through the bladder (B) and urinary contamination of the vulva. A large abnormal focus of radioiodine uptake was also in the anterior pelvis (T), which was quite separate from the gut and bladder and best seen on the (panel **A**) anterior and (panel **C**) right anterior oblique projections. On the (panel **B**) posterior projection, the focus was much fainter, indicating a relatively anterior location. The abnormal radioiodine uptake was in a large fibroid uterus, which extended out of the pelvis. (From ref. *214* with permission from Elsevier.)

Table 11
Currently Unexplained Sites of Uptake

Other Sites and Causes	Mechanisms for Radioiodine Uptake	Factors to Be Considered in Otherwise Unexplained Thoracic Radioiodine
Unexplained thymic uptake *(203–211)*	Currently unexplained	Mediastinal mass on CT scan from thymic hyperplasia
Unexplained mediastinal uptake (? normal variant) *(207–211)*	Same as above	To be considered in otherwise unexplained thoracic radioiodine
Unexplained uptake of porencephaly *(212)*	Same as above	Trauma occurred 25 yr earlier
Posttraumatic cerebral malacia *(213)*	Possible chronic inflammation of cerebral or overlying tissues	Prior surgery for cerebral abscess 25 yr earlier

Source: From ref. *214* with permission from Elsevier.

adenocarcinoma, bronchial adenocarcinoma, salivary adenocarcinoma, ovarian and other teratomas containing gastric, salivary, thyroid, and similar tissues *(47–53,55,68,167,177, 178,191–195,197–200)*.

CURRENTLY UNEXPLAINED SITES OF ARTIFACTUAL UPTAKE

A few reports remain of focal radioiodine uptake in postthyroidectomy patients for which there is no obvious physiological or pathophysiological explanation (Table 11). Radioiodine uptake in normal or hyperplastic thymic tissue is left unexplained because there does not seem to be a well-defined iodine uptake mechanism in the thymus *(203–211)*. Focal uptake of radioiodine at sites of porencephaly and cerebral malacia occurring up to 25 yr after the original cerebral injury are still in question but may relate to ongoing chronic inflammation *(212,213)*.

SUMMARY

This classification and organization of artifacts, anatomic and physiological variants, and nonthyroidal diseases causing false-positive whole-body radioiodine scans in thyroid cancer patients, and in the correct interpretation of both diagnostic and posttherapeutic radioiodine studies, provides access to an extensive and scattered literature. This chapter provides an update of our previous review of the literature, and the organizational schema is offered as a means to interpret and clarify additional future observations in this area.

ACKNOWLEDGMENT

The authors wish to thank Judith A. Csoka and Jean Lobdell for their assistance in preparation of the text.

REFERENCES

1. Bakheet SM, Hammami MM. False positive radioiodine whole-body scan in thyroid cancer patients due to unrelated pathology. Clin Nucl Med 1994; 19:325–329.
2. Berson SA, Yalow RS. Quantitative aspects of iodine metabolism: The exchangeable organic iodine pool and the rates of thyroid secretion, peripheral degradation and fecal excretion of endogenously synthesized organically bound iodine. J Clin Invest 1954; 33:1533–1552.
3. Cavalieri RR. Nuclear imaging in the management of thyroid carcinoma. Thyroid 1996; 6:485–492.

4. Datz FL. Gamuts in Nuclear Medicine, 3rd ed. St. Louis, MO: Mosby-Yearbook, 1995:14–15, 27–34.
5. Echenique R, Kasi L, Haynie TP, Glenn HJ, et al. Critical evaluation of serum thyroglobulin levels and I-131 scans in post-therapy patients with differentiated thyroid carcinoma: Concise communication. J Nucl Med 1982; 23:235–240.
6. Fogelman I, Maisey MN. The thyroid scan in the management of thyroid disease. In Freeman LM, Weissmann HS, editors. Nuclear Medicine Annual. New York: Raven Press, 1989:1.
7. Freitas JE, Gross MD, Ripley S, Shapiro B. Radionuclide diagnosis and therapy of thyroid cancer: Current status report. Semin Nucl Med 1985; 15:106–131.
8. Johnson PM. Thyroid and whole-body scanning. In Werner SC, Ingbar SH, editors. The Thyroid, A Fundamental and Clinical Text, 4th ed. Hagerston, PA: Harper & Row, 1978:247–297.
9. Maxon RH, Smith HS. Radioiodine-131 in the diagnosis and treatment of metastatic well differentiated thyroid cancer. Endocrinol Metab Clin North Am 1990; 19:685–718.
10. Ramanna L, Waxman AD, Brachman MB, Sensel N, et al. Correlation of thyroglobulin measurements and radioiodine scans in the follow-up of patients with differentiated thyroid cancer. Cancer 1985; 55:1525–1529.
11. Riggs DS. Quantitative aspects of iodine metabolism in man. Pharmacol Rev 1952; 4:283–293.
12. Sutter CW, Masilungan BG, Stadalnik RC. False-positive results of I-131 whole-body scans in patients with thyroid cancer. Semin Nucl Med 1995; 25:279–282.
13. Carlisle MR, Lu C, McDougall IR. The interpretation of ^{131}I scans in the evaluation of thyroid cancer, with an emphasis on false positive findings. Nucl Med Commun 2003; 24:715–735.
14. Mitchell G, Pratt BE, Vini L, McCready VR, et al. False positive ^{131}I whole body scans in thyroid cancer. Br J Radiol 2000; 73:627–635.
15. Zalis ED, Ellison RB, Captain MC. A diagnostic pitfall with radio-iodine scanning. Am J Roentgenol 1965; 94:837–838.
16. Wu S, Brown T, Milne N, Egbert R, et al. Iodine-131 total body scan: Extra-thyroidal uptake of radioiodine. Semin Nucl Med 1986; 16:82–84.
17. Wolff J. Iodide concentrating mechanisms. In Tall JE, Kopin IJ, Berson SA, editors. The Thyroid and Biogenic Amines: Methods in Investigative and Diagnostic Endocrinology, vol 1. Amsterdam: North-Holland Publishing Co, 1972:115–203.
18. Spitzweg C, Joba W, Eisenmenger W, Heufelder AE. Analysis of human sodium iodide symporter gene expression in extrathyroidal tissues and cloning of its complementary deoxyribonucleic acids from salivary gland, mammary gland, and gastric mucosa. J Clin Endocrinol Metab 1998; 83:1746–1751.
19. Wayne EJ, Koutras DA, Alexander WD, editors. In Clinical Aspects of Iodine Metabolism. Philadelphia, PA: Davis Company 1964; 1–303.
20. Coover LR. False positive result of a total body scan caused by benign thyroidal tissue after ^{131}I ablation. Clin Nucl Med 1999; 24:182–183.
21. Greenler DP, Klein HA. The scope of false-positive iodine-131 images for thyroid carcinoma. Clin Nucl Med 1989; 14:111–117.
22. Geatti O, Shapiro B, Orsolon PG, Mirolo R, et al. An unusual false positive scan in a patient with pericardial effusion. Clin Nucl Med 1994; 19:678–682.
23. Bakheet S, Powe J, Hammami M. Radioiodine uptake in the chest. J Nucl Med 1997; 38:984–986.
24. Bakheet S, Hammami M, Powe J. False-positive radioiodine uptake in the abdomen and the pelvis: Radioiodine retention in the kidneys and review of the literature. Clin Nucl Med 1996; 21:932–937.
25. Turlington B. Embryology and anatomy of the thyroid and parathyroid glands. In Eisenberg B, editor. Imaging of the Thyroid and Parathyroid Glands. New York: Churchill Livingstone Inc., 1991:1–8.
26. Larochelle D, Arcand P, Belzile M, Gagnon NB. Ectopic thyroid tissue: A review of the literature. J Otolaryngol 1979; 8:523–530.
27. Sloan LW, Feind CR. Clinical aspects of anomalous development. In Werner SC, Ingbar SH, editors. The Thyroid. New York: Harper & Row, 1971:317–333.
28. Weider DJ, Parker W. Lingual thyroid. Ann Otol Rhinol Laryngol 1977; 86:841–848.
29. Strain J, Oates E, Nejad A. Unusual appearance of lingual thyroid in congenital hypothyroidism. Clin Nucl Med 1998; 23:460.
30. Coover L. False-positive result of a total-body scan caused by benign thyroidal tissue after I-131 ablation. Clin Nucl Med 1999; 24:182–183.
31. Lin DS. Thyroid imaging-mediastinal uptake in thyroid imaging. Semin Nucl Med 1983; 13:395–396.
32. Leung AKC, Wong AL, Robson WLM. Ectopic thyroid gland simulating a thyroglossal duct cyst: A case report. Can J Surg 1995; 38:87–89.
33. Sironi M, Assi A, Andruccioli M, Spreafico G. Submandibular ectopic thyroid gland. Clin Nucl Med 1996; 21:585.
34. Touliopoulos P, Oates E. Autonomously functioning thyroid rests following total thyroidectomy for Graves' disease. Clin Nucl Med 1993; 18:914.
35. Dowling EA, Johnson IM, Collier FCD. Intratracheal goiter: A clinico-pathologic review. Ann Surg 1962; 156:258–267.
36. Dundas P. Intrathoracic aberrant goiter. Acta Chir Scand 1964; 128:729–736.
37. Fogelfeld L, Rubinstein U, Bar-On J, Feigl D. Severe thyrotoxicosis caused by an ectopic intrathoracic goiter. Clin Nucl Med 1986; 11:20–22.
38. Salvatore M, Gallo A. Accessory thyroid in the anterior mediastinum: Case report. J Nucl Med 1975; 16:1135–1136.
39. Salvatore M, Rufini V, Corsellow SM, Saletnich I, et al. Thyrotoxicosis due to ectopic retrotracheal adenoma treated with radioiodine. J Nucl Biol Med 1993; 37:69–72.
40. Thakore K, Vansant J. Hyperthyroidism die to toxic, intrathoracic thyroid tissue with absent cervical thyroid gland. Clin Nucl Med 1993; 18:535–536.
41. Rieser GD, Ober KP, Cowan RJ, Cordell AR. Radioiodine imaging of struma cordis. Clin Nucl Med 1988; 13:421–422.
42. Aldasouqi S, Edmondson J, Prince M. Carcinoma of thyro-glossal duct remnants: Report of three cases and a review of the literature. The Endocrinologist 1996; 6:238–244.
43. Gaby M. The role of thyroid dysgenesis and maldescent in the etiology of sporadic cretinism. J Pediatr 1962; 60:830–835.
44. Gorbman A, Dickhoff WW, Vigna SR. The thyroid gland. In Gorbman A, editor. Comparative Endocrinology. New York: John Wiley and Sons, 1983:185–202.
45. Myers EN, Pantangco IP. Intratracheal thyroid. Laryngoscope 1975; 85:1833–1840.
46. Postlethwait RN, Detmer DE. Ectopic thyroid nodule in the esophagus. Ann Thorac Surg 1975; 19:98–100.
47. Brown WW, Shetty KR, Rosenfeld PS. Hyperthyroidism due to struma ovarii: Demonstration by radioiodine scan. Acta Endocrinol 1973; 73:266–272.
48. Falsetti L, Schivardi MR, Maira G, Favret M, et al. Riscontro di struma ovarii in una paziente in trattamento per cacinoma tiroideo. Ann Ost Gin Med Perin 1985; 106:290–293.
49. March DE, Desai AG, Park CH, Hendricks PJ. Struma ovarii: Hyperthyroidism in a postmenopausal woman. J Nucl Med 1988; 29:263–265.
50. Salvatore M, Rufini V, Daudone MS. Occasional detection of "struma ovarii" in a patient with thyroid cancer. Radiol Med (Torino) 1991; 81:744–767.
51. Thomas RD, Batty VB. Metastatic malignant struma ovarii: Two case reports. Clin Nucl Med 1992; 17:577–578.
52. Yeh E-L, Meade RC, Reutz PP. Radionuclide study of struma ovarii. J Nucl Med 1973; 14:118–121.

53. Zwas ST, Heyman Z, Lieberman LM. 131-I ovarian uptake in a whole-body scan for thyroid carcinoma. Semin Nucl Med 1989; 19:340–342.
54. Ziessman HA, Bahar H, Fahey FH, Dubiansky V. Hepatic visualization on iodine-131 whole-body thyroid cancer scans. J Nucl Med 1987; 28:1408–1411.
55. Joja I, Asakawa T, Mitsumori A, Nakagawa T, et al. I-123 uptake in non-functional struma ovarii. Clin Nucl Med 1998; 23:10–12.
56. Konez O, Hanelin LG, Jenison EL, Goyal M, et al. Functioning liver metastases on a whole-body scan: a case of malignant struma ovarii. Clin Nucl Med 2000; 25:465–466.
57. Moses DC, Thompson NW, Nishiyama RH, Sisson JC. Ectopic thyroid tissue in the neck, benign or malignant? Cancer 1976; 38: 361–365.
58. Ryo UY, Stachura ME, Schneider AB, Nichols R, et al. Significance of extrathyroidal uptake of Tc-99m and I-123 in the thyroid scan: Concise communication. J Nucl Med 1981; 22:1039–1042.
59. Sud AM, Gross MD. Radioiodine uptake following thyroidectomy for thyroid cancer: Recurrence or ectopic tissue? Clin Nucl Med 1991; 16:894–897.
60. Todino V, Pacella CM, Crescenzi A. Ectopic thyroid tissue in the liver: Case report. Eur J Nucl Med 1996; 23(Abstr):1055.
61. Bakheet S, Powe J, Hammami MM, Amin TM, et al. Isolated porta hepatis metastasis of papillary thyroid cancer. J Nucl Med 1996; 37: 993–994.
62. Feuerstein IM, Harbert JC. Hypertrophied thyroid tissue in a thyroglossal duct remnant. Clin Nucl Med 1986; 11:135.
63. Freinkel N, Ingbar SH. Concentration gradients for inorganic iiodide I-131 and chloride in mixed human saliva. J Clin Invest 1953; 32:1077–1084.
64. Ahlgren L, Ivarsson S, Johansson L, Mattsson S, et al. Excretion of radionuclides in human breast milk after the administration of radiopharmaceuticals. J Nucl Med 1985; 26:1085–1090.
65. Bakheet S, Hammami MM. False positive thyroid cancer metastasis on whole body radioiodine scanning due to retained radioactivity in the oesophagus. Eur J Nucl Med 1993; 20:415–419.
66. Boxen I, Zhang M. Nasal secretion of iodine-131. Clin Nucl Med 1990; 15:610–611.
67. Coakley AJ, Mountford PJ. Nuclear medicine and the nursing mother. Br Med J 1985; 291:159–160.
68. Clode WH, Sobral JMV, Lima-Basto E. Elective uptake of radioiodine by cancer of the stomach. Surgery 1961; 50:725–727.
69. Duong RB, Fernandez-Ulloa M, Planitz MK, Maxon, HR. 123I breast uptake in a young primipara with postpartum transient thyrotoxicosis. Clin Nucl Med 1983; 8:35.
70. Ganatra RD, Atmaram SH, Sharma SM. An unusual site of radioiodine concentration in a patient with thyroid cancer (letter). J Nucl Med 1972; 13:777.
71. Hedrick WR, DiSimone RN, Keen RL. Radiation dosimetry from breast milk excretion of radioiodine and pertechnetate. J Nucl Med 1986; 27:1569–1571.
72. Honour AJ, Myant NB, Rowlands EN. Secretion of redioiodine in digestive juices and milk in man. Clin Sci (Colch) 1952; 11: 447–462.
73. Lopez OL, Maisano ER. Vascular retention of Tc-99m pertechnetate simulating ectopic or metastatic thyroid tissue. Clin Nucl Med 1983; 8:503–504.
74. Malpani BL, Samuel AM, Ray S. Defferential kinetics of parotid and submandibular gland function as demonstrated by scintigraphi means and its possible implications. Nucl Med Commun 1995; 16:706–709.
75. Mountford PJ, Coakley AJ. A review of the secretion of radioactivity in human breast milk: Data, quantitative analysis and recommendations. Nucl Med Commun 1989; 10:15–27.
76. Neutze JA, Norby EH, Van Nostrand D. Nasal radioiodine uptake: A prospective study of frequency, degree, and pattern. J Nucl Med 1987: 28:686.

77. Norby EH, Neutze J, Van Nostrand D, Burman KD, et al. Nasal radioiodine activity: A prospective study of frequency, intensity and pattern. J Nucl Med 1990; 31:52–54.
78. Park HM, Tarver RD, Schauwecker DS, Burt R. Spurious thyroid cancer metastasis: Saliva contamination artifact in high dose iodine-131 metastases survey. J Nucl Med 1986; 27:634–636.
79. Riccabona G. Differentiated thyroid carcinoma. In Murray IPC, Ell PJ, editors. Nuclear Medicine in Clinical Diagnosis and Treatment. Churchill Livingstone, 1998:941–957.
80. Romney, B, Nicholoff EF, Esser PD. Excretion of radioiodine in breast milk. J Nucl Med 1989; 30:124–126.
81. Romney BM, Nicholoff EL. Diagnostic nuclear medicine and the nursing mother. App Radiol 1987; 16:51–56.
82. Romney BM, Nickoloff EL, Esser PD. Radionuclide administration to nursing mothers: Mathematically derived guidelines. Radiology 1986; 160:549–554.
83. Schuster DM, Alazraki N. Esophageal scarring causing false-positve uptake on I-131 whole-body imaging. Clin Nucl Med 1998; 23:334.
84. Hammami MM, Bakheet S. Radioiodine breast uptake in non-breast feeding women. Clinical and scintigraphic characteristics. J Nucl Med 1996; 37:26–31.
85. Park HM, Wellman H. Hot nose after I-131 sodium iodide thyroablation therapy. Clin Nucl Med 1992; 17:130–131.
86. Allen T, Wiest P, Vela S, Hartshorne M, Crooks LA. I-131 uptake in the breast for thyroid cancer surveillance with biopsy-proven benign tissue. Clin Nucl Med 1998; 23:585–587.
87. Baemler GR, Joo KG. Radioactive iodine uptake by breasts (letter). J Nucl Med 1986; 27:149–151.
88. Watanabe N, Matsumoto M, Ohtake H, Hirano T, et al. Bilateral breast uptake of Tl-201 chloride in a nursing woman. Clin Nucl Med 1996; 21:818–819.
89. McDougall IR. Whole body scintigraphy with radioiodine-131: A comprehensive list of false-positives with some examples. Clin Nucl Med 1995; 20:869–875.
90. Robinson PS, Barker P, Campbell A, Henson P, et al. Iodine-131 in breast milk following therapy for thyroid carcinoma. J Nucl Med 1994; 35:1797–1801.
91. Bakheet S, Hammami M, Hemidan A, Powe JE, et al. Radioiodine secretion in tears. J Nucl Med 1998; 39:1452–1454.
92. Bakheet SM, Hammami MM. Patterns of radioiodine uptake by the lactating breast. Eur J Nucl Med 1994; 21:604–608.
93. Howarth DV, Forstrom LA, O'Connor MK, Thomas PA, et al. Patient-related and pitfalls artifacts in nuclear medicine imaging. Semin Nucl Med 1996; 26:295–307.
94. Achong DM, Oates E, Lee SL, Doherty FJ. Gallbladder visualization during post-therapy iodine-131 imaging of thyroid carcinoma. J Nucl Med 1991; 32:2275–2277.
95. Nishizawa K, Ohara K, Ohshima M, Maekoshi H, et al. Monitoring of iodine excretions and used materials of patients treated with 131I. Health Phys 1980; 38:467–481.
96. Daumerie C, Vynckier S, Caussin J, Jadoul M, et al. Radioiodine treatment of thyroid carcinoma in patients on maintenance hemodialysis. Thyroid 1996; 6:301–304.
97. Howard N, Glasser M. Iodine-131 ablation therapy for a patient on maintenance haemodialysis. Br J Radiol 1981; 54:259–261.
98. Mello AM, Isaacs R, Petersen J, Kronenberger S, et al. Management of thyroid papillary carcinoma with radioiodine in a patient with end-stage renal disease on hemodialysis. Clin Nucl Med 1994; 19: 776–781.
99. Morrish DW, Filipow JL, McEwan AJ, Schmidt R, et al. 131I treatment of thyroid papillary carcinoma in a patient with renal failure. Cancer 1990; 66:2509–2513.
100. Nibhanupudy JR, Hamilton W, Sridhar R, Talley GB, et al. Iodine-131 treatment of hyperthyroidism in a patient on dialysis for chronic renal failure. Am J Nephrol 1993; 13:214–217.

101. Rosenbaum RC, Johnston GS, Valente WA. Frequency of hepatic visualization during 131I imaging for metastatic thyroid carcinoma. Clin Nucl Med 1988; 13:657–660.
102. Schober B, Cohen P, Lyster D, Charron M, et al. Diffuse liver uptake of 131I (letter). J Nucl Med 1990; 31:1575–1576.
103. Nodine JH, Maldia G. Pseudostruma ovarii. Obstet Gynecol 1961; 17:460–463.
104. You DL, Tzen KY, Chen JF, Kao PF, et al. False-positive whole-body iodine-131 scan due to intrahepatic duct dilatation. J Nucl Med 1997; 38:1977–1979.
105. Chung JK, Lee YJ, Jeong JM, Lee DS, et al. Clinical significance of hepatic visualization on I-131 whole-body scan in patients with thyroid carcinoma. J Nucl Med 1997; 38:1191–1195.
106. Muherji S, Ziessman HA, Earll JM, Keyes JW. False-positive iodine-131 whole-body scan due to pectus excavatum. Clin Nucl Med 1988; 13:207–208.
107. Giuffrida D, Garofalo MR, Cacciaguerra G, Freni V, et al. False positive I-131 tatal body scan due to an ectasia of the common carotids. J Endocrinol Invest 1993; 16:207–211.
108. Abdel-Dayem HM, Halker K, El Sayed M. The radioactive wig in iodine-131 whole-body imaging. Clin Nucl Med 1984; 9:454–455.
109. Varoglu E, Yildirim M, Bayrakdar R, Kantalri AM, et al. Radioiodine pooling in dilated greater saphenous vein mimicking contamination. Clin Nucl Med 2003; 28:866–868.
110. Bakheet SM, Hammami MM. Spurious thyroid cancer bone metastases on radioiodine scan due to external contamination. Eur J Radiol 1993; 16:239–242.
111. Bakheet S, Jammami MM. Spurious lung metastases on radioiodine thyroid and whole body imaging. Clin Nucl Med 1993; 18:307–312.
112. Brodkey JS, Gibbs GE. Sweat iodide excretion in patients with cystic fibrosis of the pancreas. J Appl Physiol 1960; 15:501–502.
113. Camponovo EJ, Goyer PF, Silverman ED, Kistler AM, et al. Axillary iodine-131 accumulation due to perspiration. Clin Nucl Med 1989; 14:762–763.
114. Chandramouly BS, Scagnelli T, Burgess CK. Artifact on iodine-131 whole body scan due to contaminated handkerchief. Clin Nucl Med 1989; 14:762–763.
115. Dick C, Mudun A, Alazraki NP. False-positive images mimicking thyroid cancer metastasis: The nose ring sign. Clin Nucl Med 1995; 20:876–877.
116. Gritters LS, Wissing J, Gross MD, Shapiro B. Extensive salivary contamination due to concurrent use of chewing tobacco during I-131 radioablative therapy. Clin Nucl Med 1993; 18:115–117.
117. Ibis E, Wilson CR, Collier BD, Akansel G, et al. Iodine-131 contamination from thyroid cancer patients. J Nucl Med 1992; 33:2110–2115.
118. Pochis WT, Krasnow AZ, Isitman AT, Cerletty JM, et al. The radioactive handkerchief sign: A contamination artifact in I-131 imaging for metastatic thyroid carcinoma. Clin Nucl Med 1990; 15:491–494.
119. Carey JE, Kumpuris TM, Wrobel MC. Release of patients containing therapeutic dosages of iodine-131 from hospitals. J Nucl Med Technol 1995; 23:144–149.
120. Ryo UY, Alavi A, Collier BD, editors. The thyroid. In Atlas of Nuclear Medicine Artifacts and Variants. Chicago: Yearbook Medical Publishers, 1995:23–33.
121. Silva F, Negron JA. Unusual contamination after a therapeutic dose of iodine-131. J Nucl Med 1996; 37:70,75.
122. Ain KB, Shih WJ. False-positive I-131 uptake at a tracheostomy site: discernment with Tl-201 imaging. Clin Nucl Med 1994; 19:619–621.
123. Kirk GA, Schulz EE. Post-laryngectomy localization of I-131 at tracheostomy site on a total body scan. Clin Nucl Med 1984; 9:409–411.
124. Joyce WT, Cowan RJ. A potential false-positive post-therapy radioiodine scan secondary to I-131 excretion in perspiration. Clin Nucl Med, 1995; 20:368–369.
125. Lawes SC. 123I excretion in breast milk-additional data. Nucl Med Commun 1992; 13:570–572.
126. Weaver JC, Kamm ML, Dobson RL. Excretion of radioiodine in human milk. JAMA 1960; 173:872–875.
127. Spencer RP, Spitznagle LA, Karimeddini MK, Hosain F. Breast milk content of 131I in a hypothyroid patient. Nucl Med Biol 1986; 13:585.
128. Wiseman J. Bony metastasis from thyroid carcinoma or contamination? Clin Nucl Med 1984; 9:363.
129. Schechter D, Krausz Y, Moshe S, Rubinstein R, et al. Radioiodine hot hand sign. Clin Nucl Med 1998; 23:378–379.
130. Barzel US, Chun KJ. Artifact of I-131 whole-body scan with thoracic vertebral uptake in a patient with papillary thyroid carcinoma. Clin Nucl Med 1997; 22:855.
131. Caplan RH, Gundersen GA, Abellera M, Kisken WA. Uptake of iodine-131 by a Meckel's diverticulum mimicking metastatic thyroid cancer. Clin Nucl Med 1987; 12:760–762.
132. Ho Y, Hicks R. Hiatus hernia: A potential cause of false-positive iodine-131 scan in thyroid carcinoma. Clin Nucl Med 1998; 23:621–622.
133. Kamoi I, Nishitani H, Oshiumi Y, Ichiya Y, et al. Intrathoracic gastric cyst demonstrated by Tc-99m pertechnetate scintigraphy. AJR Am J Roentgenol 1980; 134:1080–1081.
134. McNamara M, Tsang H. Hiatal hernia with reflux resulting in false positive I-131 scan. Clin Nucl Med 1998; 23:178–179.
135. Misaki T, Iida Y, Kasayi K. First impressions: Unusual extrathyroidal uptake. J Nucl Med 1998; 39:1650.
136. Schneider JA, Divgi CR, Scott AM, Macapinlac HA, et al. Hiatal hernia on whole-body radioiodine survey mimicking metastic thyroid cancer. Clin Nucl Med 1993; 18:751–753.
137. Unal S, Oguz H, Alagol F, Cantez S. Misinterpretation of I-131 scintigraphy because of diaphragmatic hernia. Clin Nucl Med 1996; 21:151–152.
138. White JE, Flickinger FW, Morgan ME. 131I accumulation in gastric pull-up simulating pulmonary metastases on total-body scan for thyroid cancer. Clin Nuc Med 1990; 15:809–810.
139. Willis LL, Cowan RJ. Mediastinal uptake of I-131 in a hiatal hernia mimicking recurrence of papillary thyroid carcinoma. Clin Nucl Med 1993; 18:961–963.
140. Bekis R, Durak H. Intrathoracic stomach causing a pitfall on thyroid imaging. Clin Nucl Med 1998; 23:848–849.
141. Ceccarelli C, Pancini F, Lippi F, Pinchera A. An unusual case of a false-positive iodine-131 whole-body scan in a patient with papillary thyroid cancer. Clin Nucl Med 1987; 3:192–193.
142. Berquist TH, Nolan NG, Stephens DM. Radioisotope scintigraphy in diagnosis of Barrett's esophagus. AJR Am J Roentgenol 1971; 123:401–411.
143. Boulahdour H, Meignan M, Melliere D, Braga F, et al. False-positive I-131 scan induced by Zenker's diverticulum. Clin Nucl Med 1992; 17:243–244.
144. Dhawan VM, Kaess KR, Spencer RP. False positive thyroid scan due to zenker's diverticulum. J Nucl Med 1978; 19:1231–1232.
145. Kistler AM, Yudt WM, Bakalar RS, Turton DB, et al. Retained esophageal activity on iodine-131 survey in patient with benign esophageal stricture. Clin Nucl Med 1993; 18:908–909.
146. Ozdemir A, Gungor F, Ozugur S, Cubuk M, et al. Abnormal iodine-131 uptake in the mediastinum caused by achalasia. Clin Nucl Med 1998; 23:706–707.
147. Grossman M. Gastroesophageal reflux: A potential source of confusion in technetium thyroid scanning: Case report. J Nucl Med 1977; 18:548–549.
148. Nair N, Basu S, Pakhale H. Unusual uptake of radioiodine in the chest in a patient with thyroid carcinoma. Br J Radiol 2004; 77:63–67.
149. Robertson JS, Verhasselt M, Wahner HW. Use of 123-I for thyroid uptake measurements and depression of 131-I thyroid uptake by incomplete dissolution of capsule filler. J Nucl Med 1974; 15:770–774.
150. Kipper MS, Krohn LD. Increased submandibular gland uptake on thyroid scintigraphy due to Wharton's duct stone. Clin Nucl Med 1996; 21:881–882.

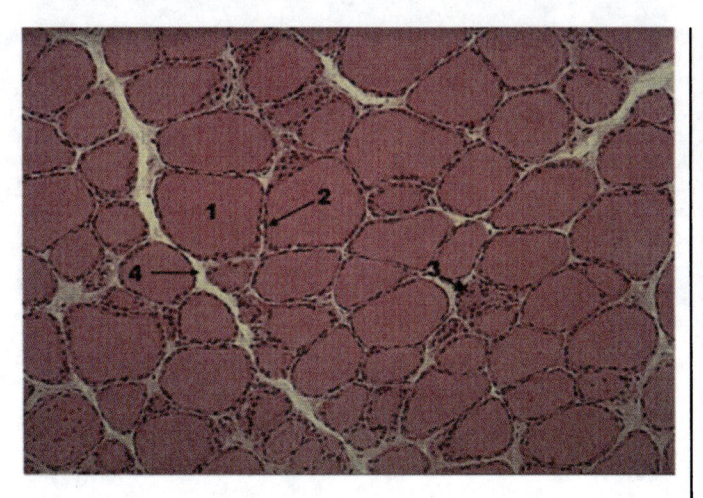

Color Plate 1, Fig. 2. Histology of normal adult thyroid gland. (*See* full caption in Ch. 1 and discussion on p. 5.)

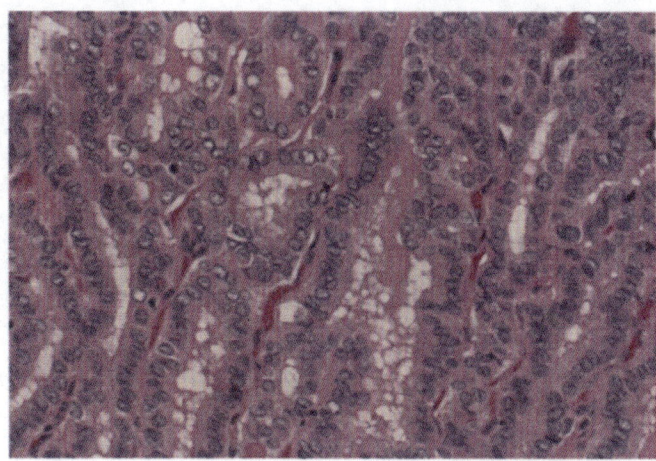

Color Plate 4, Fig. 3. Small papillae of the papillary carcinoma are crowded together, and follicular spaces are elongated (H&E stain). (*See* full caption in Ch. 25 on p. 264 and discussion on p. 263.)

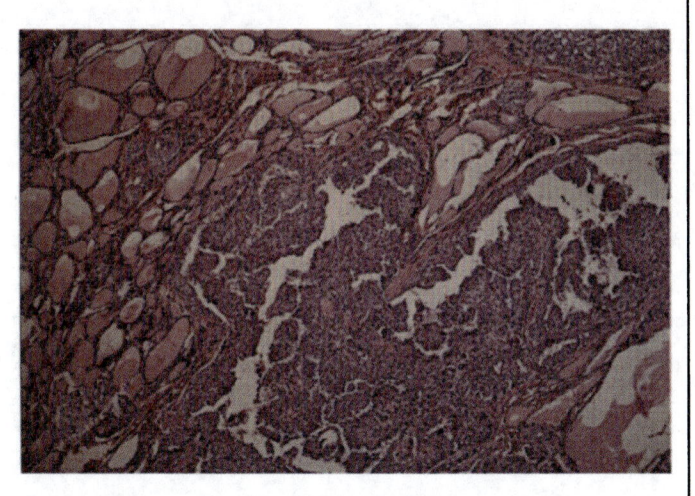

Color Plate 2, Fig. 1. Papillary carcinoma (classical pattern) invades the normal gland. (H&E stain). (*See* full caption in Ch. 25 on p. 264 and discussion on p. 263.)

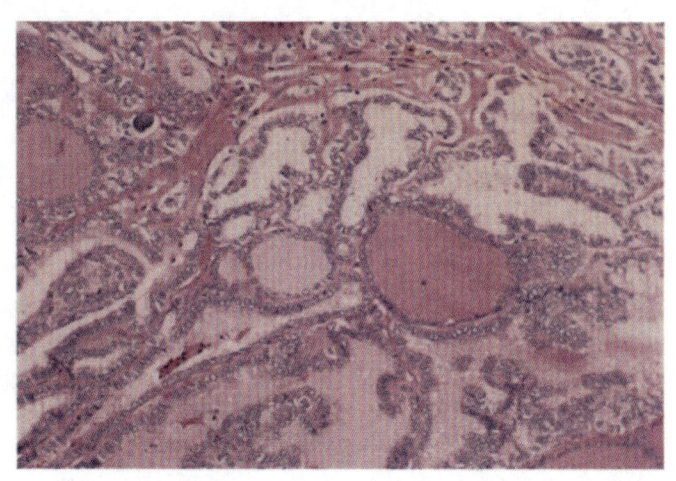

Color Plate 5, Fig. 4. A psammona body lies in the lower right of the papillary carcinoma. (H&E stain). (*See* full caption in Ch. 25 on p. 264 and discussion on p. 263.)

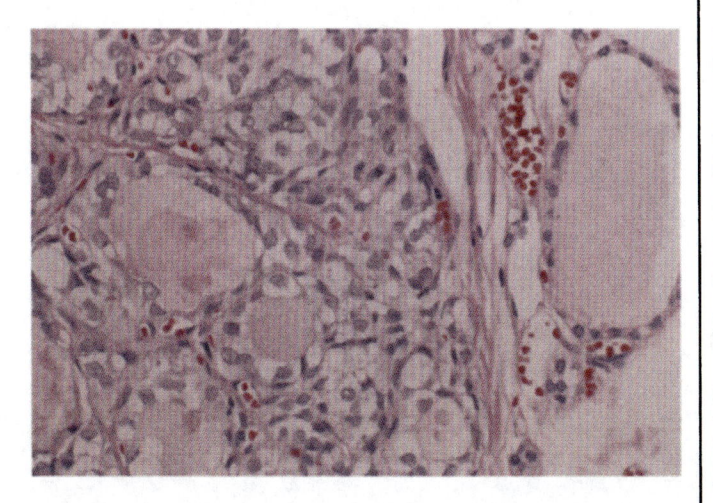

Color Plate 3, Fig. 2. Normal thyroid tissue of the papillary carcinoma lies to the right of the figure. (*See* full caption in Ch. 25 on p. 264 and discussion on p. 263.)

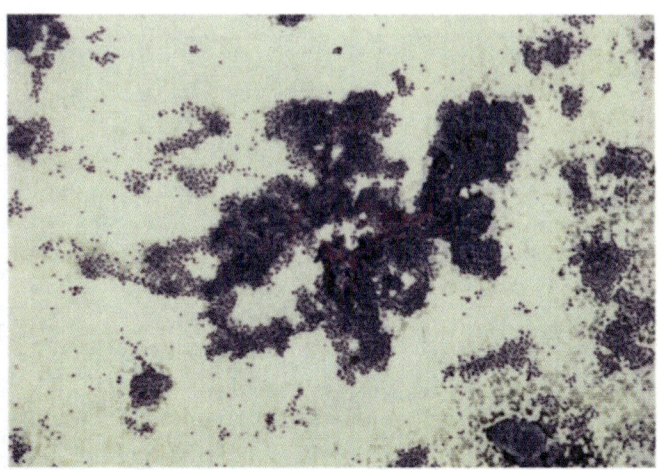

Color Plate 6, Fig. 5. Aspirate showing papillary tissue fragments of the papillary carcinoma (Diff-Quik stain). (*See* full caption in Ch. 25 on p. 264 and discussion on p. 263.)

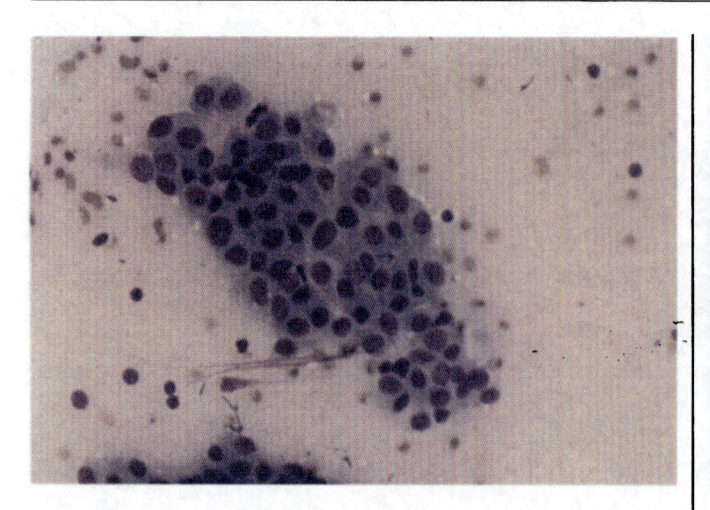

Color Plate 7, Fig. 6. Aspirate showing neoplastic cells with variation in nuclear sizes (Diff-Quik stain) in the papillary carcinoma. (*See* full caption in Ch. 25 on p. 265 and discussion on p. 264.)

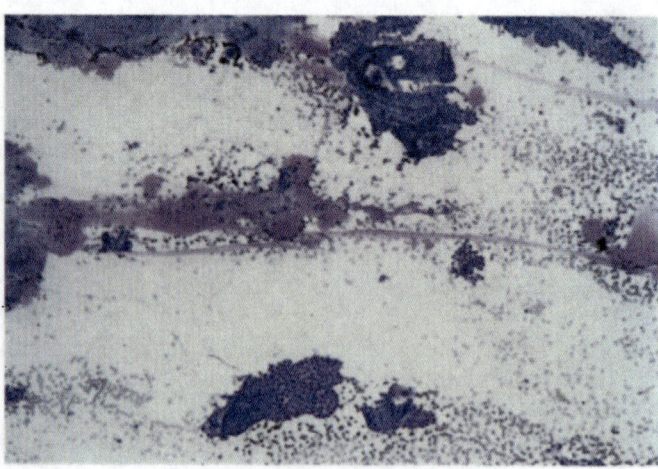

Color Plate 10, Fig. 9. Aspirate showing bubble-gum (chewing-gum or ropy) colloid (Diff-Quik stain) of the papillary carcinoma. (*See* full caption in Ch. 25 on p. 265 and discussion on p. 264.)

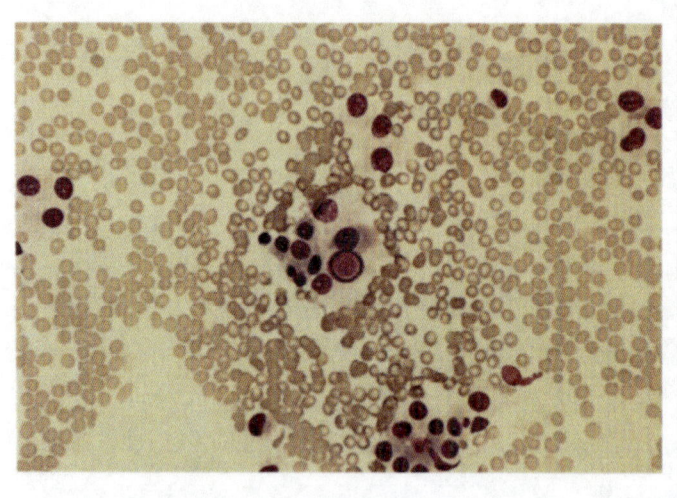

Color Plate 8, Fig. 7. Aspirate of the papillary carcinoma showing "intranuclear cytoplasmic pseudoinclusion" in large nucleus in center filed (Diff-Quik stain), low magnification. (*See* full caption in Ch. 25 on p. 265 and discussion on p. 264.)

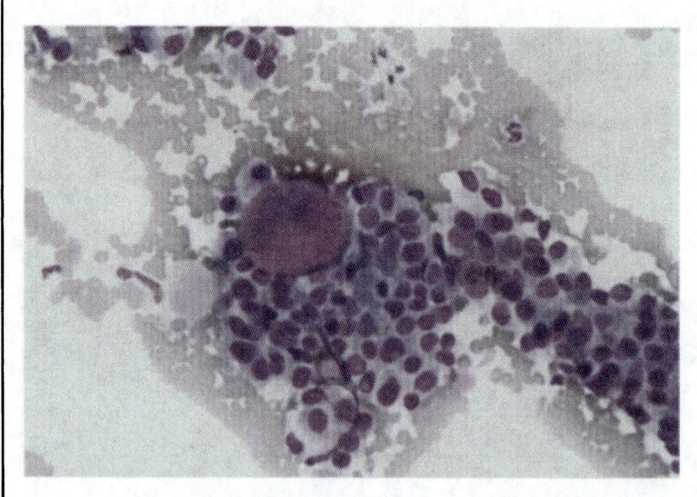

Color Plate 11, Fig. 10. Papillary carcinoma. Aspirate showing neoplastic cells surrounding colloid, which appears as a "pink ball" (Diff-Quik stain). (*See* full caption in Ch. 25 on p. 265 and discussion on p. 264.)

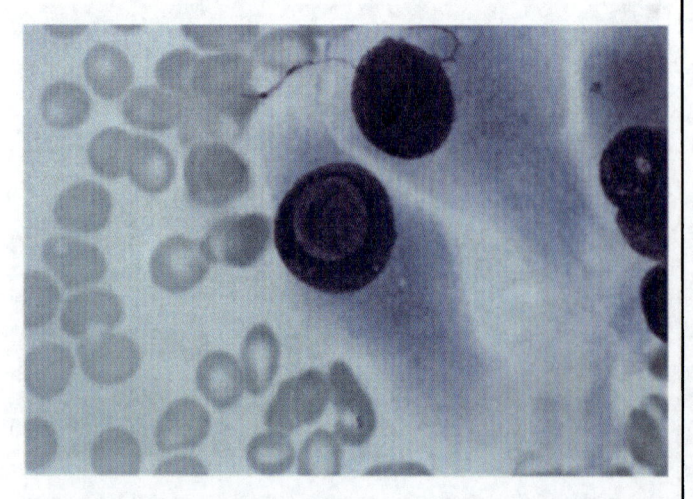

Color Plate 9, Fig. 8. Aspirate of the papillary carcinoma showing "intranuclear cytoplasmic pseudoinclusion." (*See* full caption in Ch. 25 on p. 265 and discussion on p. 264.)

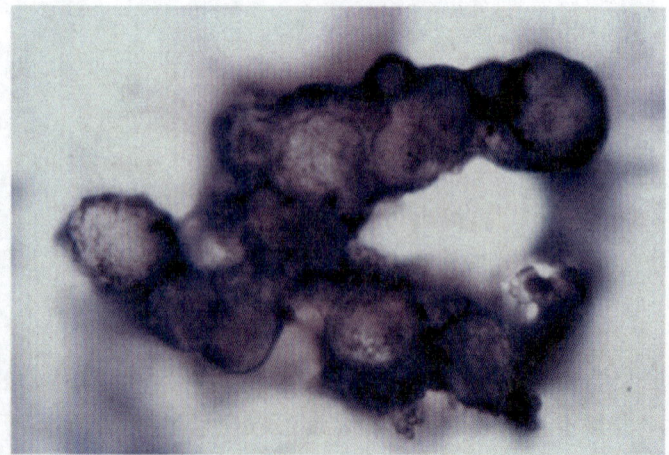

Color Plate 12, Fig. 11. Aspirate showing psammoma bodies of the papillary carcinoma (Diff-Quik stain). (*See* full caption in Ch. 25 on p. 265 and discussion on p. 264.)

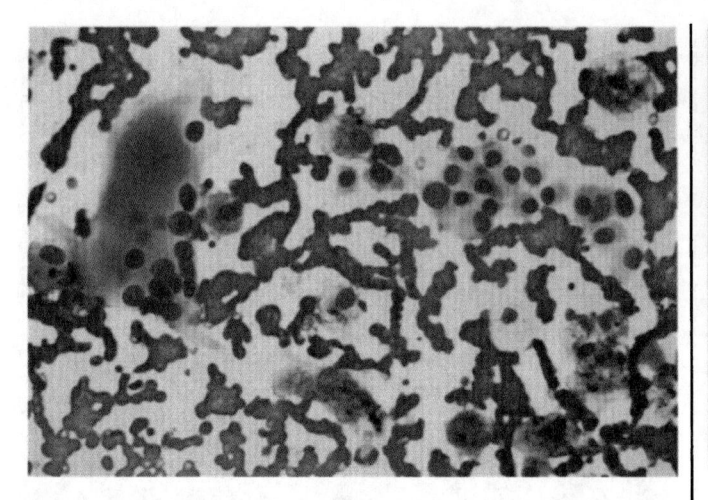

Color Plate 13, Fig. 12. Multinucleated histiocyte (on the right) and neoplastic cells of the papillary carcinoma. Many erythocytes lie in the background of the smear (Diff-Quik stain). (*See* full caption in Ch. 25 on p. 266 and discussion on p. 264.)

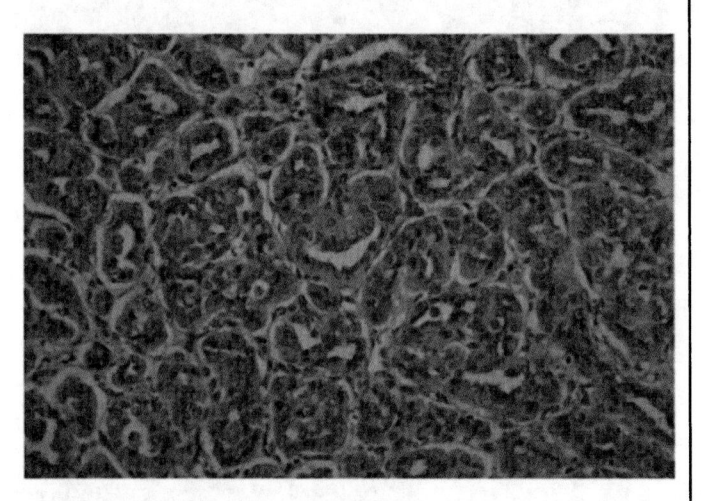

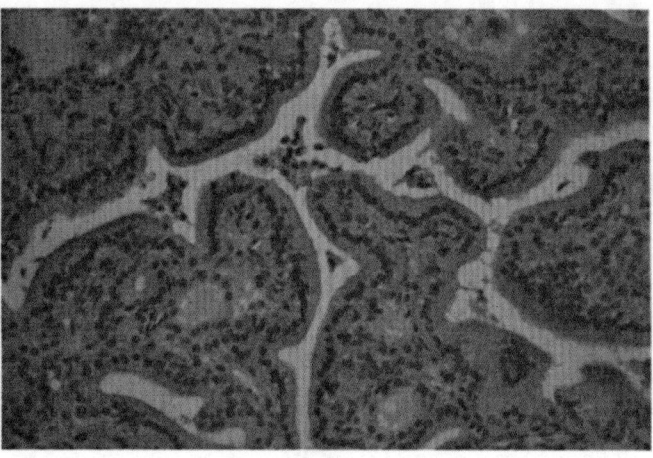

Color Plate 16, Fig. 15. Benign adenomatoid nodule with papillae. Compare these regular nuclei with those of papillary carcinoma in the other figures (H&E stain). (*See* full caption and discussion in Ch. 25 on p. 266.)

Color Plate 14, Fig. 13. Follicular pattern of the papillary carcinoma. The nuclei are irregular in shape, size, and position in the cells. Follicles are tiny and generally appear empty (H&E stain). (*See* full caption and discussion in Ch. 25 on p. 266.)

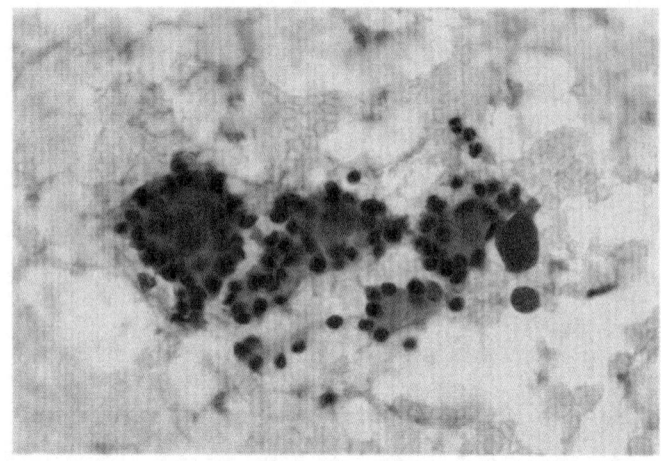

Color Plate 17, Fig. 16. Follicular variant of the papillary carcinoma. Aspirate showing multiple microfollicles with inspissated luminal colloid (Papanicolaou stain). (*See* full caption in Ch. 25 on p. 267 and discussion on p. 266.)

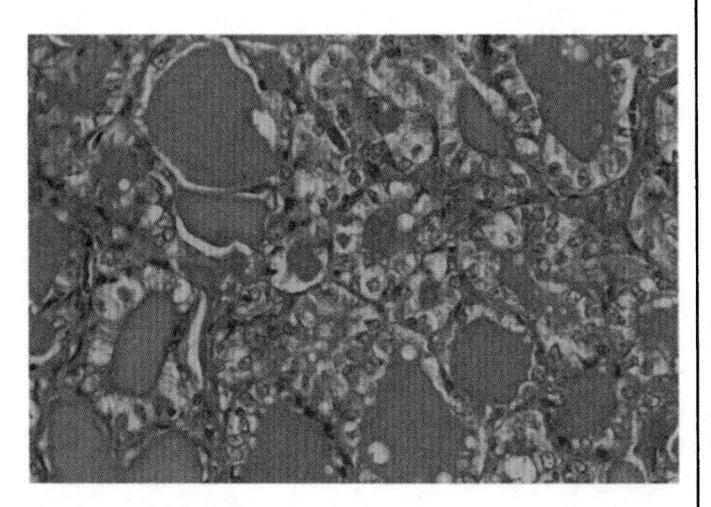

Color Plate 15, Fig. 14. Follicular pattern of the papillary carcinoma. (*See* full caption and discussion in Ch. 25 on p. 266.)

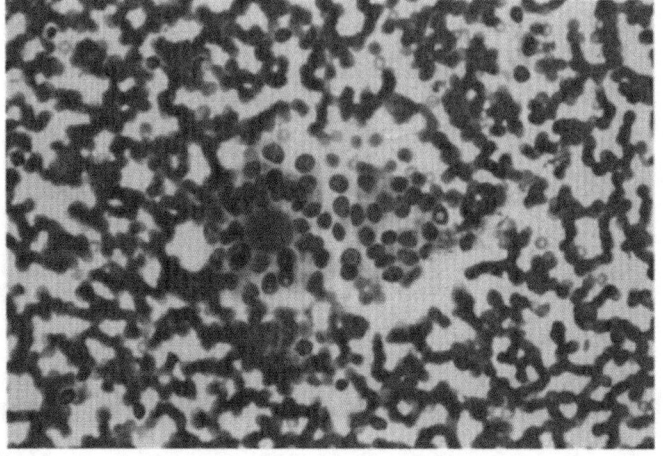

Color Plate 18, Fig. 17. Follicular variant of the papillary carcinoma. (*See* full caption in Ch. 25 on p. 267 and discussion on p. 266.)

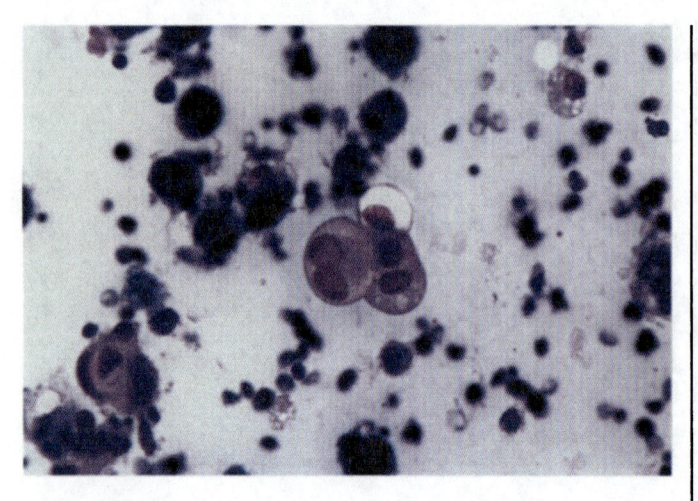

Color Plate 19, Fig. 18. Papillary carcinoma with cystic change. Aspirate showing neoplastic cells with dense well-demarcated cytoplasm and one with pale cytoplasm (Diff-Quik stain) (*See* full caption in Ch. 25 on p. 268 and discussion on pp. 267.)

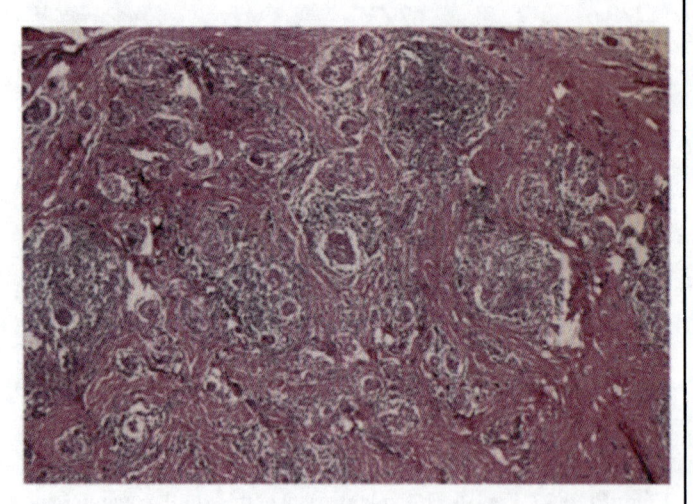

Color Plate 20, Fig. 19. Papillary carcinoma of the diffuse sclerosing type (H&E). (*See* full caption and discussion in Ch. 25 on p. 268.)

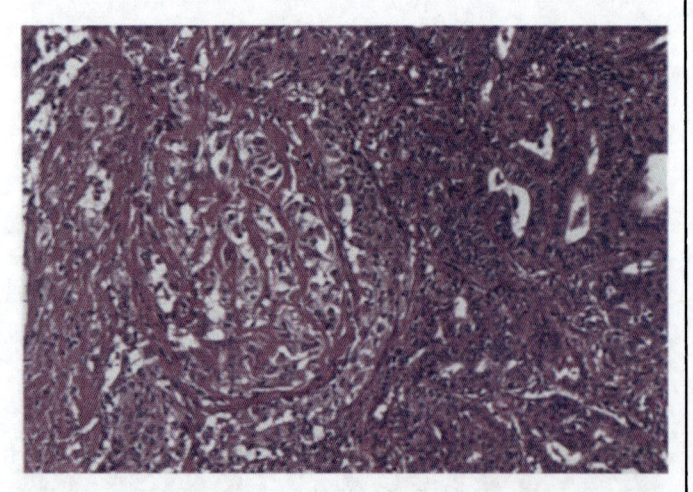

Color Plate 21, Fig. 20. Less well-defferentiated papillary carcinoma. (*See* full caption and discussion in Ch. 25 on p. 269.)

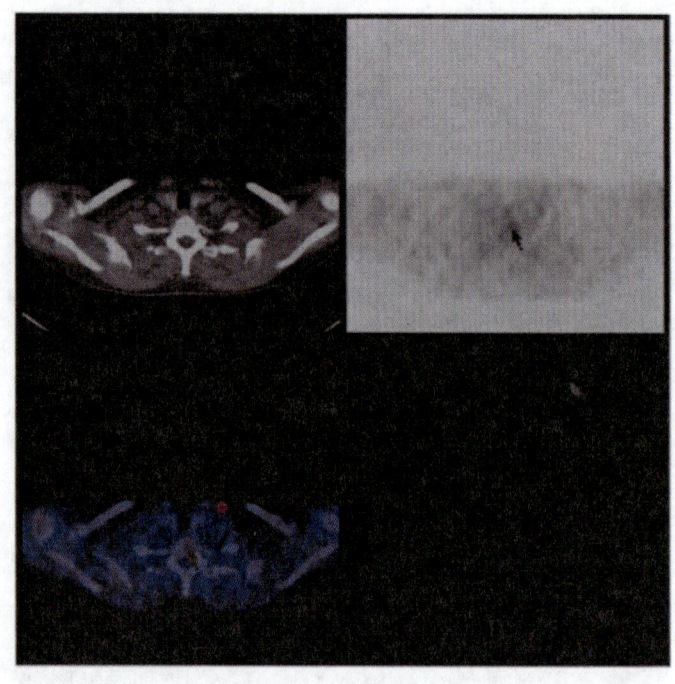

Color Plate 22, Fig. 1. A transaxial scan showing PET (upper right), CT (upper left), and combined PET and CT (lower panel). The white arrow show the thyroid on CT, and the black arrow shows a vertebra on PET scan. (*See* full caption and discussion in Ch. 34 on p. 320.)

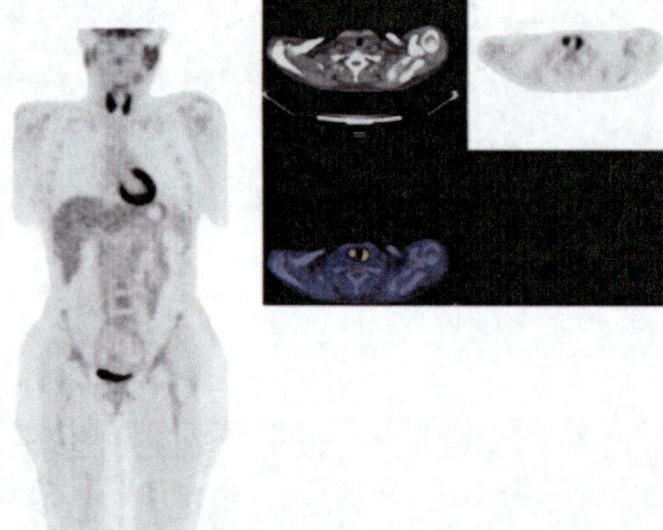

Color Plate 23, Fig. 2. A coronal PET scan (left). The image on the right is the transaxial images of the PET scan, CT, and combined PET/CT, as oriented in Fig. 1 and at the thyroid level. (*See* full caption in Ch. 34 on p. 321 and discussion on p. 320.)

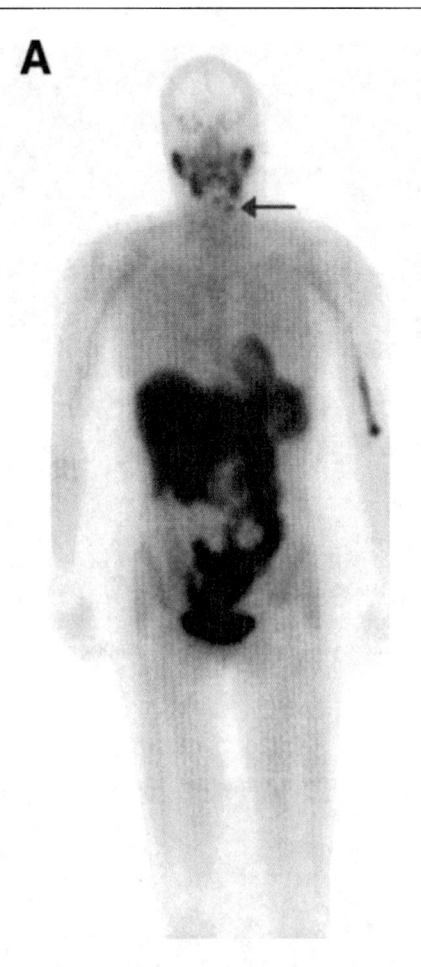

Color Plate 24, Fig. 2A. This patient is a 53-yr-old female who had papillary thyroid cancer and was ablated with radioiodine. At the time of followup and after thyroid hormone withdrawal. Whole-body ^{99m}Tc sestamibi scan. (*See* full caption in Ch. 35 on p. 331 and discussion on p. 330.)

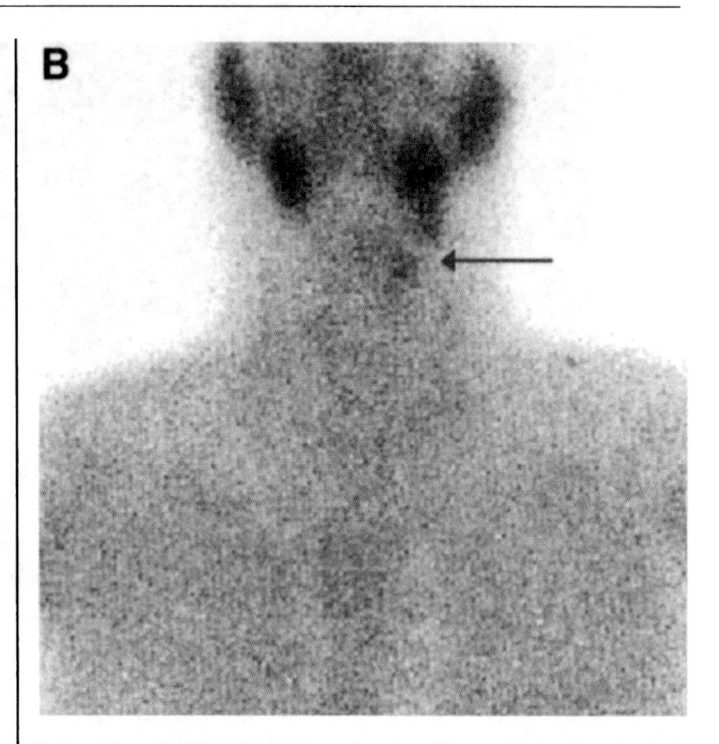

Color Plate 25, Fig. 2B. This patient is a 53-yr-old female who had papillary thyroid cancer and was ablated with radioiodine. At the time of followup and after thyroid hormone withdrawal. Demonstrated faint uptake in the left neck area. (*See* full caption in Ch. 35 on p. 331 and discussion on p. 330.)

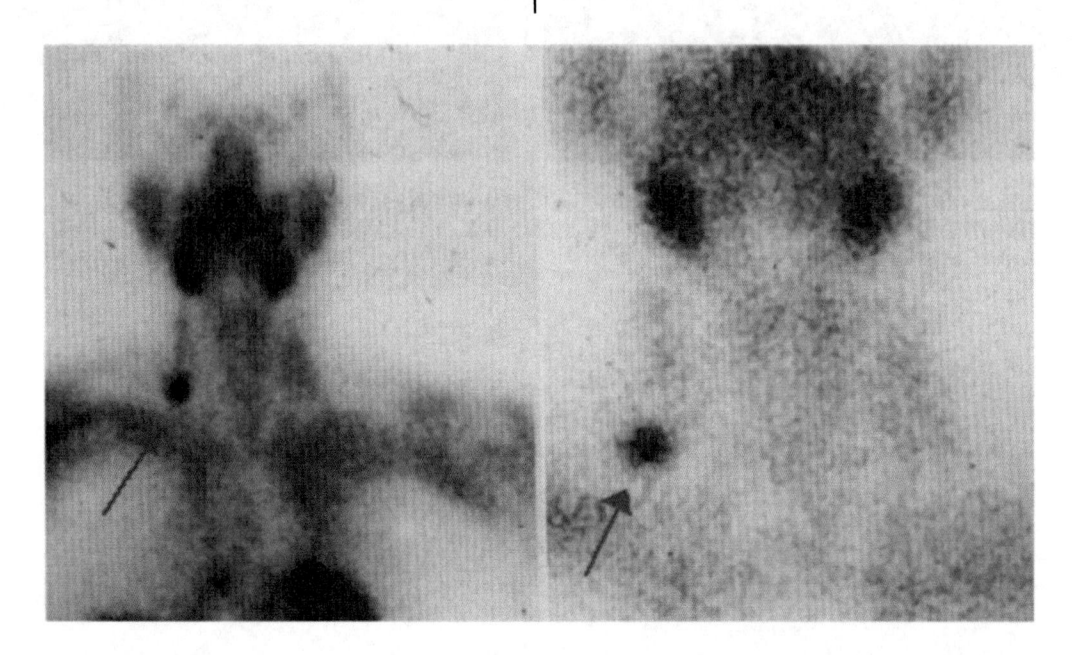

Color Plate 26, Fig. 3. This is a ^{99m}Tc sestamibi scan of a 56-yr-old patient who has had a previous thyroidectomy and negative radioiodine scan and now has an elevated serum thyroglobulin level off thyroid suppression of 50 pg/mL. (*See* full caption and discussion in Ch. 35 on p. 332.)

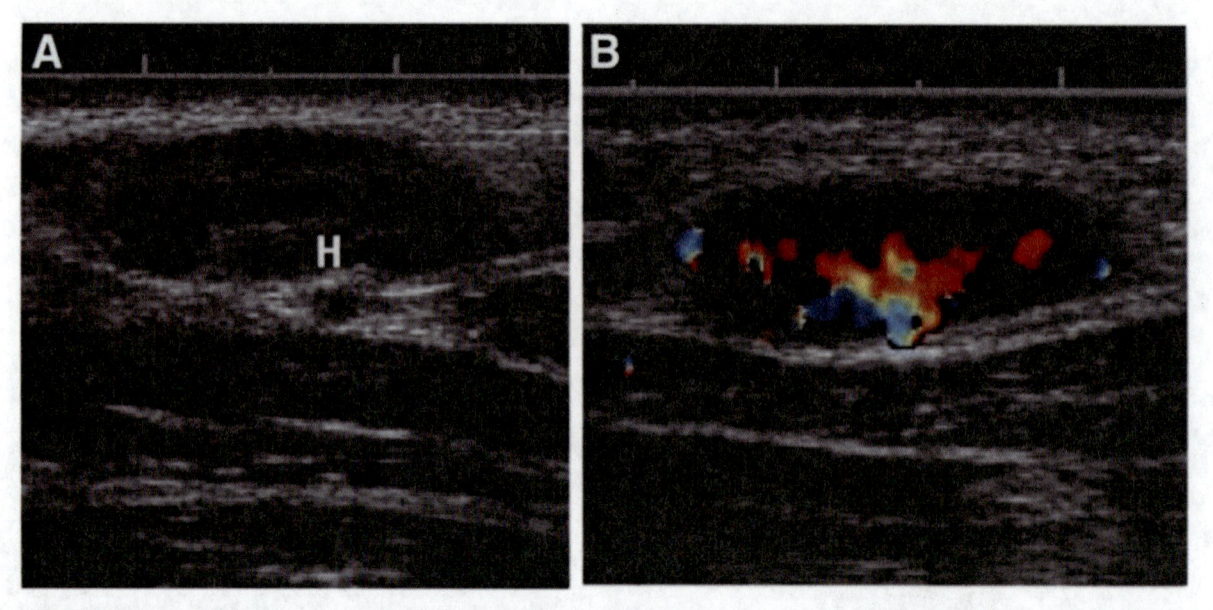

Color Plate 27, Fig. 1. Longitudinal projections of a normal lymph node on sonographic examination. (*See* full caption in Ch. 37 on p. 353 and discussion on p. 352.)

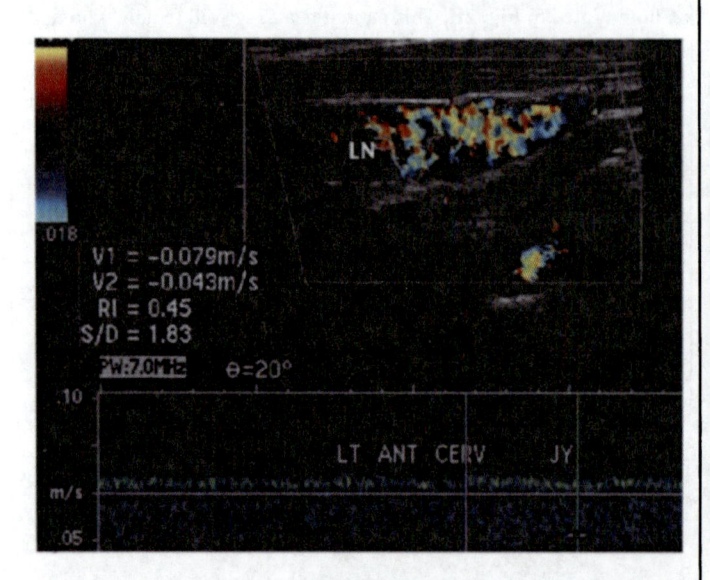

Color Plate 28, Fig. 2. Longitudinal view of a narrow, oval normal lymph node with Doppler showing physiologic vasculatlure. (*See* full caption in Ch. 37 on p. 353 and discussion on p. 352.)

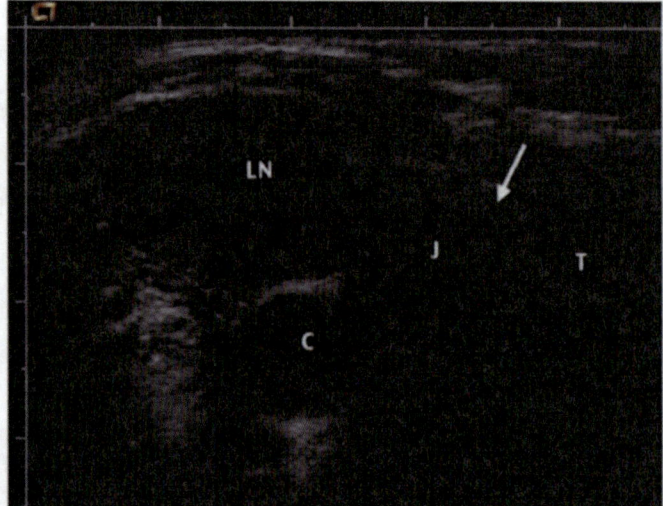

Color Plate 29, Fig. 3. Sonogram of the neck from a patient who had a total thyroidectomy for papillary cancer of the thyroid. (*See* full caption in Ch. 37 on p. 354 and discussion on p. 353.)

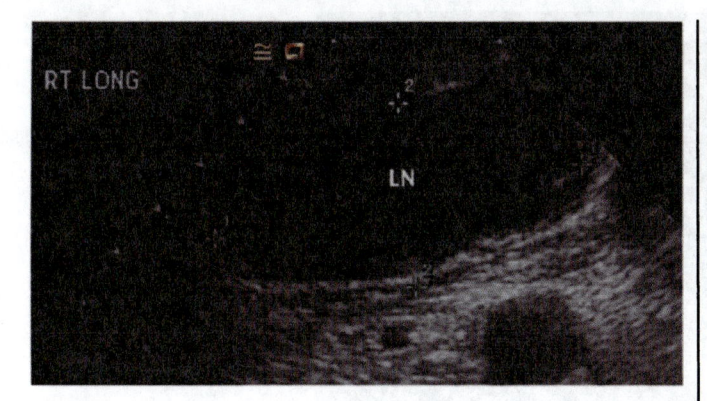

Color Plate 30, Fig. 4. Longitudinal projection of a sonogram of a plump, heterogeneous lymph node involved with metastic papillary thyroid cancer. (*See* full caption and discussion in Ch. 37 on p. 354.)

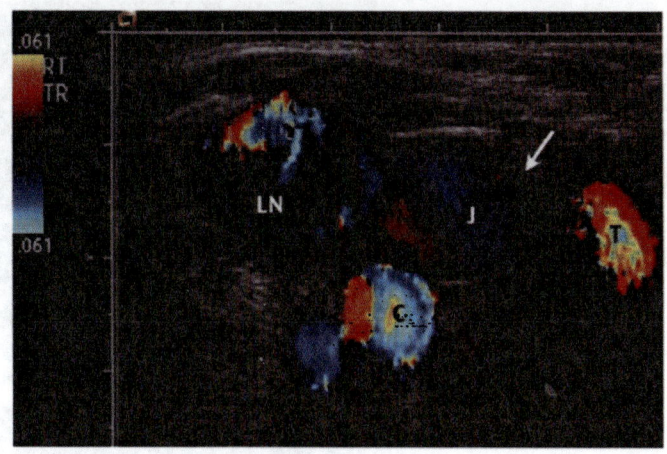

Color Plate 31, Fig. 6. Longitudinal view of a sonogram of a lymph node that was plump and was therefore deemed suspicious by the fatty hilum, suggesting benign disease. (*See* full caption and discussion in Ch. 37 on p. 354.)

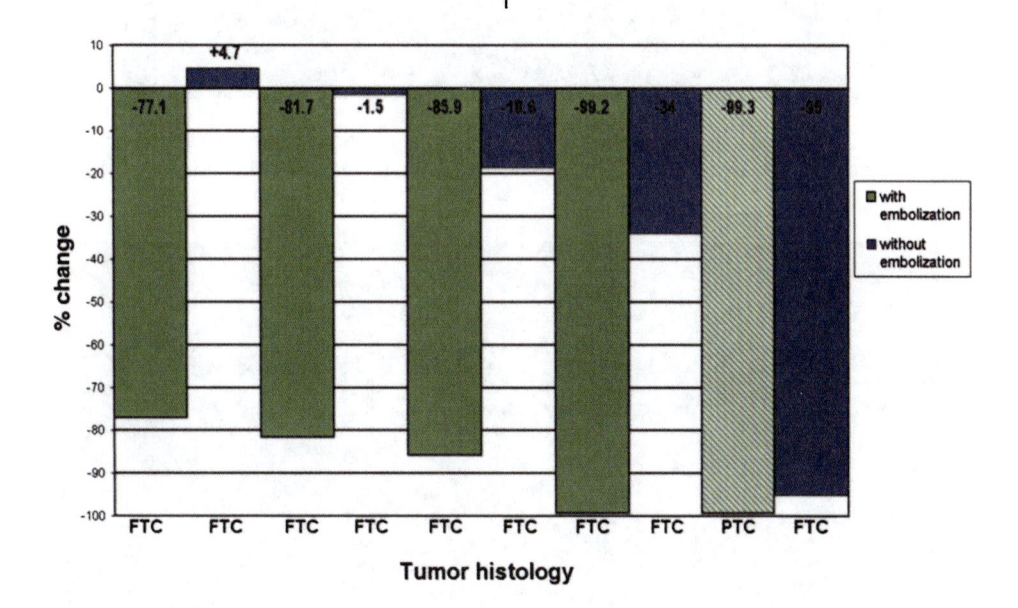

Color Plate 32, Fig. 5. Reduction of the thyroglobulin levels with and without embolization of differentiated thyroid cancer mestatases. (*See* full caption in Ch. 53 on p. 502 and discussion on p. 501.)

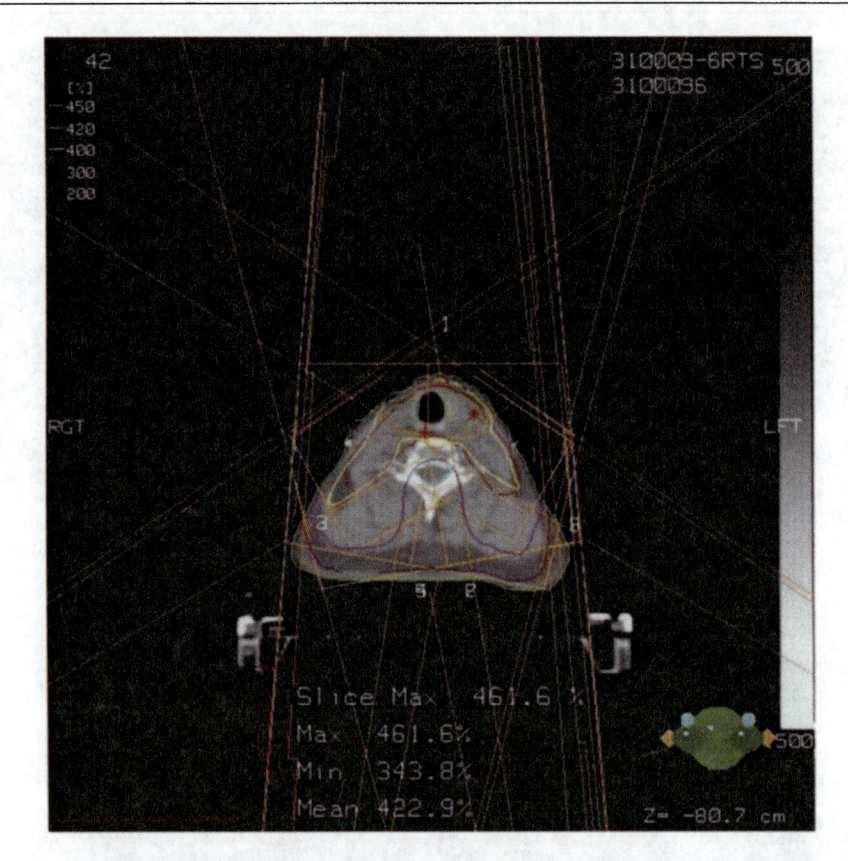

Color Plate 33, Fig. 1. These axial CT-planning images of a five-field conformal technique were used at Princess Margaret Hospital to treat the thyroid bed and adjacent regional lymph nodes. (*See* full caption in Ch. 84 on p. 654 and discussion on p. 653.)

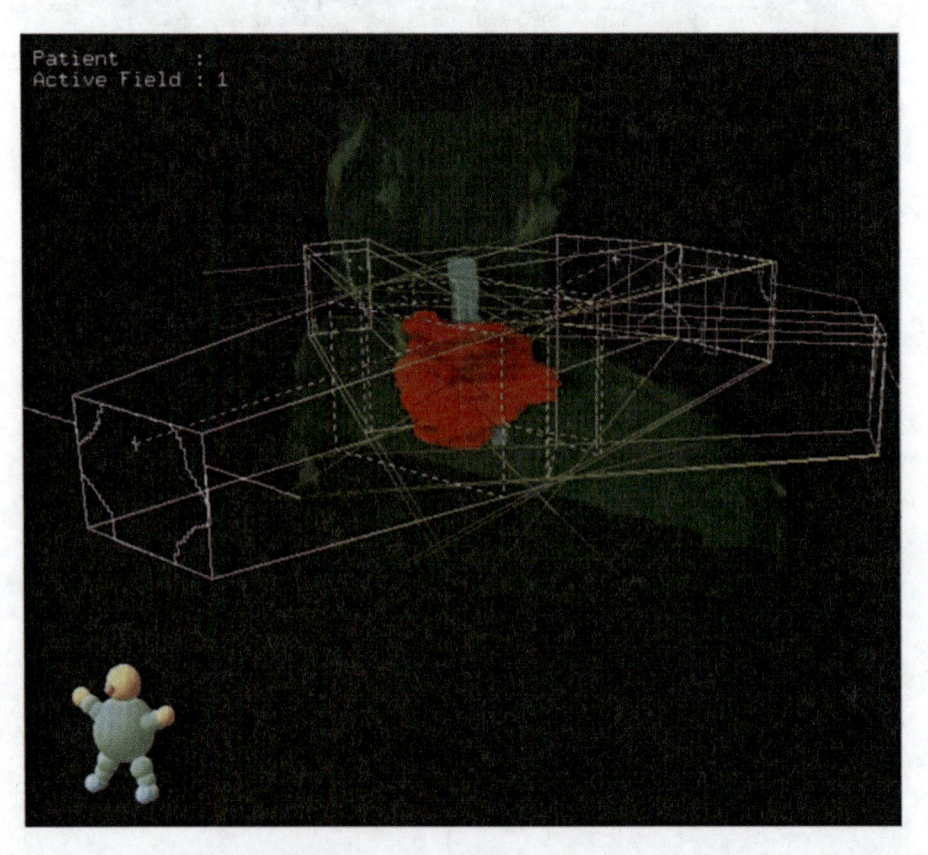

Color Plate 34, Fig. 2. The 3D view of the conformal five-field beam arrangement was designed to achieve dose uniformity for the thyroid bed CTV and spare the spinal cord. (*See* full caption in Ch. 84 on p. 655 and discussion on p. 653.)

151. Kolla IS, Alazraki NP, Watts NB. Sialoadenitis mimicking metastatic thyroid carcinoma. Clin Nucl Med 1989; 14:564–566.
152. Tyson JW, Wilkinson RH, Witherspoon LR, Goodrich JK. False-positive I-131 total body scans. J Nucl Med 1974; 15:1052–1053.
153. Wolff H, Breda DJ, DaSilva N, Hartmann AA. False-positive I-131 deposition in a parotid gland duct ectasia. Clin Nucl Med 1998; 23:257–259.
154. Wendell TJ, Wilkinson RH, Witherspoon LR. False positive ^{131}I total-body scans. J Nucl Med 1974; 15:1052–1053
155. Carlisle M, Cortes A, McDougall IR. Uptake of I-131 in the biliary tract: A potential cause of a false-positive result of scintiscan. Clin Nucl Med 1998; 23:524–527.
156. Schall GL, Temple R. Importance of proper bowel cleansing before I-131 whole body scan or retention study. J Nucl Med 1972; 13:181–182.
157. Brachman MB, Rothman BJ, Ramanna L, Tanasescu DE, et al. False-positive iodine-131 body scan caused by a large renal cyst. Clin Nucl Med 1988; 13:416–418.
158. Bakheet MS, Powe J, Hammami MM. Unilateral radioiodine breast uptake. Clin Nucl Med 1998; 23:170–171.
159. Robinson PS, Surveyor I. Response to letter: Unilateral iodine-131 uptake in the lactating breast. J Nucl Med 1995; 36:1725.
160. Grunwald F, Palmedo H, Biersack HJ. Unilateral iodine-131 uptake in the lactating breast. J Nucl Med 1995; 36:1724–1725.
161. Serafini A, Sfakianakis G, Georgiou M, Morris J. Breast cyst simulating metastases of iodine-131 imaging in thyroid carcinoma. J Nucl Med 1998; 39:1910–1912.
162. Blue PW, Dydek GJ, Ghaed N. Radiation dosimetry from breast milk excretion of iodine-123. J Nucl Med 1987; 28:544–545.
163. Nurnberger CE, Lipscomb A. Transmission of radioiodine (I-131) to infants through human maternal milk. JAMA 1952; 150:1398–1400.
164. Rubow S, Klopper J. Excretion of radioiodine in human milk following a therapeutic dose of 131I. Eur J Nucl Med 1988; 14:632–633.
165. Maslack MM, Wilson CA. Iodine-131 accumulation in a pericardial effusion (letter). J Nucl Med 1987; 28:133.
166. Silva F, Garcia L, Flores C, Storer D, et al. Pericardial effusion: Unusual complication in thyroid cancer. Clin Nucl Med 1996; 21:218–220.
167. Haubold-Reuter BG, Landolt U, Schulthess GKV, et al. Bronchogenic carcinoma mimicking metastatic thyroid carcinoma. J Nucl Med 1993; 34:809–811.
168. Kim EE, Pjura G, Gobuty A, Verani R. 131-I uptake in a benign serous cystadenoma of the ovary. Eur J Nucl Med 1984; 9:433–435.
169. Francese C, Schlumberger M, Travagli JP, Vera P, et al. Iodine-131 uptake in a pleuropericardial cyst: Case report of a false-positive radioiodine total body scan result in a patient with a thyroid cancer. Eur J Nucl Med 1991; 18:779–780.
170. Bakheet SM, Hammami MM, Powe J. Radioiodine bronchogram in acute respiratory tract infection. Clin Nucl Med 1997; 22:308–309.
171. Duque JJ, Miguel MB, Ruiz E, Castillo L, et al. False-positive ^{131}I whole-body scan in follicular thyroid carcinoma caused by frontal sinus mucocele. Clin Nucl Med 2000; 25:137–138.
172. Lungo M, Tenenbaum F, Chaumerliac P, Vons C, et al. Ovarian endometriosis cyst with iodine-131 uptake3: first case of positive uptake in the follow up for differentiated thyroid carcinoma. Ann Endocrinol (Paris) 2000; 61:147–150.
173. Bakheet SM, Hammami MM, Powe J. Radioiodine uptake in rheumatoid arthritis-associated lung disease mimicking thyroid cancer metastases. Clin Nucl Med 1998; 23:319–320.
174. Bakheet SM, Hammami MM, Powe J, Bazarbashi M, et al. Radioiodine in inactive tuberculosis. Eur J Nucl Med 1999; 26:659–662.
175. Regalbuto C, Buscema M, Arena S, Vigneri R, et al. False-positive findings on ^{131}I whole-body scans because of posttraumatic superficial scabs. J Nucl Med 2002; 43:207–209.
176. Hoschl R, Choy DHL, Grandevia B. Iodine-131 uptake in inflammatory lung disease: A potential pitfall in treatment of thyroid cancer. J Nucl Med 1988; 29:701–706.
177. Herzog G, Kisling G, Bekerman C. Diagnostic significance of dental history in the clinical evaluation of patients with thyroid carcinoma: Periodontal surgery mimicking a metastasis on I-131 whole-body survey. Clin Nucl Med 1992; 17:589–590.
178. Wadhwa SS, Mansberg R. Benign oral disease as a cause of false-positive iodine-131 scans. Clin Nucl Med 1998; 23:747–749.
179. Otsuka N, Fukunaga M, Morita K, Ono S, et al. 131I uptake in patient with thyroid cancer and rheumatoid arthritis during acupuncture treatment. Clin Nucl Med 1990; 15:29–31.
180. Matheja P, Lerch H, Schmid K, Kuwert T, et al. Frontal sinus mucocele mimicking a metastasis of papillary thyroid carcinoma. J Nucl Med 1997; 38:1022–1024.
181. Brucker-Davis F, Reynolds JC, Skarulis MC, Fraker DL, et al. False-positive iodine-131 whole-body scans due to cholecystitis and sebaceous cyst. J Nucl Med 1996; 37:1690–1693.
182. Bakheet SM, Hammami MM, Powe J, et al. Radioiodine in the head and neck. Endocr Pract 2000; 6:37–41.
183. Kinuya S, Yokoyama K, Michigishi T. I-131 accumulation in folliculitis of the scalp. Clin Nucl Med 1996; 21:807–808.
184. Froncova K. Uptake of radioiodine by myocardium following infarction. Cas Lek Cesk 1978; 103:64.
185. Turoglu HT, Naddaf S, Young I, Abel-Dayem H. Infected sebaceous cyst: A cause for false-positive total-body I-123 metastatic survey for thyroid cancer. Clin Nucl Med 1996; 23:887.
186. Naddaf S, Akisik MF, Omar WS, Young I, et al. I-123 uptake in the chest wall after needle biopsy of a pulmonary nodule. Clin Nucl Med 1997; 22:572573.
187. Langsteger W, Koltringer P, Meister E, Eber O. False-positive scans in papillary thyroid carcinoma (letter). J Nucl Med 1993; 34:2280.
188. Wu S, Kollin J, Coodley E, Lockyer T, et al. I-131 total body scan: Localization of disseminated gastric adenocarcinoma. Case report and survey of the literature. J Nucl Med 1984; 25:1204–1209.
189. Berding G, Forsting M, Georgi P. Unspezifische speichergung in J-131-Ganzkorperszintigramm bei de Nachsorgeeines metasterierienden papillaren. Schilddrusencarcinoms bedingt durch ein meningeom. Nuc Compact 1990; 21:163–164.
190. Priesman RA, Halpern SE, Shishido R, Waltz T, et al. Uptake of 131-I by a papillary meningioma. AJR Am J Roentgenol 1977; 128:349–350.
191. Acosta J, Chitkara R, Kahn F, Azueta V, et al. Radioactive iodine uptake by a large cell-undifferentiated bronchogenic carcinoma. Clin Nucl Med 1982; 7:368–369.
192. Fernandez-Ulloa M, Maxon HR, Mehta S, Sholiton L. Iodine-131 uptake by primary lung adenocarcinoma, misinterpretation of ^{131}I scan. JAMA 1976; 236:857–858.
193. Langsteger W, Lind P, Koltringer P, Beham A, et al. Misinterpretation of iodine uptake in papillary thyroid carcinoma and primary lung adenocarcinoma. J Cancer Res Clin Oncol 1990; 116:8–12.
194. Misaki T, Takeuchi R, Miyamoto S, Kasagi K, et al. Radioiodine uptake by squamous-cell carcinoma of the lung. J Nucl Med 1994; 35:474–475.
195. Burt RW. Accumulation of ^{123}I in a Warthin's tumor. Clin Nucl Med 1978; 3:155–156.
196. Harbert JC. Radio iodine therapy of differentiated thyroid carcinoma In Harbert JC, Robertson JS, Held KD, editors. Nuclear Medicine Therapy. New York: Thieme Medical Publishers Inc. 1987:37–89.
197. Wynne HMN, McCartney JC, McClendon JF. Struma ovarii. Am J Obstet Gynecol 1940; 39:263–275.
198. Willemse PHB, Oosterhuis JW, Aalders JG, Piers DA, et al. Malignant struma ovarii treated by ovariectomy, thyroidectomy and I-131 administration. Cancer 1987; 60:178–182.
199. Brenner W, Bohuslavizki KH, Wolf H, Sippel C, et al. Radiotherapy with iodine-131 in recurrent malignant struma ovarii. Eur J Nucl Med 1996; 23:91–94.
200. Lakshmanan M, Reynolds JC, DelVecchio S, Merino MJ, et al. Pelvic radioiodine uptake in a rectal wall teratoma after thyroidectomy for papillary carcinoma. J Nucl Med 1992; 33:1848–1850.
201. Wang PW, Chen HY, Li CH. Uptake of I-131 by an abdominal neurilemoma mimicking metastatic thyroid carcinoma. Clin Nucl Med 1993; 18:964–966.

202. Wilson RL, Cowan RJ. Tc-99m pertechnetate uptake in a thymoma: Case report. Clin Nucl Med 1982; 7:149–150.
203. Bestagno M, Pagliavni R, Maira G. Mediastinal uptake of 131I in patients with thyroid cancer: may it be referred to normal thymus? Eur J Nucl Med 1993; 20(Abstr):648.
204. Goldman M, Bauer SR. A comparative study of iodine uptake by thyroid and thymus glands of male and female Sprague-Dawley rats of different ages. Acta Endocrinol 1977; 85:64–70.
205. Jackson GL, Graham WP III, Flickinger FW, Kennedy TJ. Thymus accumulation of radioactive iodine. Pa Med 1979; 82:37–38.
206. Michigishi T, Mizukami Y, Shuke N, Yokoyama K, et al. Visualization of the thymus with therapeutic doses of radioiodine in patients with thyroid cancer. Eur J Nucl Med 1993; 20:75–79.
207. Veronikis IE, Simkin P, Braverman LE. Thymic uptake of iodine-131 in the anterior mediastinum. J Nucl Med 1996; 37:991–992.
208. Vermiglio F, Baudin E, Travagli JP, Caillou B, et al. Iodine concentration by the thymus in thyroid carcinoma. J Nucl Med 1996; 37:1830–1831.
209. Wilson L, Barrington SF, Kettle AG. Physiological uptake occurs in the thymus of young patients treated with radioiodine for thyroid carcinoma. J Nucl Med 1998; 38(Abstr):152P.
210. Wilson LM, Barrington SF, Morrison ID, Kettle, AG, et al. Therapeutic implications of thymic uptake of radioiodine in thyroid carcinoma. Eur J Nucl Med 1998; 25:622–628.
211. Davidson J, McDougall IR. How frequently is the thymus seen on whole-body iodine-131 diagnostic and post-treatment scans. Eur J Nucl Med 2000; 27:425–430.
212. Salvatore M, Saletmich I, Rufini V, Troncone L. Unusual false-positive radioiodine whole-body scans in patients with differentiated thyroid carcinoma. Clin Nucl Med 1997; 22:380–384.
213. Andreas J, Bruhl K, Eissmer D. False-positive I-131 whole body imaging after I-131 therapy for a follicular carcinoma. Clin Nucl Med 1997; 22:123–124.
214. Shapiro B, Rufini V, Jaruan A, Geatti O, et al. Artifacts, anatomical and physiological variants, and unrelated diseases that might cause false-positive whole-body 131-I scans in patients with thyroid cancer. Semin Nucl Med 2000; 30:115–132.

Part III
The Thyroid Nodule

17
The Thyroid Nodule
Evaluation, Risk of Malignancy, and Management

Leonard Wartofsky

INTRODUCTION

Palpable nodules of the thyroid are frequently encountered in clinical practice, and their evaluation requires the physician to be familiar with a growing number of diagnostic tools to identify those nodules representing cases of carcinoma that require surgical intervention. Under most circumstances, what constitutes optimal clinical management of nodular thyroid disease is somewhat controversial *(1–6a)*. However, major professional organizations and the authoritative National Comprehensive Cancer Network have published consensus guidelines for the diagnosis and management of thyroid nodules *(7–9)*.

PREVALENCE

Solitary nodules of the thyroid gland are present in about 6.4% of women and 1.5% of men in the United States *(1,2,6)*. Surveys in northeast England are comparable with 5.3% of adult women and 0.8% of adult men who have been found to have nodules *(10)*. The low prevalence in children (~1.5%) increases linearly with age. During a 15-yr follow-up of the Framingham population, new nodules appeared in 0.1% of patients per year *(11)*. Many single palpable nodules thought to be solitary are actually in a multinodular thyroid gland. Although autopsy studies indicate thyroid nodules in as many as 50% of consecutive necropsies, many may be small and clinically inapparent *(1,2)*. High-resolution ultrasound has identified nodules in 13–40% of patients evaluated for non-thyroid problems *(12–14)*. Indeed, nodules may be detected by ultrasound in up to 70% of adults, but most will be quite small and of uncertain clinical importance. Thus, a discrepancy exists between the true prevalence of thyroid nodules and that seen by physical exam. Generally, nodules must approach 1 cm in diameter to be recognized on palpation. The significance of nonpalpable nodules incidentally found by ultrasound, so-called "incidentalomas," is discussed below.

PATHOGENESIS

While the cause of thyroid nodules is not known, iodine deficiency and indirect evidence of thyrotropin (TSH) may have possible relationships. Cold nodules occur about 2.5 times more often in areas of low naturally occurring iodine. In rats, iodine deficiency enhances TSH secretion and the development of thyroid nodules, some of which are malignant *(15)*. The relationship to TSH is unclear, but the response of benign nodular thyroid enlargement to thyroxine *(2,16,17)*, as well as the improved prognosis of patients with papillary thyroid cancer treated with thyroxine *(18)*, suggest a role of TSH in human neoplasia.

Radiation exposure can cause thyroid neoplasia, with a linear relationship between radiation doses up to 1800 rad and the incidence of thyroid nodules and cancer. The increased risk of clinically significant thyroid cancer associated with prior radiotherapy to the head and neck given for thymic enlargement, tonsillitis, acne, and adenitis, is around 3% *(19–21)*. Radiation exposure during childhood is more likely to produce thyroid neoplasia than similar exposure at a later age, possibly related to greater cellular mitotic activity at the earlier age of insult. Among individuals in the United States who received head and neck irradiation as children, palpable nodules are found in 16–29% and carcinoma in one third of these nodules *(21,22)*. Most nodules tend to occur within 10–20 yr of exposure, but the risk may exist for over 35 yr. The irradiated thyroid gland often presents with multiple nodules; at surgery, the lesion of initial concern may prove to be benign, whereas one or more carcinomas will be found elsewhere in the gland. Thus, those nodules associated with a radiation history do not demonstrate a reduction of cancer risk when the thyroid contains multiple nodules. The dramatic increase in thyroid nodules and thyroid cancer occurring in Belarus after the 1986 Chernobyl nuclear disaster is discussed in detail in Chapter 7 by J. Figge and associates, and has been reviewed recently *(22a)*.

Higher doses of irradiation, e.g., that from external radiation therapy for Hodgkin's disease (>2000 rad) or internal radiation from ^{131}I therapy for toxic goiter, do not appear to be related to subsequent development of thyroid carcinoma. In both cases, the high-dose exposure with attendant cell destruction, fibrosis, and hypothyroidism may serve to attenuate any carcinogenic effect of lesser degrees of radiation injury.

DIFFERENTIAL DIAGNOSIS

As indicated in Table 1, the differential diagnosis of apparent thyroid nodules covers a wide range of pathology *(1–6)*. Most true intrathyroidal nodules will represent colloid adenomas (27–60%) or simple follicular adenomas (26–40%). About 5% of thyroid nodules are classified as hyperfunctioning and are "hot" on radionuclide scanning based on a relative increased ability to trap iodide. Most hot nodules are autonomously functioning and are associated with either subclinical or overt hyperthyroidism in more than half of patients over 60 yr of age. Of nodules greater than 3 cm in diameter 20% are associated with hyperthyroidism *(23)*, compared with 2% of smaller lesions. Although most toxic autonomous nodules secrete both thyroxine (T_4) and triiodothyronine (T_3), elevations of T_3 or T_4 alone occasionally may be seen. Moreover, even when T_3 and T_4 levels are "normal," low or undetectable, serum TSH by a sensitive assay ("subclinical" hyperthyroidism) may be commonly seen, suggesting supraphysiologic iodothyronine production.

Cancers are found in 10–14% of patients presenting with palpable thyroid nodules *(1–6)*. Papillary carcinomas account for about 70–75% of all thyroid cancer in Americans, with follicular as the next most common (20–25%) and anaplastic and medullary thyroid carcinomas comprising the remaining 3–5%. The thyroid gland has a rich blood supply, and a thyroid nodule occasionally may represent a secondary or metastatic neoplasm, including malignant melanoma, renal cell, breast, or bronchogenic carcinoma. In 2005, the American Cancer Society estimates that there will be approximately 25,690 new thyroid cancer cases diagnosed and 1490 thyroid cancer-related deaths in the United States *(24)*. Thyroid cancer is estimated among the top 10 leading causes of new cases of cancer in women. Autopsy studies have revealed occult thyroid cancer in 6% of autopsies in North American series *(25)*. There is general agreement that these small, occult, and mostly papillary cancers are of little or no clinical significance, and their increased prevalence does not correlate with an increase in the death rate from thyroid carcinoma *(26)*.

DIAGNOSTIC EVALUATION

As the vast majority of thyroid nodule morbidity is related to those lesions representing carcinoma, the evaluation is focused on the identification of nodules that may be malignant.

History and Physical Examination

The single most important historical risk factor for cancer is exposure to radiation. It is important to determine the age at time of exposure, exact region of the body irradiated, and if possible, the type and dose of radiation to the thyroid.

Table 1
Differential Diagnosis of Apparent Thyroid Nodules

Benign thyroid neoplasms
  Follicular adenoma
    Colloid
    Simple
    Fetal
    Embryonal
    Hurthle cell
  Papillary adenoma
  Teratoma
  Lipoma
  C-cell adenoma
  Dermoid cyst
Malignant thyroid neoplasms
  Papillary carcinoma
  Follicular carcinoma
  Medullary thyroid carcinoma
  Anaplastic carcinoma
  Metastatic carcinoma
  Sarcoma
  Lymphoma
Other thyroid abnormalities
  Thyroiditis
  Thyroid cyst
  Hemiagenetic thyroid
  Infectious Granulomatous disease (e.g., sarcoidosis)
Nonthyroidal lesions
  Lymphadenopathy
  Aneurysm
  Thyroglossal duct cyst
  Parathyroid cyst
  Parathyroid adenoma
  Laryngocele
  Cystic hygroma

Although women are more prone to thyroid nodules and cancer than men, the probability of cancer is higher among men with nodules, especially in those over age 70. The incidence of thyroid cancer increases with age, but a higher percentage of nodules in patients less than 20 yr of age will be malignant. Thus, the features regarding history and physical examination that are more suggestive of a malignant nodule include male sex, age less than 15 or greater than 70, history of irradiation of the head and neck, and associated cervical lymphadenopathy.

Thyroid lymphoma should be considered in patients with rapid thyroid enlargement and a previous diagnosis of Hashimoto's thyroiditis, especially in women over age 50. Such lesions may present as a dominant "cold" nodule, and there is often coincident diabetes mellitus. A family history of pheochromocytoma, hypercalcemia, mucosal abnormalities, or medullary thyroid carcinoma raises suspicion of the latter diagnosis as part of a multiple endocrine neoplasia (MEN) syndrome. Although family history of benign goiter may be reassuring, the rare Pendred's syndrome of familial goiter and deaf mutism is linked with a higher cancer risk *(1,3)*.

Most thyroid nodules are discovered incidentally in asymptomatic patients. Although only a solitary nodule may be detected on physical examination, as many as 50% of glands will actually harbor multiple nodules *(27)*. As noted in Table 2, many symptoms or physical findings are believed to be more common in malignant than in benign nodules, but as few as 5–10% of patients with malignancy present with symptoms. Patients with advanced disease may present with lymphadenopathy, growth of hard nodules, thyroid pain and tenderness, and vocal cord paralysis, all of which point to the likelihood of malignancy.

Laboratory Tests

Thyroid function tests are usually of little value in the evaluation of thyroid nodules, with the exception of possible toxic adenomas. Thyroglobulin levels may be elevated in patients with thyroid malignancy and are useful as a tumor marker in the routine follow-up of patients undergoing surgery for thyroid cancer *(28–30)*, but preoperative blood levels do not differentiate from those associated with benign adenomas or thyroiditis. Serum antithyroglobulin and antimicrosomal (or antithyroid peroxidase) antibodies also have limited value for initial diagnosis. However, the disappearance or reappearance of antithyroglobulin antibodies may herald cure or recurrence, respectively, of thyroid cancer *(31)*.

Special diagnostic studies are available for the detection of medullary thyroid cancer (MTC), which may present as a dominant cold nodule *per se* or as part of a MEN syndrome *(32–34)*. MENIIA is characterized by MTC with pheochromocytoma, and in some cases, hyperparathyroidism. The familial MTC of MENIIA differs from sporadic MTC in being often preceded by C-cell hyperplasia, leading to multifocal tumors. MENIIB includes MTC, pheochromocytoma, and several phenotypic abnormalities, e.g., mucosal neuromata. The *RET* proto-oncogene has been shown as the gene responsible for MENIIA and IIB, and mutations in differing codons and exons of *RET* have been identified in sporadic MTC as well. It is possible to routinely identify *RET* in material obtained by fine-needle aspiration (FNA) of a thyroid nodule. Differentiation between the mutations known for sporadic vs familial MTC provides information that helps to determine whether preoperative screening for pheochromocytoma is necessary.

MTC may secrete calcitonin, carcinoembryonic antigen (CEA), chromogranin, and other peptides *(35–37)*. As tumor markers (analogous to thyroglobulin for follicular thyroid cancer), these measurements are most useful for the detection of recurrence, rather than for initial diagnosis. Not all patients with proven MTC have elevated levels of calcitonin *(38,39)*. Pentagastrin for provocative testing is no longer available in the United States. Generally, the measurement of basal plasma calcitonin or CEA or assessment for the *RET* proto-oncogene intended to identify whether a nodule represents MTC are not cost-effective in the initial evaluation of the nodular thyroid. However, this is controversial *(40–42)* and not universally held. Screening serum calcitonin was deemed to be worthwhile in one large series of patients *(43)*, and the ostensibly earlier detection was associated with a better prognosis. False-positive elevated calcitonin may be seen in Hashimoto's disease *(44)*, in the presence of heterophile antibodies *(45)*, with renal failure *(46)*, with proton pump inhibitor drug therapy *(47)*, or in pseudohypoparathyroidism *(48)*. "Normal" individuals usually have serum calcitonin levels of less than 10 pg/mL *(42)*. Calcitonin levels correlate with MTC tumor size and preoperative calcitonin levels have been shown to correlate with prognosis *(48a)*.

Table 2
Physical and Historical Factors Increasing Risk of Carcinoma in a Thyroid Nodule

History	Physical Exam
Radiation	Cervical lymphadenopathy
Family history of MEN	Firmness
Rapid growth	Documented growth
Hoarseness	Vocal cord paralysis
Pain	Fixation
Dysphagia	Horner's syndrome
Respiratory obstructive symptoms	
Growth with thyroxine medication	

Fine-Needle Aspiration

The single best preoperative method to identify a malignancy is to obtain cells from the nodule for cytopathologic examination by a FNA technique *(49–52)*. FNA with a 22–25 gauge needle provides the highest rate of successful sampling and the lowest rate of complications, while yielding diagnostic precision that is equal or superior to other methods *(1,5)*. Both the collection technique and availability of a skilled cytopathologist are critical to the adequate collection and interpretation of specimen. As a result, the best success is achieved when both the operator and pathologist have considerable, continuous experience; false-negatives should average only 1% and false-positives 2% or less. It should be emphasized that the yield from FNA is only cells for cytologic examination and consequently does not represent a tissue biopsy. True core needle biopsy of thyroid nodules for tissue is still done in some centers with reportedly higher yields than FNA *(52a)* but is likely to have significantly more morbidity.

Several reports have indicated that FNA performed under ultrasound guidance causes a higher yield of satisfactory specimens, thereby enabling improved diagnostic accuracy *(53,54)*. The results of a FNA of a thyroid nodule is generally categorized as "benign," "suspicious," "malignant," or "inadequate for diagnosis," and the distinctions are discussed in Chapter 25 devoted to cytology and pathology by Oertel and Oertel.

Some studies have sought to use cytometric DNA analysis to improve the predictive value of FNA. Although it has not been found to be entirely successful in separating benign from malignant disease, it does correlate with the outcome and survival in patients with proven malignancy *(55,56)*. A number of biochemical and cellular markers have been identified and examined regarding their potential association with malignancy and their potential use to distinguish benign from malignant nodules *(57)*. These markers are described below in Chapter 19 by Prendergast and in a recent review *(57a)*. Of potentially great interest is the promise to one day distinguish between benign and malignant follicular neoplasms by molecular profiling *(57b)*.

FNA carries no significant risk, and reported cases of tumor seeding in the needle track are exceedingly rare *(58)*. Over the past decade, the use of FNA has had a clear salutary effect on the economics of nodule management by reducing the required frequency of surgical thyroidectomy by approximately 50% and doubling the yield of cancer in those patients undergoing operation *(55,56)*. FNA cytologic examination is also applied to the identification of carcinoma in lymph nodes, and measurement of thyroglobulin in the needle washout *(58a)* or of RT-PCR for TSH-receptor and thyroglobulin mRNA *(58b)* may prove useful adjuncts to cytology.

Thyroid Scanning

Specific aspects of radionuclide scanning are described in depth in various chapters (see Index), and this section serves only as an introduction to these procedures as they are applied to the initial evaluation of a thyroid nodule. Notably, scans reveal little about nodule size or shape and instead find their greatest utility in describing the functional state of a nodule. The majority of thyroid adenomas and carcinomas have defects in iodide accumulation and/or organification. Such defects can be demonstrated by images consistent with focal reduction in isotope accumulation (reduced trapping of radionuclide), leading to the designation of a "cold" nodule. On radionuclide scanning, about 5% of nodules are found to be "hot" (hyperfunctioning), 10% are "warm" (normal functioning), and 84% are "cold" (nonfunctioning).

The Hyperfunctioning ("Hot") Thyroid Nodule

A thyroid scan is useful in identifying hyperfunctioning nodules in patients with symptoms of hyperthyroidism, suppressed TSH levels, or biopsy results suggestive of follicular neoplasm. Hot nodules rarely represent malignancy, warm nodules carry an intermediate risk of about 5%, and cold nodules, with the highest risk *(3,6,7)* of malignancy, still represent benign pathology in more than 80% of cases. Therefore, radioisotopic scans are of low specificity despite their high sensitivity for nodules over 1 cm in diameter *(36)*. Scanning is usually done with ^{123}I or ^{99m}Tc pertechnetate (often referred to as "technetium scans"). Regardless of some limitations, the qualities of low-radiation dose, low cost, short-scanning interval, and reliability of hypofunctioning scans have led to the continued use of Tc at many centers. ^{123}I also delivers low radiation and is the preferred iodine-scanning agent but is not universally employed primarily because of its brief half-life (12 h) and the higher cost associated with its use. In addition to functional information, scans may reveal evidence of multinodularity in up to one third of clinically palpable solitary lesions—a finding that has been thought to be associated with a decreased risk of malignancy, at least in the past. Some recent studies still support this perspective *(59)*, but the majority of studies (particularly those that have utilized ultrasound to detect additional nodules) have demonstrated no difference in the frequency of malignancy in patients with single vs multiple nodules *(27,60,61)*. Moreover, thyroid cancer can arise in multiple foci within the gland as either independent tumors or on a monoclonal basis *(61a, 61b)*.

A recent vogue in Europe, which is yet to gain wide popularity in the United States, is the percutaneous injection of 95% ethanol into thyroid nodules, and in this case, specifically into a hyperfunctioning nodule *(62,63)*. This therapeutic approach has also been applied to benign thyroid cysts after aspiration, as well as to cold nodules proven initially to be benign by FNA. The procedure can be painful for the patient and has been associated with transient increases in serum thyroglobulin and thyroid hormones with self-limited thyrotoxicosis. Fever, local pain and hematomata, and vocal cord paralysis are also possible complications with inexperienced physicians. Although it has been claimed that no serious side effects of ethanol ablation have occurred, there is one case reported of fairly dramatic toxic necrosis of the larynx and overlying skin *(63a, 63b)*.

Ultrasound-guided laser photocoagulation has also been employed *(64)*.

Although hyperfunctioning nodules are rarely the seat of carcinoma, one advantage of their management by surgical excision (usually lobectomy) is the acquisition of a definitive histopathologic diagnosis, which would be lacking with management by radioiodine therapy or ethanol injection. Nevertheless, surgery is infrequently recommended for hyperfunctioning nodules because of its associated risks, the low incidence of cancer, and the proven efficacy and low morbidity of radioiodine therapy. One exception may be those very large (>4-cm diameter) nodules for which the required dose of radioiodine is so great that it increases the risk of radiation-induced neoplasia with the contralateral lobe.

The differential diagnosis for thyroid pain is quite short and includes thyroiditis, hemorrhage, and thyroid cancer. Hemorrhagic necrosis, heralded by pain, may occur during the natural history of a hyperfunctioning adenoma. With infarction of the hyperfunctioning nodule, the subsequent loss of the existing hyperfunction leads to reduced TSH suppression, return of TSH levels to normal, and resumption of function in the previously suppressed extranodular thyroid tissue. The previously hyperfunctioning nodule may then appear cold on scintiscanning, which taken together with the history of pain could be misinterpreted to represent a carcinoma. The functional state of a solitary autonomous nodule may not be sufficiently active to cause hyperthyroidism, and such patients have measurable levels of TSH, a hot nodule on the scan but with visible extranodular uptake of radionuclide, and they are euthyroid. Hot nodules enlarge with time, and there is a correlation of size with associated hyperthyroidism in approximately 4% of patients per year developing thyrotoxicosis *(65)*.

Other Scanning Modalities

Fluorescent thyroid scanning offers special advantages in childhood and pregnancy owing to minimal radiation exposure. The procedure has been reported as nearly 100% sensitive but only 64% specific when cold areas are taken as positive results. The procedure employs ^{241}Am, which has the ability to excite thyroidal iodine, causing release of X-rays that quantitatively correlate with iodine content of the imaged tissue. The required equipment is not widely available, and accumulated data remain too limited to recommend standard use of this technique.

A variety of other scanning techniques, including ^{99m}Tc-SestaMIBI *(66)*, ^{201}Tl *(67–70)*, ^{75}Sel, ^{67}Ga, and ^{131}Cs, have been investigated, and none have been proven to be reliable indicators of malignancy *(71,72)*. ^{131}I *Meta*-iodobenzylguanidine has been used successfully to image medullary carcinoma of the thyroid *(73)*. Fluorodeoxyglucose-positron emission tomography (PET) scanning has an important role in the follow-up of patients with thyroid cancer and has also been used earlier in the preoperative evaluation of thyroid nodules *(74)*.

Ultrasonography

A full discussion of thyroid ultrasound appears in Chapter 21 by Blum, and the utility of this diagnostic modality to determine which thyroid nodules might be malignant has been well described *(75–81)*. With the refinement of equipment, low cost, absence of radiation exposure, and the more universal office-based application of ultrasound, it has become arguably the most useful and important imaging technique for disorders of the thyroid gland. One putative problem with ultrasound is its increasing sensitivity, with the ability to delineate nodules as small as 1 mm *(82)*. This sensitivity raises the management problem of what to do with such little nodules, especially when found incidentally during an ultrasound study for some other purpose ("incidentalomas"), as discussed below. Although the field of view is characteristically small with conventional ultrasound, newer approaches have employed computerized modifications that allow panoramic images of the entire thyroid gland *(83)*. In contrast to radioisotopic-scanning techniques, ultrasound enables guidance for FNA, thereby improving diag-

Table 3
Potential Utility of Ultrasonography of Thyroid Nodules

Differentiation of solid vs cystic consistency
Detection of multinodularity
Detection of occult thyroid malignancy in cases of metastatic cervical lymphadenopathy from unknown primary
Monitoring nodule size, including response to suppressive therapy
Determination of solid vs hemorrhagic expansion in thyroid lesions showing rapid increase in size
Guidance for needle aspiration cytology in selected difficult cases
Guidance for therapy with ethanol or laser photocoagulation
(?) Monitoring irradiated thyroids
(?) Monitoring for local recurrence of thyroid carcinoma

nostic yield and accuracy *(53,54,60,61,84–88)* or guidance for therapeutic ablative therapy *(64,89,90)* (Table 3). Some workers have characterized the blood flow within nodules by color Doppler ultrasonography to distinguish between benign and malignant follicular neoplasms *(90a)*.

THYROID INCIDENTALOMA

Thyroid nodules discovered during routine imaging for other purposes have been termed "incidentalomas" if less than 1.5 cm in size. Because of the presumed rare occurrence of carcinoma in these small tumors, FNA with cytology has generally not been recommended for nodules of less than 1 cm; rather, it has been suggested that prudent follow-up by ultrasound examination was sufficient and more cost-effective *(91)*. However, opinions on this subject have since evolved *(92)* in view of recent literature describing early detection of malignancy in incidentalomas with PET scanning *(93–95)* and studies implying that the frequency of malignancy in small lesions is no different than that in nodules more than 1.5 cm *(79,84,94,95)*. High standardized uptake values on the PET scan appear to correlate well with the likelihood of malignancy and may prove useful to guide management in the future, specifically to determine which incidentalomas to biopsy *(94,95)*. Based on ultrasonographic criteria, the features of greatest concern that indicate possible cancer are a solid or hypoechoic appearance, irregular or blurred margins, intranodular vascularity on Doppler, and microcalcifications *(79,96)*. Based on their review of the literature, Silver and Parangi *(97)* recommended FNA of all incidentalomas seen on ultrasound that measure between 8 and 15 mm, with at least one of the telltale ultrasound features. The finding of medullary thyroid cancer in an incidentaloma represents yet another unique clinical problem. Some of these patients have had only subtotal thyroidectomy, raising the question of whether complete thyroidectomy is necessary for a small medullary tumor. Fortunately, many of these patients may do well with conservative management and close follow-up *(98)*. The risk of malignancy in incidentalomas is discussed further in Chapter 23 on papillary thyroid cancer.

THYROID HORMONE SUPPRESSION

Thyroid hormone has been used for many years to reduce the size of thyroid lesions thought to be dependent on TSH stimulation. As a diagnostic test, the assumption is that benign lesions will show preferential reduction in size. Typically, patients are given a 3–6-mo trial of L-thyroxine at a dose titrated to result in TSH suppression to, or slightly below, the lower limit of a normal sensitive TSH assay. The presumption is that growth of a nodule or lack of reduction in size during therapy raises suspicion of malignancy. This notion has been significantly challenged by the observations that even benign nodules grow with time (99,100). A greater than 75% reduction in size on L-thyroxine therapy likely occurs in only 5–10% of cases, whereas a 50% decline in size has been reported in an average of 30% of cases (1,5). Generally, those nodules that shrink with thyroxine suppression tend to enlarge again if therapy is withdrawn (101,102).

The controversy regarding whether to treat a nodule proven to be benign by FNA with thyroid hormone has been extensively discussed (16,17,103–105). Numerous trials of suppressive therapy have variably met with failure or success (103,109–114) compared to placebo (106–108), and there may be certain nodule cytological characteristics that predict responsiveness (115). Overall, long-term benefits of suppressive therapy may not be significant (108).

More carefully controlled studies of large patient populations are required to clarify the management of thyroid nodules with suppression therapy. The increasing concern about the possible risk of osteopenia after long-term suppressive doses of thyroid hormone has been somewhat allayed by careful analyses of the data (116). Use of prudent suppression doses of thyroxine has not been shown to contribute to osteopenia (117) and low-dose TSH suppression has been shown to have a comparable salutary effect on nodule size as higher dose TSH suppression in some (118), but not all (108), studies.

A trial of thyroid hormone suppression is neither sensitive nor specific but may have utility as an adjunct to other modalities of evaluation. In addition, suppressive therapy may have benefit in preventing the development of additional nodules. In a study examining recurrence rates for thyroid nodules after partial surgical thyroidectomy for benign disease in patients with a previous history of radiation, treatment with thyroid hormone postoperatively decreased the risk of benign recurrence from 36% to 8.4% (119).

Some patients given thyroxine may have concomitant autoimmune thyroid disease and/or other hyperfunctioning nonsuppressible nodules, in addition to the cold nodule being treated. These patients may require less levothyroxine because of the presence of functioning tissue that complements the exogenously administered hormone. An approximate suppressive dosage is 1.7 µg/kg body weight per day (120), which usually results in a serum T_4 at, or somewhat above, the upper limit of the normal range. The dose is incremented by 0.025 mg/d every 5–6 wk with TSH monitoring until a suppressed TSH is observed. Nodules are assessed for change in size by physical examination every 6 wk for the first 6 mo (or less frequently by ultrasound if required). The follow-up intervals may be more prolonged when significant decreases in size are observed, eventually extending to annual follow-up. Because of its long half-life, levothyroxine is administered as a single daily dose. Although the serum T_3 may be superior to the serum T_4 as an indicator of the metabolic state in the patient receiving levothyroxine, the optimal dose is best determined by clinical criteria and measurement of serum TSH by an ultrasensitive assay. An elevated serum TSH indicates that treatment is insufficient, and an elevated serum T_3 demonstrates that it is excessive. A decrease in dosage may be required with progressive emergence of autonomy and hyperfunction in a uninodular or multinodular goiter. The latter may be prompted by exposure to a high-iodine source. FNA biopsy should be repeated immediately when a nodule enlarges with suppressive therapy, and surgical exploration should be considered inevitable unless cystic fluid or hemorrhage with benign cytology is obtained. FNA should also be repeated when there is a failure to achieve a significant reduction in nodule size after 6–12 mo of suppressive therapy.

SUMMARY: APPROACH TO THE THYROID NODULE

The majority of thyroid nodules will be follicular adenomas, which are benign tumors that may occur singly or in multiples and may mimic normal thyroid function, trapping iodide, and producing thyroid hormones. On a radionuclide scan, they may be nonfunctional (cold), normally functional (warm), or hyperfunctioning (hot). Hot nodules are almost always benign. Hot nodules that cause hyperthyroidism are treated with radioiodine or surgery, whereas euthyroid patients with hot nodules may be followed without therapy, advised to avoid iodine excess, and monitored periodically with thyroid function tests. Other common benign nodules include colloid adenomas or cysts.

Concern should be raised that a thyroid nodule may be malignant in patients with a history of irradiation to the neck in childhood, associated cervical lymphadenopathy, a family history of thyroid cancer or pheochromocytoma, or recent or rapid nodule enlargement. Symptoms and signs that may be more suggestive of a malignant nodule include odynophagia, pain or pressure (compressive symptoms), vocal cord paralysis, or superior vena caval syndrome. Routine laboratory tests are insufficient to distinguish between benign and malignant nodules, but an elevated and rising level of serum thyroglobulin may be suggestive. FNA for cytology is the initial procedure of choice (49–52,121). Molecular analytical techniques to improve diagnosis of carcinoma in suspicious aspirates are being developed, such as the detection of BRAF mutations in aspirates by polymerase chain reaction-restriction fragment length polymorphism analysis

(122,123). Ultrasound for sizing, detection of cystic components, and evaluation for characteristics suggestive of cancer are likely to be beneficial, and a scintiscan to confirm functional state may be effective. Cysts or colloid adenomas demonstrated to be benign on FNA may reduce their size with levothyroxine therapy by approx 50%. L-T_4 treatment is contraindicated for autonomous hyperfunctioning adenomata.

The clinical challenge in thyroid nodule management is the formulation of the most accurate and cost-effective diagnostic protocol. Decision analysis has suggested that FNA—the most accurate single-evaluation parameter—provides a minimal advantage in quality-adjusted life expectancy over thyroid suppression. Figure 1 suggests an algorithm that may be useful in a practice where FNA is frequently utilized with experienced cytopathology support. Use of radionuclide scans as the initial step may result in increased cost, as only 5–10% of scans obviate the need for aspiration, whereas 60–80% of FNAs eliminate scan requirements. Some investigators place a greater emphasis on the role of ultrasonography in the evaluation of patients with nodules *(124)*, and a spherical shape of nodules has been shown to be highly associated with malignancy *(125)*. Others believe that because FNA predominantly identifies cystic lesions, sonography has limited initial utility but is valuable to further characterize the nodule and to follow results of suppressive therapy. However, sonography may permit identification of other nodules than the dominant nodule felt on palpation, as well as disclosing the presence of metastatic disease in lymph nodes preoperatively. For patients with proven benign nodules administered levothyroxine suppressive therapy, adequate TSH suppression is usually achieved at a dose of approx 1.7 μg/kg. Patients may be started on lower doses based on age and potential underlying cardiovascular disease, with patient reevaluations within 6 wk to monitor for symptoms of hyperthyroidism and to evaluate serum TSH levels. Starting from the initial dose, the dose is then incremented by 0.025 mg every 6 wk until TSH suppression or near suppression is documented, depending on the target TSH range desired, unless the patient has symptoms that require lowering the thyroxine dose. Nodules should be assessed for change in size every 2 mo for the first 6 mo. If the nodule significantly decreases in size, follow-up intervals may be gradually prolonged, with eventual annual follow-up. FNA may be repeated when nodules fail to respond to thyroxine suppression after 6–12 mo and sooner for any nodule that seems to be enlarging. Of repeat FNAs, 95% confirm the original diagnosis *(126)*.

Patients with a history of irradiation present a special situation. Historically, these patients have been immediately referred to surgery because of their higher cancer rate. Some clinicians now advocate FNA in the management of these patients as well, but sufficient evidence for reliability of benign results is still lacking owing to the frequent coexistence of both benign and malignant nodules *(127)*.

When surgical therapy is recommended, an ipsilateral lobectomy and isthmusectomy is the most common approach in single nodules where the preoperative diagnosis is uncertain (see Chapter 22). Frequently, frozen-section histologic evaluation is inconclusive or unreliable, and final diagnosis requires careful examination of permanent sections *(128)*. Many papillary carcinomas have multicentric growth, with tumor foci in the contralateral lobe in 30–82% of cases *(129)*. In questionable diagnostic cases, gene profiling of surgical thyroid tissue may distinguish benign follicular adenoma from carcinoma *(57a,130)*. Accordingly, when the ultimate diagnosis is carcinoma, it is customary to complete a near-total thyroidectomy within 1 wk of the first surgery. Studies have not shown any differences in survival or recurrence rates between total and near-total thyroidectomy, as well as greater morbidity associated with total thyroidectomy *(131)*. Inspection of regional lymph nodes with excision of suspicious nodes should also be conducted in all cases of thyroid cancer. Near-total thyroidectomy is the initial preferred procedure in patients with thyroid nodules and a history of thyroid irradiation because of the high incidence (54–75%) of bilateral disease *(131)*.

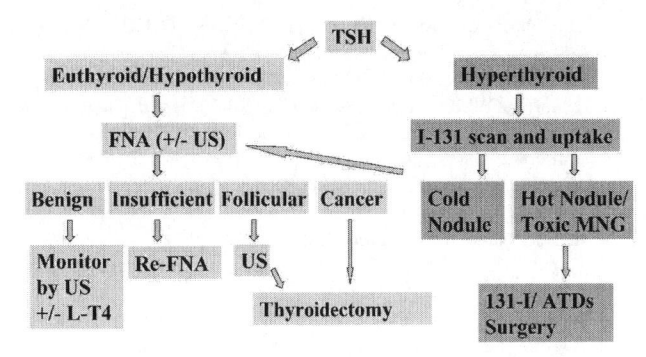

Fig. 1. Suggested algorithm for diagnosis and management of thyroid nodules, starting with serum TSH level.

REFERENCES

1. Mazzaferri EL. Management of a solitary thyroid nodule. N Engl J Med 1993; 328:553–559.
2. Burch HB. Evaluation and management of the solid thyroid nodule. Endocrin Metab Clin North Am 1995; 24:663–710.
3. Daniels GH. Thyroid nodules and nodular thyroids: A clinical overview. Comp Ther 1996; 22:239–250.
4. Ridgway EC. Clinical evaluation of solitary thyroid nodules. In Braverman LE, Utiger RD, editors. Werner & Ingbar's The Thyroid: A Fundamental and Clinical Text, 9th ed. Philadelphia: Lippincott, Williams & Wilkins, 2004.
5. Sheppard MC, Franklyn JA. Management of the single thyroid nodule. Clin Endocrinol 1992; 37:398–401.
6. Ridgway EC. Clinical review 30: clinician's evaluation of a solitary thyroid nodule. J Clin Endocrinol Metab 1992; 74:231–235.
6a. Castro MR, Gharib H. Continuing controversies in the management of thyroid nodules. Ann Intern Med 2005; 142:926–931.
7. Feld S. AACE clinical practice guidelines for the management of thyroid nodules. Endocrine Pract 1996; 2:78–84.
8. Singer PA, Cooper DA, Daniels GH, et al. Treatment guidelines for patients with thyroid nodules and well differentiated thyroid cancer. Arch Int Med 1996; 156:2165–2172.

9. National Comprehensive Cancer Network (NCCN) Thyroid Carcinoma: Clinical Practice Guidelines 2005, J Natl Comprehensive Cancer Network 2005; 3:404–457.
10. Tunbridge WMG, Evered DC, Hall R, et al. The spectrum of thyroid disease in a community: the Wichham survey. Clin Endocrinol 1977; 7:481–493.
11. Vander JB, Gaston EA, Dawber TR. The significance of nontoxic thyroid nodules: final report of a 15-year study on the incidence of thyroid malignancy. Ann Intern Med 1968; 69:537–540.
12. Hopkins CR, Reading CC. Thyroid and parathyroid imaging. Semin Ultrasound CT MR. 1995; 16:279–295.
13. Horlocker TT, Hay JE, James EM. Prevalence of incidental nodular thyroid disease detected during high resolution parathyroid ultrasonography. In Medeiros-Neto G, Gaitan E, editors. Frontiers in Thyroidology, vol. 1. New York: Plenum Press. 1986; 1309–1312.
14. Brander A, Viikinkoski P, Nickels J, Kivisaari L. Thyroid gland: ultrasound screening in a random adult population. Radiology 1991; 181: 683–687.
15. Burrow GN. The thyroid: nodules and neoplasia. In Felig P, Baxter JD, Broadus AE, Frohman LA, editors. Endocrinology and Metabolism. New York: McGraw-Hill. 1987; 473–507.
16. Richter B, Neises G, Clar C. Pharmacotherapy for thyroid nodules: A systematic review and meta-analysis. Endocrinol Metab Clin North Am 2002; 31:699–722.
17. Hegedus L, Bonnema SJ, Bennedbaek FN. Management of simple nodular goiter: Current status and future perspectives. Endocr Rev 2003; 24:102–132.
18. Mazzaferri EL, Young RL, Oertel JE, et al. Papillary thyroid carcinoma: the impact of therapy in 576 patients. Medicine 1977; 56:171–196.
19. Sarne D, Schneider AB. External radiation and thyroid neoplasia. Endocrin Metab Clin North Am 1996; 25:181–196.
20. Ron E, Kleinerman RE, Boice JD Jr, et al. A population-based case-control study of thyroid cancer, J Natl Cancer Inst 1987; 79:1–12.
21. Favus MJ, Schneider AB, Stachura ME, et al. Thyroid cancer occurring as a late consequence of head-and-neck irradiation. N Engl J Med 1976; 294:1019–1025.
22. DeGroot LJ, Reilly M, Pinnameneni K, Refetoff S. Retrospective and prospective study of radiation-induced thyroid disease. Am J Med 1983; 74:852–862.
22a. Cardis R, Kesminiene A, Ivanov V, et al. Risk of thyroid cancer after exposure to 131-I in childhood. J Natl Cancer Institute 2005; 97:724–732.
22b. Boice JD. Radiation-induced thyroid cancer—What's new? J Natl Cancer Institute 2005; 97:703–705.
23. Hamburger JI. The autonomously functioning thyroid nodule: Goetsch's Disease. Endocr Rev 1987; 8:439–447.
24. Jemal A, Murray T, Ward E, et al., Cancer statistics 2005. Ca: a Cancer Journal for Clinicians 2005; 55:10–30
25. Sampson RJ, Woolner LB, Bahn RC. Occult thyroid carcinoma in Olmsted County, Minnesota. Prevalence at autopsy compared with that in Hiroshima and Nagasaki. Cancer 1974; 34:2070–2076.
26. Sampson RJ. Prevalence and significance of occult thyroid cancer. In DeGroot LJ, Frohman LA, Kaplan EL, Refetoff S, editors. Radiation-Associated Thyroid Carcinoma. New York: Grune & Stratton. 1977; 137–143.
27. McCall A, Jarosz H, Lawrence AM. The incidence of thyroid carcinoma in solitary cold nodules and in multinodular goiters. Surgery 1986; 100:1128–1131.
28. Spencer CA, Wang C-C. Thyroglobulin measurement: Techniques, clinical benefits, and pitfalls. Endocrin Metab Clin North Am 1995; 24:841–864.
29. Whitley RJ, Ain KB. Thyroglobulin: a specific serum marker for the management of thyroid carcinoma. Clin Lab Med 2004; 24:29–47.
30. Spencer CA, LoPresti JS, Fatemi S, Nicoloff JT. Detection of residual and recurrent differentiated thyroid carcinoma by serum thyroglobulin measurement. Thyroid 1999; 9:435–441.
31. Spencer CA, Takeuchi M, Kazaroxyan M, et al. Serum thyroglobulin autoantibodies: prevalence, influence on serum thyroglobulin measurement, and prognostic significance in patients with differentiated thyroid carcinoma. J Clin Endocrinol Metab 1998; 83:1121–1127.
32. Marsh DJ, Learoyd DL, Robinson BG. Medullary thyroid carcinoma: recent advances and management update. Thyroid 1995; 5:407–424.
33. Pacini F, Fontanelli M, Fugazzola L, et al. Routine measurement of serum calcitonin in nodular thyroid diseases allows the preoperative diagnosis of unsuspected sporadic medullary thyroid carcinoma. J Clin Endocrinol Metab 1994; 78:826–829.
34. Vitale G, Caraglia M, Ciccarelli A, et al. Current approaches and perspectives in the therapy of medullary thyroid carcinoma. Cancer 2001; 91:1797–1808.
35. Wells SA Jr, Dilley WG, Farndon JA, et al. Early diagnosis and treatment of medullary thyroid carcinoma. Arch Intern Med 1985; 145: 1248–1252.
36. Hanna FWF, Ardill JES, Johnston CF, et al. Regulatory peptides and other neuroendocrine markers in medullary carcinoma of the thyroid. J Endocrinol 1997; 152:275–281.
37. Franke WG, Pinkert J, Runge R, et al. Chromogranin A: An additional tumor marker for postoperative recurrence and metastases of medullary thyroid carcinomas? Anticancer Res 2000; 20:5257–5260.
38. Redding AH, Levine SN, Fowler MR. Normal preoperative calcitonin levels do not always exclude medullary thyroid carcinoma in patients with large palpable thyroid masses. Thyroid 2000; 10:919–922.
39. Bockhorn M, Frilling A, Rewerk S, et al. Lack of elevated serum carcinoembryonic antigen and calcitonin in medullary thyroid carcinoma. Thyroid 2004; 6:468–470.
40. Hodak SP, Burman KD. Editorial: The calcitonin conundrum—Is it time for routine measurement of serum calcitonin in patients with thyroid nodules? J Clin Endocrinol Metab 2004; 89:511–514.
41. Vierhapper H, Raber W, Bieglmayer C, et al. Routine measurement of plasma calcitonin in nodular thyroid diseases. J Clin Endocrinol Metab 1997; 82:1589–1593.
42. Hahm JR, Lee MS, Min YK, et al. Routine measuement of serum calcitonin is useful for early detection of medullary thyroid carcinoma in patients with nodular thyroid diseases. Thyroid 2001; 11:73–80.
43. Elisei R, Bottici V, Luchetti F, et al. Impact of routine measurement of serum calcitonin on the diagnosis and outcome of medullary thyroid cancer: Experience in 10,864 patients with nodular thyroid disorders. J Clin Endocrinol Metab 2004; 89:163–168.
44. Karanikas G, Moameni A, Poetzi C, et al. Frequency and relevance of elevated calcitonin levels in patients with neoplastic and nonneoplastic thyroid disease and in healthy subjects. J Clin Endocrinol Metab 2004; 89:515–519.
45. Tommasi M, Brocchi A, Cappellini A, et al. False high serum calcitonin levels using a non-competitive two-site IRMA. J Endocrinol Invest 2001; 24:356–360.
46. Kotzmann H, Schmidt A, Scheuba C, et al. Basal calcitonin levels and the response to pentagastrin stimulation in patients after kidney transplantation or on chronic hemodialysis as indicators of medullary carcinoma. Thyroid 1999; 9:943–947.
47. Erdogan MF, Gullu S, Baskal N, et al. Omeprazole: calcitonin stimulation test for the diagnosis, follow-up and family screening in medullary thyroid carcinoma. J Clin Endocrinol Metab 1997; 82: 897–899.
48. Vlaeminck-Guillem V, D'Herbomez M, Pigny P, et al. Pseudo-hypoparathyroidism Ia and hypercalcitoninemia. J Clin Endocrinol Metab 2001; 86:3091–3096.
48a. Machens A, Schneyer U, Holzhausen H-J, Dralle H. Prospects of remission in medullary thyroid carcinoma according to basal calcitonin level. J Clin Endocrinol Metab 2005; 90:2029-2034.
49. Oertel YC. Fine needle aspiration and the diagnosis of thyroid cancer. Endocrin Metab Clin North Am 1996; 25:69–92.
50. Ravetto C, Colombo L, Dottorini ME. Usefulness of fine needle aspiration in the diagnosis of thyroid carcinoma: a restrospetive study in 37,895 patients. Cancer 2000; 90:357–363.
51. Gharib H, Goellner JR. Fine needle aspiration biopsy of the thyroid: an appraisal. Ann Intern Med 1993; 118:282–289.

52. Ko HM, Jhu IK, Yang SH, et al. Clinicopathologic analysis of fine needle aspiration cytology of the thyroid. A review of 1613 cases and correlation with histopathologic diagnoses. Acta Cytol 2003; 47: 727–732.

52a. Harvey JN, Parker D, De P, Shrimali RK, Otter M. Sonographically guided core biopsy in the assessment of thyroid nodules. J Clin Ultrasound 2005; 33:57–62.

53. Danese D, Sciacchitano S, Farsetti A, et al. Diagnostic accuracy of conventional versus sonography-guided fine-needle aspiration biopsy of thyroid nodules. Thyroid 1998; 8:15–21.

54. Hatada T, Okada K, Ishii H, et al. Evaluation of ultrasound-guided fine-needle aspiration biopsy for thyroid nodules. Am J Surg 1998; 175:133–136.

55. Singer PA. Evaluation and management of the thyroid nodule, Otolaryngol. Clin North Am 1996; 29:577–592.

56. Backdahl M, Wallin G, Lowhagen T, et al. Fine-needle biopsy cytology and DNA analysis: their place in the evaluation and treatment of patients with thyroid neoplasms Surg Clin North Am 1987; 67: 197–211.

57. Finley DJ, Arora N, Zhu B, et al. Molecular profiling distinguish papillary carcinoma from benign thyroid nodules. J Clin Endocrinol Metab 2004; 89:3214–3223.

57a. Finley DJ, Lubitz CC, Wei C, Zhu B, Fahey TJ III. Advancing the molecular diagnosis of thyroid nodules: Defining benign lesions by molecular profiling. Thyroid 2005; 15:562–568.

57b. Weber F, Shen L, Aldred MA, et al. Genetic classification of benign and malignant thyroid follicular neoplasia based on a three-gene combination. J Clin Endocrinol Metab 2005; 90:2512–2521.

58. Karwlowski JK, Nowels KW, McDougall IR, Weigel RJ. Needle track seeding of papillary thyroid carcinoma from fine needle aspiration biopsy. A case report. Acta Cytol 2002; 46:591–595.

58a. Baskin HJ. Detection of recurrent papillary thyroid carcinoma by thyroglobulin assessment in the needle washout after fine-needle aspiration of suspicious lymph nodes. Thyroid 2004; 14:959–963.

58b. Wagner K, Arciaga R, Siperstein A, et al. Thyrotropin receptor/thyroglobulin messenger ribonucleic acid in peripheral blood and fine-needle aspiration cytology: diagnostic synergy for detecting thyroid cancer. J Clin Endocrinol Metab 2005; 90:1921–1924.

59. Kumar H, Daykin J, Holder R, et al. Gender, clinical findings, and serum thyrotropin measuements in the prediction of thyroid neo-plasia in 1005 patients presenting with thyroid enlargement and investigated by fine-needle aspiration cytology. Thyroid 1999; 9: 1105–1109.

60. Tollin SR, Mery GM, Jelveh N, et al. The use of fine-needle aspiration biopsy under ultrasound guidance to assess the risk of malignancy in patients with a multinodular goiter. Thyroid 2000; 10:235–241.

61. Marqusee E, Benson CB, Frates MC, et al. Usefulness of ultrasonography in the management of nodular thyroid disease. Ann Intern Med 2000; 133:696–700.

61a. Shattuck TM, Westra WH, Ladenson PW, Arnold A. Independent clonal origins of distinct tumor foci in multifocal papillary thyroid carcinoma. N Engl J Med 2005; 352:2406–2412.

61b. Utiger RD. The multiplicity of thyroid nodules and carcinomas. N Engl J Med 2005; 352:2376–2378.

62. Bennedbaek FN, Hegedus L. Treatment of rrecurrent thyroid cysts with ethanol: a randomized double-blind controlled trial. J Clin Endocrinol Metab 2003; 88:5773–5777.

63. Guglielmi R, Pacella CM, Bianchini A, et al. Percutaneous ethanol injection treatment in benign thyroid lesions: Role and efficacy. Thyroid 2004; 14:125–131.

63a. Mauz PS, Stiegler M, Holderried M, Brosch S. Complications of ultrasound guided percutaneous ethanol injection therapy of the thyroid and parathyroid glands. Ultraschall in der Medizin 2005; 26:111142-5.

63b. Mauz PS, Maassen MM, Braun B, Brosch S. How safe is percutaneous ethanol injection for treatment of thyroid nodules? Report of a case of severe toxic necrosis of the larynx and adjacent skin. Acta Oto-Laryngol 2004; 124:1226–1230.

64. Dossing H, Bennedbaek FN, Hegedus L. Ultrasound-guided interstitial laser photocoagulation of an autonomous thyroid nodule: the introduction of a novel alternative. Thyroid 2003; 13:885–888.

65. Corvilain B. The natural history of thyroid autonomy and hot nodules. Ann Endocrinol 2003; 64:17–22.

66. Boi F, Lai ML, Deias C, et al. The usefulness of 99mTC-SestaMIBI in the diagnostic evaluation of thyroid nodules with oncocytic cytology. Eur J Endocrinol 2003; 149:493–498.

67. Maki K, Okumura Y, Sato S, et al. Quantitative evaluation by TI-201 scintigraphy in the diagnosis of thyroid follicular nodules. Ann Nucl Med 17:91–98.

68. Chang CT, Liu FY, Tsai JJ, et al. The clinical usefulness of dual phase 201Tl thyroid scan for false-negative fine-needle aspiration cytological diagnoses in non-functioning cold thyroid nodules. Anticancer Res 2003; 23:2965–2967.

69. Tamizu A, Okumura Y, Sato S, et al. The usefulness of serum thyroglobulin levels and Tl-201 scintigraphy in differentiating between benign and malignant thyroid follicular lesions. Ann Nucl Med 2002; 16:95–101.

70. Sinha PS, Beeby DI, Ryan P. An evaluation of thallium imaging for detection of carcinoma in clinically palpable solitary, nonfunctioning thyroid nodules. Thyroid 2001; 11:85–89.

71. Cases JA, Surks MI. The changing role of scintigraphy in the evaluation of thyroid nodules. Semin Nucl Med 2000; 30:81–87.

72. Meller J, Becker W. The continuing importance of thyroid scintigraphy in the era of high-resolution ultrasound. Eur J Nucl Med Mol Imaging 2002; 29(Suppl 2):S425–S438.

73. Asari AN, Siegel ME, DeQuattro V. Imaging of medullary thyroid carcinoma and hyperfunctioning adrenal medulla using iodine-131 metaiodobenzylguanidine. J Nucl Med 1986; 27:1858–1860.

74. Kresnik E, Gallowitsch HH, Mikosch P, et al. Fluorine-18-fluorodeoxyglucose positron emission tomography in the preoperative assessment of thyroid nodules in an endemic goiter area. Surgery 2003; 133:294–299.

75. Hegedus L. Thyroid ultrasound. Endocrinol Metab Clin North Am 2001; 30:339–360.

76. Koike E, Noguchi S, Yamashita H, et al. Ultrasonographic characteristics of thyroid nodules: prediction of malignancy. Arch Surg 2001; 136:334–337.

77. Kakkos SKl Skopa CD, Chalmoukis AK, et al. Relative risk of cancer in sonographically detected thyroid nodules with calcifications. J Clin Ultrasound 2000; 28:347–352.

78. Chung WY, Chang HS, Kim EK, Park CS. Ultrasonographic mass screening for thyroid carcinoma: a study in women scheduled to undergo a breast examination. Surg Today 2001; 31:763–767.

79. Koike E, Shiro N, Yamashita H, et al. Ultrasonographic characteristics of thyroid nodules: Prediction of malignancy. Arch Surg 2001; 136:334–337.

80. Papini E, Guglielmi R, Gianchini A, et al. Risk of malignancy in non-palpable thyroid nodules: Predictive value of ultrasound and color-Doppler features. J Clin Endocrinol Metab 2002; 87:1941–1946.

81. Rago T, Vitti P, Chiovato L, et al. Role of conventional ultrasonography and color flow-Doppler sonography in predicting malignancy in 'cold' thyroid nodules. Eur J Endocrinol 1998; 138:41–46.

82. Solbiati L, Charboneau JW, James EM, Hat ID. The thyroid gland. In Rumack CM, Wilson SR, Charboneau JW, editors. Diagnostic Ultrasound, 2nd ed. St Louis, MO: Mosby-Yearbook, 1998; 703–729.

83. Shapiro RS. Panoramic ultrasound of the thyroid. Thyroid 2003; 13: 177–181.

84. Nam-Goong IS, Kim HY, Gong G, et al. Ultrasonography-guided fine-needle aspiration of thyroid incidentaloma: correlation with pathololological findings. Clin Endocrinol 2004; 60:21–28.

85. Leenhardt L, Hejblum G, Franc B, et al. Indications and limits of ultrasound-guided cytology in the management of nonpalpable thyroid nodules. J Clin Endocrinol Metab 1999; 84:24–28.

86. Bellantone R, Lombardi CP, Raffaelli M, et al. Management of cystic or predominantly cystic thyroid nodules: The role of ultrasound-guided fine-needle aspiration biopsy. Thyroid 2004; 14:43–47.

87. Alexander EK, Heering JP, Benson CB, et al. Assessment of nondiagnostic ultrasound-guided fine needle aspirations of thyroid nodules. J Clin Endocrinol Metab 2002; 87:4924–4927.
88. Braga M, Cavalcanti TC, Collaco LM, Graf H. Efficacy of ultrasound-guided fine-needle aspiration biopsy in the diagnosis of complex thyroid nodules. J Clin Endocrinol Metab 2001; 86: 4089–4091.
89. Dossing H, Bennedbaek FN, Karstrup S, Hegedus L. Benign solitary solid cold thyroid nodules: US-guided interstitial laser photocoagulation—initial experience. Radiology 2002; 225:53–57.
90. Pacini F. Role of percutaneous ethanol injection in management of nodular lesions of the thyroid gland. J Nucl Med 2003; 44:211–212.
90a. Fukunari N, Nagahama M, Sugino K, Mimura T, Ito K, Ito K. Clinical evaluation of color Doppler imaging for the differential diagnosis of thyroid follicular lesions. World J Surg 2004; 28:1261–1265.
91. Burguera B, Gharib H. Thyroid incidentalomas. Prevalence, diagnosis, significance, and management. Endocrinol Metab Clin North Am 2000; 29:187–203.
92. Bailey Rh, Aron DC. The diagnostic dilemma of incidentalomas: Working through uncertainty. Endocrinol Metab Clin North Am 2000; 29:91–105.
93. Van den Bruel A, Maes A, De Potter T, et al. Clinical relevance of thyroid fluorodeoxyglucose-whole body positron emission tomography incidentaloma. J Clin Endocrinol Metab 2002; 87:1517–1520.
94. Cohen MS, Arslan N, Dehdashti F, et al. Risk of malignancy in thyroid incidentalomas identified by fluorodeoxyglucose-positron emission tomography. Surgery 2001; 130:941–946.
95. Kang HW, Kim S-K, Kang H-S, et al. Prevalence and risk of cancer of focal thyroid incidentaloma identified by 18F-fluorodeoxyglucose positron emission tomography for metastasis evaluation and cancer screening in healthy subjects. J Clin Endocrinol Metab 2003; 88: 4100–4104.
96. Kang HW, No JH, Chung JH, et al. Prevalence, clinical and ultrasonographic characteristics of thyroid incidentalomas. Thyroid 2004; 14:29–33.
97. Silver RJ, Parangi S. Management of thyroid incidentalomas. Surg Clin North Am 2004; 84:907–919.
98. Raffel A, Cupisti K, Krausch M, et al. Incidentally found medullary thyroid cancer: treatment rationale for small tumors. World J Surg 2004; 28:397–401.
99. Quadbeck B, Pruellage J, Roggenbuck U, et al. Long-term follow-up of thyroid nodule growth. Exp Clin Endocrinol Diab 2002; 110:348–354.
100. Alexander EK, Hurwitz S, Heering JP, et al. Natural history of benign solid and cystic thyroid nodules. Ann Intern Med 2003; 138:315–318.
101. Zelmanovitz R, Genro S, Gross JL. Suppressive therapy with levothyroxine for solitary thyroid nodules: a double-blind controlled clinical study and cumulative meta-analyses. J Clin Endocrinol Metab 1998; 83:3881–3885.
102. Gharib H, Mazzaferri EL. Thyroxine suppressive therapy in patients with nodular thyroid disease. Ann Intern Med 1998; 128:386–394.
103. Castro MR, Caraballo PJ, Morris JC. Effectiveness of thyroid hormone suppressive therapy in benign solitary thyroid nodules: a meta-analysis. J Clin Endocrinol Metab 2002; 87:4154–4159.
104. Ridgway EC. Medical treatment of benign thyroid nodules: Have we defined a benefit? Ann Intern Med 1998; 128:403–405.
105. Hoermann R. Thyroid-hormone suppressive therapy in benign thyroid nodules—is it effective? Lancet 2002; 360:1899–1900.
106. Gharib H, James EM, Charboneau JW. Suppressive therapy with levothyroxine for solitary nodules. N Engl J Med 1987; 317:70–75.
107. Reverter JL, Lucas A, Salinas I, et al. Suppressive therapy with levothyroxine for solitary thyroid nodules. Clin Endocrinol 1992; 36:25–28.
108. Papini E, Petrucci L, Guglielmi R, et al. Long term changes in nodular goiter: a 5 year prospective randomized trial of levothyroxine suppressive therapy for benign cold thyroid nodules. J Clin Endocrinol Metab 1998; 83:780–783.
109. Cheung PSY, Lee JMH, Boey JH. Thyroxine suppressive therapy of benign solitary thyroid nodules: a prospective randomized study. World J Surg 1989; 13:818–822.
110. Celani MF, Mariani M, Mariani G. On the usefulness of levothyroxine suppressive therapy in the medical treatment of benign solitary, solid, or predominantly solid thyroid nodules. Acta Endocrinol 1990; 123:603–608.
111. Papini E, Bacci V, Panunzi C, et al. A prospective randomized trial of levothyroxine suppressive therapy for solitary thyroid nodules. Clin Endocrinol 1993; 38:507–513.
112. LaRosa GL, Lupo L, Giuffrida D, et al. Levothyroxine and potassium iodide are both effective in treating benign solitary solid cold nodules of the thyroid. Ann Intern Med 1995; 122:1–8.
113. Lima N, Knobel M, Cavaliere H, et al. Levothyroxine suppressive therapy is partially effective in treating patients with benign, solid thyroid nodules and multinodular goiters. Thyroid 1997; 7:691–697.
114. Wemeau JL, Caron P, Schvartz C, et al. Effects of TSH suppression with levothyroxine in reducing volume of solitary thyroid nodules and improving extranodular nonpalpable changes. J Clin Endocrinol Metab 2002; 87:4928–4934.
115. La Rosa GL, Ippolito AM, Lupo L, et al. Cold thyroid nodule reduction with L-thyroxine can be predicted by initial nodule volume and cytological characteristics. J Clin Endocrinol Metab 1996; 81: 4385–4387.
116. Stathatos N, Wartofsky L. Effects of thyroid hormone on bone. Clin Rev Bone Mineral Metab 2004; 2:135–150.
117. Marcocci C, Golia F, Bruno-Bossio G, et al. Carefully monitored levothyroxine suppressive therapy is not associated with bone loss in premenopausal women. J Clin Endocrinol Metab 1994; 78: 818–823.
118. Koc M, Ersoz HO, Akpinar I, et al. Effect of low-and high-dose levothyroxine on thyroid nodule volume: a crossover placebo-controlled trial. Clin Endocrinol 2002; 57:621–628.
119. Fogelfeld L, Wiviott MBT, Shore-Freedman E, et al. Recurrence of thyroid nodules after surgical removal in patients irradiated in childhood for benign conditions. N Engl J Med 1989; 320:835–840.
120. Hennessey JV, Evaul JE, Tseng YL, et al. L-thyroxine dosage: A re-evaluation of therapy with contemporary preparations. Ann Intern Med 1986; 105:11–16.
121. Wartofsky L, Oertel Y. Fine needle aspiration biopsy of thyroid nodules. In Van Nostrand D, editor. Nuclear Medicine Atlas. Philadelphia: J. B. Lippincott, 1987; 193–200.
122. Hayashida N, Namba H, Kumagai A, et al. A rapid and simple detection method for the BRAFT1796A mutation in fine needle aspirated thyroid carcinoma cells. Thyroid 2004; 14:910–915.
123. Xing M, Tufano RP, Tufaro AP, et al. Detection of BRAF mutation on fine needle aspiration biopsy specimens: a new diagnostic tool for papillary thyroid cancer. J Clin Endocrinol Metab 2004; 89: 2867–2872.
124. Mandel SJ. A 64 year old woman with a thyroid nodule. JAMA 2004; 292:2632–2642.
125. Alexander EK, Marqusee E, Orcutt J, et al. Thyroid nodule shape and prediction of malignancy. Thyroid 2004; 14:953–958.
126. Hamburger JI, Hamburger SW. Fine needle biopsy of thyroid nodules: avoiding the pitfalls. NY State J Med 1986; 86:241–249.
127. Rosen IB, Palmer JA, Bain J, et al. Efficacy of needle biopsy in postradiation thyroid disease. Surgery 1983; 94:1002–1007.
128. Duek DS, Goldenberg D, Linn S, et al. The role of fine-needle aspiration and intaoperative frozen section in the surgical management of solitary thyroid nodules. Surg Today 2002; 32:857–861.
129. Lennquist S. The thyroid nodule: diagnosis and surgical treatment. Surg Clin North Am 1987; 67:213–232.
130. Finley DJ, Zhu B, Barden CB, Fahey TJ III. Discrimination of benign and malignant thyroid nodules by molecular profiling. Ann Surg 2004; 240:425–437.
131. Norton JA, Doppman JL, Jensen RT. Cancer of the endocrine system. In Devita VT Jr, Hellman L, Rosenberg SA, editors. Cancer: Principles and Practice of Oncology. Philadelphia: J. B. Lippincott, 1989; 1269–1287.

18
Fine-Needle Aspiration
Technique

Yolanda C. Oertel

INTRODUCTION

Fine-needle aspiration (FNA) is a quick, valuable, minimally invasive procedure to assess the nature of a thyroidal mass. It should not be confused with "needle biopsy," which requires a Tru-cut or Vim-Silverman needle and yields tissue fragments for histologic diagnosis. Details of the FNA technique (as we practice it) and the equipment required are described in refs. *1* and *2*. Of particular importance are the use of a syringe holder and needles with clear plastic hubs *(3)*. It is essential to use little or no suction when aspirating the lesions *(4)*.

EQUIPMENT REQUIRED

1. The syringe holder or handle is an indispensable item. We prefer the Cameco Syringe Pistol (Precision Dynamics Corporation, Burbank, CA). A less expensive, plastic handle is the Aspir Gun (The Everest Company, Linden, NJ).
2. Plastic disposable syringes: 10-cc and, rarely, 20-cc.
3. Disposable needles: 22-, 23-, and 25-gauge; 1 and 1.5 in. long; and 25-gauge, 5/8 in. long, with clear plastic hubs.
4. Plain glass slides, preferably with one frosted end.
5. Hemacytometer cover glass. This is a thick piece of glass, more narrow than the width of the regular glass microslide, which we use to smear the aspirated material on the glass slide (Fisher Scientific, Pittsburgh, PA).
6. Appropriate staining solutions. We prefer the Diff-Quik stain, a hematological stain similar to the May-Grünwald Giemsa stain.

PERFORMANCE OF THE ASPIRATION

Ask the patient if he or she knows what you are going to do. While you explain the procedure, ask the patient to hold an ice pack (for mild anesthesia) on the area to be aspirated. Then have the patient lie down on the examining table. Proceed in the following way:

1. Place the mass between the index and middle fingers of your nondominant hand in a position suitable for needling.
2. Clean the skin with a cotton swab soaked in ethyl alcohol. Dry the skin with a gauze sponge to avoid the stinging sensation caused by residual alcohol when inserting the needle. The cytotechnologist gives the aspiration device to the pathologist, then holds the patient's hand. (Patients often mention how helpful and reassuring it is for someone to hold their hands.)
3. Ask the patient to swallow. (If necessary, water can be provided through a bent straw.) After the patient has swallowed, hold down the lesion between your left index and middle fingers.
4. Pierce the needle through the skin, making sure that the syringe is in "the resting position" (plunger at the 0-cc mark).
5. Advance the needle perpendicularly into the lesion.
6. Once the needle has entered the nodule, move it back and forth in the same plane (do not vary the angle of the needle) *without applying any suction*. Do this twice; if nothing appears in the clear plastic needle hub, then apply suction gradually and gently by pulling the plunger of the syringe.
7. While inserting the needle in the lesion, keep talking to the patient: "You are doing fine." "Everything is all right." "It looks pretty good." "You are helping me beautifully." Such expressions calm the patient. As you apply suction, gradually push the needle deeper, with gentle movements back and forth in the lesion, maintaining the suction. Usually, when the plunger of the syringe is at the 2- or 3-cc mark, you should see material in the clear plastic needle hub. However, if the lesion is firm, and no material appears in the needle hub, keep applying suction until you reach the 10-cc mark. Again, move the needle back and forth with gentle jabbing movements. By now you should have hemorrhagic material in the needle hub. Release the plunger to stop the suction. Shift your fingers from the "trigger" to hold the outside of the handle.
8. Withdraw the needle.
9. Ask the patient to apply *firm* pressure at the site of the aspiration using the same piece of gauze that you used to dry the skin.
10. While the patient is still applying pressure, move quickly to prepare the smears. The cytotechnologist assists in this procedure. Because the aspirate tends to clot promptly, we cannot emphasize enough that *rapid preparation of the smears is*

extremely important. Once the smears have been prepared, and the technologist has started drying and staining one slide, the physician may help the patient sit up, and continue to apply pressure at the site of aspiration until the smear is ready for microscopic examination. Then tell the patient to apply pressure while we examine the slide under the microscope. The patient remains seated on the examining table until after we have examined the smear and decided which size needle to use in the next aspiration. These simple precautions—sitting up between aspirates (to improve the venous drainage) and applying steady pressure at the puncture site—prevent the formation of hematomas. However, if the patient feels dizzy and does not want to sit up, allow the patient to remain lying down. Also, if the patient cannot tolerate pressure on the neck (e.g., the lesion is over the trachea and pressure produces coughing), apply an ice cube to the site.

11. Once satisfied that you have sampled the lesion thoroughly, tell the patient that there are no restrictions and that he or she can go back to work or routine activities. (We seldom put a small adhesive bandage on the area that has been aspirated.)

Obtaining an adequate and representative sample is crucial for a correct diagnosis. We reiterate that the technique is deceptively simple.

Notes

1. While applying suction and moving the needle into the lesion, look at the needle hub.
   a. If fluid appears, continue applying suction until the syringe is filled or until there is no more fluid aspirated.
   b. If blood appears in the needle hub, immediately stop applying suction, whether the plunger is at the 1- or 4-cc mark.
   c. If no blood appears, continue applying suction up to the 10-cc mark on the syringe.
2. Observe your patient's face. If you see grimacing or any signs of discomfort, state that you are almost done, that it will take a little longer, to bear with you, and so on. If you notice that the patient is about to swallow, release the plunger immediately, and pull out of the lesion. Sometimes, a patient will start swallowing and surprise you; then just move along, do not offer resistance, release the plunger, and pull out of the lesion as quickly as possible.
3. *Do not forget to release the plunger.* When unexperienced, it is a common mistake to withdraw the needle from the nodule while still applying suction. This action will cause the aspirated material to flow into the syringe. To recover the material, rinse the syringe and prepare a filter specimen.

TECHNICAL HINTS

Most publications refer to the use of full suction once the needle penetrates the lesion. *We do not advocate this procedure.* After inserting the needle in the lesion, the needle should be moved up and down (if the patient is lying down) or back and forth (if the patient is sitting upright), with gentle jabbing movements and without applying any suction. There should *not* be any lateral movements. If bright red blood is seen immediately in the needle hub, the procedure should be stopped, and the needle should be withdrawn at once.

One smear should be checked under the microscope. Depending on the microscopic findings, change the needle gauge or apply more suction in the next aspirate.

Although the technique is not complicated, we have seen such a high rate of failure among internists, endocrinologists, and surgeons that this procedure is apparently more difficult than it seems. These physicians can likely palpate thyroid nodules better than the pathologist; thus, the problem probably does not derive from localizing the lesion. Often, they apply too much suction too soon.

We stain the smears with Diff-Quik, and the cytologic diagnostic criteria described are based on this staining method. Other pathologists prefer the Papanicolaou stain or hematoxylin and eosin; some diagnostic criteria are different with these stains *(5).*

REFERENCES

1. Oertel YC. Fine-needle aspiration of the thyroid. In Moore WT, Eastman RC, editors. Diagnostic Endocrinology, 2nd ed. St. Louis, MO: Mosby-Year Book, 1996; 211–228.
2. Oertel YC. Fine-needle aspiration and the diagnosis of thyroid cancer. Endocrinol Metab Clin North Am 1996; 25:69–91.
3. Oertel YC. Fine-needle aspiration: a personal view. Lab Med 1982; 13: 343–347.
4. Oertel YC. A pathologist's comments on diagnosis of thyroid nodules by fine needle aspiration. J Clin Endocrinol Metab 1995; 80: 1467–1468.
5. Kini SR, editor. Thyroid. Guides to Clinical Aspiration Biopsy, 2nd ed. New York: Igaku-Shoin; 1996.

19
Thyroid Nodules
Cellular and Biochemical Markers for Malignancy

Kathleen A. Prendergast

INTRODUCTION

Although the majority of histologic specimens obtained by fine-needle aspiration (FNA) yield a definitive diagnosis, 10–30% are deemed indeterminate. Generally, surgery is recommended for these patients, as up to one quarter of these nodules are found to be malignant. Notwithstanding that concern, 75% of patients with a benign nodule undergo an unnecessary procedure. In an effort to reduce these potentially avoidable surgeries, a number of biochemical and molecular markers have been developed to assist in the discernment of benign from malignant nodules.

GALECTIN-3

Galectin-3 (Gal-3), a 30-kDa member of the β-galactoside-binding animal lectins, is expressed in many tissues and cell types and is involved in cellular adhesion, cell cycle regulation, and apoptosis. In malignant tissues, Gal-3 is implicated in neoplastic transformation and the propensity for metastasis. Gal-3 was first proposed as a marker for thyroid malignancy by Xu et al. in 1995 *(1)*. Immunohistochemical (IHC) staining of various thyroid samples demonstrated that malignancies (both follicular and papillary) were positive for Gal-3, whereas all the benign samples were negative. Several subsequent studies have confirmed these results by analyzing Gal-3 expression, utilizing both IHC and reverse transcriptase-polymerase chain reaction (RT-PCR); *(2–6)*. On these thyroid pathology specimens, detection of Gal-3 appears to be a sensitive and specific marker for malignancy *(6a,6b,6c)*.

Given the promise of Gal-3 as a marker on surgical pathology specimens, several investigators examined its use in FNA specimens. Orlandi et al. *(7)* analyzed immunocytochemical staining on cell blocks from FNA and the corresponding histological samples. All 18 papillary thyroid carcinomas (PTC) and 14 of 17 follicular thyroid carcinomas (FTC) stained positive for Gal-3. Only 3 of 29 follicular adenomas (FA) stained positive for Gal-3. Subsequent studies *(8–12)* have confirmed that immunocytochemistry on FNA samples is useful in distinguishing malignant from benign tissues. In a prospective study on nodular thyroid lesions by Bartolazzi et al. *(10)*, the sensitivity, specificity, positive predictive value (PPV), negative predictive value (NPV) and diagnostic accuracy was determined to be 100%, 98%, 92%, 100%, and 99%, respectively. Moreover, they found that 5 of 132 well-characterized FA and 11 of 13 follicular neoplasms of indeterminate malignant behavior were positive for Gal-3, suggesting that this marker may be useful in determining lesions that may be "premalignant."

Two studies have investigated the use of Gal-3 in difficult diagnostic circumstances. Saggiorato et al. *(11)* performed Gal-3 immunocytochemistry to distinguish minimally invasive FTC from FA—a distinction that cannot be made preoperatively because it requires knowledge of the extent of invasion based on histopathologic examination. Nearly all (16 of 17) minimally invasive cancers and only 4 of 52 FAs were positive for Gal-3. In FNAs of cystic thyroid nodules prone to false-negative results owing to the low number of epithelial cells, Papotti et al. *(12)* determined that standard FNA had a sensitivity, specificity, PPV, NPV, and accuracy of 75%, 100%, 100%, 63.2%, and 82.5%, respectively. Gal-3 staining significantly improved sensitivity (89.3%) and PPV (80%).

Another technique to establish Gal-3 expression is by RT-PCR *(8,13–15)*. Unfortunately, this method appears to increase sensitivity at the expense of specificity. Bernet et al. *(14)* quantified gene expression to find out if there was a threshold above which cancer could be accurately diagnosed. Unfortunately, although the levels of Gal-3 gene expression were significantly elevated in PTC vs normal tissue, there was no significant difference between benign and malignant follicular lesions or between PTC and FA. A study in children and adolescents found that false-positive Gal-3 expression was likely to occur in the setting of Hashimoto's thyroiditis *(15)*.

From these data, it appears that Gal-3 immunostaining is a sensitive and specific method to assist in the preoperative

From: *Thyroid Cancer: A Comprehensive Guide to Clinical Management, 2/e*
Edited by: L. Wartofsky and D. Van Nostrand © Humana Press Inc., Totowa, NJ

diagnosis of thyroid malignancy. Gal-3 antibodies are commercially available, and it is anticipated that this marker will have more widespread use in the near future.

TELOMERASE

Normally found in stem cells and lymphocytes, telomerase is a RT that regenerates the ends of chromosomes (telomeres) prone to instability (16). Telomerase is important for chromosome structural integrity and protects chromosome ends from errors in recombination. At each cell division, a loss of DNA occurs at the terminus because of the inability of DNA replication to complete the lagging-strand synthesis. At a certain point, it is believed that the shortening of telomeres is a signal to cells to exit the cell cycle and become senescent. This places a restriction on the proliferative capacity of all cells. Activation of telomerase and subsequent lengthening or maintenance of telomeres would allow the cell to remain in the cell cycle and foster immortalization. Telomerase is not found in differentiated epithelial cells but can be reactivated in epithelial cancers; for this reason, it has been investigated as a possible marker of neoplastic transformation.

Two methods are available to investigate telomerase activity and expression. The telomerase repeat amplification protocol (TRAP, 17) is a PCR assay that detects the activity of the telomerase enzyme and has been shown to be positive in many epithelial malignancies. Utilizing the TRAP assay on normal and malignant thyroid tissue, Haugen et al. (18) observed no activity in benign adenomas, whereas 61% of malignancies demonstrated telomerase activity. Although not statistically significant, most invasive carcinomas were TRAP-positive, suggesting that telomerase-positive tumors were more aggressive.

Noting that 39% of malignant tissues were TRAP-negative in this study, a subsequent study on follicular neoplasms by Umbricht et al. (19) sought to improve the sensitivity of the TRAP assay. It was theorized that false-negatives were the result of inhibitory contaminants and enzymatic instability. If PCR inhibition was suspected secondary to lack of amplification of the control, a phenol extraction was performed. With this modification, the sensitivity improved to 100%, but the specificity declined to 72%, yielding a PPV of only 58%. The authors suggested that false-positives could be a result of one of two processes: (1) contaminating nonthyrocyte sources of telomerase activity, e.g., lymphocytes; or (2) in the case of specimens without lymphocytic infiltration, premalignant lesions that have acquired telomerase activity but are still histologically benign and have not yet invaded. In a pilot study investigating FNA samples, these authors found that 4 of 4 papillary cancers were TRAP-positive, whereas 2 of 2 benign adenomas were negative.

Subsequent studies both on histology (20,21) and FNA cytology (22,23) samples found wide variability in the sensitivity and specificity of the TRAP assay to distinguish benign from malignant lesions. In addition, it was recognized that assaying for enzyme activity may be more difficult because of the need for a significant amount of cellular material, which is not always available in FNA specimens. For this reason, the second method of detecting telomerase expression—RT-PCR of the catalytic component of the human telomerase (hTERT) gene—was developed (23a).

Saji et al. (24) investigated hTERT expression in 37 pathology specimens and 10 of the correlating FNA samples. The sensitivity was found to be 75%, with a 72% specificity and 74% diagnostic accuracy. If specimens with lymphocytic infiltration were excluded, the sensitivity was found to be 71%, but the specificity and diagnostic accuracy improved to 100% and 85%, respectively. RT-PCR of 10 FNA samples revealed 4 of 4 PTC-positive and 5 of 6 benign samples negative for hTERT expression.

A subsequent study further investigated hTERT expression in FNA samples. When compared to corresponding histologic specimens, Zeiger et al. (25) demonstrated a 93% sensitivity, 90% specificity, 92% accuracy, 90% NPV, and 93% PPV in samples suspicious for malignancy. Although additional studies (26–29) have failed to duplicate the superior results obtained in this report, RT-PCR for hTERT expression does appear to be a sensitive marker for malignancy. Specificity in these studies continues to be problematic, with many benign samples yielding positive results. Still, RT-PCR for the hTERT gene may serve as a useful adjunct to standard cytology in the future.

THYROID PEROXIDASE

Thyroid peroxidase (TPO) is present in all normal thyroid cells and is essential for thyroid hormone synthesis. TPO catalyzes iodide oxidation, thyroglobulin iodination, and iodothyronine coupling, and it is believed that TPO function is gradually lost as thyroid adenoma progresses to carcinoma. Therefore, unlike most of the other markers, whose presence is indicative of malignancy, it is the loss of TPO that suggests progression to carcinoma.

TPO immunostaining has been studied extensively in both surgical pathology and FNA specimens. De Micco et al. (30) established a cut-off criterion of 80%, with specimens staining more than 80% on immunocytochemistry considered benign and malignant if less than 80% of the cells stained positive for TPO. In a number of studies (31–34) on FNA specimens, this same group found that TPO staining of less than 80% was 100% sensitive for malignancy, with a specificity as high as 86.6%. In one study (31) that analyzed samples from follicular neoplasms only, the specificity was less than 68%. The false-positive FAs (i.e., with <80% staining) exhibited a significant amount of atypia. A separate study (34) correlated TPO expression on histologic samples with differentiation and tumor growth in thyroid follicular tumors. An inverse relation was found between TPO staining and the degree of cellular atypia. From this study, it was suggested that the progression from FA to follicular carcinoma was a linear process that involved further loss of the gland's normal function.

Confirming the findings of this group, other studies (35–37) determined the sensitivity of TPO immunostaining to be from 94% and 100%, with a specificity between 81% and 99%, suggesting that this marker might reliably establish malignancy. Studies investigating only indeterminant samples have not been performed. It would be interesting to ascertain the value of TPO immunochemistry in these circumstances, when discriminant staining would prove most useful. RT-PCR of the TPO gene has also been performed on postsurgical samples (38,39). TPO gene expression was found to be significantly lower in carcinomas when compared to benign lesions, as well as to correlate well with immunochemistry.

CYCLOOXYGENASE-2

Cyclooxygenase-2 (COX-2) is the inducible form of the COX enzymes, which catalyze the formation of prostaglandins from arachidonic acid (40). Although COX-1 is thought to be a housekeeping gene, COX-2 is an early response gene that is induced by growth factors, oncogenes, tumor promoters, and carcinogens. The role of COX-2 in malignancy is currently under active investigation. COX-2 is known to be upregulated in colon, stomach, pancreas, and prostate cancers. A null mutation in COX-2 is associated with a marked reduction in the number and size of intestinal polyps in APC mice—a model for familial adenomatous polyposis (FAP). Whereas the APC mutations are uncommon in thyroid cancer, increased thyroid malignancies in FAP and Gardner's syndrome are recognized. In a study by Specht et al. (41), the presence of COX-2 was studied in thyroid cancer. In surgical specimens and thyroid cancer cell lines, COX-2 mRNA and protein were increased in tumor tissue vs normal adjacent tissues and benign nodules. COX-2 IHC staining was found to be positive in malignant cells in comparison to the surrounding stroma. Lo et al. (41a) also found higher COX-2 expression in malignant than benign tissues.

CADHERINS

Cadherins are a large family of transmembrane glycoproteins that mediate cell–cell dhesion and have a significant impact in normal cell architecture. E-cadherin, a major member of this family, is thought to suppress cancer invasion and metastases. Indeed, E-cadherin has been found to be downregulated in undifferentiated or aggressive thyroid carcinomas (42,43). However, E-cadherin has proved to be more useful to determine prognosis in thyroid cancer, rather than to act as a distinguishing feature between benign and malignant tissues.

Another relevant family member, CD44, has been investigated extensively in thyroid tissue. CD44 is immunologically related to integral-membrane glycoproteins. It can be expressed on the cell surface (CD44s) and is the putative receptor for hyaluronic acid. The CD44 gene is altered in many tumors, and variable splicing of the transcript can result in many protein isoforms, yielding the CD44 variant (CD44v). Consequently, CD44v is often detected in malignant tissues and therefore may serve as a marker of malignant transformation.

Surgical pathology specimens have been analyzed for the presence of three isoforms of CD44v (v2, v3, and v6) in a study by Aogi et al. (26). Although CD44v3 had the highest sensitivity for malignancy (92%), the specificity for this marker was only 41%. CD44v2 was less sensitive (75%) but more specific (71%), and isoform v6 was 83% sensitive and 65% specific. These latter two had approx 70% diagnostic accuracy. However, other studies suggest that there is no tumor-specific isoform that could be used alone as a diagnostic marker (44,45).

This impression is supported by analyses of CD44v that have been undertaken in FNA samples (9,10,46,47). Gasbarri et al. (9) investigated CD44v6 expression in benign vs malignant tissues. Thorough analysis revealed that immunodetection of CD44v6 alone did not improve diagnostic accuracy over standard cytology, but its coexpression with Gal-3 was noted to provide a near perfect sensitivity, specificity, PPV, and NPV. A subsequent study (10) performed a similar analysis of FNA specimens. Again, CD44v6 alone had good sensitivity for malignancy, but specificity was poor. In combination with Gal-3, however, specificity improved to 98%, with a 88% sensitivity, and a 97% diagnostic accuracy. From these studies, it appears that CD44v alone is not an adequate marker, but as a component of a panel of markers, it may assist in the diagnosis of malignancy on FNA.

ONCOFETAL FIBRONECTIN

Fibronectins are high-molecular-weight adhesive glycoproteins contained in the extracellular matrix and body fluids. Oncofetal fibronectin (onfFN) contains the (normally absent) oncofetal domain and has been found to be expressed in a variety of malignant tissues. Several studies utilizing RT-PCR amplification have demonstrated significantly increased onfFN expression in papillary and anaplastic carcinoma surgical specimens (48–50) when compared to normal tissue. The expression was also noted to be 10–100-fold higher than in follicular tumors. Indeed, there is significant overlap in the level of expression between follicular carcinomas and adenomas, limiting its use in distinguishing between these two entities.

RT-PCR assays permit detection of onfFN in a small amount of starting material, such as what remains in a needle after FNA biopsy. Takano et al. have utilized this technique in several studies to determine the clinical efficacy of determining onfFN expression preoperatively *(51,52)*. The sensitivity and specificity in the diagnosis of papillary or anaplastic cancer was 96.9% and 100%, respectively *(51)*. Refining this technique further by decreasing the subjectivity of semiquantitative RT-PCR, this group developed a quantitative real-time RT-PCR assay utilizing thyroglobulin as an internal standard. In concordance with the prior study, expression of onfFN was significantly elevated in papillary and anaplastic cancer when compared to follicular neoplasm and normal tissue *(52)*. A subsequent study by Giannini et al. *(13)* demonstrated similar sensitivity (97.8%) but a lower specificity of 60%. NPV and PPV were 92.3% and 84.6%, respectively, with an accuracy of 86%. However, this study used a nonquantitative determination of onfFN expression and included follicular neoplasms in the determination of sensitivity and specificity. Because some FA do express onfFN, the specificity markedly declined. Although demonstrating that it is a useful marker in PTC, onfFN does not allow for distinction between FA and FTC.

CD97

This dimeric glycoprotein is a leukocyte early activation antigen and is believed to function in adhesion and cell-to-cell signaling processes. Aust et al. *(53)* performed IHC staining on thyroid cancer specimens. In this small study, 11 of 12 anaplastic cancers were found to express CD97 as measured by immunohistochemistry and RT-PCR; whereas in differentiated thyroid cancer, CD97 expression was either absent or low. The authors suggest that CD97 may act as a marker of dedifferentiation and lymph node metastases. More studies are needed to delineate whether weak positivity in differentiated thyroid cancer is associated with metastases. If this were the case, staining FNA samples may help establish the extent of surgery required.

RET/PTC

RET is a proto-oncogene that encodes a tyrosine kinase and is not usually expressed in normal thyroid follicular tissue. Gene rearrangements can place the *RET* gene under transcriptional control of heterologous genes normally expressed in thyroid follicular epithelium *(54)*. The *RET*/PTC mutation is specific to papillary carcinomas and has been found in up to 77% of these malignancies *(55)*. To date, 15 chimeric mRNAs have been identified, and the two most common rearrangements in humans are *RET*/PTC-1 and *RET*/PTC-3. It has been suggested that the *RET*/PTC rearrangement occurs more frequently in radiation-exposed populations, e.g., the post-Chernobyl population. A study by Elisei et al. *(56)* performed RT-PCR for *RET*/PTC-1 or *RET*/PTC-3 rearrangement and demonstrated presence in both malignant (55%) and benign (29.2%) nodules. However, because this study was designed to investigate the frequency of *RET*/PTC rearrangements after irradiation, the high prevalence of subjects who had undergone radiation in this study possibly skewed the results to demonstrate a higher frequency in benign lesions. Notably, 13.9% of the nonirradiated benign lesions were also positive for the *RET*/PTC arrangements.

Another study *(57)* analyzed IHC staining of surgical pathology specimens with borderline morphological signs of thyroid cancer for the *RET*/PTC-1 or *RET*/PTC-3 rearrangement, and 65.2% demonstrated *RET* immunoreactivity. Of the seven samples that underwent RT-PCR for mutations, five were found to have rearrangement. The authors suggested that positive samples in this setting may represent malignant transformation and may allow for earlier intervention.

In the single study on FNA specimens *(58)* RT-PCR for three *RET*/PTC gene rearrangements was performed on 73 FNA specimens that were ultimately referred for surgery. In this series, 17 cases of PTC were found to be *RET*/PTC-positive on FNA sampling with no false-positives. Papillary cancer was diagnosed from cytology on 12 FNA samples, and only 6 were found to be *RET*/PTC-positive preoperatively. However, 9 of 15 indeterminate samples on FNA diagnosed as PTC were found to be *RET*/PTC-positive.

From these studies, detection of the *RET*/PTC gene rearrangement may provide additional diagnostic information to FNA. Further research is required to determine whether the benign samples that harbor this rearrangement are, in fact, premalignant, as has been suggested in these preliminary investigations.

HBME-1

HBME-1 is a marker of mesothelial cells, and prior studies have utilized a monoclonal antibody against HBME-1 as a marker for malignant mesothelioma. On histologic sections of thyroid pathology, HBME-1 positivity suggests malignancy of follicular epithelial origin *(6b,54,59,60)*. In FNA samples, HBME-1 was found to be 100% sensitive and 80% specific in one study *(61)* but only 57% sensitive in another *(62)*, but this study did report 100% specificity. However, these studies were quite small, and larger series are needed to prove HBME-1 is a useful marker for malignancy. In a study with the largest sample size *(62a)* all papillary cancers were positive but had only a 64% PPV in discriminating follicular carcinoma from FA.

HIGH-MOBILITY GROUP I

High-mobility group I (HMGI) is a family of proteins often expressed only during embryogenesis. This protein functions to regulate chromatin organization and gene expression. *HMGI(Y)* is the gene that encodes this protein and has been generally found to be activated in malignancy and has been specifically found to be expressed in thyroid malignancies *(63)*. Chiapetta et al. *(64)* performed IHC and RT-PCR analysis of 358 histologic and cytologic samples.

Of the 126 pathology specimens histologically judged to be malignant, 121 demonstrated positive IHC staining, and 100% were positive on RT-PCR. Of 232, 45 benign lesions were also positive on IHC, with 4 of 19 positive on RT-PCR. There were 10 FNA specimens also analyzed for *HMGI(Y)* expression and showed 100% sensitivity and specificity for both IHC and RT-PCR. Clearly, more studies should be undertaken to confirm these excellent results. However, this study did analyze a large number of tissues, and this marker may be quite useful in the preoperative diagnosis of thyroid malignancy.

BRAF

Mutations in *BRAF*, a serine-threonine kinase, cause constitutive activation of RAS/RAF/mitogen-activated protein kinase pathway, leading to cell transformation and malignancy. *BRAF* mutations, particularly *BRAF*^{V599E} in which a valine-to-glutamate substitution occurs at residue 599, are specific for papillary cancer and are not found in normal thyroid or follicular neoplasms *(65)*. *BRAF* mutations may be in 40–70% of PTCs *(66,67)* and are mutually exclusive of other mutations, including *RET/PTC* or *RAS (65)*.

Cohen et al. *(68)* showed that *BRAF* mutations were present in 38% of PTC histology specimens but were more likely to be positive in conventional papillary cancers than in the follicular variant. In the FNA specimens, there was 94% concordance with histology. One specimen was initially read on histology as negative for malignancy, but after discovering the *BRAF* mutation, reanalysis of the sample determined that it was, in fact, a PTC. None of the lesions ultimately determined as benign were positive for the *BRAF* mutation. An additional study analyzed colorimetric mutation detection of *BRAF* on FNA, and 50% of the nodules ultimately found to be PTC harbored the mutation *(69)*.

Although *BRAF* mutations are seen in a minority of specimens, their presence is highly correlated with malignancy *(69a)*. If determined on FNA to harbor the mutation, the decision to proceed with thyroidectomy would be justified.

EPITHELIAL MEMBRANE ANTIGEN

Epithelial membrane antigen (EMA) is a glycoprotein expressed by malignant lesions of epithelial origin *(70)*, which has been expressed by both follicular and papillary carcinomas *(71–73)*. In a study by Cheifetz et al. *(74)*, positive EMA immunohistochemistry had a sensitivity of 75% and specificity of 90% in distinguishing follicular adenomas from carcinomas. Although 13 of 16 (81%) of papillary cancers were positive for EMA in their study, the application of EMA on FNA specimens has not yet been evaluated.

LEU-7/CD57

Leu-7 (CD57) is an antigen frequently expressed in natural killer cells and has also been in various epithelial and nonepithelial tumors, including thyroid cancer *(74,75)*. Positive immunoreactivity has been noted in up to 95% of thyroid cancers *(76)*, with normal thyroid tissue demonstrating no staining on immunohistochemistry. However, results from several studies indicate that a significant number of FAs are also positive in both pathologic *(74)* and FNA *(77)* specimens; thus, its value in differentiating FA from FTC appears marginal at this time.

PAX8-PPARγ

PAX8 is a transcription factor essential for thyroid follicular cell differentiation. Peroxisome proliferator-activated receptor γ1 (PPARγ1) is a nuclear factor that inhibits growth and induces differentiation of cancer cell lines *(78)*. Chromosomal translocation that creates the PAX8/PPARγ rearrangement has been observed and may impact follicular oncogenesis. Indeed, this rearrangement has been found in follicular but not papillary or anaplastic neoplasms *(79)*. Studies utilizing both IHC and RT-PCR have been performed to detect the gene rearrangement *(80–84)*. It has been suggested that this chromosomal translocation is more common in patients who have been irradiated *(80)*, and it has been reported in up to 56% of histological samples *(82)*. Dwight et al. *(83)* showed that only 13% of follicular carcinomas were positive for PAX8-PPARγ and hypothesized that the low incidence was owing to exclusion from the study of patients irradiated. Some authors theorize that tumors containing this gene rearrangement are more likely to be multifocal and demonstrate vascular invasion, whereas mutation-negative samples are more likely to be minimally invasive *(80)*. It should be noted that a significant number of benign neoplasms are also positive for this mutation, but it is not known whether these tumors may be premalignant.

NM23

NM23 is considered to be a metastasis suppressor gene. Depending on the tissue, *NM23* gene expression has found to be inversely correlated with the presence of metastases in several cancers (breast, hepatocellular, and melanoma). In hematological malignancies and prostate cancer, high *NM23* levels were associated with a poor prognosis. In thyroid cancer, there are conflicting results on the association of *NM23* and metastatic potential. Some studies report lower expression of *NM23* in metastatic lymph node tissue *(85–87)*; another by Zou et al. *(88)* indicates that the level of *NM23* was directly correlated with aggressiveness of malignancy. Of note, these studies primarily investigated PTC samples. In patients with FTC, Zafon et al. *(89)* illustrated that four of five patients that stained negative for *NM23* on the original pathology specimen developed distant metastases and that the 10-yr survival rate declined from 90% in *NM23*-positive tumors to 40% in those with negative tumors. Other studies have shown no correlation with

NM23 levels and propensity for metastases *(90–92)*. Whether this marker would be able to add useful information to an FNA has not yet been investigated.

CD30 ANTIGEN/LIGAND

CD30 antigen is a cytokine receptor that belongs to the tumor necrosis factor superfamily. Originally detected in Hodgkin's lymphoma, additional studies proved it to be expressed in other malignancies, including thyroid neoplasms. In a study by Trovato et al. *(93)*, coexpression of CD30 with its ligand was seen in malignant thyroid tissues. Staining in benign adenomas occurred less frequently and was always less intense than that seen in carcinomas.

AURORA B

Aurora B is a member of the Aurora family of genes that regulate cell cycle events related to chromosome dynamics that serve to maintain genetic stability *(93a,93b)*. Overexpression of Aurora B is associated with chromosome instability leading to aneuploidy as has been described in several cancer cell lines, colorectal cancers, and seminoma. Sorrentino et al. *(93a)* analyzed Aurora B expression in normal thyroid tissue and in a variety of thyroid cancers including anaplastic cancer. Aurora B was not detected in normal thyroid and signal strength was seen to correlate with the degree of differentiation of tumors with the highest signal in anaplastic cancer. Even more exciting was their demonstration that inhibition of Aurora B kinase slowed the growth of anaplastic thyroid cancer cells in culture. The authors propose that Aurora B expression could be useful as a prognostic marker as well as serving as a target for treatment. We shall await further studies with great interest.

CERULOPLASMIN/LACTOFERRIN

Lactoferrin is overexpressed in adenocarcinomas of the stomach, colon, and lung and has been implicated in carcinogenesis. Ceruloplasmin shares sequence homology with lactoferrin, and both have been found to be expressed in thyroid neoplasms *(94,95)*. In an analysis of lactoferrin immunochemistry on FNA samples *(96)*, only 1 of 30 benign samples demonstrated lactoferrin staining, whereas lactoferrin staining was in 57% and 31% of PTC and FTC samples, respectively. More research is warranted for this marker to be proven as useful in the preoperative diagnosis of thyroid cancer.

MET/HEPATOCYTE GROWTH FACTOR

Met, a 195-kd transmembrane glycoprotein, is the receptor for hepatocyte growth factor, which stimulates proliferation, motility, and morphogenesis in epithelial cells *(97)*. Met has been overexpressed in thyroid malignancies, especially PTC *(98)*. Interestingly, the level of Met expression is inversely correlated with the risk of metastases *(99)*, and it is theorized that Met expression may represent a malignant transformation, but that this is lost as cancers dedifferentiate and increase in metastatic potential. Ippolito et al. *(100)* performed immunostaining of 80 suspicious FNA lesions that underwent surgical excision. There were 30 typical PTC and 10 nodular goiters also analyzed as positive and negative controls. An estimated 85.7% of papillary cancers, 72.7% of the follicular variant of PTC, 28% of follicular, and 100% of Hurthle cell adenomas were positive for Met staining. However, none of the suspicious lesions that were determined as benign were positive, yielding a specificity of 87%. Although the sensitivity for papillary cancer was good at 85.5%, it was only 28% for follicular cancer. This marker seems to have promise in identifying PTC, but its use in distinguishing FA vs FTC appears limited. Yet, given the findings that lower Met expression is associated with a higher risk of metastases, this marker could be helpful in guiding the extent of surgery when PTC is detected on cytopathology.

HYPERMETHYLATION OF THYROID-STIMULATING HORMONE RECEPTOR

Radioiodine uptake is frequently decreased in thyroid cancers, partly considered secondary to decreased thyroid-stimulating hormone receptor (TSHR) expression. One cause of decreased TSHR expression results from epigenetic modification through DNA methylation of CpG dinucleotides in the 5′-flanking area of the TSHR gene, leading to gene silencing. Xing et al. *(10)* analyzed methylation of the TSHR gene in malignant and benign surgical specimens and showed that 49% of malignancies and none of benign specimens demonstrated TSHR gene methylation. Furthermore, FNA specimens from eight benign adenomas and 10 thyroid cancers had 100% specificity and sensitivity when analyzed for methylation. This study examined a limited number of specimens, but TSHR hypermethylation may not only serve as a useful marker but also provides insight into the molecular mechanisms of radioactive iodine-resistant tumors.

CYTOKERATIN 19 (CK19)

On pathologic specimens, IHC staining for cytokeratin 19 (CK19) has been strongly positive in PTC but is usually negative or weakly positive in follicular lesions *(54, 102–104)*.

Two studies have investigated its use in FNA specimens *(105,106)*. Nasser et al. *(106)* studied CK19 immunostaining on FNA from 73 thyroid nodules that had histologic follow-up. The authors found that 34 of 37 papillary carcinomas were strongly positive for CK19, and 35 of 36 of other lesions (4 FA, 10 multinodular goiters, 5 Hashimoto's thyroiditis,

Table 1
Potential Molecular Markers for Thyroid Cancer and Method of Detection

Name	Assay
Gal-3	Immunochemistry, RT-PCR
Telomerase	TRAP, RT-PCR
TPO	Immunochemistry, RT-PCR
COX-2	Immunochemistry, RT-PCR
CD44	Immunochemistry, RT-PCR
OnfFN	RT-PCR
CD97	Immunochemistry, RT-PCR
RET/PTC	Immunochemistry, RT-PCR
HBME-1	Immunochemistry
HMGI	Immunochemistry, RT-PCR
BRAF	RT-PCR
EMA	Immunochemistry
Leu7/CD57	Immunochemistry
PAX8-PPARγ	Immunochemistry, RT-PCR
NM23	Immunochemistry
CD30 antigen/ligand	Immunochemistry
Ceruloplasmin/lactoferrin	Immunochemistry
Met/hepatocyte growth factor	Immunochemistry
Hypermethylation of TSHR	Methylation-specific PCR
CK19	Immunochemistry
Molecular profiling	Gene chip analysis

Acronyms defined in text.

6 Hürthle cell neoplasm, and 1 follicular carcinoma) were negative. This yielded 92% sensitivity and 97% specificity. Seven of the papillary carcinomas were suggestive of, but not diagnostic for, papillary carcinoma. Six of these stained for CK19; the authors suggested that CK19 would have aided the diagnosis of PTC preoperatively in these cases.

MOLECULAR PROFILING

The use of molecular profiling by gene chips has recently been employed in thyroid tissue. With this technique, thousands of genes are screened for differential expression between benign and malignant samples. Computer software is "trained" to distinguish gene expression patterns specific for pathological subtypes. This method has been used successfully in thyroid histological specimens *(106a,106b,106c)*. In one study *(107)*, 105 genes were differentially expressed between FA's and follicular carcinomas. Application of this differential expression correctly diagnosed all five unknown specimens tested. This same group also utilized molecular profiling in PTC, particularly the follicular variant of PTC *(108)*. Again, a large number (262) of genes were differentially expressed between benign and malignant samples. In the author's analysis, molecular profiling detected cancer with a 93% sensitivity and 100% specificity. When applied to unknowns, molecular profiling correctly diagnosed all seven samples. In a subset analysis of the follicular variant of PTC vs benign nodules, the sensitivity was 91% and 100%, respectively. In the subset of PTC vs benign nodules, the sensitivity and specificity was 100%. This molecular profiling is new and has not yet been applied to FNA samples; yet, it is an exciting and promising technique in the preoperative diagnosis of thyroid cancer.

SUMMARY

Clearly, a number of markers are being developed to assist in the preoperative diagnosis of thyroid malignancies. FNA has significantly reduced the need for surgery for thyroid nodules; however, indeterminate or suspicious biopsies often lead to unnecessary thyroidectomy. Gal-3 and TPO have been extensively studied and appear to be sensitive and specific markers that can aid in the definitive diagnosis of indeterminate samples. As laboratory techniques continue to improve and experience develops, it is anticipated that more biochemical and molecular markers will be available to perfect their utility and application to FNA samples.

REFERENCES

1. Xu XC, el-Naggar AK, Lotan R. Differential expression of galectin-1 and galectin-3 in thyroid tumors. Potential diagnostic implications. Am J Pathol 1995; 147:815–822.
2. Coli A, Bigotti G, Zucchetti F, et al. Galectin-3, a marker of well-differentiated thyroid carcinoma, is expressed in thyroid nodules with cytological atypia. Histopathology 2002; 40:80–87.
3. Cvejic D, Savin S, Paunovic I, et al. Immunohistochemical localization of galectin-3 in malignant and benign human thyroid tissue. Anticancer Res 1998; 18:2637–2641.
4. Martins L, Matsuo SE, Ebina KN, et al. Galectin-3 messenger ribonucleic acid and protein are expressed in benign thyroid tumors. J Clin Endocrinol Metab 2002; 87:4806–4810.
5. Fernandez PL, Merino MJ, Gomez M, et al. Galectin-3 and laminin expression in neoplastic and non-neoplastic thyroid tissue. J Pathol 1997; 181:80–86.
6. Herrmann ME, LiVolsi VA, Pasha TL, et al. Immunohistochemical expression of galectin-3 in benign and malignant thyroid lesions. Arch Pathol Lab Med 2002; 126:710–713.
6a. Nucera C, Mazzon E, Cailou B, et al. Human galectin-3 immunoexpression in thyroid follicular adenomas with cell atypia. J Endocrinol Invest 2005; 28:106–112.
6b. Papotti M, Rodrgiuez J, DePompa R, Bartolazzi A, Rosai J. Galectin-3 and HBME-1 expression in well-differentiated thyroid tumors with follicular architecture of uncertain malignant potential. Mod Pathol 2005; 18:541–546.
6c. Oestreicher-Kedem Y, Halpern M, Roizman P, et al. Diagnostic value of galectin-3 as a marker for malignancy in follicular patterned thyroid lesions. Head & Neck 2004; 26:960–966.
7. Orlandi F, Saggiorato E, Pivano G, et al. Galectin-3 is a presurgical marker of human thyroid carcinoma. Cancer Res 1998; 58:3015–3020.
8. Aratake Y, Umeki K, Kiyoyama K, et al. Diagnostic utility of galectin-3 and CD26/DPPIV as preoperative diagnostic markers for thyroid nodules. Diagn Cytopathol 2002; 26:366–372.
9. Gasbarri A, Martegani MP, Del Prete F, et al. Galectin-3 and CD44v6 isoforms in the preoperative evaluation of thyroid nodules. J Clin Oncol 1999; 17:3494–3502.

10. Bartolazzi A, Gasbarri A, Papotti M, et al. Application of an immunodiagnostic method for improving preoperative diagnosis of nodular thyroid lesions. Lancet 2001; 357:1644–1650.
11. Saggiorato E, Cappia S, De Giuli P, et al. Galectin-3 as a presurgical immunocytodiagnostic marker of minimally invasive follicular thyroid carcinoma. J Clin Endocrinol Metab 2001; 86:5152–5158.
12. Papotti M, Volante M, Saggiorato E, et al. Role of galectin-3 immunodetection in the cytological diagnosis of thyroid cystic papillary carcinoma. Eur J Endocrinol 2002; 147:515–521.
13. Giannini R, Faviana P, Cavinato T, et al. Galectin-3 and oncofetal-fibronectin expression in thyroid neoplasia as assessed by reverse transcription-polymerase chain reaction and immunochemistry in cytologic and pathologic specimens. Thyroid 2003; 13:765–770.
14. Bernet VJ, Anderson J, Vaishnav Y, et al. Determination of galectin-3 messenger ribonucleic Acid overexpression in papillary thyroid cancer by quantitative reverse transcription-polymerase chain reaction. J Clin Endocrinol Metab 2002; 87:4792–4796.
15. Niedziela M, Maceluch J, Korman E. Galectin-3 is not an universal marker of malignancy in thyroid nodular disease in children and adolescents. J Clin Endocrinol Metab 2002; 87:4411–4415.
16. Shay JW. Telomerase in cancer: diagnostic, prognostic, and therapeutic implications. Cancer J Sci Am 1998; 4(Suppl 1):S26–S34.
17. Kim NW, Piatyszek MA, Prowse KR, et al. Specific association of human telomerase activity with immortal cells and cancer. Science 1994; 266:2011–2015.
18. Haugen BR, Nawaz S, Markham N, et al. Telomerase activity in benign and malignant thyroid tumors. Thyroid 1997; 7:337–342.
19. Umbricht CB, Saji M, Westra WH, et al. Telomerase activity: a marker to distinguish follicular thyroid adenoma from carcinoma. Cancer Res 1997; 57:2144–2147.
20. Yashima K, Vuitch F, Gazdar AF, Fahey TJ III. Telomerase activity in benign and malignant thyroid diseases. Surgery 1997; 122:1141–1145; discussion 1145–1146.
21. Matthews P, Jones CJ, Skinner J, et al. Telomerase activity and telomere length in thyroid neoplasia: biological and clinical implications. J Pathol 2001; 194:183–193.
22. Saji M, Westra WH, Chen H, et al. Telomerase activity in the differential diagnosis of papillary carcinoma of the thyroid. Surgery 1997; 122:1137–1140.
23. Aogi K, Kitahara K, Buley I, et al. Telomerase activity in lesions of the thyroid: application to diagnosis of clinical samples including fine-needle aspirates. Clin Cancer Res 1998; 4:1965–1970.
23a. Ito Y, Yoshida H, Tomoda C, et al. Telomerase activity in thyroid neoplasms evaluated by the expression of human telomerase reverse transcriptase (hTERT). Anticancer Res 2005; 25:509–514.
24. Saji M, Xydas S, Westra WH, et al. Human telomerase reverse transcriptase (hTERT) gene expression in thyroid neoplasms. Clin Cancer Res 1999; 5:1483–1489.
25. Zeiger MA, Smallridge RC, Clark DP, et al. Human telomerase reverse transcriptase (hTERT) gene expression in FNA samples from thyroid neoplasms. Surgery 1999; 126:1195–1198; discussion 1198–1199.
26. Aogi K, Kitahara K, Urquidi V, et al. Comparison of telomerase and CD44 expression as diagnostic tumor markers in lesions of the thyroid. Clin Cancer Res 1999; 5:2790–2797.
27. Siddiqui MT, Greene KL, Clark DP, et al. Human telomerase reverse transcriptase expression in Diff-Quik-stained FNA samples from thyroid nodules. Diagn Mol Pathol 2001; 10:123–129.
28. Liou MJ, Chan EC, Lin JD, Liu FH, Chao TC. Human telomerase reverse transcriptase (hTERT) gene expression in FNA samples from thyroid neoplasms. Cancer Lett 2003; 191:223–227.
29. Kammori M, Nakamura K, Hashimoto M, et al. Clinical application of human telomerase reverse transcriptase gene expression in thyroid follicular tumors by fine-needle aspirations using in situ hybridization. Int J Oncol 2003; 22:985–991.
30. De Micco C, Zoro P, Garcia S, et al. Thyroid peroxidase immunodetection as a tool to assist diagnosis of thyroid nodules on fine-needle aspiration biopsy. Eur J Endocrinol 1994; 131:474–479.
31. De Micco C, Vasko V, Garcia S, et al. Fine-needle aspiration of thyroid follicular neoplasm: diagnostic use of thyroid peroxidase immunocytochemistry with monoclonal antibody 47. Surgery 1994; 116:1031–1035.
32. De Micco C, Vassko V, Henry JF. The value of thyroid peroxidase immunohistochemistry for preoperative fine-needle aspiration diagnosis of the follicular variant of papillary thyroid cancer. Surgery 1999; 126:1200–1204.
33. Henry JF, Denizot A, Porcelli A, et al. Thyroperoxidase immunodetection for the diagnosis of malignancy on fine-needle aspiration of thyroid nodules. World J Surg 1994; 18:529–534.
34. Garcia S, Vassko V, Henry JF, De Micco C. Comparison of thyroid peroxidase expression with cellular proliferation in thyroid follicular tumors. Thyroid 1998; 8:745–749.
35. Christensen L, Blichert-Toft M, Brandt M, et al. Thyroperoxidase (TPO) immunostaining of the solitary cold thyroid nodule. Clin Endocrinol 2000; 53:161–169.
36. Pluot M, Faroux MJ, Flament JB, Patey M, Theobald S, Delisle MJ. Quantitative cytology and thyroperoxidase immunochemistry: new tools in evaluating thyroid nodules by fine-needle aspiration. Cancer Detect Prev 1996; 20:285–293.
37. Faroux MJ, Theobald S, Pluot M, et al. Evaluation of the monoclonal antibody antithyroperoxidase MoAb47 in the diagnostic decision of cold thyroid nodules by fine-needle aspiration. Pathol Res Pract 1997; 193:705–712.
38. Lazar V, Bidart JM, Caillou B, et al. Expression of the Na+/I– symporter gene in human thyroid tumors: a comparison study with other thyroid-specific genes. J Clin Endocrinol Metab 1999; 84:3228–3234.
39. Tanaka T, Umeki K, Yamamoto I, et al. Immunohistochemical loss of thyroid peroxidase in papillary thyroid carcinoma: strong suppression of peroxidase gene expression. J Pathol 1996; 179:89–94.
40. Herschman HR. Prostaglandin synthase 2. Biochim Biophys Acta 1996; 1299:125–140.
41. Specht MC, Tucker ON, Hocever M, et al. Cyclooxygenase-2 expression in thyroid nodules. J Clin Endocrinol Metab 2002; 87:358–363.
41a. Lo CY, Lam KY, Leung PP, Luk JM. High prevalence of cyclooxygenase 2 expression in papillary thyroid carcinoma. Eur J Endocrinol 2005; 152:545–550.
42. Sato H, Ino Y, Miura A, et al. Dysadherin: expression and clinical significance in thyroid carcinoma. J Clin Endocrinol Metab 2003; 88:4407–4412.
43. Smyth P, Sheils O, Finn S, et al. Real-time quantitative analysis of E-cadherin expression in ret/PTC-1-activated thyroid neoplasms. Int J Surg Pathol 2001; 9:265–272.
44. Ermak G, Gerasimov G, Troshina K, et al. Deregulated alternative splicing of CD44 messenger RNA transcripts in neoplastic and nonneoplastic lesions of the human thyroid. Cancer Res 1995; 55:4594–4598.
45. Ermak G, Jennings T, Robinson L, et al. Restricted patterns of CD44 variant exon expression in human papillary thyroid carcinoma. Cancer Res 1996; 56:1037–1042.
46. Kim JY, Cho H, Rhee BD, Kim HY. Expression of CD44 and cyclin D1 in fine needle aspiration cytology of papillary thyroid carcinoma. Acta Cytol 2002; 46:679–683.
47. Takano T, Sumizaki H, Amino N. Detection of CD44 variants in fine needle aspiration biopsies of thyroid tumor by RT-PCR. J Exp Clin Cancer Res 1997; 16:267–271.
48. Takano T, Matsuzuka F, Miyauchi A, et al. Restricted expression of oncofetal fibronectin mRNA in thyroid papillary and anaplastic carcinoma: an in situ hybridization study. Br J Cancer 1998; 78:221–224.

49. Higashiyama T, Takano T, Matsuzuka F, et al. Measurement of the expression of oncofetal fibronectin mRNA in thyroid carcinomas by competitive reverse transcription-polymerase chain reaction. Thyroid 1999; 9:235–240.
50. Takano T, Matsuzuka F, Sumizaki H, et al. Rapid detection of specific messenger RNAs in thyroid carcinomas by reverse transcription-PCR with degenerate primers: specific expression of oncofetal fibronectin messenger RNA in papillary carcinoma. Cancer Res 1997; 57: 3792–3797.
51. Takano T, Miyauchi A, Yokozawa T, et al. Accurate and objective preoperative diagnosis of thyroid papillary carcinomas by reverse transcription-PCR detection of oncofetal fibronectin messenger RNA in fine-needle aspiration biopsies. Cancer Res 1998; 58:4913–4917.
52. Takano T, Miyauchi A, Yokozawa T, et al. Preoperative diagnosis of thyroid papillary and anaplastic carcinomas by real-time quantitative reverse transcription-polymerase chain reaction of oncofetal fibronectin messenger RNA. Cancer Res 1999; 59:4542–4545.
53. Aust G, Eichler W, Laue S, et al. CD97: a dedifferentiation marker in human thyroid carcinomas. Cancer Res 1997; 57:1798–1806.
54. Cheung CC, Ezzat S, Freeman JL, et al. Immunohistochemical diagnosis of papillary thyroid carcinoma. Mod Pathol 2001; 14:338–342.
55. Sugg SL, Ezzat S, Rosen IB, et al. Distinct multiple RET/PTC gene rearrangements in multifocal papillary thyroid neoplasia. J Clin Endocrinol Metab 1998; 83:4116–4122.
56. Elisei R, Romei C, Vorontsova T, et al. RET/PTC rearrangements in thyroid nodules: studies in irradiated and not irradiated, malignant and benign thyroid lesions in children and adults. J Clin Endocrinol Metab 2001; 86:3211–3216.
57. Fusco A, Chiappetta G, Hui P, et al. Assessment of RET/PTC oncogene activation and clonality in thyroid nodules with incomplete morphological evidence of papillary carcinoma: a search for the early precursors of papillary cancer. Am J Pathol 2002; 160: 2157–2167.
58. Cheung CC, Carydis B, Ezzat S, et al. Analysis of ret/PTC gene rearrangements refines the fine needle aspiration diagnosis of thyroid cancer. J Clin Endocrinol Metab 2001; 86:2187–2190.
59. Miettinen M, Karkkainen P. Differential reactivity of HBME-1 and CD15 antibodies in benign and malignant thyroid tumours. Preferential reactivity with malignant tumours. Virchows Arch 1996; 429: 213–219.
60. Mase T, Funahashi H, Koshikawa T, et al. HBME-1 immunostaining in thyroid tumors especially in follicular neoplasm. Endocr J 2003; 50:173–177.
61. van Hoeven KH, Kovatich AJ, Miettinen M. Immunocytochemical evaluation of HBME-1, CA 19-9, and CD-15 (Leu-M1) in fine-needle aspirates of thyroid nodules. Diagn Cytopathol 1998; 18:93–97.
62. Sack MJ, Astengo-Osuna C, Lin BT, et al. HBME-1 immunostaining in thyroid fine-needle aspirations: a useful marker in the diagnosis of carcinoma. Mod Pathol 1997; 10:668–674.
62a. Ito Y, Yoshida H, Tomoda C, et al. HBME-1 expression in follicular tumor of the thyroid: an investigation of whether it can be used as a marker to diagnose follicular carcinoma. Anticancer Res 2005; 25: 179–182.
63. Chiappetta G, Bandiera A, Berlingieri MT, et al. The expression of the high mobility group HMGI (Y) proteins correlates with the malignant phenotype of human thyroid neoplasias. Oncogene 1995; 10: 1307–1314.
64. Chiappetta G, Tallini G, De Biasio MC, et al. Detection of high mobility group I HMGI(Y) protein in the diagnosis of thyroid tumors: HMGI(Y) expression represents a potential diagnostic indicator of carcinoma. Cancer Res 1998; 58:4193–4198.
65. Kimura ET, Nikiforova MN, Zhu Z, et al. High prevalence of BRAF mutations in thyroid cancer: genetic evidence for constitutive activation of the RET/PTC-RAS-BRAF signaling pathway in papillary thyroid carcinoma. Cancer Res 2003; 63:1454–1457.
66. Cohen Y, Xing M, Mambo E, et al. BRAF mutation in papillary thyroid carcinoma. J Natl Cancer Inst 2003; 95:625–627.
67. Xu X, Quiros RM, Gattuso P, et al. High prevalence of BRAF gene mutation in papillary thyroid carcinomas and thyroid tumor cell lines. Cancer Res 2003; 63:4561–4567.
68. Cohen Y, Rosenbaum E, Clark DP, et al. Mutational analysis of BRAF in fine needle aspiration biopsies of the thyroid: a potential application for the preoperative assessment of thyroid nodules. Clin Cancer Res 2004; 10:2761–2765.
69. Xing M, Tufano RP, Tufaro AP, et al. Detection of BRAF mutation on fine needle aspiration biopsy specimens: a new diagnostic tool for papillary thyroid cancer. J Clin Endocrinol Metab 2004; 89: 2867–2872.
69a. Hayashida N, Namba H, Kumagai A, et al. A rapid and simple detection method for the BRAF (T1796A) mutation in fine-needle aspirated thyroid carcinoma cells. Thyroid 2004; 14:910–915.
70. Pinkus GS, Kurtin PJ. Epithelial membrane antigen—a diagnostic discriminant in surgical pathology: immunohistochemical profile in epithelial, mesenchymal, and hematopoietic neoplasms using paraffin sections and monoclonal antibodies. Hum Pathol 1985; 16: 929–940.
71. Damiani S, Fratamico F, Lapertosa G, et al. Alcian blue and epithelial membrane antigen are useful markers in differentiating benign from malignant papillae in thyroid lesions. Virchows Arch A Pathol Anat Histopathol 1991; 419:131–135.
72. Wilson NW, Pambakian H, Richardson TC, et al. Epithelial markers in thyroid carcinoma: an immunoperoxidase study. Histopathology 1986; 10:815–829.
73. Mitselou A, Vougiouklakis TG, Peschos D, et al. Immunohistochemical study of the expression of S-100 protein, epithelial membrane antigen, cytokeratin and carcinoembryonic antigen in thyroid lesions. Anticancer Res 2002; 22:1777–1780.
74. Cheifetz RE, Davis NL, Robinson BW, et al. Differentiation of thyroid neoplasms by evaluating epithelial membrane antigen, Leu-7 antigen, epidermal growth factor receptor, and DNA content. Am J Surg 1994; 167:531–534.
75. Ghali VS, Jimenez EJ, Garcia RL. Distribution of Leu-7 antigen (HNK-1) in thyroid tumors: its usefulness as a diagnostic marker for follicular and papillary carcinomas. Hum Pathol 1992; 23:21–25.
76. Khan A, Baker SP, Patwardhan NA, Pullman JM. CD57 (Leu-7) expression is helpful in diagnosis of the follicular variant of papillary thyroid carcinoma. Virchows Arch 1998; 432:427–432.
77. Ostrowski ML, Brown RW, Wheeler TM, et al. Leu-7 immunoreactivity in cytologic specimens of thyroid lesions, with emphasis on follicular neoplasms. Diagn Cytopathol 1995; 12:297–302.
78. Suh N, Wang Y, Williams CR, et al. A new ligand for the peroxisome proliferator-activated receptor-gamma (PPAR-gamma), GW7845, inhibits rat mammary carcinogenesis. Cancer Res 1999; 59: 5671–5673.
79. Kroll TG, Sarraf P, Pecciarini L, et al. PAX8-PPARgamma1 fusion oncogene in human thyroid carcinoma [corrected]. Science 2000; 289:1357–1360.
80. Nikiforova MN, Biddinger PW, Caudill CM, et al. PAX8-PPARgamma rearrangement in thyroid tumors: RT-PCR and immunohistochemical analyses. Am J Surg Pathol 2002; 26:1016–1023.
81. Nikiforova MN, Lynch RA, Biddinger PW, et al. RAS point mutations and PAX8-PPAR gamma rearrangement in thyroid tumors: evidence for distinct molecular pathways in thyroid follicular carcinoma. J Clin Endocrinol Metab 2003; 88:2318–2326.
82. Marques AR, Espadinha C, Catarino AL, et al. Expression of PAX8-PPARgamma1 Rearrangements in both follicular thyroid carcinomas and adenomas. J Clin Endocrinol Metab 2002; 87:3947–3952.
83. Dwight T, Thoppe SR, Foukakis T, et al. Involvement of the PAX8/peroxisome proliferator-activated receptor gamma rearrangement in follicular thyroid tumors. J Clin Endocrinol Metab 2003; 88:4440–4445.

84. Cheung L, Messina M, Gill A, et al. Detection of the PAX8-PPAR gamma fusion oncogene in both follicular thyroid carcinomas and adenomas. J Clin Endocrinol Metab 2003; 88:354–357.
85. Arai T, Watanabe M, Onodera M, et al. Reduced nm 23-H1 messenger RNA expression in metastatic lymph nodes from patients with papillary carcinoma of the thyroid. Am J Pathol 1993; 142:1938–1944.
86. Arai T, Yamashita T, Urano T, et al. Preferential reduction of nm23-H1 gene product in metastatic tissues from papillary and follicular carcinomas of the thyroid. Mod Pathol 1995; 8:252–256.
87. Okubo T, Inokuma S, Takeda S, Itoyama S, Kinoshita K, Sugawara I. Expression of nm23-H1 gene product in thyroid, ovary, and breast cancers. Cell Biophys 1995; 26:205–213.
88. Zou M, Shi Y, al-Sedairy S, Farid NR. High levels of Nm23 gene expression in advanced stage of thyroid carcinomas. Br J Cancer 1993; 68:385–388.
89. Zafon C, Obiols G, Castellvi J, et al. nm23-H1 immunoreactivity as a prognostic factor in differentiated thyroid carcinoma. J Clin Endocrinol Metab 2001; 86:3975–3980.
90. Farley DR, Eberhardt NL, Grant CS, et al. Expression of a potential metastasis suppressor gene (nm23) in thyroid neoplasms. World J Surg 1993; 17:615-20; discussion 620–621.
91. Bertheau P, De La Rosa A, Steeg PS, Merino MJ. NM23 protein in neoplastic and nonneoplastic thyroid tissues. Am J Pathol 1994; 145: 26–32.
92. Luo W, Matsuo K, Nagayama Y, et al. Immunohistochemical analysis of expression of nm23-H1/nucleoside diphosphate kinase in human thyroid carcinomas: lack of correlation between its expression and lymph node metastasis. Thyroid 1993; 3:105–109.
93. Trovato M, Villari D, Ruggeri RM, et al. Expression of CD30 ligand and CD30 receptor in normal thyroid and benign and malignant thyroid nodules. Thyroid 2001; 11:621–628.
93a. Sorrentino R, Libertini S, Pallante PL, et al. Aurora B overexpression associates with the thyroid carcinoma undifferentiated phenotype and is required for thyroid carcinoma cell proliferation. J Clin Endocrinol Metab 2005; 90:928–935.
93b. Nikiforov YE. Editorial: Anaplastic carcinoma of the thyroid—Will Aurora B light a path for treatment? J Clin Endocrinol Metab 2005; 90:1243–1245.
94. Tuccari G, Barresi G. Immunohistochemical demonstration of ceruloplasmin in follicular adenomas and thyroid carcinomas. Histopathology 1987; 11:723–731.
95. Kondi-Pafiti A, Smyrniotis V, Frangou M, et al. Immunohistochemical study of ceruloplasmin, lactoferrin and secretory component expression in neoplastic and non-neoplastic thyroid gland diseases. Acta Oncol 2000; 39:753–756.
96. de Camargo R, Longatto Filho A, Alves VA, et al. Lactoferrin in thyroid lesions: immunoreactivity in fine needle aspiration biopsy samples. Acta Cytol 1996; 40:408–413.
97. Stoker M, Gherardi E, Perryman M, Gray J. Scatter factor is a fibroblast-derived modulator of epithelial cell mobility. Nature 1987; 327:239–242.
98. Di Renzo MF, Olivero M, Ferro S, et al. Overexpression of the c-MET/HGF receptor gene in human thyroid carcinomas. Oncogene 1992; 7:2549–2553.
99. Belfiore A, Gangemi P, Costantino A, et al. Negative/low expression of the Met/hepatocyte growth factor receptor identifies papillary thyroid carcinomas with high risk of distant metastases. J Clin Endocrinol Metab 1997; 82:2322–2328.
100. Ippolito A, Vella V, La Rosa GL, et al. Immunostaining for Met/HGF receptor may be useful to identify malignancies in thyroid lesions classified suspicious at fine-needle aspiration biopsy. Thyroid 2001; 11:783–787.
101. Xing M, Usadel H, Cohen Y, et al. Methylation of the thyroid-stimulating hormone receptor gene in epithelial thyroid tumors: a marker of malignancy and a cause of gene silencing. Cancer Res 2003; 63:2316–2321.
102. Erkilic S, Aydin A, Kocer NE. Diagnostic utility of cytokeratin 19 expression in multinodular goiter with papillary areas and papillary carcinoma of thyroid. Endocr Pathol 2002; 13:207–211.
103. Raphael SJ, McKeown-Eyssen G, Asa SL. High-molecular-weight cytokeratin and cytokeratin-19 in the diagnosis of thyroid tumors. Mod Pathol 1994; 7:295–300.
104. Beesley MF, McLaren KM. Cytokeratin 19 and galectin-3 immunohistochemistry in the differential diagnosis of solitary thyroid nodules. Histopathology 2002; 41:236–243.
105. Hirokawa M, Inagaki A, Kobayashi H, et al. Expression of cytokeratin 19 in cytologic specimens of thyroid. Diagn Cytopathol 2000; 22:197–198.
106. Nasser SM, Pitman MB, Pilch BZ, Faquin WC. Fine-needle aspiration biopsy of papillary thyroid carcinoma: diagnostic utility of cytokeratin 19 immunostaining. Cancer 2000; 90:307–311.
106a. Finley DJ, Lubitz CC, Wei C, Zhu B, Fahey TJ III. Advancing the molecular diagnosis of thyroid nodules: Defining benign lesions by molecular profiling. Thyroid 2005; 15:562–568.
106b. Weber F, Shen L, Aldred MA, et al. Genetic classification of benign and malignant thyroid follicular neoplasia based on a three-gene combination. J Clin Endocrinol Metab 2005; 90:2512–2521.
106c. Chevillard S, Ugolin N, Vielh P, et al. Gene expression profiling of differentiate thyroid neoplasms: diagnostic and clinical implications. Clin Cancer Res 2004; 10:6586–6597.
107. Barden CB, Shister KW, Zhu B, et al. Classification of follicular thyroid tumors by molecular signature: results of gene profiling. Clin Cancer Res 2003; 9:1792–1800.
108. Finley DJ, Arora N, Zhu B, et al. Molecular profiling distinguishes papillary carcinoma from benign thyroid nodules. J Clin Endocrinol Metab 2004; 89:3214–3223.

20
Radionuclide Imaging of Thyroid Nodules

Douglas Van Nostrand

INTRODUCTION

Thyroid scintigraphy has been used for many years to evaluate thyroid nodules. The clinical value of thyroid scintigraphy has been established based on the knowledge that (1) functioning nodules have not only increased radioiodine uptake relative to normal functioning thyroid tissue but also have a low probability of malignancy; and (2) thyroid cancers have no or very low (e.g., 1 in 100) radioiodine accumulation relative to normal thyroid tissue. This section presents an overview of thyroid scintigraphy in the evaluation of thyroid nodules (see Table 1).

RADIOPHARMACEUTICALS AND MECHANISMS

The most frequently used radiopharmaceuticals for thyroid scintigraphy have been ^{131}I, ^{99m}TcO$_4$, and ^{123}I. The physical characteristics of the various radiopharmaceuticals are shown in Table 2, and their respective advantages and disadvantages are listed in Table 3. Because of the significant radiation-absorbed dose to normal functioning thyroid tissue, ^{131}I is no longer routinely used for scanning when ^{99m}TcO$_4$ and ^{123}I are available, and the latter are widely available in the United States and many other countries. Although ^{123}I is more expensive than ^{99m}TcO$_4$, over the last several years, the cost of ^{123}I has decreased significantly. Both ^{99m}TcO$_4$ and ^{123}I result in good images; ^{123}I is slightly better. As an isotope of iodine, ^{123}I is both trapped and organified, whereas ^{99m}TcO$_4$ only reflects trapping.

IMAGING PROCEDURE

The Society of Nuclear Medicine created guidelines for thyroid scintigraphy (1). For thyroid scintigraphy, the prescribed activity of ^{123}I ranges typically between 200 and 400 uCi (7.4–14.8 MBq), with images performed 6–24 h later. The prescribed activity of ^{99m}TcO$_4$ is approx 10 mCi (370 MBq), and images were performed 20–30 min later. Images are obtained on γ camera with a pinhole collimator in the anterior, left-anterior oblique (LAO), and right-anterior oblique (RAO) positions. Markers may be placed on various landmarks, such as the suprasternal notch and chin.

After completion of the standard images, the thyroid gland should be examined, and additional images—with or without radioactive markers placed on nodules or anatomical landmarks—may need to be performed. The radioactive markers on the palpable nodule(s) help determine whether the nodule is cold, hot, warm, indeterminate, normofunctioning, or hyperfunctioning. However, when using a pinhole collimator, caution must be taken in the imaging of markers to determine the nodule function. As discussed in greater detail in Chapter 14 entitled "Radioiodine Whole-Body Imaging," pinhole collimators have the best resolution, but they may distort the location of the anatomy—a phenomenon that has been called "parallax" (2). Structures or markers located close to the face of the pinhole collimator are recorded on the final image farther toward the edge of the field of view than deeper structures. Thus, a marker placed on the skin surface near the face of the pinhole collimator, precisely over a deep, underlying nodule may appear on the images to be lateral to the cold or hot area. The only location in the field of view of a pinhole collimator where it can be determined that all the structures line up on the image, regardless of their depth, is at the center. Standard and marker images can usually be completed within 30–60 min.

RADIATION DOSIMETRY

Estimates of radiation-absorbed dose for adults for ^{123}I, ^{99m}TcO$_4$, and ^{131}I are noted in Table 4. For standard prescribed activity for imaging, ^{131}I delivers the highest radiation-absorbed dose to the thyroid, and all three radioisotopes have reasonably low whole-body radiation-absorbed doses. As noted above, and because of the absorbed radiation dose to the thyroid, ^{131}I is no longer routinely used when ^{123}I or ^{99m}TcO$_4$ is available.

TERMINOLOGY FOR NODULE FUNCTION ASSESSED ON THYROID SCINTIGRAPHY AND THE FREQUENCY OF THYROID CANCER

The terminology for describing the function of nodules on thyroid scans can be confusing. "Cold," "hypofunctioning,"

From: *Thyroid Cancer: A Comprehensive Guide to Clinical Management, 2/e*
Edited by: L. Wartofsky and D. Van Nostrand © Humana Press Inc., Totowa, NJ

Table 1

Radiopharmaceuticals and Mechanisms
Imaging Procedure
Radiation Dosimetry
Terminology for Describing the Function of Nodules Assessed
 on Thyroid Scintigraphy and the Frequency of Thyroid Cancer
Discordance of ^{123}I and ^{99m}TcO$_4$ Pertechnetate Scans
Utility of Thyroid Scintigraphy
Summary

Table 2
Radiopharmaceuticals Used for Thyroid Scintigraphy

	Decay Mode	Half-Life	γ Energy (keV)	Production Method	Typical Prescribed Activity mCi (MBq)
^{123}I	Electron capture	13.6 h	159	Cyclotron methods; one method referred to as a (p,5n) produces ^{123}I with no ^{124}I contamination and little ^{125}I. The other approach referred to as (p,2n) has a number of impurities that have high-energy γ and long half-lives. These contaminations reduce image quality and increase the radiation exposure of the patient	0.2–0.4 (1.5–3.0)
^{99m}Tc	Isomeric transition	6.02 h	140	Molybdenum 99 generator	2–10 (7.4–370)
^{131}I	β-decay	8.02 d	364	Reactor produced either from direct bombardment of a target by neutrons or from the reprocessing of spent fuel rods from a nuclear power plant	0.005 (0.185) for uptakes 1–5 (37–185) for imaging 29–1000 (1.07–37 GBq) for therapy

and "nonfunctioning" nodules have reduced radioiodine uptake relative to adjacent normal or abnormal tissue (see Fig. 1). Of note, an important adjective of this definition is the use of the word "radioiodine." Hypofunctioning nodules on radioiodine scans may not be hypofunctioning on ^{99m}TcO$_4$ scans, which is discussed further in the "Discordance of ^{123}I and ^{99m}TcO$_4$ Scans" section. Nevertheless, in a study of 2237 patients, Borner et al. (3) reported a 21% frequency of cold nodules in patients ages 15 and 16 and a 44% frequency in patients over age 65. Thyroid cancer was present in 11% of cold nodules in patients ages 45–65 and evident in 25% of patients over age 65. In a review of the literature, Ashcraft and Van Herle (4) reported that 16–21% of cold nodules harbored a malignancy.

The designations of "indeterminate," "normofunctioning," and sometimes "warm" nodules imply that there is either no abnormality on scan or the function of a palpable nodule cannot be determined. Small nodules located posteriorly in the thyroid may be obscured by radioiodine uptake in normal thyroid tissue that overlies the small thyroid nodule. Similarly, a small nodule located anteriorly may not attenuate the radioiodine from the normal underlying thyroid tissue. The half-value for attenuation by tissues of ^{123}I is approximately 6 cm, i.e., it would require a 6-cm nodule overlying normal thyroid tissue to attenuate 50% of the radioactivity from the underlying normal thyroid tissue. The half-value for attenuation of ^{99m}TcO$_4$ is approximately 5 cm. Thus, although a nodule may be truly hypofunctioning relative to normal thyroid tissue, its "cold" appearance on the scan may not be seen at all; it would be called "indeterminate," "normofunctioning," or sometimes "warm." Ashcraft and Van Herle (4) reported that 9% of intermediate nodules harbored malignancy. Sandler et al. (5) have stated that indeterminate nodules have equivalent significance as a hypofunctioning nodule.

Table 3
Comparison of ^{123}I, ^{99m}Tc, and ^{131}I

Characteristics	Advantages/Disadvantages		
	^{123}I	$^{99m}TcO_4$	^{131}I
Expense	$$	$	$
Readily available	Y	Y	Y
Reimbursed by insurance	Y	Y	Y
Image quality	Excellent	Excellent but not as good when trapping is low	Good
Mechanism of accumulation of radioactivity in the thyroid	Organification	Trapping	Organification
Esophageal or vascular radioactivity	Unlikely	Possibly	Unlikely
Patient convenience	Requires longer time between administration and imaging (6–24 h)	More rapid exam: Imaging within 30 min of administration	Imaging typically 24-h after administration
Radiation dose to thyroid	Depends on method of production*	Low	Significant
Ability to obtain 24-h uptake	Y	N (Can obtain a 20-min trapping)	Y
Risk to personnel handling patient and radionuclide	Very low	Very low	Low
Necessity of radiation safety precautions for the patient and public	N	N	Y

*Although the radiation absorbed dose to the thyroid from ^{123}I is low, the presence of contaminants of ^{124}I and ^{125}I in the preparation of ^{123}I can result in higher radiation absorbed doses to the thyroid, and the presence of contaminants depends on the method of ^{123}I production. ^{123}I produced by the (p,5n) cyclotron method has no contaminants of ^{124}I and little contaminants of ^{125}I. ^{123}I produced by the (p,2n) cyclotron method can have significant contaminants of ^{124}I and ^{125}I.

Table 4
Absorbed Radiation Dose in Adults for ^{123}I, ^{99m}Tc, and ^{131}I

	^{123}I	$^{99m}TcO_4$	^{131}I
Activity administered	0.2–0.6 mCi (7.4–25 MBq)	1–10 mCi (37–370 MBq)	0.05–0.2 mCi (1.85–7.4 MBq)
Organ receiving the largest radiation-absorbed dose	Thyroid	Upper large intestine	Thyroid
Thyroid	7.7 rad/0.4 mCi* (77 mGy/14.8 MBq)	0.390 rad/3 mCi 3.9 mGy/111 MBq	78 rad/0.1 mCi* (780 mGy/3.7 MBq)
Total body	0.014 rad/0.4 mCi* (0.14 mGy/14.8 MBq)	0.042 rad/3 mCi 0.42 mGy/111 MBq	0.047 rad/0.1 mCi* (0.47 mGy/3.7 MBq)

*Thyroid uptake of 15%.

"Hot" or "hyperfunctioning" nodules indicate significant increased radioiodine uptake relative to normal thyroid tissue, with or without suppression of the remaining thyroid tissue (see Figs. 2 and 3). Sometimes "warm" has also been used to describe the latter, which again is an area on the scan that has slightly increased radioiodine uptake in association with adjacent normal thyroid tissue. Frequently, "hot" or "hyperfunctioning" tacitly imply that the nodules are

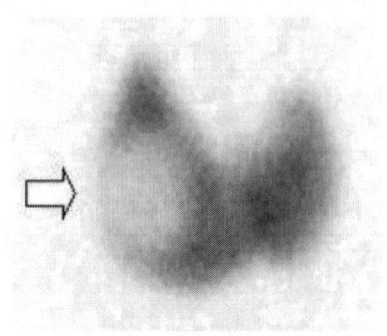

Fig. 1. A prominent, "cold," or hypofunctioning area in the mid-aspect of the right lobe (white arrow). Reproduced with permission from Keystone Press, Inc. *(32)*.

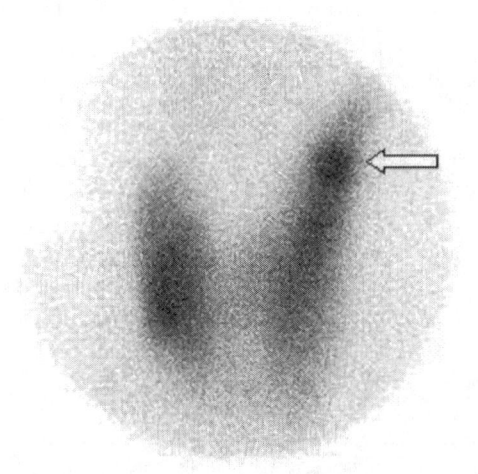

Fig. 2. A small area of increased activity ("warm" or hyperfunctioning) in the upper pole of the left lobe of the thyroid (white arrow). No significant suppression of the remaining thyroid is apparent. This finding is the most consistent with a hypertrophic area, which is not autonomous (under the regulation of TSH), not toxic, and does not suppress the remainder of the thyroid tissue. However, the scan cannot exclude the less likely possibility that the small hyperfunctioning area is autonomous but is not yet toxic and produces enough thyroid hormone to suppress the TSH. Reproduced with permission from Keystone Press, Inc. *(32)*.

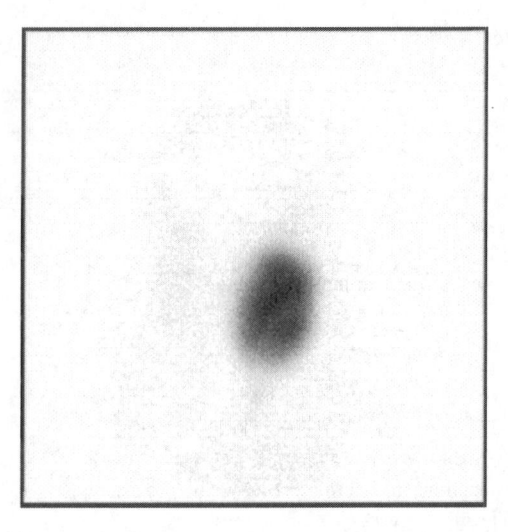

Fig. 3. A single, prominent "hot" or hyperfunctioning area with no visualization of the remaining thyroid. This is consistent with an autonomous and toxic hyperfunctioning thyroid nodule with suppression of the TSH and the remainder of the thyroid tissue. These images were contributed by Elmo Acio, MD, Division of Nuclear Medicine, Department of Medicine, Washington Hospital Center.

autonomous, but this is not part of the definition. A "hot" or "hyperfunctioning" nodule may either be "hypertrophic" and under the regulation of thyrotropin (TSH) or "autonomous" and not under the regulation of TSH.

Relative to the frequency of malignancy in cold thyroid nodules, there is a limited number of cases documenting the presence of malignancy in a hyperfunctioning nodule *(6–21)*. Ashcraft and Van Herle reported that 1–4% of hyperfunctioning nodules harbored malignancy, and this rate may depend on the definition of "coexisting thyroid cancer and hyperfunctioning nodules *(4)*." Lupi *(22)* has described several possible conditions regarding the coexistence of thyroid carcinoma and hyperfunctioning tissue and are provided as follows. Coexistence of thyroid carcinoma and hyperfunctioning thyroid tissue may occur (1) in the same gland but in different locations; (2) in a hyperfunctioning nodule but adjacent to the hyperfunctioning adenoma; (3) in a true hyperfunctioning thyroid carcinoma; and (4) in "the presence of such a large tumor mass that the large tumor mass competes with normal tissue for radioiodine uptake, despite being hormonogentically ineffective in itself *(22)*."

Lupi suggested that the coexistence of carcinoma and focally hyperfunctioning tissue in the same gland in different locations is uncommon. However, he also suggested that the incidence of thyroid carcinoma coexisting in a different part of the thyroid, which has a hyperfunctioning nodule without autonomy and suppression, may be more frequent and near the incidence of thyroid carcinoma that exists without a hyperfunctioning thyroid nodule. Thyroid carcinoma coexisting and adjacent to a hyperfunctioning adenoma represents the majority of reports *(6,9–16,18,23–26)*, but documented true hyperfunctioning thyroid carcinomas are rare *(19,20)*. Ghose et al. *(19)* confirmed high radioiodine uptake in the thyroid carcinoma by autoradiography, and Sandler et al. *(20)* showed low in vitro iodine content by X-ray fluorescence. Regarding Lupi's fourth possibility above, Lupi stated this is unlikely.

Finally, the descriptive phrase, "owl's eye" has been used to denote a cold area within an autonomous hyperfunctioning area *(5)*. In the appropriate clinical situation, the cold area often represents cystic degeneration, hemorrhage, or both in an autonomously functioning thyroid nodule.

DISCORDANCE OF ^{123}I AND ^{99m}TCO$_4$ SCANS

As discussed above, radioiodine scans demonstrate organification of the iodine, and ^{99m}TcO$_4$ scans show only trapping of the ^{99m}TcO$_4$. As a result, discordant findings on ^{123}I and ^{99m}TcO$_4$ scans may be observed. Kusic et al. *(27)* found six different discordant ^{123}I and ^{99m}TcO$_4$ patterns, and the overall incidence of discordance was 5–8%. These patterns were: ^{99m}Tc hot/^{123}I normal, ^{99m}Tc hot/^{123}I cold, ^{99m}Tc normal/^{123}I cold, ^{99m}Tc normal/^{123}I hot, ^{99m}Tc cold/^{123}I normal, and ^{99m}Tc cold/^{123}I hot. Although Kusic reported thyroid cancer in 4% (12 of 16) of patients, none of the patients with thyroid cancer had a discordant pattern. Ryo et al. *(28)* reported a discordance of 33% (40 of 122) of patients, many of which had a functioning or "warm" nodule on ^{99m}TcO$_4$ scanning and a hypofunctioning nodule on ^{123}I scanning. Erjaec et al. *(29)* reported disparate results in 31% (18 of 58) of patients; of the 18 patients, 78% (14 of 18) had cancer. Turner and Spencer *(30)* reviewed the literature until about 1976 and determined that a discordant pattern of ^{123}I and ^{99m}TcO$_4$ scanning with cancer would occur in approx 1 of 30 studies.

Therefore, should thyroid scans be performed only with radioiodine, or if ^{99m}TcO$_4$ is used, does a radioiodine scan need to be performed in those patients with hyperfunctioning or warm nodules on the ^{99m}TcO$_4$ scan? Certainly, arguments exist that support the recommendation that only ^{123}I scans should be performed to obtain the slightly superior quality of ^{123}I images, to eliminate the potential discordance of a hot nodule on ^{99m}Tc scan/cold nodule on subsequent ^{123}I scan, and/or to obtain a 6- or 24-h uptake.

However, counter arguments also exist for the preference of ^{99m}TcO$_4$ scans as either the only scan or as the first scan followed by a sub-sequent ^{123}I scan to assess a hot nodule on the ^{99m}TcO$_4$ scan *(31)*. The reasons for this latter approach are that ^{99m}TcO$_4$ is inexpensive, provides good images, and allows imaging within 30 min, rather than 6–24 h after administration of ^{123}I. With a theoretical example, the cost and inconvenience of performing ^{123}I scans can be put in perspective in all patients (group A) vs the alternative approach of first employing ^{99m}TcO$_4$ with subsequent ^{123}I scans for hot nodules on ^{99m}TcO$_4$ scans (group B). If 100 ^{99m}Tc scans are performed, and 5% of these scans have hot nodules, then group A would have had 100 scans performed with ^{123}I, whereas group B would have had 100 scans performed with ^{99m}TcO$_4$, in addition to five scans performed with ^{123}I scans. If the radioisotope costs for $250 for ^{123}I, the cost of ^{99m}TcO$_4$ is $10, and the cost of the scans for either radioisotope is considered equal, then group A would have spent $25,000 vs $2250 for group B (100 doses of ^{99m}TcO$_4$ plus five doses of ^{123}I). Additionally, patients in group A would have had to come to the imaging facility 200 times, whereas patients in group B would have had to come to the imaging facility for 110 visits (100 for the ^{99m}TcO$_4$ scan, 10 visits for the five ^{123}I scans).

However, if only ^{99m}TcO$_4$ scans are performed with no subsequent ^{123}I scan to evaluate hot nodules on the ^{99m}TcO$_4$ scan, how many cancers would be missed? Again, a theoretical example helps put this into perspective. If 1000 ^{99m}Tc scans are performed, 5% of these scans have hot nodules; 10% of these hot nodules are cold on ^{123}I scans; and 20% of these cold nodules harbor cancer, then one thyroid cancer would be missed out of 1000 patients if only ^{99m}TcO$_4$ scans had been conducted.

In summary, because of the radiation absorbed dose to the thyroid from ^{131}I, this isoform is not recommended when ^{123}I and ^{99m}TcO$_4$ are available. However, if thyroid scintigraphy is to be performed, then both ^{99m}TcO$_4$ and ^{123}I are reasonable alternatives, each with their own strengths and weaknesses.

UTILITY OF THYROID SCINTIGRAPHY

The major roles of thyroid scintigraphy have been threefold:

1. The evaluation of the function of nodules (e.g., hot and cold) to help triage patients for fine-needle aspiration or surgery.
2. The demonstration of other nodules (e.g., multinodular goiter), which may reduce the risk of malignancy.
3. The identification of hyperfunctioning nodules in patients with symptoms of hyperthyroidism, suppressed TSH levels, equivocal biopsy, and/or biopsy results that are suggestive of follicular neoplasm.

SUMMARY

Historically, thyroid scintigraphy has been a valuable imaging modality in the evaluation and characterization of the function of thyroid nodules. ^{123}I and ^{99m}TcO$_4$ are the preferred radioisotopes, and the thyroid scintigraphic procedure is simple to perform. Most palpable nodules are hypofunctioning or have indeterminate function, and despite good sensitivity of thyroid scintigraphy for cancer, the specificity is low. A hypofunctioning or indeterminate nodule is associated with a 10–30% chance of harboring cancer. Functioning nodules are less frequent and are rarely associated with thyroid cancer.

However, despite the historical utility of thyroid scintigraphy, its role in the evaluation of thyroid nodules has been significantly altered with the ease, safety, and reliability of fine-needle aspiration (see Chapters 17 and 18) and the refinement of ultrasound (see Chapter 21). The evaluation of nodule function (e.g., hot and cold) is no longer sufficient help in the triage of patients for fine-needle aspiration or surgery. Fine-needle aspiration is easy, safe, and cost-effective. The demonstration of other nodules in the thyroid (e.g., multinodular goiter) is no longer of significant utility. Ultrasound can provide efficacious images, does not use radiation, and costs about the same or possibly less than radionuclide scanning. However, a thyroid scan may still be useful in the evaluation of patients with signs or symptoms of hyperthyroidism, suppressed TSH, an equivocal biopsy, or a biopsy suggestive of follicular neoplasm. Nevertheless, it is time to look for "smarter" radiolabeled molecular tracers that will help differentiate benign from malignant nodules.

REFERENCES

1. Society of Nuclear Medicine Procedure Guideline for Thyroid Scintigraphy, version 2.0, approved February 7, 1999. Procedure Guidelines Manual, Society of Nuclear Medicine, 2003:29–32.
2. McKitrick WL, Park HM, Kosegi JE. Parallax error in pinhole thyroid scintigraphy: a critical consideration in the evaluation of substernal goiters. J Nucl Med 1985; 26:418–420.
3. Borner W, Lautsch M, et al. Die diagnostiche bedeutung des "kalten Knotens" im schilddrusenszintigramm. Med Welt 1965; 17:892–897.
4. Ashcraft MW, Van Herle AJ. Management of thyroid nodules. II. Scanning techniques, thyroid suppressive therapy, and fine needle Laspiration. Head Neck Surg 1981; 3:296–322.
5. Sandler MP, Coleman RE, Patton JA, et al. Diagnostic Nuclear Medicine, 4th ed. Philadelphia, PA: Lippincott Williams & Wilkins, 2003.
6. Freitas JE, Gross MD, Ripley S, et al. Radionuclide diagnosis and therapy of thyroid cancer: current status report. Semin Nucl Med 1985; 15:106–131.
7. Appetecchia M, Ducci M. Hyperfunctioning differentiated thyroid carcinoma. J Endocrinol Invest 1998; 21:189–192.
8. Mulnar GD, Childs DS, Wollner LB. Histologic evidence of malignancy in a thyroid gland bearing a "hot" nodule. J Clin Endocrinol Metab 1958; 18:1132–1134.
9. Becker FO, Economou PG, Schwartz TB. The occurrence of carcinoma in "hot" thyroid nodules: report of two cases. Ann Intern Med 1963; 58:877–882.
10. Dische S. The radioscope scan applied to the detection of carcinoma in thyroid swellings. Cancer 1964; 17:473–495.
11. McLaughlin RP, Scholz DA, McConahey WM, et al. Metastatic thyroid carcinoma with hyperthyroidism: two cases with functioning metastatic follicular thyroid carcinoma. Mayo Clin Proc 1970; 45:328–335.
12. Meier DA, Hamburger JI. An autonomously functioning thyroid nodule, cancer, and prior radiation. Arch Surg 1971; 103:759–761.
13. Fujimoto YU, Oka A, Nagataki S. Occurrence of papillary carcinoma in hyperfunctioning thyroid nodule; report of a case. Endocrinol Jpn 1972; 19:371–374.
14. Hamburger JI. Solitary autonomously functioning thyroid lesions. Am J Med 1975; 58:740–749.
15. Wolfstein RS. Enigma of the "hyperfunctioning" thyroid carcinoma resolved? J Nucl Med 1978; 19:441–442.
16. Abdel-Razzak M, Christie JH. Thyroid carcinoma in an autonomously functioning nodule. J Nucl Med 1979; 20:1001–1002.
17. Blitzer A, Son ML. Thyroid carcinoma in a patient with a coexisting functional adenoma. Otolaryngol Head Neck Surg 1979; 887:768–774.
18. Khan O, Ell PJ. Maclennan KA, et al. Thyroid carcinoma in a autonomously hyperfunctioning thyroid nodule. Postgrad Med J 1981; 57:172–175.
19. Ghose MK, Genuth SM, Abellera RM, et al. Functioning primary thyroid carcinoma and metastases producing hyperthyroidism. J Clin Endocrinol Metab 1971; 33:639–646.
20. Sandler MP, Fellmeth B, Salhany KE, et al. Thyroid carcinoma masquerading as a solitary benign hyperfunctioning nodule. Clin Nucl Med 1988; 13:410–415.
21. Iwata M, Kasagi K, Hatabu H, et al. Causes of appearance of scintigraphic hot areas on thyroid scintigraphy analyzed with clinical features and comparative ultrasonographic findings. Ann Nuc Med 2002; 164:279–287.
22. Lupi A, Orsolon P, Cerisara D, et al. "Hot" carcinoma of the thyroid. Case reports and comments on the literature." Minerva Endocrinologica 2002; 27:53–57.
23. Livada DP, Kotoulas OB, Bouropoulos V, et al. The coexistence of thyroid malignancy with autonomous hot nodules of the thyroid. Clin Nucl Med 1997; 2:350–351.
24. Kahn O, Ell PJ, Maclennan KA, et al. Thyroid carcinoma in an autonomously hyperfunctioning thyroid nodule. Postgrad Med J 1981; 57:172–175.
25. Sato Y, Sakurai A, Miyamoto T, et al. Hyperfunctioning thyroid adenoma concomitant with papillary thyroid carcinoma, follicular thyroid adenoma and primary hyperparathyroidism. Endocr J 1998; 45:61–67.
26. Rubenfeld S, Wheeler TM. Thyroid cancer presenting as a hot thyroid nodule: report of a case and review of the literature. Thyroidology 1988; 1:63–68.
27. Kusic Z, Becker DV, Saenger EL, et al. Comparison of technetium-99m and iodine-123 imaging of thyroid nodules: correlation with pathologic findings. J Nucl Med 1990; 31:393–399.
28. Ryo UY, Vaidya PV, Schneider AB, et al. Thyroid imaging agents: a comparison of I-123 and Tc-99m pertechnetate. Radiology 1983; 148:819–822.
29. Erjavec M, Movrin T, Auersperg M, Golough R. Comparative accumulation of 99mTc and 131-I in thyroid nodules: case report. J Nucl Med 1977; 18:346–347.
30. Turner JW, Spencer RP. Thyroid carcinoma presenting as a pertechnetate "hot" nodule, but without 131-I uptake: case report. J Nucl Med 1976; 17:22–23.
31. Dos Remedios LV, Weber PM, Jasko IA. Thyroid scintiphotography in 1,000 patients: rational use of 99mTC and 131-I compounds. J Nucl Med 1971; 12:673–677.
32. Wartofsky L. Thyroid nodules. In Van Nostrand D, Bloom G, Wartofsky L, editors. Thyroid Cancer: A Guide for Patients. Baltimore, MD: Keystone Press Inc., 2004, pp. 15–31.

21
Ultrasonic Imaging of the Neck in Patients with Thyroid Cancer

Manfred Blum

This chapter discusses the clinical relevance of ultrasonic imaging of the neck in patients in whom thyroid cancer is suspected or in those with a history of thyroid cancer and ultrasound-guided percutaneous fine-needle aspiration biopsy.

THE CLINICAL BASIS OF DIAGNOSIS

The approach to the diagnosis of thyroid cancer consists of two aspects. Initially, the physician must determine if a thyroid nodule is benign or malignant. Then, after a thyroid cancer has been surgically removed, residual or recurrent cancer must be detected early, accurately, and safely. However, recent societal economic constraints on medicine and the greater acceptability of uncertainty in clinical practice may be perceived to suggest a lower diagnostic standard (1). This perception should not be the case. While uncertainty is and always has been inescapable, it should be minimized with knowledge about the disease process and with the use of clinical skills and judgment. The economy can be enhanced by the optimal use of current technology for imaging thyroid cancer, i.e., ultrasonography.

Although thyroid nodules are common, fewer than 5% are malignant. Considerable time, money, and health care resources are spent to identify this small number of patients with cancer and to spare the approx 4–7% of all people who have benign thyroid nodules from needless operations. From the perspective of economists and those who fund health care, the cost of thyroid cancer management is particularly important because these tumors are uncommon, generally slow-growing, rarely result in death, and are usually cured by the initial surgical procedure. Furthermore, recurrence of this malignancy is also not typical and rarely leads to death. Yet, for the patient and family who are insured members of a managed care system seeking medical attention for this problem, cost containment is not a great concern at the time of illness. The clinician is challenged to meet the expectations of both the patient and payer, as well as to uncover those few who actually have thyroid cancer and the even fewer who need additional treatment after a thyroidectomy. Ultrasonography can aid the physician to rise to the challenge in both situations. The procedure can simplify the diagnosis of thyroid nodules by facilitating aspiration biopsy and in patients who have had thyroid cancer surgery, it can identify persistent or even nonpalpable recurrent disease.

IMAGING PROCEDURES AND THEIR CORRELATION WITH THE CLINICAL SITUATION

The diagnosis of thyroid nodules is beyond the scope of this chapter (see Chapters 17–20), but a brief discussion follows because similar principles apply to both benign and cancerous nodules (2,3).

The medical history and clinical examination alert the clinician to the problem and direct the selection of testing. In the past, it was perceived that a solitary nodule had the highest risk of cancer. Now there appears to be controversy among experts about the cancer risk of a solitary nodule in an otherwise normal-feeling thyroid gland, opposed to a nodule in a goiter. The perception of the controversy clouds the issue and confuses the clinician. Multiple benign thyroid nodules are common, increasingly so with age, particularly in women. Modern technology, especially ultrasonography, has revealed that approx 30–50% of people have small nodules that have been called "incidentalomas" and are not palpable or discoverable by scintiscanning (4). Therefore, many patients with an apparently solitary nodule actually have multiple nodules. The chance that any particular subclinical nodule in a clinical goiter or in a nonpalpable thyroid gland is cancerous is exceedingly small unless clinical characteristics suggest a high cancer risk. The clinical implication is that a palpable nodule or a micronodule in a goiter may not require immediate diagnostic or therapeutic attention because of the benign nature of most goiters and the low virulence of most thyroid tumors. However, the nodule cannot be ignored because it could be malignant.

Historical and physical factors that are associated with an increased risk that a specific nodule is cancerous have been identified but are less reliable than cytological examination of the tissue. There are certain characteristics of nodules that are the most suspicious for thyroid cancer, either

From: *Thyroid Cancer: A Comprehensive Guide to Clinical Management, 2/e*
Edited by: L. Wartofsky and D. Van Nostrand © Humana Press Inc., Totowa, NJ

presurgery or when a new nodule appears after a prior thyroid cancer had been removed. These include a history of therapeutic irradiation to the head or neck, hard consistency, coexistent lymphadenopathy, and evidence of invasion. Another suspicious characteristic is enlargement of a nodule, making it a dominant mass in a goiter. A nodule may be associated with a 10% risk of cancer if it does not accumulate radioiodine as efficiently as the rest of the thyroid gland (i.e., a "cold" nodule), less than 1% risk if it accumulates the isotope more avidly ("hot"), and 30% risk if there is a history of radiation therapy. A nodule is much more likely to be malignant in a male than a female and in a child than an adult. Furthermore, because of the multifocal tendency of thyroid cancer, there is a greater-than-average risk of cancer when a nodule emerges in the contralateral thyroid tissue after surgical lobectomy for cancer. Additionally, the cancer risk is particularly high when a nodule grows during a course of therapy with L-thyroxine that has resulted in suppression of thyrotropin (TSH) and exceedingly high when there is persistent, painless, regional lymphadenopathy after partial or complete thyroidectomy for cancer.

Clinical methods, such as visual inspection and palpation, along with the history, can provide adequate clues about the thyroid region and may be sufficient for diagnosis and a therapeutic decision. It is appropriate to proceed to imaging procedures when these data are not diagnostically adequate. The optimal test must then be chosen to achieve the diagnosis safely, expeditiously, and economically. A working knowledge of the imaging methods and an understanding of the regional anatomy of the thyroid gland are required for the clinician to suggest the examination best designed to resolve the patient's specific condition.

However, risks exist when the neck is imaged to diagnose a thyroid nodule or recurrent cancer. To diminish this danger, a precise question must be relayed to the radiologist for the images to be interpreted in context. Imaging data alone may be misleading unless integrated with the remaining factors of the clinical situation. It is important when interpreting images to be aware of the principles of statistics and the limitations inherent in the method. The beauty and apparent detail of the images of the thyroid gland and its surroundings are simultaneously a promise for enhanced diagnosis and a hazard for misinformation; overinterpretation may lead to the wrong diagnosis. Synthesizing the images with various techniques provides enhanced anatomic information and avoids the errors and controversies that occur all too frequently when the diverse data and images are analyzed independently and without meticulous attention to the clinical problem.

Although the most cost-effective diagnostic tool for a nodule in the thyroid region of the neck is fine-needle aspiration biopsy and cytologic analysis, regional imaging can also provide useful ancillary information that will place the cytology into an accurate perspective. It may also alert the clinician to false-positive or false-negative interpretations. For instance, a scintiscan (see Chapters 14–16) can improve the utility of biopsy by revealing a "hot" nodule, in which case malignancy is unlikely, even if the cytology is classified as atypical, cellular (the cancer cannot be excluded), or nondiagnostic. In addition, after a thyroidectomy for cancer has been performed, radionuclide scanning can facilitate biopsy by identifying tissue that is iodine-avid, thus revealing that a nodule contains thyroid follicular cells. Another example is that ultrasonography may enhance cytology, as it can depict the regional anatomy accurately, safely, and economically. Furthermore, ultrasound can identify the solid component of a complex nodule, provide an anatomic guide for fine-needle aspiration, and document the comparative size of nodules in patients being observed (especially when administered TSH-suppressive therapy). Ultrasound can also detect a small nodule in patients who were exposed to therapeutic irradiation of the head or neck and reveal even nonpalpable recurrent thyroid cancer after surgery. In contrast, the more costly sectional imaging methods, computed tomography (CT) and magnetic resonance imaging (MRI; see Chapter 38) have no impact in the management of a patient with an average thyroid nodule. However, CT and MRI may be important to meet specific clinical goals:

1. To evaluate patients with an invasive nodule.
2. To depict the gross anatomy when there are cryptic symptoms, confusing findings on palpation, conflicting results from other imaging tests, or altered anatomy after other regional operations.
3. To identify metastatic malignancy, especially in regions blind to sonography.

ULTRASONOGRAPHY (SONOGRAPHY)

Ultrasonography has a significant role in the thyroid gland's diagnostic evaluation because of its safety, low cost, clear images displayed in real time, remarkable resolving power, and wide availability (5–8). Sonography has gained the primary imaging method for the thyroid region in patients with thyroid cancer. Figure 1 shows a postoperative thyroid bed that is free of tumor, and Fig. 2 illustrates a local recurrence of cancer after surgery even before the lesion is palpable. Figure 3 shows ultrasound imaging of regional nonpalpable adenopathy.

Principles and Method

Gray-Scale Ultrasonography

Ultrasonography involves the intermittent generation of a pulse of sound energy and the reception of the reflected echoes to produce a tissue image that has been traversed by the sound. Current technology produces high-resolution thyroid images by employing sound frequencies between 5 and

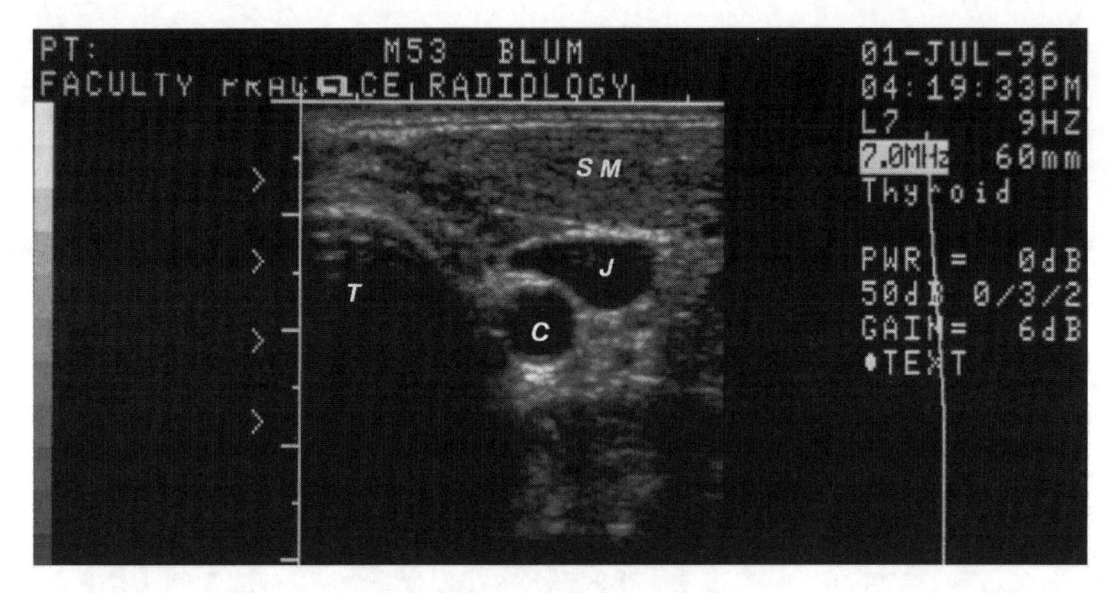

Fig. 1.

15 million MHz. These frequencies are well above the range audible by the human ear. The sound waves penetrate tissues, and a portion of the energy is reflected at tissue interfaces up to a 5-cm depth using typical equipment. The superficial location in the neck of the thyroid gland or regional metastases is well within this limitation. Current clinical equipment provides high resolution of structures as small as 2 mm. By contrast, all of the other imaging methods are considerably less sensitive. Linear array transducers are preferred to sector transducers because they minimize distortion, produce superior images from the superficial portions, and facilitate correlation with images derived by other techniques. Some factors limiting the usefulness of sonography include attenuation of the high-frequency sound waves in deeper tissues (which may be an issue with very large tumors), distortion by air-filled structures (e.g., trachea), blockade of the ultrasound by calcified deposits, and inaccessibility of substernal tumor.

The process of producing an optimal ultrasound image requires an operator who is familiar with the anatomy and the suspected pathology. Ultrasound scanning is a subjective art; skill improves with experience. A diligent search for the solution to the clinical problem is required. If the clinical question is poorly thought-out, ill-conceived, or not transmitted to the sonographer, an efficient answer cannot be expected. Furthermore, the average technician cannot optimally perform the procedure and then submit the films for later interpretation. Rather, the efficacy of the procedure can be helped with a well-trained and experienced sonography technician, active participation by a qualified radiologist or sonologist, and input by the clinician. Many clinicians conduct their own sonograms during the patient's visit. Unfortunately, this may pose a dilemma. The clinician may be tempted to acquire suboptimal equipment for economic reasons. The author would advise that state-of-the-art equipment with Doppler capability and an experienced examiner willing to devote the time required for a thorough evaluation, performed in multiple planes are necessary. Primitive apparatus with transducers below 10 MHz and interpretation by a clinician who lacks specific knowledge and experience cannot be expected to yield optimal diagnostic information.

Images are best obtained with the patient lying supine with the neck maximally extended, consistent with comfort. Patience and attention to positioning, body habitus, and specific factors (e.g., arthritis) are rewarded with improved images. Anatomic landmarks, the thyroid gland, and abnormalities must be carefully palpated, and their locations should be noted. Particularly in patients with thyroid cancer, the entire region must be completely examined in both the transverse and longitudinal planes, beginning in the midline and extending laterally to encompass nodal regions. Scanning must be done from the sternal notch to the chin. The entire length of the carotid sheath must be explored to identify enlarged lymph nodes. The esophagus can be differentiated from adenopathy when the patient sips water and is made possible because images are obtained in real time.

Color Flow Doppler Imaging

Color flow Doppler imaging of the thyroid gland adds dynamic flow information to a static gray-scale image. Color-encoded signals are superimposed on real-time gray-

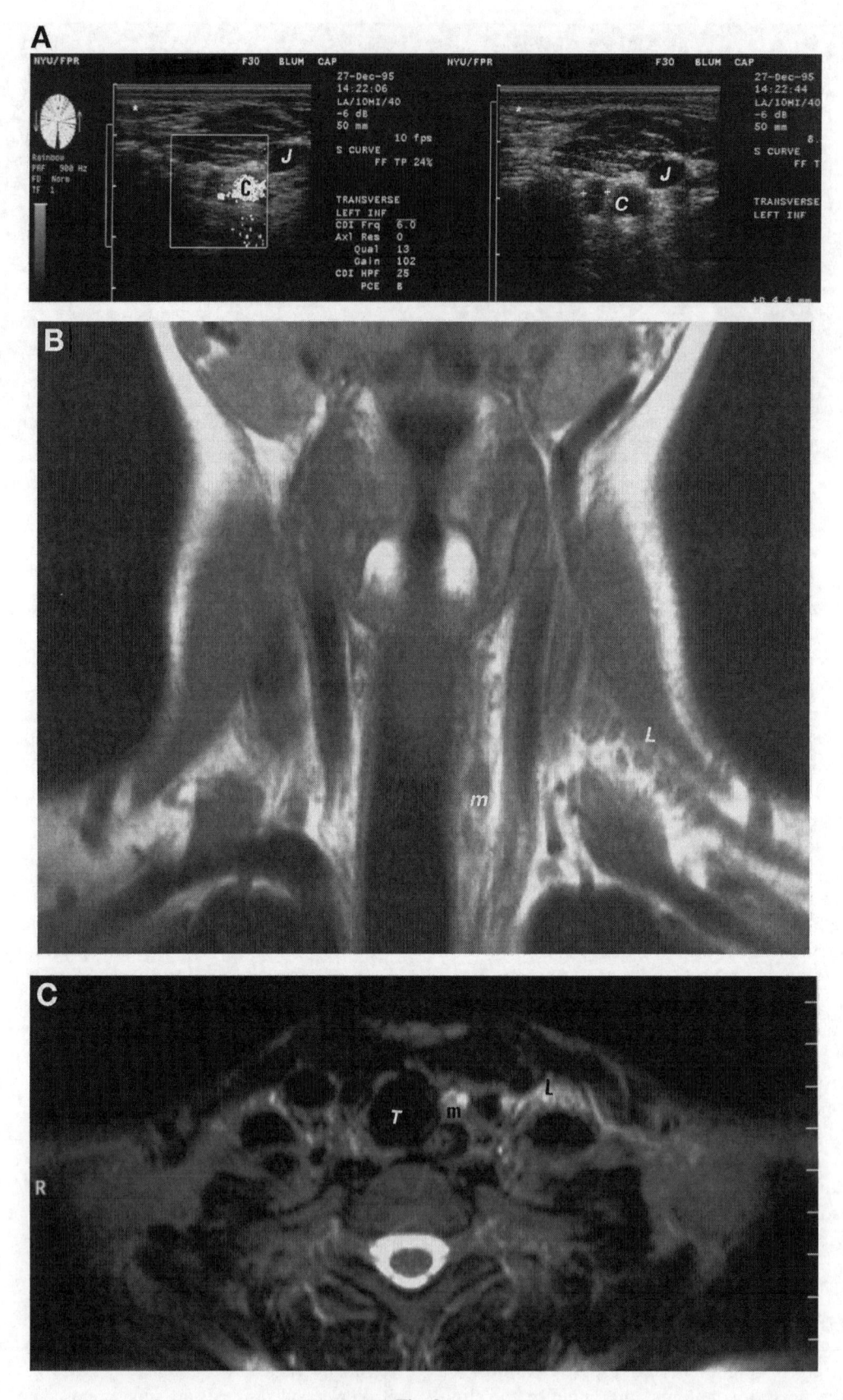

Fig. 2.

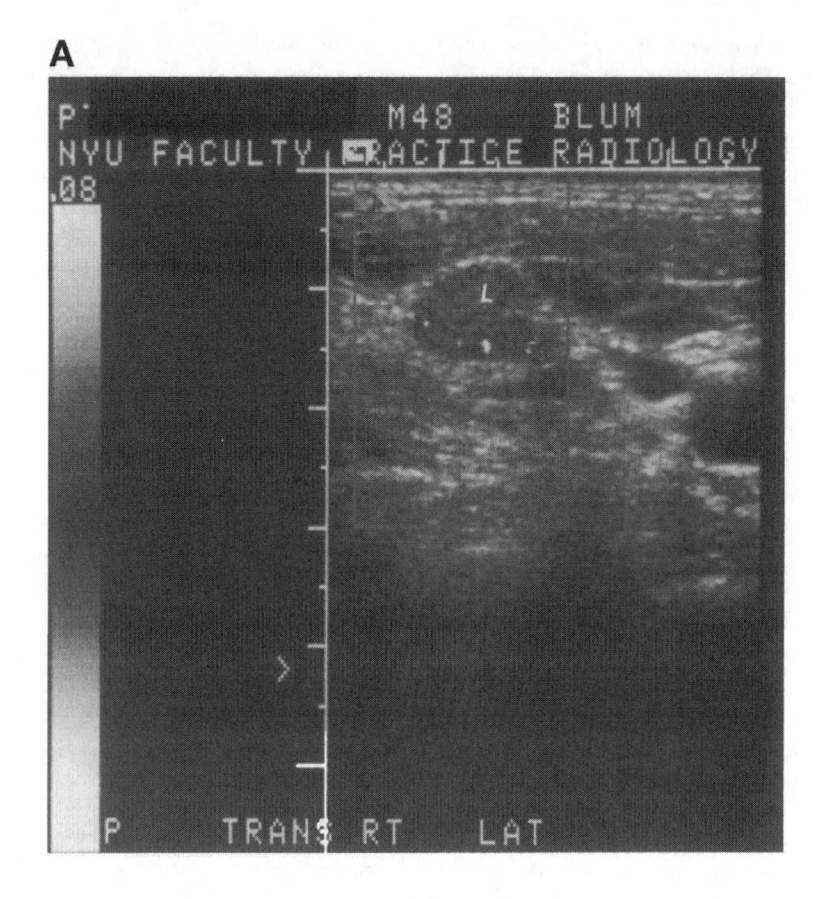

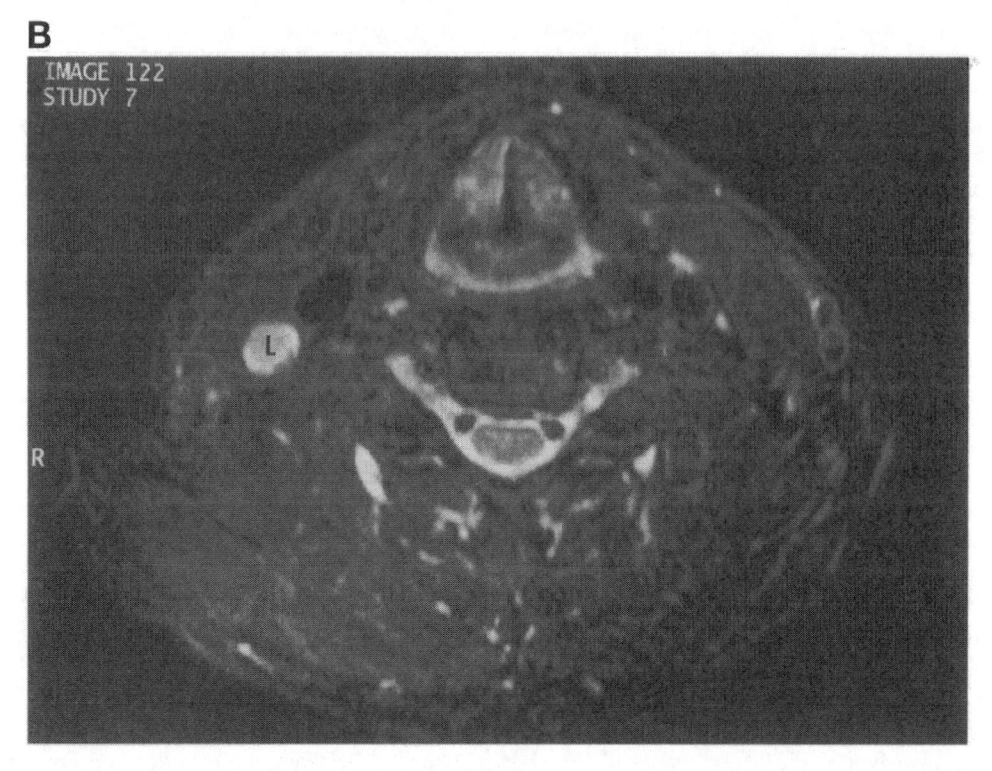

Fig. 3.

scale images to indicate both the direction (phase shift) and velocity (frequency shift) of blood flow. They are also useful in depicting the degree of vascularity *(9,10)*, which may be diagnostically effective in identifying blood vessels in contrast to a cystic space in a nodule and in differentiating a hypoechoic nodule from a blood vessel (Fig. 2).

Correlation of the Ultrasonic Properties of Thyroid Nodules and Goiters With Pathology and Its Applicability in Clinical Management

This discussion is derived from experience with the current commercially available high-resolution ultrasound equipment using a 7.5–14-MHz transducer and a review of the literature. At this time, correlation of sonic images and histopathology is limited but sometimes clinically useful. It seems safe to anticipate that enhanced images and better correlation with pathology will occur with higher-resolution devices, scanners with a mechanized drive, and video-spatial depiction of the signal that is quickly digitalized and reconstructed by the computer to produce three-dimensional images.

Sonography merely depicts the anatomy from the perspective of sound waves that are reflected by tissue interfaces. However, the correlation of the ultrasonic properties of tissues and histopathology is tentative. Benign and malignant lesions are not reliably differentiated. Nevertheless, certain associations with diseases can be made using state-of-the-art equipment. However, these associations are relatively weak statistical probabilities that have been drawn from comparatively small numbers of patients and offer limited insight into a single person's problem.

Even the partial correlations between the ultrasound image and pathology can be clinically helpful. For instance, relatively unique thyroid ultrasound patterns have been recognized in patients with subacute thyroiditis or lymphocytic thyroiditis *(11–17)*. Furthermore, an ultrasonically unique area in a patient with a goiter or thyroiditis can alert the clinician to a coexisting pathological entity, including cancer or lymphoma *(18)*.

However, analysis of the criteria suggestive of identifying thyroid cancer among thyroid nodules have yielded conflicting results *(17,18)*. These criteria are not useful either preoperatively when cancer is suspected or postoperatively in the residual thyroid tissue after cancer has been removed from another part of the gland. The sonographic characteristics of nodules examined for their correlation with malignancy include: echo intensity, nodular shape *(18a)*, boundary sharpness, the presence of a "halo," calcifications, internal structure, and blood flow *(9,19)*.

Although many thyroid cancers are less echogenic than the surrounding normal thyroid tissue (Figs. 2 and 4), many benign nodules are also hypoechoic. Most, but not all, hyperechoic nodules are benign. Regarding boundary sharpness, some grossly invasive nodules may exhibit a poorly defined margin in the invaded area, but many benign nodules may have an indistinct border.

In addition to simple margin, some nodules are partly or completely surrounded by a sonolucent "halo." Some echographers have suggested that a thin "halo" may be more likely associated with benign disease; a thick, partial "halo" may be more often linked with malignant disease. However, some have not been able to confirm either of these conclusions *(20)*. The "halo" can be considered as an interface between two different types of thyroid tissue that represents a capsule in some cases. In others, it signifies compressed or atrophic thyroid tissue and can also represent local inflammation or edema. Color flow Doppler imaging has shown that the "halo" is often vascular and may designate capsular vessels. The nodule's internal structure has not been a useful indicator of malignancy. Cancers may be sonographically solid tissue or complex in nature, experiencing cystic or hemorrhagic degeneration, or both, which is a common occurrence in large nodules. Similarly, cystic degeneration may be seen in cancerous regional lymph nodes. Indeed, it has been reported that cystic degeneration of a pathologic cervical node indicates papillary thyroid cancer because other head and neck cancers do not undergo such deterioration *(21)*. (I would view that assertion with caution because it is based on a small sample, and some chronically infected lymph nodes undergo degeneration, e.g., tuberculous adenopathy.)

Calcifications commonly occur in benign or malignant nodules, as well as lymph nodes, and are usually not predictive of histopathology. However, some information about the pathology can be derived from the nature of a calcification in a thyroid nodule or pathological lymph node. The most diagnostically useful calcification is pinpoint in size. It correlates significantly with psammoma bodies in papillary thyroid carcinoma (Fig. 4) but may be observed in benign disease. In contrast, a peripheral rim or eggshell-like calcification is suggestive of chronicity, which favors the benign nature of a nodule but may occur in cancers. Coarse, scattered calcifications may be seen in benign or malignant nodules that have undergone hemorrhage. Notably, large calcifications can be effective as indicators of medullary thyroid cancer. Clinically, this correlation is useful only in patients who may have medullary carcinoma because they have an increased concentration of calcitonin or in the clinical setting of familial multiple endocrine neoplasia.

Because ultrasonography cannot reliably diagnose or exclude thyroid cancer, it is not cost-effective to routinely perform a sonogram on patients with a thyroid nodule before thyroid surgery. However, preoperative sonography can be useful in selected patients to answer specific questions about a nodule or goiter, or it is efficacious to detect gross evidence of invasion or encasement of regional structures with a large nodule. Ultrasonography after surgery for thyroid cancer will be discussed below.

Ultrasonic Imaging of the Neck

these lesions may indicate occult thyroid cancer, and its incidence in patients varies from a small percentage in the United States to possibly as much as 20% in other areas of the world. Data suggest that these lesions are of no clinical consequence in most patients, and their discovery during echography may cause needless concern and therapy. Yet, some incidentalomas are clinical carcinomas, a few of which metastasize, and rarely may cause death (10). Therefore, finding an incidentaloma cannot be dismissed.

The ultrasonographic characteristics of an incidentaloma may reveal factors about the pathology, as with a palpable nodule. In an investigation of 402 patients with 8–15-mm nonpalpable nodules, the cancers were most likely to be hypoechoic and solid, with microcalcifications, irregular borders, or central blood flow (22). As only 125 (31%) of all nodules met those criteria, the investigators inquired if biopsy could be limited to micronodules with these chacteristics. There were 31 cancers, only 13% of which lacked suspicious sonographic features and would have been missed unless biopsies had been done without regard to the ultrasound appearance of the nodule. Thus, relying on the sonographic characteristics provided a useful but imperfect triage. When there is an incidentaloma and an increased risk of cancer, such as a history of irradiation, the ultrasound-guided aspiration biopsy may be appropriate when it is feasible, as is discussed below.

Papini et al. reported that among 31 cancers in a population of 402 incidentalomas, the cancer prevalence, adenopathy, and extra-capsular growth were similar in nodules 8–10 mm in diameter when compared to those 10–15 mm. Cancer was perhaps slightly more common among "solitary" micronodules (18 of 195, 9.2%) than when there was evidence of a multinodular thyroid (13 of 207, 6.3%; 22).

Routine sonographic cervical screening of those with a low risk of thyroid cancer does not seem to be cost-effective. The detection rate for thyroid cancer was 2.6% of 1401 women who were scheduled to undergo either a breast examination or follow-up examination for breast cancer and who had thyroid ultrasonography (23). Therefore, there is a small benefit and relatively large cost to detect a few low-virulence tumors. Yet, the size of the cancers detected by ultrasound screening was significantly smaller than those that were clinically detected ($p < 0.05$). It is unknown if small tumors will metastasize as often as larger tumors, or if they will invade as often; thus, the value of screening requires additional study.

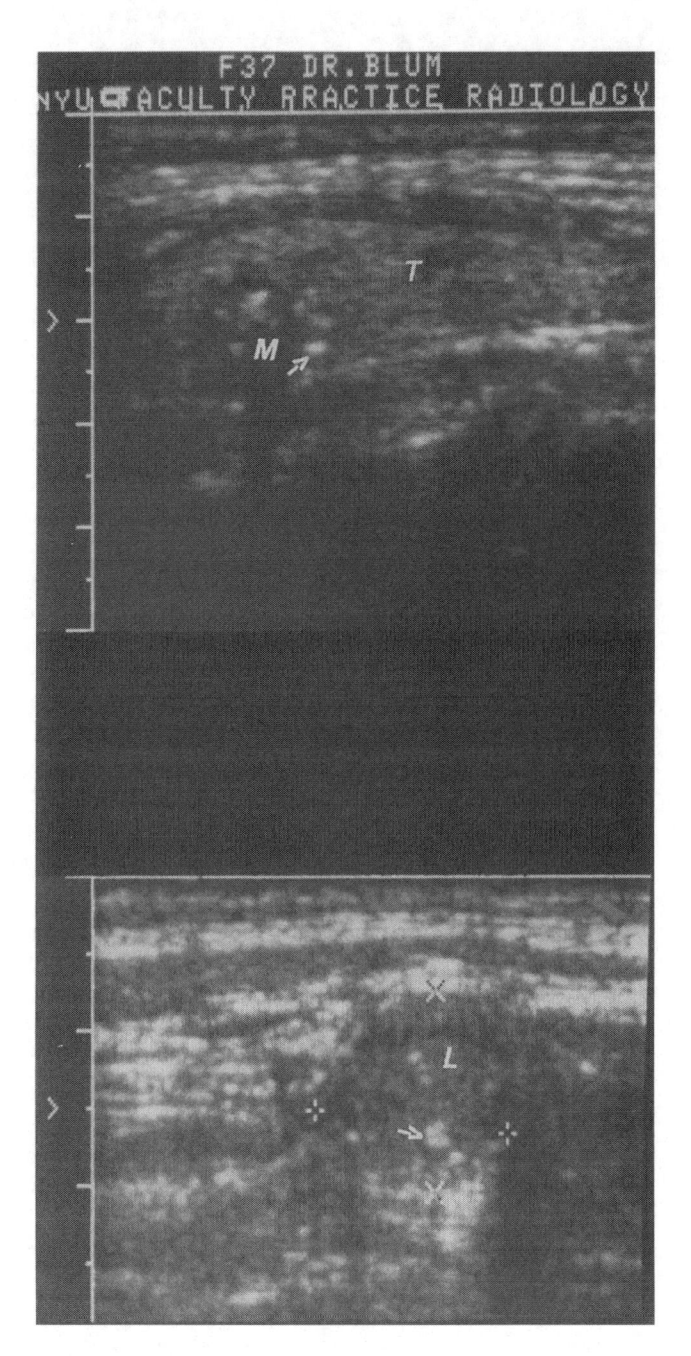

Fig. 4.

Sonography and the Micronodule ("Incidentaloma") (See Chapter 17)

Technological advances enable the recognition of nodules in the millimeter range, which is an enormous advance but is also the source of a dilemma in clinical management (5). Sonography can detect nonpalpable micronodules—"incidentalomas"—that are of indeterminate significance but are usually benign and do not require therapy. Some of

Sonography in Patients With Lymphadenopathy

Ultrasonography may offer diagnostic insights for patients who have palpable or impalpable lymphadenopathy before a thyroidectomy or after surgery for thyroid cancer—the topic discussed in Chapter 37.

Sonography in Patients With Thyroid Cancer

Finding Small Lesions in Thyroid Cancer Patients With High-Resolution Ultrasonography

Sonography has become the most frequently used imaging procedure in the management of thyroid cancer. Its value was recognized even before the advent of current high-resolution equipment *(7)*. More recently, in a study of 100 patients with thyroid carcinoma, Simeone and colleagues *(19)* reported that sonography is actually the preferred method for evaluating postoperative thyroid tissue after partial thyroidectomy. Periodic sonography may discover recurrent carcinoma in the thyroid bed after surgery, the contralateral lobe, or in lymph nodes even before it has grown sufficiently to be palpable (Fig. 2). Sonography is highly efficient in detecting a thyroid mass in patients with cervical adenopathy owing to thyroid cancer, but the primary lesion is not palpable, even if the scintiscan is normal (Fig. 4). Furthermore, sonography can demonstrate much smaller lesions than any other imaging methods. The procedure can be done during replacement or suppressive therapy, avoiding the inconvenience and risks of hypothyroidism necessary for scintillation scanning, at a much lower expense than CT or MRI (see Chapter 38).

Sonography during about a month after surgery for thyroid cancer may give misleading results. During this time, there may be noncancerous, enlarged lymph nodes, and edematous or inflammatory postoperative changes that appear as heterogeneous and usually sonodense focal structures. These findings should not be confused with tumors and can be avoided by delaying the examination for 3 mo or more.

After partial removal of the gland (lobectomy or subtotal thyroidectomy) has revealed cancer, the discovery of a nodule by sonogram in the residual thyroid tissue, even if there is no palpable nodule, may be considered a strong indication when deciding whether a completion thyroidectomy is necessary. The role of ultrasound-guided fine-needle aspiration biopsy in this circumstance is controversial. Cytological identification of malignant cells would suggest additional surgery, but sampling errors and limitations inherent in cytological examination of thyroid nodules require caution in interpreting the significance of a "negative" aspiration.

Ultrasound-Assisted Fine-Needle Aspiration Biopsy

Many clinically detected and palpable thyroid nodules may be punctured directly; ultrasound guidance is not needed and makes the procedure more complicated, adding to the expense. Direct ultrasound guidance for percutaneous biopsy is generally reserved for certain conditions *(24–29)*:

1. Unusually deep nodules, particularly in the obese, muscular, or large-framed patient.
2. Very small nodules.
3. Nonpalpable nodules.
4. Ultrasonically detected incidentalomas that are associated with cancer risk factors.
5. Some complex degenerated nodules.
6. Nonpalpable adenopathy.

Ultrasound-guided biopsy is very useful when prior aspirations have been nondiagnostic.

The most simple and frequently used method for ultrasound-assisted aspiration biopsy for palpable nodules is to locate the lesion on the film or screen, taking note of the nodule's solid and cystic components relative to palpable or visual land marks. The operator then estimates the proper location on the skin to puncture the nodule to sample solid tissue. For small nodules, where this approach is not possible or has not been successful, real-time ultrasound may be employed to observe the insertion of a needle, free hand or using a special needle guide attached to the transducer. The free-hand technique offers greater flexibility. The transducer is placed at some distance from the point of needle insertion. In our practice, the nodule is identified ultrasonically, and the skin above it is indented using a blunt millimeter-diameter wooden dowel as the insertion marker. After the skin has been cleansed and punctured, the needle path is observed on the screen in more than one plane, while the operator maneuvers the needle to pierce the target. Transducers that are fitted with a needle guide are preferred by some physicians but require considerable practice and need special attention for sterile technique. Some ultrasound units have computer-generated grids, which map the path of the needle and estimate the distance to the target. Ultrasound biopsy probes for intraoperative use are available, although not widely employed now, but may have wider use in the future.

Cytology on minute nodules can be obtained (with good fortune). However, there are unresolved questions about puncturing micronodules. How often is the procedure accurate with nonpalpable nodules smaller than 1 cm in size? How certain can one be that the end of the needle is within the nodule at the time of sampling? What is the clinical impact of the information? These questions cannot be currently answered critically. However, it would appear that the success rate, accuracy, and reliability are significantly higher when experienced investigators and seasoned operators do ultrasound-guided biopsy, rather than sonographers and clinicians who only occasionally conduct the procedure. The central point is that the presence of a malignancy is persuasive, but the absence of cytological evidence of malignancy should be interpreted with caution.

The clinical diagnostic role of ultrasound-guided aspiration of incidentalomas is under investigation. The success rate appears to be limited for subcentimeter nodules. Boland and coworkers *(29)* showed 91% sensitivity (102 of 112 masses). The failure rate was 10% among 29 nodules less than 1 cm

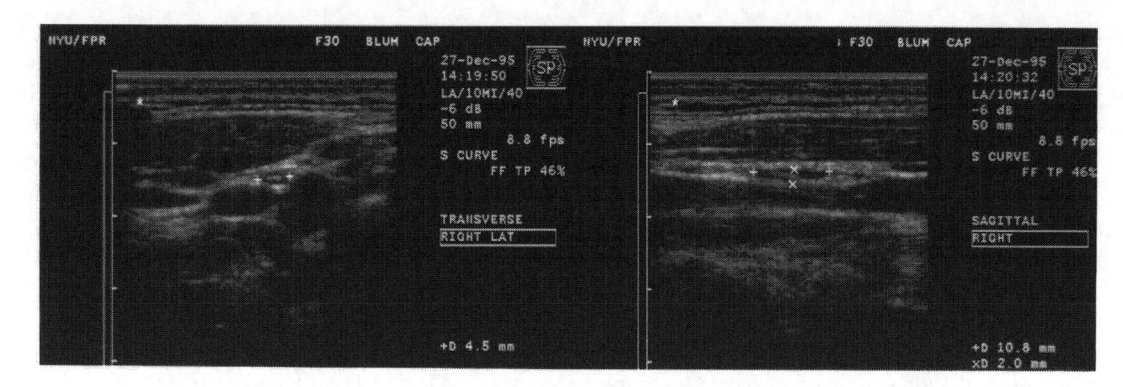

Fig. 5.

in diameter and 5% among 83 larger lesions. There were seven nondiagnostic punctures: four in complex nodules and three in nodules that were 0.8–0.9 cm in diameter. It is noteworthy that the failures with large nodules occurred when there was evidence of cystic or hemorrhagic degeneration. Most importantly, sonography was useful to aspirate the 71 nodules that had been imaged but not clearly palpated and was effective when prior nonguided biopsy attempts were unsuccessful, as was the case in 16 nodules in this series. Another study reported success in detecting small thyroid cancers in endemic goiters when thyroid nodules were selected for aspiration biopsy based on their ultrasound characteristics, rather than palpability (30). The investigators selected for ultrasound-guided aspiration those nodules with a hypoechoic pattern, a blurred perinodular halo microcalcifications, or an enhanced intranodular color Doppler signal. Of the 27 histologically malignant nodules identified in this way, 12 (45%) were not palpable, and 52% were found only with the aid of ultrasound guidance.

When interpreting the results of thyroid biopsies of micronodules and any nodule within a goiter, it is critical to be aware that multiple punctures improve the diagnostic yield (however, that increases the risk of a "bloody" specimen that is difficult to diagnose), and one should not be convinced that a nodule has been sampled adequately unless malignancy is detected. Furthermore, even when the cytology does not reveal malignancy, growth of a nodule, particularly during the course of suppressive therapy, should be viewed with suspicion.

Therapy of Inoperable Thyroid Cancer Using Ultrasound-Assisted Percutaneous Puncture

Thyroid nodules can be treated by percutaneous ultrasound-guided injection of ethanol or sclerosing agents. The size and function of autonomous nodules (31–34) have been successfully reduced in this manner (35). Ethanol injection has also been reported to reduce the size of metastases from thyroid carcinomas not amenable to surgery (36), which could be beneficial in the management of patients with bulky cancers that do not concentrate sufficient ^{131}I for therapeutic efficacy. Percutaneous biopsy of pathological lymph nodes is discussed in Chapter 37.

Applications of Color Doppler Imaging

To date, the clinical usefulness of color Doppler is best exemplified by the detection of diffuse hyperemia in the thyroid gland of patients with Graves' disease (37). However, an increased vascularity on color Doppler has been reported in some focal lesions, especially autonomous "hot" nodules where the risk of cancer is small (38). The value of color Doppler thyroid imaging in the diagnosis of cancer is currently being investigated (38a). One area of study is the diagnostic significance of a sonographic halo around a nodule, as discussed above. Criteria for altered vascularity in the halo, the implications of the halo interruption, and correlation with pathological findings have not been well defined. Investigation with color flow Doppler in cervical lymph nodes has shown vascular patterns that are significantly different in benign and malignant lymphadenopathy, with a reported 93% sensitivity, an 86% specificity, and an 89% accuracy (39).

Intraoperative Thyroid Ultrasonography After Thyroidectomy

Surgical resection of recurrent thyroid cancer after thyroidectomy is a therapeutic option when well-differentiated thyroid cancer does not trap radioiodine. However, it may be difficult for the surgeon to locate the lesions even if they were readily identified by preoperative ultrasonography. In one study of such patients, intraoperative ultrasonography facilitated the localization of nonpalpable recurrent thyroid cancer, particularly in patients who had previous external-beam radiotherapy (40). Most importantly, intraoperative sonography reportedly identified small tumor nodules that were invasive or adherent to the airway. The authors of this investigation contend that intraoperative ultrasonography may allow a "complete resection." They reported that in 10 of 11 patients who had detectable serum thyroglobulin preoperatively, the level declined, and became undetectable in 7 after the nonpalpable nodules had been removed with ultrasound guidance.

Ultrasonography may be helpful to investigate the outcome of surgical and isotopic treatments of patients with thyroid carcinoma (41,42).

Enhanced Ultrasound Imaging

Exciting advances in technology augur for a greater role of ultrasonography in the diagnosis and management of patients with thyroid cancer. Image quality has improved considerably, and the instruments have become simultaneously more simple, sophisticated, and affordable. Enhanced sensitivity of Doppler technology may provide greater understanding of tumor vasculature and blood circulation as an index of pathology. Greater objectivity may be gained from higher resolution scanners with a mechanized drive and videospatial depiction of the signal that is quickly digitalized and reconstructed by computer to produce three-dimensional images. Sonographic contrast agents currently in experimental stages suggest the potential for insights and more specific characterization of tumors and lymph nodes. Correlation of images with histopathology may improve but appears to have inherent limitations. Rather ultrasound-guided percutaneous aspiration of specimens for biochemical, serologic, or genetic analysis seems to have more diagnostic potential. Intraoperative ultrasound may improve surgical management of small deposits of cancer and lymphadenopathy. However, fiscal constraints may deter the clinician from acquiring state-of-the-art equipment in favor of more primitive instruments within their means. As a result, full advantage of the progress in the field may not be achieved quickly, except in specialized centers.

Epidemiologic Use of Ultrasonography

Systematic screening with ultrasound has been reported as useful for early detection of thyroid carcinoma in populations who were exposed to radiation (42a) such as those in Belarus after the Chernobyl accident (43). It is presumed, albeit speculative, that the discovery and treatment of these cancers before they became palpable or otherwise clinically manifest will be beneficial to the patients and translate into fewer metastases or surgical cure.

SECTIONAL IMAGING AND SCINTISCANNING RELATIVE TO ULTRASONOGRAPHY

The sectional imaging techniques, CT and MRI, are discussed in Chapter 38, and scintiscanning is discussed in Chapters 14–16.

Because they are pertinent to ultrasonography, a personal perspective is given about the clinical role and utility of these techniques. The efficacy of CT and MRI reflects their ability to accurately define the regional anatomy of the neck and superior mediastinum (18,44–46). However, ultrasonography can detect even smaller lesions and is a less costly test. Therefore, other imaging modalities have been relegated to a secondary role. Furthermore, sectional imaging may have a negative impact on the management of patients with thyroid cancer.

Usefulness of Sectional Imaging in Clinical Management

Sectional imaging techniques should not be used to search for thyroid pathology or to evaluate the usual thyroid nodule or goiter because they are too expensive and insufficiently specific to be useful in the initial diagnosis (18). Sectional methods become necessary only when the results of other methods are inadequate. Nevertheless, thyroid lesions may be noted incidentally on CT or MRI examinations of the cervical spine or other regional structures, leading to further investigation.

Because MRI does not require ionizing radiation or iodinated contrast agents to produce its images, it is often assumed that MRI is "better" than CT scans in patients with thyroid cancer. However, CT scans provide greater spatial resolution than MRI. In contrast, MRI offers several advantages in the assessment of suspected thyroid pathology. Direct sagittal, coronal, and axial images may be obtained with the patient supine. This multiplanar capability facilitates neoplasm localization (47; Figs. 2 and 3). MRI is superior to CT in the differentiation of postoperative scar from recurrent tumor (48). MRIs are not degraded by the "shoulder artifact" commonly found on CT (49). In contrast, CT offers its own advantages in the assessment of thyroid disease. CT is more sensitive than MRI in detecting small metastases (≤1.5-cm diameter) to cervical or mediastinal lymph nodes (50). CT is currently more reliable than MRI in the detection of small nodules, especially pulmonary (51,52). The total examination time for CT is shorter than MRI—an important consideration in unstable or claustrophobic patients. Patients with cardiac pacemakers or other biomechanical devices can be assessed with CT, not MRI (53). Access to CT examinations is greater than to MRIs because there are more scanners available. Importantly, the cost of a CT examination is considerably lower than MRI. Mainly because of the consequences of iodine containing contrast dye, many thyroidologists consider CT a complementary examination to MRI. CT without iodine-containing intravenous contrast is sometimes adequate, e.g., for the lungs, but it is insufficient for the thyroid gland or cervical lymph adenopathy.

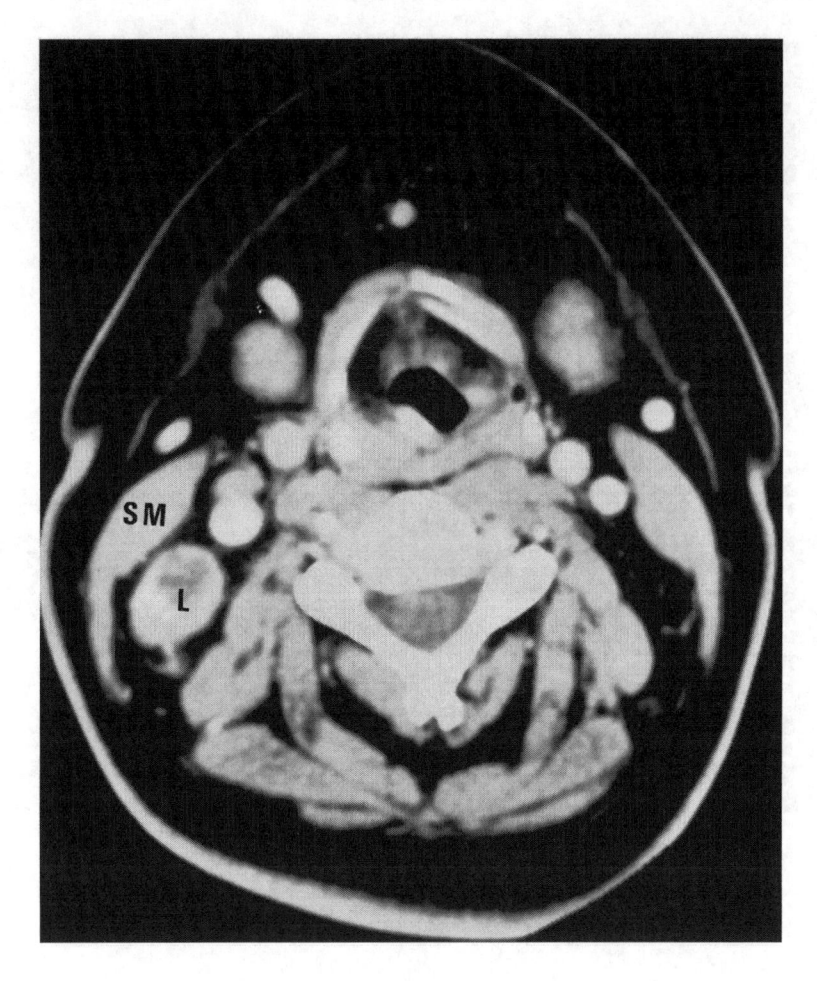

Fig. 6.

Isotope studies, when necessary, should be done before contrast-enhanced CT to avoid contamination with iodine (Fig. 6). This issue is especially important in patients with thyroid cancer who may need an ^{131}I whole-body scan or therapy with ^{131}I. Iodide from the contrast agent blocks the radioiodine uptake by normal thyroid tissue or cancer, even if TSH is high, thereby delaying or precluding testing and therapy. In patients taking suppressive therapy with a thyroid hormone, and in whom a contrast CT is required, it is best to continue the medication for several days after the CT until iodide from the dye is excreted to minimize the effects of excessive iodine on any thyroid tissue. Alteration of thyroid function by iodide is also a serious issue. If the patient has not had a thyroidectomy, the excessive iodide may cause either hyperthyroidism or hypothyroidism, depending on the underlying thyroid condition. It is imperative for the radiologist and clinician to discuss these aspects prior to the performance of a contrast CT and to consider a noncontrast study, which, although not optimal, may be adequate to address the clinical problem. Iodinated dye is not used for MRI examinations—a distinct advantage.

A preoperative sectional imaging examination is useful for a thyroid nodule for specific situations. When the clinical examination demonstrates a mass that is fixed to surrounding tissue or when extra-thyroid masses are palpated, the study may provide a guide for surgery or may demonstrate that total excision is precluded. This allows an appropriate plan for a palliative procedure or the need for a specialized surgeon. MRI or CT is useful when there is an unusually large mass that obstructs the thoracic inlet and impinges on other structures or extends substernally. Important information may be obtained about tracheal compression or invasion *(53a)*, even when conventional radiographs fail to demonstrate such evidence (Fig. 7). Evaluating substernal or retrotracheal extension may lead to involving a chest surgeon, but a cervical approach is adequate in most cases. In one report, the results of CT caused the surgeon to alter the surgical plan in 5 of 19 patients who had intrathoracic extension of a thyroid

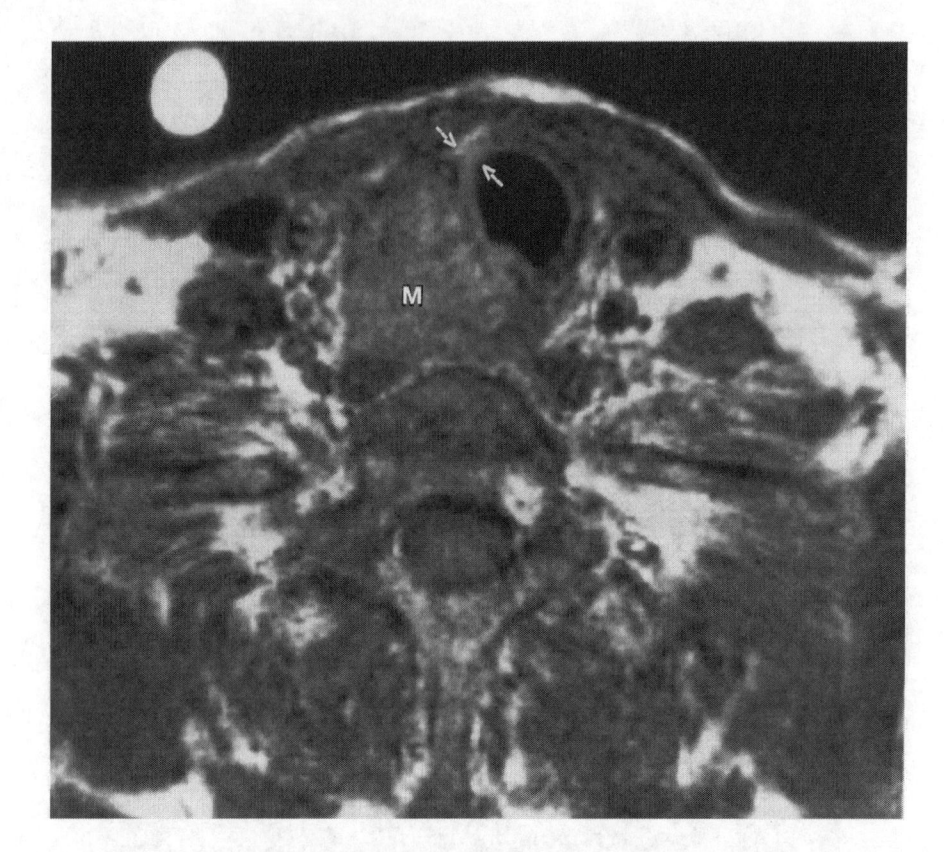

Fig. 7.

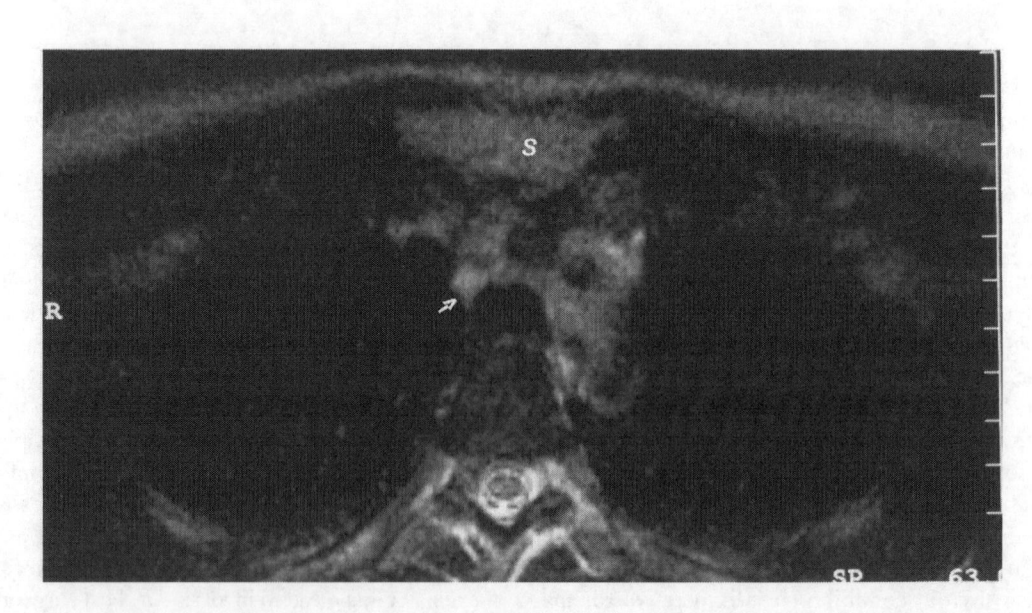

Fig. 8.

Table 1
Role of Nonisotopic Imaging in Clinical Management when Thyroid Cancer is Suspected but Undiagnosed

Clinical Circumstance	Role of Sonogram	Role of MRI	Role of CT
Is "solitary" thyroid nodule malignant?	Minimal, if any and may show lymphadenopathy	None	None
Dominant nodule in a diffuse or nodular goiter or goiters of Hashimoto's or Graves' disease	May disclose region with unique-appearing ultrasound texture that is suspicious, may have "halo" around nodule and may demonstrate psammoma bodies	None	None
History of exposure to radiation therapy during youth but no palpable nodule	May show one or more nodules (some say a source of confusion, others say useful)	None	None
History of surgery for benign disease (adenoma) that may have malignant potential	May show new nodule in contralateral lobe and may show lymphadenopathy	None	None
Worrisome chemical marker: elevated thyroglobulin or calcitonin	May show nodule that has not been palpated and may show lymphadenopathy	None	None

tumor and in 3 of 19 with laryngeal or esophageal invasion *(54)*. Sectional imaging is valuable to detect recurrent thyroid cancer located in the mediastinum, but sonography is useless in this region (Fig. 8).

Sectional imaging procedures have been particularly effective in the assessment and management of patients after thyroid cancer surgery. The MRI characteristics of recurrent thyroid carcinoma may allow discrimination of thyroid tumor, scarring in the thyroid bed, or postsurgical inflammation *(55)*. In one study, CT correlated with tumor invasion of the carotid artery (7 of 7) internal jugular vein (9 of 10), larynx (5 of 6), trachea (8 of 10), esophagus (4 of 5), mediastinum (5 of 5), and regional lymph nodes (14 of 16; *56*). Tumor, scar, tissue deformity, displaced normal structures, and cryptic findings may be elucidated.

The major uses of sectional imaging in thyroid cancer patients are to detect the following:

1. Recurrent thyroid cancer.
2. Cervical or mediastinal lymphadenopathy.
3. Regional metastases.
4. New masses that have been palpated.
5. Evaluating cryptic findings on palpation, sonography, or scintiscan.

PERFORMING NONISOTOPIC IMAGING STUDIES: A PERSONAL PERSPECTIVE

How often and under what circumstances is it necessary to perform nonisotopic imaging studies when there is a history of thyroid cancer? Should any tests be used routinely? Is it enough to examine the patients clinically? How do these examinations relate to isotope scanning and other studies, such as thyroglobulin assays? The answers to these questions are a matter of judgment, as certain issues have not been, and may never be, evaluated critically. Some current insights are tentative and intuitive, but they will evolve with experience, the outcome of investigation, and technologic advances.

For most patients whose tumor is not progressing rapidly, clinical evaluation with patient history, palpation, and assaying thyroglobulin (especially after an injection of Thyrogen® may be done at annual intervals or when there are new complaints or findings. This frequency of testing is probably adequate to detect cancer recurrence in a timely manner. It is unknown if there is an additional benefit from performing nonisotopic imaging studies to detect subclinical lesions. After partial or complete thyroidectomy for cancer, sonography is the most cost-effective, sensitive, and accurate method available for identifying persistent or recurrent cancer. Therefore, sonographic annual examination of the neck is appropriate for the first decade when most recurrences occur. Thereafter, it seems prudent to repeat a sonogram every 5–10 yr for life, as late recurrence (or undetected persistence) of thyroid cancer has been reported many years after an apparent cure. The patient should be carefully assessed if it becomes necessary to unclamp TSH by reducing suppressive therapy because of concern regarding risk of osteoporosis or cardiac disease *(57)*.

CT or MRI should be selectively employed to augment sonography to elucidate distorted anatomy, resolve conflicting medical opinions, or expose the origin of tumor markers, such as the elevation of calcitonin or thyroglobulin when sonography does not reveal the responsible site. PET scanning has become very important, as discussed in Chapter 34.

It is usually not necessary to further localize anatomically a lesion that takes up ^{131}I. Indeed, sometimes lesions that accumulate radioactive iodine are too small to be detected

Table 2
Role of Nonisotopic Imaging in Detecting Persistent or Recurrent Thyroid Cancer Shortly After the Initial Surgery for Cancer

Clinical Circumstance	Role of Sonogram	Role of MRI*	Role of CT*
After lobectomy or nodule removal	May show nodule in contralateral lobe that has not been palpated and may show lymphadenopathy	None	None
After near-total thyroidectomy	May show unsuspected residual tissue and may show lymphadenopathy	None	None
After complete thyroidectomy	May show unsuspected residual tissue and may show lymphadenopathy	None	None
After removal of thyroid cancer in a lymph node or discovery of distant thyroid metastasis	May disclose primary thyroid lesion	Rarely adds information to sonogram	Rarely adds information to sonogram
After surgery for inoperable cancer	Documents baseline anatomy objectively	If sonogram is cryptic documents baseline anatomy objectively	If sonogram is cryptic and MRI is not available or cannot be used (pacemaker) documents baseline anatomy objectively

Editors' Note: The opinions in this chapter may be at variance with those expressed in Chapter 38.

Table 3
Role of Nonisotopic Imaging in the Follow-Up Evaluation of Patients with a History of Thyroid Cancer and No Known Residual Tumor

Clinical Circumstance	Role of Sonogram	Role of MRI*	Role of CT*
After less than total thyroidectomy	Annual to detect early a new nodule in the contralateral lobe or lymphadenopathy	None	None
After total thyroidectomy	Annual to detect recurrence or lymphadenopathy	None	None

Editors' Note: The opinions in this chapter may be at variance with those expressed in Chapter 38.

by nonisotopic imaging, including ultrasonography. However, it may be useful to assess the actual volume of a mass in the neck or its extent of regional structures. For these purposes, sonography is usually sufficient, but sectional imaging, avoiding iodinated contrast medium, may be required.

Imaging in selected circumstances is outlined in Tables 1–4.

SUMMARY

Imaging the neck has an important role in the management of patients with thyroid cancer. The imaging tests are expensive and for cost efficiency, they must be selectively employed to answer specific questions posed by the clinical problem. Sonography has become the most frequently used

Table 4
Role of Nonisotopic Imaging in the Follow-Up Evaluation of the Patient with Known Residual Thyroid Cancer

Clinical Circumstance	Role of Sonogram	Role of MRI*	Role of CT*
Thyroid is intact (no thyroidectomy, thyroid primary not found) after removal of adenopathy or discovery of distant thyroid metastasis	May disclose primary thyroid lesion that was not previously seen; may show lymphadenopathy	None	None
Residual tumor after partial or complete thyroidectomy	Shows change from baseline anatomy objectively	Usually not needed; if sonogram is cryptic shows change from baseline anatomy objectively	Usually not needed; if sonogram is cryptic and MRI is not available or can't be used (pacemaker) shows change from baseline anatomy objectively
Evaluating new masses that have been palpated	Documents change from baseline anatomy objectively	Usually not needed; if is cryptic documents change from baseline anatomy objectively	Usually not needed; if sonogram is cryptic, and MRI is not available or cannot be used (pacemaker) documents change from baseline anatomy objectively
Evaluating local recurrence or metastases that were discovered by whole body ^{131}I scan	Usually not needed	Usually not needed	Usually not needed
Evaluating disease that was discovered by elevated thyroglobulin or calcitonin	May disclose primary thyroid lesion that was not previously seen, may show lymphadenopathy	Usually not needed; if sonogram is cryptic may disclose lesion	Usually not needed; if sonogram is cryptic, and MRI is not available or cannot be used (pacemaker) may disclose lesion
Search for nonpalpated regional metastases	May disclose primary thyroid lesion that was not previously seen, may show lymphadenopathy	None	None
Evaluating substernal extension or obstruction of the thoracic inlet	Not useful	Usually not needed; if sonogram is cryptic, may disclose lesion	Usually not needed; if sonogram is cryptic, and MRI is not available or cannot be used (pacemaker) may disclose lesion
Evaluating findings on palpation or imaging studies that are cryptic	Sometimes useful	Usually not needed; if sonogram is cryptic, may disclose lesion	Usually not needed; if sonogram is cryptic, and MRI is not available or cannot be used (pacemaker) may disclose lesion

MRI, magnetic resonance imaging: CT, computed tomography
Editors' Note: The opinions in this chapter may be at variance with those expressed in Chapter 38.

imaging procedure in the thyroid cancer patient to depict the regional anatomy accurately, safely, and economically. The major use is to reveal nonpalpable recurrent thyroid cancer, including adenopathy, after surgery. Ultrasound also provides an anatomic guide for fine-needle aspiration biopsy, and it documents the comparative size of nodules and lymph nodes during a particular time period. In addition, ultrasonography can guide the instillation of sclerosing medication into nodules or isolated metastatic cancers and can intraoperatively identify small nonpalpable cancerous nodules for excision. MRI or CT becomes necessary only when palpation and ultrasonography are inadequate. They can identify metastatic malignancy in regions that are blind to sonography and further define the anatomy when there are cryptic symptoms, confusing findings, conflicting results, or altered anatomy after regional operations. MRI offers the advantage that does not require iodinated contrast agents.

REFERENCES

1. Logan RL, Scott PJ. Uncertainty in clinical practice: implications for quality and costs of health care. Lancet 1996; 347:595–598.
2. Van Herle AJ, Rich P, Ljung BME, et al. The thyroid nodule. Ann Intern Med 1982; 96:221–232.
3. Molitch ME, Beck JR, Dreisman M, et al. The cold thyroid nodule: an analysis of the diagnostic and therapeutic options. Endocr Rev 1984; 5:185–199.
4. Brander A, Viikinkoski P, Nickels J, Kivisaari L. Thyroid ultrasound screening in a random adult population. Radiology 1991; 181:683–687.
5. Blum M, Goldman AB, Herskovic A, Hernberg J. Clinical applications of thyroid echography. N Engl J Med 1972; 287:1164–1169.
6. Leopold GR. Ultrasonography of superficially located structures. Radiol Clin North Am 1980; 18:161–173.
7. Butch RJ, Simeone JF, Mueller PR. Thyroid and parathyroid ultrasonography. Radiol Clin North Am 1985; 23:57–71.
8. Blum M. Ultrasonography and computed tomography of the thyroid gland. In Ingbar SH, Braverman LE, editors. Werner's the Thyroid, 5th ed. New York: Lippincott, 1986:576–591.
9. James EM, Charboneau JW, Hay ID. The thyroid. In Rumack CM, Wilson SR, Charboneau JW, editors. Diagnostic Ultrasound, vol. 1. St. Louis, MO: Mosby Year Book, 1991:507–523.
10. Foley WD. Physical principles and instrumentation. In Foley WD, editor. Color Doppler Flow Imaging, Boston, MA: Andover Medical Publishers, Inc., 1991:3–13.
11. Boehm TM, Rothouse L, Wartofsky L. Metastatic occult follicular thyroid carcinoma with a solitary slowly growing metastasis. JAMA 1976; 235:2420–2421.
12. Blum M, Passalaque AM, Sackler J, Pudiowski R. Thyroid echography of subacute thyroiditis. Radiology 1977; 124:795–799.
13. Espinassse P. L'echographie thyroidienne dans les thyroidites lymphocytaires chroniques autoimmunes. J Radiol 1983; 64:537–544.
14. Hayashi N, Tamaki N, Konishi J, et al. Sonography of Hashimoto's thyroiditis. J Clin Ultrasound 1986; 14:123–126.
15. Jayaran G, Marwaha RK, Gupta RK, Sharma SK. Cytomorphologic aspects of thyroiditis: a study of 51 cases with functional, immunologic and ultrasonographic data. Acta Cytol 1987; 31:687–693.
16. Gutenkust R, Hafermann W, Mansky T, Scriba PC. Ultrasonography related to clinical and laboratory findings in lymphocytic thyroiditis. Acta Endocrinol 1989; 121:129–135.
17. Marcocci C, Vitti P, Cetani F, et al. Thyroid ultrasonography helps to identify patients with diffuse lymphocytic thyroiditis who are prone to develop hypothyroidism. J Clin Endocrinol Metabol 1991; 72: 209–213.
18. Blum M. Evaluation of thyroid function: sonography, computed tomography and magnetic resonance imaging. In Becker KL, editor. Principles and Practice of Endocrinology and Metabolism. Philadelphia, PA: Lippincott, 1990: 289–293.
18a. Alexander EK, Marqusee E, Orcutt J, et al. Thyroid nodule shape and prediction of malignancy. Thyroid 2004; 14:953–958.
19. Simeone JF, Daniels GH, Hall DA, et al. Sonography in the follow-up of 100 patients with thyroid carcinoma. AJR Am J Roentgenol 1987; 148:45–49.
20. Propper RA, Skolnick ML, Weinstein BJ, Decker A. The nonspecificity of the "halo" sign. J Clin Ultrasound 1980; 8:129–132.
21. Kessler A, Rappaport Y, Blank A, et al. Cystic appearance of cervical lymph nodes is characteristic of metastatic papillary thyroid carcinoma. J Clin Ultrasound 2003; 31:21–25.
22. Papini E, Guglielmi R, Bianchini A, et al. Risk of malignancy in nonpalpable thyroid nodules: predictive value of ultrasound and color-Doppler features. J Clin Endocrinol Metab 2002; 87:1941–1946.
23. Chung WY, Chang HS, Kim EK, Park CS. Ultrasonographic mass screening for thyroid carcinoma: a study in women scheduled to undergo a breast examination. Surg Today 2001; 31:763–767.
24. Sutton RT, Reading CC, Charboneau JW, et al. US-guided biopsy of neck masses in preoperative management of patients with thyroid cancer. Radiology 1988; 168:769–772.
25. Vassallo P, Wernecke K, Roos N, Peters PE. Differentiation of benign from malignant superficial lymphadenopathy: the role of high-resolution US. Radiology 1992; 183:215–220.
26. Solbiati L, Osti V, Cova L, Tonolini M. Ultrasound of thyroid, parathyroid glands and neck lymph nodes. Europ Radiol 2001; 11:2411–2424.
27. Rizzatto G, Solbiati L, Croce F, Derci LE. Aspiration biopsy of superficial lesions: ultrasonic guidance with a linear-array probe. AJR Am J Roentgenol 1987; 148:623–625.
28. Matalón TAS, Silver B. US guidance of interventional procedures. Radiology 1990; 174:43–47.
29. Boland GW, Lee MJ, Mueller PR, et al. Efficacy of sonographically guided biopsy of thyroid masses and cervical lymph nodes. AJR Am J Roentgenol 1993; 161L:1053–1056.
30. Deandrea M, Mormile A, Veglio M, et al. Fine-needle aspiration biopsy of the thyroid: comparison between thyroid palpation and ultrasonography. Endocr Pract 2002; 8:282–286.
31. Ozdemir H, Ilgit ET, Yucel C, et al. Treatment of autonomous thyroid nodules: safety and efficacy of sonographically guided percutaneous injection of ethanol. AJR Am J Roentgenol 1994; 163:929–932.
32. Brkljacic B, Sucic M, Bozikov V, et al. Treatment of autonomous and toxic thyroid adenomas by percutaneous ultrasound-guided ethanol injection. Acta Radiol 2001; 42:477–481.
33. Janowitz P, Ackmann S. Long-term results of ultrasound-guided ethanol injections in patients with autonomous thyroid nodules and hyperthyroidism. Medizinische Klinik 2001; 96:451–456.
34. Del Prete S, Russo D, Caraglia M, et al. Percutaneous ethanol injection of autonomous thyroid nodules with a volume larger than 40 ml: three years of follow-up. Clin Radiol 2001; 56:895–901.
35. Cho YS, Lee HK, Ahn IM, et al. Sonographically guided ethanol sclerotherapy for benign thyroid cysts: results in 22 patients. AJR Am J Roentgenol 2000; 174:213–216.
36. Lewis BD, Hay ID, Charboneau JW, et al. Percutaneous ethanol injection for treatment of cervical lymph node metastases in patients with papillary thyroid carcinoma. AJR Am J Roentgenol 2002; 178:699–704.
37. Rails PW, Mayekawa DS, Lee K, et al. Color-flow Doppler sonography in Graves' disease: "thyroid inferno." Am J Roentgenol 1988; 150:781–784.

38. Fobbe F, Finke R, Reichenstein E, et al. Appearance of thyroid diseases using colour-coded duplex sonography. Eur J Radiol 1989; 9: 29–31.
38a. Fukunari N, Nagahama M, Sugino K, et al. Clinical evaluation of color Doppler imaging for the differential diagnosis of thyroid follicular lesions. World J Surg 2004; 28:1261–1265.
38b. Frates MC, Benson CB, Doubilet PM, et al. Can color Doppler sonography aid in the prediction of malignancy of thyroid nodules? J Ultrasound Med 2003; 22:127–131.
39. Tschammler A, Wirkner H, Ott G, Hahn D. Vascular patterns in reactive and malignant lymphadenopathy. Eur Radiol 1996; 6: 473–480.
40. Karwowski JK, Jeffrey RB, McDougall IR, Weigel RJ. Intraoperative ultrasonography improves identification of recurrent thyroid cancer. Surgery 2002; 132:924–928.
41. Arora P, Wang L, Blum M. Outcome analysis of the predictive value of initial age and tumor positive lymph nodes on subsequent neck recurrences in post surgical differentiated thyroid cancer. Annual Meeting of the Endocrine Society, San Francisco, CA, 2002.
42. Arora P, Wang L, Blum M. Outcome analysis of neck recurrences in differentiated thyroid carcinoma by neck uptake in post surgical whole body scan and RAI therapy. Annual Meeting of the Endocrine Society, San Francisco, CA, 2002.
42a. Kopecky KJ, Onstad L, Hamilton TE, Davis S. Thyroid ultrasound abnormalities in persons exposed during childhood to 131-I from the Hanford nuclear site. Thyroid 2005; 15:604–613.
43. Reiners C. Systematic ultrasound screening as a significant tool for early detection of thyroid carcinoma in Belarus. J Pediatr Endocrinol Metab 2002; 15:979–984.
44. Blum M, Reede DL, Seltzer TF, et al. Computerized axial tomography in the diagnosis and management of thyroid and parathyroid disorders. Am J Med Sci 1984; 287:34–39.
45. Bashist B, Ellis K, Gold RP. Computed tomography of intrathoracic goiters. AJR Am J Roentgenol 1983; 140:455–460.
46. Higgins CB, Auffermann W. MR imaging of thyroid and parathyroid glands: a review of current status. AJR Am J Roentgenol 1988; 151: 1095–1106.
47. Mancuso AA, Dillon WP. The neck. Radiol Clin North Am 1989; 27: 407–434.
48. Glazer HS, Niemeyer JH, Balfe DM, et al. Neck neoplasms: MR imaging. Part II. Posttreatment evaluation. Radiology 1986; 160: 349–354.
49. Freeman M, Toriumi DM, Mafee MF. Diagnostic imaging techniques in thyroid cancer. Am J Surg 1988; 155:215–223.
50. Yousem DM, Som PM, Hackney DB, et al. Central nodal necrosis and extracapsular neoplastic spread in cervical lymph nodes: MR imaging versus CT. Radiology 1992; 182:753–759.
51. Webb WR, Sostman HD. MR imaging of thoracic disease: clinical uses. Radiology 1992; 182:621–630.
52. Davis SD. CT evaluation of pulmonary metastases in patients with extrathoracic malignancy. Radiology 1991; 180:1–12.
53. Shellock FG. MR imaging of metallic implants and materials: a compilation of the literature. AJR Am J Roentgenol 1988; 15:811–814.
53a. Wang J-C, Takashima S, Takayama F, et al. Tracheal invasion by thyroid carcinoma: Prediction using MR imaging. Amer J Roentgenol 2001; 177:929–936.
54. Auffermann W, Clark OH, Thurner S, et al. Recurrent thyroid carcinoma: characteristic on MR images. Radiology 1988; 168:753–757.
55. Takashima S, Morimoto S, Ikezoe J, et al. CT evaluation of anaplastic thyroid carcinoma. Am J Neuroradiol 1990; 11:361–367.
56. Cooper JC, Nakielny R, Talbot CH. The use of computered tomography in the evaluation of large multinodular goiters. Ann R Coll Surg Engl 1991; 73:32–35.
57. Blum M, Perlman S. Reducing suppressive therapy in patients with a history of thyroid cancer. Ann Intern Med 1995; 123:808–809.

22
Thyroid Nodules and Cancer Risk
Surgical Management

Orlo H. Clark

RISKS OF THYROID CANCER

Patients with thyroid nodules are selected for thyroidectomy if they have been diagnosed with cancer or are at risk of cancer, experience related symptoms, or have cosmetic abnormalities. As about 4% of the US population has thyroid nodules (determined by the Framingham studies), and yet only 40 patients per million have clinical thyroid cancer, a selective approach must be used to determine who will benefit from thyroidectomy *(1)*. Factors that increase the risk that a thyroid nodule may be cancerous are listed in Table 1.

Patients with a family history of thyroid cancer are much more likely to develop thyroid cancer. Thus, about 25% of patients with medullary thyroid cancer (MTC) have familial rather than sporadic disease *(2)*. This familial disease occurs in four forms:

1. Familial MTC without other endocrinopathies.
2. Familial medullary cancer with multiple endocrine neoplasia, type IIA (MENIIA), such as MTC, hyperparathyroidism, and pheochromocytomas. Some patients also have cutaneous lichen amyloidosis with a pruritic plaquelike skin rash over the scapular region and/or concurrent Hirschsprung's disease.
3. Familial MTC with MENIIB (pheochromocytomas, marfanoid habitus, mucosal neuromas, and ganglioneuromatosis).
4. Familial MTC as well as papillary thyroid cancer (PTC; *3–5*). Patients with familial MTC can now be diagnosed by a blood test for RET germline point mutations *(3–6)*.

RET somatic mutations are present in about half of sporadic MTCs, and specific mutations appear to correlate with tumor behavior *(7,8)*.

About 5% of patients with papillary and Hürthle cell cancer have familial thyroid cancer, but follicular thyroid cancer is rarely familial *(9,10)*. Patients with autosomal dominant disorders that cause disseminated gastrointestinal polyposis or Gardner syndrome (large and small bowel tumors, desmoid tumors, lipomas, and epidermoid cysts) and Cowden syndrome (multiple hemartomas, breast cancer, colon cancer, and nodular goiter) have an increased risk of thyroid cancer *(10,11)*. Thyroid cancer also appears to be more common in patients with MENI and with familial hyperparathyroidism without MENI *(12,13)*. Loss of genetic material at or close to the MENI centromeric region on chromosome 11 has been documented in some sporadic thyroid cancers of follicular cell origin *(14)*. Patients with other thyroid pathology also appear to be predisposed to develop thyroid cancer *(15,16)*.

Exposure to low or moderate doses of therapeutic radiation also dramatically increases the risk of thyroid cancer *(17)*. There does not appear to be a threshold dose, because exposure to as little as 6 cGy of radiation appears to increase the risk of thyroid cancer sixfold *(18)*. An almost linear increase in cancer frequency occurs as the dose of radiation increases from 6 to 2000 cGy. Higher doses of radiation, such as 5000–6000 cGy, can cause hypothyroidism, but thyroid cancer does not appear to increase appreciably likely because the thyroid cells are destroyed *(17)*. Thyroid cancer is more likely to occur in younger children after radiation exposure. A hereditary predisposition to the increased frequency of thyroid cancer after exposure to low-dose therapeutic radiation or radiation fallout seems to be present *(19,20)*. Thus, after exposure to low-dose therapeutic radiation, or after exposure to radiation from the Chernobyl nuclear accident, thyroid cancer developed in several members of some families, but in other neighboring families, tumors did not develop *(19)*. Sporadic PTCs may have somatic *BRAF* of *RET/PTC* mutations. PAX-8/PPAR8 and *ras* mutations occur most often in follicular thyroid cancers *(20)*.

Thyroid nodules that develop in those younger than 20 or over 60 yr are more likely to be cancerous, as are nodules associated with vocal cord paralysis and hoarseness, rapidly growing nodules, hard solitary nodules fixed nodules, or nodules associated with palpable ipsilateral lymphadenopathy. In my experience, nodules that ache or are minimally painful are more likely to be MTC.

From: *Thyroid Cancer: A Comprehensive Guide to Clinical Management, 2/e*
Edited by: L. Wartofsky and D. Van Nostrand © Humana Press Inc., Totowa, NJ

Table 1
Increased Risks of Thyroid Cancer

Family history of thyroid cancer
MTC or MENII
Familial nonmedullary thyroid cancer
Cowden syndrome
Familial polyposis (Gardner syndrome)
MENI or familial hyperparathyroidism
Exposure to low- or moderate-dose therapeutic radiation
External radiation
Nuclear fallout
Hard thyroid nodule
New thyroid nodule in young person (<20 yr) or older person (>60 yr)
Thyroid nodule with adjacent lymphadenopathy
History of hoarseness with vocal cord paralysis

CYTOLOGIC DIAGNOSIS

Regardless of the risk of cancer, fine-needle aspiration (FNA) for cytological examination helps determine the histological nature of a nodule. FNA requires an experienced cytologist to interpret the aspirate. A cytological examination can help establish whether a thyroid nodule is benign (95% reliability), malignant (99% reliability), or suspicious (~20% cancerous), or whether the cytologic specimen is inadequate and requires a repeat aspiration (21,22). When cytologic examination suggests MTC, the specimen should be stained for amyloid, calcitonin, and carcinoembryonic antigen. Patients with possible MTC should also have a blood test for calcitonin and a plasma and urine test for catecholamines and metanephrine to rule out a coexistent pheochromocytoma. FNA is often unreliable in patients with a thyroid nodule who have been exposed to low-dose therapeutic radiation because of the multifocal nature of the tumors in these patients (23). Around 40% of these patients will have thyroid cancer somewhere in the thyroid gland, and the dominant nodule is the cancer in these patients only 60% of the time. Thus, there is a high false-negative rate (23). Consequently, we recommend total or near-total thyroidectomy for these patients rather than needle biopsy. Patients with follicular neoplasms, follicular variants of PTC, and Hürthle cell neoplasms usually have thyroid nodules that are interpreted as suspicious by cytological examination. When these nodules are "cold" by radioiodine scanning, about 20% will be malignant; thus removal is recommended in most patients (22). When nodules are suspicious for PTC, repeat FNA biopsy may help clarify the cytologic diagnosis, and ultimately approx 50% of these tumors are found to be malignant (24).

OPERATIVE APPROACH

Considerable controversy continues relating to the most appropriate treatment of patients with thyroid cancer. Because there are no prospective studies comparing various surgical or postsurgical therapies, this debate will probably continue. Most surgeons and endocrinologists agree that the minimal thyroid operation that should be done for a thyroid nodule that might be malignant is an ipsilateral total thyroid lobectomy and isthmusectomy (24a,24b). The reason for this recommendation is that, if further surgery is needed, one does not have to operate in an area of scar tissue; thus, there should be no appreciable increased risk of complications, such as hypoparathyroidism or recurrent laryngeal nerve injury (25). It is also more difficult to remove all of the remaining thyroid gland after a partial thyroidectomy because the remaining thyroid tissue is often adherent to the surrounding structures when less than a thyroid lobectomy has been performed.

One reason for the debate concerning the extent of thyroidectomy required is that most patients with PTC have an excellent prognosis. Thus, patients with occult (<1 cm) PTCs without nodal involvement have a 6–8% recurrence rate but only a 0.2% mortality rate (26,27). Therefore, it is difficult to improve with these numbers. When lymph node metastases are present, or when there is angioinvasion within the occult PTC, the recurrence and death rates are higher (26,27). We recommend total or near-total thyroidectomy for virtually all patients with PTC larger than 1 cm. The mortality rate of patients considered to be at low risk by the TNM, AGES, AMES, or MACIS classifications is less than 5%, and about 75% of all patients with thyroid cancer would be classified at low risk (28). However, if this mortality rate can be lowered further, it is advisable, unless the improvement in survival rate is countered by a high complication rate. It is also important to mention that the AGES, AMES, and MACIS classifications are postoperative classifications. For example, local invasion, tumor differentiation, resectability, and even distant metastases are not often recognized until after the operation or after a postoperative ^{131}I scan and serum thyroglobulin determination. Grant and colleagues (29) also reported that recurrent cancer is less common after bilateral thyroid operations in both low- and high-risk patients, as determined by the AGES classification. DeGroot and coworkers (30) and Mazzaferri and Jhiang (31) also reported fewer recurrences and improved survival in patients after total or near-total thyroidectomy.

The major reasons we recommend total thyroidectomy is that the use of serum thyroglobulin levels and radioactive scanning can help determine if all tumor has been removed, or if residual tumor needs to be ablated with radioiodine (32–35). Why not wait to see if patients will develop recurrent disease, as most patients do not develop recurrent tumor? The problem with this approach is that once the recurrent tumor becomes clinically evident, or is evident on a chest radiograph, the chance of curative therapy with ^{131}I decreases from approx 70% to about 7% in tumors that take up radioiodine *(33,34)*. Other reasons to perform a total thyroidectomy are as follows:

1. It removes multifocal or bilateral disease that occurs in 30–87% of patients.
2. It lowers the recurrence rate.
3. It likely improves survival, as one third to half of patients who develop recurrent thyroid cancer die of thyroid cancer *(32–34)*.

The easiest time to conduct a total thyroidectomy is also at the initial operation.

Near-total thyroidectomy, leaving less than 1 g of thyroid tissue, rather than total thyroidectomy, should be done when the surgeon is concerned about the viability of the parathyroid glands or the recurrent laryngeal nerve during the initial dissection on the side of the tumor. Leaving a small remnant of normal thyroid tissue on the contralateral side to the tumor that can subsequently be ablated with ^{131}I is preferable in this situation. Numerous retrospective studies report that total or near-total thyroidectomy followed by ^{131}I ablation and thyrotropin suppressive therapy results in the fewest recurrences and the best survival *(30–32)*. Before thyroidectomy, ultrasonography of the neck is recommended to evaluate both the thyroid and cervical lymph nodes. During the initial thyroid operation, the surgeon should also carefully look and palpate for enlarged lymph nodes adjacent to the thyroid tumor and medial or lateral to the carotid sheath. All nodes in the central neck should be removed, and patients with palpable nodes in the lateral neck benefit from an ipsilateral modified radical neck dissection.

For most patients today, the histology of the thyroid tumor is known preoperatively because of information gained from a FNA performed before the operative procedure. Cytologic interpretation of an aspirate is accurate for papillary, medullary, and anaplastic thyroid cancers but cannot differentiate between a follicular or Hürthle cell adenoma and a follicular or Hürthle cell carcinoma *(35a)*. After needle biopsy, the surgeon can usually plan the definitive operation and discuss what will be done with the patient preoperatively. At operation in patients with follicular or Hürthle cell neoplasms by cytological examination, the surgeon should look for lymph nodes and, if present, remove them for frozen-section examination. About half of patients with follicular neoplasms, confirmed by cytological examination to have thyroid cancer, have a follicular variant of PTC. Nodal involvement is common in these patients, whereas fewer than 10% of patients with follicular cancer have nodal involvement *(36)*. Frozen-section examination is unfortunately not that effective in differentiating between benign or malignant follicular or Hürthle cell neoplasms. However, those follicular and Hürthle cell neoplasms that are larger than 4 cm or occur in older patients are more likely to be malignant. In patients with follicular or Hürthle cell neoplasms, the author usually performs a thyroid lobectomy, as most patients will have benign disease. The various options should also be discussed with the patient before surgery, including that in about 10% of cases, a second operation (completion total thyroidectomy) may be necessary if cancer is diagnosed only by permanent histological examination. Patients who have solitary follicular adenomas usually do not require thyroxine postoperatively because recurrent follicular adenomas are rare.

REFERENCES

1. Vander JB, Gaston EA, Dawber TR. The significance of nontoxic thyroid nodules: final report of a 15-year study of the incidence of thyroid malignancy. Ann Intern Med 1968; 69:537–540.
2. Wohllk N, Cote GJ, Evans DB, et al. Application of genetic screening information to the management of medullary thyroid carcinoma and multiple endocrine neoplasia type 2. Endocrinol Metab Clin North Am 1996; 25:1–25.
3. Donis-Keller H, Dou S, Chi D, et al. Mutations in the RET protooncogene are associated with MEN 2A and FMTC. Hum Mol Genet 1993; 2:851–856.
4. Mulligan LM, Kwok JB, Healey CS, et al. Germ-line mutations of the RET proto-oncogene in multiple endocrine neoplasia type 2A. Nature 1993; 363:458–460.
5. Carlson KM, Dou S, Chi D, et al. Single missense mutation in the tyrosine kinase catalytic domain of the RET protooncogene is associated with multiple endocrine neoplasia type 2B. Proc Natl Acad Sci USA 1994; 91:1579–1583.
6. Jimenez C, Dang GT, Schultz PN, et al. A novel point mutation of the RET protooncogene involving the second intracellular tyrosine kinase domain in a family with medullary thyroid carcinoma. J Clin Endocrinol Metab 2004; 89:3521–3526.
7. Jhiang SM, Fithian L, Weghorst CM, et al. RET mutation screening in patients with familial and sporadic medullary thyroid carcinoma disease and a discovery of a novel mutation in a sporadic disease. Thyroid 1996; 6:115–121.
8. Grossman RF, Tu SH, Duh QY, et al. Familial nonmedullary thyroid cancer: an emerging entity that warrants aggressive treatment. Arch Surg 1995; 130:892–899.
9. Ozaki O, Ito K, Kobayashi K, et al. Familial occurrence of differentiated, nonmedullary thyroid carcinoma. World J Surg 1988; 12:565–571.
10. Alsanea O, Clark OH. Familial thyroid cancer. Curr Opin Oncol 2001; 13:44–51.
11. Weary PE, Gorlin RJ, Gentry WC Jr, et al. Multiple hamartoma syndrome (Cowden's disease). Arch Dermatol 1972; 106:682–690.
12. Huang SM, Duh QY, Shaver J, et al. Familial hyperparathyroidism without multiple endocrine neoplasia. World J Surg 1997; 21:22–29.
13. Lips CJ, Vasen HF, Lamers CB. Multiple endocrine neoplasia syndromes. Crit Rev Oncol Hematol 1984; 2:117–184.
14. Matsuo K, Tang SH, Fagin JA. Allelotype of human thyroid tumors: loss of chromosome 11q13 sequences in follicular neoplasms. Mol Endocrinol 1991; 5:1873–1879.
15. Ron E, Kleinnerman RA, Boice JD Jr, et al. A population-based case-control study of thyroid cancer. J Natl Cancer Inst 1987; 79:1–12.
16. D'Avanzo B, La Vecchia C, Franceschi S, et al. History of thyroid diseases and subsequent thyroid cancer risk. Cancer Epidemiol Biomarkers Prev 1995; 4:193–199.
17. Greenspan FS. Radiation exposure and thyroid cancer. JAMA 1977; 237:2089–2091.
18. Modan B, Ron E, Werner A. Thyroid cancer following scalp irradiation. Radiology 1977; 123:741–744.
19. Baiter M. Chernobyl's thyroid cancer toll [news]. Science 1995; 270:1758–1759.

20. Puxeddu E, Moretti S, Elisei R. BRAF V^{599E} Mutation is the leading genetic event in adult sporadic papillary thyroid carcinomas. J Clin Endocrinol Metab 2004; 89:2414–2420.
21. Lowhagen T, Granberg PO, Lundell G, et al. Aspiration biopsy cytology (ABC) in nodues of the thyroid gland suspected to be malignant. Surg Clin North Am 1979; 59:3–18.
22. Kikuchi S, Perrier ND, Ituarte PH, et al. Accuracy of fine-needle aspiration cytology in patients with radiation-induced thyroid neoplasms. Br J Surg 2003; 90:755–758.
23. Kebebew K, Clark OH. Differentiated thyroid cancer: "complete" rational approach. World J Surg 2000; 24:942–951.
24. Zieger MA, Chen H, Clark D, et al. Papillary thyroid cancer: can operative management be solely based on fine needle aspiration? San Francisco, CA: Paper presented at the American College of Surgeons, 82nd Annual Clinical Congress, October 7, 1996.
24a. National Comprehensive Cancer Network (NCCN) Thyroid Carcinoma: Clinical Practice Guidelines 2005, J Natl Comprehensive Cancer Network 2005; 3:404–457.
24b. Kouvaraki MA, Shapiro SE, Lee JE, Evans DB, Perrier ND. Surgical management of thyroid carcinoma. J Natl Comprehensive Cancer Network 2005; 3:458–466.
25. Levin KE, Clark AH, Duh QY, et al. Reoperative thyroid surgery. Surgery 1992; 111:604–609.
26. Mazzaferri EL, Jhiang SM. Differentiated thyroid cancer long-term impact of initial therapy. Trans Am Clin Climatol Assoc 1994; 106: 151–170.
27. Mazzaferri EL. Papillary thyroid carcinoma: factors influencing prognosis and current therapy. Semin Oncol 1987; 14:315–332.
28. Hay ID. Papillary thyriod carcinoma. Endocrinol Metab Clin North Am 1990; 19:545–576.
29. Grant CS, Hay ID, Gough IR, et al. Local recurrence in papillary thyroid carcinoma: is extent of surgical resection important? Surgery 1988; 104:954–962.
30. DeGroot LJ, Kaplan EL, McCormick M, Straus FH. Natural history, treatment, and course of papillary thyroid carcinoma. J Clin Endocrinol Metab 1990; 71:414–424.
31. Mazzaferri EL, Jhiang SM. Long-term impact of initial surgical and medical therapy on papillary and follicular thyroid cancer. Am J Med 1994; 97:418–428.
32. Loh K-C, Miller TR, Greenspan FS. Differentiated thyroid cancer. In Clark OH, Duh QY, Perrier ND, Jahan TM, editors. Endocrine Tumors. Hamilton, Ontario: BC Decker Inc., 2003:23–36.
33. Clark OH, Levin K, Zeng QH, et al. Thyroid cancer: the case for total thyroidectomy. Eur J Cancer Clin Oncol 1988; 24:305–313.
34. Schlumberger M, Tubiana M, De Vathaire F, et al. Long-term results of treatment of 283 patients with lung and bone metastases from differentiated thyroid carcinoma. J Clin Endocrinol Metab 1986; 63: 960–967.
35. Casara D, Rubello D, Saladini G, et al. Different features of pulmonary metastases in differentiated thyroid cancer: natural history and multivariate statistical analysis of prognostic variables. J Nucl Med 1993; 34:626–1631.
35a. Chao T-C, Lin J-D, Chen M-F. Surgical treatment of Hurthle cell tumors of the thyroid. World J Surg 2005; 29:164–168.
36. Emerick GT, Duh QY, Siperstein AE, et al. Diagnosis, treatment, and outcome of follicular thyroid carcinoma. Cancer 1993; 72:3287–3295.
37. D'Avanzo A, Ituarte P, Treseler P, et al. Prognostic scoring systems in patients with follicular thyroid cancer: A comparison of different staging systems in predicting the patient outcome. Thyroid 2004; 14: 453–458.

Part IV
Well-Differentiated Thyroid Cancer: Papillary Carcinoma
Presentation

23
Papillary Carcinoma
Clinical Aspects

Leonard Wartofsky

INTRODUCTION

Papillary thyroid carcinoma (PTC) is a cancer of the thyroid follicular epithelium; like follicular carcinoma, it is the more highly differentiated of all of the classes of thyroid malignancy. The biological behavior of PTC varies widely, from small (<1.0 cm) tumors found at autopsy with surprisingly high frequency that show little evidence of invasion, to rapidly growing, locally invasive tumors that may be resistant to radioiodine therapy, eventually metastasizing and can cause death. To date, it has not been possible in a given patient to predict which course the tumor may take until several years, or even decades, of follow-up have elapsed. Fortunately, the overwhelming majority of tumors less than 1.5 cm in diameter tend to behave in a more biologically benign manner and can be completely cured with definitive therapy. This reflects the importance of tumor size on prognosis and risk of recurrence or death. Although PTC tends to affect women more often than men (~2:1), the risk of cancer in thyroid nodules in men is equally, if not more, significant because of the much lower frequency of any type of thyroid disease in men. This chapter deals with several clinical aspects of these tumors and descriptions of pathology and management appear in the immediate chapters that follow.

EPIDEMIOLOGY

According to 2004 data from the American Cancer Society, thyroid cancer is one of the top 10 leading causes of new cases of cancer in women, representing 3% of all cancers in women, about 1% in men (1), and approx 1.4% of all cancers in children. They estimate 25,690 new cases of thyroid cancer in 2005 (6500 in men; 19,190 in women), with an estimated 1490 deaths from thyroid cancer. Because most patients with thyroid cancer are followed for a long time, it is estimated that there are approx 300,000 patients with the disease in the United States. The frequency of thyroid cancer has been increasing each year of the past decade. The reasons for this rise are not clear and may relate to earlier diagnosis owing to the ever-increasing use of ultrasound and fine-needle aspiration (FNA), but many believe that it is because of exposure to ionizing radiation, such as from the nuclear tests of the 1950s and 60s.

Thyroid cancer is the most common malignancy of the endocrine system, and papillary carcinoma is the most common type of thyroid malignancy, accounting for 65–80% of all thyroid cancers (2,3). The frequency of papillary cancer appears to increase relative to the incidence of follicular thyroid cancer, which has been attributed to the higher iodine content of the American diet. Incidence of follicular cancer has not declined in geographic areas with relative iodine deficiency. PTC tends to occur in younger patients, most commonly in the third and fourth decades of life, and has the best prognosis of all the varieties of thyroid malignancy. There is a weak association with breast cancer in that white (but not black) women with a history of thyroid cancer have a somewhat greater risk (relative risk [RR] = 1.42) of developing breast cancer, but women with breast cancer do not have a greater risk of developing thyroid cancer (4).

A number of clinical and pathological characteristics have been evaluated as predictors of tumor behavior and ultimate patient prognosis. The more useful of these parameters are described in Chapter 9 on Staging and Prognosis. As described in Chapter 7, exposure to radiation is a risk factor for PTC, where the risk of malignancy in a thyroid nodule rises from 5–10% up to 30–50% (5). This chapter discusses general aspects of typical papillary carcinoma, but the discussion also applies to the follicular variant of papillary carcinoma (FVPTC). FNA cytology may not be sufficiently sensitive to distinguish between PTC and FVPTC preoperatively (6,7). Some studies have indicated that the FVPTC may be less invasive and associated with a lower frequency of neck node metastases (6,8), but it may present with larger original tumor size and higher tumor stage (8). Experts have proposed that clear-cut histopathologic features should be present to make

From: *Thyroid Cancer: A Comprehensive Guide to Clinical Management, 2/e*
Edited by: L. Wartofsky and D. Van Nostrand © Humana Press Inc., Totowa, NJ

the diagnosis of FVPTC (9). Other variants of papillary carcinoma, such as the tall-cell variant, columnar variant, and insular variant may behave in a more aggressive or invasive manner (10–13) and are discussed in Chapter 65.

Annual incidence rates for well-differentiated thyroid cancer range from 1 to 10 cases per 100,000 population, and a detailed description of the epidemiology of these tumors appears in Chapter 2. One of the largest cohorts of patients with PTC was followed up at the Mayo Clinic and reviewed by Hay (14). Of 1500 patients, two thirds were women (2:1 ratio), and age at diagnosis ranged widely from only 5 yr to 93 yr. Most patients presented between ages 30 and 60. There are major differences in frequencies of PTC in other ethnic groups. For example, the female-to-male ratio among Japanese has been reported as high as 13:1 (15).

CLINICAL PRESENTATION

In most patients, the first clinical presentation of PTC is that of a thyroid nodule, discovered during routine physical examination by a physician or noted as a lump in the neck by a friend or relative. The diagnostic evaluation of the nodule (see Chapters 17–21) virtually always includes FNA cytology, which can demonstrate the tumor's pathognomonic features. Use of new molecular biologic techniques that may distinguish benign from malignant cytologies are under intensive study (see Chapter 19). A survey of clinical thyroid specialists indicated fair consensus regarding the diagnostic evaluation of such patients and the need for subsequent thyroidectomy and radioiodine ablation with surgically proven PTC; however, there were several areas of controversy (16). Guidelines for management of thyroid nodules in respect to the diagnosis of thyroid cancer and its initial evaluation have been published by several authoritative sources (17–20).

As many as one third of patients will have some underlying thyroid disease, such as Hashimoto's disease or multinodular or adenomatoid goiter. In one series of 596 PTC patients from the Mayo Clinic (14), 40% had other benign thyroid disease, 33% had coexistent thyroid nodules, and 20% had Hashimoto's thyroiditis. Underlying Hashimoto's disease appears to be a favorable prognostic factor for both reduced rates of recurrence and increased survival (21,22). This may relate to a lymphocyte-mediated immune response against the cancer (23). Some familial papillary cancers occur in association with Hashimoto's thyroiditis (24,25), and a family history of thyroid cancer could be highly relevant at presentation, either indicating a possible medullary carcinoma or a familial type of PTC (26). Indeed, in one study, the RR of thyroid cancer was 10 times higher in relatives of thyroid cancer patients than in controls (27).

In some of the cancer literature, papillary tumors have been classified as occult, intrathyroidal, or extrathyroidal. An occult tumor is typically be less than 1.0 cm in size, an intrathyroidal tumor is more than 1.0 cm in size but confined to the thyroid gland, and an extrathyroidal tumor demonstrates extension to the soft tissues or lymph nodes of the neck. A first presentation to a physician of PTC as cervical lymphadenopathy is fairly common, and this evaluation then leads to detection of the primary thyroid tumor (28). The lymphadenopathy is from local metastases of the tumor, and the most frequent presentation is to nodes on the ipsilateral side of the tumor's neck, as well as down into the superior mediastinum. Metastases to the contralateral cervical chains of nodes occur with either more advanced or more aggressive disease. This may be related to initial intrathyroidal seeding via the thyroidal lymphatic system because microscopic to macroscopic foci of papillary carcinoma are often found in the contralateral thyroid lobe.

In the Mayo series (14,29) of 1500 patients, the primary tumor was confined to one lobe in 71%, bilateral in 19%, and with multicentric lesions in 26%. Cervical lymph node involvement was diagnosed in 38% (573 of 1500; median number of nodes = 4), and 2% (32 of 500) had distant metastases at time of initial diagnosis. These findings are comparable to the series reported by Mazzaferri and Jhiang (30) in which 32% of the tumors were multicentric and 43% had nodal involvement. When the papillary cancer is more aggressive, as evident by vascular invasion (30a) or widespread involvement throughout the thyroid gland, the likelihood of lymph node metastases is approx 75%. This was seen frequently in the series of 129 patients reported by DeJong and associates (28) in whom 34% had metastases to the ipsilateral jugular nodes, 41% had bilateral jugular nodes, and 81% had metastasis in the central compartment. In their total series of 243 patients with PTC, DeJong's group found that 21% actually presented with lateral cervical nodes and no palpable thyroid nodule(s).

Patients presenting with palpable cervical lymph nodes at varying intervals after their original thyroidectomy should be evaluated for metastases. The extent of the lymphadenopathy can be assessed by computed tomography (CT) or magnetic resonance imaging (MRI) scans of the neck and mediastinum, and such recurrent disease is usually, but not always (31), suggested by rising levels of serum thyroglobulin (Tg). The lymph node metastases may be indicated by increasing serum levels of Tg either basally or after recombinant human thyrotropin (rhTSH) administration (32,32a) or by Tg measurement in FNA aspirates of suspicious lymph nodes (33). Enlarged palpable lymph nodes can be readily aspirated with or without ultrasound guidance for cytological examination and Tg measurement. To confirm metastasis, polymerase chain reaction amplification of TSH receptor and Tg mRNA transcripts in blood, thyroid nodule (33a) or lymph node aspirate have also been employed (34). Some workers have also had measured success with the measurement of Tg mRNA in serum (35), especially in those patients with thyroid autoantibodies that interfere with the Tg assay.

Because these tumors are so frequently detected incidentally, it is obvious that most are asymptomatic. Symptoms arise only from increasing size and/or invasion. Symptoms commonly include a sense of fullness or pressure in the neck, as well as cough, dysphagia, or odynophagia. Occasionally, patients complain of an aching in the area of the involved lobe. The differential diagnosis of pain in the thyroid gland is fairly short, consisting of only three entities: invasive thyroid cancer, subacute thyroiditis, and hemorrhage within a nodule or cyst.

Young (≤17 years old) patients may have metastases of PTC to the lungs *(36–38)*. Patients with lung metastases may present with hemoptysis or dyspnea at rest or upon exertion. Pulmonary metastases were confirmed in one report by cytological examination after bronchoalveolar lavage *(39)*. Although PTC can metastasize to the lungs, follicular thyroid carcinoma is more likely to invade blood vessels and appear in distant sites, such as bone and lung, and present with symptoms of local bone pain or dyspnea, respectively *(18,40–42)*. Pulmonary metastases of PTC are typically difficult to completely eradicate with radioiodine therapy *(43)*, and the best results were seen in younger patients with positive radioiodine uptake on scan *(44; see also Chapters 45 and 53)*. More rare sites for metastasis of PTC include the eyes and skin *(45)*.

Patients with PTC only rarely present with local thyroid or cervical pain, in contrast to the patients with less differentiated thyroid cancers. Involvement of the recurrent laryngeal nerve results in palsy of the ipsilateral vocal cord and hoarseness. The texture or consistency of a malignant thyroid nodule may be no different from that of a benign follicular adenoma; the classic, firm-to-hard consistency of a nodule of papillary cancer may be related to the nodule's content of calcium (psammoma bodies). Medullary cancers (in which calcifications are frequent) or anaplastic carcinoma are much more hard on palpation than are well-differentiated tumors. The diagnostic evaluation for patients presenting with a mass in the thyroid is described (Chapters 17–21) and may include FNA cytology and ultrasound imaging. The tumors are almost always solid on ultrasound scans. Although purely cystic nodules rarely contain malignancy, large, mixed cystic/solid nodules pose a greater risk that demand closer management. Other imaging techniques, such as CT or MRI (Chapter 38), are rarely required but can demonstrate the extent of metastatic lymphadenopathy either before or after surgery. It is common for a patient to present with a thyroid mass because a CT scan or MRI was performed for another unrelated problem.

MANAGEMENT

Mazzaferri and Kloos have provided a concise summary of the issues involved with the management of PTC *(46)*, and Ringel and Ladenson have written an excellent analysis of the controversies underlying management *(47)*. Virtually all patients with PTC presenting as a thyroid nodule are euthyroid; hence there is little need for routine thyroid function tests. Occasional patients with underlying Hashimoto's disease may have associated hypothyroidism, which is coincidental and not related to the tumor *per se*, as it is only the more aggressive anaplastic forms of cancer that replace so much normally functioning thyroid parenchyma to cause thyroid hypofunction. In patients undergoing thyroidectomy for benign causes, there may be some advantage in knowing the preoperative levels of serum TSH and free thyroxine to have target levels for subsequent levothyroxine replacement therapy. However, such information is rarely pragmatic for postoperative management of patients with malignant disease. The dosage of thyroxine therapy is selected to be suppressive, rather than for replacement; the preoperative hormone levels are thus irrelevant.

Once the diagnosis is established, surgical thyroidectomy is the next step, which is usually a near-total to total thyroidectomy with exploration for enlarged lymph nodes, especially on the side ipsilateral to the nodule, as described in Chapters 22 and 24. Total thyroidectomy is associated with greater risk of complications (recurrent laryngeal nerve trauma with subsequent hoarseness or temporary to permanent hypoparathyroidism) but is more likely to result in a lower rate of recurrence, presumably from the removal of bilateral or multifocal foci of tumor *(19,36,47a)*. Patients who undergo only lobectomy or subtotal thyroidectomy may have a 2.5-fold risk of death compared to those undergoing total thyroidectomy *(48)*. Modeling for life expectancy and quality-adjusted life years indicates that total thyroidectomy is the preferred procedure in both low- and high-risk patients with PTC *(49)*. Dackiw and Zeiger *(50)* summarized the benefits of total thyroidectomy as:

- Radioiodine may be used to find and treat residual tissue or metastases.
- Serum Tg measurements can be used more effectively with all normal thyroid tissue excised.
- There is a 50–85% chance of microscopic cancer in the contralateral lobe.
- Residual tumor could dedifferentiate into anaplastic cancer.
- Frequency of recurrence is reduced.
- Without total thyroidectomy, recurrence occurs in 7% of patients, and 50% of patients with recurrence may die from their disease.
- Improved survival statistics.
- Later surgery for recurrence is associated with more complications.

Clearly, there are compelling arguments for total thyroidectomy. However, patients with tumors of 1.5-cm diameter or less usually have an excellent prognosis after only a lobectomy with isthmusectomy, without postoperative radioiodine ablation of the residual contralateral thyroid lobe *(5,19,51–56)*. This includes the so-called incidental "microcarcinomas" (discussed below) that may be found in a thyroid gland resected for some other indication, such as Graves' disease or nodular goiter, and that tend to have an excellent prognosis. These tumors are often found in the thyroid at postmortem examination. Based on the findings at surgery, tentative staging may be considered, but the full assignment of stage is based on both the extent of disease, as determined by clinical, radiological, and pathological examinations, and patient age at presentation *(57)*. Appropriate staging is critical to optimal patient management. Staging of papillary cancer is discussed in Chapter 9.

Following thyroidectomy for papillary lesions more than 1.5 cm, most physicians employ radioiodine in doses of 30–100 mCi to ablate residual tissue and facilitate follow-up monitoring *(58,59)*, as discussed in Chapters 26, 27, and 36. The degree of success with ablation depends on the dose of radioiodine administered *(60)*. Early series of patients have indicated that ^{131}I ablation of thyroid remnants was followed by a significantly lower recurrence rate *(52)*; this has been confirmed in a more recent review and meta-analysis *(61)*. However, the belief that such management is necessary and actually improves prognosis has been disputed *(14)* and remains a matter of some controversy *(62,63)*. One retrospective analysis of 700 patients suggested that patients that were not treated with radioiodine ablation had a 2.1-fold greater risk of recurrence of their malignancy ($p = 0.0001$) but no difference in death rates *(48)*. Several studies have been done and more are currently underway to assess the efficacy of rhTSH preparation for ablation, rather that ablation during traditional thyroid hormone withdrawal and hypothyroidism *(63a*; see Chapter 27). Standard low-ablation doses of 30 mCi have been found to be adequate for ablation in one study *(64)* but not another *(65)*. Higher doses are likely to be required because of the more rapid renal clearance of isotope in the euthyroid patient receiving rhTSH in comparison to the slowed renal clearance in hypothyroidism. Satisfactory ablation under rhTSH stimulation can be achieved with higher ^{131}I dosage, particularly with dosimetry *(66,67)*, but it is not possible to achieve the same degree of iodide depletion in these patients because of the contribution to dietary iodine of the iodine in their levothyroxine or L-triiodothyronine medications.

The postoperative follow-up of patients regarding thyroxine suppressive therapy and monitoring with periodic radioisotopic scans and serum Tg measurement is discussed in Chapters 28–35. Increasingly sensitive assays for Tg have revolutionized the approach to monitoring these patients *(68,69)*. Highly predictive insights into the risk of residual or recurrent tumors are provided by assays for Tg postoperatively and at 6–12 mo subsequently *(70)*. Measurement of serum Tg is not always feasible, however, because of the high prevalence of interfering anti-Tg antibodies in serum *(71)*. Some investigators have found the use of assays for Tg mRNA to be useful in such patients *(35,72–74)*, but the results have not been uniform *(75)*, and others decry the low specificity of such assays *(76)*. When basal Tg levels are undetectable on levothyroxine suppressive therapy, 18–26% of patients may still have occult tumor, which may be uncovered by Tg measurement after rhTSH stimulation *(77)*. Indeed, rhTSH-stimulated Tg is sufficiently sensitive that abandonment of diagnostic scanning has been advocated by some *(78,79)* but not all *(80)* centers and is especially useful when coupled with ultrasound of the neck *(81)*.

Detection of significantly measurable serum Tg or residual uptake with isotopic imaging generally leads to a search to better delineate the presence of tumors, e.g., additional imaging, to determine whether additional therapy is needed and the appropriate approach to further therapy. Guidelines for these evaluations are described in Chapters 28, 30, 31, 39, and 45. Because residual or recurrent papillary carcinoma presents most often in the neck, ultrasound examination of the neck has become the first choice for surveillance monitoring in both adults *(17,19,20)* and children *(82,83)*. Detection of residual or recurrent tumor prompts consideration for additional radioactive iodine therapy (see Chapters 45–49). Most centers employ relatively standard or empiric dosage of radioiodine, whereas a few more highly specialized thyroid cancer treatment centers also employ ^{131}I dosage dosimetrically determined with either ^{131}I *(84,85)* or ^{124}I *(86*; see Chapter 45). Dosimetric approaches have also been characterized in association with rhTSH administration *(87*; see Chapter 46).

Unfortunately too often, tumor is identified but found not to trap tracer radioiodine, thereby likely excluding the possibility of therapy with radioiodine, although empiric therapy with radioiodine may be attempted *(87a,87b)*. The clue to the presence of disease in such cases may be detectable or rising levels of serum thyroglobulin, and the management of the "radioisotope scan negative but thyroglobulin positive" patient is discussed in Chapter 39. The negative scans and iodine uptake in these patients is presumed to be the result of dedifferentiation and loss of the sodium iodide symporter (NIS). An active area of current research involves attempts to restore NIS and thus enable therapy in these patients. Approaches to this "redifferentiation therapy" are the subject of some excellent reviews *(88–90)* and are discussed in Chapter 86. External radiation therapy *(91,92)* has been used with variable success for tumors that do not trap radioiodine or are resistant to such therapy, as discussed in Chapter 51. Chemotherapy is another alternative in such patients *(93–95)* and is discussed in Chapter 52. The availability of rhTSH (Thyrogen; *96–98*) has radically altered routine follow-up evaluations for residual or recurrent disease of patients after their initial management by thyroidectomy and radioiodine ablation. Its use is fully discussed in Chapter 11.

MALIGNANT THYROID INCIDENTALOMA

With the increasing use of imaging procedures of the head and neck, such as ultrasound, CT, or MRI, a large number of small thyroid nodules are being detected. These so-called "incidentalomas" (because of their incidental discovery during an imaging procedure) may be benign nodules or papillary thyroid microcarcinomas. These tumors may also be found during thyroidectomy performed for an indication other than tumor and can range in size from 2 mm to 1.5 cm in diameter and are usually nonencapsulated (99). These small tumors have been thought to have a clearly different natural history than larger lesions, appearing to remain biologically silent with minimal morbidity. This impression was supported by studies, e.g., Hay and colleagues (100), representing a review of 535 microcarcinoma cases, of which 99% were histologically grade 1 tumors with no local invasion apparent in 98% of the patients. However, 32% had positive nodes at presentation that correlated with higher risk of recurrence, but the prognosis was nevertheless excellent after near-total thyroidectomy alone, irrespective of whether radioiodine remnant ablation was done. The low frequency of malignancy in incidentally discovered small thyroid nodules and the excellent prognosis even if malignant, as was implied by the experience of Hay et al., led to some complacency and the development of fairly nonaggressive guidelines for management of incidental nodules (14). These guidelines may have been proven to be too conservative on the basis of more recent studies, particularly those employing positron emission tomography (PET) scanning.

PET scanning with ^{18}F-fluoro-deoxyglucose (see Chapters 34 and 39) has proven to be a useful procedure for the detection of residual or recurrent malignancy (100a) and is based on the presence of an increased number of Glut transporters in cancer cells. With the increasing use of PET scans, incidental thyroid cancers are being detected at a greater frequency (101,102), raising questions about the wisdom of a conservative approach to small thyroid nodules detected incidentally. Moreover, a recent retrospective review of 299 patients with microcarcinoma (103) should allow the reevaluation of the management of these tumors. During follow-up, persistent disease was found in 77 of 292 (26%), 68 patients had locoregional metastases, and 10 had distant metastases. Fortunately, no patients died of their disease during follow-up, and, not surprisingly given their small size, tumor size was *not* predictive of relapse. Although the management of cancers less than 1.5 cm has often been either subtotal thyroidectomy or near-total thyroidectomy but without radioiodine ablation, the authors and those of an accompanying editorial (104) make a good case for total thyroidectomy followed by radioiodine ablation. Based on their experience, ablation would be warranted in those patients who were more likely to have recurrent or residual disease after thyroidectomy and included those with multicentric tumors, positive lymph node metastases, or vascular or capsular invasion. Also instructive in this regard is a study from Japan in which 162 patients with papillary microcarcinoma on FNA elected to be conservatively followed without surgery, and 70% had stable tumors during a follow-up period of just under 4 years (105). It has been suggested that optimal management strategies that take all relevant factors into account (including costs of evaluation and therapy vs benefits of earlier cancer diagnosis) are not available; properly controlled randomized studies are needed (106).

REFERENCES

1. Jemal A, Murray T, Ward E, et al. Cancer Statistics, 2005. Ca: a Cancer Journal for Clinicians 2005; 55:10–30.
2. Ain KB. Papillary thyroid carcinoma: etiology, assessment, and therapy. Endocr Metab Clin N Am 1995; 24:711–760.
3. Schlumberger MJ. Papillary and follicular thyroid carcinoma. N Engl J Med 1998; 338:297–306.
4. Chen AY, Levy L, Goepfert H, et al. The development of breast carcinoma in women with thyroid carcinoma. Cancer 2001; 92:225–231.
5. Robbins J, Merino MJ, Boice JD, et al. Thyroid cancer: a lethal endocrine neoplasm. Ann Intern Med 1991; 115:133–147.
6. Jain M, Khan A, Patwardhan N, et al. Follicular variant of papillary thyroid carcinoma: a comparative study of histopathologic features and cytology results in 141 patients. Endocr Pract 2001; 7:79–84.
7. Kesmodel SB, Terhune KP, Canter RJ, et al. The diagnostic dilemma of follicular variant of papillary thyroid carcinoma. Surgery 2003; 134:1005–1012.
8. Birmingham AR, Krishnan J, Davidson BJ, et al. Papillary and follicular variant of papillary carcinoma of the thyroid: Initial presentation and response to therapy. Submitted for publication.
9. Lloyd RV, Erickson LA, Casey MB, et al. Observer variation in the diagnosis of follicular variant of papillary thyroid carcinoma. Am J Surg Path 2004; 28:1336–1340.
10. van den Brekel MWM, Hekkenberg RJ, Asa SL, et al. Prognostic featues in tall cell papillary carcinoma and insular thyroid carcinoma. Laryngoscope 1997; 107:254–259.
11. Prendiville S, Burman KD, Ringel MD, et al. Tall cell variant: An aggressive form of papillary thyroid carcinoma. Otolaryngol Head Neck Surg 2000; 122:352–357.
12. Volante M, Landolfi S, Chiusa L, et al. Poorly differentiated carcinomas of the thyroid with trabecular, insular, and solid patterns: a clinicopathologic study of 183 patients. Cancer 2004; 100:950–957.
13. Chao T-C, Lin J-D, Chen M-F. Insular carcinoma: infrequent subtype of thyroid cancer with aggressive clinical course. World J Surg 2004; 28:393–396.
14. Hay ID. Papillary thyroid carcinoma. Endocrinol Metab Clin North Am 1990; 19:545–576.
15. Ito J, Noguchi S, Murakami T, et al. Factors affecting the prognosis of patients with carcinoma of the thyroid. Surg Gynecol Obstet 1980; 150:539.
16. Solomon BL, Wartofsky L, Burman KD. Current trends in the management of well differentiated papillary thyroid carcinoma. J Clin Endocrinol Metab 1996; 81:333–339.

17. AACE/AAES Medical/Surgical guidelines for clinical practice: management of thyroid carcinoma. Endocrine Practice 2001; 7:1–19.
18. Singer PA, Cooper DA, Daniels GH, et al. Treatment guidelines for patients with thyroid nodules and well differentiated thyroid cancer. Arch Int Med 1996; 156:2165–2172.
19. National Comprehensive Cancer Network (NCCN) Thyroid Carcinoma: Clinical Practice Guidelines 2005, J Natl Comprehensive Network 2005; 3:404–457.
20. British Thyroid Association. Guidelines for the management of differentiated thyroid cancer in adults. Available at: www.british-thyroid-association.org/guidelines.htm, 2002.
21. Kashima K, Yokoyama S, Noguchi S, et al. Chronic thyroiditis as a favorable prognostic factor in papillary thyroid carcinoma. Thyroid 1998; 8:197–202.
22. Loh K-C, Greenspan FS, Dong F, et al. Influence of lymphocytic thyroiditis on the prognostic outcome of patients with papillary thyroid carcinoma. J Clin Endocrinol Metab 1999; 84:458–463.
23. Modi J, Patel A, Terrell R, et al. Papillary thyroid carcinomas from young adults and children contain a mixture of lymphocytes. J Clin Endocrinol Metab 2003; 88:4418–4425.
24. Mechler C, Bounacer A, Suarez H, et al. Papillary thyroid carcinoma: 6 cases from 2 families with associated lymphocytic thyroiditis harbouring RET/PTC rearrangements. Brit J Cancer 2001; 85:1831–1837.
25. Uchino S, Noguchi S, Kawamoto H, et al. Familial nonmedullary thyroid carcinoma characterized by multifocality and a high recurrence rate in a large study population. World J Surg 2002; 26:897–902.
26. Alsanea O, Clark OH. Familial thyroid cancer. Current Opin Oncol 2001; 13:44–51.
27. Pal T, Vogl FD, Chappuis PO, et al. Increased risk for nonmedullary thyroid cancer in the first degree relatives of prevalent cases of nonmedullary thyroid cancer: a hospital-based study. J Clin Endocrinol Metab 2001; 86:5307–5312.
28. DeJong S, Demeter J, Jarosz H, et al. Primary papillary thyroid carcinoma presenting as cervical lymphadenopathy. Am Surg 1993; 59:172–177.
29. McConahey WM, Hay ID, Woolner LB, et al. Papillary thyroid cancer treated at the Mayo Clinic, 1946 through 1970: initial manifestations, pathologic findings, therapy, and outcome. Mayo Clin Proc 1986; 61:978–996.
30. Mazzaferri EL, Jhiang SM. Long-term impact of initial surgical and medical therapy on papillary and follicular thyroid cancer. Am J Med 1994; 97:418–428.
30a. Falvo L, Catania A, D'Andrea V, et al. Prognostic importance of histologic vascular invasion in papillary thyroid carcinoma. Ann Surg 2005; 241:640–646.
31. Miller JH, Marcus CS. Metastatic papillary thyroid carcinoma with normal thyroglobulin level. Clin Nutr Med 1988; 9:652.
32. Robbins RJ, Srivastava S, Shaha A, et al. Factors influencing the basal and recombinant human thyrotropin-stimulated serum thyroglobulin in patients with metastatic thyroid carcinoma. J Clin Endocrinol Metab 2004; 89:6010–6016.
32a. Kohlfuerst S, Igerc I, Lind P. Recombinant human thyrotropin is helpful in the follow-up and 131-I therapy of patients with thyroid cancer: A report of the results and benefits using recombinant human thyrotropin in clinical routine. Thyroid 2005; 15:371–376.
33. Baskin HJ. Detection of recurrent papillary thyroid carcinoma by thyroglobulin assessment in the needle washout after fine-needle aspiration of suspicious lymph nodes. Thyroid 2004; 14:959–963.
33a. Wagner K, Arciaga R, Siperstein A, et al. Thyrotropin receptor/thyroglobulin messenger ribonucleic acid in peripheral blood and fine-needle aspiration cytology: Diagnostic synergy for detecting thyroid cancer. J Clin Endocrinol Metab 2005; 90:1921–1924.
34. Arturi F, Russo D, Giuffrida D, et al. Early diagnosis by genetic analysis of differentiated thyroid cancer metastases in small lymph nodes. J Clin Endocrinol Metab 1997; 82:1638–1641.
35. Ringel MD, Ladenson PW, Levine MA. Molecular diagnosis of residual and recurrent thyroid cancer by amplification of thyroglobulin messenger ribonucleic acid in peripheral blood. J Clin Endocrinol Metab 1998; 83:4435–4442.
36. Thompson GB, Hay ID. Current strategies for surgical management and adjuvant treatment of childhood papillary thyroid carcinoma. World J Surg 2004; 28:1187–1198.
37. McClellan DR, Francis GL. Thyroid disease in children, pregnant women, and patients with Graves' disease. Endocrin Metab Clin North Am 1996; 25:27–48.
38. Zimmerman D, Hay ID, Gough IR, et al. Papillary thyroid carcinoma in children and adults: follow-up of 1039 patients conservatively treated at one institution during three decades. Surgery 1988; 104: 1157–1166.
39. Mello CJ, Veronikis I, Fraire AE, et al. Metastatic papillary thyroid carcinoma to lung diagnosed by bronchoalveolar lavage. J Clin Endocrinol Metab 1996; 81:406–410.
40. Goldman ND, Coniglio JU, Falk SA. Thyroid cancers I: Papillary, follicular, and Hürthle cell. Otolaryngol Clin North Am 1996; 29: 593–609.
41. Cooper DS, Schneyer CR. Follicular and Hürthle cell carcinoma of the thyroid. Endocr Metab Clin North Am 1990; 19:577–592.
42. Grebe SKG, Hay ID. Follicular thyroid cancer. Endocr Metab Clin North Am 1995; 24:761–802.
43. Sisson JC, Jamadar DA, Kazerooni EA, et al. Treatment of micronodular lung metastases of papillary thyroid cancer: are the tumors too small for effective irradiation from radioiodine? Thyroid 1998; 8: 215–221.
44. Ronga G, Filesi M, Montesano T, et al. Lung metastases from differentiated thyroid carcinoma. A 40 years' experience. Quart J Nucl Med 2004; 48:12–19.
45. Avram AM, Gielczyk R, Su L, et al. Choroidal and skin metastas from papillary thyroid cancer: Case and a review of the literature. J Clin Endocrinol Metab 2004; 89:5303–5307.
46. Mazzaferri EL, Kloos RT. Current approaches to primary therapy for papillary and follicular thyroid cancer. J Clin Endorinol Metab 2001; 86:1447–1461.
47. Ringel MD, Ladenson PW. Controversies in the follow-up and management of well differentiated thyroid cancer. Endocr Relat Cancer 2004; 11:97–116.
47a. Kouvaraki MA, Shapiro SE, Lee JE, Evans DB, Perrier ND. Surgical management of thyroid carcinoma. J Natl Comprehensive Cancer Network 2005; 3:458–466.
48. Loh K-C, Greenspan FS, Gee L, et al. Pathological tumor-node-metastasis (pTNM) staging for papillary and follicular thyroid carcinomas: a retrospective analysis of 700 patients. J Clin Endocrinol Metab 1997; 82:3553–3562.
49. Esnaola NF, Cantor SB, Sherman SI, et al. Optimal treatment strategy in patients with papillary thyroid cancer: A decision analysis. Surgery 2001; 130:921–930.
50. Dackiw APB, Zeiger M. Extent of surgery for differentiated thyroid cancer. Surg Clin N Am 2004; 84:817–832.
51. Simpson WJ, McKinney SE, Carruthers JS, et al. Papillary and follicular thyroid cancer: prognostic factors in 1578 patients. Am J Med 1987; 83:479–488.
52. Mazzaferri EL. Thyroid remnant 131-I ablation for papillary and follicular thyroid carcinoma. Thyroid 1997; 7:265–271.
53. Mazzaferri EL, Young RL, Oertel JE, et al. Papillary thyroid carcinoma: the impact of therapy in 576 patients. Medicine 1977; 56:171–196.
54. Mazzaferri EL, Young RL. Papillary thyroid carcinoma: A 10 year follow-up report of the impact of therapy in 576 patients. Am J Med 1981; 70:511–518.
55. Gilliland FD, Hunt WC, Morris DM, Key CR. Prognostic factors for thyroid carcinoma: a population based study of 15698 cases from the surveillance, epidemiology and end results (SEER) program 1973-1991. Cancer 1997; 79:564–573.

56. Samaan NA, Schultz PN, Hickey RC, et al. Well differentiated thyroid carcinoma and the results of various modalities of treatment: a retrospective review of 1599 cases. J Clin Endocrinol Metab 1992; 75: 714–720.
57. American Joint Committee on Cancer. The Thyroid Gland. In AJCC Cancer Staging Manual, 6th Edition, Springer, New York, NY, 2002; pp. 77–87.
58. Sweeney DC, Johnston GS. Radioiodine therapy for thyroid cancer. Endocr Metab Clin North Am 1995; 24:803–840.
59. Heufelder AE, Gorman CA. Radioiodine therapy in the treatment of differentiated thyroid cancer: guidelines and considerations. Endocrinologist 1991; 1:273–280.
60. Bal CS, Kumar A, Pant GS. Radioiodine dose for remnant ablation in differentiated thyroid carcinoma: a randomized clinical trial in 509 patients. J Clin Endocrinol Metab 2004; 89:1666–1673.
61. Sawka AM, Thephamongkhol K, Brouwers M, et al. A systematic review and metaanalysis of the effectiveness of radioactive iodine remnant ablation for well differentiated thyroid cancer. J Clin Endocrinol Metab 2004; 89:3668–3676.
62. Mazzaferri E. Editorial: A randomized trial of remnant ablation—in search of an impossible dream? J Clin Endocrinol Metab 2004; 89: 3662–3664.
63. Haugen BR. Editorial: patients with differentiated thyroid carcinoma benefit from radioiodine remnant ablation. J Clin Endocrinol Metab 2004; 89:3665–3667.
63a. Luster M, Lippi F, Jarzab B, et al. rhTSH-aided radioiodine ablation and treatment of differentiated thyroid carcinoma: a comprehensive review. Endocrine-Related Cancer 2005; 12:49–64.
64. Barbaro D, Boni G, Meucci G, et al. Radioiodine treatment with 30 mCi after recombinant human thyrotropin stimulation in thyroid cancer: Effectiveness for postsurgical remnants ablation and possible role of iodine content in L-thyroxine in the outcome of ablation. J Clin Endocrinol Metab 2003; 88:4110–4115.
65. Pacini F, Molinaro E, Castagna MG, et al. Ablation of thyroid residues with 30 mCi 131-I: A comparison in thyroid cancer patients prepared with recombinant human TSH or thyroid hormone withdrawal. J Clin Endocrinol Metab 2002; 87:4063–4068.
66. Robbins RJ, Tuttle RM, Sonenberg M, et al. Radioiodine ablation of thyroid remnants after preparation with recombinant human thyrotropin. Thyroid 2001; 11:865–869.
67. Robbins RJ, Larson SM, Sinha N, et al. A retrospective review of the effectiveness of recombinant human TSH as a preparation for radioiodine thyroid remnant ablation. J Nucl Med 2002; 43: 1482–1488.
68. Spencer CA. New insights for using serum thyroglobulin (Tg) measurement for managing patients with differentiated thyroid carcinomas. Thyroid International 2003; 4:1–14.
69. Whitley RJ, Ain KB. Thyroglobulin: a specific serum marker for the management of thyroid carcinoma. Clinics Lab Med 2004; 24:29–47.
70. Toubeau M, Touzery C, Arveux P, et al. Predictive value for disease progression of serum thyroglobulin levels measured in the postoperative period and after (131)I ablation therapy in patients with differentiated thyroid cancer. J Nucl Med 2004; 45:988–994.
71. Ligabue A, Possgioli MC, Zacchini A. Interference of specific autoantibodies in the assessment of serum thyroglobulin. J Nucl Biol Med 1993; 37:273–279.
72. Ringel MD, Balducci-Silano PL, Anderson JS, et al. Quantitative reverse transcription polymerase chain reaction of circulating thyroglobulin messenger ribonucleic acid for monitoring patients with thyroid carcinoma. J Clin Endocrinol Metab 1999; 84:4037–4042.
73. Chinnappa P, Taguba L, Arciaga R, et al. Detection of thyrotropin-receptor messenger ribonucleic acid (mRNA) and thyroglobulin mRNA transcripts in peripheral blood of patients with thyroid disease: sensitive and specific markers for thyroid cancer. J Clin Endocrinol Metab 2004; 89:3704–3709.
74. Li D, Butt A, Clarke S, Swaminathana R. Real-time quantitative PCR measurement of thyroglobulin mRNA in peripheral blood of thyroid cancer patients and healthy subjects. Ann NY Acad Sci 2004; 1022: 147–151.
75. Spencer CA. Editorial: Challenges of serum thyroglobulin (Tg) measurement in the presence of Tg autoantibodies. J Clin Endocrinol Metab 2004; 89:3702–3704.
76. Elisei R, Vivaldi A, Agate L, et al. Low specificity of blood thyroglobulin messenger ribonucleic acid assay prevents its use in the follow-up of differentiated thyroid cancer patients. J Clin Endocrinol Metab 2004; 89:33–39.
77. Mazzaferri EL, Robbins RJ, Spencer CA, et al. A consensus report of the role of serum thyroglobulin as a monitoring method for low-risk patients with papillary thyroid carcinoma. J Clin Endocrinol Metab 2003; 88:1433–1441.
78. Wartofsky L. Editorial: Using baseline and recombinant human TSH-stimulated Tg measurements to manage thyroid cancer without diagnostic 131-I scanning. J Clin Endocrinol Metab 2002; 87: 1486–1489.
79. Mazzaferri EL, Kloos RT. Is diagnostic iodine-131 scanning with recombinant human TSH useful in the follow-up of differentiated thyroid cancer after thyroid ablation? J Clin Endocrinol Metab 2002; 87: 1490–1498.
80. Robbins RJ, Chon JT, Fleisher M, et al. Is te serum thyroglobulin response to recombinant human thyrotropin sufficient, by itself, to monitor for residual thyroid carcinoma? J Clin Endocrinol Metab 2002; 87: 3242–3247.
81. Pacini F, Molinaro E, Castagna MG, et al. Recombinant human thyrotropin-stimulated serum thyroglobulin combined with neck ultrasonography has the highest sensitivity in monitoring differentiated thyroid carcinoma. J Clin Endocrinol Metab 2003; 88:3668–3673.
82. Antonelli A, Miccoli P, Fallahi P, et al. Role of neck ultrasonography in the follow-up of children operated on for thyroid papillary cancer. Thyroid 2003; 13:479–484.
83. Hung W, Sarlis NJ. Current controversies in the management of pediatric patients with well-differentiated nonmedullary thyroid cancer: A review. Thyroid 2002; 12:683–702.
84. Van Nostrand D, Atkins F, Yeganeh F, et al. Dosimetrically determined doses of radioiodine for the treatment of metastatic thyroid carcinoma. Thyroid 2002; 12:121–134.
85. Dorn R, Kopp J, Vogt H, et al. Dosimetry-guided radioactive iodine treatment in patients with metastatic differentiated thyroid cancer: Largest safe dose using a risk-adapted approach. J Nucl Med 2003; 44: 451–456.
86. Sgouros G, Kolbert KS, Sheikh A, et al. Patient specific dosimetry for 131-I thyroid cancer therapy using 124-I PET and 3-dimensional-internal dosimetry (3D-ID) software. J Nucl Med 2004; 45: 1366–1372.
87. de Keizer B, Hoekstra A, Konijnenberg MW, et al. Bone marrow dosimetry and safety of high 131-I activities given after recombinant human thyroid-stimulating hormone to treat metastatic differentiated thyroid cancer. J Nucl Med 2004; 45:1549–1554.
87a. Mazzaferri EL. Empirically treating high serum thyroglobulin levels. J Nucl Med 2005; 46:1079–1088.
87b. Ma C, Xie J, Kuang A. Is empiric 131-I therapy justified for patients with positive thyroglobulin and negative 131-K whole-body scanning results? J Nucl Med 2005; 46:1164–1170.
88. Park J-W, Clark OH. Redifferentiation therapy for thyroid cancer. Surg Clin N Am 2004; 84:921–943.
89. Braga-Basaria M, Ringel MD. Beyond radioiodine: a review of potential new therapeutic approaches for thyroid cancer. J Clin Endocrinol Metab 2003; 88:1947–1960.
90. Spitzweg C, Morris JC. Gene therapy for thyroid cancer: current status and future prospects. Thyroid 2004; 14:424–434.
91. Tubiana M, Haddad E, Schlumberger M, et al. External radiotherapy in thyroid cancers. Cancer 1985; 55:2062–2071.

92. Simpson WJ, Carruthers JS. The role of external radiation in the management of papillary and follicular thyroid cancer. Am J Surg 1978; 136:457.
93. Ahuja S, Ernst H. Chemotherapy of thyroid carcinoma. J Endocrinol Invest 1987; 10:303.
94. Shimaoka K, Schoenfeld DA, DeWys WD, et al. A randomized trial of doxorubicin versus doxorubicin plus cisplatin in patients with advanced thyroid carcinoma. Cancer 1985; 56:2155–2160.
95. Kim JH, Leeper RD. Treatment of locally advanced thyroid carcinoma with a combination of doxorubicin and radiation therapy. Cancer 1987; 60:2372–2375.
96. Mazzaferri EL. An overview of the management of papillary and follicular thyroid cancer. Thyroid 1999; 9:421–427.
97. Ladenson PW. Strategies for thyrotropin use to monitor patients with treated thyroid carcinoma. Thyroid 1999; 9:429–433.
98. Robbins RJ, Robbins AK. Recombinant human thyrotropin and thyroid cancer management. J Clin Endocrinol Metab 2003; 88: 1933–1938.
99. Burguera B, Gharib H. Thyroid incidentalomas. Prevalence, diagnosis, significance, and management. Endocrin Metab Clin N Am 2000; 29: 187–203.
100. Hay ID, Grant CS, van Heerden JA, et al. Papillary thyroid microcarcinoma: a study of 535 cases observed in a 50-year period. Surgery 1992; 112:1139–1147.
100a. Nahas Z, Goldenberg D, Fakhry C, et al. The role of positron emission tomography/computed tomography in the management of recurrent papillary thyroid carcinoma. Laryngoscope 2005; 115: 237–243.
101. Cohen MS, Arslan N, Dehdashti F, et al. Risk of malignancy in thyroid incidentalomas identified by fluorodeoxyglucose-positron emission tomography. Surgery 2001; 130:941–946.
102. Kang HW, Kim S-K, Kang H-S, et al. Prevalence and risk of cancer of focal thyroid incidentaloma identified by 18F-fluorodeoxyglucose positron emission tomography for metastasis evaluation and cancer screening in healthy subjects. J Clin Endocrinol Metab 2003; 88: 4100–4104.
103. Pellegriti G, Scollo C, Lumera G, et al. Clinical behavior and outcome of papillary thyroid cancers smaller than 1.5 cm in diameter: Study of 299 cases. J Clin Endocrinol Metab 2004; 89:3713–3720.
104. Pearce EN, Braverman LE. Editorial: Papillary thyroid microcarcinoma outcomes and implications for treatment. J Clin Endocrinol Metab 2004; 89:3710–3712.
105. Ito Y, Uruno T, Nakano K, et al. An observation trial without surgical treatment in patients with papillary microcarcinoma of the thyroid. Thyroid 2003; 13:381–387.
106. Silver RJ, Parangi S. Management of thyroid incidentalomas. Surg Clin N Am 2004; 84:907–919.

24
Surgical Approach to Papillary Carcinoma

Orlo H. Clark

General aspects for the approach for patients with thyroid nodules proven to be malignant are discussed earlier in this volume. Without prospective studies comparing various surgical or postsurgical therapies, the debate over which procedure to select is likely to continue. Most thyroid surgeons agree that the minimal operation for a thyroid nodule suspicious for malignancy is a total thyroid lobectomy and isthmectomy on the side of the nodule. The reason for this recommendation is that if further surgery is needed, one does not have to operate in an area of scar tissue, and risks of complications (e.g., hypoparathyroidism or recurrent laryngeal nerve injury) should be minimized (1). Furthermore, thyroid tissue remaining after a partial thyroidectomy may be difficult to remove during a second procedure because of its adherence to the surrounding structures. This chapter addresses aspects of the surgical management of papillary thyroid carcinoma, and special considerations regarding follicular, medullary, and anaplastic carcinoma of the thyroid are discussed in later chapters of this volume.

One reason for the controversy about the extent of thyroidectomy required is that most patients with papillary thyroid cancer have a good prognosis. Consequently, patients with occult papillary thyroid cancers less than 1 cm without nodal involvement have a 6–8% recurrence rate but only a 0.2% mortality rate (2,3). Therefore, it is difficult to improve on with these numbers. When lymph node metastases are present, or when there is angioinvasion within the occult papillary thyroid cancer, the recurrence and death rates are higher (2,3). We recommend total or near-total thyroidectomy for nearly all patients with papillary thyroid cancer more than 1 cm. The mortality rate of patients considered to be at low risk by the TNM (tumor, lymph nodes, distant metastases), AGES, AMES, or MACIS classifications (see Chapter 9 on staging) is less than 5%, and approx 75% of all patients with thyroid cancer would be classified at low risk (4). Yet, if this mortality can be decreased further, it is advisable, unless the improvement in survival rate is countered by a high complication rate. Notably, the AGES, AMES, and MACIS are postoperative classifications. For example, local invasion, tumor differentiation, resectability, and even distant metastases are not often recognized until after the operation or after a postoperative ^{131}I scan and serum thyroglobulin determination. Grant and colleagues (5) also reported that recurrent cancer is less common after bilateral thyroid operations in both low- and high-risk patients, as established by the AGES classification. DeGroot and colleagues (6) and Mazzaferri and Jhiang (7) also indicated fewer recurrences and improved survival in patients after total or near-total thyroidectomy.

The primary reasons a total thyroidectomy is recommended is because the use of serum thyroglobulin levels and radioactive scanning can help determine if all tumor has been removed, or if residual disease should be treated with radioiodine (8–10). Why not wait to conduct a completion thyroidectomy and see if patients will develop recurrent disease, as most patients do not develop recurrent tumor? The problem with this approach is that once the recurrent tumor becomes clinically evident, or is evident on a chest radiograph, the chance of curative therapy with ^{131}I decreases from about 70% to 7% in tumors that take up radioiodine (9–11). Other reasons for total thyroidectomy include that it removes multifocal or bilateral disease that occurs in 30–87% of patients, it lowers the recurrence rate, and it probably improves survival, because one third to half of patients who develop recurrent thyroid cancer die of thyroid cancer (8–10). Technically, the most simple time for a total thyroidectomy is also at the initial operation. This approach applies to papillary thyroid cancer, and recommendations will differ for other thyroid cancers (11a).

Near-total thyroidectomy, leaving less than 1 g of thyroid tissue, rather than total thyroidectomy, should be done when the surgeon is concerned about the viability of the parathyroid glands or the recurrent laryngeal nerve during the initial dissection on the side of the tumor. In this case, a small remnant of normal thyroid tissue should be left on the contralateral side to the tumor that can subsequently be ablated with ^{131}I. Numerous retrospective studies report that total or near-total thyroidectomy followed by ^{131}I ablation and thyrotropin suppressive therapy results in the least number of recurrences and the best survival (6–8). Prior to thyroidectomy, ultrasonography of the neck is helpful to identify

From: *Thyroid Cancer: A Comprehensive Guide to Clinical Management, 2/e*
Edited by: L. Wartofsky and D. Van Nostrand © Humana Press Inc., Totowa, NJ

multiple abnormalities in the thyroid and lymphadenopathy *(12)*. During the thyroid operation, the surgeon should monitor carefully and palpate for enlarged lymph nodes adjacent to the thyroid tumor and medial or lateral to the carotid sheath. All nodes in the central neck should be removed, and patients with palpable nodes in the lateral neck benefit from an ipsilateral modified radical neck dissection, as has been advocated for medullary thyroid cancer *(13)*. Neck levels 2, 3, and 4 are most frequently involved.

For most patients today, the histology of the thyroid tumor is known preoperatively because a fine-needle aspiration (FNA) cytology is usually done before the operative procedure. FNA cytology is accurate for papillary, medullary, and anaplastic thyroid cancers but cannot differentiate between a follicular or Hürthle cell adenoma and a follicular or Hürthle cell carcinoma. After the FNA, the surgeon can usually plan the definitive operation and discuss what will be done with the patient preoperatively. Surgical management of thyroid cancer in children does not differ significantly *(13a)*. At operation in patients with follicular or Hürthle cell neoplasms by cytological examination, the surgeon should look for lymph nodes and, if present, remove them for frozen-section examination. About half of patients with follicular neoplasms by cytological examinations who are found to have thyroid cancer have a follicular variant of papillary thyroid cancer. Nodal involvement is common in these patients, but only about 10% of patients with follicular cancer have nodal involvement *(14)*.

Frozen-section examination is unfortunately not that effective in differentiating between benign or malignant follicular or Hürthle cell neoplasms. However, follicular and Hürthle cell neoplasms larger than 4 cm or that occur in older patients are more likely to be malignant. In patients with follicular or Hürthle cell neoplasms, the author usually performs a thyroid lobectomy, as most patients will have benign disease. The various situations should be discussed with the patient before surgery, and they should be informed that in about 10%, a second operation—completion total thyroidectomy—may be necessary if cancer is only diagnosed by permanent histological examination. As with follicular thyroid cancer *(15)*, staging of the patient with papillary cancer can occur after surgical pathology and the first postoperative scan results are known (see Chapter 9). Patients who have had a lobectomy and isthmusectomy for a benign solitary follicular adenoma usually do not require thyroxine postoperatively because recurrent follicular adenomas are rare.

REFERENCES

1. Levin KE, Clark AH, Duh QY, et al. Reoperative thyroid surgery. Surgery 1992; 111:604–609.
2. Mazzaferri EL, Jhiang SM. Differentiated thyroid cancer long-term impact of initial therapy. Trans Am Clin Climatol Assoc 1994; 106: 151–170.
3. Pearce EN, Braverman LE. Editorial: Papillary thyroid microcarcinoma outcomes and implications for treatment. J Clin Endocrinol Metab 2004; 89:3710–3712.
4. Hay ID. Papillary thyroid carcinoma. Endocrinol Metabol Clin North Am 1990; 19:545–576.
5. Grant CS, Hay ID, Gough IR, et al. Local recurrence in papillary thyroid carcinoma: is extent of surgical resection important? Surgery 1988; 104:954–962.
6. DeGroot LJ, Kaplan EL, McCormick M, Straus FH. Natural history, treatment, and course of papillary thyroid carcinoma. J Clin Endocrinol Metab 1990; 71:414–424.
7. Mazzaferri EL, Jhiang SM. Long-term impact of initial surgical and medical therapy on papillary and follicular thyroid cancer. Am J Med 1994; 97:418–428.
8. Loh K-C, Miller TR, Greenspan FS. Differentiated thyroid carcinomas. In Clark OH, Duh QY, Perrier ND, Jahan TM, editors. Endocrine Tumors. Hamilton, Ontario: BC Decker Inc., 2003:23–36.
9. Clark OH, Levin K, Zeng QH, et al. Thyroid cancer: the case for total thyroidectomy. Eur J Cancer Clin Oncol 1988; 24:305–313.
10. Schlumberger M, Tubiana M, De Vathaire F, et al. Long-term results of treatment of 283 patients with lung and bone metastases from differentiated thyroid carcinoma. J Clin Endocrinol Metab 1986; 63:960–967.
11. Casara D, Rubello D, Saladini G, et al. Different features of pulmonary metastases in differentiated thyroid cancer: natural history and multivariate statistical analysis of prognostic variables. J Nucl Med 1993; 34:1626–1631.
11a. Kouvaraki MA, Shapiro SE, Lee JE, Evans DB, Perrier ND. Surgical management of thyroid carcinoma. J Natl Comprehensive Cancer Network 2005; 3:458–466.
12. Kouvaraki MA, Shapiro SE, Fornage BD, et al. Role of preoperative ultrasonography in the surgical management of patients with thyroid cancer. Surgery 2003; 134:946–955.
13. Scollo C, Baudin E, Travagli J-P, et al. Rationale for central and bilateral lymph node dissection in sporadic and hereditary medullary thyroid cancer. J Clin Endocrinol Metab 2003; 88:2070–2075.
13a. Thompson GB, Hay ID. Current strategies for surgical management and adjuvant treatment of childhood papillary carcinoma. World J Surg 2004; 28:1187–1198.
14. Emerick GT, Duh QY, Siperstein AE, et al. Diagnosis, treatment, and outcome of follicular thyroid carcinoma. Cancer 1993; 72:3287–3295.
15. D'Avanzo A, Ituarte P, Treseler P, et al. Prognostic scoring systems in patients with follicular thyroid cancer: A comparison of different staging systems in predicting the patient outcome. Thyroid 2004; 14: 453–458.
16. Besic N, Zgajnar J, Hocevar M, Frkovic-Grazio S. Is patient's age a prognostic factor for follicular thyroid carcinoma in the TNM classification system? Thyroid 2005; 15:439–448.

25
Papillary Carcinoma
Cytology and Pathology

Yolanda C. Oertel and James E. Oertel

INTRODUCTION

Papillary carcinoma is the most common thyroid cancer, constituting 75–85% of the malignant thyroid lesions in regions where iodine-deficient goiter is no longer present *(1)*. It represents most of the thyroid cancers that occur in children and young adults, whether idiopathic or related to radiation. A small proportion is familial. Generally, papillary carcinomas grow slowly and spread mostly by lymphatic vessels. The majority are infiltrative, without a capsule. Both gross and microscopic features are varied, depending on cellularity, amount and type of stroma, and the content of colloid *(2)*. Nondiploid papillary cancers *(3)* and those having N-ras mutations are more likely to have metastases and to cause death *(4)*. Furthermore, cyclo-oxygenase-2 and matrix metalloproteinase-2 expression have been reported to be significantly higher in older patients with more aggressive papillary carcinomas *(5,6)*. Cytologic and pathologic features of the more common variants of papillary carcinoma are described in this chapter and in Chapter 66 with clinical descriptions in Chapter 66.

CLASSICAL PATTERN

The not otherwise specified (NOS) papillary carcinoma (classical pattern) is a mixture of neoplastic papillae (Fig. 1) and follicles, sometimes with several tiny solid regions. Minor cystic changes are common. The gross appearance is a firm opaque mass, usually poorly defined and with a granular or finely nodular-cut surface. Irregular scarring is typical, and foci of calcification can be found frequently. If part of the tumor is rich in colloid, this is translucent and gelatinous and has some resemblance to normal thyroid tissue or an adenomatoid nodule. If there are numerous psammoma bodies, the tissue feels gritty, and it should be decalcified.

In histological sections, the cells are larger than normal follicular cells and are cuboidal to low columnar (Fig. 2). The cytoplasm is typically amphophilic to slightly eosinophilic. Nuclei are relatively large (but vary somewhat in size), ovoid, and subtly irregular in shape and in their positions in the cells. Nuclear indentations and round intranuclear inclusions of cytoplasm are common, but these vary in number and degree in different tumors and in different parts of the same tumor. Nucleoli are usually close to the nuclear membranes, along with the heterochromatin, thereby causing the nuclear membrane to seem "thick" and much of the interior of the nucleus to be "pale," "empty," "clear," or "ground glass" in appearance. Follicles may be colloid-filled or empty and range from tiny to large. Many are abnormally shaped and may be elongated (almost tubular; Fig. 3). Papillae differ greatly in size and complexity (Fig. 1). Each papilla consists of a fibrovascular core that is covered by a single layer of cuboidal to low columnar cells. The longer papillae are typically twisted and slightly irregular.

Nearly all these cancers contain immunoreactive thyroglobulin and keratins. Psammoma bodies occur in about 40% *(2)*. Foci of irregular calcification (even ossification) are moderately common. The colloid may be dense or thin; dense colloid often appears "stringy" or globular. Fibrosis occurs in an erratic pattern, often as trabeculae or nodules of dense collagenous tissue *(7)*. A latticework of dense fibrous tissue often is present.

There may be many chronic inflammatory cells, mostly lymphocytes, within and around a papillary neoplasm. The papillae may be filled with lymphocytes and/or histiocytes, often foamy histiocytes. Presumably, this inflammatory response is a reflection of the high incidence of the deposition of immunoglobulin G and complement factors on the cells of papillary carcinoma *(8)*. Histiocytes in the tumor may contain lipofuscin and/or hemosiderin, particularly when hemorrhage and/or cystic change are present.

Foreign-body-type giant cells (multinucleated histiocytes) are moderately frequent in the classic papillary carcinomas. Some may be closely associated with psammoma bodies (Fig. 4). Multiple foci of cancer cells are common in the thyroid, both as spread through the lymphatic vessels and

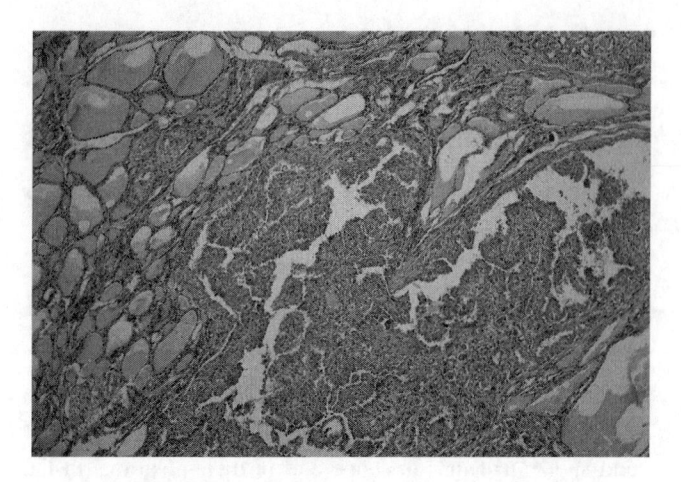

Fig. 1. Papillary carcinoma (classical pattern) invades the normal gland (H&E stain).

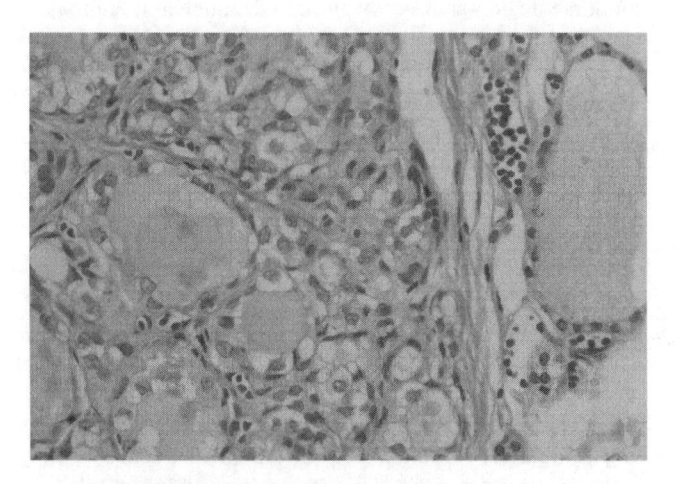

Fig. 2. Normal thyroid tissue lies to the right in the figure. Note that the cells of the cancer are much larger than the normal follicular epithelial cells (H&E stain).

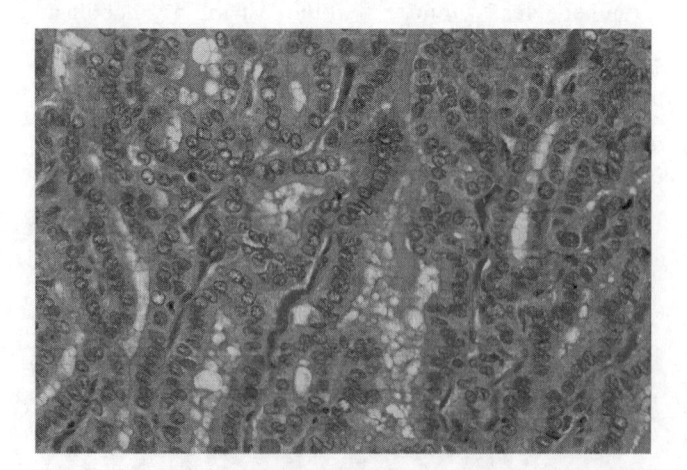

Fig. 3. Small papillae of the papillary carcinoma are crowded together, and follicular spaces are elongated (H&E stain).

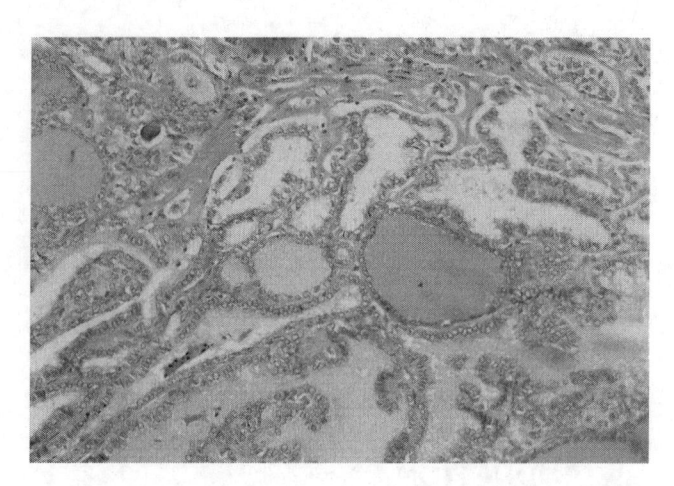

Fig. 4. A psammoma body lies in the upper left of the figure (H&E stain).

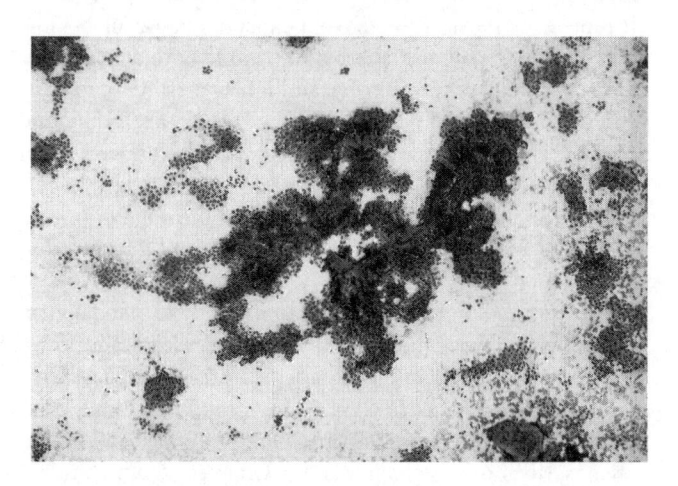

Fig. 5. Aspirate showing papillary tissue fragments of the papillary carcinoma (Diff-Quik stain).

as several simultaneous primary sites. Cervical lymph nodes are the most typical sites of metastatic foci.

The cytologic smears contain large numbers of cells ("tumor cellularity"). Tight clusters of neoplastic cells—some in a papillary arrangement (Fig. 5)—and single cells are observed. These cells have enlarged nuclei (at least twice the size of red blood cells; Fig. 6), dense chromatin, sharp nuclear borders, and variable shapes (round, ovoid, and triangular). Nucleoli are seldom seen. Nuclear "grooves" are rarely evident in smears stained with Diff-Quik. Intranuclear cytoplasmic inclusions are seen frequently (Figs. 7 and 8). The cytoplasm is usually dense and well demarcated. Colloid may range from scarce to abundant, appearing as thick strands ("ropy" or "bubble-gum" colloid) (Figs. 9 and 10), irregular masses, or dense balls that stain bright pink (Fig. 10) to lavender. Psammoma bodies often are seen (Fig. 11). Multinucleated histiocytes are commonly a conspicuous feature (*11*; Fig. 12).

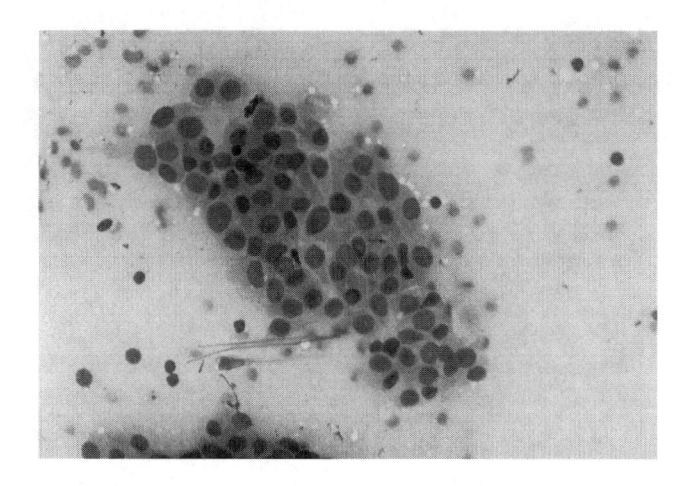

Fig. 6. Aspirate of a papillary carcinoma showing neoplastic cells with variation in nuclear sizes (Diff-Quik stain).

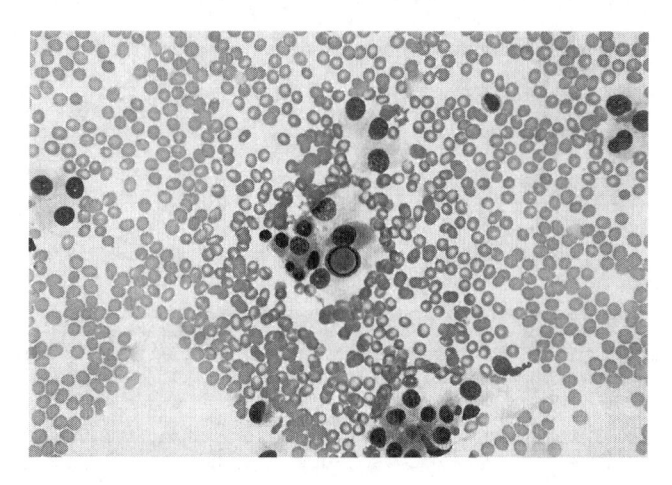

Fig. 7. Aspirate of a papillary carcinoma showing "intranuclear cytoplasmic pseudoinclusion" in large nucleus in the center of the field (Diff-Quik stain, low magnification).

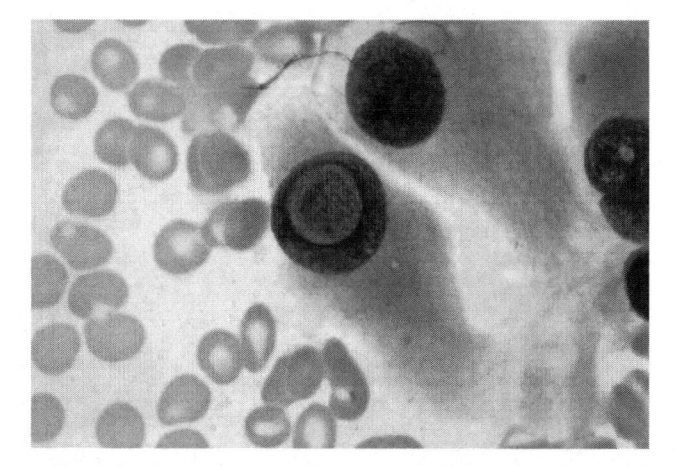

Fig. 8. Aspirate of a papillary carcinoma showing "intranuclear cytoplasmic pseudoinclusion" (Diff-Quik stain, high magnification).

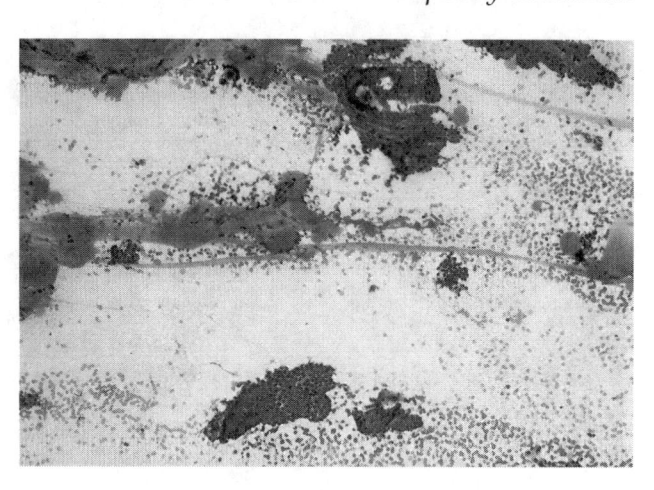

Fig. 9. Aspirate of a papillary carcinoma showing bubble-gum (chewing-gum or ropy) colloid (Diff-Quik stain).

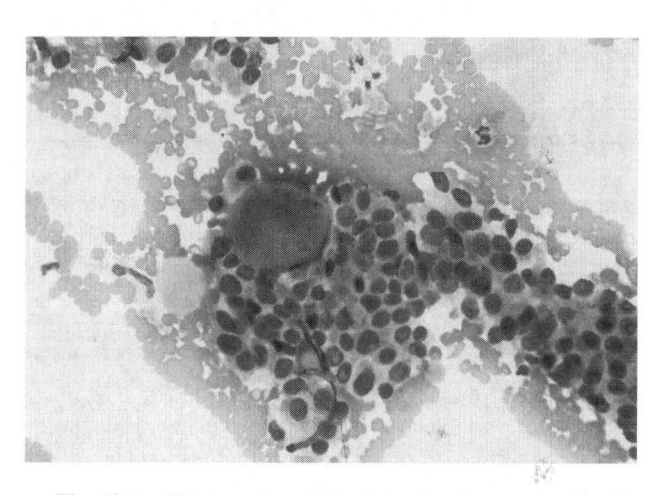

Fig. 10. Papillary carcinoma. Aspirate showing neoplastic cells surrounding colloid, which appears as a "pink ball" (Diff-Quik stain).

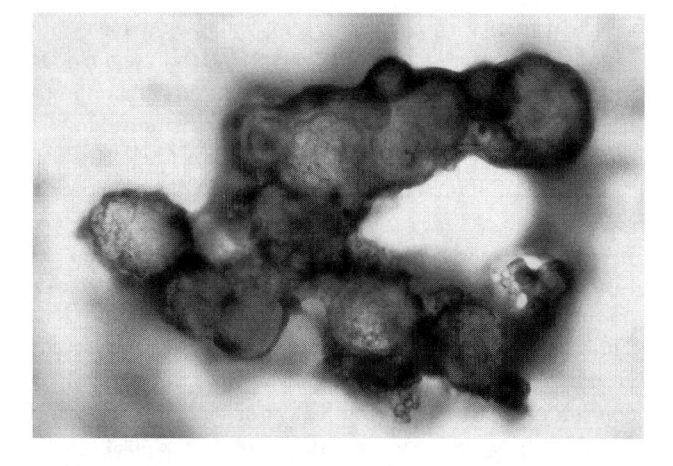

Fig. 11. Papillary carcinoma aspirate showing psammoma bodies (Diff-Quik stain).

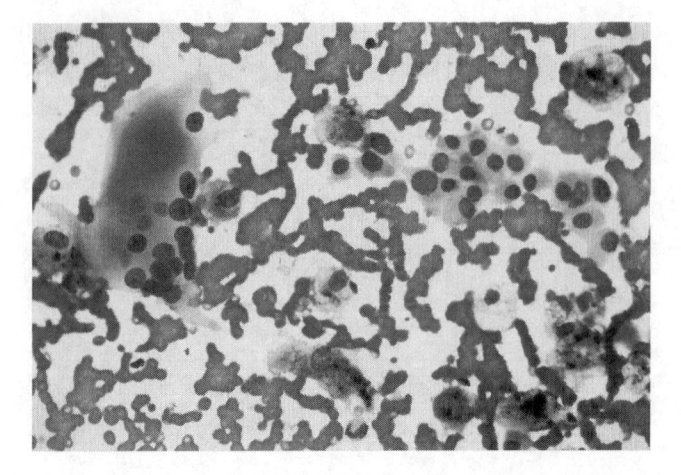

Fig. 12. Multinucleated histiocyte (on the left) and neoplastic cells of a papillary carcinoma. Many erythrocytes lie in the background of the smear (Diff-Quik stain).

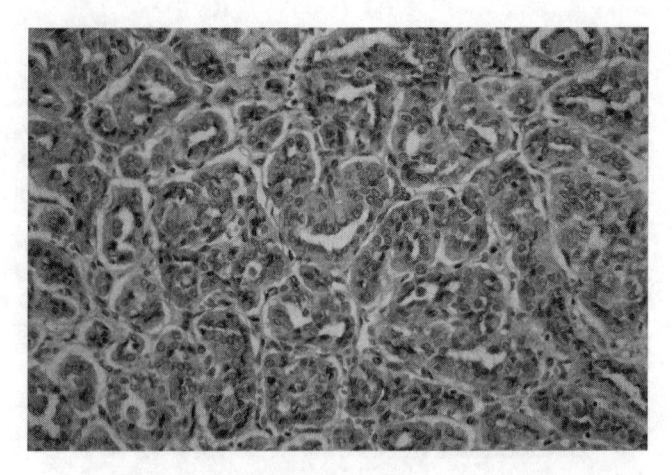

Fig. 13. Papillary carcinoma, follicular pattern. The nuclei are irregular in shape, size, and in their position in the cells. Follicles are tiny and generally appear empty (H&E stain).

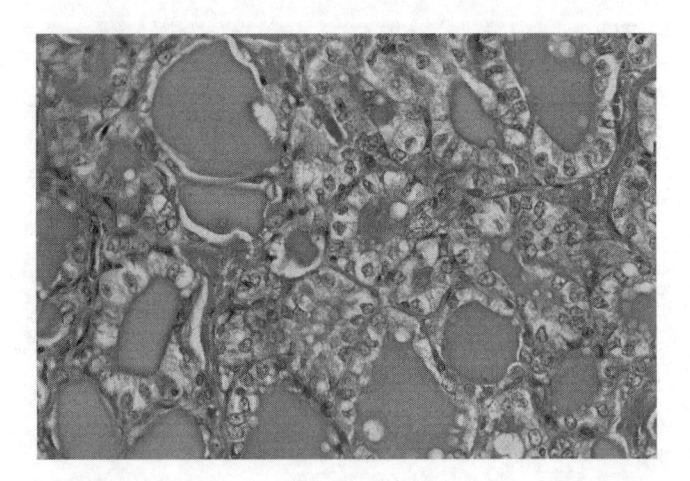

Fig. 14. Papillary carcinoma, follicular pattern. Much colloid is present, and the irregularity of the nuclei is readily apparent (H&E stain).

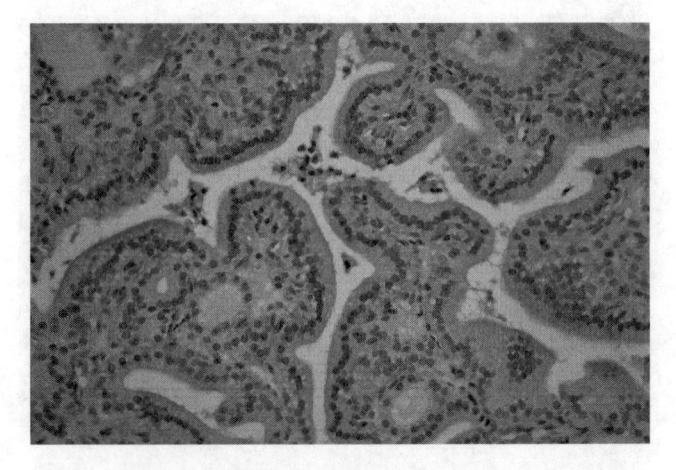

Fig. 15. Benign adenomatoid nodule with papillae. Compare these regular nuclei with those of papillary carcinoma in the other figures (H&E stain).

FOLLICULAR VARIANT

A diagnosis of the follicular variant of papillary carcinoma may be made when more than 70% of the histological pattern is composed of neoplastic follicles (Fig. 13). Such neoplasms are often small and are usually less fibrotic or cystic than the papillary carcinomas NOS, but the amount of colloid present and size of the follicles vary considerably. If follicles are small and contain little colloid, and if papillae are tiny and scarce, the tumor will appear fleshy and opaque on gross examination; it may be misclassified as a follicular adenoma or follicular carcinoma on microscopic examination. If most follicles are medium-sized to large, and there is abundant colloid (Fig. 14), then the tumor resembles an adenomatoid nodule or macrofollicular adenoma, both grossly and microscopically; it may be mistaken for an adenomatoid nodule (Fig. 15). This is the diffuse follicular variant or the macrofollicular variant. Psammoma bodies and multinucleated histiocytes are usually sparse.

The follicular variant is characterized by frequent encapsulation of the tumor, by a relatively low rate of lymph nodal metastases in comparison to the classic papillary carcinoma, frequent *RAS* point mutations, and by a low prevalence of *ret/PTC* and PAX8-PPAR γ rearrangements *(12)*.

Smears from fine-needle aspiration (FNA) are markedly cellular. The enlarged neoplastic cells form small follicles with well-demarcated lumina (Fig. 16) or lie in clusters, forming rosettes and tubules. Occasionally, papillary tissue fragments may be seen. The nuclei are dark-staining, have smooth contours, and differ in size and shape; a few are triangular, resembling arrowheads. Pink-staining colloid appears inside follicles (Fig. 17) or as balls and masses of variable shapes in close proximity to the neoplastic cells. Intranuclear cytoplasmic inclusions, psammoma bodies, and multinucleated histiocytes are less frequent than in the classic type of papillary carcinoma *(13)*.

Papillary Carcinoma

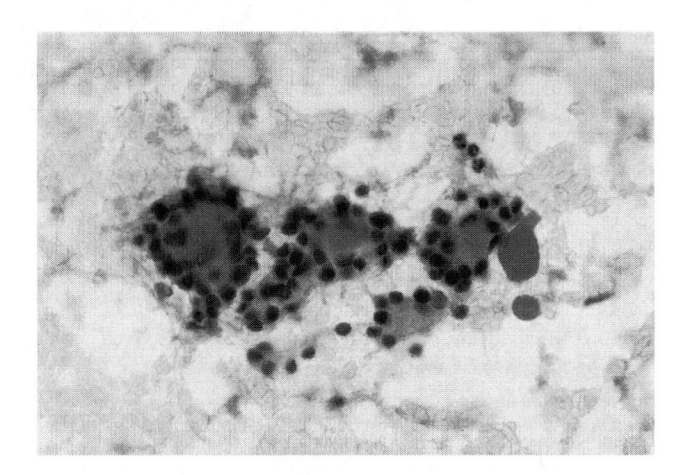

Fig. 16. Papillary carcinoma, follicular variant. Aspirate showing multiple microfollicles with inspissated luminal colloid (Papanicolaou stain).

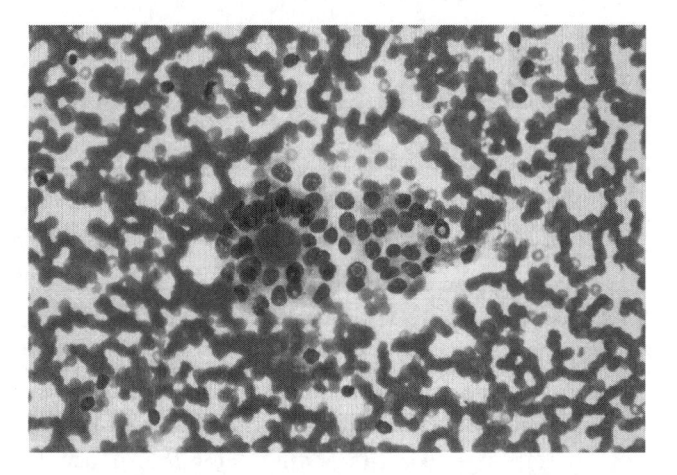

Fig. 17. Papillary carcinoma, follicular variant. Aspirate showing a rosette (on the right) and a microfollicle with "pink colloid" in its lumen (Diff-Quik stain).

ENCAPSULATED VARIANT

About 10–20% of the papillary cancers that are not microcarcinomas are encapsulated variants. Some are cystic and encapsulated; thus, the gross appearance is extremely varied. Capsules range from delicate to thick. These neoplasms have a lower incidence of nodal metastases than the other types, but careful search of the periphery of such a tumor usually reveals microscopic evidence of penetration of its capsule or foci of neoplastic cells in the thyroid tissue just outside the tumor's capsule. Therefore, gross evidence of invasion is often absent, but microscopic evidence of aggressiveness is usually present.

Many papillary carcinomas have irregular and dense fibrous tissue that accompanies their infiltrating cells, producing a "pseudocapsule" around part of the neoplasm. This should be differentiated from the well-organized, continuous, real capsule just described. Cytologic smears are diagnosed as classic papillary carcinoma on FNA.

A few papillary carcinomas are composed almost exclusively of papillae, and neoplastic follicles are rare. The cytologic smears are those of the classic papillary carcinoma.

CYSTIC CARCINOMA

Tiny cystic foci are fairly common in papillary carcinoma, but a few cancers include one or two cysts that occupy most of the lesion. The fluid often contains bits of tissue and flecks of calcific material, and papillary fronds may be visible to the naked eye. Sometimes, there is so little epithelium that the tumor appears as a fluid-filled sac. These cancers are often encapsulated, suggesting a reduced risk of metastases.

Aspiration yields at least 1.0 mL of fluid, often a larger amount, typically thin and pale yellow, greenish, brown, or thick and brown. The fluid may reaccumulate rapidly. If a residual mass can be detected after fluid evacuation and collapse of the cyst, this should be aspirated. It is important to remember that most cystic thyroid masses are benign *(14)*.

Direct smears and smears from sediment after centrifugation of the fluid should be prepared. Large numbers of hemosiderin-laden histiocytes and considerable cellular debris are present. Sheets of intact follicular cells may be seen, which resemble those from cellular adenomatoid nodules *(15)*; however, these may be neoplastic cells. In a benign cystic lesion, such epithelial cells should be shrunken and degenerate, and the presence of apparently well-preserved cells is therefore a warning of a possible neoplasm. These cells are slightly larger than normal follicular cells, their cytoplasm is denser, they lack paravacuolar granules, and their nuclei are larger than normal nuclei and are not pyknotic. Some groups of larger cells with clear cytoplasm and dense, convex cellular borders also are seen. The edges of these cellular clusters have a scalloped appearance *(16;* Fig. 18*)*. In other cases, the predominant cell type resembles a histiocyte with clear cytoplasm and an enlarged atypical nucleus; these are presumably partly degenerated neoplastic epithelial cells *(17)*. Dense globules of pink-staining colloid ("pink balls") may be present.

EXTENSIVELY FIBROTIC CARCINOMA

Extensively fibrotic tumors are rare and typically infiltrative. Little epithelium is present, and the stroma may be dense, myxomatous *(18)*, or fasciitis-like *(3)*. The gross appearance depends on the amount and density of the stroma. The authors have not made this diagnosis on cytological smears.

DIFFUSE PAPILLARY CARCINOMA

In diffuse papillary carcinoma, most of a lobe or the entire thyroid gland is involved, and the tissue is firm, pale, and opaque. Usually, no discrete mass can be found. The lymphatic vessels of the gland are permeated by the cancer, and

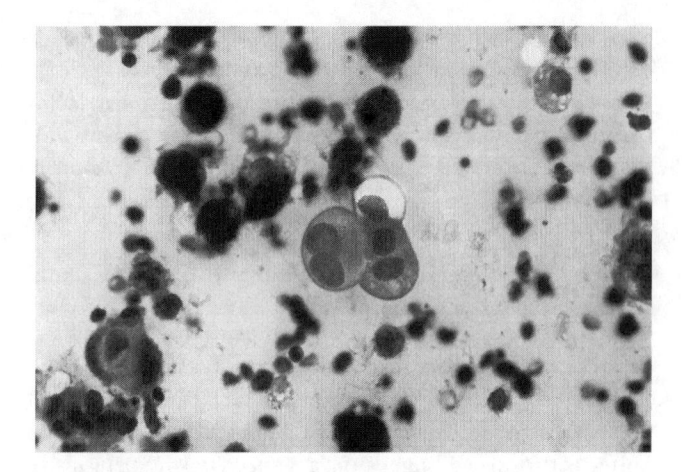

Fig. 18. Papillary carcinoma with cystic change. Aspirate showing neoplastic cells with dense well-demarcated cytoplasm and one with pale cytoplasm (Diff-Quik stain).

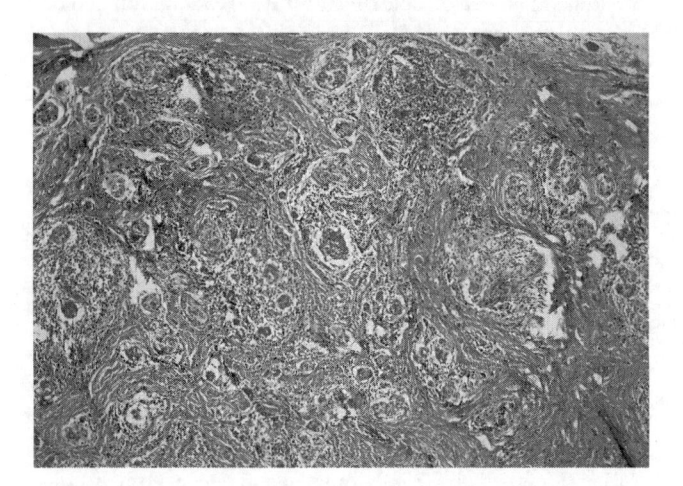

Fig. 19. Papillary carcinoma of the diffuse sclerosing type (H&E stain).

typical autoimmune thyroiditis is often present (19). Frequently, there is diffuse fibrosis throughout (Fig. 19) but not always. Psammoma bodies and foci of squamous metaplasia in the cancer are common. Adjacent lymph nodes often are involved, and metastatic spread to the lungs is common, but these features do not necessarily portend short survival, as many of the patients are young women. Cytological smears from these cases have been diagnosed as classic papillary carcinoma by the authors.

MICROCARCINOMA

Small papillary carcinomas were identified as 1.5 cm or less in diameter and considered "occult" (1,20). Because this size is now regarded as too large to be occult, carcinomas may be labeled as such if each tumor is 1.0 cm or less in diameter. A carcinoma that is only a few millimeters in diameter is palpable if it is fibrotic and on the anterior surface of the gland; therefore, it is not truly "occult." These tiny lesions could be called "microcarcinomas" or "minimal carcinomas."

OXYPHILIC PAPILLARY CARCINOMA

Only a small number of papillary carcinomas with oxyphilic cells occur; only a few have been studied, and they may be infiltrative or encapsulated. Some pathologists believe this variant is considerably more aggressive than the usual papillary carcinoma (21). Others have not been able to detect any clear differences, allowing for the other prognostic factors also present (22). Aspirates may be misdiagnosed as follicular neoplasms of the Hürthle cell type because of the cytoplasmic characteristics. In the oxyphilic papillary carcinoma, nucleoli are rarely visible, intranuclear cytoplasmic inclusions are common, and multinucleated histiocytes are seen frequently.

CLEAR-CELL PAPILLARY CARCINOMA

A few cells with clear cytoplasm are present in a modest proportion of papillary carcinomas. Only a few cancers have many or most of their cells with clear cytoplasm. This feature does not have any known prognostic significance. We have limited experience with this type of neoplasm on aspirations.

TALL-CELL VARIANT

The tall-cell variant of papillary carcinoma is uncommon and has a poor prognosis, with a greater tendency to recur or metastasize (23,24). The neoplastic cell has a height two times as great as its width. Cytoplasm is usually eosinophilic. Many tumors are large, extensively papilliferous, and occur mostly in middle-aged or elderly persons (unfavorable prognostic features). Trabecular patterns have been reported (24). In a small series, all tall-cell examples were positive for Leu Ml—a myelomonocytic marker from cluster designation group 15 (CD 15; 24). The tumors may fit with the less well-differentiated group. The prognosis may be better when the tumor is heavily infiltrated by lymphocytes and plasma cells (25).

Recently, some attempts have been made to establish diagnostic criteria for the recognition of this variant in cytologic smears (26–29). These reports are based on a small number of cases in retrospective studies; therefore, conflicting statements have been made. Harach and Zusman (26) described the presence of papillary fronds in their three cases, Bocklage and colleagues (29) found them in only one case, Kaw (27) did not find their presence in his case, and Gamboa-Dominguez and colleagues (28) did not even mention papillary fronds as diagnostic features. Some common characteristics have been reported: larger cells with

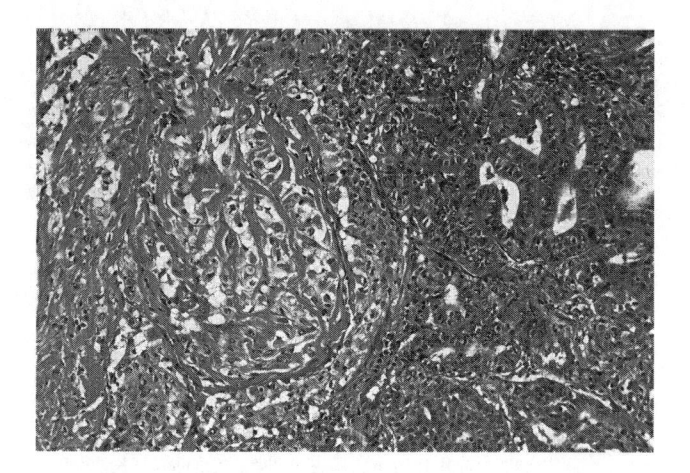

Fig. 20. Less well-differentiated papillary carcinoma. Relatively tall and irregular cells are on the left; a trabecular pattern with tall cells is on the right. Almost no colloid is visible (H&E stain).

abundant oxyphilic cytoplasm, more frequent intranuclear cytoplasmic inclusions, and fewer psammoma bodies than in classic papillary carcinoma.

LESS WELL-DIFFERENTIATED PAPILLARY CARCINOMAS

Less well-differentiated papillary cancers are classified as grades 2 and 3 by the Mayo Clinic Broders' classification and are described as "moderately differentiated papillary carcinoma" *(30)*, i.e., papillary carcinoma with marked atypia (multilayered epithelium, notable variations in size and shape of the cells and nuclei, and nuclei with hyperchromatism and abnormal chromatin distribution; *31*). Other investigators include the tall-cell and columnar-cell cancers as less well-differentiated papillary carcinomas (*23*; Fig. 20).

An extensive trabecular pattern of growth has been stated to indicate a worse prognosis *(32)*, but such cases may overlap with the tall-cell variant *(24)*. Patterns of solid growth might not be significant, especially in young persons *(3)*. Focal necrosis and invasion of blood vessels may also indicate a higher grade of malignancy *(33)*.

When follicles are empty and closed, or when papillae or trabeculae are pressed together, a neoplasm may appear solid, without actually having a solid diffuse pattern of growth. True solid regions are moderately typical in papillary carcinoma but are usually only a minor component. Sometimes the solid foci are the result of focal squamous metaplasia; this is often not a significant feature. The entire neoplasm is only solid or predominantly solid in a few instances. Aspirates may show malignant features without specifically resembling a papillary thyroid carcinoma. We have diagnosed a few of these cases as "carcinoma, cannot further classify."

COLUMNAR-CELL CARCINOMA

Columnar-cell papillary carcinoma is rare, occuring in adults of all ages. It is usually a solid, nodular, light-colored mass, either encapsulated or infiltrative, and contains tall, slender, columnar cells arranged in patterns that are papillary or trabecular *(34–37)*. Solid regions may present with small polygonal and/or spindled cells. Follicles of multiple sizes may be present. An alveolar pattern is sometimes suggested. Cytoplasm is usually clear, sometimes eosinophilic or amphophilic, and is scanty. Nuclei are hyperchromatic, rarely pale, elongated in the tall cylindrical cells, and may contain longitudinal grooves; intranuclear cytoplasmic inclusions are rare. These elongated nuclei differ sufficiently in their positions in the cells to produce a stratified or pseudostratified appearance. Nucleoli are inconspicuous, and there are many mitotic figures *(37)*. The cells contain glycogen, thyroglobulin, and sometimes keratin. A few psammoma bodies may be found.

Neoplasms have been reported where the columnar-cell pattern was mixed with tall-cell papillary carcinoma *(38,39)*, as well as with solid regions of typical papillary carcinoma *(36,39,40)*. Also, we have seen extensive insular and trabecular patterns adjacent to the columnar-cell pattern.

Reports suggest that the locally infiltrative tumors are usually fatal *(34,38,39,41)*, but those that are encapsulated may be resected successfully *(36,37)*. We have no personal experience with aspirates from this neoplasm. One report has described papillary fragments composed of pseudostratified columnar cells crowded together *(42)*. The neoplastic cells had oval to elongated nuclei and resembled respiratory epithelial cells. The background of the smears was devoid of colloid.

REFERENCES

1. Rosai J, Carcangiu ML, DeLellis RA. Tumors of the thyroid gland. In Rosai J, Sobin LJ, editors. Atlas of Tumor Pathology, 3rd ed. Washington, DC: A. F. I. P., 1992.
2. LiVolsi VA. Surgical pathology of the thyroid. Major Probl Pathol 1990; 22:136–172.
3. Nishida T, Nakao K, Hamaji M, et al. Overexpression of p53 protein and DNA content are important biologic prognostic factors for thyroid cancer. Surgery 1996; 119:568–575.
4. Hara H, Fulton N, Yashiro T, et al. N-Ras mutation: an independent prognostic factor for aggressiveness of papillary thyroid carcinoma. Surgery 1994; 116:1010–1016.
5. Siironen P, Ristimäki A, Nordling S, et al. Expression of COX-2 is increased with age in papillary thyroid cancer. Histopathology 2004; 44:490–497.
6. Stephenson TJ. Papillary carcinoma of the thyroid: difficult yet fascinating model of oncogenesis and tumour progression. Histopathology 2004; 44:498–500.
7. Isarangkul W. Dense fibrosis: another diagnostic criterion for papillary thyroid carcinoma. Arch Pathol Lab Med 1993; 117:645–646.
8. Lucas SD, Karlsson-Parra A, Nilsson B, et al. Tumor-specific deposition of immunoglobulin G and complement in papillary thyroid carcinoma. Hum Pathol 1996; 27:1329–1335.

9. Löwhagen T, Willems J-S, Lundell G, et al. Aspiration biopsy cytology in diagnosis of thyroid cancer. World J Surg 1981; 5:61–73.
10. Abele JS, Miller TR. Fine-needle aspiration of the thyroid nodule: clinical applications. In Clark OH, editor. Endocrine Surgery of the Thyroid and Parathyroid Glands, 1st ed. St. Louis, MO: CV Mosby, 1985; 293–366.
11. Kini SR, Miller JM, Hamburger JI, Smith MJ. Cytopathology of papillary carcinoma of the thyroid by fine needle aspiration. Acta Cytol 1980; 24:511–521.
12. Zhu Z, Gandhi M, Nikiforova MN, et al. Molecular profile and clinical-pathologic features of the follicular variant of papillary thyroid carcinoma. An unusually high prevalence of ras mutations. Am J Clin Pathol 2003; 120:71–77.
13. Gallagher J, Oertel YC, Oertel JE. Follicular variant of papillary carcinoma of the thyroid: fine-needle aspirates with histologic correlation. Diagn Cytopathol 1997; 16:207–213.
14. de los Santos ET, Keyhani-Rofagha S, Cunningham JJ, Mazzaferri EL. Cystic thyroid nodules: the dilemma of malignant lesions. Arch Intern Med 1990; 150:1422–1427.
15. Busseniers AE, Oertel YC. "Cellular adenomatoid nodules" of the thyroid: review of 219 fine-needle aspirates. Diagn Cytopathol 1993; 9:581–589.
16. Oertel YC. Fine-needle aspiration and the diagnosis of thyroid cancer. Endocrinol Metab Clin North Am 1996; 25:69–91.
17. Droese M. Atlas and Manual: Aspiration Cytology of the Thyroid, 2nd ed. Stuttgart: Schat-Tauer, 1995.
18. Ostrowski MA, Asa CL, Chamberlain D, et al. Myxomatous change in papillary carcinoma of thyroid. Surg Pathol 1989; 2:249–256.
19. Gómez-Morales M, Alvaro T, Muñoz M, et al. Diffuse sclerosing papillary carcinoma of the thyroid gland: immunohistochemical analysis of the local host immune response. Histopathology 1991; 18:427–433.
20. Rosen IB, Azadian A, Walfish PG. Adverse aspects of small thyroid cancer and need for treatment. Head Neck 1995; 17:373–376.
21. Schroder S. Pathological and Clinical Features of Malignant Thyroid Tumours: Classification, Immunohistology, Prognostic Criteria. New York: Gustav Fischer, 1988.
22. Beckner ME, Heffess CS, Oertel JE. Oxyphilic papillary thyroid carcinomas. Am J Clin Pathol 1995; 103:280–287.
23. Pilotti S, Collini P, Manzari A, et al. Poorly differentiated forms of papillary thyroid carcinoma: distinctive entities or morphological patterns? Semin Diagn Pathol 1995; 12:249–255.
24. Ostrowski ML, Merino MJ. Tall cell variant of papillary thyroid carcinoma: a reassessment and immunohistochemical study with comparison to the usual type of papillary carcinoma of the thyroid. Am J Surg Pathol 1996; 20:964–974.
25. Ozaki O, Ito K, Mimura T, et al. Papillary carcinoma of the thyroid: tall-cell variant with extensive lymphocyte infiltration. Am J Surg Pathol 1996; 20:695–698.
26. Solomon A, Gupta PK, LiVolsi VA, Baloch ZW. Distinguishing tall cell variant of papillary thyroid carcinoma from usual variant of papillary thyroid carcinoma in cytologic specimens. Diagn Cytopathol 2002; 27:143–148.
27. Kaw YT. Fine needle aspiration cytology of the tall cell variant of papillary carcinoma of the thyroid. Acta Cytol 1994; 38:282–283.
28. Gamboa-Dominguez A, Candanedo-González F, Uribe-Uribe NO, Angeles-Angeles A. Tall cell variant of papillary thyroid carcinoma: a cytohistologic correlation. Acta Cytol 1997; 41:672–676.
29. Bocklage T, DiTomasso JP, Ramzy I, Ostrowski ML. Tall cell variant of papillary thyroid carcinoma: cytologic features and differential diagnostic considerations. Diagn Cytopathol 1997; 17:25–29.
30. Tscholl-Ducommun J, Hedinger CE. Papillary thyroid carcinomas: morphology and prognosis. Virchows Arch A Pathol Anat Histopathol 1982; 396:19–39.
31. Tennvall J, Biörklund A, Möller T, et al. Prognostic factors of papillary, follicular and medullary carcinomas of the thyroid gland: retrospective multivariate analysis of 216 patients with a median follow-up of 11 years. Acta Radiol Oncol 1985; 24:17–24.
32. Mizukami Y, Noguchi M, Michigishi T, et al. Papillary thyroid carcinoma in Kanazawa, Japan: prognostic significance of histological subtypes. Histopathology 1992; 20:243–250.
33. Akslen LA. Prognostic importance of histologic grading in papillary thyroid carcinoma. Cancer 1993; 72:2680–2685.
34. Evans HL. Columnar cell carcinoma of the thyroid: a report of two cases of an aggressive variant of thyroid carcinoma. Am J Clin Pathol 1986; 85:77–80.
35. Hwang TS, Suh JS, Kim YI, et al. Poorly differentiated carcinoma of the thyroid: retrospective clinical and morphologic evaluation. J Korean Med Sci 1990; 5:47–52.
36. Ferreiro JA, Hay ID, Lloyd RV. Columnar cell carcinoma of the thyroid: report of three additional cases. Hum Pathol 1996; 27:1156–1160.
37. Evans HL. Encapsulated columnar-cell neoplasms of the thyroid: a report of four cases suggesting a favorable prognosis. Am J Surg Pathol 1996; 20:1205–1211.
38. Akslen LA, Varhaug JE. Thyroid carcinoma with mixed tall-cell and columnar-cell features. Am J Clin Pathol 1990; 94:442–445.
39. Mizukami Y, Nonomura A, Michigishi T, et al. Columnar cell carcinoma of the thyroid gland: a case report and review of the literature. Hum Pathol 1994; 25:1098–1101.
40. Gaertner EM, Davidson M, Wenig BM. The columnar cell variant of thyroid papillary carcinoma: case report and discussion of an unusually aggressive thyroid papillary carcinoma. Am J Surg Pathol 1995; 19:940–947.
41. Sobrinho-Simoes M, Nesland JM, Johannessen JV. Columnar-cell carcinoma: another variant of poorly differentiated carcinoma of the thyroid. Am J Clin Pathol 1988; 89:264–267.
42. Jayaram G. Cytology of columnar-cell variant of papillary thyroid carcinoma. Diagn Cytopathol 2000; 22:227–229.

Part IV
Well-Differentiated Thyroid Cancer
Initial Management

26
Prescribed Activity for Radioiodine Ablation

Douglas Van Nostrand

INTRODUCTION

Radioiodine or remnant ablation refers to the destruction of residual macroscopically normal thyroid tissue in the thyroid bed after near-total thyroidectomy in patients with well-differentiated thyroid carcinoma.

Five objectives have been proposed for radioiodine ablation (1–3) (1) to increase the sensitivity of detecting metastatic disease on subsequent radioiodine whole-body scans for patient follow-up; (2) to facilitate the interpretation of serum thyroglobulin levels for follow-up; (3) to obtain postablation whole-body scans, which have higher sensitivity than diagnostic scans; (4) to decrease the rate of recurrence; and (5) to increase survival.

Most authors agree that ablation achieves the first three objectives, which are discussed briefly in the first sections of this chapter. The last two objectives are controversial and are discussed in more detail. Two additional matters of debate are also examined: (1) If radioablation is performed, how much radioiodine should be used? (2) What is considered "successful" radioablation?

INCREASING THE SENSITIVITY OF METASTATIC DISEASE DETECTION

A large intense focus of radioiodine uptake may make it difficult to demonstrate more subtle foci of uptake in an *adjacent* area (see Fig. 28 in Chapter 15). This is especially true for whole-body or individual images obtained with a parallel-hole collimator. The longer that an intense focus of activity is imaged, the larger the apparent area of radioactivity is on the scan. This is frequently called "blooming" or "blossoming," and may obscure adjacent, less intense areas of radioiodine uptake. If the images are obtained for a shorter period of time, the number of counts may not be sufficient to demonstrate the second less intense area. This phenomenon was a larger problem with older analog imaging systems (not part of this discussion) but may also occur with newer digital imaging systems. In addition, a focus of tissue with intense uptake will compete for the radioiodine and may therefore reduce the radioiodine available for uptake elsewhere. At least theoretically, this may reduce visualization of more distant functioning metastases. Finally, even a small amount of residual thyroid tissue can produce enough thyroid hormone to interfere with the patient's ability to increase their endogenous thyrotropin (TSH), and thus also reduce TSH stimulation of potential uptake of radioiodine by the tumor. By ablating all or most of the residual functioning thyroid tissue, one may (1) better assess the area that initially had uptake from the residual thyroid tissue; (2) eliminate or reduce competition between residual normal thyroid tissue and metastatic carcinoma for radioiodine for future diagnostic scans or therapies; and (3) enhance tumor visualization when thyroid hormone withdrawal is used to increase endogenous TSH production.

FACILITATING THE INTERPRETATION OF SERUM THYROGLOBULIN LEVELS

Normal residual functioning thyroid tissue produces thyroglobulin that can make the use and interpretation of serum thyroglobulin levels more problematic as a marker for metastatic thyroid cancer. However, radioiodine ablation of residual thyroid tissue can eliminate (in most cases) this source of thyroglobulin from nonmalignant cells, thereby allowing the interpretation of serum thyroglobulin levels to be easier and more reliable. Nevertheless, this objective of radioiodine ablation is also somewhat controversial. Schlumberger (2) suggests that thyroglobulin measurements taken while the patient is on thyroid suppression can be accurately followed even if the residual thyroid tissue is not ablated. Within this context, radioiodine ablation may only be indicated in those patients who have detectable thyroglobulin levels while on thyroid suppression. With the increasingly routine use of periodic recombinant human (rh) TSH-stimulated thyroglobulin levels to assess the presence of disease, prior radioiodine ablation would also be useful in these patients to facilitate the subsequent interpretation of serum thyroglobulin levels.

OBTAINING INFORMATION FROM POSTABLATION WHOLE-BODY SCANS

Scans performed after radioablation have higher sensitivity for the detection of functioning thyroid metastases than diagnostic scans because the prescribed activities are much greater *(4–9)*. The information obtained from the postablative scan may have prognostic value, which then may alter the schedule for follow-up, subsequent management, or both.

EFFECTS OF RADIOABLATION ON RECURRENCE AND SURVIVAL

A reduced recurrence rate and increased survival is achieved—at least theoretically—by (1) ablating functioning or nonfunctioning cancer within the residual thyroid tissue; (2) ablating functioning metastases outside the thyroid bed; and (3) ablating normal thyroid cells in the residual thyroid tissue that are destined to become malignant *(10)*. However, whether these theoretical mechanisms actually result in reduced recurrence rate and increased survival is still debatable *(1,2,11–26)*.

Sawka et al. *(11)* performed a review of 1543 English references to determine whether remnant ablation decreases the risk of recurrence or thyroid cancer–related death after bilateral thyroidectomy for papillary or follicular thyroid cancer. Out of this group, only 23 studies met their inclusion/exclusion criteria for review. Of these 23 studies, 13 cohort studies employed multivariate analyses that were statistically adjusted to a variable degree for prognostic factors or cointerventions, whereas 18 cohort studies reported unadjusted data.

In the 13 statistically adjusted cohort studies, rates of *recurrences* of thyroid cancer–related outcomes were significantly *decreased* as follows:

- One of seven studies examining thyroid cancer–related mortality.
- Three of six studies evaluating tumor recurrence.
- Three of three studies analyzing locoregional recurrence.
- Two of three studies examining distant metastases.

For thyroid cancer–related mortality, only one study reported a statistically significant benefit for radioiodine ablation. Six studies, each examining between 135 and 2282 patients, reported no mortality advantage. For tumor recurrence, the two largest studies of 1501 and 1599 patients, as well as a smaller study of 187 patients, showed a decrease in disease-specific mortality after radioiodine ablation. For locoregional recurrence, three studies of 135, 1587, and 382 patients revealed a reduction. For distant metastases, two studies (1510 and 1587 patients) showed a decrease.

In the 18 cohort studies in which there was no statistical adjustment for prognostic variables or cointervention, the benefit of radioiodine in reducing thyroid cancer–related recurrence and mortality was inconsistent. A pooled analysis suggested that ablation might decrease locoregional recurrence and distant metastases. Sawka et al. *(11)* concluded "that the effectiveness of radioiodine ablation decreasing recurrence and possibly mortality in low-risk patients with well-differentiated thyroid carcinoma, although suspected, cannot be definitively verified by summarizing the current body of observational patient data *(11)*."

Despite the comprehensive analysis by Sawka et al., the controversy over the efficacy of ablation continued with the belief that analysis may be more significant after risk stratification of patients. Thus, by dividing the patient population based on the size of the primary tumor and other factors determining tumor stage, the decision-making process regarding ablation for an individual patient may be facilitated.

Impact of Primary Tumor Size

In patients who have a single primary tumor of less than 1.5-cm diameter, no local invasion, no positive nodes, and no distant metastasis, the prognosis is excellent without a significant survival benefit gained from postoperative radioiodine ablation *(12,15–18)*.

In patients with a primary tumor of more than 1.5 cm in diameter, with or without residual disease or extension, the controversy persists. Separating the published data for the rates of recurrence and survival by the presence or absence of residual disease and extension is problematic, as already demonstrated by Sawka. Nevertheless, several selected studies are briefly discussed below to present the spectrum of the data involving this debate.

For patients with a primary tumor greater than 1.5 cm who have undergone near-total thyroidectomy, it has been generally accepted that radioablation improves recurrence rates and survival, based on an early study by Mazzaferri et al. *(21)*. In 1994, Mazzaferri *(18)* reported on 1004 patients in whom not only was the tumor recurrence rate about threefold lower ($p < 0.001$), but also fewer patients developed distant metastases ($p < 0.002$) after thyroid remnant ablation than after other forms of postoperative treatment in patients with primary tumors 1.5 cm or more. Similarly, there were fewer cancer deaths after thyroid remnant ablation than after the other treatment strategies ($p < 0.001$) in patients over age 40 with primary tumors 1.5 cm or greater.

Mazzaferri subsequently updated his data in 2001 *(1)*. In this study, remnant ablation was performed in 230 patients, whereas 789 patients had only thyroid hormone suppression, and 163 patients received no medical therapy. The mean follow-up in each of these groups was 14.7, 20.8, and 21.2 yr, respectively. The recurrence rate for the suppression-alone group was four times higher than that of the ablation group ($p < 0.0001$), and the rate of distant recurrence was five times higher ($p < 0.02$) then that after thyroid ablation (see Fig. 1A,B). Based on regression modeling of 1510 patients without distant metastases at the time of initial therapy, Mazzaferri reported that remnant ablation was an independent

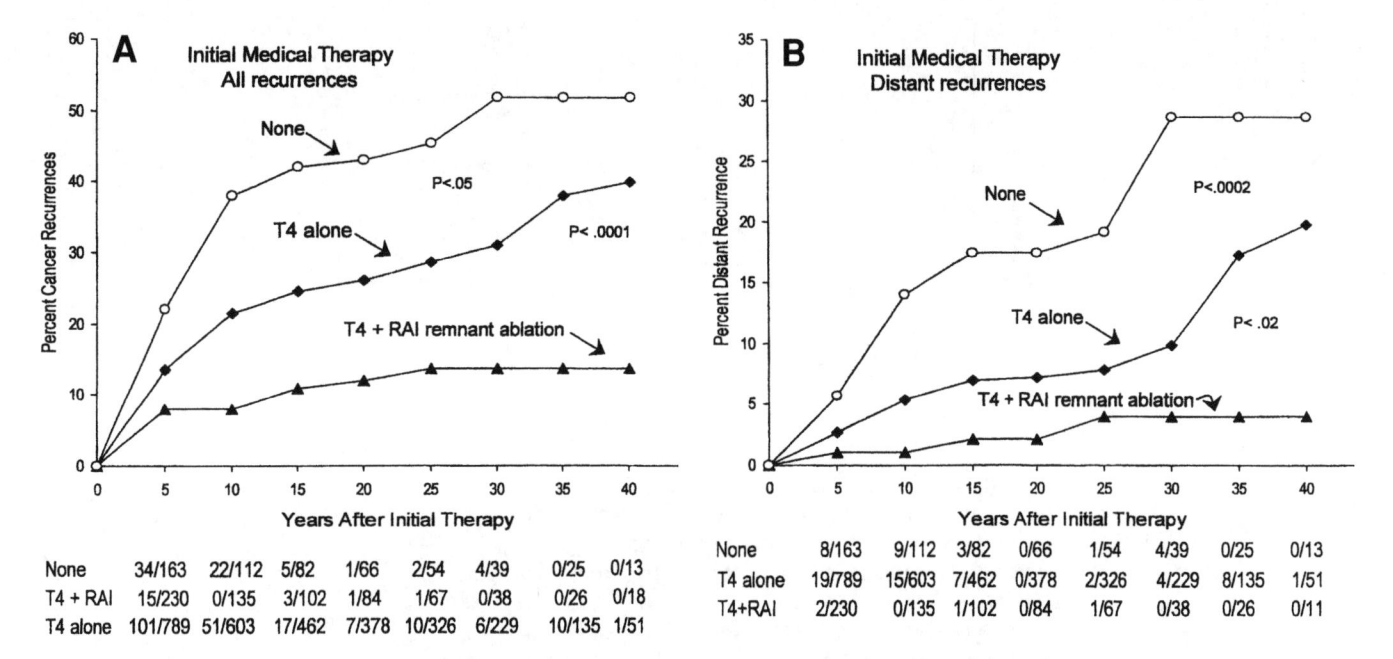

Fig. 1. Tumor recurrence 16.7 yr (median) after thyroid surgery and ^{131}I ablation of uptake in the thyroid bed compared with those treated with thyroid hormone alone. The numerator is the number of patients with recurrence, and the denominator is the number of patients in each time interval. **(A)** All recurrences. **(B)** Distant metastases recurrences. P values are the log rank statistical analysis of 40-yr life-table data *(1)*. Reproduced with permission from EL Mazzaferri, MD and the Endocrine Society.

variable that reduced cancer recurrence, distant recurrences, and cancer death (see Fig. 2).

DeGroot et al. *(16)* reported that remnant ablation decreased recurrence of tumors larger than 1 cm, including those predicted to have a good prognosis (patients with stage I or II disease). However, remnant ablation reduced the risk of death only in patients with more advanced disease (stage III or IV disease).

Massin et al. *(22)* reported that the rates of pulmonary metastases among 58 patients with well-differentiated thyroid cancer were 11% after partial thyroidectomy, 5% after subtotal thyroidectomy and ^{131}I, 3% after total thyroidectomy, and 1.3% after total thyroidectomy and ^{131}I.

Tsang et al. reported that total thyroidectomy and ^{131}I radioablation in 382 patients was associated with a significantly lower rate of local relapse, independent of tumor stage *(23)*.

Using data obtained from 13 Canadian hospitals, Simpson et al. *(20)* reviewed 1578 patients of whom 201 patients had postoperative external radiotherapy, 214 had radioiodine therapy, and 107 had both. In patients with no residual disease (i.e., no cancer observed close to the resection margins), neither radiotherapy nor radioiodine ablation significantly improved local control (see Table 1). In a group of 244 patients with microscopic residual disease (defined as disease within 2 mm of the margin), the local cancer was controlled more often after ^{131}I therapy, with or without postoperative external radiotherapy, than with thyroid hormone alone (Table 2). However, the interpretation of Simpson's data has been debated *(2)*. Schlumberger and Hay *(2)* cited Simpson's data as evidence that the difference between the recurrence rates reported by Mazzaferri *(17,18,21)* and Grebe *(25)* at the Mayo Clinic were owing to the extent and completeness of the surgery, not radioiodine ablation. However, Wartofsky *(2)* interprets Simpsons' data as demonstrating a "benefit from radioiodine ablation." The potential benefit is (1) the ablation of microscopic residual disease that the physician may not be aware of and (2) the maximization of the utility of subsequent radioiodine scans, serum thyroglobulin levels, or both.

In a group of 94 patients, Hay *(24)* reported recurrence rates of 9.6% for those treated with surgery alone ($n = 726$) and 13.3% for patients who also received radioiodine ablation ($n = 220$). Cause-specific mortality rates at 10 yr were 2.0% and 3.0% in the surgical and radioiodine treatment groups, respectively.

Grebe and Hay *(25)* reported that the recurrence rates at 30 yr were comparable for both the radioiodine ablation group (16.6%) and the nonradioiodine ablation group (19.1%; $p = 0.89$). Similarly, the death rates for the two groups (5.9% and 7.8%, respectively) were not statistically different ($p = 0.43$). Schlumberger and Hay proposed that the variations between their results and those of Simpson's may be related to the extent and completeness of the surgical excision in the two groups, but this also has been debated *(2)*.

The data and utility of radioiodine treatment for patients with a primary tumor more than 1.5 cm, with significant extension and metastasis, are discussed further in Chapter 45 entitled "Radioiodine Treatment."

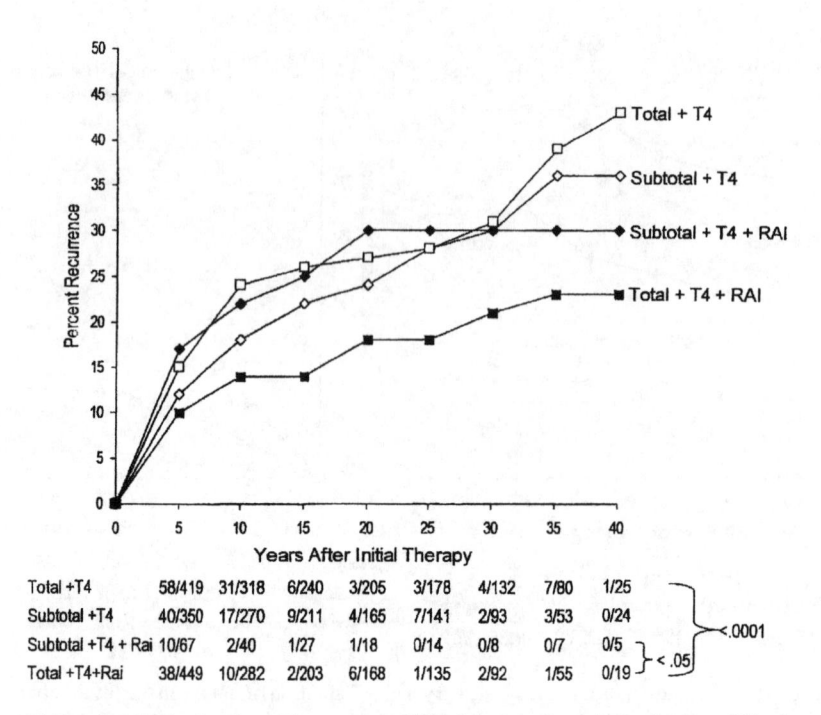

[Graph showing Percent Recurrence vs Years After Initial Therapy with four curves: Total + T4, Subtotal + T4, Subtotal + T4 + RAI, Total + T4 + RAI]

Total +T4	58/419	31/318	6/240	3/205	3/178	4/132	7/80	1/25
Subtotal +T4	40/350	17/270	9/211	4/165	7/141	2/93	3/53	0/24
Subtotal +T4 + Rai	10/67	2/40	1/27	1/18	0/14	0/8	0/7	0/5
Total +T4+Rai	38/449	10/282	2/203	6/168	1/135	2/92	1/55	0/19

Fig. 2. Tumor recurrence 16.7 yr (median) after thyroid surgery and ^{131}I ablation of uptake in the thyroid bed compared with those treated with thyroid hormone alone. The numerator is the number of patients with recurrence; the denominator is the number of patients in each time interval. **(A)** All recurrences. **(B)** Distant metastases recurrences. P values are the log rank statistical analysis of 40-yr life-table data *(1)*. Reproduced with permission from EL Mazzaferri, MD and the Endocrine Society.

Table 1
Frequency of Local Control in Patients With No Residual Disease*

Treatment	Papillary	Follicular
Surgery ± thyroid hormone	86% (535 patients)	85% (209 patients)
Surgery + radiotherapy	86% (56 patients)	90% (21 patients)
Surgery + radioiodine	90% (61 patients)	86% (57 patients)
Surgery + radiotherapy + radioiodine	100% (12 patients)	90% (10 patients)
	$p = 0.46$	$p = 0.87$

*No residual disease was defined as no cancer close to resection margins. Cancer within 2 mm of resection margin was considered microscopic residual disease. Adapted from ref. *20*.

Table 2
Frequency of Local Control in Patients With Microscopic Residual Disease*

Treatment	Papillary	Follicular
Surgery ± thyroid hormone	26% (38 patients)	38% (21 patients)
Surgery + radiotherapy	90% (52 patients)	53% (15 patients)
Surgery + radioiodine	82% (39 patients)	77% (13 patients)
Surgery + radiotherapy + radioiodine	86% (43 patients)	70% (23 patients)
	$p = 0.00001$	$p = 0.079$

*Residual disease was defined as disease extending to the margin or within 2 mm of the resected margin. Adapted from ref. *20*.

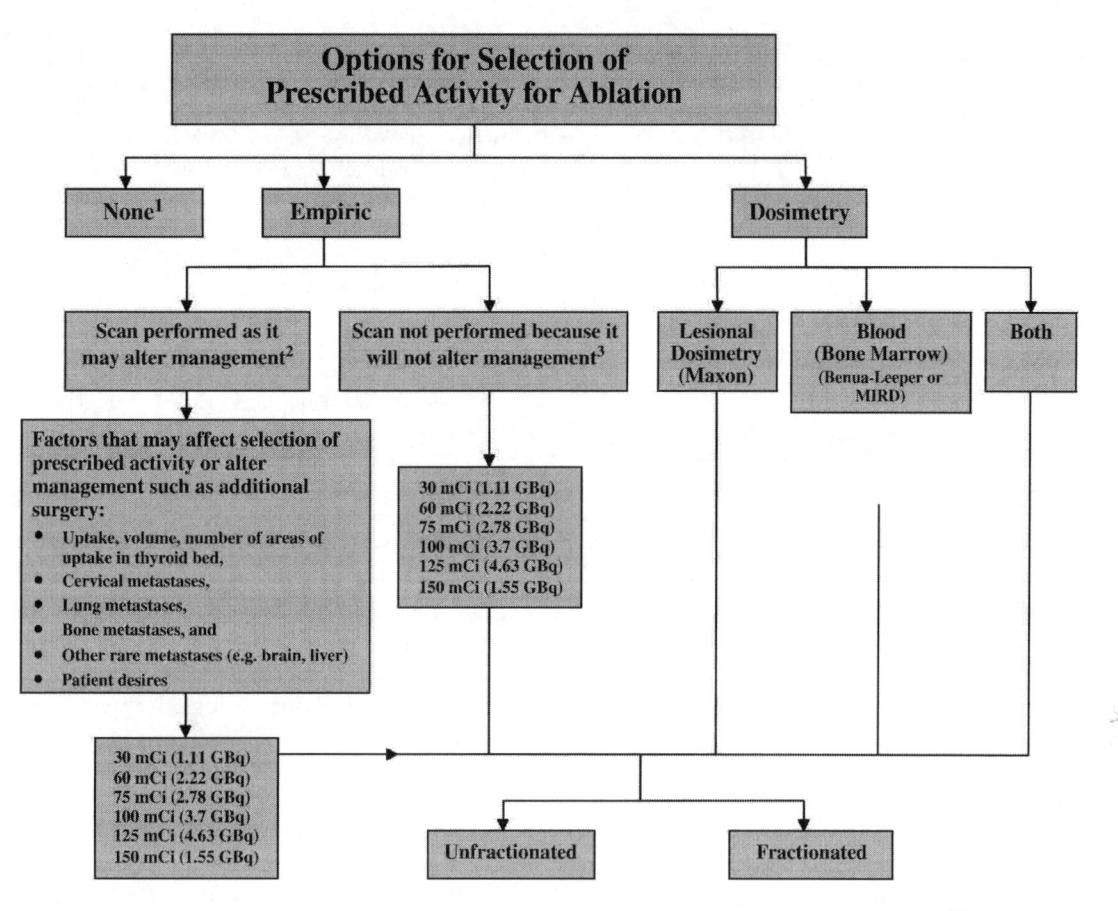

Fig. 3. This algorithm displays an overview of most of the options for the selection of prescribed activity of ^{131}I for ablation.

[1]If the primary tumor is less than 1.5 cm in diameter, with no local invasion, no positive nodes, and no distant metastasis, no administration of radioiodine.

[2]For further discussion, see Chapter 14. For metastatic disease, empiric prescribed activity for initial ablation (treatment) with higher than 150 mCi (1.55 GBq) of radioiodine has been advocated and used. See Chapter 45.

[3]See text in this chapter.

SELECTING THE PRESCRIBED ACTIVITY FOR RADIOABLATION

Many approaches for the selection of the radioiodine prescribed activity for ablation have been proposed and are currently being used (see Fig. 3). One option is to use prescribed activity that is selected empirically, which is defined by *Webster's New World Dictionary* as "relying or based on practical experience without reference to scientific principles."

One such set of empiric values for prescribed activities was proposed by Beierwaltes et al. *(26)*. Empiric prescribed activities for radioiodine ablation may range from 29 to 150 mCi (1.07–5.55 GBq). Although many facilities use one empiric prescribed activity for all patients (a fixed-standard empiric prescribed activity), other facilities alter the empiric prescribed activity (if needed) based on a number of variables. These factors include the patient's level of risk, uptake in the thyroid bed, number of foci of uptake in the thyroid bed,

patient weight, body surface area, the patient's fear regarding radiation, and regulations in terms of hospitalization. However, there are no standardized rules by which these adjustments in the empiric prescribed activity can be made quantitatively and objectively. Prescribed activities have also been administered in two or more fractions given at weekly intervals *(27,28,28a)*. The prescribed activity of radioiodine ablation may also be determined for each individual patient based on lesional dosimetry *(29)*, whole-body dosimetry *(30)*, or both. These are discussed in Chapter 47 entitled "Dosimetry."

Some issues that influence the selection of prescribed activity for ablation are noted in Table 3. Within the United States, prescribed activity 30 mCi or less (1.11 GBq) does not require hospitalization. More recent regulations permit some patients to receive prescribed activities from 75 to over 100 mCi (2.8 to >3.7 GBq) as part of outpatient care. These patients must be willing and able to comply with specific instructions designed to minimize exposure to both family members and the general public below specific reg-

Table 3
Factors Affecting Selections of Prescribed Activity for Radioiodine Ablation

Expense
Public risk
Patient convenience
Potential side effects
Rate of successful ablation
Hospitalization

Table 4
Factors That Impact the Results of Ablation

Extent of surgery
Percent uptake of radioiodine in residual thyroid tissue
Volume of residual thyroid tissue
Effective half-life of ^{131}I in the residual thyroid tissue
Geometrical shape of residual thyroid tissue
Patient compliance with low-iodine diet
Value of low-iodine diet
Level of TSH
Previous diagnostic prescribed activity of ^{131}I
Stunning
Definition of "successful" thyroid bed ablation

Table 5
Society Guidelines for Prescribed Activity of Radioiodine for Ablation in Patients With Thyroid Cancer

Society of Nuclear Medicine Procedure Guideline for Therapy of Thyroid Disease With ^{131}I
"A variety of approaches have been used to select the amount of administered activity. General guidelines are: For postoperative ablation of thyroid bed remnants, activity in the range of 75–150 mCi (2.75–5.5 GBq) is typically administered, depending on the RAIU and amount of residual functioning tissue present."

European Association of Nuclear Medicine Procedure Guidelines for Therapy With ^{131}I
"For thyroid malignancy . . . for patients undergoing ablation of thyroid remnant, administered activities in the range of 100–150 mCi (3700–5500 MBq) are usually given."

Quotes taken from refs. 48–50. RAIU, radioactive iodine uptake.

ulatory limits. Obviously, outpatient treatments are more convenient for patients and reduce health care costs.

Specific factors that confound the interpretation of the data regarding these various methods to select the prescribed activity for ablation are presented in Table 4. The current guidelines recommended by the Society of Nuclear Medicine and the European Association of Nuclear Medicine are summarized in Table 5.

As noted above, the selection of an empiric prescribed activity remains controversial. Many articles suggest that prescribed activities in the lower range, e.g., 30–50 mCi (1.11–1.85 GBq), are as effective as prescribed activities in the higher range, e.g., 100–150 mCi (3.7–5.55 GBq), and vice versa. DeGroot et al. *(31)* compared the utility of 30 mCi (1.11 GBq) with higher 50–60 mCi (1.85–2.22 GBq) of prescribed activities of ^{131}I. Of the 18 patients who had received the lower prescribed activity, 15 had successful ablation, whereas all 30 patients who received the higher prescribed activity had successful ablation. Mazzaferri *(1)* noted no difference in success of ^{131}I ablation between two stratified groups. For patients with prescribed activities of 29–50 mCi (1.97–1.85 GBq) and 51–200 mCi (1.88–7.4 GBq), similar 30-yr recurrence rates of 4% and 6% ($p < 0.1$) were observed, respectively. Kuni et al. *(32)* reported successful ablation in only 1 of 13 patients after an initial prescribed activity between 25 and 29.9 mCi (925–1106 MBq) of ^{131}I. Bal et al. *(33)* observed complete ablation in 17 of 27 (63%) remnants after 30 mCi (1.11 GBq); 42 of 54 (78%) after 50 mCi (1.85 GBq); 28 of 38 (74%) after 90 mCi (3.33 GBq); and 23 of 30 (77%) after 155 mCi (9.4 GBq). Thus, they concluded that the dose–response curve reached a plateau after 50 mCi (1.85 GBq). Bal et al. *(34)* further evaluated prescribed activities between 15 and 50 mCi (555–1850 MBq) in 509 patients. Ablation was successful in 78% of the patients (395), but the success rate was only 60% in patients who took 15–20 mCi (555–740 MBq) and 80% in patients receiving 25–50 mCi (925–1850 MBq). Prescribed activities higher than 50 mCi (1850 MBq) were not administered.

This chapter could continue to review the many other studies that either support lower or higher prescribed activities for radioiodine ablation. Doi and Woodhouse *(35)* performed a meta-analysis of 19 studies published between January 1966 and June 1999 that evaluated various prescribed activities of radioiodine for ablation. Eleven of these studies met Doi and Woodhouse's criteria for inclusion in a comparative analysis, and they added two of their own cohort studies. The prescribed activities were categorized as "high" (75–100 mCi [2.78–3.7 GBq]) and "low" (29–30 mCi [1.074–1.11 GBq]). The average failure of a single low-prescribed activity was 46% ± 28%. Meta-analysis revealed (1) a statistically significant advantage for a single high prescribed activity over a single low-prescribed activity and (2) a pooled reduction in the relative risk of failure of the high-prescribed activity of approx 27% ($p < 0.01$). From this data, Doi and Woodhouse estimated that for every seven patients treated, one additional patient would be ablated when a high, rather than low, prescribed activity was administered. Based on this multistudy analysis, Doi and Woodhouse concluded that high-prescribed activities were more efficient than low-prescribed activities for remnant ablation, which was particularly true after near total thyroidectomy. The debate is likely to continue.

As noted above, fractionated ablative radioiodine treatments have also been proposed. Arad et al. *(27)* achieved successful ablation in 75% (9 of 12). In 99 patients, Wang et al. *(28)* achieved successful ablation in 72% (71 patients). However, fractionated prescribed activities may result in stunning, partial treatment, or both. Consequently, the first "treatment" could significantly reduce the uptake of the second "treatment," which would most likely result in less absorbed radiation dose to the residual thyroid tissue or cancer for essentially the same amount of absorbed radiation dose to the bone marrow, salivary glands, and other organs. Stunning, partial treatment, or both may also occur even when the second treatment is administered as early as 1 wk after the first prescribed activity. In addition, fractioned ablations result in lower radiation absorbed dose rates, and Samuel et al. *(36)* demonstrated the importance of dose rate. In 87 patients, the initial dose rate was significantly higher in patients who had complete ablation of residual thyroid tissue than in those patients who had only partial ablation ($0.05 > p > 0.02$). Samuel concluded that the higher the radiation absorbed dose rate in the first 24–48 h, the higher the success rate of ablation. Again, fractionated ablations reduce the dose rate. Although the administration of fractionated treatments might be a potential option in a country where regulatory or facility constraints prevent patients from receiving an unfractionated treatment, this author believes that unless there is a compelling reason, ablative treatments should not be fractionated. If the ablative radioiodine must be fractionated, then the interval between treatments could be shortened to 1 or 2 d *(37)*.

Empiric prescribed activities may also be modified by other factors. Numerous reports have demonstrated a relationship between the success of ablation and (1) the mass of residual tissue *(36)*, (2) the radioiodine uptake *(26,29, 37–44,44a)*, and (3) effective half-time of ^{131}I in tissue *(29,38,39)*. Samuel et al. *(36)* demonstrated the importance of the tissue mass size as an important determinant for successful ablation of residual thyroid tissue. For patients taking an initial dose rate of 300 rad/h (cGy/h), complete ablation was achieved in 87% of patients when the size of the residual tissue was less than 5 g and 52% when the size was more than 5 g. Regarding uptake, Hodgson et al. *(40)* reported that patients who had lower radioiodine uptake on postoperative thyroid scans could receive lower activities of ^{131}I while maintaining the same ablation rate.

Maxon et al. *(39)* initially reported that there was no association between the amount of ^{131}I administered and uptake pertaining to success of the ablation. They subsequently showed that the two most important factors impacting successful ablation were the mass of residual tissue ($p < 0.001$) and the effective half-time of ^{131}I in the thyroid tissue ($p < 0.05$) *(38)*. However, in this study, the radioiodine uptake was also important; as the uptake increased, the success rate decreased. Although it might be expected that the

Table 6
Modification Factors of Prescribed Activity for Childhood Ablation

Factor	Body Weight (kg)	Body Surface Area (m^2)
0.2	10	0.4
0.4	25	0.8
0.6	40	1.2
0.8	55	1.4
1.0	77	1.7

Body surface area = $0.1 \times$ (Weight in kg)$^{0.67}$. Adapted from refs. *45* and *46*.

higher the uptake, the higher the success rate, this would be true only if the thyroid tissue mass was the same. However, Maxon showed that the uptake correlated highly—and was inseparable—from the mass of residual thyroid tissue *(37)*. Thus, size of the residual tissue (mass), effective half-time, and/or uptake possibly as a surrogate marker for the size of thyroid tissue) could be used to modify the empiric prescribed activity. The larger the residual tissue (mass) and/or as the uptake increases, the higher the empiric prescribed activity that is needed; the longer the effective half-time, the lower the empiric prescribed activity that is required. Logically, this is expected and is the foundation of the quantitative lesional dosimetry described and used by Thomas and Maxon *(29,38,39)*.

Regarding other possible factors considered when determining the ablative prescribed activity, Reynolds et al. *(45)* noted the absorbed radiation dose for children had a linear relationship with body weight and body surface area. They proposed factors based on these parameters for reducing the prescribed activity (see Table 6). For example, if the intended adult prescribed activity is 100 mCi (3.7 GBq), and the child weighed 25 kg, then the Reynolds' factor would reduce the child's prescribed activity to 40 mCi (1.48 GBq) (0.4 factor × 100 mCi) *(46)*.

The lesional and whole-body dosimetry for the selection of the prescribed activity for radioiodine ablation are again discussed in Chapter 47 entitled, "Dosimetry." Maxon *(38)* performed lesional dosimetry according to the method described by Thomas *(29)*. In 142 thyroid remnants in 70 patients, ^{131}I ablation was successful in 81% (57) of patients and 86% (122) of foci of residual thyroid tissue. Although whole-body dosimetry could be performed to limit the maximal permissible prescribed activity for radioiodine ablation, it is infrequently done. When a radioiodine whole-body scan does not demonstrate any evidence of functioning metastases, such as diffuse pulmonary metastases, the likelihood that an empiric prescribed activity in the range of 30–100 mCi (1.11–3.7 GBq) would exceed 200 rad (200 cGy) to the blood—a surrogate for the bone marrow—would be low *(27a)*. It would not (in this author's opinion)

Table 7
Various Criteria Used to Define "Successful" or "Adequate" Radioablation of the Thyroid Bed

No visible radioiodine accumulation above background in the thyroid bed
If visible radioiodine accumulation is above background in the thyroid bed, then an uptake of <0.1%, <0.2%, <0.5%, or <1.0% at variable time intervals from dosing at 24, 48, or 72 h
TSH-stimulated thyroglobulin undetectable of <1, <2, or <5 ng/mL
Whole-body retention at 7 d of <3%
Various combinations of the above

An Algorithm for the Selection of Prescribed Activity for Radioiodine Ablation

Low risk patient*
- No scan or ablation

Moderate to high risk patient**
- Perform an I-123 whole body post-operative pre-ablation scan with 24-hour thyroid bed uptake.

Known metastatic disease
- Manage on an individual basis.
- Lesional and whole body dosimetry to determine initial radioiodine prescribed activity

Findings in thyroid bed most consistent with normal residual thyroid tissue

*Findings suggesting metastatic disease or ≥ 4 foci of uptake in thyroid bed****

Pediatric
- Ablate with reduced empiric prescribed activity.
- Use Reynolds' modification factors as guidelines (See Table 6).
- Frequently in the range of 30-75 mCi (1.11-2.8 GBq) depending upon the body weight and/or surface areas.

Adult

- Modify management on an individual basis such as discussed in Table 6 of Chapter 14 entitled Radioiodine Whole Body Imaging and Chapter 45 entitled Radioiodine Treatment.
- Lesional and whole body dosimetry

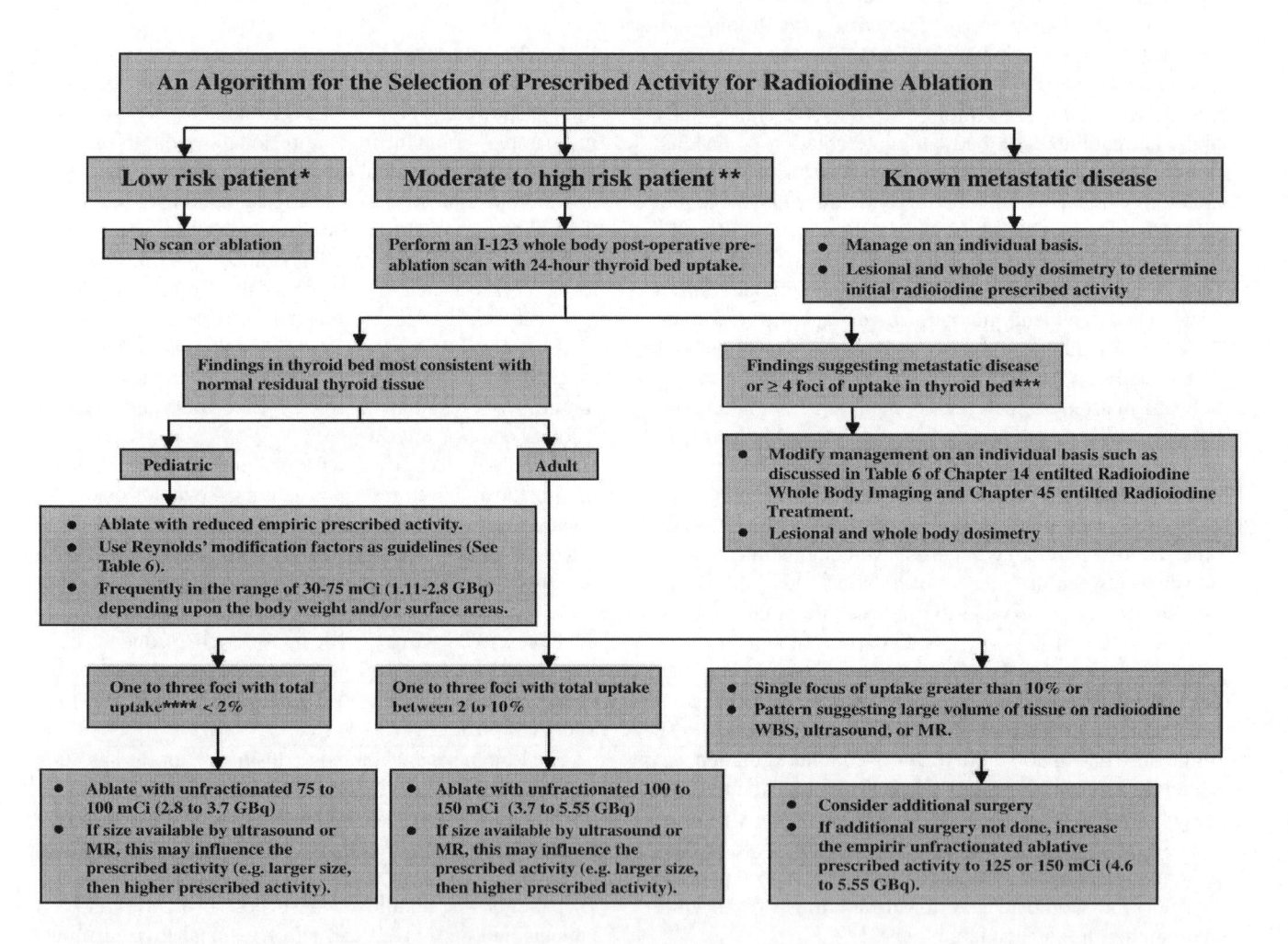

One to three foci with total uptake** < 2%**
- Ablate with unfractionated 75 to 100 mCi (2.8 to 3.7 GBq)
- If size available by ultrasound or MR, this may influence the prescribed activity (e.g. larger size, then higher prescribed activity).

One to three foci with total uptake between 2 to 10%
- Ablate with unfractionated 100 to 150 mCi (3.7 to 5.55 GBq)
- If size available by ultrasound or MR, this may influence the prescribed activity (e.g. larger size, then higher prescribed activity).

- Single focus of uptake greater than 10% or
- Pattern suggesting large volume of tissue on radioiodine WBS, ultrasound, or MR.
  - Consider additional surgery
  - If additional surgery not done, increase the empiric unfractionated ablative prescribed activity to 125 or 150 mCi (4.6 to 5.55 GBq).

Fig. 4. *A low-risk patient is defined for this algorithm as a patient who has a primary of <1.5-cm diameter, no invasion, no positive nodes, no distant metastasis, two or less microscopic foci, and well-differentiated thyroid cancer without histopathology associated with a worse prognosis (e.g., tall-cell variant or Hurthle cell carcinoma).
**Anybody that is not in the low-risk group.
***The number of separate foci of residual normal thyroid tissue in the thyroid bed depends on the individual surgeon. However, with our surgeons, there are typically only one or two areas of thyroid tissue left in the thyroid bed. As the number of foci increases over three in our patients, the likelihood of metastases significantly increases, such that metastatic thyroid carcinoma to lymph nodes or metastasis in the soft tissue must be considered. (See Chapter 15 entitled "Primer and Atlas of Radioiodine Whole-Body Imaging," Fig. 15.)
****Although it is expected that the higher the uptake, the lower the required prescribed activity of radioiodine, the uptake in this case is most likely a surrogate marker for the volume of the residual thyroid tissue (see text; 46).

Table 8
"Successful" Ablation

Ideal

No visible radioiodine accumulation above background in the thyroid bed on:
- A pinhole image obtained 24 h or later after the administration of 4 mCi (148 MBq) of ^{123}I with an acquisition time of at least 10 min and with a TSH >25 or rhTSH injections on the 2 d prior to the day of radioiodine dosing *or*
- A pinhole image obtained 48 h or later after the administration of 1 mCi (74 MBq) of ^{131}I using a pinhole collimator with acquisition time of at least 10 min and with a TSH >25 or two rhTSH injections on the 2 d prior to the day of radioiodine dosing

Acceptable

If one or two visible foci of radioiodine accumulation are noted above the background in the thyroid bed, then the 24-h uptake of thyroid bed is ≤0.5%, *and*
TSH-stimulated thyroglobulin level <2 ng/mL (controversial)

---

warrant the extra (1) inconvenience for the patient, (2) work for the facility, and (3) cost. However, for pediatric or small patients, dosimetry may be appropriate.

RADIOABLATION OF RESIDUAL NORMAL THYROID TISSUE

Various criteria have been used to define what constitutes a successful or adequate radioiodine ablation of residual function thyroid tissue in the thyroid bed. Several of these criteria are listed in Table 7.

Several years ago, Wartofsky et al. *(2)* had proposed that for low-to-moderate risk patients, ablative therapy would not be required with a baseline thyroglobulin level of less than 5 ng/mL and a postoperative radioactive iodine uptake of less than 0.5%. This recommendation is likely to be different today, as better assays for thyroglobulin are allowing detection of thyroglobulin levels down to 0.3 ng/mL, which then prompt more aggressive therapy. Another popular criterion for ablation that has been suggested is the absence of any visible thyroid bed uptake, or if visible, then less than 0.1% of the tracer-prescribed activity, coupled with a secondary criteria of no visible uptake and TSH-stimulated thyroglobulin lower than 2 ng/mL. This was the criterion for a randomized, controlled, open-label, multinational trial to evaluate rhTSH and thyroid hormone withdrawal as preparation for thyroid remnant ablation in differentiated thyroid carcinoma *(47)*. No data are available to confirm whether one criteria, or a combination, is superior to another.

SUMMARY AND RECOMMENDATIONS

Radioiodine ablation has been advocated and used for many years, and it is generally successful in accomplishing a number of objectives. These include (1) increasing the sensitivity of detecting metastatic disease on subsequent radioiodine whole-body scans for patient follow-up, (2) facilitating the interpretation of serum thyroglobulin levels for follow-up, and (3) providing a postablation whole-body scan with higher sensitivity than a diagnostic scan. However, the debate continues regarding not only whether these three objectives warrant the cost, radiation exposure, and inconvenience of radioiodine ablation, but also whether radioiodine ablation actually improves the rate of recurrence and survival.

At this time, this author's algorithm for selecting the prescribed activity for radioiodine ablation is noted in Fig. 4, and the criteria for successful ablation are noted in Table 8. As with any algorithm or criteria, neither is absolute. Rather, they both represent one individual's guidelines, which must be modified based on the specific details of each individual patient. Of course, as new data become available, these guidelines will likely be modified.

REFERENCES

1. Mazzaferri EL, Kloos RT. Current approaches to primary therapy for papillary and follicular thyroid cancer. J Clin Endocrinol Metab 2001; 86:1447–1463.
2. Wartofsky L, Sherman SI, Gopal J, et al. Therapeutic Controversy: The use of radioactive iodine in patients with papillary and follicular thyroid cancer. J Clin Endocrinol Metab 1998; 83:4195–4203.
3. Klain M, Ricard M, Leboulleux S, et al. Radioiodine therapy for papillary and follicular thyroid carcinoma. Eur J Nucl Med 2002; 29 (Suppl 2):S479–S485.
4. Nemec J, Rohling S, Zamarazil V, Pohunkova D. Comparison of the distribution of diagnostic and thyroablative I-131 in the evaluation of differentiated thyroid cancers. J Nucl Med 1979; 20:92–97.
5. Balachandran S, Sayle BA. Value of thyroid carcinoma imaging after therapeutic doses of radioiodine. Clin Nucl Med 1981; 6:162–167.
6. Sherman SI, Tielens ET, Sostre S, et al. Clinical utility of post treatment radioiodine scans in the management of patients with thyroid carcinoma. J Clin Endocrinol Metab 1994; 78:629–634.
7. Spies WG, Wojtowicz CH, Spies SM, et al. Value of post-therapy whole-body I-131 imaging in the evaluation of patients with thyroid carcinoma having undergone high-dose I-131 therapy. Clin Nucl Med 1989; 14:793–800.
8. Fatourechi V, Hay ID, Mullan BP, et al. Are post therapy radioiodine scans informative and do they influence subsequent therapy of patients with differentiated thyroid cancer? Thyroid 2000; 10:573–577.
9. Pineda JD, Lee T, Ain K, et al. Iodine-131 therapy for thyroid cancer patients with elevated thyroglobulin and negative diagnostic scan. J Clin Endocrinol Metab 1995; 80:1488–1492.
10. Sugg SI, Ezzat S, Rosen IB, et al. Distinct multiple RET/PTC gene rearrangements in multifocal papillary thyroid neoplasia. J Clin Endocrinol Metab 1998; 83:4116–4122.
11. Sawka AM, Thephamongkhol K, Brouwers M, et al. A systematic review and meta-analysis of the effectiveness of radioactive iodine remnant ablation for well-differentiated thyroid cancer. J Clin Endocrinol Metab 2004; 89:3668–3676.
12. Dulgeroff AJ, Hershman JM. Medical therapy for differentiated thyroid carcinoma. Endocr Rev 1994; 15:500–515.
13. Heufelder AE, Gorman CA. Radioiodine therapy in the treatment of differentiated thyroid cancer: Guidelines and considerations. Endocrinologist 1991; 1:273–280.
14. Samaan NA, Schultz PN, Hickey RD, et al. The results of various modalities of treatment of well-differentiated thyroid carcinoma: a ret-

rospective review of 1599 patients. J Clin Endocrinol Metab 1992; 75: 714–720.
15. Hay ID, Bergstralh EJ, Goellner JR, et al. Predicting outcome in papillary thyroid carcinoma: development of a reliable prognostic scoring system in a cohort of 1779 patients surgically treated at one institution during 1980 though 1989. Surgery 1993; 114:1050–1058.
16. DeGroot KJ, Kaplan EL, McCormick M, Straus FH. Natural history, treatment, and course of papillary thyroid carcinoma. J Clin Endocrinol Metab 1990; 71:414–424.
17. Mazzaferri EL, Jhiang SM. Long-term impact of initial surgical and medical therapy on papillary and follicular thyroid cancer. Am J Med 1994; 97:418–428.
18. Mazzaferri EL. Thyroid remnant 131-I ablation for papillary and follicular thyroid carcinoma. Thyroid 1997; 7:265–271.
19. Hay ID, Grant CS, Van Heerden JA, et al. Papillary thyroid microcarcinoma: a study of 535 cases observed on a 50-year period. Surgery 1992; 112:1139–1147.
20. Simpson WJ, Panzarella T, Carruthers JS, et al. Papillary and follicular thyroid cancer: impact of treatment in 1578 patients. Int J Radiat Oncol Biol Phys 1988; 104:1063–1075.
21. Mazzaferri EL, Young RI, Oertel JE, et al. Papillary thyroid carcinoma: the impact of therapy in 576 patients. Medicine 1977; 56:171–196.
22. Massin JP, Savoie JC, Garnier H, et al. Pulmonary metastases in differentiated thyroid carcinoma: study of 58 cases with implications for the primary tumor treatment. Cancer 1984; 53:982–992.
23. Tsang TW, Brierley JD, Simpson WJ, et al. The effects of surgery, radioiodine, and external radiation therapy on the clinical outcome of patients with differentiated thyroid carcinoma. Cancer 1998; 82: 375–388.
24. Hay ID. Papillary thyroid carcinoma. Endocrinol Metab Clin North Am 1990; 19:545–576.
25. Grebe SKG, Hay ID. Follicular cell-derived thyroid carcinomas. In Arnold A, editor. Endocrine Neoplasm. Kluwer Academic Publishers, 1997: 91–140.
26. Beierwaltes WH, Rabbani R, Dmuchowski C, et al. An analysis of ablation of thyroid remnants" with I-131 in 511 patients from 1947–1984: experience at University of Michigan. J Nucl Med 1984; 25:1287–1293.
27. Arad E, Flannery K, Wilson GA, O'Mara R. Fractionated doses of radioiodine for ablation of postsurgical thyroid tissue remnants. Clin Nuc Med 1990; 10:676–677.
27a. Atkins F, Van Nostrand D, Kulkarni K, et al. The frequency with which empiric amounts of radioiodine "over" and "under" treat patients with metastatic well-differentiated thyroid cancer. J Nucl Med 2005; 46:129P.
28. Wang SJ, Liu TJ. Use of fractionated doses of iodine-131 for ablation of thyroid remnants. Chinese Med J 2002; 65:336–340.
28a. Hung Gu, Tu ST, Wu IS, et al. Comparison of the effectiveness between a single low dose and fractionated doses of radioiodine in ablation of post-operative thyroid remnants. Jpn J Clin Onc 2004; 34:469–471.
29. Thomas SR, Maxon HR, Kereiakes JG, Saenger EL. Quantitative external counting techniques enabling improved diagnostic and therapeutic decisions in patients with well-differentiated thyroid cancer. Radiology 1997; 122:731–737.
30. Benua RS, Cicale NR, Sonenberg M, Rawson RW. The relation of radioiodine dosimetry to results and complications in the treatment of metastatic thyroid cancer. Am J Roentgenol Radium Ther Nucl Med 1962; 87:171–182.
31. DeGroot L, Reily M. Comparison of 30- and 50-mCi of doses of iodine-131 for thyroid ablation. Annals Intern Med 1992; 96:51–53.
32. Kuni CC, Klingensmith WC. Failure of low doses of I-131 to ablate residual thyroid tissue following surgery for thyroid cancer. Radiology 1980; 137:773–774.
33. Bal C, Padhy AK, Jana S, et al. Prospective randomized clinical trial to evaluate the optimal dose of I-131 for remnant ablation in patients with differentiated thyroid carcinoma. Cancer 1996; 77:2574–2580.
34. Bal CS, Kumar A, Pant GS. Radioiodine doses of 25 to 50 mCi are equally effective for thyroid remnant ablation in patients with thyroid carcinoma. J Clin Endocrinol Metab 2004; 89:1666–1673.
35. Doi SAR, Woodhouse NJY. Ablation of the thyroid remnant and 131 dose in differentiated thyroid cancer. Clin Endocrinol 2000; 52:765–773.
36. Samuel AM, Rajashekharrao B. Radioiodine therapy for well-differentiated thyroid cancer: A quantitative dosimetric evaluation for remnant thyroid ablation after surgery. J Nucl Med 1994; 35: 1944–1950.
37. Sisson JC. Applying the radioactive eraser: I-131 to ablate normal thyroid tissue in patients from whom thyroid cancer has been resected. J Nucl Med 1983; 24:743–745.
38. Maxon HR, Englaro EE, Thomas SR, et al. Radioiodine-131 therapy for well differentiated thyroid cancer—a quantitative radiation dosimetric approach: Outcome and validation in 85 patients. J Nucl Med 1992; 33:1132–1136.
39. Maxon HR, Thomas SR, Hertzberg VS, et al. Relation between effective radiation dose and outcome of radioiodine therapy for thyroid cancer. N Engl J Med 1983; 309:937–941.
40. Hodgson DC, Brierley JD, Tsang RW, Panzarella T. Prescribing 131-I iodine based on neck uptake produces effective thyroid ablation and reduced hospital stay. Radiother Oncol 1998; 47:325–330.
41. Comtois R, Theriault C, Del Vecchio P. Assessment of the efficacy of iodine-131 for thyroid ablation. J Nucl Med 1993; 34:1927–1930.
42. Leung SF, Law MWM, Ho SKW. Efficacy of low-dose iodine-131 ablation of postoperative thyroid remnants: a study of 69 cases. Br J Radiol 1992; 65:905–909.
43. Logue JP, Tang RW, Brierley JD, et al. Radioiodine ablation of residual tissue in thyroid cancer: relationship between administered activity, neck uptake and outcome. Br J Radiol 1994; 67:1127–1131.
44. Ramacciotti C, Pretorius HT, Line B, et al. Ablation of non-malignant thyroid remnants with low doses of radioactive iodine: concise communication. J Nucl Med 1982; 23:483–489.
44a. Verkooijen RB, Stokkel MPM, Smit JWA, et al. Radioactive I-131 in differentiated thyroid cancer: a retrospective analysis of an uptake-related ablation strategy. Eur J Nucl Med 2004; 31:499–506.
45. Reynolds JC. Comparison of I-131 absorbed radiation doses in children and adults; a tool for estimating therapeutic I-131 doses in children. In Robbins J, editor. Treatment of Thyroid Cancer in Children. Springfield, VA: US Department of Commerce Technology Administration, National Technical Information Service, 1994: 127–135.
46. Maxon HR. Quantitative radioiodine therapy in the treatment of differentiated thyroid cancer. Q J Nucl Med 1999; 43:313–323.
47. Pacini F. Options for ablating thyroid remnants. Vancouver, Canada: Presentation at the 2004 American Thyroid Association Meeting, 2004.
48. Society of nuclear medicine procedure guideline for therapy of thyroid disease with iodine-131 (sodium iodide). Procedure Guidelines Manual, Society of Nuclear Medicine, 2002: 159–164.
49. Meier DA, Brill DR, Becker DV, et al. Procedure guideline for therapy of thyroid disease with I-131. J Nucl Med 2002; 43:856–861.
50. EANM procedure guidelines for therapy with iodine-131. Eur J Nucl Med 2003; 30:BP27–BP31.

27
Thyroid Remnant Radioiodine Ablation with Recombinant Human Thyrotropin

R. Michael Tuttle and Richard J. Robbins

INTRODUCTION

The primary treatment modalities for most patients with differentiated thyroid cancer include total thyroidectomy and radioactive iodine (RAI) remnant ablation (RRA; *1*). The goal of RRA is to eliminate not only normal thyroid cells but also to destroy any residual microscopic thyroid carcinoma that may remain following total thyroidectomy and appropriate lymph node dissection. As reviewed in Chapters 14, 26, 32, and 88, RAI uptake into thyroid cells is enhanced by a low-iodine diet and thyrotropin (TSH) stimulation. For the past 40–50 yr, endogenous TSH production was stimulated by several weeks of thyroid hormone withdrawal prior to RAI dosing. However, thyroid hormone withdrawal often results in hypothyroid symptoms that are not well tolerated by many patients.

Exogenous TSH (bovine TSH) was used to stimulate RAI uptake in thyroid cancer patients over 40 yr ago but fell out of favor due to the development of neutralizing antibodies and allergic reactions with repeated exposures (*2–6*). As reviewed in Chapter 11, the FDA approved recombinant human TSH (rhTSH, Thyrogen®, Genzyme Corporation) in 1998 for diagnostic whole-body RAI scanning and stimulated thyroglobulin measurements in the follow-up of patients with differentiated thyroid cancer (*7,8*). Although currently FDA approved only for diagnostic purposes, several investigators began to explore the utility of rhTSH as an alternative preparation for thyroid remnant ablation that would avoid thyroid hormone withdrawal. This chapter reviews the published data on rhTSH-stimulated RAI for remnant ablation and describes how rhTSH is used for RRA in clinical practice.

rhTSH AS PREPARATION FOR RRA

Before rhTSH became commercially available in December 1998, many patients received rhTSH-stimulated RAI treatments as part of the Genzyme Corporation's Compassionate Use Program (*9–11*). Although most of these patients were receiving RAI for treatment of recurrent/persistent disease, rhTSH was used for RRA in at least 15 patients. These reports provided information on safety and RAI uptake into the thyroid remnants at the time of remnant ablation but with little information on results of the follow-up diagnostic scans.

In addition to diagnostic whole-body RAI scanning, our initial patients at Memorial Sloan Kettering Cancer Center who received rhTSH stimulation were offered whole-body and blood dosimetry studies to determine the maximal tolerable activity (MTA) of RAI therapy that could be administered if a therapy was required. As dosimetry studies conducted with rhTSH were significantly different from those with hypothyroid withdrawal, it was not possible to use the MTA calculations using rhTSH to predict a safe maximum dose of RAI following thyroid hormone withdrawal. Therefore, we offered selected patients the option of rhTSH-assisted RRA based on their individual dosimetry results as an alternative to repeating the dosimetry studies in the hypothyroid state before proceeding with RRA.

Each of these initial patients received 0.9 mg of rhTSH for two consecutive days during week 1 to allow for full rhTSH-stimulated dosimetry studies and two additional rhTSH injections during week 2 to prepare for RRA (see Fig. 1). Complete absence of visible thyroid bed uptake on a follow-up diagnostic scan done 5–13 mo after administering a mean activity of 110 mCi (range 30–250 mCi) was reported in all 10 patients in our initial series (*12*). Although RAI activity in the thyroid bed was the primary endpoint of this initial study, two patients had uptake outside of the thyroid bed (presumably cervical lymph node metastases), which was no longer visible at the time of the follow-up diagnostic whole-body scan.

In a subsequent nonrandomized retrospective analysis, we directly compared RRA following thyroid hormone withdrawal ($n = 42$) with rhTSH simulation ($n = 45$; *13*). In this larger patient cohort, complete resolution of visible thyroid bed uptake on the 1-yr follow-up whole-body diagnostic RAI scan was seen in 84% of those prepared with rhTSH and 81%

From: *Thyroid Cancer: A Comprehensive Guide to Clinical Management, 2/e*
Edited by: L. Wartofsky and D. Van Nostrand © Humana Press Inc., Totowa, NJ

	Mon	Tue	Wed	Thur	Fri	Sat
Wk 1	rhTSH	rhTSH	RAI Tracer	D	D	D WBS
Wk 2	rhTSH	rhTSH	Ablation			
Wk 3			Post-Rx WBS			

rhTSH: 0.9 mg IM, Tracer: 2-5 mCi ^{131}I, D: blood and body dosimetry measurements, Ablation: 75-150 mCi ^{131}I, WBS: diagnostic whole body scan

Fig. 1. Full whole body and blood dosimetry in preparation for rhTSH-stimulated RRA *(12)*. rhTSH, 0.9 mg IM; tracer, 2–5 mCi ^{131}I; D, blood and body dosimetry measurements, ablation, 75–150 mCi ^{131}I, WBS, diagnostic whole-body scan.

prepared with thyroid hormone withdrawal (p = ns). The mean administered ^{131}I activity after rhTSH preparation was 110 ± 65 mCi (range 30–330 mCi) compared to 129 ± 74 mCi (range 30–300 mCi) following thyroid hormone withdrawal.

In 2002, Pacini et al. reported the results of a nonrandomized, consecutive block design study comparing the effectiveness of 30 mCi of ^{131}I after thyroid hormone withdrawal or rhTSH as preparation for RRA *(14)*. The rate of successful RRA (defined by absence of uptake in the thyroid bed on the 1-yr diagnostic whole-body scan) was significantly higher in the 50 patients prepared with thyroid hormone withdrawal (84%), compared to euthyroid patients prepared with rhTSH (54%, $p < 0.01$). A third cohort prepared with both thyroid hormone withdrawal and rhTSH administration demonstrated successful RRA rates similar to standard thyroid hormone withdrawal (78.5% vs 84%, respectively). Unlike previously published studies in which the RAI was administered 24 h after the second rhTSH injection, the ablative dose of RAI was given 48 h after the second injection of rhTSH.

To assess the impact of the obligate intake of stable iodine associated with the continuation of levothyroxine supplementation during rhTSH-stimulated RRA, Barbaro et al. designed a study to evaluate the effect of short-term levothyroxine withdrawal (4 d) at the time of RAI dosing for RRA *(15)*. In the rhTSH-stimulated RRA arm, levothyroxine therapy was initiated at the time of total thyroidectomy and discontinued 24 h prior to the first injection of rhTSH (0.9 mg for two consecutive days). The ablative dose of 30 mCi of ^{131}I was administered 24 h after the second injection of rhTSH. Levothyroxine therapy was restarted 24 h after administration of the ablative dose of RAI. At the 1-yr follow-up diagnostic whole-body scan, no visible uptake in the thyroid bed was seen in 88% (14 of 18) of patients prepared with rhTSH and 4-d levothyroxine withdrawal, compared to 75% (18 of 24) of patients prepared with traditional thyroid hormone withdrawal.

When successful RRA ablation was defined as absence of uptake in the thyroid bed and undetectable serum thyroglobulin, similar success rates were reported (81% with rhTSH, 75% with thyroid hormone withdrawal; p = not significant). The urinary iodine values were significantly lower in the rhTSH with 4-d levothyroxine withdrawal group (47 ± 4 μg/L) and the thyroid hormone withdrawal group (39 ± 4 μg/L) than in an additional control group undergoing diagnostic rhTSH scanning without discontinuation of levothyroxine (76 ± 9 μg/L).

The preliminary results of the first prospective randomized trial examining traditional thyroid hormone withdrawal vs rhTSH stimulation in low-risk differentiated thyroid cancer patients for RRA was reported by Ladenson at the American Thyroid Association Annual Meeting in 2004 *(16)*. This multicenter study enrolled 63 patients in 9 centers in Europe, Canada, and the United States. All patients received approx 100 mCi of ^{131}I for RRA. At the follow-up diagnostic rhTSH whole-body scan 1 yr later, all patients in both arms had less than 0.1% uptake in the thyroid bed. A more careful analysis of these data will be necessary once the study is submitted for a peer-reviewed publication.

VARIATIONS IN THE PUBLISHED DATA

Several important differences in study design are likely to account for the alterations in the effectiveness of rhTSH as preparation for RRA in the published reports *(12–15*; see Table 1). Most studies have defined successful RAI ablation as the absence of visible uptake in the thyroid bed on the 1-yr follow-up diagnostic whole-body scan.

Pacini et al. reported the lowest published success rates with rhTSH-assisted RRA by administering a lower amount of ^{131}I (30 mCi) 48 h following the second injection of rhTSH *(14)*. It is likely that this smaller activity of RAI given at a time when the serum TSH was declining resulted in less radiation to the thyroid remnant than was achieved when higher activities of RAI were given 24 h after the second injection. The other important factor to consider is that Pacini et al. used a traditional thyroid hormone withdrawal whole-body diagnostic scan as their endpoint for complete ablation, which may be more sensitive for detecting minimal thyroid remnants than rhTSH diagnostic scanning, used in the other published series *(13,15)*.

Levothyroxine therapy was continued throughout RRA in each of the studies except that of Barbaro et al. *(15)*. Although short-term discontinuation of levothyroxine prior to RRA did result in a statistically lower urine iodine excretion (47 ± 4 μg/L vs 76 ± 9 μg/L), the clinical significance of this small decrease remains to be defined. Likely, low-level stable iodine contamination resulting from continued use of levothyroxine may be a more important confounder when lower administered activities (e.g., 30 mCi) are used for RRA. Larger administered activities (e.g., 80–100 mCi

Table 1
Variations in Published Reports

Study Characteristics	Pacini et al. (13)	Robbins et al. (12)	Barbaro et al. (14)	Prospective Randomized
Successful rhTSH-stimulated RRA	54% (27/50)	84% (38/45)	88% (14/18)	100%
Definition of successful RRA	No visible uptake on follow-up diagnostic WBS	No visible uptake on follow-up diagnostic WBS	No visible uptake on follow-up diagnostic WBS	Less than 0.1% uptake on follow-up diagnostic WBS
Administered activity (^{131}I)	30 mCi	110 ± 65 mCi	30 mCi	80 mCi
Timing of RAI administration	48 h after second rhTSH injection	24 h after second rhTSH injection	24 h after second rhTSH injection	24 h after second rhTSH injection
Follow-up diagnostic WBS	Thyroid hormone withdrawal WBS	rhTSH diagnostic WBS	rhTSH diagnostic WBS	rhTSH diagnostic WBS
Levothyroxine therapy	Continued	Continued	Suspended for 4 d	Continued

WBS, whole-body scan.

of ^{131}I) appear to result in successful RRA even when levothyroxine therapy is continued throughout the time of ablation.

A Note of Caution

A large body of evidence is mounting that rhTSH stimulation can be used as a viable alternative to traditional thyroid hormone withdrawal for the destruction of normal thyroid remnants after total thyroidectomy. However, it is important to note that none of the published studies provide sufficient follow-up to compare disease recurrence rates among the two approaches. Until long-term recurrence studies are available, interim studies are needed to carefully evaluate suppressed and stimulated serum thyroglobulin values during follow-up of patients who had RRA after either rhTSH or traditional thyroid hormone withdrawal.

CURRENT APPROACH

Following total thyroidectomy for differentiated thyroid cancer, patients at Memorial Sloan Kettering Cancer Center are offered the option of traditional thyroid hormone withdrawal or rhTSH stimulation as preparation for RRA. A low-iodine diet is recommended for all patients for 1 wk prior to RRA.

In patients without evidence for distant metastases based on initial clinical staging parameters, a simplified regimen is offered that does not require full dosimetry (see Fig. 2). This approach uses 0.9 mg of rhTSH administered intramuscularly on two consecutive days in conjunction with a diagnostic whole-body scan with ^{123}I prior to administration of a therapeutic dose of ^{131}I. The ^{123}I diagnostic scan is not mandatory, but it allows the identification of patients who have a large thyroid remnant and may need less ^{131}I for ablation. Occasionally, the ^{123}I scan may disclose unexpected distant metastatic lesions, which may result in an increase in the amount of ^{131}I to be administered. This simplified approach incorporates a high-quality diagnostic whole-body scan with ^{123}I into the standard 3-d rhTSH-stimulated RRA ablation. The administered activity of ^{131}I at our center is typically in the 75–150 mCi range depending on the severity of the disease and other patient risk factors.

- Day 1
  o rhTSH 0.9 mg IM
- Day 2
  o rhTSH 0.9 mg IM
  o 3-4 hours later: 1.5 mCi ^{123}I is administered orally
- Day 3
  o Diagnostic whole body scan (about 16 hours after ^{123}I dosing)
  o 75-150 mCi ^{131}I administered
- Day 10
  o Post therapy whole body scan

Fig. 2. A simplified approach to rhTSH-stimulated RRA ablation in low-risk patients.

SUMMARY

Even though not approved by the FDA for therapeutic use, the available preliminary data suggest that rhTSH (0.9 mg for two consecutive days followed by 75–100 mCi ^{131}I on day 3) can be used as an alternative to traditional thyroid hormone withdrawal for destruction of normal thyroid remnants following total thyroidectomy. As this is an off-label use of rhTSH, patients must be informed that the long-term outcomes are not well defined using this method of preparation for ablation. This is an important issue because the primary long-term goals of RRA are destruction of microscopic residual thyroid cancer cells and reduction in recurrence rates.

More data are needed to determine the optimal dose of RAI required, the precise time interval between rhTSH administration and RAI dosing, and the potential importance of a short period of thyroid hormone withdrawal to minimize stable iodine intake at the time of RAI dosing.

REFERENCES

1. Mazzaferri EL, Kloos RT. Clinical review 128: Current approaches to primary therapy for papillary and follicular thyroid cancer. J Clin Endocrinol Metab 2001; 86:1447–1463.
2. Benua R, et al. An 18 year study of the use of beef thyrotropin to increase I-131 uptake in metastatic thyroid cancer. J Nucl Med 1964; 5:796–801.
3. Kirkpatrick CH, Meek JC, Rich RR. Mechanism of allergy to components of commercial bovine thyrotropin. J Allergy Clin Immunol 1973; 51:296–302.
4. Melmed S, Harada A, Hershman JM, Krishnamurthy GT, Bland WH. Neutralizing antibodies to bovine thyrotropin in immunized patients with thyroid cancer. J Clin Endocrinol Metab 1980; 51: 358–363.
5. Robbins J. Pharmacology of bovine and human thyrotropin: an historical perspective. Thyroid 1999; 9:451–453.
6. Seidlin S, Oshry E, Yallow A. Spontaneous and experimentally induced uptake of radioactive iodine in metastases from thyroid carcinoma. J Clin Endocrinol Metab 1948; 8:423–425.
7. Woodmansee WW, Haugen BR. Uses for recombinant human TSH in patients with thyroid cancer and nodular goiter. Clin Endocrinol 2004; 61:163–173.
8. Robbins RJ, Robbins AK. Clinical review 156: Recombinant human thyrotropin and thyroid cancer management. J Clin Endocrinol Metab 2003; 88:1933–1938.
9. Perros P. Recombinant human thyroid-stimulating hormone (rhTSH) in the radioablation of well-differentiated thyroid cancer: preliminary therapeutic experience. 1999:30–34.
10. Berg G, et al. Radioiodine ablation and therapy in differentiated thyroid cancer under stimulation with recombinant human thyroid-stimulating hormone. J Endocrinol Invest 2002; 25:44–52.
11. Luster M, Lassmann M, Haenscheid H, et al. Use of recombinant human thyrotropin before radioiodine therapy in patients with advanced differentiated thyroid carcinoma. J Clin Endocrinol Metab 2000; 85: 3640–3645.
12. Robbins RJ, et al. Radioiodine ablation of thyroid remnants after preparation with recombinant human thyrotropin. Thyroid 2001; 11: 865–869.
13. Robbins RJ, et al. A retrospective review of the effectiveness of recombinant human TSH as a preparation for radioiodine thyroid remnant ablation. J Nucl Med 2002; 43:1482–1488.
14. Pacini F, et al. Ablation of thyroid residues with 30 mCi (131)I: a comparison in thyroid cancer patients prepared with recombinant human TSH or thyroid hormone withdrawal. J Clin Endocrinol Metab 2002; 87:4063–4068.
15. Barbaro D, et al. Radioiodine treatment with 30 mCi after recombinant human thyrotropin stimulation in thyroid cancer: effectiveness for postsurgical remnants ablation and possible role of iodine content in L-thyroxine in the outcome of ablation. J Clin Endocrinol Metab 2003; 88:4110–4115.
16. Ladenson PW, Pacini F, Schlumberger M, et al. Thyroid remnant ablation: A randomized comparison of thyrotropin alfa and thyroid hormone withdrawal. New Orleans, LA: 86th Annual Meeting, The Endocrine Society, June 16–19, 2004, Program S35-1, p. 45.

Part IV
Well-Differentiated Thyroid Cancer
Surveillance

28
Follow-Up Strategy in Papillary Thyroid Cancer

Henry B. Burch

INTRODUCTION

Effective surveillance for recurrent papillary thyroid cancer begins with an assessment of the risk of recurrence or death from disease, depending on individual characteristics of patients and their tumor. This information is used to determine an appropriate level of follow-up, which may vary from as little as an annual neck examination on replacement thyroid hormone therapy for occult lesions, to annual or semiannual thyrotropin (TSH) stimulated whole-body scan (WBS) and thyroglobulin (Tg) measurement for high-risk patients. Effective follow-up is also contingent upon a current understanding of the strengths and limitations of the tools available for thyroid cancer surveillance. This chapter focuses on the rationale used to determine the method and frequency of follow-up for patients with papillary thyroid cancer and reviews current guidelines regarding surveillance for persistent or recurrent disease.

DEFINING THE RISK LEVEL

The factors used to determine a given patient's risk category and, hence, an appropriate level of surveillance are specific patient characteristics. These include age and sex, tumor features (e.g., size), histological grade or subtype, and presence of extrathyroidal extension or distant metastases, as well as the extent of prior surgery and radioiodine therapy. A number of scoring and staging systems have been derived from retrospective analysis of large patient cohorts studying differentiated thyroid cancer (see Chapter 9). Although it is tempting to assign a numerical score to an individual patient, and use this to design an appropriate level of surveillance, realistically, patients from all stages of disease may experience recurrence and death (1), and the onus is therefore on the clinician to provide an adequate approach to detect not only the typical but the atypical patient as well.

LEVEL OF SURVEILLANCE

The rate of persistent or recurrent differentiated thyroid cancer is relatively high. One large cohort of 1528 patients was found to have an overall recurrence rate of 23.5% at a median of 16.6 yr (1). A great deal of variability exists among thyroidologists in the level and frequency of follow-up in patients with papillary thyroid cancer (2). However, this evaluation should be individualized, with more rigorous and frequent monitoring in those patients deemed likely to experience a recurrence or death from disease and less intense surveillance for patients with a low risk of an adverse outcome. Generally, patients with one or more poor prognostic factors (see Chapters 23, 40) tend to be given a higher dose of remnant ablation and undergo more frequent surveillance. A common approach to patients with papillary thyroid cancers larger than 1.5 cm in diameter is to recommend near-total thyroidectomy, followed by radioiodine ablation with 30–150 mCi of ^{131}I (2), and then serial surveillance for recurrent disease. As discussed below, the appropriate modalities and frequency of surveillance are currently undergoing reevaluation owing to the introduction of recombinant human (rh)TSH and a changing view of the relative value of the WBS in patients with low-risk differentiated thyroid cancer.

A CHANGING ROLE FOR WBS

Recently, it has been suggested that the WBS adds little information to the stimulated Tg level in patients with differentiated thyroid cancer (3,4), particularly in low-risk patients whose last WBS was negative (5). In a French study, among 256 patients with differentiated thyroid cancer undergoing withdrawal scanning 6–12 mo after thyroidectomy and remnant ablation, the WBS did not detect disease outside the thyroid bed in a single case, including 46 patients with stimulated serum Tg levels greater than 1 ng/mL (3). In a smaller US study, among 108 patients 1–35 yr after initial therapy, a rhTSH WBS using 3–5 mCi of ^{131}I showed no activity outside the thyroid bed, including 20 patients with stimulated serum Tg levels more than 2.0 ng/nL (4). Conversely, a third study examined rhTSH scanning in 109 low-risk differentiated thyroid cancer patients and found WBS evidence of metastatic disease in 8% of cases, with a stimulated serum Tg level of less than 2.0 ng/mL (5).

From: *Thyroid Cancer: A Comprehensive Guide to Clinical Management, 2/e*
Edited by: L. Wartofsky and D. Van Nostrand © Humana Press Inc., Totowa, NJ

However, when these authors confined their analysis to those patients whose last WBS was negative, the current WBS was never informative if the stimulated Tg level was less than 2.0 ng/mL.

The proposed diminished role for the WBS is somewhat self-fulfilling, attributable at least partly to the use of a progressively lower ^{131}I-scanning dose due to fear of the stunning phenomenon, as well as a greater reliance on rhTSH scanning, which provides slightly inferior scanning images compared to withdrawal scanning. Concerns over this phenomenon *(6–10)* have led many centers to reduce the scanning dose from 10 mCi of ^{131}I to 2–5 mCi, whereas other centers have supplanted the ^{131}I WBS altogether with the ^{123}I WBS *(11)*. Although the application of rhTSH to thyroid cancer surveillance represents a major quality-of-life improvement for patients with thyroid cancer *(12,13)*, the slightly diminished quality of the rhTSH-stimulated WBS is apparent from phase III trial data. In the 11% of patients with discordant rhTSH and withdrawal scans in the second phase III trial, the withdrawal scan was twice as likely to give superior results for the entire group and four times more likely to give superior results in patients with known metastatic disease *(13)*.

The use of rhTSH-stimulated Tg alone to manage patients with low-risk differentiated thyroid cancer was examined by Wartofsky and colleagues in a multicenter study *(14)*. Patients with prior near-total thyroidectomy and remnant ablation, with a thyroid hormone suppressive therapy (THST)-Tg of less than 5.0 ng/mL, were enrolled. At baseline, 89% of 300 eligible patients had THST-Tg levels of less than 1.0 ng/mL. For the whole group, 53 of 300 (18%) had Tg increments of more than 2 ng/mL after rhTSH administration. Among these patients, WBS was positive (thyroid bed or metastases) in approx 50%. Patients with American Joint Commission on Cancer (AJCC) stage III disease were more likely to have positive stimulated Tg values than were lower stage patients. Interestingly, among 14 patients with a stimulated Tg less than 2, but in whom WBS was also obtained, 9 had positive WBS, including 5 with metastatic disease. Considered together, these data suggest that elevated rhTSH-stimulated Tg levels greater than 2 ng/mL frequently signify persistent or recurrent disease, whereas a negative Tg response does not guarantee that the patient is disease-free *(14)*.

There are important factors to consider before omitting the WBS from a given patient's surveillance regimen. First, the patient may not have anti-Tg antibodies—a caveat that immediately excludes approx 25% of differentiated thyroid cancer patients *(15)*. Second, the Tg assay must have sufficient sensitivity to detect low levels of Tg elevation (a functional sensitivity of 1.0 ng/mL is recommended; *16*). Third, the patient should have had a negative WBS on the last (or preferably last two) WBS *(5,17)*. Finally, the patient should be in a group with a low-pretest probability of metastatic disease, i.e., a low-risk group, as discussed above *(16)*.

CLINICAL PRACTICE GUIDELINES

Over the past several years, many groups have released clinical practice guidelines (CPGs) to assist the management of patients with thyroid cancer *(17–19)*. The American Association of Clinical Endocrinologists, in conjunction with the American Association of Endocrine Surgeons, released guidelines regarding this disease in 2001 *(18)*. These guidelines provided an overview of current practices, reviewed clinical features affecting decisions about initial therapy and subsequent surveillance, pinpointed areas of ongoing controversy, and identified limitations in the evidence currently available in these areas. Trends toward less extensive THST and greater use of rhTSH testing were discussed as well.

The National Comprehensive Cancer Network (NCCN) CPGs, updated annually and available online *(17)*, provide the most organized, specific, and evidence-based recommendations for the management of thyroid cancer. These guidelines were developed by experts from many large cancer centers in the United States and provide separate sections for the treatment of patients with papillary, follicular, Hürthle cell, and medullary thyroid cancer. According to the NCCN guidelines, routine follow-up for a patient with papillary thyroid cancer who has had near-total thyroidectomy and remnant ablation should consist of a neck exam every 3–6 mo for 2 yr, Tg and anti-Tg antibody measurement at 6 and 12 mo and annually thereafter if disease-free, and a WBS every 12 mo until one negative scan arises. The guidelines do not stipulate the point at which rhTSH-stimulated Tg testing may be safely replaced by the less sensitive method of measuring Tg while a patient is taking THST.

A consensus statement on the role of serum Tg as a primary monitoring method for low-risk patients with papillary thyroid cancer was published in 2003 *(16)*. This group of thyroid cancer experts addressed such issues as the minimal acceptable Tg assay standards, a comparison of the sensitivity of the WBS with the stimulated Tg level, and whether THST-Tg alone is sufficiently sensitive to either detect persistent disease initially or to follow patients once they are noted to have a negative-stimulated Tg test. A low-risk patient was defined as generally having AJCC stage I or II disease, no distant metastases, a prior total thyroidectomy with remnant ablation, no clinical evidence of disease, and a THST-Tg level less than 1 ng/mL. It was concluded that Tg assays used to follow thyroid cancer patients should have a functional sensitivity of 1 ng/mL, and that the WBS generally added little to the information provided by a stimulated Tg level. THST-Tg was deemed too insensitive to detect persistent disease, but in low-risk patients with a prior stimulated Tg level less than 1 ng/mL, the consensus was that an *annual* stimulated Tg level was not necessary. The group was unable to determine how often, if at all, stimulated Tg testing was required in this group of patients once a single negative-stimulated Tg level is obtained *(16)*. Other

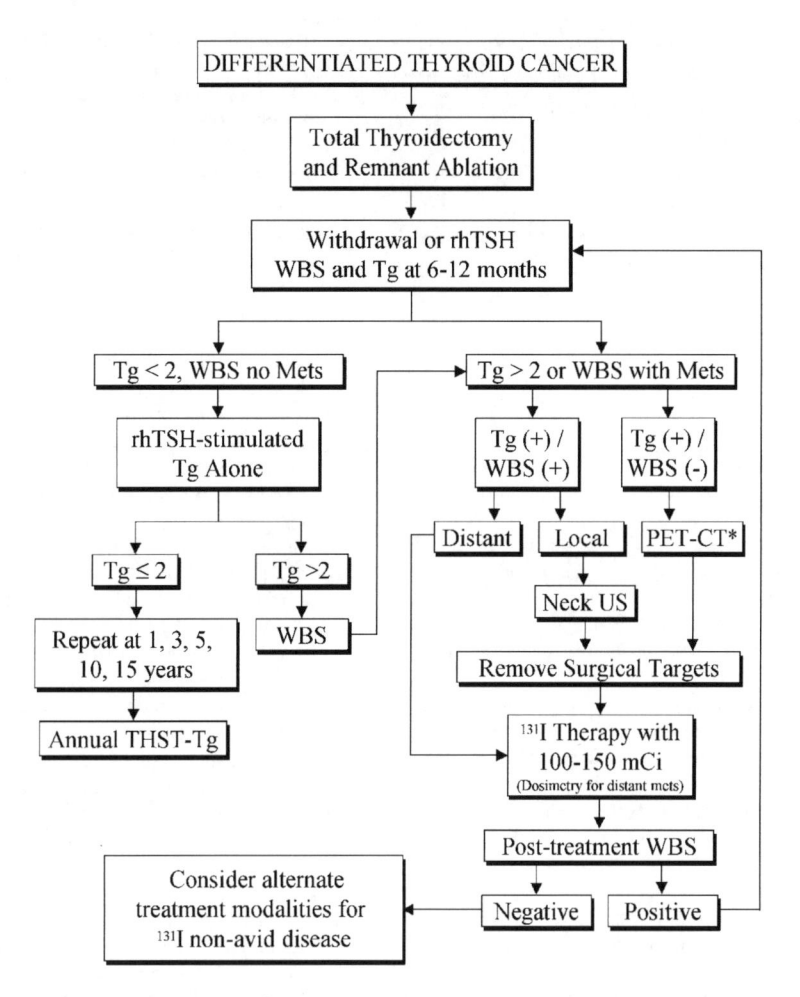

```
                    DIFFERENTIATED THYROID CANCER
                                 │
                                 ▼
                        Total Thyroidectomy
                        and Remnant Ablation
                                 │
                                 ▼
                        Withdrawal or rhTSH     ◄──────────┐
                        WBS and Tg at 6-12 months          │
                                 │                         │
                 ┌───────────────┴───────────────┐         │
                 ▼                               ▼         │
         Tg < 2, WBS no Mets           Tg > 2 or WBS with Mets
                 │                       │               │
                 ▼                       ▼               ▼
         rhTSH-stimulated             Tg (+)/         Tg (+)/
             Tg Alone                 WBS (+)         WBS (-)
                 │                       │               │
          ┌──────┴──────┐          ┌─────┼──────┐        ▼
          ▼             ▼          ▼     ▼      ▼      PET-CT*
        Tg ≤ 2        Tg > 2    Distant Local
          │             │               │
          ▼             ▼             Neck US
    Repeat at 1, 3, 5, WBS              │
      10, 15 years                      ▼
          │                      Remove Surgical Targets
          ▼                              │
     Annual THST-Tg                      ▼
                                  ¹³¹I Therapy with
                                    100-150 mCi
                                (Dosimetry for distant mets)
                                         │
                                         ▼
                                 Post-treatment WBS
                                    │        │
         Consider alternate         ▼        ▼
         treatment modalities for ◄─Negative  Positive
         ¹³¹I non-avid disease
```

Fig. 1. An algorithmic approach to the follow-up of differentiated thyroid cancer after a near-total thyroidectomy and remnant ablation therapy. Patients with negative serum Tg levels and WBS at 6–12 mo are followed with rhTSH-stimulated Tg levels alone, which is ultimately supplanted by annual THST-Tg monitoring. Patients with evidence of persistent disease at 12 mo are distinguished on the basis of Tg and WBS status. Tg-positive/WBS-negative patients are assessed for surgical targets using fluorodeoxyglucose positron emission tomography (PET) uptake, which is the most sensitive when Tg levels are higher than 10 ng/mL. Tg-positive/WBS-positive patients require further evaluation to assess for surgical targets (WBS uptake in the neck), followed by radioiodine ablation, or they are treated with high-dose radioiodine directly if distant metastases are seen on WBS. US, ultrasound; CT, computed tomography.

workers *(19a)* also have found that a WBS added very little to information provided by rhTSH-stimulated thyroglobulin levels.

Because most recurrences from papillary thyroid cancer occur within the first 15 yr of diagnosis *(20–22)*, it seems prudent to continue to perform stimulated Tg testing at increasing intervals until the risk of recurrence is low enough to justify the use of TSHT-Tg as a primary screening method. Figure 1 reviews an algorithmic approach to the follow-up of differentiated thyroid cancer, applicable to patients who have undergone near-total thyroidectomy and remnant ablation. Withdrawal or rhTSH scanning and Tg measurement is performed at 12 mo (6 mo for patients in high-risk categories). The majority of patients will have stimulated Tg less than 2 ng/mL and a negative WBS for metastatic disease.

These patients may be managed with serial rhTSH-stimulated Tg alone, which is performed at 3, 5, 10, and 15 yr, after which surveillance consists of neck exam and THST-Tg administration. Patients deemed to be at low risk (younger patients with small primary tumors and negative initial testing) may be advanced to THST-Tg testing alone earlier in this course (e.g., after the 5-yr stimulated testing). According to this algorithm, patients with stimulated Tg levels greater than 2 ng/dL or who have metastatic disease on WBS are considered as Tg-positive/WBS-positive or Tg-positive/WBS-negative. Patients in the former group with cervical lymph node metastases on scan and surgical targets identified on neck ultrasound should be referred for neck dissection, followed by radioiodine therapy. Patients with distant metastases are generally treated with higher doses of radioiodine, which may be determined using dosimetry. Tg-positive/scan-negative patients with Tg levels greater than 10–15 ng/mL are candidates for fluorodeoxyglucose positron emission tomography scanning *(23–26)*, preferably with computed tomography colocalization, with the objective of identifying and removing surgical targets *(27)*. By definition, these patient's tumors have less iodine avidity and are unlikely to respond to radioiodine *(28)*. A negative posttherapy WBS in patients with known persistent or recurrent disease should prompt consideration of other treatment modalities, such as external radiation therapy *(17)*.

REFERENCES

1. Mazzaferri EL, Kloos RT. Clinical review 128: Current approaches to primary therapy for papillary and follicular thyroid cancer. J Clin Endocrinol Metab 2001; 86:1447–1463.
2. Solomon BL, Wartofsky L, Burman KD. Current trends in the management of well differentiated papillary thyroid carcinoma. J Clin Endocrinol Metab 1996; 81:333–339.
3. Cailleux AF, Baudin E, Travagli JP, et al. Is diagnostic iodine-131 scanning useful after total thyroid ablation for differentiated thyroid cancer? J Clin Endocrinol Metab 2000; 85:175–178.
4. Mazzaferri EL, Kloos RT. Is diagnostic iodine-131 scanning with recombinant human TSH useful in the follow-up of differentiated thyroid cancer after thyroid ablation? J Clin Endocrinol Metab 2002; 87:1490–1498.
5. Robbins RJ, Chon JT, Fleisher M, et al. Is the serum thyroglobulin response to recombinant human thyrotropin sufficient, by itself, to monitor for residual thyroid carcinoma? J Clin Endocrinol Metab 2002; 87:3242–3247.
6. Bajen MT, Mane S, Munoz A, Garcia JR. Effect of a diagnostic dose of 185 MBq ^{131}I on postsurgical thyroid remnants. J Nucl Med 2000; 41:2038–2042.
7. Kao CH, Yen TC. Stunning effects after a diagnostic dose of iodine-131. Nuklearmedizin. 1998; 37:30–32.
8. Lees W, Mansberg R, Roberts J, et al. The clinical effects of thyroid stunning after diagnostic whole-body scanning with 185 MBq ^{131}I. Eur J Nucl Med Mol Imaging 2002; 29:1421–1427.
9. Leger FA, Izembart M, Dagousset F, et al. Decreased uptake of therapeutic doses of iodine-131 after 185-MBq iodine-131 diagnostic imaging for thyroid remnants in differentiated thyroid carcinoma. Eur J Nucl Med 1998; 25:242–246.
10. Park HM, Park YH, Zhou XH. Detection of thyroid remnant/metastasis without stunning: an ongoing dilemma. Thyroid 1997; 7:277–280.
11. Mandel SJ, Shankar LK, Benard F, et al. Superiority of iodine-123 compared with iodine-131 scanning for thyroid remnants in patients with differentiated thyroid cancer. Clin Nucl Med 2001; 26:6–9.
12. Ladenson PW, Braverman LE, Mazzaferri EL, et al. Comparison of administration of recombinant human thyrotropin with withdrawal of thyroid hormone for radioactive iodine scanning in patients with thyroid carcinoma. N Engl J Med 1997; 337:888–896.
13. Haugen BR, Pacini F, Reiners C, et al. A comparison of recombinant human thyrotropin and thyroid hormone withdrawal for the detection of thyroid remnant or cancer. J Clin Endocrinol Metab 1999; 84:3877–3885.
14. Wartofsky L. Management of low-risk well-differentiated thyroid cancer based only on thyroglobulin measurement after recombinant human thyrotropin. Thyroid. 2002; 12:583–590.
15. Torrens JI, Burch HB. Serum thyroglobulin measurement. Utility in clinical practice. Endocrinol Metab Clin North Am 2001; 30:429–467.
16. Mazzaferri EL, Robbins RJ, Spencer CA, et al. A consensus report of the role of serum thyroglobulin as a monitoring method for low-risk patients with papillary thyroid carcinoma. J Clin Endocrinol Metab 2003; 88:1433–1441.
17. National Comprehensive Cancer Network (NCCN) Thyroid Carcinoma: Clinical Practice Guidelines 2005, J Natl Comprehensive Cancer Network 2005; 3:404–457.
18. AACE/AAES medical/surgical guidelines for clinical practice: management of thyroid carcinoma. American Association of Clinical Endocrinologists. American College of Endocrinology. Endocr Pract 2001; 7:202–220.
19. Kendall-Taylor P. Guidelines for the management of thyroid cancer. Clin Endocrinol 2003; 58:400–402.
19a. David A, Blotta A, Rossi R, et al. Clinical value of different responses of serum thyroglobulin to recombinant human thyrotropin in the follow-up of patients with differentiated thyroid carcinoma. Thyroid 2005; 15:267–273.
20. Ain KB. Papillary thyroid carcinoma. Etiology, assessment, and therapy. Endocrinol Metab Clin North Am 1995; 24:711–760.
21. Mazzaferri EL. Long-term outcome of patients with differentiated thyroid carcinoma: effect of therapy. Endocr Pract 2000; 6:469–476.
22. Hay ID. Papillary thyroid carcinoma. Endocrinol Metab Clin North Am. 1990; 19:545–576.
23. Grunwald F, Schomburg A, Bender H, et al. Fluorine-18 fluorodeoxyglucose positron emission tomography in the follow-up of differentiated thyroid cancer. Eur J Nucl Med 1996; 23:312–319.
24. Sisson JC, Ackermann RJ, Meyer MA, Wahl RL. Uptake of 18-fluoro-2-deoxy-D-glucose by thyroid cancer: implications for diagnosis and therapy. J Clin Endocrinol Metab 1993; 77:1090–1094.
25. Chung JK, So Y, Lee JS, et al. Value of FDG PET in papillary thyroid carcinoma with negative ^{131}I whole-body scan. J Nucl Med 1999; 40:986–992.
26. Chin BB, Patel P, Cohade C, et al. Recombinant human thyrotropin stimulation of fluoro-D-glucose positron emission tomography uptake in well-differentiated thyroid carcinoma. J Clin Endocrinol Metab 2004; 89:91–95.
27. Yeo JS, Chung JK, So Y, et al. F-18-fluorodeoxyglucose positron emission tomography as a presurgical evaluation modality for I-131 scan-negative thyroid carcinoma patients with local recurrence in cervical lymph nodes. Head Neck 2001; 23:94–103.
28. Wang W, Larson SM, Fazzari M, et al. Prognostic value of [18F] fluorodeoxyglucose positron emission tomographic scanning in patients with thyroid cancer. J Clin Endocrinol Metab 2000; 85:1107–1113.

29
Levothyroxine Therapy and Thyrotropin Suppression

Leonard Wartofsky

INTRODUCTION

Levothyroxine (L-T4) is arguably the most prescribed medication in the United States, with its primary therapeutic indication for hypothyroidism from chronic thyroiditis or Hashimoto's disease. Such patients are candidates for so-called replacement dosage, with the administered dosage of L-T4 titrated to a target thyrotropin (TSH) level within the normal range of 0.4–2.0 mU/L. Patients with thyroid cancer who have had near-total to total thyroidectomy are usually candidates for suppressive levothyroxine dosage, which is "so-called" because the aim of therapy is to give a slightly supraphysiologic dosage of thyroxine to suppress TSH. The rationale for suppressive therapy is based on studies indicating that TSH stimulation enhances tumor growth, TSH serving as a growth factor or mitogen for thyroid malignancies with observations of more rapid tumor growth seen clinically after thyroxine withdrawal. The growth-promoting property of TSH is presumed to be from the presence of TSH receptors on thyroid cancer cells (1); however, non-TSH receptor–mediated growth is certainly a property of undifferentiated thyroid cancers.

An early study by Mazzaferri and Jhiang (2) demonstrated that thyroid hormone therapy had a salutary effect on the survival of patients with papillary thyroid cancer. Although a clear relationship between the magnitude of TSH suppression and mortality has not been definitively shown, observational studies tend to suggest lower rates of both tumor recurrence and cancer-specific death in patients on suppressive dosage. One retrospective study concluded that improved prognosis and outcome was associated with full TSH suppression, in contrast to outcomes in patients with lesser degrees of TSH suppression (3). Those patients with TSH levels of less than 0.5 mU/L had more prolonged disease-free intervals than those with a higher mean TSH level, making the TSH level an independent predictive factor for recurrence. The National Comprehensive Cancer Network guidelines (4) do not stipulate what degree of TSH suppression should be achieved, whereas the British Thyroid Association guidelines advocate suppression to less than 0.1 mU/L or to undetectable levels in a sensitive assay (5).

Only once-daily levothyroxine therapy is required because of the long (6–7 d) half-life of thyroxine. Other thyroid hormone preparations are available and include desiccated thyroid extract USP, a tri-iodothyronine (T3) preparation, and a mixture of thyroxine (T4) and T3 (liotrix). Although once in popular use, the desiccated thyroid extract preparation is not generally recommended because of its T3 content, which is so rapidly absorbed that the resultant high-serum T3 can cause tachycardias or arrhythmias in elderly patients or those with underlying cardiac disease. The T4 products are more stable with a longer and more predictable shelf-life. As T4 is converted to T3, near-normal concentrations of serum T3 can be restored ultimately by administering T4 alone.

Target goals for TSH suppression vary within clinical centers and among thyroid cancer experts but are generally linked to risk stratification, stage of disease, and the presence or absence of residual or recurrent tumor. If not indicated, oversuppression should be avoided because of the known deleterious effects of excessive thyroid hormone levels on both the heart (6–9) and bone mineral density (10,11). Even in thyroid cancer patients who have evidence of residual cancer, there should be careful dosage titration and avoidance of overjudicious suppression, particularly in elderly patients with underlying cardiovascular disease, osteopenia, or osteoporosis. Moreover, there is a subpopulation of patients who, for unknown reasons, appear to be extremely sensitive to minor fluctuations (either increases or decreases) in their L-T4 levels. For all of these reasons, it is important for patients to be taking L-T4 tablets of precise levothyroxine content, potency, and bioequivalence (12,13). The Thyroid Foundation of America has warned patients of potential untoward effects of a change or "switch" in L-T4 preparations that are not truly bioequivalent (14), along with the American Thyroid Association, Endocrine Society, and the American Association of Clinical Endocrinologists (15). These organizations recommend that patients remain on the same branded levothyroxine preparation and are not prescribed generic levothyroxine because pharmacists dispense different generics as refills from one month to the next, preparations that have not been proven bioequivalent to each other. If a change in brand is necessary, the professional organizations recommend remeasurement of TSH in 6 wk and retitration of the levothyroxine dose to the desired level.

For most individuals, a normal metabolic state is associated with normalization of the TSH level to the range of 0.5–1.5 mU/L; on average, this equates to a daily dose of L-T4 of approx 1.7 µg/kg. Patients who have had a total thyroidectomy, e.g., for thyroid malignancy, especially when surgery was followed by radioiodine ablation, will have no residual thyroid tissue, and their requirement will be closer to 2.1 µg/kg/d. Clearly, dosage adjustments should not be based solely on such approximations and are best determined by clinical criteria and TSH measurement. In high-risk patients with evidence of residual disease, we would generally prescribe dosage targeted to keep TSH levels at less than 0.02 mU/L, whereas somewhat lower risk patients with the possibility of residual disease might be kept between 0.05 and 0.1 mU/L. Within the first 5 yr of diagnosis, thyroid cancer patients at low risk of recurrence and who have been proven free of residual disease do not need to have their TSH levels fully suppressed and may have their L-T4 dose reduced to the replacement level range of 0.2–0.6 mU/L. Finally, patients with negative recombinant human TSH-stimulated thyroglobulin levels isotope scans, and imaging more than 5 yr since diagnosis may have their dosage reduced to achieve normal-range TSH levels of 0.3–1.5 mU/L. In either case, careful and precise L-T4 dose titration is mandatory to achieve a specific end point for the therapy, whether it is a normal-range level of TSH or is just suppressed into the undetectable range.

Although there are no specific studies designed to assess what degree of TSH suppression may be required for individual patients with thyroid cancer, the analysis by Cooper et al. *(16)* of 683 patients with differentiated thyroid cancer provided useful insights into this issue. Examination of patient records of a multicenter thyroid cancer registry revealed that most patients did not have fully suppressed TSH levels at all visits, but suppression appeared to be more uniform for patients with follicular thyroid cancer. Importantly, no relationship between cancer progression and degree of TSH suppression was found for stage I or stage II papillary cancer, the staging indicating that the risk of recurrence was low; hence, the degree of TSH suppression should not matter. However, this was not the case for stage III or IV patients, whose outcomes were improved by greater degrees of TSH suppression. These data serve to provide guidelines based on risk stratification on how aggressive to be with TSH suppression.

In some circumstances, a previously stable dosage of levothyroxine may have to be increased or decreased for a variety of reasons. Of course, the most common explanation for an inappropriately high TSH is nonadherence to the prescribed regimen, but occasionally, there may be other explanations. For example, a rising TSH could signal a reduction in gastrointestinal thyroxine absorption. This could be owing to concomitant ingestion of L-T4 with food or certain other pharmacologic agents that interfere with gastrointestinal absorption (e.g., calcium, cholestyramine, colestipol, kayexalate, antacids, sucralfate, iron, and so on) or that enhance the metabolic clearance of levothyroxine (e.g., carbamazepine and phenytoin).

Most manufacturers of levothyroxine products provide a wide range of dosage strengths: 25, 50, 75, 88, 100, 112, 125, 137, 150, 175, 200, and 300 µg per tablet. Theoretically, the availability of these multiple-dosage strengths allow the clinician to precisely titrate a given patient's levothyroxine requirement to a desired metabolic and serum TSH level. Recent changes in regulations governing bioavailability and bioequivalence of the levothyroxine preparations by the US Food and Drug Administration (FDA) has led to a flurry of new L-T4 preparations, including generic or nonbranded forms of L-T4 with presumed therapeutic interchange of one preparation for another *(13)*. In the current era of pressures on clinicians for the most cost-effective medicine, a lower cost preparation is obviously desirable but is acceptable only if shown to be of proven equivalent potency and pharmacodynamics. Some older studies have suggested similar bioequivalence between various levothyroxine preparations, whereas other reports have found differences. Practical application of the conclusions, or definitive interpretation of the results, taken from these earlier reports is difficult because of methodologic defects in patient selection or study design that have become appreciated only in retrospect.

Apart from factors of cost and industry competition, the issue of therapeutic equivalence is obviously important regarding the quality of patient care. The American Thyroid Association (ATA) and the American Association of Clinical Endocrinologists (AACE) have published management guidelines, indicating that the various levothyroxine products may not be therapeutically equivalent *(15,17,18)*. The literature is replete with examples of the lack of interchangeability and varying potency of the different preparations, available as either branded and generic formulations. Consequently, repetitive measurements of serum TSH and appropriate dosage retitration are recommended by the ATA and other experts when patients or their physicians may decide to switch from one preparation to another *(17,18)*. The costs and inconvenience of retesting and retitration understandably may vitiate any cost savings from switching to a less expensive preparation. Hence, for an alternative product to be affirmed as cost-effective, proof of bioequivalence would be required. The ATA recommendation for retitration after switching preparations implies that the various levothyroxine preparations have not been shown to be therapeutically equivalent and interchangeable.

THE QUESTIONABLE ROLE OF T3 THERAPY

Recent interest in combined T3 and T4 therapy for hypothyroidism is based on the longstanding concern whether hypothyroid patients can be optimally replaced by treatment with T4 alone. This topic has been reviewed in two excellent editorials (19,20), and similar questions often arise in patients with thyroid cancer. To more closely mimic thyroidal T3 secretion and normal blood levels, oral supplements of triiodothyronine would need to be given in frequent and divided dosage—a regimen that makes patient compliance problematic. Moreover, convincing arguments or data demonstrating benefit of concomitant T3 administration are lacking. A small fraction of patients continue to complain of persistent nonspecific symptoms, such as easy fatigue, and these complaints tend to be more prominent in patients with autoimmune thyroid disease (Hashimoto's thyroiditis or Graves' disease postablative therapy) than in thyroidectomized thyroid cancer patients. Depending on patient responses to symptom questionnaires, studies indicate that patients tend to feel better, at least transiently, when mildly thyrotoxic, whether by T4 therapy (21) or by T3 (22). Perhaps thyroid cancer patients complain less because higher doses of thyroxine are administered to suppress their TSH levels.

Much interest in the concept that concomitant T3 therapy was necessary to restore euthyroidism at the tissue level was the result of the experimental rat studies by Escobar-Morreale et al. (23) who examined whether T4 therapy alone might provide insufficient intracellular levels of T3, irrespective of serum levels of either T3 or TSH. They found that no dose of T4 by itself simultaneously normalized both T4 and T3 levels in tissues, but there are no precisely comparable studies in humans. The same group (23a) did perform a crossover clinical trial of combination T3/T4 versus T4 alone in humans, and although many of the patients preferred the combination, there was no objective advantage observed. A clinical study that ostensibly demonstrated a greater clinical benefit from combined T3/T4 therapy than that achieved with T4 alone was reported by Bunevicius and coworkers (22). In that study, 33 patients (16 with autoimmune thyroid disease and hypothyroidism, 17 on suppression for thyroid cancer) were being treated with an average daily dose of 0.175 mg T4. Irrespective of the dosage (some took as little as 75 µg daily), 12.5 µg of T3 was substituted for 50 µg of T4, with the patients treated in a randomized crossover sequence of 5-wk duration. Based on their observations, the authors concluded that "partial substitution of T3 for T4 may have more salutary effects on the brain and perhaps other tissues than those of equivalent doses of T4." Possible deficiencies in their study design and criticism of their methods and conclusions have been published (19,20,24). Analysis of the data indicates that it was the thyroid cancer patients, not the Hashimoto's patients, who seemed to derive benefit from the T3 combination, suggesting that it was the overdosage that was responsible, as seen in other studies. The validity of subsequent skepticism in their results appears supported by five more recent reports of studies, all of which indicated no benefit with combined L-T4 and L-T3 therapy (25–29).

In most cases, the study designs in these clinical trials did not provide optimally physiologic doses of T3. For thyroxine, thyroidal T4 secretion approximates 56 µg/m^2/d, which amounts to 100 µg of T4/d, given an average surface area of 1.78 m^2. With an approx 80% effective gastrointestinal absorption, the optimal T4 replacement dose to deliver 100 µg would be 112–125 µg/d. With thyroidal secretion of T3, there are 3.3 µg/m^2/d produced that, for a body surface area of 1.78 m^2, amounts to only 5.9 µg/d, far less than the 10–25 µg given in most of the reported trial. Thus, we cannot invoke inadequate T3 dosage as the explanation for the failure of these trials to prove a benefit of T3 combination therapy. Of circulating T3, 80% is derived from the monodeiodination of T4 in peripheral tissues; thus, of a total daily T3 production rate of 25–30 µg/d, 19–24 µg are derived from T4 and only 6 µg are from the thyroid gland.

The argument can be readily made that those patients showing some ostensible benefit from T3 coadministration received supraphysiologic dosage of T3. The most recently published study on combination T4/T3 therapy did examine the question of possible benefit in doses given in a more appropriate molar ratio, i.e., 14:1 (30), but again, the authors concluded that there was no benefit to T4/T3 and potential risk from subclinical hyperthyroidism. The ideal combination T3/T4 therapy might occur if given in the correct molar ratio, such as a tablet containing 112 µg of T4 and 6 µg of T3 and one that is not given in a "bolus" form but in a delayed-release vehicle. The 112 µg of T4 would provide 22 µg of T3 via deiodination for a total of 30 µg of T3 production daily. A delayed-release vehicle for the T3 could provide a real test of efficacy of combined L-T3/L-T4 therapy. Current preparations are problematic because using current T3 preparations to achieve a premorbid normal profile of thyroid function tests might require administering the T3 as 5 µg TID or perhaps 2.5 µg QID, certainly not an optimal regimen for thyroid cancer patients. As a result of missing the occasional second daily dose, patients will ingest less than that required for the desired suppression of their TSH levels, with resultant inadequately treated cancer and greater risk of recurrence.

For all of these reasons, we do not believe that there is any current role in thyroid cancer patients for combined T3/T4 therapy. Rather, the evidence of therapeutic benefit from the administration of exogenously administered T3 vs endogenous T3 derived from T4 is intriguing but unconvincing. Clearly, the earlier Bunevicius study (22) has not been confirmed, and the reported symptomatically beneficial clinical responses are likely to have been from transient relative T3 excess (24–30). Imprecise dosing with current T3 preparations is undesirable considering the risks of underdosage of a thyroid cancer patient in whom full suppression is indicated or the risk of overdosage when not warranted, causing subclinical hyperthyroidism. Availability of a more physiologic slow-release T3 product may prove to be of interest, but at the present time, the best management for both thyroid hormone replacement and TSH suppression in thyroid cancer patients continues to be L-T4 alone. Despite the risks to the heart and bone of full thyrotropin suppression, outcome analysis suggests that suppression therapy is associated with a reduction in adverse clinical events (31).

REFERENCES

1. Carayon P, Thomnas-Morvan C, Castan E, Tubiana M. Human thyroid cancer: Membrane thyrotropin binding and adenylate cyclase activity. J Clin Endocrinol Metab 1980; 51:915–920.
2. Mazzaferri EL, Jhiang SM. Long-term impact of initial surgical and medical therapy on papillary and follicular thyroid cancer. Am J Med 1994; 97:418–428.
3. Pujol P, Daures J-P, Nsakala N, et al. Degree of thyrotropin suppression as a prognostic determinant in differentiated thyroid cancer. J Clin Endocrinol Metab 1996; 81:4318–4322.
4. National Comprehensive Cancer Network (NCCN) Thyroid Carcinoma: Clinical Practice Guidelines 2005, J Natl Comprehensive Cancer Network 2005; 3:404–457.
5. British Thyroid Association. Guidelines for the management of differentiated thyroid cancer in adults. Available at: www.british-thyroid-association.org/guidelines.htm, 2002.
6. Sawin CT, Geller A, Wolf PA, et al. Low serum thyrotropin concentrations as a risk factor for atrial fibrillation in older persons. N Engl J Med 1994; 331:1249–1252.
7. Parle JV, Maisonneuve P, Sheppard MC, et al. Prediction of all-cause and cardiovascular mortality in elderly people from one low serum thyrotropin result: a 10-year cohort study. Lancet 2001; 358:861–865.
8. Fazio S, Palmieri EA, Lombardi G, Biondi B. Effects of thyroid hormone on the cardiovascular system. Recent Prog Horm Res 2004; 59: 31–50.
9. Biondi B, Palmieri EA, Lombardi G, Fazio S. Effects of subclinical thyroid dysfunction on the heart. Ann Intern Med 2002; 137:904–914.
10. Stathatos N, Wartofsky L. Effects of thyroid hormone on bone. Clin Rev Bone Mineral Metab 2004; 2:135–150.
11. Mikosch P, Obermayer-Pietsch B, Jost R, et al. Bone metabolism in patients with differentiated thyroid carcinoma receiving suppressive levothyroxine treatment. Thyroid 2003; 13:347–356.
12. Katz M, Rosen DL, Wartofsky L. Issues in bioequivalence and therapeutic equivalence of levothyroxine products. US Pharm 2003; 9(Suppl):2–14.
13. Wartofsky L. Levothyroxine: Therapeutic use and regulatory issues related to bioequivalence. Expert Opin Pharmacother 2002; 3:727–732.
14. Thyroid Foundation of America. Advice to patients from the Thyroid Foundation of America. Thyroid 2004; 14:487.
15. American Thyroid Association, Endocrine Society, American Association of Clinical Endocrinologists. Joint Statement on the U.S. Food and Drug Administration's decision regarding bioequivalence of levothyroxine sodium. Thyroid 2004; 14:486.
16. Cooper DS, Specker B, Ho M, et al. Thyrotropin suppression and disease progression in patients with differentiated thyroid cancer: Results from the National Thyroid Cancer Treatment Cooperative Registry. Thyroid 1998; 9:737–744.
17. AACE/AAES Medical/Surgical guidelines for clinical practice: management of thyroid carcinoma. Endocr Pract 2001; 7:1–19.
18. Singer PA, Cooper DA, Daniels GH, et al. Treatment guidelines for patients with thyroid nodules and well differentiated thyroid cancer. Arch Int Med 1996; 156:2165–2172.
19. Cooper DS. Combined T4 and T3 therapy—back to the drawing board. JAMA 2003; 290:3002–3004.
20. Kaplan MM, Sarne DH, Schneider AB. Editorial: In search of the impossible dream? Thyroid hormone replacement therapy that treats all symptoms in all hypothyroid patients. J Clin Endocrinol Metab 2003; 88:4540–4542.
21. Carr D, McLeod DT, Parry G, et al. Fine adjustment of thyroxine replacement dosge: comparison of thyrotrophin releasing hormone test using a sensitive thyrotrophin assay with measurement of free thyroid hormones and clinical assessment. Clin Endocrinol 1988; 28: 325–333.
22. Bunevicius R, Kazanavicius G, Zalinkevicius R, Prange AJ, Jr. Effects of thyroxine as compared with thyroxine plus triiodothyronine in patients with hypothyroidism. N Engl J Med 1999; 340: 424–429.
23. Escobar-Morreale HF, Escobar del Rey FE, Obregon MJ, Morreale de Escobar G. Only the combined treatment with thyroxine and triiodothyronine ensures euthyroidism in all tissues of the thyroidectomized rat. Endocrinology 1996; 137:2490–2502.
23a. Escobar-Morreale HF, Botella-Carretero JI, Gomez-Bueno M, et al. Thyroid hormone replacement therapy in primary hypothyroidism: A randomized trial comparing L-thyroxine plus liothyronine with L-thyroxine alone. Ann Intern Med 2005; 142:412–424.
24. Toft AD. Thyroid hormone replacement—one hormone or two? N Engl J Med 1999; 340:469–470.
25. Clyde PW, Harari AE, Getka EJ, Shakir KMM. Combined levothyroxine plus liothyronine compared with levothyroxine alone in primary hypothyroidism. JAMA 2003; 290:2952–2958.
26. Levitt A, Silverberg J. T4 plus T3 treatment for hypothyroidism: a double-blind comparison with usual T4. Los Angeles, CA: Program 74th Annual Meeting, American Thyroid Association, 2002, 112.
27. Sawka AM, Gerstein HC, Marriott MJ, et al. Does a combination regimen of thyroxine (T4) and 3,5,3'-triiodothyronine improve depressive symptoms better than T4 alone in patients with hypothyroidism? Results of a double-blind, randomized, controlled trial. J Clin Endocrinol Metab 2003; 88:4551–4555.
28. Walsh JP, Shiels L, Lim EM, et al. Combined thyroxine/liothyronine treatment does not improve well-being, quality of life, or cognitive function compared to thyroxine alone: a randomized controlled trial in patients with primary hypothyroidism. J Clin Endocrinol Metab 2003; 88:4543–4550.
29. Cassio A, Cacciari E, Cicognani A, et al. Treatment for congenital hypothyroidism: thyroxine alone or thyroxine plus triiodothyronine? Pediatrics 2003; 111:1055–1060.
30. Siegmund W, Spieker K, Weike AI, et al. Replacement therapy with levothyroxine plus triiodothyronine (bioavailable molar ratio 14:1) is not superior to thyroxine alone to improve well-being and cognitive performance in hypothyroidism. Clin Endocrinol 2004; 60: 750–757.
31. McGriff NJ, Csako G, Gourgiotis L, et al. Effects of thyroid hormone suppression therapy on adverse clinical outcomes in thyroid cancer. Ann Med 2002; 34:554–564.

30
Thyroglobulin and Thyroglobulin Antibodies
Measurement and Interferences

D. Robert Dufour

THYROGLOBULIN AND ITS MEASUREMENT

Thyroglobulin

Thyroglobulin, an approximately 670-kDa glycopeptide, is the major protein product of thyroid follicular cells; its rate of synthesis is increased by thyrotropin (TSH). After synthesis, it is modified by the attachment of iodine to selected tyrosine residues, which undergo rearrangement to form iodothyronines, particularly thyroxine (T4) and, to a lesser extent, thysonine (T3). Other modifications of thyroglobulin also occur, including glycation and sulfation *(1)*. The degree of TSH stimulation affects the extent of branching of carbohydrate side chains *(2)*. There is variable processing of thyroglobulin, creating a family of proteins with different molecular structures around a common core peptide backbone. Interestingly, there is less variability in thyroglobulin structure in thyroid cancer than in other thyroid diseases *(3)*. Reduced iodine content in thyroglobulin exists in patients with thyroid malignancy *(4)*, which can lead to different recognition by monoclonal antibodies *(5)*. This structural heterogeneity creates a challenge for thyroglobulin immunoassays, and results often differ significantly when using different thyroglobulin methods *(6)*.

Normally, only small amounts of intact thyroglobulin reach the circulation in proportion to thyroid mass. It has been estimated that 1 g of thyroid tissue increases serum thyroglobulin by 1 µg/L (ng/mL) under normal TSH stimulation and 0.5 µg/L (ng/mL) during suppression of TSH. Reference intervals for thyroglobulin based on healthy ambulatory individuals with normal iodide intake typically range from 3 to 40 µg/mL (ng/L). Increased thyroglobulin is also released in response to inflammation, as in thyroiditis. Other factors that increase serum thyroglobulin include low-iodide intake, trauma to the thyroid (e.g., fine-needle aspiration), and cigarette smoking. After complete thyroidectomy and remnant ablation by radioactive iodine, thyroglobulin concentration should be below the detection limit of the assay. This forms the basis for use of thyroglobulin as a marker for residual differentiated thyroid cancer.

Thyroglobulin Assays

Thyroglobulin is measured in the laboratory by use of antibodies to thyroglobulin. There are two principal assay formats: competitive (single antibody) and sandwich (double antibody) methods. Generally, the laboratory procedure does not indicate the type of assay used on its reports. It is important for the endocrinologist to be aware of the method(s) used by the laboratory, especially for thyroglobulin measurements *(7)*. The two types of assay formats vary in the lowest amount of thyroglobulin detectable, the risk of interference from antithyroglobulin antibodies and other potentially interfering substances (particularly heterophile antibodies and rheumatoid factor), and the direction of change in apparent concentration caused by these interferences.

To measure thyroglobulin by immunoassay, the amount of thyroglobulin-bound antibody in a patient sample is compared to that in samples with known amounts of a standard thyroglobulin preparation. The process of comparing the amount of antibody bound to samples containing the standard preparation of thyroglobulin is termed "assay calibration." Because of the varying structures of thyroglobulin, it is critical that assays use the same "standard" preparation of thyroglobulin for calibration. Currently, a Certified Reference Material (CRM-457; *8*), available through the Community Bureau of Reference, Commission of the European Communities, is considered the preferred standard preparation *(9)*. One potential drawback to this standard is that it is derived from normal thyroid tissue and may not accurately reflect forms found in those with thyroid malignancy *(10)*.

Development of Thyroglobulin Antibodies

The process of developing antibodies to use in the assay involves immunization of animals with thyroglobulin. As a large complex molecule, thyroglobulin has many epitopes that can be recognized by the immune system of the

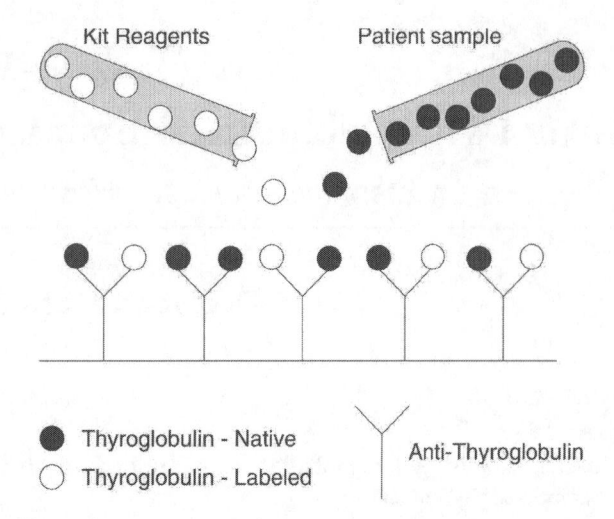

Fig. 1. Principle of competitive immunoassay for thyroglobulin. The principle of the assay is to use a limited amount of antibody to thyroglobulin, along with a limited amount of a labeled form of thyroglobulin; the label can be a radioactive isotope, an enzyme, or a fluorescent compound. By adding known amounts of unlabeled thyroglobulin, a calibration curve is created in which the amount of labeled thyroglobulin bound to the antibody is inversely related to the amount of unlabeled thyroglobulin in the sample tested. Unknown patient samples are then evaluated using the calibration curve to determine their concentration of thyroglobulin.

injected animal. Each host genetic structure allows varying recognition of differing epitopes. Antibodies produced are harvested and processed in one of two main methods. In the simplest, serum from the animal is processed by absorbing with human samples devoid of thyroglobulin and tested for its ability to react with thyroglobulin. Strongly reacting animals can then be bled repetitively (after booster injections with thyroglobulin) as a source of antibody. This creates a mixture of antibodies produced by several clones of plasma cells (polyclonal antibody) to different epitopes on thyroglobulin. A single animal produces the same relative mixture of polyclonal antibodies that recognize varying epitopes differently. Nonidentical animals, even from the same species, produce different mixtures of antibodies that may have varying recognition of different thyroglobulin epitopes. Combined with the varying structures of thyroglobulin molecules, this creates different binding of thyroglobulin to antibody in kits containing antibody from different animals. This will be true even of kits from the same manufacturer because the antibody used in the kits will differ as one animal dies and is replaced by another.

Alternatively, plasma cells from the injected animal are harvested, and individual cells are fused with myeloma cell lines to produce hybridomas; each hybridoma creates a monoclonal antibody product. The monoclonal immunoglobulins derived from cell culture supernates of the hybridoma line are then absorbed with thyroglobulin-deficient human samples and tested for reactivity against thyroglobulin. The advantages of monoclonal antibodies include reproducible production of antibody by the immortalized cell line and recognition of only a single epitope of the molecule, thereby minimizing differences between kits prepared by the same manufacturer. Kits from different companies employ different monoclonal antibodies.

The result of differences in antibodies used leads to measurable differences in thyroglobulin concentration between assays when testing a single sample. Several studies have documented up to a fourfold difference in concentration between methods, even when CRM-457 is used in method calibration (11–13). It is therefore critical that endocrinologists treating patients with thyroid cancer have an effective working relationship with their laboratory. If the laboratory switches assays for thyroglobulin, it is essential that patient samples be tested in parallel with both the old and new method (6). This testing allows determination of the expected difference to be seen and prevents unnecessary action based solely on the varying recognition of the patient's thyroglobulin by the assay. It has been suggested that laboratories save samples and run old samples at the same time as those that are new to enable better detection of differences in concentration (13), but this is impractical for most laboratories.

Competitive Immunoassays for Thyroglobulin

The earliest assays for measuring thyroglobulin were based on competitive immunoassay formats, as illustrated in Fig. 1. In general, competitive immunoassays cannot detect low concentrations of thyroglobulin as well as sandwich methods. In a review of thyroglobulin assays, the functional sensitivity (defined as the level at which reproducibility between repeated measurements of the same sample was at an acceptable limit of 20%) of competitive assays ranged from 0.7 to 2.0 µg/L (ng/mL). The functional sensitivity of sandwich assays ranged from 0.2 to 0.6 µg/L (ng/mL; 9). Competitive assays are relatively free from interference by the rheumatoid factor and heterophile antibodies, which can cause falsely elevated results in sandwich assays (9). Competitive assays may produce falsely high results in the presence of antithyroglobulin antibodies, as discussed in more detail below and illustrated in Fig. 2.

Sandwich Immunometric Assays for Thyroglobulin

Most current thyroglobulin assays are based on sandwich or immunometric assays, as illustrated in Fig. 3. The two major advantages of sandwich assays are enhanced ability to detect low concentrations of thyroglobulin and the ability to measure a wide range of concentrations without the need for sample dilution. Most sandwich assays also use at least two monoclonal antibodies, allowing more reproducible measurement of thyroglobulin over time with use of the same manufacturer's method. Sandwich assays are subject to interference by the presence of heterophile antibodies and the

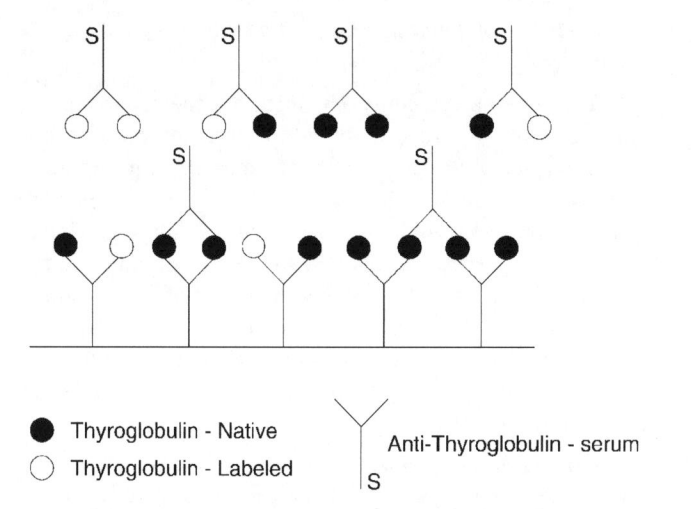

Fig. 2. Mechanism of interference of thyroglobulin antibodies in competitive immunoassay for thyroglobulin. Thyroglobulin antibodies likely interfere with competitive assays by one or both mechanism(s). Thyroglobulin levels in the bloodstream increase because of reduced clearance when bound to antibody. Additionally, free antibody can bind labeled thyroglobulin in the reagent. Both phenomena reduce the amount of labeled thyroglobulin bound to the reagent antibody, falsely increasing reported thyroglobulin concentration.

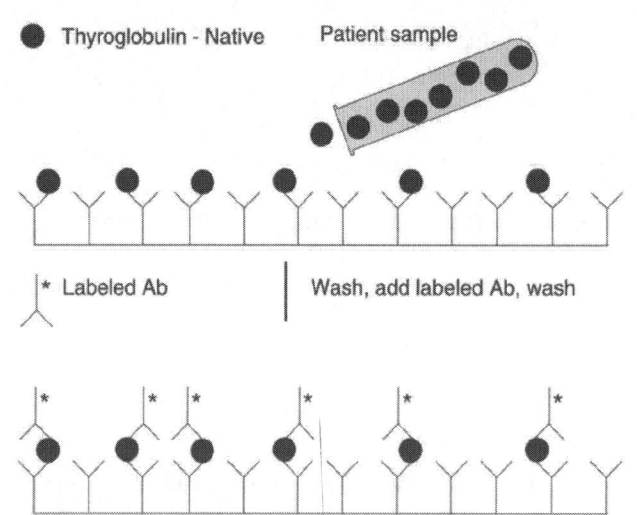

Fig. 3. Principle of sandwich immunometric assays for thyroglobulin. A known excess amount of antibody to thyroglobulin is fixed to a solid support. Known calibrators or unknown patient samples are incubated with the antibody-labeled support, which is then washed to remove any unbound thyroglobulin. A second antithyroglobulin antibody (often directed against a separate part of the thyroglobulin molecule), labeled with a radioactive isotope, enzyme, or fluorescent compound, is then added to the solid support. The amount of label remaining on the solid support (after a second wash) is directly related to the number of antigen–antibody complexes formed. Because the quantity of antigen–antibody complexes decreases when the amount of antigen exceeds the amount of antibody, sandwich assays may produce falsely low results at high thyroglobulin concentrations—a phenomenon known as the "high-dose hook effect."

rheumatoid factor, producing falsely high results *(14–17)*. One study found such interference in 3% of samples tested for thyroglobulin *(18)*. Although manufacturers have modified their kits to minimize heterophile antibody interference, the efficacy of such modifications is variable, including in kits from the same manufacturer *(19)*. Some laboratories use tubes that absorb these heterophile antibodies. One multicenter study of sandwich assays (usually not for thyroglobulin) found that use of binding tubes (along with the manufacturer's approaches to minimize interference) failed to prevent 49% of clinically important interferences *(20)*. As illustrated in Fig. 4, and discussed in more detail later, antithyroglobulin antibodies in a patient sample cause falsely low results in sandwich assays.

Issues in Thyroglobulin Measurement

Numerous other issues limit the utility of thyroglobulin measurements for monitoring thyroid cancer. In addition to the interferences from thyroglobulin and heterophile antibodies, two other major issues exist in thyroglobulin measurement, as outlined recently by Spencer *(13)*, variation between thyroglobulin methods and detection limits of assays for identifying recurrent cancer.

Assay Differences in Thyroglobulin Level

Currently, there are four kits to perform thyroglobulin measurement that are commercially available in North America. In testing 88 euthyroid normal volunteers who are negative for thyroglobulin antibodies, the mean thyroglobulin concentration varied between 8.9 and 16.9 µg/L (ng/L), but the average difference was 30%. Thus, there is a possible cause for misinterpretation of results when individual patients are seen at institutions that utilize different thyroglobulin methods. No data are provided on variations in patients with thyroid cancer, which may differ in magnitude based on differences in the structure of thyroglobulin produced by different tumors.

Lower Limit of Detection of Assays

Spencer also advocates adopting new approaches to evaluate a method's ability to detect low levels of thyroglobulin *(13)*. Although functional sensitivity represents a reasonable approach to evaluate methods, all current methods have less than a one-log difference between the lower end of the reference interval and the functional sensitivity limit. Spencer proposes to employ the concept of "generations," which are currently used to describe the functional sensitivity of TSH assays. In this nomenclature, current assays would be termed "first generation," whereas those with a 1–2 log difference between the lower reference limit and functional sensitivity

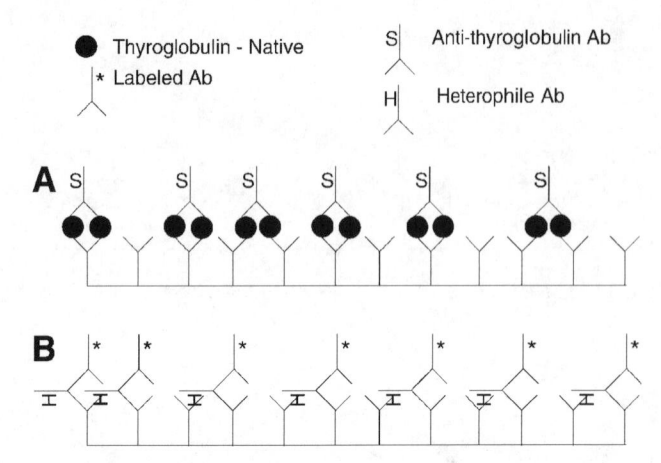

Fig. 4. Mechanisms of interference in sandwich immunometric assays for thyroglobulin. **(A)** Thyroglobulin antibody interference. Thyroglobulin antibodies likely interfere in sandwich assays by attaching to thyroglobulin linked to the bound antibody. This leads to steric inhibition of binding by the labeled antibody and falsely low thyroglobulin concentrations. **(B)** Heterophile antibody interference. Heterophile antibodies are human antibodies that react with the Fc portion of immunoglobulin molecules of other species; most commonly, anti-mouse antibodies are the cause of interference, as mouse cells are used to produce most monoclonal antibodies. (In the figure, for space reasons, the antibodies are shown as if they attach to the Fab portion of the antibody molecule.) After attaching to the bound antibody, they retain one binding site to which the labeled antibody can attach, producing falsely high values. While less commonly encountered, rheumatoid factor (which attaches to the Fc portion of human and animal immunoglobulins) can produce the same pattern of interference.

would be termed "second generation" and those with a 2–3 log difference, "third generation." Currently, it is not clear whether lower detection limits will improve the ability to recognize residual thyroid cancer or will prove too sensitive to detect minute amounts of residual normal thyroid tissue.

In one study using an assay with a detection limit of 0.18 ng/mL (µg/L), compared to an assay with a detection limit of 1.0 ng/mL (µg/L), the more sensitive assay detected 11 additional patients (29%) with positive basal thyroglobulin on suppression. In addition, 20% of patients with undetectable baseline thyroglobulin showed an increase using the more sensitive assay that was not detected by the other assay *(21)*. Use of an even more sensitive assay, with a detection limit of 0.03 µg/L (ng/mL) vs a conventional assay with a detection limit of 0.6 µg/L (ng/mL), found increased basal thyroglobulin in 7 of 139 with the conventional assay but 106 of 139 with the more sensitive assay. None of these individuals had evidence of residual thyroid tissue, even using the positron emission tomography scan *(22)*. Although more studies using highly sensitive assays are clearly needed, it is not clear at this time that they will be more clinically useful.

Guidelines for Laboratories Performing Thyroglobulin Assays

The National Academy of Clinical Biochemistry has published extensive recommendations for laboratories performing thyroid-related tests, including several pertaining to thyroglobulin *(9)*. These guidelines were extensively peer-reviewed, not only by the laboratory community, but by all of the international thyroid societies. Laboratories that perform thyroglobulin measurement should be aware of these state-of-the-art recommendations, and endocrinologists should assure that their laboratories are following these recommendations. The most important of these guidelines are summarized here *(6)*.

- There is no "normal" range for thyroglobulin for a thyroidectomized patient; it is misleading to cite the "normal" euthyroid reference interval for thyroidectomized patients.
- Serum thyroglobulin values for antithyroglobulin-positive specimens should not be reported if the method gives inappropriately undetectable values.
- Recovery tests should be eliminated (to detect thyroglobulin antibody interference); discordance between immunoassay and immunometric assay suggests interference (if values are concordant in antibody-negative specimens).
- If laboratories change their thyroglobulin method, they should consult the physician and compare results between the old and new method in both thyroglobulin antibody–negative and– positive patients. If results are more than 10% different between methods in antibody-negative patients, physicians should be notified to allow retesting (rebaselining) critical patients.
- If thyroglobulin results are reported for antibody-positive patients, an appropriate cautionary comment should be displayed on each laboratory report.

THYROGLOBULIN ANTIBODIES

Prevalence of Thyroglobulin Antibodies in Differentiated Thyroid Cancer

Thyroglobulin antibodies are commonly encountered autoantibodies, both in the general population and in patients with thyroid cancer. At the time of diagnosis, thyroglobulin antibodies are found in a greater proportion of patients with thyroid cancer than in the general population, with an average prevalence of 25% *(23)*; however, some studies have found the prevalence to be as low as 10% *(24)*. With successful eradication of thyroid cancer, titers of thyroglobulin antibodies decrease and usually become undetectable at a median of 3 yr after treatment *(25)*, whereas titers may rise with recurrence *(24)*. The presence of high-titer antithyroglobulin also suggests presence of residual thyroid cancer. Two studies found a much higher incidence of residual thyroid cancer in those with thyroglobulin antibodies (or high-titer antibodies) than in those with negative or low-titer antibody *(24,26)*. Loss of thyroglobulin antibodies is associated with a favorable prognosis and a low risk of recurrent or metastatic thyroid cancer *(23)*.

Thyroglobulin Antibody Interference in Thyroglobulin Measurement

As discussed earlier, thyroglobulin antibodies are a major cause for erroneous thyroglobulin results. Thyroglobulin antibodies should be measured routinely when thyroglobulin is ordered for thyroid cancer monitoring, even if the antibodies were previously undetectable. Recovery experiments involve adding a known amount of thyroglobulin to a serum sample and measuring the increase of thyroglobulin compared to the expected increase. Some studies have suggested that recovery close to 100% of added thyroglobulin can predict levels of antibody that do not interfere with thyroglobulin measurement *(27,28)*. Unfortunately, samples that show high recovery often still demonstrate significantly higher thyroglobulin with immunoassays than with sandwich assays, indicating a clinically important interference *(23,29, 30)*. Reaction strength, either in titer or the relative signal in enzyme-linked immunoabsorbent assays (ELISA), has also failed to predict samples that yield erroneous results. Some samples with high-titer antibodies show no difference between immunoassays and sandwich assays, but some samples with weakly positive antibodies (even below the detection limit of some assays) show clinically significant differences *(31)*. As most laboratories do not perform thyroglobulin levels using two different methods, it is reasonable to assume that results may be inaccurate in samples with thyroglobulin antibodies. The approach for a thyroid cancer patient with thyroglobulin antibodies is discussed in more detail in Chapter 31.

Measurement of Thyroglobulin Antibodies

There are two primary methods for measurement of thyroglobulin antibodies. Historically, hemagglutination inhibition (HAI) was the main method, but has been largely replaced by immunoassay methods, including radioimmunoassay and ELISA formats. The immunoassay methods are more sensitive and have good reproducibility *(32)*, making them suitable for detecting level changes after the removal of a thyroid cancer. They also frequently detect antibodies when HAI methods are negative *(33)*. Current guidelines do not recommend the use of HAI for detection of thyroglobulin antibodies *(9)*.

THYROGLOBULIN IN DIFFERENTIATED THYROID CANCER

Current treatment for differentiated thyroid cancer (total or near-total thyroidectomy, followed by radioiodine ablation) should eradicate thyroglobulin production. Thyroglobulin is thus a highly sensitive marker for recurrent or metastatic thyroid cancer. Rarely, thyroid tumors may fail to produce thyroglobulin. In one study, 1% of 1143 patients with thyroid cancer had undetectable thyroglobulin despite recurrent cancer *(34)*. Because thyroglobulin was measured by the sandwich assay, and HAI was used as the method to measure thyroglobulin antibodies in this study, it is possible that the undetectable thyroglobulin results were from antibody interference in some cases.

There are several potential situations where thyroglobulin measurement could be useful in the diagnosis and management of thyroid cancer, as discussed in detail below. The diagnostic utility of thyroglobulin measurement is impaired in those with thyroglobulin antibodies; therefore, thyroglobulin measurements should always be accompanied by tests for thyroglobulin antibodies. As a practical matter, results of thyroglobulin measurement in the presence of thyroglobulin antibodies can be interpreted accurately (as to the presence or absence of residual thyroid tumor) in some circumstances. For example, a detectable thyroglobulin by the sandwich assay in a person with thyroglobulin antibodies indicates residual thyroid tumor, whereas undetectable stimulated thyroglobulin supports complete ablation of thyroid tumor when measured by immunoassay *(9)*. Because changes in titer affect the degree of interference, it is not possible to use serial thyroglobulin measurement to assess changes in tumor volume or response to therapy until such time as thyroglobulin antibodies become undetectable. As discussed earlier, falling titers indicate a favorable prognosis, and rising titers suggest recurrent thyroid malignancy.

Thyroglobulin Before Surgery

Thyroglobulin is produced by most differentiated thyroid cancers. Although guidelines do not recommend thyroglobulin for preoperative diagnosis of thyroid cancer *(35)*, there may be limited benefit to preoperative thyroglobulin measurement. Thyroid cancers tend be associated with higher preoperative thyroglobulin levels than benign thyroid nodules, particularly when interpreted relative to nodule size *(36–38)*; however, the predictive value of preoperative thyroglobulin measurement is low. One retrospective case-control study found a relative risk of 7 for the development of differentiated thyroid cancer in patients with elevated thyroglobulin measured up to 23 yr before diagnosis *(39)*. However "normal" thyroglobulin in a thyroglobulin antibody–negative individual preoperatively may indicate that the tumor does not produce thyroglobulin and demonstrate the need for other approaches to follow thyroid cancer *(9)*.

Thyroglobulin During TSH Suppression

After resection of thyroid cancer, thyroglobulin falls with a half-life of 65 h and thyroglobulin levels become undetectable after about 1 mo *(40)*. When TSH is suppressed below the lower limits of "normal" by thyroid hormone, thyroglobulin production indicates residual or metastatic disease with a high degree of specificity. Several studies have shown that individuals with detectable thyroglobulin in this setting almost always have residual thyroid cancer, even when tested as early as 1 mo after surgery *(41–43)* and may predict which patients are likely to recur *(43a)*. Measurements are still useful in patients who have not undergone complete thyroidectomy but are more difficult to interpret *(44,45)*. As discussed in more detail below, undetectable thyroglobulin in such situations is not reliable in excluding the presence of residual cancer.

TSH-Stimulated Thyroglobulin

The most sensitive method for detecting residual thyroid cancer is to measure thyroglobulin during TSH stimulation. This is particularly true for low-risk patients, in whom sensitive testing is important to detect the relatively small number of patients who need additional treatment. Several studies have shown that about 20–25% of those with undetectable thyroglobulin during TSH suppression will show a rise in thyroglobulin to 2.0 µg/L (ng/mL) or more under TSH stimulation *(7,46,46a)*. Historically, TSH stimulation was achieved by withdrawing thyroid hormone therapy to produce hypothyroidism. With the availability of recombinant human TSH (rhTSH), its administration is an alternative approach. Consensus shows that this is now the preferred method to evaluate patients for residual thyroid cancer if nonstimulated thyroglobulin is undetectable *(7)*.

While thyroid hormone withdrawal produces greater increases in TSH and thyroglobulin than the administration of rhTSH *(47,48)*, an analysis of eight comparison studies showed equivalent sensitivity of the two approaches for detecting residual cancer *(7)*. In the recommended protocol, 0.9 mg of rhTSH is given on days 1 and 2 (typically Monday/Tuesday), and thyroglobulin is measured on day 5 (Friday). Although one study suggests that this is not always the time of peak TSH or thyroglobulin, and that weight-based dosing may be more accurate *(48)*, consensus guidelines suggest the simpler protocol. Failure of thyroglobulin to rise to detectable levels following TSH stimulation indicates a group of patients with virtually no chance of developing recurrent thyroid cancer if maintained on thyroxine suppression *(49)*. For such individuals, consensus guidelines recommend periodic monitoring of thyroglobulin on suppressive therapy, but there is no need to perform stimulated thyroglobulin testing *(7)*, including in patients who are not at low risk for recurrence *(50)*. Minor increases in thyroglobulin ranging between the detection limit and 2.0 µg/L (ng/mL) are of undetermined significance and require further evaluation *(7)*.

SUMMARY

Thyroglobulin—the major protein product of thyroid follicular cells—is not produced by other cells in the body. Thyroglobulin antibodies, found frequently in the general population, have a high prevalence in those with thyroid cancer. Two principal immunoassay formats exist to measure thyroglobulin, and each is affected in different ways by the presence of thyroglobulin antibodies and other interfering substances. Most laboratories currently use double-antibody (sandwich) methods, which can reliably detect lower concentrations of thyroglobulin, can measure higher values without dilution, and have lower risks of interference from cross-reactive substances. These assays will give falsely low results in the presence of thyroglobulin antibodies but can produce falsely increased results in the presence of heterophile antibodies or the rheumatoid factor. Older competitive immunoassays have a limited ability to detect low concentrations of thyroglobulin, must be diluted at high concentrations, and are potentially subject to interference from similar molecules in the circulation. When antithyroglobulin antibodies are present, results tend to be falsely increased; however, interference from heterophile antibodies and the rheumatoid factor is minimal or absent. While preoperative thyroglobulin has no clinical utility, thyroglobulin measurements are commonly used to detect residual thyroid tissue or tumor in the follow-up of patients with differentiated thyroid cancer who lack thyroglobulin antibodies. Increased thyroglobulin while on thyroid hormone suppression indicates a high chance of residual or metastatic thyroid cancer but is insensitive as a sole test. Stimulation of thyroglobulin production by administration of rhTSH or thyroid hormone withdrawal detects almost all patients with residual or metastatic disease.

REFERENCES

1. van de Graaf S, Ris-Stalpers C, Pauws E, et al. Up to date with human thyroglobulin. J Endocrinol 2001; 170:307–321.
2. Di Jeso B, Liguoro D, Ferranti P, et al. Modulation of the carbohydrate moiety of thyroglobulin by thyrotropin and calcium in Fisher rat thyroid line-5 cells. J Biol Chem 1992; 267:1938–1944.
3. Druetta L, Croizet K, Bornet H, Rousset B. Analyses of the molecular forms of serum thyroglobulin from patients with Graves' disease, subacute thyroiditis or differentiated thyroid cancer by velocity sedimentation on sucrose gradient and Western blot. Eur J Endocrinol 1998; 139:498–507.
4. Schneider A, Ikekubo K, Kuma K. Iodine content of serum thyroglobulin in normal individuals and patients. J Clin Endocrinol Metab 1983; 57:1251–1256.
5. Kohno Y, Tarutani O, Sakata S, Nakajima H. Monoclonal antibodies to thyroglobulin elucidate differences in protein. J Clin Endocrinol Metab 1985; 61:343–350.
6. Spencer CA, Wang C. Thyroglobulin measurement. Techniques, clinical benefits, and pitfalls. Endocrinol Metab Clin North Am 1995; 24:841–863.
7. Mazzaferri E, Robbins R, Spencer C, et al. A consensus report of the role of serum thyroglobulin as a monitoring method for low-risk patients with papillary thyroid carcinoma. J Clin Endocrinol Metab 2003; 88:1433–1441.
8. Feldt-Rasmussen U, Profilis C, Colinet E, et al. Human thyroglobulin reference material (CRM 457). 2nd Part Physicochemical characterization and certification. Ann Biol Clin 1996; 54:343–348.
9. Demers L, Spencer C. Laboratory support for the diagnosis and monitoring of thyroid disease. Thyroid 2003; 13:3–126.

10. Whitley RJ, Ain KB. Thyroglobulin: a specific serum marker for the management of thyroid carcinoma. Clin Lab Med 2004; 24:29–47.
11. Ferrari L, Biancolini D, Seregni E, et al. Critical aspects of immunoradiometric thyroglobulin assays. Tumori 2003; 89:537–539.
12. Spencer CA, Takeuchi M, Kazarosyan M. Current status and performance goals for serum thyroglobulin assays. Clin Chem 1996; 42:164–173.
13. Spencer CA. New insights for using serum thyroglobulin (Tg) measurement for managing patients with differentiated thyroid carcinomas. Thyroid Int 2003:3–14.
14. Kricka L. Human anti-animal antibody interferences in immunological assays. Clin Chem 1999; 45:942–956.
15. Levinson S, Miller J. Towards a better understanding of heterophile (and the like) antibody interference with modern immunoassays. Clin Chim Acta 2002; 325:1–15.
16. Ward G, McKinnon L, Badrick T, Hickman P. Heterophilic antibodies remain a problem for the immunoassay laboratory. Am J Clin Pathol 1997; 108:417–421.
17. Weber T, Kapyaho K, Tanner P. Endogenous interference in immunoassays in clinical chemistry. A review. Scand J Clin Lab Invest Suppl 1990; 201:77–82.
18. Preissner C, O'Kane D, Singh R, et al. Phantoms in the assay tube: heterophile antibody interferences in serum thyroglobulin assays. J Clin Endocrinol Metab 2003; 88:3069–3074.
19. Marks V. False-positive immunoassay results: a multicenter survey of erroneous immunoassay results from assays of 74 analytes in 10 donors from 66 laboratories in seven countries. Clin Chem 2002; 48: 2008–2016.
20. Marks V. False-positive immunoassay results: a multicenter survey of erroneous immunoassay results from assays of 74 analytes in 10 donors from 66 laboratories in seven countries. Clin Chem 2002; 48:2008–2016.
21. Fugazzola L, Mihalich A, Persani L, et al. Highly sensitive serum thyroglobulin and circulating thyroglobulin mRNA evaluations in the management of patients with differentiated thyroid cancer in apparent remission. J Clin Endocrinol Metab 2002; 87:3201–3208.
22. Wunderlich G, Zophel K, Crook L, et al. A high-sensitivity enzyme-linked immunosorbent assay for serum thyroglobulin. Thyroid 2001; 11:819–824.
23. Spencer CA, Takeuchi M, Kazarosyan M, et al. Serum thyroglobulin autoantibodies: prevalence, influence on serum thyroglobulin measurement, and prognostic significance in patients with differentiated thyroid carcinoma. J Clin Endocrinol Metab 1998; 83:1121–1127.
24. Hjiyiannakis P, Mundy J, Harmer C. Thyroglobulin antibodies in differentiated thyroid cancer. Clin Oncol (R Coll Radiol) 1999; 11: 240–244.
25. Chiovato L, Latrofa F, Braverman L, et al. Disappearance of humoral thyroid autoimmunity after complete removal of thyroid antigens. Ann Intern Med 2003; 139:346–351.
26. Chung J, Park Y, Kim T, et al. Clinical significance of elevated level of serum antithyroglobulin antibody in patients with differentiated thyroid cancer after thyroid ablation. Clin Endocrinol (Oxf) 2002; 57: 215–221.
27. Bourrel F, Hoff M, Regis H, et al. Immunoradiometric assay of thyroglobulin in patients with differentiated thyroid carcinomas: need for thyroglobulin recovery tests. Clin Chem Lab Med 1998; 36:725–730.
28. Erali M, Bigelow R, Miekle A. ELISA for thyroglobulin in serum: recovery studies to evaluate autoantibody interference and reliability of thyroglobulin value. Clin Chem 1996; 42:766–770.
29. Mariotti S, Barbesino G, Caturegli P, et al. Assay of thyroglobulin in serum with thyroglobulin autoantibodies: an unobtainable goal? J Clin Endocrinol Metab 1995; 80:468–472.
30. Massart C, Maugendre D. Importance of the detection method for thyroglobulin antibodies for the validity of thyroglobulin measurements in sera from patients with Graves' disease. Clin Chem 2002; 48: 102–107.
31. Cubero J, Rodriguez-Espinosa J, Gelpi C, Estorch M, Corcoy R. Thyroglobulin autoantibody levels below the cut-off for positivity can interfere with thyroglobulin measurement. Thyroid 2003; 13:659–661.
32. Gilmour J, Brownlee Y, Foster P, et al. The quantitative measurement of autoantibodies to thyroglobulin and thyroid peroxidase by automated microparticle based immunoassays in Hashimoto's disease, Graves' disease and a follow-up study on postpartum thyroid disease. Clin Lab 2000; 46:57–61.
33. Lindberg B, Svensson J, Ericsson U, et al. Comparison of some different methods for analysis of thyroid autoantibodies: importance of thyroglobulin autoantibodies. Thyroid 2001; 11:265–269.
34. Westbury C, Vini L, Fisher C, Harmer C. Recurrent differentiated thyroid cancer without elevation of serum thyroglobulin. Thyroid 2000; 10:171–176.
35. Sager P, Cooper D, Daniels G, et al. Treatment guidelines for patients with thyroid nodules and well-differentiated thyroid cancer. Arch Intern Med 1996; 256:2165–2172.
36. Tamizu A, Okumura Y, Sato S, et al. The usefulness of serum thyroglobulin levels and Tl-201 scintigraphy in differentiating between benign and malignant thyroid follicular lesions. Ann Nucl Med 2002; 16:95–101.
37. Hocevar M, Auersperg M. Role of serum thyroglobulin in the preoperative evaluation of follicular thyroid tumours. Eur J Surg Oncol 1998; 24:553–557.
38. Sharma A, Sarda A, Chattopadhyay T, Kapur M. The role of estimation of the ratio of preoperative serum thyroglobulin to the thyroid mass in predicting the behaviour of well differentiated thyroid cancers. J Postgrad Med 1996; 42:39–42.
39. Hrafnkelsson J, Tulinius H, Kjeld M, et al. Serum thyroglobulin as a risk factor for thyroid carcinoma. Acta Oncol 2000; 39:973–977.
40. Hocevar M, Auersperg M, Stanovnik L. The dynamics of serum thyroglobulin elimination from the body after thyroid surgery. Eur J Surg Oncol 1997; 23:208–210.
41. Lima N, Cavaliere H, Tomimori E, et al. Prognostic value of serial serum thyroglobulin determinations after total thyroidectomy for differentiated thyroid cancer. J Endocrinol Invest 2002; 25:110–115.
42. Lin J, Huang M, Hsu B, et al. Significance of postoperative serum thyroglobulin levels in patients with papillary and follicular thyroid carcinomas. J Surg Oncol 2002; 80:45–51.
43. Ronga G, Filesi M, Ventroni G, et al. Value of the first serum thyroglobulin level after total thyroidectomy for the diagnosis of metastases from differentiated thyroid carcinoma. Eur J Nucl Med 1999; 26:1448–1452.
43a. Kim TY, Kim WB, Kim ES, et al. Serum Thyroglobulin levels at the time of 131-I remnant ablation just after thyroidectomy are useful for early prediction of clinical recurrence in low-risk patients with differentiated thyroid carcinoma. J Clin Endocrinol Metab 2005; 90:1440–1445.
44. Van Wyngaarden K, McDougall I. Is serum thyroglobulin a useful marker for thyroid cancer in patients who have not had ablation of residual thyroid tissue? Thyroid 1997; 7:343–346.
45. Grunwald F, Menzel C, Fimmers R, et al. Prognostic value of thyroglobulin after thyroidectomy before ablative radioiodine therapy in thyroid cancer. J Nucl Med 1996; 37:1962–1964.
46. Baudin E, Do Cao C, Cailleux A, et al. Positive predictive value of serum thyroglobulin levels, measured during the first year of follow-up after thyroid hormone withdrawal, in thyroid cancer patients. J Clin Endocrinol Metab 2003; 88:1107–1111.
46a. David A, Blotta A, Rossi R, et al. Clinical value of different responses of serum thyroglobulin to recombinant human thyrotropin in the follow-up of patients with differentiated thyroid carcinoma. Thyroid 2005; 15:267–273.
47. Pacini F, Molinaro E, Castagna M, et al. Recombinant human thyrotropin-stimulated serum thyroglobulin combined with neck

ultrasonography has the highest sensitivity in monitoring differentiated thyroid carcinoma. J Clin Endocrinol Metab 2003; 88: 3668–3673.
48. Pellegriti G, Scollo C, Regalbuto C, et al. The diagnostic use of the rhTSH/thyroglobulin test in differentiated thyroid cancer patients with persistent disease and low thyroglobulin levels. Clin Endocrinol (Oxf) 2003; 58:556–561.
49. Pacini F, Capezzone M, Elisei R, et al. Diagnostic 131-iodine whole-body scan may be avoided in thyroid cancer patients who have undetectable stimulated serum Tg levels after initial treatment. J Clin Endocrinol Metab 2002; 87:1499–1501.
50. Wartofsky L. Using baseline and recombinant human TSH-stimulated Tg measurements to measurements to manage thyroid cancer without diagnostic 131-I scanning. J Clin Endocrinol Metab 2002; 87: 1486–1489.

31
Diagnosis of Recurrent Thyroid Cancer in Patients with Antithyroglobulin Antibodies

Matthew D. Ringel

INTRODUCTION

Whole-body radioiodine scanning, measurement of serum thyroglobulin, and various radiographic methods are used to monitor patients with thyroid cancer for the risk of recurrence. Over the past decade, substantial improvements in thyroglobulin immunoassays and a greater recognition of the limitations of ^{131}I scanning, particularly regarding its relatively low sensitivity for neck recurrences, have led to recommendations that rely greatly on accurate thyroglobulin measurements and neck ultrasound (1,2). However, significant limitations of current thyroglobulin immunoassays include inadequate sensitivity during levothyroxine (L-T4) therapy and the presence of interfering antithyroglobulin antibodies in approx 20% of patients. The latter issue, circulating antithyroglobulin antibodies, is especially difficult to circumvent and has been largely ignored in current monitoring recommendations. Indeed, the early and accurate detection of recurrence or tumor progression is difficult in this population. This chapter discusses potential alternative peripheral blood markers. The use of imaging modalities in thyroid cancer is only briefly reviewed, as they are unaffected by antithyroglobulin antibodies. However, various imaging methods are part of a general approach to monitor patients and are discussed in detail in other sections of the book (see Chapters 14–16, 21, 32–35, 37, and 38).

THYROGLOBULIN ANTIBODIES

Thyroglobulin is a thyroid-specific 660-kDa protein that serves as a precursor and storage protein in thyroid hormone biosynthesis. It is thyroid-specific, but not thyroid cancer–specific; thus, its detection only in athyreotic patients who have had thyroidectomy and ^{131}I therapy implies the presence of recurrent or residual thyroid cancer. Patients with a history of thyroid cancer who are not athyreotic may have detectable levels that reflect the presence of remaining normal thyroid tissue. Moreover, the quantitative amount of circulating thyroglobulin usually correlates with the extent of disease and amount of residual or recurrent tissue, enhancing the clinical usefulness of the assay (3). Similar to ^{131}I uptake, thyroglobulin production and release are regulated by thyrotropin (TSH). Consequently, to maximize sensitivity in recently diagnosed or high-risk patients, TSH-stimulated thyroglobulin measurements are frequently performed. In this setting, the assay retains its specificity and becomes even more sensitive for disease detection. For these reasons, thyroglobulin monitoring has become an essential part of monitoring for thyroid cancer over the past 10–20 years.

Circulating antithyroglobulin antibodies are the major limitation of modern thyroglobulin immunoassays. Thyroglobulin is a large protein with numerous antigenic epitopes, many of which can induce antibody formation within an individual patient (4). Significant efforts have been made by investigators to circumvent the effects of these heterogenic antibodies on the thyroglobulin assays, but none have proven successful thus far. Consequently, it is recommended that antithyroglobulin antibodies are measured on the same serum sample as thyroglobulin to assess the accuracy of the thyroglobulin measurement, helping confirm that the measurement clinicians receive is correct. Therefore, the validity of the measurement of both thyroglobulin and the antithyroglobulin antibodies essentially relies on the accuracy of the antithyroglobulin antibody measurement—a topic that is receiving increased scrutiny over the past few years. Most laboratories now measure antibody presence using a sensitive immunoassay and a standard antibody preparation, rather than determining antibody titers (3). Some authors have advocated the use of "recovery" assays to measure the degree of interference by antithyroglobulin antibodies in particular samples, as not all antibodies may interfere with thyroglobulin measurement. Another approach is to perform both the radioimmunoassay (RIA) and immunoradiometric assay on the same sample to identify discordant results. However, because the majority of antithyroglobulin antibodies appear to interfere with measurement (5), recovery assays and the use of multiple types of thyroglobulin assays on patient samples are either not recommended (3,5) or not routinely performed.

From: *Thyroid Cancer: A Comprehensive Guide to Clinical Management, 2/e*
Edited by: L. Wartofsky and D. Van Nostrand © Humana Press Inc., Totowa, NJ

Antithyroglobulin autoantibodies are excellent markers of autoimmune thyroid disease in patients who are hypo- or hyperthyroid, and they are highly prevalent in the general population. Their presence was recently reported in 4–10% of unselected women and 1–3% of unselected men in a large US population *(6,7)*. For uncertain and highly debated reasons, patients with thyroid cancer have a much greater incidence of detectable antithyroglobulin antibodies, with most studies reporting an incidence of approx 20% *(2,8)*. In addition, one recent study reported the presence of interfering heterophilic antithyroglobulin antibodies in up to 3% of thyroglobulin antibody–negative thyroid cancer serum samples *(9)*. In some cases, the presence of circulating antithyroglobulin antibodies correlates with the presence of intrathyroidal autoimmunity, as shown by chronic lymphocytic thyroiditis or a peritumoral lymphocytic infiltration on histopathology of the thyroid gland. The correlation between antithyroglobulin antibodies and thyroid autoimmunity has led to speculation that patients with detectable antithyroglobulin antibodies may have a better prognosis owing to an enhanced antithyroid cancer cell immune response; however, correlation studies have reported inconsistent results *(10–12)*.

ALTERNATIVE LABORATORY TESTS FOR THYROID CANCER

Thyroglobulin Antibody Levels

Because thyroglobulin antibodies represent a response to a thyroid-specific antigenic stimulus, it has been speculated that the reduction and/or disappearance of antithyroglobulin antibodies in peripheral blood would correlate with a reduced antigenic burden, i.e., the remission and/or cure of thyroid cancer in patients with antithyroglobulin antibodies. In support of this concept, several studies have correlated the reduction and disappearance of antithyroglobulin antibodies with decreased tumor burden *(5,8,13,14)*. The quantitative nature of the reduction and the short-term association of antibody with remission are promising. Several areas require further study prior to the recommendation of this monitoring method for all patients, particularly the standardization of the antithyroglobulin assay method or use of a standard control preparation to allow for reliable assay quantitation. Studies also need to address whether patients with underlying Hashimoto's thyroiditis with a genetic predisposition to thyroid autoimmunity differ from patients with perimalignancy lymphocytic infiltration regarding this association. Despite these issues, it appears that the loss of detectable antithyroglobulin antibodies in patients with differentiated thyroid cancer who have circulating antithyroglobulin antibodies reflects an improvement in disease burden and enhances the ability to accurately measure thyroglobulin. Therefore, it is reasonable to monitor thyroglobulin and antithyroglobulin antibodies in these patients.

Serum Levels of Other Cancer-Related Proteins

There has been growing interest in the development of new markers for recurrent thyroid cancer because of antibody interference, TSH dependency, lack of cancer specificity, and the loss of thyroglobulin production in some poorly differentiated cancers. A number of growth factors are crucial to thyroid cancer growth and progression, including basic fibroblast growth factor (bFGF) and vascular endothelial growth factor (VEGF). Expression of bFGF and VEGF has been described in thyroid cancer and is associated with tumor aggressiveness *(15–17)*. Thus, several groups have evaluated the utility of serum levels of these two proteins in the peripheral blood of patients with thyroid cancer. Serum VEGF levels appear to be elevated in patients with progressive and metastatic thyroid cancer in comparison to those free of clinically detectable disease *(18–21)*. In these studies, the response of serum VEGF levels to recombinant human TSH administration was reported to be either unchanged or reduced. Similar results, although from fewer groups, have been reported for serum bFGF levels and also for levels of matrix metalloproteinase-9 *(18)* and intracellular adhesion molecule-1 *(22)*.

Another approach to serum markers is to identify global changes in serum protein expression in patients with metastatic cancer, either from tumor cells or from responses to metastatic cancer. Indeed, it has been recently reported that circulating protein samples taken from patients with metastatic cancer differ substantially from those of patients with no cancer or cured cancer *(23)*. Although not fully tested in thyroid cancer, this more global analysis may hold diagnostic promise independently or help in identifying a novel panel of markers that might be appropriate for thyroid cancer detection in peripheral blood.

RNA-Based Assays

Because of antibody interference, and the potential for enhanced assay sensitivity, there has been an interest in developing RNA-based assays for thyroid cancer monitoring using reverse-transcription polymerase chain reaction (RT-PCR). These types of assays do not rely on antibody to detect protein and are thus unaltered by antithyroglobulin antibodies and are more sensitive than immunoassays. The sensitivity of these assays is because of the inherent nature of RT-PCR, which logarithmically amplifies the target RNA to allow for sensitive measurement. More recently, the ability to accurately quantify RT-PCR reactions using probes specific for the gene being detected (real-time RT-PCR) has generated even greater interest in these techniques. The potential for RNA-based detection for thyroid cancer has been mirrored for many other hematologic and solid malignancies for similar reasons. Because of its high inherent sensitivity, the principal issues in developing accurate thyroid-specific or thyroid cancer–specific RNA-based assays relate to specificity, as well as the stability of isolated RNA, which are notoriously unstable using standard laboratory practices.

Studies from a large number of international groups have been performed using several thyroid-specific markers, e.g., thyroglobulin, thyroid peroxidase, and TSH receptor mRNA, along with thyroid cancer–specific markers, such as RET/PTC expression. Using qualitative methods, initial studies demonstrated that the presence of circulating thyroglobulin mRNA correlated with the presence of thyroid cancer and was absent in the setting of a normal thyroid (24,25). Follow-up studies demonstrated that thyroglobulin mRNA could be detected in most patients with thyroid tissue (benign or malignant) but rarely in patients who were athyreotic (26). The differences in results are likely from enhanced assay sensitivity, alternative PCR primer design, or other methodologic differences, as reviewed in detail elsewhere (27). The subsequent results from multiple investigators have been highly varied, some supporting a relationship with thyroid cancer and others demonstrating no relationship (28–32). More recently, one group has reported utility in the preoperative diagnosis of thyroid cancer using their TSH receptor and thyroglobulin mRNA method (28,33,33a).

To determine whether patients with greater tumor burden or extent of disease can be distinguished based on their thyroid mRNA levels, several groups have attempted to quantify circulating thyroid mRNA transcripts (30,34–39). Overall, the results of these studies are also highly varied. Some studies demonstrate a good correlation between an increased thyroid mRNA level and greater tumor burden, with thyroglobulin immunoassay levels, whereas others do not. However, in all published reports, there is considerable overlap between patients with different stages of disease. Furthermore, all studies using the highly sensitive techniques of real-time RT-PCR have unequivocally demonstrated the presence of low levels of thyroglobulin mRNA variants in patients without evidence of thyroid tissue, leading to questions regarding the specificity of "thyroid-specific" transcripts when detected using this highly sensitive method.

There are several important caveats about these data: (1) It appears that the many primer sequences utilized are able to not only detect thyroglobulin but also splice variants that may not reflect production from thyroid cells (28,38). (2) The methods of quantitative normalization differ between groups (27). (3) The method of cell isolation and RNA stabilization is inconsistent between groups. Methods that may further enhance the specificity of RT-PCR peripheral blood assays for thyroid cancer include the use of RNA-stabilizing solutions in blood tubes, enriching the cellular population for epithelial cells using separation methods, and careful avoidance of primers that amplify splice variants of thyroglobulin that seem more easily detected in patients without evidence of thyroid cancer. These types of methodologic modifications may create a "second generation" of thyroid cancer RT-PCR assays that could determine if this approach will have clinical usefulness.

DISEASE MONITORING FOR PATIENTS WITH ANTITHYROGLOBULIN ANTIBODIES

Because of the difficulties in reliable serum testing for thyroid cancer monitoring in patients with antithyroglobulin antibodies, there is a greater reliance on radiographic testing. This includes the use of ^{131}I scanning, neck ultrasound, and chest computed tomography (CT). In addition, for patients with aggressive tumors, positron emission tomography (PET) with fluorodeoxyglucose also has a potentially important role. The utility of these studies is not different in patients with antithyroglobulin antibodies and is discussed in detail in other chapters in this text. However, it is important to recognize that current proposed algorithms that rely heavily on the measurement of serum thyroglobulin exclude patients with circulating antithyroglobulin antibodies and therefore do not apply to this population. As a result, one approach is to monitor patients with both quantitative thyroglobulin and antithyroglobulin antibody measurements as tumor markers and to perform neck ultrasonography and ^{131}I scanning annually for several years after diagnosis, depending on the initial extent of tumor. Additional radiographic studies, e.g., chest CT and PET, may be needed in high-risk patients. Because RIAs for thyroglobulin are generally falsely elevated by antithyroglobulin levels, their use in this situation may be advantageous as the reduction of thyroglobulin concentrations has been reported to parallel the quantitative reduction or rise of antithyroglobulin antibodies. The utility of making treatment recommendations on antithyroglobulin antibodies alone has not yet been studied. Advances in the evaluation of alternative serum markers, the global analysis of peripheral blood proteins, and molecular diagnostics are promising areas of future research to aid the management of patients with antithyroglobulin antibodies.

REFERENCES

1. Schlumberger M, Berg G, Cohen O, et al. Follow-up of low-risk patients with differentiated thyroid carcinoma: a European perspective. Eur J Endocrinol 2004; 150:105–112.
2. Mazzaferri EL, Robbins RJ, Spencer CA, et al. A consensus report of the role of serum thyroglobulin as a monitoring method for low-risk patients with papillary thyroid carcinoma. J Clin Endocrinol Metab 2003; 88:1433–1441.
3. Baloch Z, Carayon P, Conte-Devolx B, et al. Laboratory medicine practice guidelines. Laboratory support for the diagnosis and monitoring of thyroid disease. Thyroid 2003; 13:3–126.
4. Benvenga S, Burek CL, Talor M, et al. Heterogeneity of the thyroglobulin epitopes associated with circulating thyroid hormone autoantibodies in hashimoto's thyroiditis and non-autoimmune thyroid diseases. J Endocrinol Invest 2002; 25:977–982.
5. Spencer CA, Takeuchi M, Kazarosyan M, et al. Serum thyroglobulin autoantibodies: prevalence, influence on serum thyroglobulin

measurement, and prognostic significance in patients with differentiated thyroid carcinoma. J Clin Endocrinol Metab 1998; 83: 1121–1127.
6. Hollowell JG, Staehling NW, Flanders WD, et al. Serum TSH, T(4), and thyroid antibodies in the United States population (1988 to 1994): National Health and Nutrition Examination Survey (NHANES III). J Clin Endocrinol Metab 2002; 87:489–499.
7. Canaris GJ, Manowitz NR, Mayor G, Ridgway EC. The Colorado thyroid disease prevalence study. Arch Intern Med 2000; 160:526–534.
8. Hjiyiannakis P, Mundy J, Harmer C. Thyroglobulin antibodies in differentiated thyroid cancer. Clin Oncol (R Coll Radiol) 1999; 11: 240–244.
9. Preissner CM, O'Kane DJ, Singh RJ, et al. Phantoms in the assay tube: heterophile antibody interferences in serum thyroglobulin assays. J Clin Endocrinol Metab 2003; 88:3069–3074.
10. McConahey WM, Hay ID, Woolner LB, et al. Papillary thyroid cancer treated at the Mayo Clinic, 1946 through 1970: initial manifestations, pathologic findings, therapy, and outcome. Mayo Clin Proc 1986; 61: 978–996.
11. Kumar A, Shah DH, Shrihari U, et al. Significance of antithyroglobulin autoantibodies in differentiated thyroid carcinoma. Thyroid 1994; 4:199–202.
12. Kebebew E, Treseler PA, Ituarte PH, Clark OH. Coexisting chronic lymphocytic thyroiditis and papillary thyroid cancer revisited. World J Surg 2001; 25:632–637.
13. Spencer CA. Editorial: Challenges of Serum thyroglobulin measurement in the presence of Tg Autoantibodies, J Clin Endocrinol Metab 2004; 89:3702–3704.
14. Chung JK, Park YJ, Kim TY, et al. Clinical significance of elevated level of serum antithyroglobulin antibody in patients with differentiated thyroid cancer after thyroid ablation. Clin Endocrinol (Oxf) 2002; 57:215–221.
15. Klein M, Vignaud J-M, Hennequin V, et al. Increased expression of the vascular endothelial growth factor is a pejorative prognosis marker in papillary thyroid carcinoma. J Clin Endocrinol Metab 2001; 86: 656–840.
16. Viglietto G, Romano A, Manzo G, et al. Upregulation of the angiogenic factors PlGF, VEGF and their receptors (Flt-1, Flk-1/KDR) by TSH in cultured thyrocytes and in the thyroid gland of thiouracil-fed rats suggest a TSH-dependent paracrine mechanism for goiter hypervascularization. Oncogene 1997; 15:2687–2698.
17. Hung CJ, Ginzinger DG, Zarnegar R, et al. Expression of vascular endothelial growth factor-C in benign and malignant thyroid tumors. J Clin Endocrinol Metab 2003; 88:3694–3699.
18. Lin SY, Wang YY, Sheu WH. Preoperative plasma concentrations of vascular endothelial growth factor and matrix metalloproteinase 9 are associated with stage progression in papillary thyroid cancer. Clin Endocrinol (Oxf) 2003; 58:513–518.
19. Pasieka Z, Stepien H, Komorowski J, et al. Evaluation of the levels of bFGF, VEGF, sICAM-1, and sVCAM-1 in serum of patients with thyroid cancer. Recent Results Cancer Res 2003; 162:189–194.
20. Sorvillo F, Mazziotti G, Carbone A, et al. Recombinant human thyrotropin reduces serum vascular endothelial growth factor levels in patients monitored for thyroid carcinoma even in the absence of thyroid tissue. J Clin Endocrinol Metab 2003; 88:4818–4822.
21. Tuttle RM, Fleisher M, Francis GL, Robbins RJ. Serum vascular endothelial growth factor levels are elevated in metastatic differentiated thyroid cancer but not increased by short-term TSH stimulation. J Clin Endocrinol Metab 2002; 87:1737–1742.
22. Pasieka Z, Kuzdak K, Czyz W, et al. Soluble intracellular adhesion molecules (sICAM-1, sVCAM-1) in peripheral blood of patients with thyroid cancer. Neoplasma 2004; 51:34–37.
23. Petricoin EF, III, Ornstein DK, Paweletz CP, et al. Serum proteomic patterns for detection of prostate cancer. J Natl Cancer Inst 2002; 94: 1576–1578.
24. Ditkoff BA, Marvin MR, Yemul S, et al. Detection of circulating thyroid cells in peripheral blood. Surgery 1996; 120:959–965.
25. Tallini G, Ghossein RA, Emanuel J, et al. Detection of thyroglobulin, thyroid peroxidase, and RET/PTC1 mRNA transcripts in the peripheral blood of patients with thyroid disease. J Clin Oncol 1998; 16: 1158–1166.
26. Ringel MD, Ladenson PW, Levine MA. Molecular diagnosis of residual and recurrent thyroid cancer by amplification of thyroglobulin messenger ribonucleic acid in peripheral blood. J Clin Endocrinol Metab 1998; 83:4435–4442.
27. Ringel MD. Molecular detection of thyroid cancer: differentiating "signal" and "noise" in clinical assays. J Clin Endocrinol Metab 2004; 89:29–32.
28. Chinnappa P, Taguba L, Arciaga R, et al. Detection of thrytropin-receptor messenger ribonucleic acid (mRNA) and thyroglobulin mRNA transcripts in peripheral blood of patients with thyroid disease: sensitive and specific markers for thyroid cancer. J Clin Endocrinol Metab 2004; 89:3705–3709.
29. Fugazzola L, Mihalich A, Persani L, et al. Highly sensitive serum thyroglobulin and circulating thyroglobulin mRNA evaluations in the management of patients with differentiated thyroid cancer in apparent remission. J Clin Endocrinol Metab 2002; 87:3201–3208.
30. Span PN, Sleegers MJ, Van Den Broek WJ, et al. Quantitative detection of peripheral thyroglobulin mRNA has limited clinical value in the follow-up of thyroid cancer patients. Ann Clin Biochem 2003; 40: 94–99.
31. Bojunga J, Kustere K, Schumm-Draeger P-M, Usadel K-H. Polymerase chain reaction in the detection of tumor cells: New approaches in diagnosis and follow-up of patients with thyroid cancer. Thyroid 2002; 12: 1097–1107.
32. Grammatopoulos D, Elliott Y, Smith SC, et al. Measurement of thyroglobulin mRNA in peripheral blood as an adjunctive test for monitoring thyroid cancer. Mol Pathol 2003; 56:162–166.
33. Gupta M, Taguba L, Arciaga R, et al. Detection of circulating thyroid cancer cells by reverse transcription-PCR for thyroid-stimulating hormone receptor and thyroglobulin: the importance of primer selection. Clin Chem 2002; 48:1862–1865.
33a. Wagner K, Arciaga R, Siperstein A, et al. Thyrotropin receptor/thyroglobulin messenger ribonucleaic acid in peripheral blood and fine-needle aspiration cytology: Diagnostic synergy for detecting thyroid cancer. J Clin Endocrinol Metab 2005; 90:1921–1924.
34. Ringel MD, Balducci-Silano PL, Anderson JS, et al. Quantitative reverse transcription-polymerase chain reaction of circulating thyroglobulin messenger ribonucleic acid for monitoring patients with thyroid carcinoma. J Clin Endocrinol Metab 1999; 84:4037–4042.
35. Savagner F, Rodien P, Reynier P, et al. Analysis of Tg transcripts by real-time RT-PCR in the blood of thyroid cancer patients. J Clin Endocrinol Metab 2002; 87:635–639.
36. Bellantone R, Lombardi CP, Bossola M, et al. Validity of thyroglobulin mRNA assay in peripheral blood of postoperative thyroid carcinoma patients in predicting tumor recurrences varies according to the histologic type: results of a prospective study. Cancer 2001; 92:2273–2279.
37. Elisei R, Vivaldi A, Agate L, et al. Low specificity of blood thyroglobulin messenger ribonucleic acid assay prevents its use in the follow-up of differentiated thyroid cancer patients. J Clin Endocrinol Metab 2004; 89:33–39.
38. Eszlinger M, Neumann S, Otto L, Paschke R. Thyroglobulin mRNA quantification in the peripheral blood is not a reliable marker for the follow-up of patients with differentiated thyroid cancer. Eur J Endocrinol 2002; 147:575–582.
39. Wingo ST, Ringel MD, Anderson JS, et al. Quantitative reverse transcription-PCR measurement of thyroglobulin mRNA in peripheral blood of healthy subjects. Clin Chem 1999; 45:785–789.

32
Surveillance Radioiodine Whole-Body Scans

Douglas Van Nostrand

INTRODUCTION

Surveillance radioiodine whole-body scans have been used for many years in the follow-up of patients with well-differentiated thyroid cancer. However, the term "surveillance whole body scan" has been used in different ways. This short chapter (1) differentiates surveillance scans from pretreatment scans; (2) presents the objectives of surveillance scans and pretreatment scans; (3) reviews the literature for the utility of surveillance scans; and (4) presents one set of guidelines.

SURVEILLANCE VS PRETREATMENT SCANS

Surveillance whole-body scans or total-body scans should be differentiated from pretreatment scans. A surveillance scan is a radioiodine whole-body scan performed at a routine interval, which is typically 6 mo to 1–2 yr after radioiodine ablation or treatment. Its primary objective is to *screen* for metastatic functioning well-differentiated thyroid cancer in patients who may be in clinical remission. Clinical remission is meant here as undetectable serum thyroglobulin levels on thyroid hormone suppression with no antithyroglobulin antibodies and no evidence of disease on physical exam.

A pretreatment scan is a radioiodine whole-body scan performed in "anticipation" of a radioiodine treatment in patients who have evidence or a high risk of recurrent local or metastatic thyroid cancer. The objectives of a pretreatment scan are to:

1. Localize as many sites of metastasis as possible.
2. Localize lesions for possible fine-needle aspiration or biopsy.
3. Localize lesions for possible surgery.
4. Determine whether radioiodine is a therapeutic option (e.g., in those facilities that use visual uptake as a criteria for treatment).
5. Identify patterns of radioiodine uptake that would alter prescribed activity for treatment (e.g., diffuse lung metastases, brain metastasis, and bone metastasis).
6. Perform lesional dosimetry, whole-body dosimetry, or both, which could alter prescribed activity for treatment.

Regarding surveillance whole-body scans as defined above, strong arguments have been presented that surveillance scans are no longer cost-effective (*1–7*). These arguments are further strengthened when thyroid hormone withdrawal is used to prepare the patient for the surveillance scan, and the patient must undergo a prolonged period of hypothyroidism. As a result, fewer and fewer facilities perform routine surveillance scans for screening low-risk patients with no evidence of disease on physical exam and undetectable serum thyroglobulin levels on thyroid hormone suppression.

However, the use of surveillance scans in several other scenarios is more controversial and suggests the need for further consideration. For example, would one surveillance scan at 6 mo or 1 yr postradioiodine ablation be cost-effective? Such a surveillance scan would serve as a baseline evaluation that may be useful in patients who subsequently require a radioiodine scan for possible recurrence. Of course, this again depends on the treatment approach at a specific facility. Second, it should be considered if surveillance scans at periodic intervals would be cost-effective in patients who are (1) at higher risk for recurrence (e.g., Hürthle cell carcinoma); (2) have antithyroglobulin antibodies that affect the interpretation of serum thyroglobulin levels; and/or (3) are already scheduled to have a routine recombinant human thyrotropin (rhTSH)-stimulated serum thyroglobulin level measured.

Mazzaferri and Kloos *(3)* suggested that a surveillance scan added little to no diagnostic information to rhTSH-stimulated thyroglobulin levels, even in high-risk patients. This study needs confirmation; alternatively, it is important not to overestimate the absorbed radiation dose and patient inconvenience of a radioiodine surveillance scan. Both are modest, and when a surveillance scan is performed with a routine rhTSH-stimulated serum thyroglobulin level, the issue of symptomatic hypothyroidism is eliminated. In addition, the cost can also be modest relative to rhTSH-stimulated thyroglobulin. In the United States, the cost for an rhTSH-stimulated serum thyroglobulin measurement ranges between $2000 and $3000. The reimbursement for

From: *Thyroid Cancer: A Comprehensive Guide to Clinical Management, 2/e*
Edited by: L. Wartofsky and D. Van Nostrand © Humana Press Inc., Totowa, NJ

Table 1
Guidelines for Surveillance and Pretreatment Scans

If	Then
Low-risk patients who received no initial scan or radioiodine ablation	No surveillance scan
Patient who received radioiodine ablation	One ^{123}I or ^{131}I surveillance scan performed 1 yr after radioiodine ablation at the same time as scheduled rhTSH-stimulated thyroglobulin levels. This will be a baseline scan for comparison of any future scan for suspected recurrence
Low-risk patient who received radioiodine ablation, has normal physical exam, has undetectable or low (<1.0 ng/mL) serum thyroglobulin on thyroid hormone suppression, and no thyroglobulin antibodies	No further surveillance scan after the 1-yr baseline surveillance scan
Low-risk patient who received radioiodine ablation, has normal physical exam, has serum thyroglobulin levels of 1–2.0 ng/mL on thyroid hormone suppression, and/or thyroglobulin antibodies that may affect the interpretation of serum thyroglobulin levels	Consider ^{123}I or ^{131}I surveillance scan with rhTSH stimulation at periodic[a] intervals
High-risk patient[a]	^{123}I or ^{131}I surveillance scan with rhTSH stimulation at periodic[a] intervals
Suspected recurrence[b]	Pretreatment scan performed with (1) either withdrawal or rhTSH stimulation, (2) 1–2 mCi of ^{131}I, and (3) whole-body dosimetry in anticipation of treatment with ^{131}I.

[a]Individualized

[b]Based on such factors as (1) elevated serum thyroglobulin level on suppression or after rhTSH stimulation (e.g., >2 ng/mL); (2) mass on physical exam; (3) abnormal computed tomography without contrast, magnetic resonance, ultrasound, or fluorodeoxyglucose positron emission tomography; (4) fine-needle aspiration; and/or (5) surgery.

the performance and interpretation of a radioiodine whole-body scan, such as in the District of Columbia by Medicare, is approx $500. Nevertheless, further evaluation is needed to determine the incremental information relative to the costs of a surveillance scan in patients who are at a higher risk of recurrence, who have thyroglobulin antibodies, and/or who are already scheduled for rhTSH-stimulated serum thyroglobulin levels.

The utility of pretreatment scans depends on the approach at each given facility for the evaluation and treatment of patients who have documented metastatic disease or have a high chance of recurrent or distant metastases. For example, for those facilities that only provide treatment if the metastasis shows radioiodine uptake, then a pretreatment scan is obviously mandatory and completely useful. For those facilities that provide treatment with a fixed empiric prescribed activity, regardless of whether or not there is radioiodine uptake, a pretreatment scan has no value (1). For those facilities that modify fixed empiric prescribed activity based on findings, patterns, and/or uptake on radioiodine whole-body scans, a pretreatment scan may have value. Finally, for those facilities that administer treatment with a prescribed activity based on whole-body dosimetry, regardless of the findings on scan, then pretreatment dosimetry is necessary.

CONCLUSION

In summary, surveillance scans must be differentiated from pretreatment scans, and the roles of both scans vary in different facilities and continue to be defined. In addition, the choice of radioiodine (e.g.,^{131}I or ^{123}I) and patient preparation (e.g., withdrawal or rhTSH stimulation) will vary and continue to be addressed. This author's general guidelines at his institution are presented in Table 1. Primarily, these are guidelines and must be individualized to each patient's specific case.

REFERENCES

1. Cailleux AF, Baudin E, Travagli JP, Schlumberger RM. Is diagnostic iodine-131 scanning useful after total thyroid ablation for differentiated thyroid cancer? J Clin Endocrinol Metab 2000; 85:175–178.
2. Wartofsky L and the rhTSH-Stimulated Thyroglobulin Study Group. Management of low risk well differentiated thyroid cancer based only upon thyroglobulin measurement after recombinant human thyrotropin. Thyroid 2002; 12:583–592.
3. Mazzaferri EL, Kloos RT. Is diagnostic iodine-131 scanning with recombinant human TSH useful in the follow-up of differentiated

thyroid cancer after thyroid ablation? J Clin Endocrinol Metab 2002; 87:1490–1498.
4. Wartofsky L. Using baseline and recombinant human TSH-stimulated Tg measurements to manage thyroid cancer without diagnostic I-131 scanning. J Clin Endocrin Metab 2002; 87:1486–1489.
5. Pacini F, Capezzone M, Elisei R, et al. Diagnostic 131-iodine whole body scan may be avoided in thyroid cancer patients who have undetectable stimulated serum Tg levels after initial treatment. J Clin Endocrinol Metab 2002; 87:1499–1501.
6. Fatemi S, Nicoloff J, Lo Presti J, Spencer S. TSH-stimulated serum thyroglobulin in the 1-10 ng/ml range suggests a low long-term recurrence risk for papillary thyroid cancer (PTC). Washington, DC: Program of the 73rd Annual Meeting of the American Thyroid Association, 2001, 290 (Abstract 194).
7. Pacini F, Molinaro E, Lippi F, et al. Prediction of disease status by recombinant human TSH-stimulated serum thyroglobulin in the post surgical follow-up of differentiated thyroid carcinoma. J Clin Endocrinol Metab 2001; 86:5686–5690.

33
Radionuclide Imaging and Treatment of Thyroid Cancer in Children

Gary L. Francis

Radioactive iodine (RAI) was first proposed as a specific treatment for thyroid cancer by Seidlin et al. in 1946 *(1)*. Since then, RAI has been incorporated into treatment protocols for adults and children with differentiated thyroid cancer (DTC; *2*). Adjunctive RAI therapy improves disease-free survival in young adults (including some adolescents) with disease similar in histology and extent to that commonly found in children *(3)*. Until recently, however, studies specifically examining the benefits of RAI in children have been difficult to perform because the number of patients is small and the prognosis is favorable for almost all children, regardless of adjunctive therapy *(4–15)*. The American Thyroid Association and American Association of Clinical Endocrinologists have published practice guidelines for the management of thyroid cancer in adults, but the treatment of thyroid cancer in children remains controversial *(2,16)*. A number of questions are left unresolved regarding the use of RAI in children. (1) Which children are most likely to benefit from RAI therapy? (2) What is the optimal dose of RAI for children? (3) What are the long-term risks and complications from RAI use in young patients? (4) What are acceptable end points for RAI therapy in children?

INTRODUCTION

DTCs arise from the follicular epithelium and are generally divided into papillary (PTC) and follicular (FTC) variants. Although the histologic features of PTC and FTC are similar across all ages, the prognosis is much more favorable for children than for adults with similar histology and extent of disease *(4–15)*. At diagnosis, the majority of childhood thyroid cancers (70%) have invaded beyond the thyroid capsule or into the regional lymph nodes, and 10–28% of patients already have pulmonary metastases *(5–7,17–22)*. Despite such widespread disease, children are less likely to die from PTC than are adults, with overall mortality ranging from 1% to 12% *(4–15)*. Most importantly, about half of children with pulmonary metastases persist with stable disease following treatment *(9,10)*. These favorable outcomes are major factors that lead to the debate about RAI therapy and its use in children with DTC.

WHICH CHILDREN ARE MOST LIKELY TO BENEFIT FROM RAI THERAPY?

Although children are less likely to die from DTC than adults, 20–40% will develop recurrent disease despite therapy *(4–15)*. Attempts to determine if adjunctive RAI therapy will improve these outcomes in children have generally failed to show benefit, but all the studies were limited by small patient populations and by the reliance on retrospective analyses in which the majority of children received RAI treatment *(4–15)*. For these reasons, there have not been evidence-based analyses with sufficient statistical proof to address the use of RAI specifically in the pediatric population.

A recent study by Chow et al. has shown statistically significant reductions in the risk of recurrence for children at high risk when treated with RAI *(23)*. In their study, 60 patients less than 21 yr old were followed for an average of 14 yr. These high-risk patients included those with tumors more than 1 cm in diameter, extrathyroidal extension, residual neck disease, or distant metastases. RAI improved local–regional failure-free survival from 71.9% to 86.5% ($p = 0.04$). With additional treatment (surgery and/or RAI), 10 of 12 patients with local recurrence and 5 of 9 patients with distant metastases were rendered free from disease.

Although the impact of RAI on mortality cannot be determined from these data, these and other studies of young adults (including some adolescents) have shown that recurrence risks can be reduced by RAI ablation *(3)*. The study by Chow et al. has now shown this to be true for children with high-risk tumors *(23)*. If administration of RAI therapy was given only to children at high risk, how could this be reasonably achieved?

It is difficult to determine the extent of disease in children without performing a standardized neck dissection and RAI whole-body scan (WBS). Most children (70% in many series) have disease in the regional lymph nodes, but only about 50% of involved lymph nodes can be identified by palpation during surgery (4–15,24). Thus, it is difficult to identify patients with lymph node involvement unless they undergo a standardized neck dissection. Another 10–28% of children have pulmonary metastases at diagnosis, but microscopic pulmonary metastases can be frequently visualized only by a RAI WBS. The WBS is only sensitive enough to detect microscopic disease if the child has undergone total thyroidectomy and has limited RAI uptake in the neck (5–7,17–22). To achieve such limited uptake, most children require at least one dose of RAI to ablate any residual thyroid remnant (22). Therefore, from a practical perspective, most children require RAI in some quantity to determine if they are high-risk patients.

The dose of RAI prescribed to ablate thyroid remnants has been reduced over the last several years to allow for outpatient ablation. Most young patients have been successfully ablated with a single dose of 75 mCi, whereas an outpatient dose of 29 mCi has resulted in the frequent need for repeat administration (22). From a practical viewpoint, most children would be treated with total thyroidectomy, neck dissection, and as much as 75 mCi of RAI prior to determining the extent of disease.

Based on the high prevalence of cervival node involvement and pulmonary metastases in children, as well as the high risk of recurrence, many authors recommend total thyroidectomy, standardized lymph node dissection, and RAI ablation for all children with clinically evident DTC (more than occult microscopic disease; 24,25). At least one retrospective analysis supports the validity of this approach. In a small study, children who were believed to have disease confined to the gland on clinical grounds (DeGroot class 1) had a higher risk of recurrence when treated with lobectomy alone (26). These data underscore the importance of an aggressive approach that includes RAI therapy for all children with clinically evident DTC, and it is this author's opinion that such an approach is warranted throughout the pediatric age range. Treatment that involves total thyroidectomy, lymph node dissection, and RAI ablation also allows serum thyroglobulin (Tg) levels to be used for disease surveillance (27,28).

WHAT IS THE OPTIMAL DOSE OF RAI FOR CHILDREN?

Optimal single and cumulative doses of RAI have not yet been established for children. In adults, individual doses more than 200 mCi, or cumulative doses greater than 1.05 Ci have not improved disease-free survival when compared to lower doses (20,29). Similar studies have not been performed in children, but several authors suggest individual doses for older children and adolescents of 100 mCi for uptake in the thyroid bed, 150 mCi for uptake in the regional nodes, and 175–200 mCi for pulmonary metastases (13,30). However, there is not a consensus on these doses or on what distinguishes an "older" child.

In attempts to standardize the use of RAI across the pediatric age range, Maxon theorized that doses of radiation delivered to the target tissue would correlate with outcome (21). He found that 8000 rad delivered to individual metastases eradicated 98% of all lesions, whereas absorbed doses below 3500 rad failed to destroy any lesion, and absorbed doses between 3500 and 8000 rad eliminated some but not all lesions (21).

Reynolds proposed a relative scale for determining the RAI dose for children with thyroid cancer. In his model, the dose of RAI was calculated to deliver radioactivity to the target tissue equivalent to what would have been received by an adult given 100 mCi. This would require approx 35 mCi for a 20-kg child (average weight for a 5–6-yr-old child of either gender) and 80 mCi for a child weighing 55 kg (average weight for a 14–15-yr-old boy or a 17–18-yr-old girl; 31).

Despite these calculations, caution is advised in applying these "standard" doses, particularly in small children. For children with large amounts of residual tumor and a high-RAI uptake, it is possible for a dose as small as 35 mCi to exceed the maximum tolerable dose (32). This maximal dose is based on years of clinical experience at Memorial Sloan Kettering Cancer Center in New York (33). Their data suggest bone marrow exposures less than 2 Gy and whole-body retention below 4.44 GBq (<120 mCi) at 48 h do not cause permanent bone marrow suppression (33). The exact calculation of this amount of radioactivity can only be determined by whole-body dosimetry (Chapters 47, 48).

Unfortunately, dosimetry also has limitations and disadvantages. Dosimetry requires administering a small dose of RAI a few days before ablation. Based on blood levels and whole-body retention, the exposure of each organ, especially the bone marrow, is calculated using simulations based on adult models. One limitation in the application of dosimetry for children is that the models might not accurately reflect the RAI distribution in children. Children have different lean body/fat mass ratios at all ages and generally distribute charged ions differently than adults. This difference might induce error into the calculations of organ exposure using the current dosimetry programs.

The major concern with dosimetry, however, is the potential for stunning (see Chapter 36), which would reduce the efficacy of follow-up treatment doses (34,35). Regardless of these limitations and drawbacks, it is the author's personal practice and that of several others to recommend dosimetry to determine the maximal safe doses of RAI in young patients and those with metastatic disease (36). Dosimetry will then provide a "best guess" as to the highest dose of RAI that could be prescribed based on short-term toxicity.

WHAT ARE THE LONG-TERM RISKS AND COMPLICATIONS FROM RAI USE IN YOUNG PATIENTS?

One of the major unknown factors in using RAI therapy for children with DTC is the paucity of data concerning long-term risks. It is important to remember that the dosimetry calculations outlined above are based on short-term toxicity, not long-term risks. A "safe" dose as defined by dosimetry might still have an unacceptably high risk of long-term complications.

Several clinical observations and in vitro data bring doubt into the debate concerning the long-term safety of RAI therapy in children. Although RAI use in adults has rarely been associated with second malignancies or leukemia, the thyroid (and presumably other tissues) in children is more susceptible to radiation-induced injury, especially in those under 10 yr of age *(37–39)*.

A recent study by Rubino et al. followed approx 6000 patients with thyroid cancer from combined Swedish, Italian, and French tumor registries. They reported a significant and dose-dependent increase in the risk of second malignancy among patients treated with RAI *(40)*. In their study, 344 patients were less than 20 yr of age at diagnosis. Thirteen developed second malignancies, among which the risks for all cancers (relative risk [RR] = 2.5), specifically breast cancers (RR = 3.4), were significantly increased when compared to the general population. Overall, 61% of the young patients received RAI, suggesting that RAI might have a role in this rise. However, when the patients who received RAI were compared to those who did not, there was no added risk from RAI administration (RR = 1.1). Unfortunately, the number of subjects (n = 344) may have been too small to identify an increase in the incidence of rare complications, such as second malignancy. Additional study of young patients is clearly warranted to better define the age-specific risks of second malignancy following RAI therapy.

In concert with these clinical observations, chromosomal analyses indicate that RAI therapy can induce specific genetic aberrations *(41–43)*. A highly significant increase in the number of dicentric chromosomes was observed in peripheral lymphocytes during the first week after RAI therapy. More importantly, chromosomal aberrations involving chromosomes 1, 4, and 10 were more prevalent even after 4 years *(41)*. The long-term implications of these alterations are not yet known, but they do raise questions about the potential of late genetic effects from RAI therapy.

Other possible side effects from RAI include direct damage to tissues that take up RAI, such as salivary glands. Sialadenitis, xerostomia, caries, stomatitis, and oral candidiasis have all been reported *(44)*. Other tissues in the head and neck may be affected, inducing edema, ocular dryness, and nasolacrimal obstruction *(45,46)*. (See Chapter 50.)

Gonadal damage has been reported in both women (temporary ovarian failure) and men (oligospermia with elevated follicular-stimulating hormone [FSH] levels; *47,48*). The risk of ovarian failure appeared to increase with age, suggesting that young patients might be less susceptible. A study by Smith et al. is particularly relevant to the use of RAI in children *(49)*. They evaluated 35 women who received RAI for thyroid remnant ablation during childhood or adolescence. Patients received an average RAI dose of 148.5 mCi (range 77.2–250 mCi) and were followed from 5.6 to 39.8 yr. Three developed infertility (8.6%). Unfortunately, two children were born to this cohort with fatal birth defects, and both had been conceived within 1 yr of RAI therapy. From these data, the authors suggested that the risks of infertility and birth defects were similar to the general population, but they cautioned against conception during the first year after RAI therapy. Although fertility appeared to be intact in this cohort, long-term follow-up would be required to determine if late complications (e.g., premature menopause) might develop as treated children approach middle age and beyond.

Elevated serum FSH levels have been reported in males after as little as 50 mCi of RAI, and only partial recovery of gonadal function was seen in a single patient after more than 2 years of follow-up *(48)*. Collectively, these data suggest that adolescents and younger children might be at risk for gonadal damage. Consideration should be given to the possibility of sperm banking, especially in those patients who require more than a single dose of RAI.

WHAT ARE ACCEPTABLE ENDPOINTS FOR RAI THERAPY IN CHILDREN?

Given the potential risks of RAI therapy, and the probability that many children with pulmonary metastases will develop stable but persistent disease over many years, what should be the ultimate goal for RAI administration? Should one strive for undetectable serum Tg levels and no evidence of disease, or should one settle for stable but persistent disease? It will be obvious from the previous discussions that the answers to these questions are not yet known.

Advocates for rendering patients free from disease, as evidenced by undetectable serum Tg, base this recommendation on theoretical concerns involving RAI uptake by tumor cells, risks of dedifferentiation, and the physics of tissue destruction that correlate with RAI incorporation/gram of malignant tumor *(21)*. Intuitively, RAI should be more effective early in therapy, when the tumor burden is small and tumor cells demonstrate avid RAI uptake and incorporation *(22)*. However, in a series of articles, Vassilopoulou-Sellin et al. showed that children can persist with stable disease despite therapy, and that death from disease was no more frequent than death from complications of therapy (50–52). Yet, this study used external-beam radiation therapy in a number of patients, which may have contributed to the mortality associated with treatment. For this reason, most authors recommend against external-beam radiation therapy for children and young patients with DTC.

It would seem prudent to suggest that treatment of children with repeated doses of RAI should be considered on an individual basis. For the majority of children and adolescents, initial therapy that includes total thyroidectomy, lymph node dissection, and RAI remnant ablation is adequate to render the patient free from disease *(9,10,22,23,52a)*. Long-term follow-up is indicated to detect potential recurrence that can be effectively treated in most cases by surgery (accessible nodal disease) or RAI (pulmonary metastases or inoperable disease; *23,53*). For patients with persistent pulmonary metastases, increasing caution is suggested as the total cumulative RAI dose exceeds 500 mCi, especially as it approaches 1000 mCi. Ideally, efficacy should be documented for each individual RAI treatment by a decrease in serum Tg level, a decrease in RAI uptake over the lung fields, or a decrease in tumor mass by other imaging techniques. In the absence of such evidence, or in the case of a detectable serum Tg level with negative RAI WBS, continued treatment of young patients is controversial *(9,10)*.

RADIONUCLIDE IMAGING

RAI scans are generally unable to distinguish benign from malignant lesions during the preoperative evaluation of children with thyroid neoplasia *(54–57)*. However, the RAI WBS has been the "gold standard" for detecting residual thyroid cancer after thyroidectomy in adults and children *(5,6)*. Recent data in adults have shown that serum Tg levels are a more sensitive indicator of disease, particularly when obtained following stimulation with synthetic recombinant human thyrotropin (rhTSH; *27,28,57a–57e*). Because rhTSH is not yet approved for use in children, similar comparative studies of rhTSH-stimulated serum Tg and WBS are lacking in the pediatric age group. Yet, we believe that serum Tg levels will be a sensitive and specific marker of persistent or recurrent DTC in children. Whether the WBS will provide additional benefit in the follow-up of children with treated DTC remains to be seen. In general, however, WBS continues to be useful for monitoring the anatomic location, treatment response and extent of disease in children.

Ultrasound has long been used in the successful preoperative evaluation of thyroid lesions in children *(57)*. However, neck ultrasound has also been introduced into patient follow-up with DTC *(58,59)*. A study by Frasoldati et al. found that neck ultrasound was the most sensitive procedure for detecting local–regional recurrence in the neck of patients with DTC *(59)*. The sensitivity of ultrasound (94%) was superior to that of either serum Tg values (57%) or WBS (45%). Based on the general availability, sensitivity, and noninvasive characteristics of ultrasonography, neck ultrasound may prove to be of great benefit in the long-term follow-up of children with DTC.

Children with detectable serum Tg, but negative RAI WBS are particularly vexing. Attempts have been made to identify and localize recurrent or persistent disease using computerized tomographic imaging, magnetic resonance imaging and more recently, [^{18}F]-2-fluoro-2-deoxy-2-D-glucose (FDG) positron emission tomography (PET). In adults with thyroid cancer, FDG-PET had a 71–93.9% sensitivity and similar specificity *(60–66a)* (see Chapters 34, 61). Unfortunately, reactive lymphadenopathy can also be imaged with this technique, resulting in false-positive localization in many cases *(66–68)*. These findings suggest the need for additional study in children before this technique could be strongly recommended.

SUMMARY

In summary, RAI has been widely used for the adjunctive treatment of children and adolescents with DTC. A recent study has now shown that RAI ablation improves outcomes specifically for children and adolescents with DTC who are at high risk, including those with tumors more than 1 cm in diameter, lymph node involvement, incomplete resection, or distant metastases. Another study found that the combination of total thyroidectomy and RAI ablation reduced the risks of recurrence for children with disease that was thought to be confined to the gland. Together, these data support the use of RAI ablation in essentially all children with clinically evident DTC. However, controversy surrounds the use of RAI therapy for children with occult, microscopic, or stable but persistent DTC. The long-term risks and benefits of RAI therapy require continued evaluation, and multicenter studies should be developed to appropriately address these concerns.

Although mortality is low, children with DTC are at risk for recurrent disease and require lifelong follow-up. The optimal means by which to survey for the risk of recurrence is not yet known, but this will probably be based on programs that offer decreasing intensity of evaluation as the patients accumulate years of disease-free follow-up. Hopefully, rhTSH will be approved for use in children and allow rhTSH-stimulated serum Tg values to be used as an indicator of disease. Even with this improvement, RAI WBS and now neck ultrasound will be used in localizing recurrent or persistent DTC in children. Both methods will be integral parts of the decision-making process for the selection of either repeat surgery or additional RAI treatment.

REFERENCES

1. Seidlin SM, Marinelli LD, Oshry E. Radioactive iodine therapy: effect on functioning metastases of adenocarcinoma of thyroid. JAMA 1946; 132:838–847.
2. Singer PA, Cooper DS, Daniels GH, et al. Treatment guidelines for patients with thyroid nodules and well-differentiated thyroid cancer. American Thyroid Association. Arch Intern Med 1996; 1996: 2165–2172.

3. DeGroot LJ, Kaplan EL, McCormick M, Straus FH. Natural history, treatment, and course of papillary thyroid carcinoma. J Clin Endocrinol Metab 1990; 71:414–424.
4. Gorlin JB, Sallan SE. Thyroid cancer in childhood. Endocrinol Metab Clin North Am 1990; 19:649–662.
5. Welch Dinauer CA, Tuttle RM, Robie DK, et al. Clinical features associated with metastasis and recurrence of differentiated thyroid cancer in children, adolescents and young adults. Clin Endocrinol (Oxf) 1998; 49:619–628.
6. McClellan DR, Francis GL. Thyroid cancer in children, pregnant women, and patients with Graves' disease. Endocrinol Metab Clin North Am 1996; 25:27–48.
7. Feinmesser R, Lubin E, Segal K, Noyek A. Carcinoma of the thyroid in children—a review. J Pediatr Endocrinol Metab 1997; 10:561–568.
8. Geiger JD, Thompson NW. Thyroid tumors in children. Otolaryngol Clin North Am 1996; 29:711–719.
9. LaQuaglia M, Telander R. Differentiated and medullary thyroid cancer in children and adolescence. Semin Pediatr Surg 1997; 6:42–49.
10. LaQuaglia M, Black T, Holcomb G, et al. Differentiated thyroid cancer: clinical characteristics, treatment, and outcome in patients under 21 years of age who present with distant metastases. A report from the Surgical Discipline Committee of the Children's Cancer Group. J Pediatr Surg 2000; 35:955–959.
11. Landau D, Vini L, AHern R, Harmer C. Thyroid cancer in children: the Royal Marsden Hospital experience. Eur J Cancer 2000; 36:214–220.
12. Newman KD, Black T, Heller G, et al. Differentiated thyroid cancer: determinants of disease progression in patients <21 years of age at diagnosis: a report from the Surgical Discipline Committee of the Children's Cancer Group. Ann Surg 1998; 227:533–541.
13. Poth M. Thyroid cancer in children and adolescents. In Wartofsky L, editor. Thyroid Cancer: A Comprehensive Guide to Clinical Management. Totowa, NJ: Humana Press, 2000:121–128.
14. Skinner MA. Cancer of the thyroid gland in infants and children. Semin Pediatr Surg 2001; 10:119–126.
15. Tronko MD, Bogdanova TI, Komissarenko IV, et al. Thyroid carcinoma in children and adolescents in Ukraine after the Chernobyl nuclear accident: statistical data and clinicomorphologic characteristics. Cancer 1999; 86:149–156.
16. Thyroid Carcinoma Task Force. AACE/AAES medical/surgical guidelines for clinical practice: management of thyroid carcinoma. American Association of Clinical Endocrinologists. American College of Endocrinology. Endocr Pract 2001; 7:202–220.
17. Harness JK, Thompson NW, McLeod MK, et al. Differentiated thyroid carcinoma in children and adolescents. World J Surg 1992; 16:547–553.
18. Fassina AS, Rupolo M, Pelizzo MR, Casara D. Thyroid cancer in children and adolescents. Tumori 1994; 80:257–262.
19. Samuel AM, Sharma SM. Differentiated thyroid carcinomas in children and adolescents. Cancer 1991; 67:2186–2190.
20. Samuel AM, Rajashekharrao B, Shah DH. Pulmonary metastases in children and adolescents with well-differentiated thyroid cancer. J Nucl Med 1998; 39:1531–1536.
21. Maxon HR. The role of radioiodine in the treatment of childhood thyroid cancer—a dosimetric approach. In Jacob Robbins M, editor. Treatment of Thyroid Cancer in Childhood. Bethesda, MD: NIDDK, National Institutes of Health, 1992:109–126.
22. Yeh SD, La Quaglia MP. 131I therapy for pediatric thyroid cancer. Semin Pediatr Surg 1997; 6:128–133.
23. Chow S, Law S, Mendenhall W, et al. Differentiated thyroid carcinoma in childhood and adolescence—clinical course and role of radioiodine. Pediatr Blood Cancer 2004; 42:176–183.
24. Tisell LE, Nilsson B, Molne J, et al. Improved survival of patients with papillary thyroid cancer after surgical microdissection. World J Surg 1996; 20:854–859.
25. Scheumann GF, Gimm O, Wegener G, et al. Prognostic significance and surgical management of locoregional lymph node metastases in papillary thyroid cancer. World J Surg 1994; 18:559–567.
26. Welch Dinauer CA, Tuttle RM, Robie DK, et al. Extensive surgery improves recurrence-free survival for children and young patients with class I papillary thyroid carcinoma. J Pediatr Surg 1999; 34:1799–1804.
27. Robbins RJ, Chon JT, Fleisher M, et al. Is the serum thyroglobulin response to recombinant human thyrotropin sufficient, by itself, to monitor for residual thyroid carcinoma? J Clin Endocrinol Metab 2002; 87:3242–3247.
28. Mazzaferri EL, Kloos RT. Is diagnostic iodine-131 scanning with recombinant human TSH useful in the follow-up of differentiated thyroid cancer after thyroid ablation? J Clin Endocrinol Metab 2002; 87:1490–1498.
29. McCowen KD, Adler RA, Ghaed N, et al. Low dose radioiodide thyroid ablation in postsurgical patients with thyroid cancer. Am J Med 1976; 61:52–58.
30. Samaan NA, Schultz PN, Hickey RC, et al. The results of various modalities of treatment of well differentiated thyroid carcinomas: a retrospective review of 1599 patients. J Clin Endocrinol Metab 1992; 75:714–720.
31. Reynolds JC. Comparison of I-131 absorbed radiation doses in children and adults: a tool for estimating therapeutic I-131 doses in children. In Jacob Robbins M, editor. Treatment of Thyroid Cancer in Childhood. Bethesda, MD: NIDDK, National Institutes of Health, 1992:127–135.
32. Dorn R, Kopp J, Vogt H, et al. Dosimetry-guided radioactive iodine treatment in patients with metastatic differentiated thyroid cancer: largest safe dose using a risk-adapted approach. J Nucl Med 2003; 44:451–456.
33. Benua R, Leeper R. A method and rationale for treating thyroid carcinoma with the largest safe dose of I-131. In Meideiros-Neto G, Gaitan E, editors. Frontiers in Thyroidology. New York, NY: Plenum, 1986:1317–1321.
34. Leger FA, Izembart M, Dagousset F, et al. Decreased uptake of therapeutic doses of iodine-131 after 185-MBq iodine-131 diagnostic imaging for thyroid remnants in differentiated thyroid carcinoma. Eur J Nucl Med 1998; 25:242–246.
35. Kao CH, Yen TC. Stunning effects after a diagnostic dose of iodine-131. Nuklearmedizin 1998; 37:30–32.
36. Hung W, Sarlis NJ. Current controversies in the management of pediatric patients with well-differentiated nonmedullary thyroid cancer: a review. Thyroid 2002; 12:683–702.
37. Schlumberger M, De Vathaire F. 131 iodine: medical use. Carcinogenic and genetic effects. Ann Endocrinol 1996; 57:166–176.
38. Shore RE. Issues and epidemiological evidence regarding radiation-induced thyroid cancer. Radiat Res 1992; 131:98–111.
39. Thompson DE, Mabuchi K, Ron E, et al. Cancer incidence in atomic bomb survivors. Part II: Solid tumors, 1958-1987. Radiat Res 1994; 137(2 Suppl):S17–S67.
40. Rubino C, F de Vathaire, ME Dottorini, et al. Second primary malignancies in thyroid cancer patients. Br J Cancer 2003; 89:1638–1644.
41. Puerto S, Marcos R, Ramirez M, et al. Equal induction and persistence of chromosome aberrations involving chromosomes 1, 4, and 10 in thyroid cancer patients treated with radioactive iodine. Mutation Res Gene Toxicol Environ Mutagenesis 2000; 469:147–158.
42. Richter HE, Lohrer HD, Hieber L, et al. Microsatellite instability and loss of heterozygosity in radiation-associated thyroid carcinomas of Belarussian children and adults. Carcinogenesis 1999; 20:2247–2252.
43. Baugnet-Mahieu L, Lemaire M, Leonard E, et al. Chromosome aberrations after treatment with radioactive iodine for thyroid cancer. Radiat Res 1994; 140:429–431.
44. Mandel SJ, Mandel L. Radioactive iodine and the salivary glands. Thyroid 2003; 13:265–271.

45. Goolden AW, Kam K, Fitzpatrick M, Munro A. Oedema of the neck after ablation of the thyroid with radioactive iodine. Br J Radiol 1986; 59:583–586.
46. Kloos R, Duvuuri V, Jhiang S, et al. Nasolacrimal drainage system obstruction from radioactive iodine therapy for thyroid carcinoma. J Clin Endocrinol Metab 2002; 87:5817–5820.
47. Raymond JP, Izembart M, Marliac V, et al. Temporary ovarian failure in thyroid cancer patients after thyroid remnant ablation with radioactive iodine. J Clin Endocrinol Metab 1989; 69:186–190.
48. Handelsman DJ, Turtle JR. Testicular damage after radioactive iodine (I-131) therapy for thyroid cancer. Clin Endocrinol (Oxf) 1983; 18: 465–472.
49. Smith MB, Xue H, Takahashi H, et al. Iodine 131 thyroid ablation in female children and adolescents: long-term risk of infertility and birth defects. Ann Surg Oncol 1994; 1:128–131.
50. Vassilopoulou-Sellin R, Schultz PN, Haynie TP. Clinical outcome of patients with papillary thyroid carcinoma who have recurrence after initial radioactive iodine therapy. Cancer 1996; 78:493–501.
51. Vassilopoulou-Sellin R, Goepfert H, Raney B, Schultz PN. Differentiated thyroid cancer in children and adolescents: clinical outcome and mortality after long-term follow-up. Head Neck 1998; 20: 549–555.
52. Vassilopoulou-Sellin R. Long-term outcome of children with papillary thyroid cancer. Surgery 2001; 129:769.
52a. Thompson GB, Hay ID. Current strategies for surgical management and adjuvant treatment of childhood papillary thyroid carcinoma. World J Surg 2004; 28:1187–1198.
53. Powers PA, Dinauer CA, Tuttle RM, Francis GL. Treatment of recurrent papillary thyroid carcinoma in children and adolescents. J Pediatr Endocrinol Metab 2003; 16:1033–1040.
54. Belfiore A, Giuffrida D, La Rosa GL, et al. High frequency of cancer in cold thyroid nodules occurring at young age. Acta Endocrinol (Copenh) 1989; 121:197–202.
55. Hopwood NJ, Kelch RP. Thyroid masses: approach to diagnosis and management in childhood and adolescence. Pediatr Rev 1993; 14: 481–487.
56. Hung W, Anderson KD, Chandra RS, et al. Solitary thyroid nodules in 71 children and adolescents. J Pediatr Surg 1992; 27:1407–1409.
57. Lugo-Vicente H, Ortiz VN. Pediatric thyroid nodules: insights in management. Bol Asoc Med P R 1998; 90:74–78.
57a. Mazzaferri EL, Robbins RJ, Spencer CA, et al. A consensus report of the role of serum thyroglobulin as a monitoring method for low-risk patients with papillary thyroid carcinoma. J Clin Endocrinol Metab 2003; 88:1433–1441.
57b. Wartofsky L. Editorial: Using baseline and recombinant human TSH-stimulated Tg measurements to manage thyroid cancer without diagnostic 131-I scanning. J Clin Endocrinol Metab 2002; 87:1486–1489.
57c. Mezzaferri EL, Kloos RT. Is diagnostic iodine-131 scanning with recombinant human TSH useful in the follow-up of differentiated thyroid cancer after thyroid ablation? J Clin Endocrinol Metab 2002; 87:1490–1498.
57d. Robbins RJ, Chon JT, Fleisher M, Larson SM, Tuttle RM. Is the serum thyroglobulin response to recombinant human thyrotropin sufficient, by itself, to monitor for residual thyroid carcinoma? J Clin Endocrinol Metab 2002; 87:3242–3247.
57e. David A, Blotta A, Rossi R, et al. Clinical value of different responses of serum thyroglobulin to recombinant human thyrotropin in the follow-up of patients with differentiated thryoid carcinoma. Thyroid 2005; 15:267–273.
58. Pacini F, Molinaro E, Castagna MG, et al. Recombinant human thyrotropin-stimulated serum thyroglobulin combined with neck ultrasonography has the highest sensitivity in monitoring differentiated thyroid carcinoma. J Clin Endocrinol Metab 2003; 88: 3668–3673.
59. Frasoldati A, Pesenti M, Gallo M, et al. Diagnosis of neck recurrences in patients with differentiated thyroid carcinoma. Cancer 2003; 97: 90–96.
60. Wang W, Larson SM, Fazzari M, et al. Prognostic value of [18F]-fluorodeoxyglucose positron emission tomographic scanning in patients with thyroid cancer. J Clin Endocrinol Metab 2000; 85: 1107–1113.
61. Robbins RJ, Hill RH, Wang W, et al. Inhibition of metabolic activity in papillary thyroid carcinoma by a somatostatin analogue. Thyroid 2000; 10:177–183.
62. Wang W, Macapinlac H, Larson SM, et al. [18F]-2-fluoro-2-deoxy-D-glucose positron emission tomography localizes residual thyroid cancer in patients with negative diagnostic (131)I whole body scans and elevated serum thyroglobulin levels. J Clin Endocrinol Metab 1999; 84:2291–2302.
63. Yeo JS, Chung JK, So Y, et al. F-18-fluorodeoxyglucose positron emission tomography as a presurgical evaluation modality for I-131 scan-negative thyroid carcinoma patients with local recurrence in cervical lymph nodes. Head Neck 2001; 23:94–103.
64. Chung JK, So Y, Lee JS, et al. Value of FDG PET in papillary thyroid carcinoma with negative 131I whole-body scan. J Nucl Med 1999; 40: 986–992.
65. Alnafisi NS, Driedger AA, Coates G, et al. FDG PET of recurrent or metastatic 131I-negative papillary thyroid carcinoma. J Nucl Med 2000; 41:1010–1015.
66. Schluter B, Bohuslavizki KH, Beyer W, et al. Impact of FDG PET on patients with differentiated thyroid cancer who present with elevated thyroglobulin and negative 131I scan. J Nucl Med 2001; 42: 71–76.
66a. Nahas Z, Goldenberg D, Fakhry C, et al. The role of positron emission tomography/computed tomography in the management of recurrent papillary thyroid carcinoma. Laryngoscope 2005; 115:237–243.
67. Frilling A, Tecklenborg K, Gorges R, et al. Preoperative diagnostic value of [(18)F] fluorodeoxyglucose positron emission tomography in patients with radioiodine-negative recurrent well-differentiated thyroid carcinoma. Ann Surg 2001; 234:804–811.
68. Frilling A, Gorges R, Tecklenborg K, et al. Value of preoperative diagnostic modalities in patients with recurrent thyroid carcinoma. Surgery 2000; 128:1067–1074.

34
Positron Emission Tomography in Well-Differentiated Thyroid Cancer

I. Ross McDougall

INTRODUCTION

Positron emission tomography (PET) is a diagnostic technique that has become an important method in oncology. The basis for this test is the injection of a positron-emitting radionuclide that localizes in cancers and allows imaging. A positron is a positive electron, and when emitted, travels a few millimeters before contacting an electron, which has a negative charge. These particles of equal mass and opposite charges annihilate one another. The mass of the two electrons produces two photons each with an energy of 511 keV. This is derived from the equation, $e = mc^2$. The photons travel in opposing directions at an angle of 180°. A positron camera usually consists of a ring of detectors that are designed to identify photons interacting at precisely the same time on opposite positions on the ring (180°).

These occurrences are called "coincident events"; millions can be reconstructed into images of the distribution of the positron-emitting radiopharmaceutical within the patient. Coincident photons arising from different parts of the patient travel through different lengths of the body to reach the ring of detectors. For example, when a positron is emitted from a lesion in the skin of the left shoulder, one photon travels through millimeters of tissue and then strikes the detector. The other photon has to travel through the width of the patient before interacting with the opposing detector. There must be correction for attenuation of the photons by the tissues of the body. Traditionally, this has been obtained by repeating the scan using a source of radiation, such as gadolinium, outside of the patient. Therefore, the complete scan requires imaging the PET radiopharmaceutical from the inferior margin of the brain to the mid-thigh. Then, the attenuation correction scan is obtained over the same region, and that data is used to produce the final or attenuation-corrected images.

Recently, improved technology has resulted in a PET scanner that has been combined with computed tomography (CT) (PET/CT). The CT images can be used for attenuation correction and for providing an anatomic correlation along with the functional PET images. Because the detector is 15 cm long, six or seven bed positions are required to cover the head, neck, and trunk. A PET scan takes approx 30–40 min to complete. The extrinsic attenuation correction requires another 20–30 min, but this time is reduced to about 1–2 min for combined PET/CT. Therefore, the combined PET/CT scan provides additional anatomic information more quickly, allowing increased throughput of patients.

For several years, companies that produced scintigraphic cameras promoted the sale of *hybrid* cameras. These were conventional whole-body cameras with two detectors whose primary functions were to produce anterior and whole-body scintiscans or single-photon tomographic images. The two heads could also be used for detecting coincident incidents and thus could be used for PET imaging *(1)*. There are several disadvantages; the most important is the reduced counting ability of two detectors vs the ring format of a dedicated PET instrument. Second, hybrid cameras have a significantly poorer resolution. One important benefit of PET is the excellent resolution. In the immediate future, the greatest utility will be dedicated PET scanner combined with CT.

RADIOPHARMACEUTICALS FOR PET

In oncology, the radiopharmaceutical that is employed almost exclusively is ^{18}F-fluoro-deoxyglucose (FDG). FDG is taken into cells by Glut transporters, where it is acted on by hexokinase. Thereafter, it is not metabolized as rapidly as glucose and remains trapped within the cells. Most cancer cells have an increase in Glut transporters and hexokinase. Images are obtained 1–2 h after intravenous injection of FDG and demonstrate cells that have trapped and retained this agent. Statistically, the greatest number of PET studies using FDG is for patients with other types of tumors. These include scans performed to differentiate a benign from malignant lung nodule and for staging and evaluating the response to therapy of nonsmall cell lung cancer, lymphoma, head and neck cancer, esophageal and recurrent colorectal cancer, or breast cancer *(2–4)*. PET of the brain is also important, not only for cancers, but in the diagnosis of degenerative diseases

From: *Thyroid Cancer: A Comprehensive Guide to Clinical Management, 2/e*
Edited by: L. Wartofsky and D. Van Nostrand © Humana Press Inc., Totowa, NJ

Table 1
Positron-Emitting Radionuclides for Thyroid Studies

Characteristic	^{18}F	^{124}I	^{120}I	^{122}I
Half-life	110 min	4.18 d	1.35 h	3.6 min
B⁺ yield (%)	97	23	46	77
E_{B^+}	635 KeV	1.5 MeV	4.6 MeV	3.1 MeV
Daughter product	^{18}O	^{124}Te	^{120}Te	^{122}Te

(e.g., Alzheimer's, multi-infarct dementia, and Parkinson's disease). PET has a role in defining whether ischemic myocardium is viable.

In the management of patients with well-differentiated thyroid cancer, its main role is for those patients who have an elevated thyroglobulin (Tg) level and a negative whole-body ^{131}I or ^{123}I diagnostic scan and/or ^{131}I posttreatment scan, or it is for those patients with antithyroglobulin antibodies that preclude the accurate measurement of thyroglobulin. PET is approved for this purpose in the United States. Other uses are differentiating a benign from a malignant thyroid nodule and preoperative staging of patients with newly diagnosed cancer.

Pertaining to thyroid cancer, there is a second positron emitter (^{124}I) that has valuable properties and has an increasing impact in management by PET. ^{120}I and ^{122}I are also positron emitters but have not been introduced into clinical practice (5). Table 1 provides the physical characteristics of these positron emitters.

METHODS

FDG is injected intravenously, and imaging is started after a delay of 1 h. The patient should fast for at least 6 h before the injection and preferably should have no food after midnight the evening before the study. The patient should also not exercise vigorously for 24 h prior to the study. In the United States, most authorities recommend measuring serum glucose prior to the injection of FDG because high values alter the distribution of the radiopharmaceutical and lower the sensitivity of the test. In countries where the incidence of latent and prediabetic patients is low, this is not necessary.

After injection of FDG, the patient should be in a quiet, warm, and comfortable room for the hour between the injection of FDG and imaging. The patient should not talk or chew. The reason for these precautions is that active muscles trap FDG, and uptake can cause difficulty in interpretation, resulting in a false-positive scan (as discussed below). Some authorities delay scanning for 90–120 min. The extra time allows more of the background activity to be excreted through the kidneys, thus making the lesions easier to detect. For thyroid cancer, this is seldom necessary, and the 1-h delay is the best compromise for accuracy and efficiency, as well as for a steady throughput of patients.

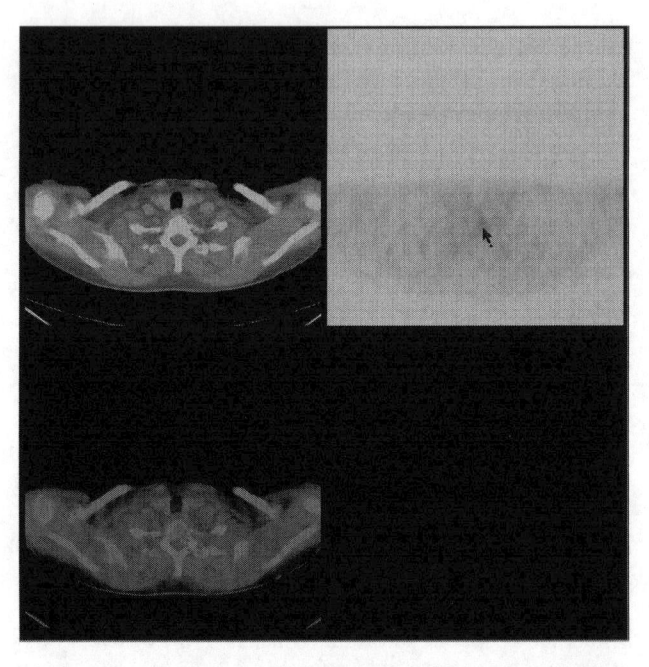

Fig. 1. A transaxial scan showing PET (upper right), CT (upper left), and combined PET and CT (lower panel). The white arrow shows the thyroid on CT, and the black arrow shows a vertebra on PET scan. The thyroid has no uptake of FDG scan. (Illustration appears in color in insert following p. 198.)

NORMAL FINDINGS AND VARIATIONS

Although the thyroid is a metabolically active gland, somewhat surprisingly, the normal thyroid is not seen or is faintly seen on FDG scan 1 h after injection. PET/CT allows the thyroid anatomy to be defined by CT; in patients being scanned for nonthyroidal cancer, frequently, the normal thyroid cannot be identified on PET (Fig. 1). When there is diffusely increased uptake in the thyroid, the patient usually has an autoimmune thyroid disease that is most often chronic lymphocytic thyroiditis and less frequently, Graves' hyperthyroidism (Fig. 2; 6–9). In the occasional patient with autoimmune thyroid disease, the uptake of FDG can be focal and misinterpreted as a malignancy in the thyroid (9).

Focal uptake of FDG in a patient being evaluated for a nonthyroidal disease has about a 25–45% chance of being evidence of a thyroid cancer. In an analysis of more than

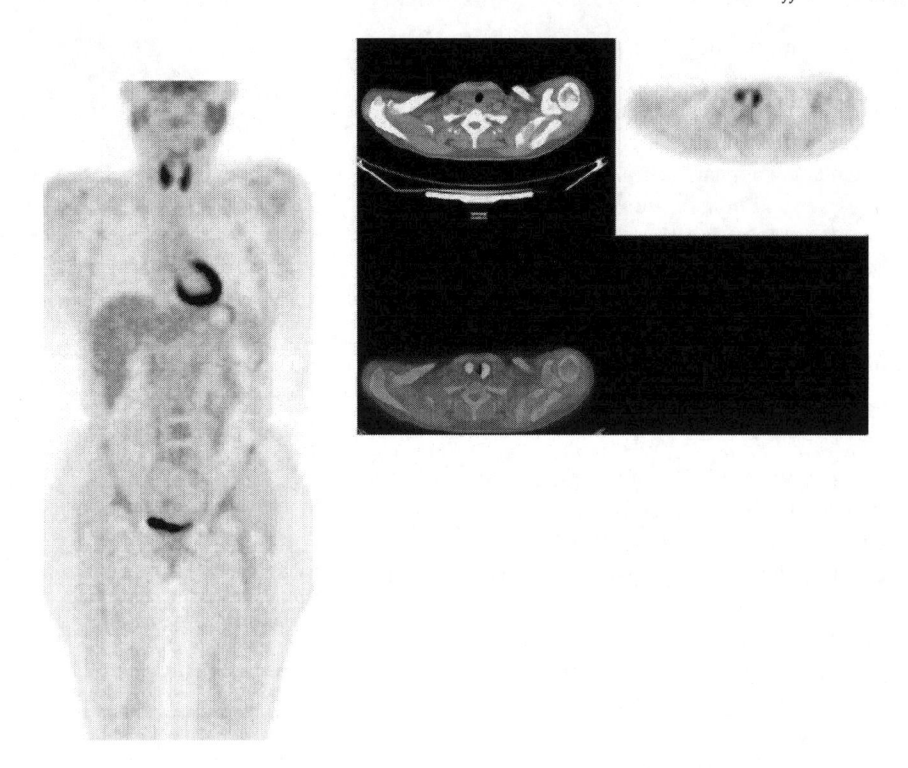

Fig. 2. A coronal PET scan (left). The image on the right is the transaxial images of the PET scan, CT, and combined PET/CT, as oriented in Fig. 1 and at the thyroid level. The thyroid has intense uptake of FDG. The patient had Hashimoto's thyroiditis. (Illustration appears in color in insert following p. 198.)

4500 PET scans, 2.3% showed some abnormality in the thyroid (10). In 87 patients, this was not pursued because of the severity of their primary cancer, but 15 patients had a biopsy, and 7 (47%) of these were thyroid cancer. These thyroid nodules found incidentally or "incidentalomas" had a 2.2% frequency of scans in a series reported by Kang et al. (11). Some areas of uptake were diffuse and consistent with thyroiditis, but 4 of 15 (27%) focal lesions were malignant. Several reports indicate a 50% risk of cancer or greater (12). In an interinstitutional collaborative study, we identified 15 focally "hot" lesions with 9 patients referred for operation, of which 8 cancers were diagnosed histologically (Fig. 3). Because undiagnosed thyroid cancer appears hot on FDG scan, there was hope that PET would differentiate a malignant from a benign nodule. However, the technology is expensive and, even if perfect, would not replace fine-needle aspiration (FNA). Although, theoretically, PET might have a role in the indeterminate microfollicular lesion, the data do not support its use. In a small study of nodules in nine patients, three cancers were PET-positive, but four of six benign lesions showed focal uptake (13). Using a standardized uptake value (SUV) of 5.0 Uematsu et al. were able to separate four cancerous nodules from six benign nodules, but one patient with thyroiditis had an SUV of 6.3 (14). Therefore, not all focal PET-positive lesions in the thyroid are cancerous, and an FNA or ultrasound-guided FNA is

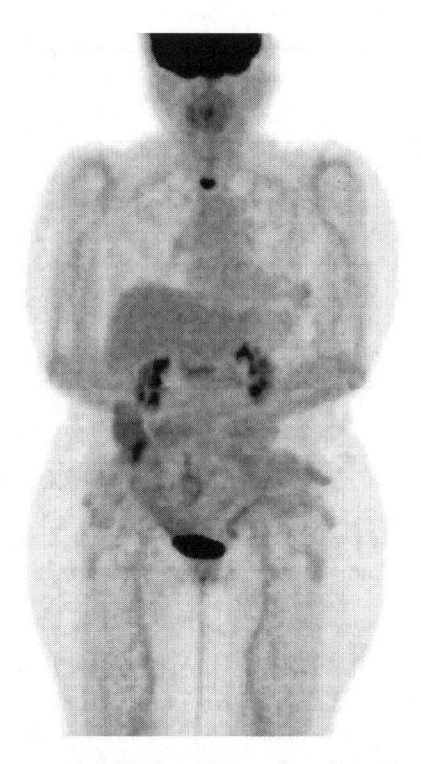

Fig. 3. A coronal projection showing a focal lesion in the thyroid that concentrates FDG. This was confirmed as an unsuspected papillary cancer. (Illustration appears in color in insert following p. 198.)

appropriate to establish the diagnosis in most patients *(15,16)*.

There is a high concentration of FDG in the brain, which depends on glucose for function. The kidneys are also noted to excrete FDG, and the bladder appears hot on scan. Varying uptake exists in the muscles and myocardium. However, in a patient who has fasted and been inactive, with a normal fasting glucose, these structures should have modest uptake and allow anatomic correlation, without interfering with the interpretation. There is diffuse concentration of FDG in the liver. These findings are shown in Figs. 2 and 3.

INTERPRETATION OF PET SCANS

Regions of abnormal uptake of FDG in recurrent or metastatic cancer are usually easy to identify. Combined PET/CT allows the exact anatomic site to be defined. Many authorities simply report on the scan findings. The optimal results are obtained by interpreting the data while at a computer terminal and viewing systematically the coronal, sagittal, and transaxial projections. It is helpful to scroll through images of regions where an abnormality is identified or suspected. Some experts use a quantitative numeric result, which determines the uptake in the lesions compared to the amount of radiopharmaceutical injected. This result is the SUV. A lesion with an SUV more than 2.5 is generally accepted as likely owing to cancer; however, in the study discussed above, the cut-off between cancerous and benign was 5.0. Consequently, in practice, the SUV is not that helpful to establish sites of thyroid cancer, and it has also been referred to as the "silly uptake value" *(17)*. More practically, the SUV can be used as a baseline for comparison with subsequent scans to judge the response to treatment. It also has a prognostic value, as discussed below. Other investigators use the ratio of uptake in the cancer to background activity. When a comparison of quantitative measurements is made between two studies, it is important to ensure that both were conducted under identical conditions.

FALSE-POSITIVE RESULTS

Any malignant or active cells can trap FDG, and several etiologies may cause false-positive interpretation *(18,19)*. It would be unusual but not impossible for a patient with thyroid cancer to also have another form of cancer. The distribution of abnormal uptake should be carefully evaluated to ensure that it is consistent with the expected spread of thyroid cancer. The common site of residual cancer would be the thyroid bed; for metastases, the regional lymph nodes in the neck and mediastinum; and distant metastases, the lungs and skeleton. Inflammatory conditions, e.g., tuberculosis and sarcoidosis, show abnormal uptake, but the distribution is not likely to be confused with thyroid cancer.

Three specific conditions are important in the interpretation of PET conducted for thyroid cancer. The first is FDG

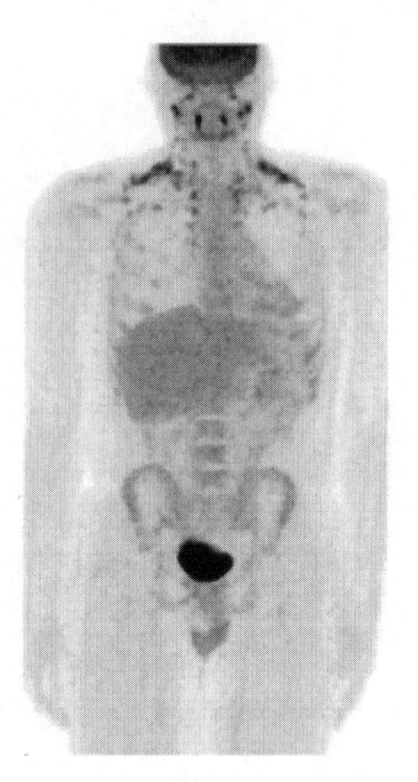

Fig. 4. A coronal section made 1 h after injection of 15 mCi (550 MBq) of FDG, showing symmetric uptake in the supraclavicular areas as a result of uptake in brown fat.

uptake in active neck muscles. Although the muscles are linear structures, its uptake can result in apparently globular uptake similar to a lymph node because of tomographic slices across muscle bellies. This finding is more common in patients who are nervous and trembling or shivering. This condition was first identified by Barrington et al., and they advise diazepam prior to injection of the radiopharmaceutical *(20)*. This requires knowledge *a priori* of the patients likely to be that stressed to have these behaviors. In the United States, the physician prescribing the tranquilizer is responsible for the patient's well-being. When the physician conducting the scan prescribes the drug, he or she must have all the requirements for conscious sedation in place. As a result, the physician is usually reluctant to take this step. Moreover, not all physicians have found that anxiety-reducing medications lower the number of false-positives *(21)*.

A poor response to anxiolytic medication is likely to indicate a different cause of a false-positive, i.e., uptake of FDG in brown fat (Fig. 4; *22–25*). Superficially, this uptake looks similar to the muscle uptake, but the distribution follows the shape of the neck, more narrow at the chin level and wider at the thoracic inlet. In contrast, the muscle uptake follows the contour of the sternocleidomastoid and is therefore more narrow at the manubrium. Uptake in brown fat is thought to increase in cold temperature *(23)*. Our experience is that it is more common in thin women. A recent laboratory study in rats confirms that the FDG uptake is increased by cold temperature, and it could be reduced by propranolol or reserpine *(26)*.

The third abnormality is asymmetric uptake in the functional muscles of one vocal cord with damage to the contralateral nerve during thyroidectomy *(27,28)*. A similar finding has been reported in a granulomatous foreign-body reaction around a Teflon implant to improve a paralyzed vocal cord *(29)*. There can be uptake of FDG in the thymus *(30–35)*, which is more typical in younger patients and those who have been recently treated with chemotherapy. Although the bilobed shape is characteristic, this can be misinterpreted as mediastinal metastases, and PET/CT would allow easy differentiation.

ROLE IN TG-POSITIVE IODINE-NEGATIVE PATIENTS

There is consensus that the optimal treatment for well-differentiated thyroid cancer is total or near-total thyroidectomy and ^{131}I treatment in selected patients. This treatment removes all functioning thyroid tissue and allows for follow-up using measurement of serum Tg and, in selected patients, whole-body scan with either ^{131}I or ^{123}I radioiodine. When the treatment has been successful, both follow-up studies are negative. If there is residual or recurrent disease, both tests are usually abnormal and enable a decision to be made whether to retreat with ^{131}I. In 15–30% of patients with residual or recurrent disease, a discrepancy exists between the tests, with measurable Tg and the negative diagnostic scan. The reasons for this discrepancy could be that there are too few cells to be identified, or that there is a defect in the function or location of the sodium iodide symporter (NIS). This difficult and trying problem for the patient and physician has led to different philosophies about management. Some recommend a therapeutic dose of ^{131}I even with negative ^{131}I uptake, hoping that sufficient radiation will be delivered to localize and kill the cells producing Tg *(36,37)*. However, not all physicians accept this approach *(38–41)*. An alternative method is to employ imaging tests that are not dependent on the NIS to identify the thyroid tissue. Such imaging could include neck ultrasound, CT, magnetic resonance imaging (MRI), and a range of nuclear medicine procedures (see Chapter 39).

The various imaging modalities with the nuclear medicine tests are briefly addressed in the sequence of their historical application. ^{201}Tl is a large atom trapped by the sodium potassium channel of cells and is valuable for evaluating myocardial perfusion. Serendipitously, it was found to be trapped by some cancers, including thyroid cancer, and became popular for imaging patients with thyroid cancer *(42–45)*. Because of the emitted photons' low energy and the high absorbed radiation, the small injected activity results in ^{201}Tl images that are poor in comparison to those made with radiopharmaceuticals containing ^{99m}Tc. Consequently, ^{201}Tl is now used infrequently in patients with thyroid cancer. When ^{99m}Tc-labeled radiopharmaceuticals were developed for studying myocardial perfusion, they were subsequently investigated in cancer patients and found to be efficient in identifying sites of metastatic thyroid cancer. The images are superior to ^{201}Tl because the emitted photons have a higher energy that is suited for current γ cameras. In addition, a larger quantity of radioactivity, 20 mCi (740 MBq) vs 0.5 mCi (18.5 MBq), can be injected.

There are two of these radiopharmaceuticals: sestamibi and tetrafosmin *(46)*. In one report of 110 scans in 99 patients, the sestamibi scans paralleled with the Tg measurements in 96%. However, in most patients, both tests were negative. Only 16 patients had abnormal results with a whole-body radioiodine scan. In four (25%) of these patients, sestamibi demonstrated a lesion unseen on ^{131}I images. Similarly, tetrafosmin has been found to identify iodine-negative cancer. Gallowitsch et al. identified 39 of 44 lesions with tetrafosmin compared to 19 on whole-body ^{131}I *(48)*. Subsequent publications from these and other investigators confirm these findings *(49–52)*. There are somatostatin receptors in thyroid cancer *(53)*; ^{111}in-octreotide has also been used, but the sensitivity does not make it a powerful test *(54–59)*.

Surprisingly, the first report of a FDG-PET scan for thyroid cancer dates as early as 1987 *(56)*. There was nearly a decade of delay before several reports appeared. Since then, many studies have been published addressing the role and value of FDG-PET in adult patients who have measurable Tg but negative studies with radioiodine *(57–64)*. Several editorials and reviews attest to the value of PET *(65–68)*. In addition, we and other authors have found PET to be valuable in children *(69)*. The images are superior to scans from all the other radiopharmaceuticals discussed briefly above. Generally, the interpretation can be reached with confidence. Using combined PET/CT imaging, abnormal FDG uptake can be correlated with the anatomy, and this approach should reduce the amount of false-positive interpretations. Apparently, the less well-differentiated the cancer is, the more likely the PET scan will be positive. Very well-differentiated cancers can show less FDG uptake. This has been called a "flip-flop" *(56,70)* and was illustrated by the comparison of FDG-PET scans and ^{131}I scans in 47 lesions *(71)*. Thirty-three lesions were iodine-positive, but 20 (61%) of these were PET-negative. Conversely, there were 9 PET-positive lesions from 14 (64%) iodine-negative sites.

Earlier studies on FDG-PET for thyroid cancer evaluated a spectrum of patients: some had a remnant after surgery, some had metastases that could be imaged with radioiodine, and others had negative scans using radioiodine but had measurable Tg levels. These studies indicated that the overall sensitivity of PET was low, and the test was not useful for "all-comers" *(72)*. However, when the Tg-positive iodine-negative patients were analyzed separately, the

Table 2
Sensitivity of PET Scan in Tg-Positive Iodine-Negative Patients

Reference	Number of Patients	Women (%)	Men (%)	Ages	Sensitivity (%)	Specificity (%)	Altered Treatment (%)
Alnafasi et al. (59)	11	73	27	19–66	100		64
Chung et al. (94)	54	78	22	24–72	94	95	
Dietlin et al. (95)	58	74	26	19–72	82		
Goshen et al. (75)	20	75	25	19–77	94		30
Grunwalt et al. (96)	222	68	32	NA	75	90	
Grunwalt et al. Tg >5 (96)					76	100	
Grunwalt et al. (96)					85	90	
McDougall	76	76	24	7–79	63		
Wang et al. (97)	37	62	38	16–83	71		51
Stokkel et al. (98)	11	55	45	26–73	100	100	

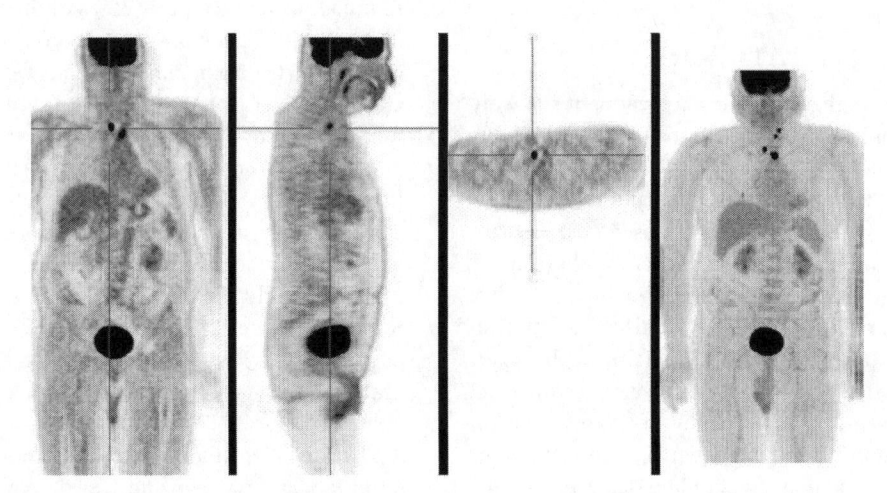

Fig. 5. Coronal, sagittal, and transaxial projections made 1 hour after injection of 15 mCi (550 MBq) of FDG. The patient was Tg-positive radioiodine-negative; four sites of abnormal FDG uptake are present. By identifying the abnormality on one projection, the images also show how it can be automatically seen on the other two projections.

sensitivity increased and specificity remained powerful (Table 2). The sensitivity varies from about 60% to as high as 100%. The high sensitivities are most likely owing to the small number of patients studied who had extensive disease. As the test has become more widely used, patients with lesser volumes of cancer are being studied, and it is not surprising that the sensitivity has fallen. It is not possible to determine the specificity in many reports because all the patients studied had an elevated Tg, i.e., there were no patients who could be defined as being disease-free. Our group has utilized more than 100 PET scans, including PET/CT, in 76 patients, and the sensitivity was 63%. No difference was found in age or gender of those with negative vs positive scans. The average ages were 41.5 ± 14.4 vs 48.9 ± 14.8 yr, and 76% and 69% were women, respectively. The earlier experience has been published (73). In many reports, there is a relationship to the level of Tg, but there is no cut-off above or below that designate all PET scans as positive or negative. The current approved indication for FDG-PET uses a Tg value of 10 ng/mL or greater. Fig. 5 demonstrates a FDG-positive PET scan in a patient who had positive Tg levels and a negative radioiodine whole-body scan.

False-negative findings occur in well-differentiated cancer, as well as in lesions that are too small to be resolved with modern dedicated cameras less than about 5–6 mm.

PROGNOSTIC VALUE OF FDG-PET SCANS

A significantly abnormal PET scan with lesions showing a high SUV signifies a bad outcome (74). In a study of 125 patients followed for 41 mo, 14 died from thyroid cancer. The most important predictor was PET positivity with a volume of cancer greater than 125 mL. In those patients with smaller tumor volumes, the 3-yr survival was 96%, and even patients with distant metastases who were PET-negative all survived, again reflecting the "flip-flop" phenomenon.

Well-differentiated cells trap iodine and are amenable to ^{131}I therapy; less well-differentiated cancer do not trap iodine but do concentrate FDG. In contrast, patients who are both iodine-negative and PET-negative appear to have a good prognosis. In our experience with the latter patients, no one has died and the recurrence rate is low.

A positive FDG scan can alter management. Alnafisi et al. changed management in 7 of 11 patients, Goshen et al. in 6 of 20 *(59,75)*. The identification of a focal lesion allows surgery to be an option. Discovery of a lesion in a vertebral body can lead to the consideration of surgical or external-beam radiation. Our approach for neck lesions identified using PET is to obtain an ultrasound for precise anatomic localization and for potential ultrasound-guided FNA. The patient can then be operated on using intraoperative ultrasound to reidentify the site and to ensure that it is excised *(76)*. In this series, all patients had a drop in Tg, and 64% achieved undetectable values.

ROLE OF THYROTROPIN IN FDG SCANNING

The vast majority of FDG studies in oncology, including patients with thyroid cancer, are conducted in the euthyroid or even biochemically hyperthyroid condition. Anecdotally reported cases studied when euthyroid, and then again with an elevated thyrotropin (TSH), showed no difference in FDG uptake *(77,78)*. However, in contrast, Sisson et al. reported increased uptake under TSH stimulus *(79)*. Several publications have since confirmed this finding, in line with in vitro studies that show TSH increases glucose uptake into thyroid cells *(80)*.

In a study of 17 patients imaged when TSH was less than 0.05 µU/mL then again when the TSH was more than 22 µU/mL (on average, 42 d later), the lesion-to-background ratio increased by a median of 63.1% *(81)*, and new lesions were identified in 3 of 10 patients. In a similarly conducted study, 30 patients who had negative or equivocal ^{131}I scintiscans and abnormal or equivocal serum Tg levels were studied before and after an injection of recombinant human (rh) TSH *(82)*. When the TSH was low, a total of 45 lesions were seen in 9 patients; after rhTSH administration, 78 lesions were seen in 19 patients. Therefore, many more lesions were diagnosed, some PET-negative patients became PET-positive, and an increased SUV or lesion-to-background ratio was observed. In a smaller study, only one of seven patients was PET-positive after an rhTSH injection.

These results present a problem. Should all patients be studied with an elevated TSH? If so, should they be hypothyroid or injected with rhTSH? rhTSH has not been approved for PET. A possible method is to obtain a TSH-stimulated PET scan when the patient receives rhTSH for diagnostic imaging with a radionuclide of iodine. For example, the injections could be given on Monday and Tuesday; the PET scan could be obtained on Wednesday morning after a 6-h fast, and then the tracer of radioiodine could be administered. Neither test would interfere with the other. TSH stimulated PET scan could also be obtained at a time when TSH is low or undetectable and there is a high risk for disease that has not been identified or localized by PET imaging when the patient was euthyroid.

^{124}I PET SCANNING

^{124}I has a half-life ($T_{1/2P}$) of 4.2 d and can be employed for PET analogous to the use of ^{123}I and ^{131}I for planar and single-photon tomographic imaging *(83)*. PET always provides tomographic information, and the images have superior resolution and can be used to determine volume with accuracy. In addition, ^{124}I PET scans can be fused with CT and MRI *(83a)*. There was a theoretical concern that the high-energy positrons and complex decay scheme with high-energy γ photons of ^{124}I would not allow high-quality images to be obtained. Experimental studies with phantoms show that high-quality well-resolved images of ^{124}I are possible using a dedicated PET camera *(84,85)*.

^{124}I has been efficient in benign conditions of the thyroid, e.g., to obtain an accurate measurement of the volume of thyroid to allow calculation of a specific radiation-absorbed dose when treating Graves' disease *(86–88)*. One study showed an excellent correlation to the volume as determined by ultrasound *(89)*. PET has the advantage of demonstrating the volume of functioning tissue, rather than total volume.

The role of ^{124}I in thyroid cancer management is in development, but there is considerable potential because volumetric calculation of lesions can be obtained, and the 4.2 $T_{1/2P}$ would allow measurements to be made of total-body clearance and $T_{1/2E}$ in metastases over time. One study compared the uptake and clearance of ^{124}I and ^{131}I that were administered simultaneously, and there was good concordance *(90)*.

^{124}I PET may permit more specific dosimetric determinations as well *(91)*, as shown in recent case reports and analyses of small patient groups with thyroid cancer *(92,93)*. A total of 12 patients were imaged 24 h after an average dose of 2.2 mCi (84 MBq) of ^{124}I. The patients had PET, combined PET/CT, CT, and posttherapy of ^{131}I. The detectability of lesions was 87%, 100%, 56%, and 83%, respectively.

^{124}I has also been used to label peptides and antibodies for positron imaging *(90)*.

SUMMARY

PET with FDG is a valuable test to help manage patients who have an elevated Tg level with cancers that cannot trap iodine. The test can identify cancer sites and lead to a change in therapy in 30–60%. Newer PET radionuclides, such as ^{124}I, will have a significant impact in providing accurate dosimetry prior to treatment with ^{131}I.

REFERENCES

1. Patton J, Turkington TG. Coincidence imaging with a dual-head scintillation camera. J Nucl Med 1999; 40:432–441.
2. Huebner RH, Park KC, Shepherd JE, et al. A meta-analysis of the literature for whole-body FDG PET detection of recurrent colorectal cancer. J Nucl Med 2000; 41:1177–1189.
3. Weihrauch MR, Dietlein M, Schicha H, et al. Prognostic significance of 18F-fluorodeoxyglucose positron emission tomography in lymphoma. Leuk Lymphoma 2003; 44:15–22.
4. Schiepers C, Filmont JE, Czernin J. PET for staging of Hodgkin's disease and non-Hodgkin's lymphoma. Eur J Nucl Med Mol Imaging 2003; 30(Suppl 1):S82–S88.
5. Moerlein SM, Mathis CA, Brennan KM, Budinger TF. Synthesis and in vivo evaluation of 122I- and 131I-labelled iodoperidol, a potential agent for the tomographic assessment of cerebral perfusion. Int J Rad Appl Instrum B 1987; 14:91–98.
6. Yasuda S, Ide M, Takagi S, Shohtsu A. Cancer screening with whole-body FDG PET. Kaku Igaku 1996; 33:1065–1071.
7. Yasuda S, Shohtsu A, Ide M, et al. Chronic thyroiditis: Diffuse uptake of FDG at PET. Radiology 1998; 207:775–778.
8. Borner AR, Voth E, Wienhard K, et al. F-qi-FDG PET of the thyroid gland in Graves' disease. Nuklearmedizin 1998; 37:227–233.
9. Schmid DT, Kneifel S, Stoeckli SJ, et al. Increased 18F-FDG uptake mimicking thyroid cancer in a patient with Hashimoto's thyroiditis. Eur Radiol 2003; 13:2119–2121.
10. Cohen MS, Arslan N, Dehdashti F, et al. Risk of malignancy in thyroid incidentalomas identified by fluorodeoxyglucose-positron emission tomography. Surgery 2001; 130:941–946.
11. Kang KW, Kim SK, Kang HS, et al. Prevalence and risk of cancer of focal thyroid incidentaloma identified by 18F-fluorodeoxyglucose positron emission tomography for metastasis evaluation and cancer screening in healthy subjects. J Clin Endocrinol Metab 2003; 88:4100–4104.
12. Ramos CD, Chisin R, Yeung HW, et al. Incidental focal thyroid uptake on FDG positron emission tomographic scans may represent a second primary tumor. Clin Nucl Med 2001; 26:193–197.
13. Adler LP, Bloom AD. Positron emission tomography of thyroid masses. Thyroid 1993; 3:195–200.
14. Uematsu H, Sadato N, Ohtsubo T, et al. Fluorine-18-fluorodeoxyglucose PET versus thallium-201 scintigraphy evaluation of thyroid tumors. J Nucl Med 1998; 39:453–459.
15. Gianoukakis AG, Karam M, Cheema A, Cooper JA. Autonomous thyroid nodules visualized by positron emission tomography with (18)f-fluorodeoxyglucose: a case report and review of the literature. Thyroid 2003; 13:395–399.
16. Park CH, Lee EJ, Kim JK, et al. Focal F-18 FDG uptake in a nontoxic autonomous thyroid nodule. Clin Nucl Med 2002; 27:136–137.
17. Keyes JW, Jr. SUV: standard uptake or silly useless value? J Nucl Med 1995; 36:1836–1839.
18. Cook G, Maisey MN, Fogelman I. Normal variants, artefacts and interpretative pitfalls in PET with 18-fluoro-2-deoxyglucose and carbon-11 methionine. Normal variants, artefacts and interpretative pitfalls in PET with 18-fluoro-2-deoxyglucose and carbon-11 methionine. Eur J Nucl Med 1999; 26:1363–1378.
19. Cook G, Wegner EA, Fogelman I. Pitfalls and artifacts in 18FDG PET and PET/CT oncologic imaging. Semin Nucl Med 2004; 34:122–133.
20. Barrington S, Maisey MN. Skeletal muscle uptake of fluorine-18 FDG: effect of oral diazepam. J Nucl Med 1996; 37:1127–1129.
21. Dobert N, Menzel C, Hamscho N, et al. Atypical thoracic and supraclavicular FDG-uptake in patients with Hodgkin's and non-Hodgkin's lymphoma. Q J Nucl Med 2004; 48:33–38.
22. Hany TF, Gharehpapagh E, Kamel EM, et al. Brown adipose tissue: a factor to consider in symmetrical tracer uptake in the neck and upper chest region. Eur J Nucl Med Mol Imaging 2002; 29: 1393–1398.
23. Cohade C, Mourtzikos KA, Wahl RL. "USA-Fat": prevalence is related to ambient outdoor temperature-evaluation with 18F-FDG PET/CT. J Nucl Med 2003; 44:1267–1270.
24. Cohade C, Osman M, Pannu HK, Wahl RL. Uptake in supraclavicular area fat ("USA-Fat"): description on 18F-FDG PET/CT. J Nucl Med 2003; 44:170–176.
25. Yeung HW, Grewal RK, Gonen M, et al. Patterns of (18)F-FDG uptake in adipose tissue and muscle: a potential source of false-positives for PET. J Nucl Med 2003; 44:1789–1796.
26. Tatsumi M, Engles JM, Ishimori T, et al. Intense (18)F-FDG uptake in brown fat can be reduced pharmacologically. J Nucl Med 2004; 45: 1189–1193.
27. Igerc I, Kumnig G, Heinisch M, et al. Vocal cord muscle activity as a drawback to FDG-PET in the followup of differentiated thyroid cancer. Thyroid 2002; 12:87–89.
28. Zhu Z, Chou C, Yen TC, Cui R. Elevated F-18 FDG uptake in laryngeal muscles mimicking thyroid cancer metastases. Clin Nucl Med 2001; 26:689–691.
29. Yeretsian RA, Blodgett TM, Branstetter BFT, et al. Teflon-induced granuloma: a false-positive finding with PET resolved with combined PET and CT. AJNR Am J Neuroradiol 2003; 24:1164–1166.
30. Alibazoglu H, Alibazoglu B, Hollinger EF, et al. Normal thymic uptake of 2-deoxy-2[F-18]fluoro-D-glucose. Clin Nucl Med 1999; 24: 597–600.
31. Kawano T, Suzuki A, Ishida A, et al. The clinical relevance of thymic fluorodeoxyglucose uptake in pediatric patients after chemotherapy. Eur J Nucl Med Mol Imaging 2004; 31:831–836.
32. Rini JN, Leonidas JC, Tomas MB, et al. FDG uptake in the anterior mediastinum. Physiologic thymic uptake or disease? Clin Positron Imaging 1999; 2:332.
33. Wittram C, Fischman AJ, Mark E, et al. Thymic enlargement and FDG uptake in three patients: CT and FDG positron emission tomography correlated with pathology. AJR Am J Roentgenol 2003; 180:519–522.
34. Nakahara T, Fujii H, Ide M, et al. FDG uptake in the morphologically normal thymus: comparison of FDG positron emission tomography and CT. Br J Radiol 2001; 74:821–824.
35. Patel PM, Alibazoglu H, Ali A, et al. Normal thymic uptake of FDG on PET imaging. Clin Nucl Med 1996; 21:772–725.
36. Pineda J, Lee T, Ain K, et al. Iodine-131 therapy for thyroid cancer patients with elevated thyroglobulin and negative diagnostic scan. J Clin Endocrinol Metab 1995; 80:1488–1492.
37. Schlumberger M, Mancusi F, Baudin E, Pacini F. 131I therapy for elevated thyroglobulin levels. Thyroid 1997; 7:273–276.
38. Wartofsky L. Management of scan negative thyroglobulin positive differentiated thyroid carcinoma. J Clin Endocrinol Metab 1998; 83: 4195–4199.
39. McDougall I. 131I treatment of 131I negative whole body scan, and positive thyroglobulin in differentiated thyroid carcinoma: What is being treated? Thyroid 1997; 7:669–672.
40. Fatourechi V, Hay ID, Javedan H, et al. Lack of impact of radioiodine therapy in tg-positive, diagnostic whole-body scan-negative patients with follicular cell-derived thyroid cancer. J Clin Endocrinol Metab 2002; 87:1521–1526.
41. McDougall IR. Management of thyroglobulin positive/whole-body scan negative: is Tg positive/131I therapy useful? J Endocrinol Invest 2001; 24:194–198.
42. Hoefnagel B, Delprat CC, Marcuse HR, Vijlder JJM. Role of thallium-201 total-body scintigraphy in follow-up of thyroid carcinoma. J Nucl Med 1986; 27:1854–1857.
43. Iida Y, Hidaka A, Hatabu H, et al. Follow-up study of postoperative patients with thyroid cancer by thallium-201 scintigraphy and serum thyroglobulin measurement. J Nucl Med 1991; 32:2098–2100.
44. Nakada K, Katoh C, Kanegae E, et al. Thallium-201 scintigraphy to predict therapeutic outcome of iodine-131 therapy of metastatic thyroid carcinoma. J Nucl Med 1998; 39:807–810.

45. Brandt-Mainz K, Muller SP, Reiners C, Bockisch A. Relationship between thyroglobulin and reliability of thallium 201 scintigraphy in differentiated thyroid cancer. Nuklearmedizin 2000; 39:20–25.
46. Yen TC, Lin HD, Lee CH, et al. The role of technetium-99m sestamibi whole-body scans in diagnosing metastatic Hurthle cell carcinoma of the thyroid gland after total thyroidectomy: a comparison with iodine-131 and thallium-201 whole-body scans. Eur J Nucl Med 1994; 21: 980–983.
47. Almeida-Filho P, Ravizzini GC, Almeida C, Borges-Neto S. Whole-body Tc-99m sestamibi scintigraphy in the follow-up of differentiated thyroid carcinoma. Clin Nucl Med 2000; 25:443–436.
48. Gallowitsch H, Mikosch P, Kresnik E, et al. Thyroglobulin and low-dose iodine-131 and technetium-99m-tetrofosmin whole-body scintigraphy in differentiated thyroid carcinoma. J Nucl Med 1998; 39: 870–875.
49. Lind P, Gallowitsch HJ, Langsteger W, et al. Technetium-99m-tetrofosmin whole-body scintigraphy in the follow-up of differentiated thyroid carcinoma. J Nucl Med 1997; 38:348–352.
50. Lind P. Multi-tracer imaging of thyroid nodules: is there a role in the preoperative assessment of nodular goiter? Eur J Nucl Med 1999; 26: 795–797.
51. Lind P, Gallowitsch HJ, Mikosch P, et al. Comparison of different tracers in the follow up of differentiated thyroid carcinoma. Acta Med Austriaca 1999; 26:115–117.
52. Drac-Kaniewska J, Kozlowicz-Gudzinska I, Tomaszewicz-Kubasik H, et al. 99mTc Tetrofosmin in diagnosis of distant metastases from differentiated thyroid cancer. Wiad Lek 2001; 54(Suppl 1):357–362.
53. Ahlman H, Tisell LE, Wangberg B, et al. The relevance of somatostatin receptors in thyroid neoplasia. Yale J Biol Med 1997; 70: 523–533.
54. Sarlis NJ, Gourgiotis L, Guthrie LC, et al. In-111 DTPA-octreotide scintigraphy for disease detection in metastatic thyroid cancer: comparison with F-18 FDG positron emission tomography and extensive conventional radiographic imaging. Clin Nucl Med 2003; 28:208–217.
55. Baudin E, Schlumberger M, Lumbroso J, et al. Octreotide scintigraphy in patients with differentiated thyroid carcinoma; contribution for patients with negative radioiodine scans. J Clin Endocrinol Metab 1996; 81:2541–2544.
56. Joensuu H, Ahonen A. Imaging of metastases of thyroid carcinoma with fluorine-18 fluorodeoxyglucose. J Nucl Med 1987; 28:910–914.
57. Adams S, Baum RP, Hertel A, et al. Comparison of metabolic and receptor imaging in recurrent medullary thyroid carcinoma with histopathological findings. Eur J Nucl Med 1998; 25:1277–1283.
58. Adams S, Baum R, Rink T, et al. Limited value of fluorine-18 fluorodeoxyglucose positron emission tomography for the imaging of neuroendocrine tumours. Eur J Nucl Med 1998; 25:79–83.
59. Alnafisi N, Driedger AA, Coates G, et al. FDG PET of recurrent or metastatic 131I-negative papillary thyroid carcinoma. J Nucl Med 2000; 41:1010–1015.
60. Altenvoerde G, Lerch H, Kuwert T, et al. Positron emission tomography with F-18-deoxyglucose in patients with differentiated thyroid carcinoma, elevated thyroglobulin levels, and negative iodine scans. Langenbecks Arch Surg 1998; 383:160–163.
61. Berger F, Knesewitsch P, Tausig A, et al. [18F] Fluorodeoxyglucose hybrid PET in patients with differentiated thyroid cancer: Comparison with dedicated PET. Paris, France: Eur Ass Nucl Med Congress, 2000.
62. Boer A, Szakall S, Jr., Klein I, et al. FDG PET imaging in hereditary thyroid cancer. Eur J Surg Oncol 2003; 29:922–928.
63. Boerner AR, Petrich T, Weckesser E, et al. Monitoring isotretinoin therapy in thyroid cancer using 18F-FDG PET. Eur J Nucl Med Mol Imaging 2002; 29:231–236.
64. Brandt-Mainz K, Muller SP, Gorges R, et al. The value of fluorine-18 fluorodeoxyglucose PET in patients with medullary thyroid cancer. Eur J Nucl Med 2000; 27:490–496.
65. Macapinlac HA. Clinical usefulness of FDG PET in differentiated thyroid cancer. J Nucl Med 2001; 42:77–78.
66. Wong CO, Dworkin HJ. Role of FDG PET in metastatic thyroid cancer. J Nucl Med 1999; 40:993–934.
67. Khan N, Oriuchi N, Higuchi T, et al. PET in the follow-up of differentiated thyroid cancer. Br J Radiol 2003; 76:690–695.
68. Crippa F, Alessi A, Gerali A, Bombardieri E. FDG-PET in thyroid cancer. Tumori 2003; 89:540–543.
69. Armstrong S, Worsley D, Blair GK. Pediatric surgical images: PET evaluation of papillary thyroid carcinoma recurrence. J Pediatr Surg 2002; 37:1648–1649.
70. Fiene ULR, Hanke JP, Wohrle H, Muller-Schauenburg W. 18FDG whole-body PET in differentiated thyroid carcinoma. Flipflop in uptake patterns of 18FDG and 131I. Nuclearmedizin 1995; 34: 127–134.
71. Shiga T, Tsukamoto E, Nakada K, et al. Comparison of (18)F-FDG, (131)I-Na, and (201)Tl in diagnosis of recurrent or metastatic thyroid carcinoma. J Nucl Med 2001; 42:414–419.
72. Dietlein M, Moka D, Scheidhauer K, et al. Follow-up of differentiated thyroid cancer: comparison of multiple diagnostic tests. Nucl Med Commun 2000; 21:991–1000.
73. McDougall IR, Davidson J, Segall GM. Positron emission tomography of the thyroid, with an emphasis on thyroid cancer. Nucl Med Commun 2001; 22:485–492.
74. Wang W, Larson SM, Fazzari M, et al. Prognostic value of [18F]fluorodeoxyglucose positron emission tomographic scanning in patients with thyroid cancer. J Clin Endocrinol Metab 2000; 85:1107–1113.
75. Goshen E, Cohen O, Rotenberg G, et al. The clinical impact of 18F-FDG gamma PET in patients with recurrent well differentiated thyroid carcinoma. Nucl Med Commun 2003; 24:9599–9561.
76. Karwowski J, Jeffrey RB, McDougall IR, Weigel RJ. Intraoperative ultrasonography improves identification of recurrent thyroid cancer. Surgery 2002; 132:924–928.
77. Wang W, Macapinlac H, Larson SM, et al. [18F]-2-fluoro-2-deoxy-D-glucose positron emission tomography localizes residual thyroid cancer in patients with negative diagnostic (131)I whole body scans and elevated serum thyroglobulin levels. J Clin Endocrinol Metab 1999; 84:2291–2302.
78. Grunwald F, Schomburg A, Bender H, et al. Fluorine-18 fluorodeoxyglucose positron emission tomography in the follow-up of differentiated thyroid cancer. Eur J Nucl Med 1996; 23:312–319.
79. Sisson JC, Ackermann RJ, Meyer MA, Wahl RL. Uptake of 18-fluoro-2-deoxy-D-glucose by thyroid cancer: implications for diagnosis and therapy. J Clin Endocrinol Metab 1993; 77:1090–1094.
80. Filetti S, Damante G, Foti D. Thyrotropin stimulates glucose transport in cultured rat thyroid cells. Endocrinology 1987; 120: 2576–2581.
81. Moog F, Linke R, Manthey N, et al. Influence of thyroid-stimulating hormone levels on uptake of FDG in recurrent and metastatic differentiated thyroid carcinoma. J Nucl Med 2000; 41:1989–1995.
82. Petrich T, Borner AR, Otto D, et al. Influence of rhTSH on [(18)F] fluorodeoxyglucose uptake by differentiated thyroid carcinoma. Eur J Nucl Med Mol Imaging 2002; 29:641–647.
83. Lambrecht RM, Woodhouse N, Phillips R, et al. Investigational study of iodine-124 with a positron camera. Am J Physiol Imaging 1988; 3:197–200.
83a. Nahas Z, Goldenberg D, Fakhry C, et al. The role of positron emission tomography/computed tomography in the management of recurrent papillary thyroid carcinoma. Laryngoscope 2005; 115:237–243.
84. Pentlow KS, Graham MC, Lambrecht RM, et al. Quantitative imaging of I-124 using positron emission tomography with applications to radioimmunodiagnosis and radioimmunotherapy. Med Phys 1991; 18:357–366.
85. Pentlow KS, Graham MC, Lambrecht RM, et al. Quantitative imaging of iodine-124 with PET. J Nucl Med 1996; 37:1557–1562.
86. Flower M, Al-Saadi A, Harmer CL, et al. Dose response study on thyrotoxic patients undergoing positron emission tomography and radioiodine therapy. Eur J Nucl Med 1994; 21:531–536.

87. Frey P, Townsend D, Jeavons A, Donath A. In vivo imaging of the human thyroid with a positron camera using I-124. In vivo imaging of the human thyroid with a positron camera using I-124. Eur J Nucl Med 1985; 10:472–476.
88. Frey P, Townsend D, Flattet A, et al. Tomographic imaging of the human thyroid using 124I. J Clin Endocrinol Metab 1986; 63: 918–927.
89. Crawford DC, Flower MA, Pratt BE, et al. Thyroid volume measurement in thyrotoxic patients: comparison between ultrasonography and iodine-124 positron emission tomography. Eur J Nucl Med 1997; 24:1470–1478.
90. Eschmann SM, Reischl G, Bilger K, et al. Evaluation of dosimetry of radioiodine therapy in benign and malignant thyroid disorders by means of iodine-124 and PET. Eur J Nucl Med Mol Imaging 2002; 29:760–767.
91. Sgouros G, Kolbert KS, Sheikh A, et al. Patient specific dosimetry for 131-I thyroid cancer therapy using 124-I PET and 3-dimensional-internal dosimetry (3D-ID) software. J Nucl Med 2004; 45: 1366–1372.
92. Freudenberg LS, Antoch G, Gorges R, et al. Combined PET/CT with iodine-124 in diagnosis of spread metastatic thyroid carcinoma: a case report. Eur Radiol 2003; 13(Suppl 4):L19–L23.
93. Freudenberg LS, Antoch G, Jentzen W, et al. Value of (124)I-PET/CT in staging of patients with differentiated thyroid cancer. Eur Radiol 2004; 14:2092–2098.
94. Chung J-K, So Y, Lee JS, et al. Value of FDG PET in papillary thyroid carcinoma with negative 131I whole-body scan. J Nucl Med 1999; 40: 486–492.
95. Dietlein M, Scheidhauer K, Voth E, et al. Fluorine-18 fluorodeoxyglucose positron emission tomography and iodine-131 whole-body scintigraphy in the follow-up of differentiated thyroid cancer. Eur J Nucl Med 1997; 24:1342–1348.
96. Grunwald F, Kalicke T, Feine U, et al. Fluorine-18 fluorodeoxyglucose positron emission tomography in thyroid cancer: results of a multicentre study. Eur J Nucl Med 1999; 26:1547–1552.
97. Wang W, Macapinlac H, Larson SM, et al. [18F]-2-fluoro-2-deoxy-D-glucose positron emission tomography localizes residual thyroid cancer in patients with negative diagnostic (131)I whole body scans and elevated serum thyroglobulin levels. J Clin Endocrinol Metab 1999; 84:2291–2302.
98. Stokkel MP, de Klerk JH, Zelissen PM, et al. Fluorine-18 fluorodeoxyglucose dual-head positron emission tomography in the detection of recurrent differentiated thyroid cancer: preliminary results. Eur J Nucl Med 1999; 26:1606–1609.

35
Alternative Thyroid Imaging

Anca M. Avram, Karen C. Rosenspire, Stewart C. Davidson, John E. Freitas, and Milton D. Gross

INTRODUCTION

Radioiodine (^{131}I and ^{123}I) remains the most frequently used radionuclide for thyroid imaging in the diagnosis and treatment of well-differentiated thyroid cancer (WDTC). However, an estimated 20–30% of WDTCs do not accumulate radioiodine at the time of initial clinical presentation, and many WDTCs that are initially radioiodine-avid will dedifferentiate and lose their ability to concentrate radioiodine. This is especially true following radioiodine therapy. In addition, medullary and anaplastic thyroid carcinomas do not accumulate radioiodine.

Because many thyroid cancers are not radioiodine-avid, other radiopharmaceuticals that have different mechanisms of accumulation have been used for thyroid cancer imaging (Table 1). Although many radiopharmaceuticals have been studied as potential thyroid cancer–imaging agents with variable success, this discussion is limited to ^{201}Tl chloride, ^{99m}Tc sestamibi, ^{99m}Tc tetrafosmin, and ^{111}In pentetreotide as alternative thyroid-imaging agents.

^{201}TL CHLORIDE

^{201}Tl chloride, a potassium analog, is accumulated in thyroid tissues by an active transport mechanism—the Na$^+$/K$^+$ ATPase transporter (1). This transport mechanism is present in many normal tissues, particularly the myocardium, but the ATPase transporter has been identified in a wide variety of neoplasms, including thyroid, breast, liver, and esophageal cancer, as well as lymphoma (2). Differential accumulation and washout of ^{201}Tl in malignant thyroid tissues, compared to adjacent benign thyroid nodules, has been used to distinguish these entities (3). Tumor uptake of ^{201}Tl is because of multiple factors, e.g., increased blood flow, tumor type, and Na$^+$/K$^+$ transporter, among others (4).

Despite the potential role for ^{201}Tl as an imaging agent for WDTC, the reported sensitivity of ^{201}Tl uptake varies significantly even in WDTC. Sensitivities range from 45% to 94%, with consistently high specificities ranging from 84% to 94%, and imaging is performed 10–90 min after the ^{201}Tl injection (2,5). Washout of ^{201}Tl from tumor tissue does occur with time, and shorter time intervals from injection to imaging tend to achieve better sensitivity for all sites.

^{201}Tl has been used to evaluate the extent of recurrent or metastatic disease. Because ^{201}Tl has lower uptake than ^{131}I in normal residual thyroid tissue (5,6), ^{201}Tl may help differentiate recurrent from normal residual thyroid tissue. It may also be help detect nodal metastasis, with a sensitivity of 66%–68% (7). Although ^{131}I is superior to ^{201}Tl in the detection of lung metastasis, ^{201}Tl may detect metastases not visualized with ^{131}I, and the sensitivity of planar ^{201}Tl may be improved with single-photon emission computed tomography (SPECT) from 60% vs 85% sensitivity. Nevertheless, lesions of less than 1.5 cm are rarely seen with either radionuclide (8). The lack of ^{201}Tl uptake in posttherapy scans has been shown to be a good predictor of response to radioiodine therapy (9). Intense ^{201}Tl uptake (>2.1 tumor-to-background ratio) in known metastases, regardless of ^{131}I uptake, predicts a failure of subsequent ^{131}I therapy. Conversely, if ^{201}Tl uptake is low with intense ^{131}I uptake, most patients (88%) responded to ^{131}I therapy. This may be similar to the findings with ^{18}F-fluoro-2-deoxyglucose positron emission tomography (FDG-PET) (see Chapter 34).

Imaging with ^{201}Tl has been of value when ^{131}I scans are negative in the presence of known thyroid cancer. ^{201}Tl has been shown to be useful in following patients with WDTC and elevated serum thyroglobulin levels, despite a negative ^{131}I scan (9). Furthermore, ^{201}Tl has been demonstrated as valuable in localizing metastases from medullary thyroid cancer, which typically does not accumulate ^{131}I (2).

Both ^{201}Tl and ^{99m}Tc sestamibi can visualize thyroid tissue in patients who are taking thyroid hormone with suppressed serum thyrotropin (TSH; 10). Whereas radioiodine imaging of thyroid tissue necessitates either thyroid hormone withdrawal or the use of recombinant TSH stimulation, imaging with ^{201}Tl can be accomplished without either requirement.

From: *Thyroid Cancer: A Comprehensive Guide to Clinical Management, 2/e*
Edited by: L. Wartofsky and D. Van Nostrand © Humana Press Inc., Totowa, NJ

Table 1
Alternative Thyroid-Imaging Agents

Well-differentiated thyroid cancer	^{201}Tl chloride
	^{99m}Tc sestamibi
	^{111}In octreotide
	^{99m}Tc tetrofosmin
	^{99m}Tc pertechnetate
	^{99m}Tc HMPAO
Medullary thyroid cancer	^{111}In octreotide
	^{131}I MIBG
	^{99m}Tc (V) DMSA
	^{111}In or ^{99m}Tc CCK
	^{131}I or ^{99m}Tc CEA
	^{201}Tl chloride
Anaplastic thyroid cancer	^{67}Ga citrate
Hürthle cell cancer	^{131}I or ^{99m}Tc CEA
	^{111}In pentetreotide
	^{99m}Tc sestamibi

HMPAO, hexamethylpropyleneamineoxime; MIBG, metaiodobenzylguanidine; DMSA, dimercaptosuccinic acid; CCK, cholecystokinin; CEA, carcinoembryonic antigen.

Multiple studies have compared ^{201}Tl with other agents, such as ^{99m}Tc sestamibi, ^{99m}Tc tetrafosmin, and FDG *(11,12)*. Although these agents all compared favorably in detecting thyroid cancer, the image quality of ^{99m}Tc radiopharmaceuticals and FDG is significantly better than ^{201}Tl.

SESTAMIBI

^{99m}Tc sestamibi is a cationic, lipophilic complex developed for myocardial perfusion imaging, which has been reported to accumulate in thyroid, lung, brain, breast, parathyroid, and bone tumors *(13–24)*. Although ^{99m}Tc sestamibi accumulates in WDTC, it is not specific for WDTC and may accumulate in Graves' disease, thyroid lymphoma, thyroid adenoma, and medullary thyroid carcinoma *(24)*. Uptake has been suggested as related to abundant mitochondria and is influenced by tumor blood flow and vascularization, cellular metabolism, and tissue viability. ^{99m}Tc sestamibi is a substrate for the membrane efflux pumps—permeability glycoprotein and multidrug resistance protein—and may influence cellular retention *(25)*. Generally, the procedure involves injection of 10–15 mCi (370–555 MBq) of ^{99m}Tc sestamibi with whole-body and planar imaging at 30 min, but some authors have suggested immediate imaging to detect lesions that have rapid washout *(23)*.

^{99m}Tc sestamibi has many advantages relative to other radionuclides and conventional imaging. Unlike radioiodine (and as already noted), ^{99m}Tc sestamibi does not require withdrawal of thyroid hormone or recombinant TSH stimulation. However, improved ^{99m}Tc sestamibi uptake in patients who are hypothyroid has been observed *(26)*. In comparison to both ^{201}Tl and ^{131}I, ^{99m}Tc sestamibi has a photon energy that is more suitable for γ cameras, and ^{99m}Tc frequently achieves higher tumor-to-background ratios than ^{131}I, which enables SPECT imaging. ^{99m}Tc sestamibi has lower radiation exposure than ^{131}I. Compared to conventional imaging, such as computed tomography (CT), magnetic resonance imaging (MRI), and ultrasound, ^{99m}Tc sestamibi whole-body scintigraphy may help differentiate viable tumor from fibrotic tissue. ^{99m}Tc sestamibi has also been used to assess thyroid nodules in the thyroid gland, but ^{99m}Tc sestamibi uptake is not specific for malignancy, and its utility is limited *(27–31)*. Foldes et al. studied 58 patients with 77 nodules and showed no relationship between ^{99m}Tc sestamibi uptake and malignancy, indicating uptake depended mainly on tissue viability *(27)*. Nakahara et al. found ^{99m}Tc sestamibi and ^{201}Tl to be less sensitive than aspiration cytology in differentiating malignant from benign nodules *(28)*. Kresnik et al. *(29)* and Wie et al. *(30)* reported similar results, suggesting increased ^{99m}Tc sestamibi uptake is more likely to represent thyroid adenoma than malignant tumor. Casara et al. recommended ^{99m}Tc sestamibi imaging should be reserved for those patients who had (1) a high-pretest probability of malignancy and nondiagnostic cytology; (2) doubtful cytology and high-operative risk; and (3) a large locally aggressive tumor with the need to determine preoperative chemotherapy *(31)*. Hürthle cell tumors are rich in mitochondria, and Vattimo et al. and Boi et al. reported intense, persistent uptake of ^{99m}Tc sestamibi in Hürthle cell tumors (Fig. 1), but the specificity was low *(32–34)*.

Numerous studies have investigated the role of ^{99m}Tc sestamibi in both ^{131}I avid and nonavid WDTC *(13–23,26, 35–39)*. Ng et al. compared ^{99m}Tc sestamibi and ^{131}I scintigraphy in 360 patients with WDTC and found that ^{131}I whole-body scintigraphy detected more abnormalities than ^{99m}Tc sestamibi whole-body scintigraphy. ^{131}I particularly detected more thyroid remnants, as well as bone and lung metastases *(36)*. In comparing ^{131}I and ^{99m}Tc sestamibi whole-body scintigraphy, Dadparvar et al. found poor sensitivity (36%) and high specificity (89%) for ^{99m}Tc sestamibi *(14)*. Low sensitivity of ^{99m}Tc sestamibi for pulmonary metastases, along with high sensitivity for lymph node metastases, has been confirmed by numerous studies *(20,21,26,35,38,39)*.

Despite the superiority of ^{131}I, ^{99m}Tc sestamibi is an alternative to radioiodine for detecting nonradioiodine-avid metastases (Figs. 2, 3; *13–23*). Nemec et al. studied 200 patients with ^{131}I negative thyroid cancer patients with ^{99m}Tc sestamibi. The sensitivity and specificity were 100% and 99%, for bone metastases, 95% and 95% for lung metastases, and 81% and 71% for locoregional disease, respectively *(15)*. Seabold et al. compared ^{99m}Tc sestamibi and ^{201}Tl after a negative or an equivocal ^{131}I whole-body scan (WBS). Sensitivity, specificity, and accuracy for both were 53%, 100%, and 69%, with a positive predictive value of 100% and a negative predictive value of 51%. Interestingly, three patients converted from negative to positive ^{99m}Tc sestamibi or ^{201}Tl scans after

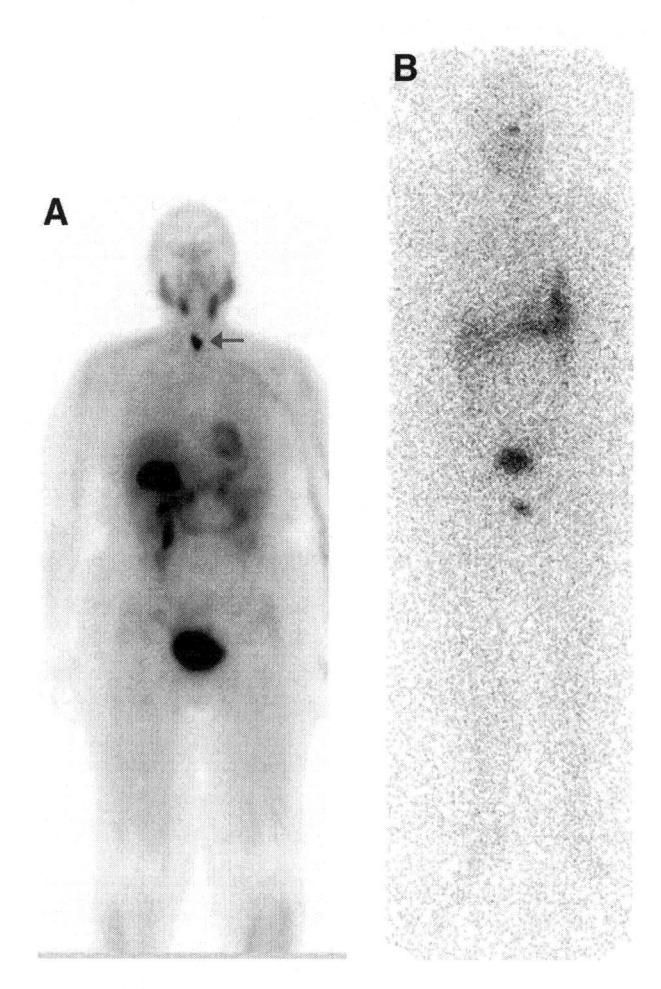

Fig. 1. This patient is a 69-yr-old female with Hürthle cell carcinoma and recurrence in the neck area. Her ^{99m}Tc sestamibi anterior WBS (**A**) was performed 30 min after injection, and the patient was on thyroid hormone suppression. Intense ^{99m}Tc sestamibi uptake is present in the neck in the area of the recurrence (arrow). However, her radioiodine scan (**B**), which was performed 48 h after the administration of 2.5 mCi (92.5 MBq) ^{131}I and after thyroid hormone withdrawal, demonstrated no radioiodine accumulation. Surgical resection was subsequently performed. (Illustration **A** appears in color in insert following p. 198.)

induction of a hypothyroid state, suggesting that TSH stimulation improves lesion detection in some patients (26). Rubello et al. performed dual-phase ^{99m}Tc sestamibi scintigraphy, neck ultrasound, CT (87 patients), or MRI (35 patients) in 122 patients who had high serum thyroglobulin and negative high-dose (100 mCi [3.7 GBq]) ^{131}I scan. Positive or suspicious cases underwent fine-needle aspiration cytology. The combination of ^{99m}Tc sestamibi and ultrasound had a combined sensitivity of 98% in detecting cervical lymph node metastases, and ^{99m}Tc sestamibi showed higher sensitivity (100%) than CT/MRI (58%) for detecting mediastinal lymph node metastases (38,39).

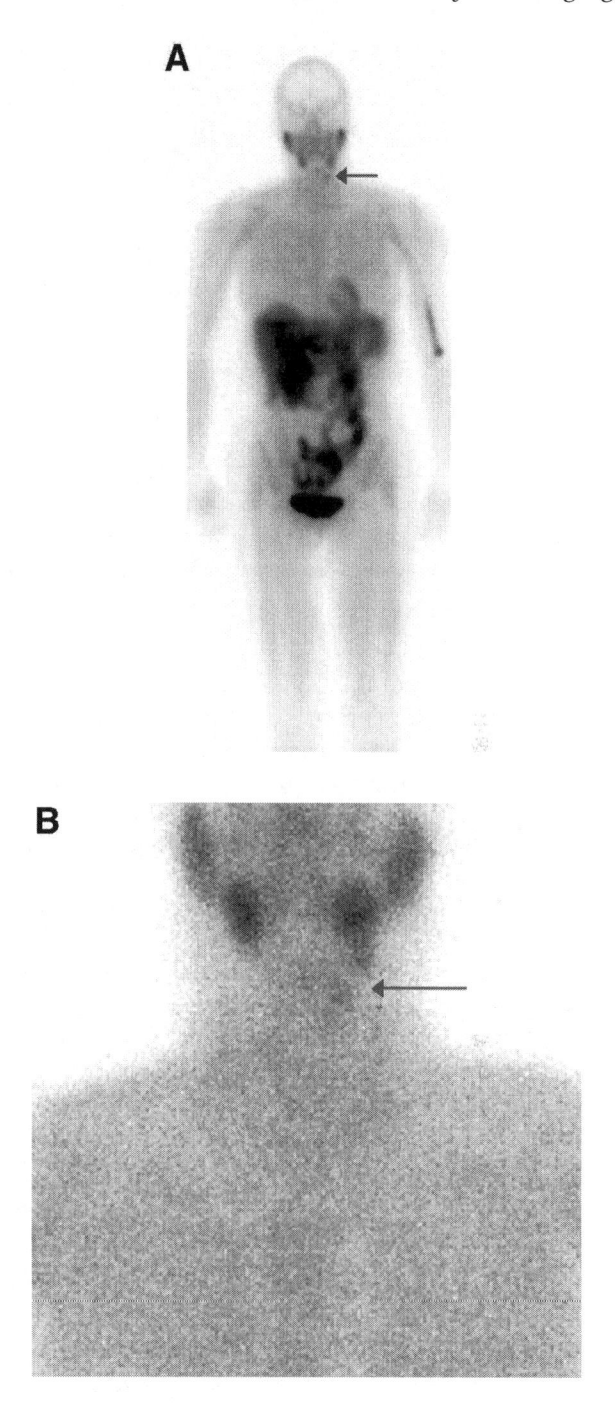

Fig. 2. This patient is a 53-yr-old female who had papillary thyroid cancer and was ablated with radioiodine. At the time of follow-up and after thyroid hormone withdrawal, her serum thyroglobulin was elevated (26 ng/mL), and her radioiodine scan was negative (not shown). However, her whole-body ^{99m}Tc sestamibi scan (**A**) demonstrated faint uptake in the left neck area (**B**). A camera "spot" view better demonstrated this abnormal uptake in the left neck region (arrow), which was surgically removed using a γ probe and confirmed as a 0.6-cm recurrence of thyroid cancer. The ^{99m}Tc sestamibi was instrumental in the localization of this recurrence. (Illustration appears in color in insert following p. 198.)

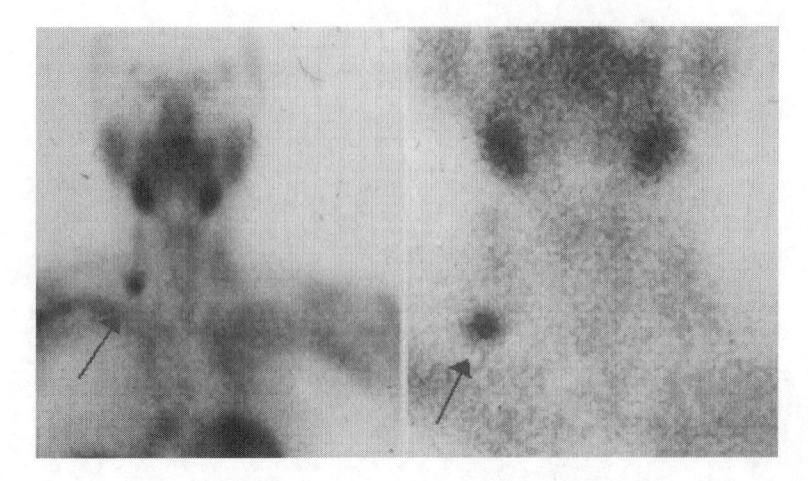

Fig. 3. This is a ^{99m}Tc sestamibi scan of a 56-yr-old patient who has had a previous thyroidectomy and negative radioiodine scan and now has an elevated serum thyroglobulin level off thyroid suppression of 50 pg/mL. The scan demonstrates a focus of ^{99m}Tc sestamibi uptake in the neck that corresponds to a metastasis of papillary thyroid cancer (arrow). (Illustration appears in color in insert following p. 198.)

^{99m}Tc sestamibi has also been used for radioguided surgery in patients with radioiodine-negative metastases (Fig. 2). Following initial evaluation and confirmation that the radioiodine-negative metastasis accumulates ^{99m}Tc sestamibi scintigraphy, an additional 1 mCi (37 MBq) of ^{99m}Tc sestamibi is injected immediately prior to surgery. During the surgery, the metastasis is localized with the help of the intraoperative γ probe. A prompt decline in neck activity after excision has been associated with normalization of elevated thyroglobulin levels (40). A similar technique using ^{111}In has also been described in medullary thyroid carcinoma (41,42).

TETROFOSMIN

^{99m}Tc tetrofosmin is a lipophilic phosphine used for myocardial perfusion imaging and has similar biodistribution and imaging qualities to ^{99m}Tc sestamibi. The few reported studies on the role of ^{99m}Tc tetrofosmin in thyroid cancer suggest results similar to ^{99m}Tc sestamibi (43–47).

SOMATOSTATIN RECEPTOR SCINTIGRAPHY

In the past 10 yr, somatostatin receptor scintigraphy (SRS) has been used for the imaging of radioiodine-negative metastatic WDTC, as well as to explore the option of somatostatin receptor–mediated therapy (see Chapter 70).

The molecular basis of SRS in WDTC is the expression of somatostatin receptors (sstr) on normal thyroid cells and thyroid carcinoma cells. Five human somatostatin receptor subtypes have been identified, and these interact with different G-proteins to mediate effects via inhibition of adenylate cyclase activity. In vitro studies have demonstrated the presence of all subtypes (sstr-1–sstr-5) on Hürthle cell carcinoma tumors, but normal thyroid tissue selectively lacked sstr-2 (48). Ain et al. reported that normal thyroid tissue has a high expression of sstr-3 and sstr-5 and a significantly weak expression of sstr-1 and -2. The sstr-2 was only found in medullary and Hürthle cell carcinomas. Papillary and follicular thyroid carcinomas demonstrated a high expression of sstr-3, -4, and -5 (49).

^{111}In pentetreotide is a somatostatin analog that displays a high affinity for sstr-2, a lower affinity for sstr-3 and -5, and notably weak affinity for sstr-1 and -4 (50). Several groups have reported the use of SRS using ^{111}In pentetreotide (octreotide) to detect residual or recurrent disease in WDTC. Baudin et al. reported a sensitivity of 80% (20 of 25) in patients, regardless of whether the radioiodine scan was positive or negative. In patients who had radioiodine-negative scans, the octreotide scans were positive in 75% (12 of 16). In patients with radioiodine-positive scans, the octreotide scans were positive in 89% (8 of 9; 51). Postema et al. reported a 75% sensitivity of SRS for the detection of metastatic WDTC (52). These results are confirmed by more recent studies by Stokkel et al., who prospectively evaluated the diagnostic and prognostic value of ^{111}In pentetreotide scintigraphy in 23 patients with progressive thyroid carcinoma (53). There were 13 papillary, 8 follicular, and 2 Hürthle cells carcinomas; 19 of 23 patients had advanced disease as defined by T3 and T4 tumor stage and/or presence of distant metastases (M1). All patients had radioiodine-negative metastases, indicated by absent or minimal ^{131}I uptake on posttherapy ^{131}I WBS, which were performed after 200 mCi (7.4 GBq) of ^{131}I. The radioactivity in metastatic tumor foci on ^{111}In pentetreotide scans was visually quantified and scored ranging from 0 (no uptake) to 4 (intense uptake). The overall sensitivity of SRS for detection of metastases was 74%. The sensitivity was better in patients in whom posttherapy ^{131}I WBS did not show any abnormal radioiodine uptake (82%) than those with minimal uptake (50%). Additionally, this study demonstrated that ^{111}In pentetreotide uptake inversely correlated with survival. The 10-yr survival rate was 33% in patients with moderate-to-intense uptake (radioactivity scores of 2–4), compared to 100% in patients with absent or slight uptake (radioactivity scores of 0 or 1). These results suggest that WDTC tumors with a high level of sstr expression display a more aggressive behavior.

In a recent report by Gorges et al., 50 scintigraphic studies with ^{111}In pentetreotide in 48 patients with metastatic WDTC were described (50). The histopathology was papillary in 9, follicular in 9, insular (poorly differentiated) in 1, and Hürthle cell in 29 patients. Radioiodine scintigraphy results of diagnostic (10–27 mCi [370–999 MBq]) or posttherapeutic (80–270 mCi [2.96–9.99 GBq]) ^{131}I WBS were available for 45 patients. There were 15 patients with radioiodine-negative tumors in which SRS was performed as an alternative imaging modality to help select patients for radionuclide therapy with Y-90-DOTA-D-Phe-1-Thy-3-octreotide (Y-90-DOTATOC). There were 30 patients with radioiodine-positive metastases in whom the results of ^{111}In pentetreotide and ^{131}I scans were compared. The sensitivity of ^{111}In pentetreotide scintigraphy was 74% (37 of 50 patients). For localization of metastatic disease, ^{111}In pentetreotide scintigraphy demonstrated a sensitivity of 87% for skeletal metastases, 79% for cervical and mediastinal lymph nodal metastases, 68% for pulmonary or distant soft-tissue metastases, and 56% for abdominal or retroperitoneal metastases. ^{111}In pentetreotide accumulation did not correlate with tumor size. The smallest visualized tumor sites were about 8 mm in diameter.

The sensitivity of ^{111}In pentetreotide scintigraphy for detection of metastatic disease was associated with tumor burden assessed by serum thyroglobulin levels that were measured when the patient was on thyroxine suppressive therapy. In patients with thyroglobulin less than 10 ng/mL, ^{111}In pentetreotide scintigraphy was positive in 27% of patients, whereas in patients with thyroglobulin more than 10 ng/mL SRS was positive in 85% of patients. The maximal uptake was observed in Hürthle cell carcinomas, and 95% of scans were positive when the thyroglobulin exceeded 10 ng/mL. The ^{111}In pentetreotide scan was positive in 45% of papillary thyroid carcinomas and 78% of follicular thyroid carcinomas. In one patient with poorly differentiated (insular) thyroid cancer, a large proportion of the metastasis was visualized with ^{111}In pentetreotide.

This study also reported the results of Y-90-DOTATOC therapy (up to 9.3 GBq/250 mCi per four cycles) in three patients with negative ^{131}I WBS and progressive metastatic disease. Y-90-DOTATOC displays sstr affinity profile similar to diagnostic ^{111}In pentetreotide and delivers β particles with a maximum range of 10 mm and mean range of 2.8 mm in targeted tumor tissues. Unfortunately, tumor progression, as demonstrated by a continuous rise in thyroglobulin levels and progressive radiological changes, could not be stopped in any patients treated with Y-90-DOTATOC.

The sensitivity of ^{111}In pentetreotide scintigraphy was compared with FDG-PET and conventional radiographic imaging (CRI) in 21 patients with metastatic thyroid carcinoma (54). CRI included noncontrast CT, MRI from head to pelvis, neck ultrasonography, and bone radiographic survey. A total of 105 lesions were detected by the combined use of CRI, FDG-PET, and SRS imaging in 21 patients. The lesion detection rates (sensitivity) for each method was as follows: CRI, 76.2%; FDG-PET, 67.6%; and SRS, 49.5%. In 9.5% (2 of 21) of patients, SRS detected five unexpected lesions, which were not seen by either CRI or FDG-PET (4.8% of all lesions). These unexpected lesions were initially negative on ^{131}I diagnostic WBS but confirmed as functioning metastatic thyroid tissue on posttherapy radioiodine scans. Thus, FDG-PET imaging was superior to SRS for the detection of metastatic radioiodine-negative WDTC, but SRS did reveal unexpected lesions and can be used in conjunction with conventional radiologic techniques for follow-up of patients with clinical and biochemical evidence of progression.

Although not a primary modality for imaging WDTC, SRS has an important role in the evaluation of radioiodine-negative tumors, with a sensitivity ranging from 50% to 85%, depending on the patient selection, thyroglobulin levels, and histopathology of the primary tumor. The highest sensitivity was reported for Hürthle cell carcinomas, which are less frequently visualized with ^{131}I scintigraphy. In approx 65% of patients with radioiodine-negative metastatic WDTC, the disease is limited to the neck or mediastinum (53), and localization of metastatic deposits with alternative thyroid-imaging modalities is essential in guiding surgical intervention.

REFERENCES

1. Kishida T, Knazawa K, Nagano K, et al. Na+, K+ ATPase activity in thyroid nodules. Mechanism of thallium-201 accumulation in the thyroid gland. J Clin Exp Med 1986; 139:527–528.
2. Hoefnagel CA, Delprat CC, Marcuse HR, de Vijlder JJM. Role of thallium-201 total-body scintigraphy in follow-up of thyroid carcinoma. J Nucl Med 1986; 27:1854–1857.
3. Yada H, Hozumi Y, Kanazawa K, Nagai H. Quantitative estimation and clinical significance of accumulation and washout of thallium-201 chloride in follicular thyroid neoplasm. Endocrine J 2002; 49:55–60.
4. Waxman AD. Thallium-201 in nuclear oncology. In Freeman LM, editor. Nuclear Medicine Annual. New York, NY: Raven, 1991:193–209.
5. Carril JM, Quirce R, Serrano J, et al. Total-body scintigraphy with thallium-201 and iodine-131 in the follow-up of differentiated thyroid cancer. J Nucl Med 1997; 38:686–692.
6. Ramanna L, Waxman A, Braunstein GD. Thallium-201 scintigraphy in differentiated thyroid cancer. Comparison with radioiodine scintigraphy and serum thyroglobulin determinations. J Nucl Med 1991; 32:441–446.
7. Brendl AJ, Guyot M, Jeandot R, et al. Thallium-201 imaging in the follow-up of differentiated thyroid carcinoma. J Nucl Med 1988; 29:1515–1520.

8. Charkes ND, Vitti RA, Brooks K. Thallium-201 SPECT increases detectability of thyroid cancer metastases. J Nucl Med 1990; 31:147–153.
9. Maxon HR. Detection of residual and recurrent thyroid cancer by radionuclide imaging. Thyroid 1999; 9:443–446.
10. Erdil, TY, Onsel C, Kanmaz B, et al. Comparison of Tc-99m-methoxyisobutyl isonitrile and Tl-201 scintigraphy in visualization of suppressed thyroid tissue. J Nucl Med 2000; 41:1163–1167.
11. Shiga T, Tsukamoto E, Nakada K, et al. Comparison of F-18 FDG, I-131 Na, and Tl-201 in diagnosis of recurrent or metastatic thyroid carcinoma. J Nucl Med 2001; 42:414–419.
12. Klain M, Maurea D, Cuocola A, et al. Tc-99m tetrofosmin imaging in thyroid diseases: comparison with Tc-99m pertechnetate, thallium-201 and Tc-99m methoxyisobutylisonitrile scans. Eur J Nucl Med 1996; 23:1568–1574.
13. Yen TC, Lin HD, Lee CH, et al. The role of technetium-99m sestamibi whole-body scans in diagnosing metastatic Hürthle cell carcinoma of the thyroid gland after total thyroidectomy: a comparison with iodine-131 and thallium-201 whole-body scans. Eur J Nucl Med 1994; 21:980–983.
14. Dadparvar S, Chevres A, Tulchinsky M, et al. Clinical utility of technetium-99m methoxyisobutylisonitrile imaging in differentiated thyroid carcinoma: comparison with thallium-201 and iodine-131 Na scintigraphy, and serum thyroglobulin quantitation. Eur J Nucl Med 1995; 22:1330–1338.
15. Nemec J, Nyvltova O, Blazek T, et al. Positive thyroid cancer scintigraphy using technetium-99m methoxyisobutylisonitrile. Eur J Nucl Med 1996; 23:69–71.
16. Dietlein M, Scheidhauer K, Voth E, et al. Follow-up of differentiated thyroid cancer: what is the value of FDG and sestamibi in the diagnostic algorithm? Nuklearmedizin 1998; 37:12–17.
17. Elser H, Henze M, Hermann C, et al. 99m-Tc-Sestamibi for recurrent and metastatic differentiated thyroid carcinoma. Nuklearmedizin 1997; 36:7–12.
18. Fridrich L, Messa C, Landoni C, et al. Whole-body scintigraphy with 99Tcm-Sestamibi, 18F-FDG and 131I in patients with metastatic thyroid carcinoma. Nucl Med Commun 1997; 18:3–9.
19. Grunwald F, Menzel C, Bender H, et al. Comparison of 18FDG-PET with 131iodine and Tc-99m-sestamibi scintigraphy in differentiated thyroid cancer. Thyroid 1997; 7:327–335.
20. Miyamoto S, Kasagi K, Misaki T, et al. Evaluation of technetium-99m-Sestamibi scintigraphy in metastatic differentiated thyroid carcinoma. J Nucl Med 1997; 38:352–356.
21. Kobayashi M, Mogami T, Uchiyama M, et al. Usefulness of Tc-99m-Sestamibil SPECT in the metastatic lesions of thyroid cancer. Nippon Igaku Hoshasen Gakkai Zasshi 1997; 57:127–132.
22. Ugur O, Kostakoglu L, Caner B, et al. Comparison of 201Tl, Tc-99m-Sestamibi and I-131 imaging in the follow-up of patients with well-differentiated thyroid carcinoma. Nucl Med Commun 1996; 17:373–377.
23. Almeida-Filho P, Ravizzini GC, Almeida C, Borges-Neto S. Whole-body Tc-99m sestamibi scintigraphy in the followup of differentiated thyroid carcinoma. Clin Nucl Med 2000; 25:443–446.
24. Sarikaya A, Huseyinova G, Irfanoglu ME, et al. The relationship between Tc-99m sestamibi uptake and ultrastructural cell types of thyroid tumors. Nucl Med Commun 2001; 22:39–44.
25. Van de Wiele C, Rottey S, Goethals I, et al. Tc-99m sestamibi and Tc-99m tetrofosmin scintigraphy for predicting resistance to chemotherapy: a critical review of clinical data. Nucl Med Commun 2003; 24:945–950.
26. Seabold JE, Gurll N, Schurrer, et al. Comparison of Tc-99m methoxyisobutyl isonitrile and Tl-201scintigraphy for detection of residual thyroid cancer after I-131 ablative therapy. J Nucl Med 1999; 40:1434–1440.
27. Foldes I, Levay A, Stotz G. Comparative scanning of thyroid nodules with technetium-99m pertechnetate and technetium-99m methoxyisobutylisonitrile. Eur J Nucl Med 1993; 20:330–333.
28. Nakahara H, Noguchi S, Murakami N, et al. Technetium-99m-sestamibi scintigraphy compared with thallium-201 in evaluation of thyroid tumors. J Nucl Med 1996; 37:901–904.
29. Kresnik E, Gallowitsch HJ, Mikosch P, et al. Technetium-99m-Sestamibi scintigraphy of thyroid nodules in an endemic goiter area. J Nucl Med 1997; 38:62–65.
30. Wei JP, Burke GJ. Characterization of the neoplastic potential of solitary solid thyroid lesions with Tc-99m-pertechnetate and Tc-99m-sestamibi scanning. Ann Surg Oncol 1995; 2:233–237.
31. Casara D, Rubello D, Saladini G. Role of scintigraphy with tumor-seeking agents in the diagnosis and preoperative staging of malignant thyroid nodules. Biomed Pharmacother 2000; 54:334–336.
32. Vattimo A, Bertelli P, Cintorino M, et al. Identification of Hürthle cell tumor by single-injection, double-phase scintigraphy with technetium-99m-sestamibi. J Nucl Med 1995; 36:778–782.
33. Vattimo A, Bertelli P, Cintorino M, et al. Hürthle cell tumor dwelling in hot thyroid nodules: preoperative detection with technetium-99m-Sestamibi dual-phase scintigraphy. J Nucl Med 1998; 39:822–825.
34. Boi F, Lai ML, Deias C, et al. The usefulness of Tc-99m-Sestamibi scan in the diagnostic evaluation of thyroid nodules with oncocytic cytology. Eur J Endocrinol 2003; 149:493–498.
35. Dietlein M, Scheidhauer K, Voth E, et al. Follow-up of differentiated thyroid cancer: what is the value of FDG and sestamibi in the diagnostic algorithm? Nuklearmedizin 1998; 37:12–17.
36. Ng DCE, Sundram FX, Sin AE. Tc-99m sestamibi and I-131 whole-body scintigraphy and initial serum thyroglobulin in the management of differentiated thyroid carcinoma. J Nucl Med 2000; 41:631–635.
37. Rubello D, Saladini G, Carpi A, Casara D. Nuclear medicine imaging procedures in differentiated thyroid carcinoma patients with negative iodine scan. Biomed Pharmacother 2000; 54:337–344.
38. Casara D, Rubello D, Saladini G, et al. Clinical approach in patients with metastatic differentiated thyroid carcinoma and negative I-131 whole body scintigraphy: importance of Tc-99m Sestamibi scan combined with high resolution neck ultrasonography. Tumori 1999; 85:122–127.
39. Rubello D, Mazzarotto R, Casara D. The role of technetium-99m methoxyisobutylisonitrile scintigraphy in the planning of therapy and follow-up of patients with differentiated thyroid carcinoma after surgery. Eur J Nucl Med 2000; 27:431–440.
40. Rubello D, Piotto A, Pagetta C, et al. 99m Tc-Sestamibi radio-guided surgery for recurrent thyroid carcinoma: technical feasibility and procedure, and preliminary clinical results. Eur J Nucl Med Mol Imaging 2002; 29:1201–1205.
41. Waddington WA, Kettle AG, Heddle RM, Coakley AJ. Intraoperative localization of recurrent medullary carcinoma of the thyroid using indium-111 pentetreotide and a nuclear surgical probe. Eur J Nucl Med 1994; 21:363–364.
42. Boz A, Arici C, Gungor F, et al. Gamma probe-guided resection and scanning with TC-99m Sestamibi of a local recurrence of follicular thyroid carcinoma. Clin Nucl Med 2001; 26:820–822.
43. Klain M, Maurea S, Cuocolo A, et al. Technetium-99m tetrofosmin imaging in thyroid diseases: comparison with Tc-99m-pertechnetate, thallium-201 and Tc-99m-methoxyisobutylisonitrile scans. Eur J Nucl Med 1996; 23:1568–1574.
44. Unal S, Menda Y, Adalet I, et al. Thallium-201, technetium-99m-tetrofosmin and iodine-131 in detecting differentiated thyroid carcinoma metastases. J Nucl Med 1998; 39:1897–1902.
45. Kanmaz B, Erdil TY, Yardi OF, et al. The role of Tc-99m-tetrofosmin in the evaluation of thyroid nodules. Nucl Med Commun 2000; 21:333–339.

46. Nishiyama Y, Yamamoto Y, Ono Y, et al. Comparison of Tc-99m-tetrofosmin with Tl-201 and I-131 in the detection of differentiated thyroid cancer metastases. Nucl Med Commun 2000; 21:917–923.
47. Wu HS, Liu FY, Huang WS, et al. Technetium-99m tetrofosmin single photon emission computed tomography to detect metastatic papillary thyroid carcinoma in patients with elevated human serum thyroglobulin levels but negative I-131 whole body scan. Clin Radiol 2003; 58: 787–790.
48. Tisell LE, Ahlman H, Wangberg B, et al. Expression of somatostatin receptors in oncocytic (Hürthle cell) neoplasia of the thyroid. Br J Cancer 1999; 79:1579–1582.
49. Ain KB, Taylor KD, Tofiq S, Venkataraman G. Somatostatin receptor subtype expression in human thyroid and thyroid carcinoma cell lines. J Clin Endocrinol Metab 1997; 82:1857–1862.
50. Gorges R, Kahaly G, Muller-Brand J, et al. Radionuclide-labeled somatostatin analogues for diagnostic and therapeutic purposes in non-medullary thyroid cancer. Thyroid 2001; 11:647–659.
51. Baudin E, Schlumberger M, Lumbroso J, et al. Octreotide scintigraphy in patients with differentiated thyroid carcinoma: contribution for patients with negative radioiodine scan. J Clin Endocrinol Metab 1996; 81:2541–2544.
52. Postema PT, de Herder WW, Reubi JC, et al. Somatostatin receptor scintigraphy in non-medullary thyroid cancer. Digestion 1996; 57(Suppl 1):36–37.
53. Stokkel MP, Verkooijen RB, Smith JW. Indium-111 octreotide scintigraphy for the detection of non-functioning metastases from differentiated thyroid cancer: diagnostic and prognostic value. Eur J Nucl Med Mol Imaging 2004; 31:950–957.
54. Sarlis NJ, Gourgiotis L, Guthrie LC, et al. In-111 DTPA-octreotide scintigraphy for disease detection in metastatic thyroid cancer: comparison with F-18 FDG positron emission tomography and extensive conventional radiographic imaging. Clin Nucl Med 2003; 28: 208–217.

36 PART A
Stunning

Untoward Effect of ^{131}I Thyroid Imaging Prior to Radioablation Therapy

Hee-Myung Park and Stephen K. Gerard

INTRODUCTION

Thyroid stunning is a radiobiological phenomenon. It may be defined as a temporary suppression of iodine, trapping function of the thyrocytes and thyroid cancer cells as a result of the radiation given off by the scanning (or first) dose of ^{131}I. The tissue-absorbed radiation dose from the scanning is often sufficient to cause hypofunction but usually not enough to destroy the target cells. The stunned cells may not be able to take up the ensuing therapeutic radioiodine-131 to the degree of their original unaffected capacity. It may lead to an incomplete ablation of the thyroid remnant or metastatic lesion. Stunning is radiation dose–dependent, i.e., the higher the radiation-absorbed dose to the target tissue, the greater the stunning effect. Stunning is a matter of quantity, not quality, and certainly is not an "all or none" phenomenon; there is a spectrum of severity. When severe, there is often a visually apparent reduction in uptake of the therapy dose of ^{131}I in the target lesion when the diagnostic and posttherapy scans are compared. When mild, it may be noticeable only when the thyroid iodide uptake function is measured. However, the visual evidence of decreased radioiodine uptake caused by stunning could be confounded by one or more uncontrolled differences in technical and/or physiologic constraints between the diagnostic and posttreatment scans. Such differences might relate to the postdose imaging time, differential radioiodine washout, nonlinear camera response between low and high doses of radioiodine, the thyrotropin (TSH) level, and the extent of iodine depletion at the time of dose administration.

Moreover, calculating the thyroid uptake a second time using ^{131}I is not an easy task because of the presence of high residual ^{131}I activity in the thyroid tissue. This difficulty is especially apparent after a large scanning dose (or after the first portion in a fractionated treatment regimen) is administered. Nevertheless, several investigators have succeeded in measuring it using various methods, proving that the radiation from the diagnostic doses of ^{131}I indeed suppressed the iodide uptake of the target tissues.

To avoid stunning, another isotope of iodine can be used. With all factors considered, ^{123}I seems to be the ideal scanning agent among the 24 possible isotopes of iodine *(1)*.

Park et al. first noticed this phenomenon in patients with thyroid cancers, when liberal amounts (up to 10 mCi [370 MBq] of ^{131}I were commonly used as a scanning dose. When treatable lesions were found, the patients were admitted to the hospital and received ^{131}I therapy (100–150 mCi [3.7–5.55 GBq]). Posttherapy whole-body scans were obtained initially at 24–48 h when the retained ^{131}I activity fell below 30 mCi (1.1 GBq), before the patients were discharged from the hospital. Those images often unexpectedly showed little or no apparent uptake of the therapy dose of ^{131}I in the remnant that had been iodine-avid on diagnostic scans. Systematic review revealed the stunning effect *(2)*. The evidence indicating that stunning was radiation-induced was especially convincing when they noticed the effect was dose-dependent. The frequency of stunning was 40%, 67%, and 89% after 3, 5, and 10 mCi (111, 185, and 370 MBq) doses of ^{131}I, respectively *(3)*. A few illustrative cases of thyroid stunning are shown in Figs. 1–4.

The time of recovery from stunning is not known and is difficult to determine because it requires repetitive whole-body scanning with necessary patient preparation, which can be quite burdensome to patients. In a few patients who underwent repeat diagnostic scanning, the thyroid showed no uptake and thus no evidence of recovery after 2 wk, 27 d, 40 d, and even 7 mo, respectively *(4)*. A diagnostic dose may be lethal if the absorbed tissue dose is sufficient.

PHYSICAL PROPERTIES OF ^{131}I AND THYROID RADIATION DOSE

Radioiodine-131 emits β particles and has a half-life of 8 d. The radiation-absorbed dose to the thyroid tissue increases daily until the ^{131}I loses all of its radioactivity. The ultimate absorbed tissue dose is reached at 8–10 wk. Most of the radiation-absorbed dose, however, is absorbed during the first few days.

From: *Thyroid Cancer: A Comprehensive Guide to Clinical Management,* 2/e
Edited by: L. Wartofsky and D. Van Nostrand © Humana Press Inc., Totowa, NJ

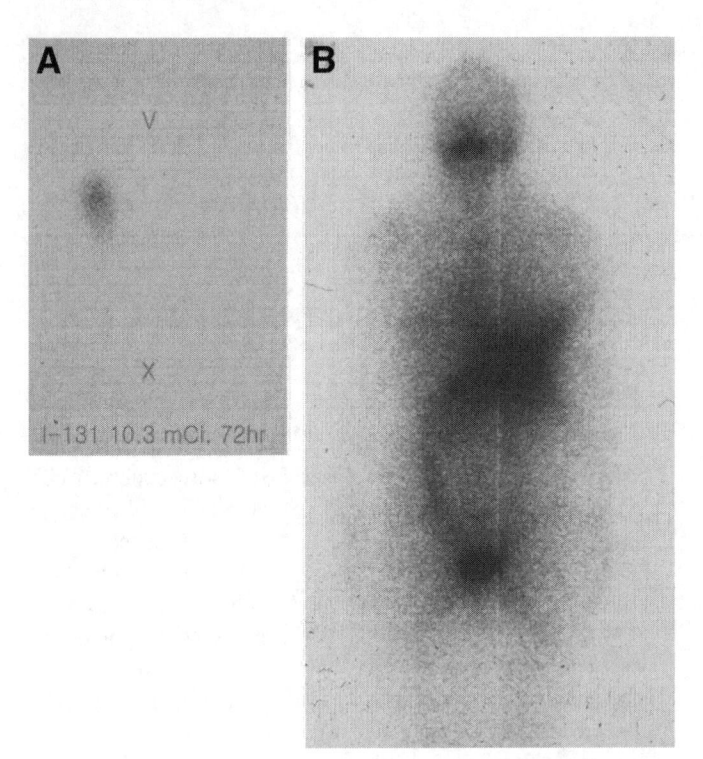

Fig. 1. Stunning from 10-mCi ^{131}I scanning. A follow-up 10-mCi (370 MBq) ^{131}I scan 1 yr after ablation therapy in a 37-yr-old female showed a persistent remnant in the right upper pole (**A**). Because of the patient's family situation, the patient received 100 mCi (3.7 GBq) of ^{131}I therapy (her second) 6 wk later. The 24-h whole-body scan shows no discernible uptake of the therapy dose in the remnant (**B**). The target tissue was undoubtedly stunned by the scanning dose and lost iodide-trapping function. Radioiodine is distributed physiologically in the stomach, gastrointestinal tract, and urinary bladder.

How much radiation would thyroid tissue receive from a scanning dose of ^{131}I? How does it compare with that from the ^{131}I therapy given for hyperthyroidism? When 1 uCi of ^{131}I is deposited in 1 g of thyroid tissue and is allowed to decay completely, the tissue would have received approx 100 rad (100 cGy). It is believed that approximately 10,000 rad (100 Gy, or 100 uCi of ^{131}I/g) are needed to treat Graves' disease. In a postoperative thyroid cancer patient, if the weight of a thyroid remnant is 1 g and the iodine uptake is 1%, a 10-mCi (370 MBq) scanning dose of ^{131}I would have delivered 100 μCi (0.1 mCi, 3.7 MBq) to the thyroid tissue. The remnant would have received approx 10,000 rad—a therapeutic dose for Graves' disease. Therefore, it becomes obvious why such irradiated thyroid tissue may not function normally and cannot fully trap the ensuing therapeutic dose.

The threshold radiation dose, below which no functional changes would occur, is not clearly known. In terms of administered quantity of ^{131}I, a 2-mCi (7.4 MBq) diagnostic dose, according to McDougall, did not cause visually apparent stunning except in 2 of 147 cases (5). However, Medvedec et al. measured the changes in uptake values and found that 2 mCi (7.4 MBq) of ^{131}I lowered the uptake by 40% (6,7). Moreover, McMenemin et al. showed that a potentially significant decrease caused by stunning may not be visually apparent in the posttreatment images (8). For three thyroid cancer patients treated with ^{131}I, a reduction in posttherapy uptake of 86%, 59%, and 40% of the pretreatment value was not seen by visual comparison of the scans. Therefore, qualitative comparison of diagnostic and posttherapy scans may be an insensitive indicator of stunning.

EVIDENCE OF STUNNING

Numerous studies have documented proof of stunning. Quantitative studies more consistently identify the stunning effect (9–12,14–16) than qualitative visual assessment reports (5,13,13a), which are likely less sensitive. Sabri et al. studied the effect of the first half of a therapy dose to the thyroid uptake function. In 171 patients with benign thyroid conditions (toxic diffuse goiter and toxic multinodular goiter), they found that the first dose (11.7 ± 6.2 mCi, with a range of 6.6–32.7 mCi) reduced thyroid uptake by 31.7% (on average) when measured 4 d later. They also found that the stunning effect was dependent on the radiation-absorbed tissue dose (14). Postgard et al. performed an elegant in vitro study using a monolayer of porcine thyrocytes in a culture medium (12). When the cells were irradiated with ^{131}I added to the medium and received 300 rad (3 Gy), their iodide transport function was reduced by 50%, with a precipitous dose–response curve for higher exposures. In a clinical situation, 300 rad would be equivalent to the absorbed tissue dose received by 1 g of thyroid tissue trapping 0.1% of a 3-mCi (111 MBq) scanning dose of ^{131}I. Gerard et al. analyzed 11 published articles on thyroid stunning and found a total of 1412 patients with thyroid cancers reported to have thyroid tissues stunned by diagnostic doses of ^{131}I ranging from 0.5 to 10 mCi (18.5–370 MBq; 17). Koch et al. also reported similar findings (18).

A recent study by Lassman et al. quantified the stunning effect of a repeat 2-mCi (7.4 MBq) ^{131}I diagnostic dose in six patients approx 5 wk following the initial diagnostic dose (15). The average reductions in both uptake and half-life for the second ^{131}I administration were 44% and 51%, respectively ($p < 0.001$ for both). Decreased fractional uptake and biological half-life would both contribute to decreases in the absorbed tissue dose in the interval between the first and second diagnostic scans in this study. These intervals were longer than those typical in clinical practice in the United States. This greater "lag time" between the two doses may amplify the stunning effect from the longer residence time of the first dose prior to the administration of the second dose. Particularly, some have advocated that keeping this dose interval as short as possible will avoid the effects of stunning (5,13). However, Medvedec et al.

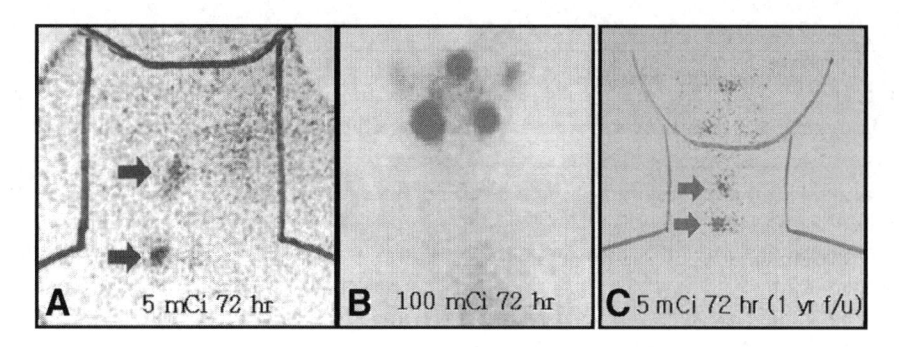

Fig. 2. Stunning from 5/mCi (185 MBq) ^{131}I scanning. After a total thyroidectomy in a 53-yr-old male with papillary cancer, two foci of thyroid remnant were identified on a 5-mCi (185 MBq) ^{131}I 72-h scan (**A**, black arrows). After 4 wk, a 100-mCi (3.7 GBq) ^{131}I ablation therapy dose was given, and a 72-h posttherapy scan showed no evidence of uptake of the dose indicative of severely stunned remnant tissues (**B**). A 1-yr follow-up scan showed the same remnant tissue present in the same locations (**C**, black arrows). The therapy dose was evidently wasted and obviously failed to ablate the target tissues.

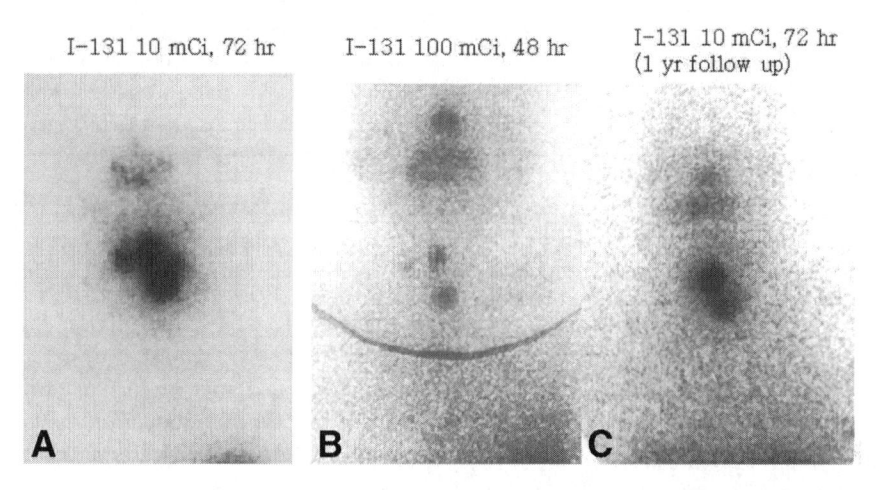

Fig. 3. Stunning from 10-mCi ^{131}I scanning. This is a 44-yr-old male with papillary thyroid cancer, and an ^{131}I scan performed 72 h after the administration of 10 mCi (370 MBq) demonstrated iodine-avid thyroid remnants (**A**). The patient received 100 mCi (3.7 GBq) of ^{131}I for ablation on the day of scanning, and a posttherapy scan performed 48 h later showed unexpectedly low ^{131}I radioactivity in the thyroid remnant tissues. These images strongly suggest that little of the therapy dose was taken up by the thyroid remnant tissue (**B**), which is again indicative of stunning. A 1-yr follow-up scan showed significant persistent remnant indicative of failure of the ablation (**C**).

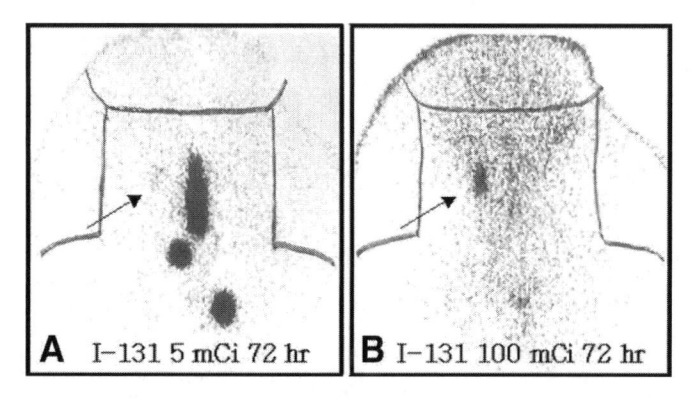

Fig. 4. The greater the uptake, the more the stunning. A postoperative thyroid scan performed after the administration of 5 mCi (185 MBq) of ^{131}I showed several foci of thyroid remnant tissue, including a vertical pyramidal lobe. The arrow points to an additional area of minimal radioiodine uptake that is probably a nodal metastasis (**A**). The 72-h posttherapy scan after 100 mCi (3.7 GBq) of ^{131}I therapy showed more uptake in the node (arrow) than the other radioiodine-avid remnant tissues, which is again indicative of significant stunning (**B**).

reported no difference in the degree of stunning by decreasing this dose interval from a mean of 8.5 d to a mean of 4.3 d *(16)*. These data suggest that most of the damage is already done at 4.3 d, and although reducing the dose interval should be helpful to decrease further stunning, it may not avoid it completely. Apparently, the waiting period after administration of the scanning dose should be shortened to reduce the stunning. The usual waiting period of 72 h would allow the β particles to bombard the thyroid tissue for just as many hours. The thyroid tissue would have received 72.7% of the ultimate total radiation dose at 72 h when the total effective half-life is 2 d or 54.1% when the total effective half-life is 4 d *(4)*. Thyroid tissue receives much less radiation if the scan is done after 24 h instead.

STUNNING EFFECT ON THE OUTCOME OF ABLATION THERAPY

The outcome-based evidence for stunning is perhaps most compelling, as it may not be a function of technical variables that confound comparisons of diagnostic and post-therapy scans. Park et al. reported that there was a lower success rate of ablation after ^{131}I scans than after ^{123}I scans (56% vs 72%) in 47 and 43 patients, respectively *(19)*. Muratet et al. examined 229 patients and found that successful outcome was significantly less frequent after a scanning dose of 3 mCi (5.55 MBq) than after 1 mCi (37 MBq) of ^{131}I (50% vs 76%, $p < 0.001$). Even 1 mCi (37 MBq) of ^{131}I caused stunning in a few cases *(20)*. Lees et al. reported a 47% ablation success rate in the ^{131}I (5 mCi, 185 MBq) scan group vs 86% in the ^{123}I (20 mCi, 740 MBq) scan group divided equally among 72 patients ($p < 0.005$) *(21)*. Morris et al. reported no difference in the success rates between an ^{131}I-scanned group and the nonscanned group when the success was based on follow-up scans obtained at 4–42 mo *(22)*. The discrepancy between these conflicting results may arise from the lack of uniform protocols for ^{131}I scanning and treatment, as well as the lack of criteria for successful ablation between the reporting institutions. More data using the same protocol with a larger patient population is needed to show significant differences. Likely, at least 12 mo should elapse before an attempt is made to determine the outcome. Stunned lesions with no uptake on earlier scans may show up after recovery on the later scans. Therapeutic effect depends on the amount of radiation absorbed by the thyroid tissue from any ^{131}I dose. In a few patients, we have observed that the scanning dose of ^{131}I was later found to be actually lethal to the target tissue *(4)*.

CONSIDERATIONS IN FRACTIONATED ^{131}I THERAPY

Similar to the case in the United States until 1997, nuclear regulations in many countries still limit the amount of ^{131}I that can be given to outpatients. In certain areas, hospitals are required to have a specifically designed stainless-steel septic tank large enough to hold ^{131}I waste from the patients to allow near-complete decay of ^{131}I.

Understandably, fractionated dosing is a common practice to circumvent such strict nuclear regulations. The longer the interval between the divided doses in fractionated ^{131}I treatment, the greater the absorbed radiation dose would be from the first dose, and the lesser the uptake would be from the subsequent ^{131}I doses. The therapeutic contribution of the second or third dose must be lower than the first dose because the amount of ^{131}I taken up by the stunned thyroid tissue (from the first dose) should be smaller, decreasing the cumulative radiation-absorbed dose. "Satisfactory" results were indicated with fractionated therapy in treating benign thyroid conditions and thyroid cancer. However, a paucity of reports analyzed the therapeutic effect of the first dose and subsequent doses separately partially because the full effect of the first dose may not become evident for up to 12 mo. Such a study would not be justifiable in patients with thyroid cancer because the consequence of probable incomplete treatment may be harmful.

USE OF ^{123}I VS ^{131}I AS A SCANNING AGENT

Radioiodine-123 emits γ rays but not β particles and has a half-life of 13 h. The radiation-absorbed tissue dose from pure ^{123}I is only 1% of that from ^{131}I *(23)*. No stunning has been observed after the use of pure ^{123}I (Fig. 5). Notably, depending on the production methods, some ^{123}I preparations contain ^{124}I as a contaminant, which will raise the absorbed tissue dose.

In nuclear imaging studies, it is generally known that a higher scanning dose provides better image quality. Waxman showed that higher ^{131}I doses gave greater sensitivity *(24)*. ^{131}I scans using a 100-mCi (3.7 GBq) therapy dose that are obtained 7 d later (when the background is low) may be considered as the "gold standard," provided that no pretreatment diagnostic ^{131}I was used. The accuracy of diagnostic scans may be compared to this standard. Gerard et al. demonstrated that the sensitivity of ^{123}I (3–5 mCi, 111–185 MBq) compared with the early post-^{131}I treatment scans was 86.7%, and that good-quality images can be obtained up to 48 h after administration *(25)*. Gulzar et al. showed that ^{123}I scans (5 mCi, 185 MBq) had a 92.6% concordance rate between the 24-h ^{123}I scan and the post-therapy ^{131}I scan. The quality of 24-h ^{123}I scans was found to be slightly better than 4-h ^{123}I images *(26)*.

Comparing diagnostic ^{123}I scans with diagnostic ^{131}I scans, Mandel et al. reported that ^{123}I (1.2–1.5 mCi, 44.4–55.5 MBq, 5-h scan) was slightly superior to ^{131}I (3 mCi, 111 MBq, 48-h scan) for whole-body imaging. ^{123}I scans showed 35 foci, whereas ^{131}I scans showed 32 foci *(27)*.

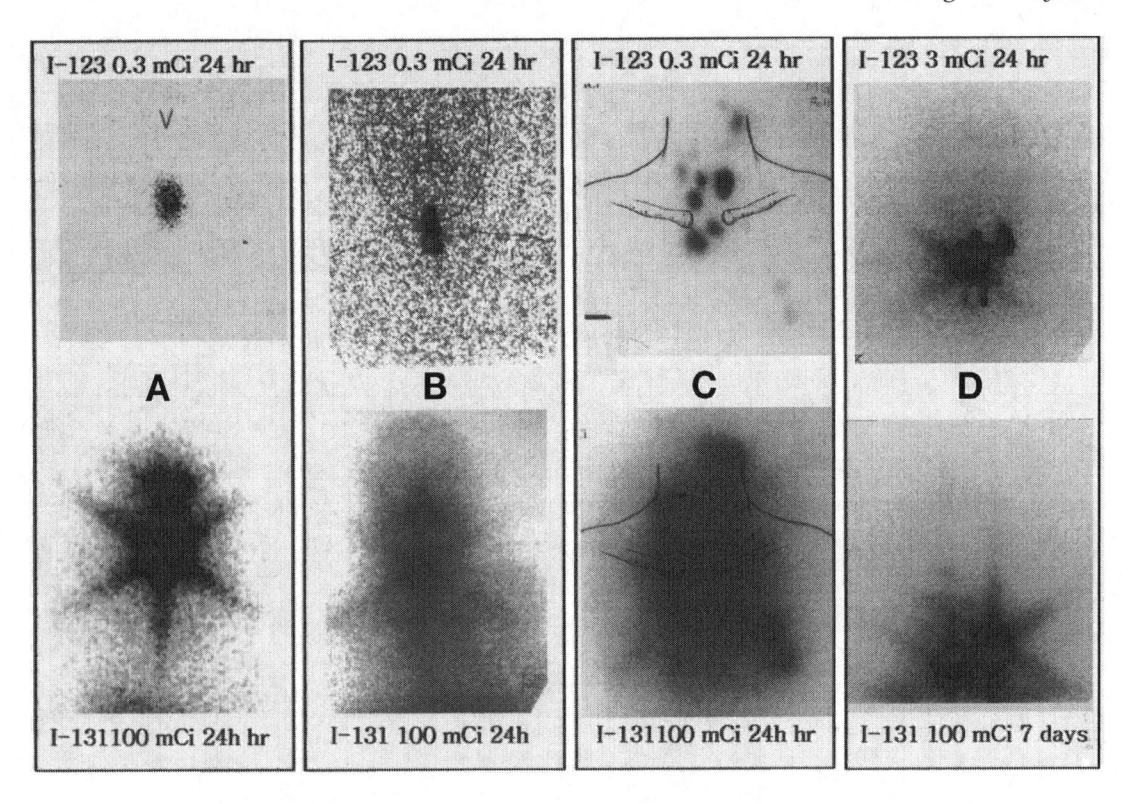

Fig. 5. Excellent uptake of therapeutic ^{131}I by unstunned thyroid. In the top row **(A–D)**, four postoperative ^{123}I scans from four different patients are shown. "V" denotes the thyroid cartilage. The images in the bottom row are the corresponding images after ^{131}I therapy, and each demonstrates markedly increased uptake of the therapy dose in the target tissues. The star artifact is caused by the penetration of the collimator's septa by the γ rays from the high uptake of therapeutic ^{131}I in the target tissues.

Owing to the relatively short half-life, ^{123}I scans are commonly done at 24 h, whereas the ^{131}I scans are obtained at 72 h. Some slow-functioning lesions may show up only on the scans obtained much later. Sarkar et al. reported four cases in which 24-h ^{123}I scans (2–3.5 mCi, 74–129.5 MBq) missed metastases that were seen on the 72–96 h ^{131}I scans (3–5 mCi, 111–185 MBq). In one patient, both the 24-h ^{123}I and 24-h ^{131}I scans missed some of the metastases, which were seen by the 96-h ^{131}I scan. This result emphasized the benefit of delayed imaging and washout of background activity to raise the target-to-background ratios. The 24-h ^{123}I images, however, showed all of the postoperative remnants present in nine patients *(28)*. Alternatively, Bautovich et al. reported superior detection of metastases from diagnostic scans using a large ^{123}I dose (27 mCi, 1 GBq) and 48-h imaging in 8 of 10 previously ablated patients compared to that with 5 mCi (185 MBq of ^{131}I) *(29)*. The ^{131}I diagnostic scans missed 13 more foci than were seen with ^{123}I, in comparison to the post-^{131}I ablation scans as the gold standard. Admittedly, routine use of such large doses could be cost-prohibitive. However, larger ^{123}I doses in combination with 48-h delayed imaging may afford competitive or superior sensitivity without the associated risks of stunning vs diagnostic ^{131}I scanning.

On a dose-for-dose basis, ^{123}I scans seem to offer equal or higher sensitivity in diagnostic scanning as do ^{131}I scans for the detection of thyroid remnant *(27,30)*. Gerard and Cavalieri have shown that ^{123}I scans obtained at 48 h are good quality when doses of at least 5 mCi (185 MBq; *25*) are used, as shown also by others *(21,29,31*; Figs. 6–8). Thus, a growing body of literature indicates that ^{123}I is preferred for whole-body imaging in thyroid cancer metastasis screening *(32)*.

The disadvantages of ^{123}I include limited availability, the higher cost necessitated by production at a cyclotron facility, as well as its short half-life, which is problematic for long-distance shipping and quantitative dosimetry. The cost of a 5-mCi (185 MBq) dose can be reduced by ordering the tracer directly from the manufacturer and administering it orally as a liquid *(25,33)*. We believe that the additional cost of ^{123}I is justified to avoid a suboptimal therapeutic outcome. One caveat in ^{123}I imaging is to recognize that salivary activity is present in the esophagus at 24 h. Repeat scanning after allowing the patient to drink a glass of water clears this activity.

Early experience using recombinant human TSH (rhTSH) for diagnostic ^{123}I scanning suggests comparable sensitivity

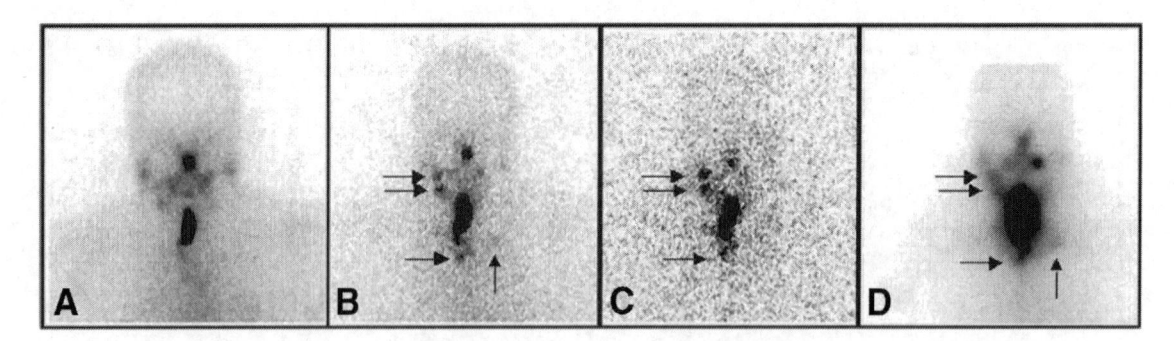

Fig. 6. Increased target to background activity in ^{123}I images performed at 6, 24, and 48 h. A 40-yr old female with multi-focal invasive papillary thyroid cancer had a postoperative scan performed after the administration of 4.9 mCi (181.3 MBq) of ^{123}I. The anterior view performed 6, 24, and 48 h after administration of the ^{123}I are shown in **A**, **B**, and **C**, respectively. The patient was treated with 201 mCi (7.44 GBq) of ^{131}I. The 3-d posttreatment anterior image is shown in **D**. The horizontal arrows in **B**, **C**, and **D** identify two upper right cervical lymph nodes (the two upper arrows) and one or two sites of thyroid remnant tissue (lower single arrow), which are below the vertical pyramidal lobe. These images show a progressive increase in ^{123}I target-to-background radioactivity ratio from 6 to 24 h and again from 24 to 48 h. The vertical arrow in **D** identifies a faint area of posttreatment ^{131}I accumulation, probably representing a lymph node metastasis. This focus was identified only in hindsight in the 24-h ^{123}I image (vertical arrow in **B**).

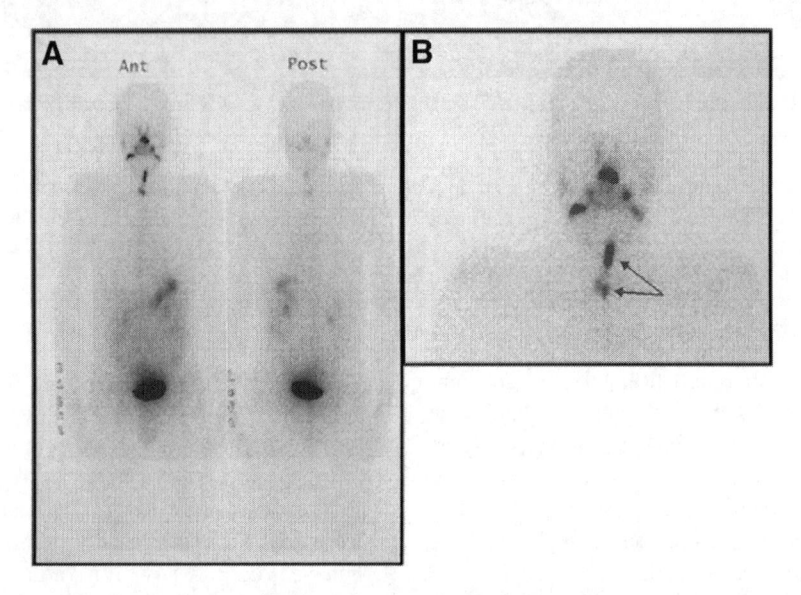

Fig. 7. ^{123}I 24-h whole-body imaging with rhTSH. A 51-yr-old male with papillary thyroid cancer underwent whole-body imaging postoperatively with 7.6 mCi (281 MBq) of ^{123}I administered after rhTSH. The 24-h images are shown in **A**; an enlarged image of the anterior head and neck is shown in **B**. The arrows in **B** showed two or three foci in the low neck and a higher midline pyramidal lobe. These sites were confirmed in the posttherapy scan (not shown). Of interest, the patient's serum thyroglobulin measured 72 h following the second intramuscular rhTSH injection was only 0.8 ng/mL, with a TSH level of 69 µU/mL on the day of ^{123}I administration. The serum thyroglobulin level at the time of treatment following full withdrawal preparation was similar—only 1.7 ng/mL. Antithyroid antibodies were negative. This case represents an example of the complementary role of radioiodine imaging and serum thyroglobulin measurement for the detection of residual differentiated thyroid tissue. If the practice had been only to measure serum thyroglobulin levels, then a decision to defer radioiodine ablation might have been made inappropriately.

to that with thyroid hormone withdrawal *(34;* Gerard SK, unpublished results (see Chapters 27, 46). Recently, it has been reported that ^{131}I therapy with rhTSH for thyroid cancer ablation may be as efficacious as therapy with thyroid withdrawal *(35–38)*. With further validation, the option to avoid the morbidity of severe hypothyroidism could be applied more routinely to both diagnostic scanning and therapy. This opportunity highlights the potential need to validate rhTSH diagnostic scanning using ^{123}I to avoid stunning by ^{131}I. Some evidence shows that thyroidal iodine residence time with rhTSH may be longer compared to that in the withdrawal setting *(39)*, which could potentiate the stunning effect. Examples of rhTSH ^{123}I whole-body scans are shown in Figs. 7 and 8.

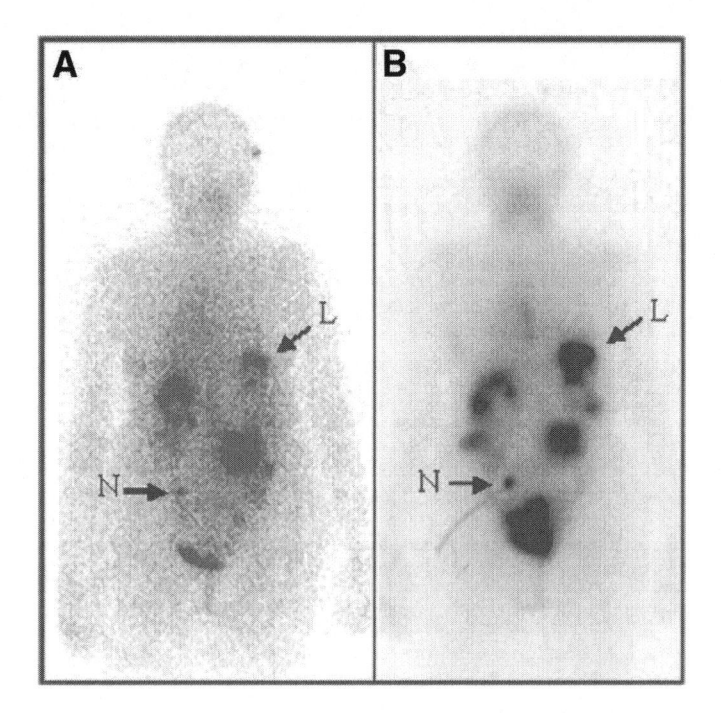

Fig. 8. ^{123}I diagnostic scan and early ^{131}I posttherapy scan with rhTSH. An 82-yr-old female with history of metastatic follicular thyroid cancer had an rhTSH-stimulated ^{123}I scan (6.3 mCi, 233 MBq) performed, followed by an rhTSH-stimulated ^{131}I treatment. The patient received rhTSH stimulation because the TSH elevation after thyroid hormone withdrawal was inadequate. The patient had a known metastasis to the liver with thyroglobulin levels more than 30,000, and the failure of the TSH to increase was attributed to significant hormone production from a functioning liver metastasis. **A** is the posterior diagnostic scan performed 24 h after administration of the ^{123}I, and **B** is the posterior view of the posttreatment scan performed 3 d after administration of 151 mCi (5.59 GBq) of ^{131}I. This demonstrated the sites of liver metastasis (arrow labeled with "L") and retroperitoneal lymph node metastasis (arrow labeled with "N"). Both metastasis sites were also confirmed in the 8-d posttherapy image (not shown). Intense renal radioactivity is seen. The posttherapy scan also showed modest esophageal activity in the low-midline area of the thorax. The spot of activity in the diagnostic scan on the right side of the head is surface contamination at the site of the patient's hair clip.

USING LOW-DOSE ^{131}I WHEN ^{123}I IS UNAVAILABLE

In places where ^{123}I is not available, the only choice may be to use ^{131}I as the imaging agent. It would be prudent to lower the administered dose as much as possible to prevent stunning prior to planned ^{131}I therapy. However, other factors may reduce stunning: (1) to scan early, e.g., at 24 h instead of 72 h, to decrease the interval between diagnostic dose and time of scanning; (2) to administer the ^{131}I treatment dose soon after scanning, preferably on the same day, noting that the stunning effect increases over time. The 72-h scans may have slightly higher sensitivity, but a clinical decision to treat can often be made on the 24-h scans. If the 24-h scan shows no lesion, further delayed scans should be obtained.

DISCUSSION

Generally, to successfully ablate the target tissues, a sufficient dose of ^{131}I should be administered at once to "hit them hard the first time." As early as 1951, Rawson et al. warned against giving a "noncancericidal" dose of ^{131}I, which results in inadequate therapy for differentiated thyroid cancers *(40)*. Efforts are continuously made to improve the radioiodine uptake by the target cells to their maximum capacity before radioablation therapy. Most physicians involved with ^{131}I therapy prepare the patients with T4 withdrawal or rhTSH injection to raise the serum TSH level. Patients are placed on a low-iodine diet to decrease the body iodide pool as low as possible to allow the target cells to take up as much administered ^{131}NaI as possible *(41)*. Some suggest the use of lithium to increase the resident time of ^{131}I in thyroid tissue; others are developing methods to increase sodium iodide symporter (NIS) gene expression in the thyroid cancer cells. In line with these efforts, stunning of the thyroid target cells should be avoided or minimized. Stunning the thyroid cells, or making them temporarily nonfunctional or less functional prior to the intended radioablation therapy, will work against most of our other efforts to improve the radioiodine uptake with the thyroid remnant or metastatic thyroid cancer cells.

To avoid thyroid stunning altogether, or to increase patient convenience, some suggest administering ^{131}I therapy blindly to all postoperative patients without conducting a diagnostic survey scan. Unfortunately, this practice may end up giving a large amount of ^{131}I to a few patients without treatable lesions. Moreover, diagnostic whole-body radioiodine scanning for thyroid cancer, although not perfect, is the best imaging test for staging the extent of disease prior to treatment. This data is often included in the treatment algorithm for determination of the ^{131}I dose.

Sodium ^{123}I is available or may soon become available in many parts of the world. Using it for scanning will alleviate the problem of stunning, and a lower therapeutic dose may be needed to treat lesions that are not stunned. Then, if the current therapy dose of ^{131}I is lowered, can the same ablation success rate still be achieved? What other factors are required to achieve the success rate of 100%? These are some questions that need to be answered by future research.

SUMMARY

Thyroid stunning is a predictable, verifiable radiobiological suppressive phenomenon that occurs when a scanning dose of ^{131}I deposits a sufficient radiation dose to the target tissue to temporarily reduce its iodide-trapping function. The stunned cells are unable to take up the ensuing therapeutic dose of ^{131}I to the degree of their prior unaffected maximal capacity, and the intended ablation may become incomplete. There must be factors other than stunning that account for some ^{131}I ablation failures. Nevertheless, stunning is one of the known causes of reduced ^{131}I uptake by the target cells and may negate all other efforts to increase the ^{131}I uptake before radioablation therapy.

Radioiodine-123 has many desirable characteristics as a thyroid imaging agent and does not stun the target cells. Wherever available, it would be prudent to utilize ^{123}I for scanning purposes before ^{131}I therapy in the management of well-differentiated thyroid cancers. When ^{131}I must be used as a diagnostic scanning agent, efforts should be made to minimize the stunning effect by administering a minimum dose and by keeping the time between the diagnostic and treatment doses as short as possible.

ACKNOWLEDGMENTS

The authors are grateful to Drs. Richard Schnute, Christine Park, and Trudy Lionel for reviewing this article and rendering helpful suggestions, as well as Dr. S. Bae of Koshin University, Korea, for providing images for the Figs. 2 and 4.

REFERENCES

1. Park HM. I-123: Almost a designer radioiodine for thyroid scanning. J Nucl Med 2002; 43:77–78.
2. Park HM. Potential adverse effect of high survey dose of I-131 administered prior to I-131 therapy in the management of differentiated thyroid cancers. In Schmidt H, Van Der Schoot JB, editors. Nuclear Medicine: The State of the Art of Nuclear Medicine in Europe. Schattauer, Stuttgart, Germany, 1991:340–342.
3. Park HM, Perkins OW, Edmondson JW, et al. Influence of diagnostic radioiodines on the uptake of ablative dose of I-131. Thyroid 1994; 4:49–54.
4. Park HM. The stunning effect in radioiodine therapy of thyroid cancer. Nucl Med Ann 2001; 49–67.
5. McDougall IR. 74 MBq I-131 does not prevent uptake of therapeutic doses of I-131 in differentiated thyroid cancer. Nucl Med Comm 1997; 18:505–512.
6. Medvedec M, Pavlinovic Z, Dodig D. 74 MBq radioiodine I-131 does prevent uptake of therapeutic activity of I-131 in residual thyroid tissue. Eur J Nucl Med 1999; 26:1013.
7. Huic D, Medvedec M, Dodig D, et al. Radioiodine uptake in thyroid cancer patients after diagnostic application of low-dose 131I. Nucl Med Comm 1996; 17:839–842.
8. McMenemin RM, Hilditch TE, Dempsey MF, Reed NS. Thyroid stunning after 131I diagnostic whole-body scanning. J Nucl Med 2001; 42:986–987.
9. Jeevanram RK, Shah DH, Sharma SM, Ganatra RD. Influence of initial large dose on subsequent uptake of therapeutic radioiodine in thyroid cancer patients. Nucl Med Biol 1986; 13:277–279.
10. Huic D, Medvedec M, Dodig D, et al. Radioiodine uptake in thyroid cancer patients after diagnostic application of low-dose I-131. Nucl Med Comm 1996; 17:839–842.
11. Leger FA, Izembart M, Dagousset F, et al. Decreased uptake of therapeutic doses of I-131 after 185 MBq I-131 diagnostic imaging for thyroid remnants in differentiated thyroid carcinoma. Eur J Nucl Med 1998; 25:242–246.
12. Postgard P, Himmelman J, Lindencrona L, et al. Stunning of iodide transport by I-131 irradiation in cultured thyroid epithelial cells. J Nucl Med 2002; 43:828–834.
13. Cholewinski S, Yoo K, Klieger P, O'Mara R. Absence of thyroid stunning after diagnostic whole-body scanning with 185 MBq I-131. J Nucl Med 2000; 41:1198–1202.
13a. Dam HQ, Kim SM, Lin HC, Intenzo CM. ^{131}I therapeutic efficacy is not influenced by stunning after diagnostic whole-body scanning. Radiology 2004; 232:527–533.
14. Sabri O, Zimny M, Schreckenberger M, et al. Does thyroid stunning exist? A model with benign thyroid disease. Eur J Nucl Med 2000; 27:1591–1597.
15. Lassmann M, Luster M, Hänscheid H, Reiners C. Impact of 131I diagnostic activities on the biokinetics of thyroid remnants. J Nucl Med 2004; 45:619–625.
16. Medvedec M, Grosev D, Loncaric S, et al. As soon as possible is already too late. J Nucl Med 2001; 42:322P.
17. Gerard S. The role of I-123 in the management of differentiated thyroid cancer. CME symposium presented at the 74th Annual Meeting of the American Thyroid Association, October 11, 2002.
18. Koch W, Knesewitsch P, Tatsch K, Hahn K. Stunning effects in radioiodine therapy of thyroid carcinoma: existence, clinical effects and ways out. Nuclearmedizin 2003; 42:10–14.
19. Park H, Park Y, Zhou X. Detection of thyroid remnant/metastasis without stunning: An ongoing dilemma. Thyroid 1997; 7:277–280.
20. Muratet J, Daver A, Minier J, Larra F. Influence of scanning doses of I-131 on subsequent first ablative treatment outcome in patients operated on for differentiated thyroid carcinoma. J Nucl Med 1998; 39:1556–1550.
21. Lees W, Mansberg R, Roberts J, et al. The clinical effects of thyroid stunning after diagnostic whole-body scanning with 185 MBq I-131. Eur J Nucl Med 2002; 29:1421–1427.
22. Morris LF, Waxman AD, Braunstein GD. The non-impact of thyroid stunning: Remnant ablation rates in I-131-scanned and non-scanned individuals. J Clin Endocrinol Metab 2001; 86:3507–3511.
23. MIRD (Medical Internal Radiation Dose) Committee Report #5. Summary of current radiation dose estimates to humans from ^{123}I, ^{124}I, ^{125}I, ^{126}I, ^{130}I, ^{131}I, and ^{132}I as sodium iodide. J Nucl Med 1975; 16:857–860.
24. Waxman A, Ramanna L, Chapman N, et al. Significance of I-131 scan dose in patients with thyroid cancer: determination of ablation: concise communication. J Nucl Med 1981; 22:861–865.
25. Gerard SK, Cavalieri RR. I-123 diagnostic thyroid tumor whole-body scanning with imaging at 6, 24, and 48 hours. Clin Nucl Med 2002; 27:1–8.
26. Gulzar Z, Jana S, Young I, et al. Neck and whole-body scanning with a 5 mCi (185 MBq) dose of I-123 as diagnostic tracer in patients with well-differentiated thyroid cancer. Endocr Pract 2001; 7:244–249.
27. Mandel SJ, Shankar LK, Benard F, et al. Superiority of iodine-123 compared with iodine-131 scanning for thyroid remnants in patients with differentiated thyroid cancer. Clin Nucl Med 2001; 26:6–9.
28. Sarkar SD, Kalapparambath TP, Palestro CJ. Comparison of I-123 and I-131 for whole-body imaging in thyroid cancer. J Nucl Med 2002; 43:632–634.
29. Bautovich GJ, Towson JE, Eberl S, et al. Comparison of iodine-123 and iodine-131 as a scanning agent for the detection of metastatic thyroid cancer. J Nucl Med 1997; 38:150P–151P.
30. Shankar LK, Yamamoto AJ, Alavi A, Mandel SJ. Comparison of 123I scintigraphy at 5 and 24 hours in patients with differentiated thyroid cancer. J Nucl Med 2002; 43:72–76.
31. De Geus-Oei LF, Pauwels EKJ, Stokkel MPM. A comparison between low and high dose I-123 WBS in the follow-up of thyroid cancer. Eur J Nucl Med 2000; 27(Suppl):931.
32. Kalinyak JE. I-123 as a diagnostic tracer in the management of thyroid cancer. Editorial. Nucl Med Comm 2002; 23:509–511.
33. Berbano R, Naddaf S, Echemendia E, et al. Use of iodine-123 as a diagnostic tracer for neck and whole-body scanning in patients with well-differentiated thyroid cancer. Endocr Pract 1998; 4:11–16.

34. Anderson GS, Fish S, Nakhoda K, et al. Comparison of I-123 and I-131 for whole-body imaging after stimulation by recombinant human thyrotropin: a preliminary report. Clin Nucl Med 2003; 28: 93–96.
35. Perros P. Recombinant human thyroid-stimulating hormone (rhTSH) in the radioablation of well-differentiated thyroid cancer: preliminary therapeutic experience. J Endocrinol Invest 1999; 22:30–34.
36. Berg G, Lindstedt G, Suurkula M, Jansson S. Radioiodine ablation and therapy in differentiated thyroid cancer under stimulation with recombinant human thyroid-stimulating hormone. J Endocrinol Invest 2002; 25:44–52.
37. Robbins RJ, Larson SM, Sinha N, et al. A retrospective review of the effectiveness of recombinant human TSH as a preparation for radioiodine thyroid remnant ablation. J Nucl Med 2002; 43:1482–1488.
38. Jarzab B, Handkiewicz-Junak D, Roskosz J, et al. Recombinant human TSH-aided radioiodine treatment of advanced differentiated thyroid carcinoma: a single-centre study of 54 patients. Eur J Nucl Med Mol Imaging 2003; 30:1077–1086.
39. Luster M, Sherman SI, Skarulis MC, et al. Comparison of radioiodine biokinetics following the administration of recombinant human thyroid stimulating hormone and after thyroid hormone withdrawal in thyroid carcinoma. Eur J Nucl Med Mol Imaging 2003; 30:1371–1377.
40. Rawson RW, Rall JE, Peacock W. Limitations and indications in the treatment of cancer of the thyroid with radioactive iodine. J Clin Endocrinol Metab 1951; 11:1128–1131.
41. Pluijmen MJHM, Eustatia-Rutten C, Goslings BM, et al. Effects of low-iodide diet on postsurgical radioiodide ablation therapy in patients with differentiated thyroid carcinoma. Clin Endocrinol 2003; 58:428–435.

36 PART B
Stunning Is Not a Problem

I. Ross McDougall

INTRODUCTION

To "stun" has been defined in several ways. The Webster dictionary provides synonyms of "to make senseless," "to daze or stupefy," or "to shock deeply." The adjective form also means excellent or attractive. None of these definitions accurately represent "stunning" in relation to the treatment of thyroid cancer. Stunning entails that a diagnostic dose of radioiodine (^{131}I) can sufficiently damage the thyroid, making follicular cells incapable of trapping subsequent therapeutic ^{131}I (1,2). It is true that some of us were stupefied when the concept was first presented. Early reports implied that there would be no uptake of therapy. Thus, when a pretreatment diagnostic scan was compared to a posttherapy scan, the latter showed absence of uptake at one or more sites. Subsequently, the term was expanded to include the possibility that the percentage uptake of the therapeutic dose would be less than that of the prior diagnostic scintiscan, i.e., a quantitatively different finding. Lastly, the term "stunning" was expanded to include a poorer outcome after treatment than when there was no diagnostic dose prescribed or when an alternative imaging agent, such as ^{123}I, is used in place of ^{131}I (3,4). Whether stunning actually occurs has divided opinion into two perspectives, generating considerable debate (5–10). This section presents data arguing against the concept of stunning.

The first argument opposing stunning is self-evident. Diagnostic whole-body scanning with ^{131}I has been employed for four decades; yet, the treatment of thyroid cancer with ^{131}I has been remarkably successful (11). Second, it has been accepted practice to obtain a diagnostic and posttherapy scan for more than 20 yr. Indeed, many publications demonstrate that posttherapy scans show more lesions than the corresponding diagnostic images. Nemec et al. were probably the first to report on this issue in 1979 (12). They used a small diagnostic dose of ^{131}I (0.5 mCi, 18.5 MBq); however, the posttherapy scan taken after 100 mCi (3.7 GBq) showed 25% more lesions. Waxman et al. compared the therapeutic scan with diagnostic images obtained with 10 mCi (370 MBq) of ^{131}I (13). When 30 mCi (1.1 GBq) of ^{131}I was prescribed as treatment, 5 of 9 patients showed more lesions, and when 100 mCi (3.7 GBq) of ^{131}I was used, 5 of 10 patients showed more abnormalities on the posttherapy scintiscans. A third report also found 40% more lesions on the posttherapy scan (14). The posttherapy scan can show the site of thyroglobulin production when the diagnostic scan is negative or faintly positive (15–17). These reports do not provide evidence of reduced or absent uptake of therapeutic ^{131}I as a result of the diagnostic dose of ^{131}I.

Many authors researching this topic cite the 1951 publication by Rawson et al.—the first publication to recognize this phenomenon (18). These investigators point out that administration of ^{131}I can reduce the efficacy of subsequent therapeutic ^{131}I. However, they reported on this finding after 25 mCi (925 MBq) of ^{131}I was administered as a treatment dose. There is no discussion of diagnostic or posttreatment rectilinear images or scintiscans, and the altered response after treatment was judged indirectly by the percentage of radioactive iodine excreted in the urine. This does not fit the essential definition of stunning described earlier. If stunning is a true finding, it is more likely to occur after a large dose of radiation, a fact addressed below.

In those publications that directly compare the pre- and posttherapy scans, several show little or no effect of the diagnostic dose. These reports cover a range of diagnostic doses of ^{131}I. A total of 122 patients were treated by Cholewinski et al. (19). The investigators prescribed a diagnostic dose of 5 mCi (185 MBq) with patients scanned after a delay of 72 h. The treatment doses covered a range from 30 to 200 mCi (1.1–7.4 GBq), but 85% of the patients received 150 mCi (5.55 GBq). The treatment was administered on the same day as the diagnostic scan. There were no areas of absent uptake on the posttreatment scintiscans that were also imaged on the 72-h images. The authors then evaluated the outcome of the ^{131}I treatment by follow-up scan. In this analysis, they separated the patients into two groups: those who had a total thyroidectomy and those who had a lobectomy. In the first group, which consisted of 92 patients, 84% were successfully ablated. The authors concluded: "Diagnostic whole-body scanning can be performed effectively with a 5-mCi (185-MBq) dose of ^{131}I 72 hours before radioiodine ablation without concern for thyroid stunning."

Investigators from the Mayo Clinic compared diagnostic and posttherapy scans in a study designed to determine whether the latter provided additional information (20). Their data also allow the question of stunning to be assessed. Diagnostic doses of ^{131}I ranged from 1 to 3 mCi (37–111 MBq), with a mean of 96 MBq, and imaging was conducted after 48 h. The authors do not specify when therapy was administered, but posttreatment scans were obtained after 3–5 d. They found reduced uptake in only 4% (5 of 117) of posttreatment scans. In four of these five cases, they identified an alternate reason from stunning to explain the reduced uptake. Regarding these five patients they commented that, "A stunning effect might have been the cause . . . although it appears unlikely." Of their patients' scans, 96% showed no evidence of stunning.

One publication used by some authors to strengthen the argument for stunning may actually support the opposite. In the report by Bajen et al., the posttreatment scan showed less uptake in 78 (21%) of 373 patients (21). A dose of 5 mCi (185 MBq) was administered for the diagnostic scan. Follow-up scans were conducted in 76 of the 78 patients and were negative in 68 (89%). Thyroglobulin (Tg) was less than 3 ng/mL in 61 of 68 patients. Of the remaining eight patients, seven had an improved follow-up scan and low Tg values. These investigators concluded, "Our data suggests that a stunning effect does not exist for doses of 5 mCi (185 MBq) ^{131}I."

For several decades, physicians at the Memorial Sloan Kettering Cancer Center have employed dosimetric measurements prior to treatment with ^{131}I. The aim is to ensure that the bone marrow does not receive a 200-rad (2-Gy) or more radiation-absorbed dose. The measurements require scans and blood measurements over 4 d, which can be achieved only with ^{131}I as the half-life of ^{123}I is too short. They used 1–5 mCi (37–185 MBq) of ^{131}I for diagnostic measurements. The researchers compared the uptake of the therapeutic dose to the diagnostic one, stating, "We did not observe a strong correlation between administered activity and the magnitude of stunning" (22).

This author has compared diagnostic and posttherapy scans in 305 patients. The diagnostic scans were usually obtained 66–72 h after 2 mCi (74 MBq) of ^{131}I (patients received the test dose on a Friday and were scanned on the following Monday). Treatment was administered as soon as possible after the information from the diagnostic scan was reviewed; 40% were treated on the same day and an additional 34% within 24 h. Post-therapy scans were obtained after an average of 8 d. Reduced uptake was identified on 10 (3.3%) of these scans. Follow-up scan and Tg measurements were negative in 8 of these 10 patients. Earlier results from this investigation have been published (23).

Because of data indicating that ^{123}I is a better radionuclide for whole-body scanning (3), our group has employed ^{123}I when the logistics were advantageous. Surprisingly, we found posttreatment scans that showed reduced uptake in 13% (4 of 30 who were treated with ^{131}I shortly after the diagnostic ^{123}I scan (24). It is not probable—indeed, not possible—that 2 mCi (74 MBq) of ^{123}I could deliver sufficient radiation to cause stunning. When a region shows reduced uptake on a delayed scan, the cause should not immediately be assumed to be stunning. It has long been recognized that cancerous thyroid traps iodine less efficiently, with more rapid turnover; this is the likely explanation.

The articles above compare the diagnostic and posttreatment scan findings and show no evidence of stunning, and several publications also demonstrate no loss of therapeutic efficacy. One criticism of the literature is the lack of quantitative comparisons. In defense of this missing information, the question remains of reliability of uptake measurements of large therapeutic doses and the relevance of a difference between a 48–72-h diagnostic value and a 7–8 d posttherapy result.

Two additional studies address therapy outcome in relationship to diagnostic scanning. The fear of stunning has led to a drift away from obtaining a diagnostic scan, and some physicians now proceed directly to therapy (25). The goal of this section is not only to argue against stunning but also to promote the value of high-quality diagnostic scanning. Morris et al. were able to compare the outcome in two well-matched patient groups. One group had a prior diagnostic scan using doses of 3–5 mCi (111–185 MBq) of ^{131}I, and the other did not (26). No difference in outcome was seen; 65% of the former group was ablated vs 67% of the latter group. Treatment was administered 2–5 d after the diagnostic scan.

A retrospective multivariate analysis of factors that influence the success of ^{131}I ablation in 389 patients found that the most important factor was the size of the therapeutic dose (27). They concluded: "Higher diagnostic doses were not associated with higher rates of ablation failure."

Park and colleagues were the first to use the term "stunning" (1), derived from a review of posttherapy scans in patients who had preliminary diagnostic scans with 3, 5, or 10 mCi (111, 185, or 370 MBq) of ^{131}I. The number of patients was small, but there was a linear relationship of dosage to stunning and the quantity of ^{131}I administered. Significantly, the same investigators in a later publication stated, "Since the scanning dose has been reduced to 2–3 mCi (74–111 MBq), we have not observed stunning."

Dosimetric evidence against stunning can be from the knowledge of how much radiation is required to ablate thyroid tissue. Maxon et al. calculated that 30,000 rad (300 Gy) has to be delivered for reliable success (28,29). Some authorities suggest a similar dose could be required for 100% success in treating hyperthyroidism. The viability of cells is dependent on nuclear function, and the nucleus is the most sensitive component of cells. Therefore, it seems reasonable that the dose required to cause stunning would have to be significant. Two reasonable examples should be considered. The first example is a patient with a 1-g remnant who has 1% uptake and is scanned after 72 h. The dose of ^{131}I administered for testing is 2 mCi (74 MBq), and treatment was prescribed soon after the diagnostic scan. Assuming almost instantaneous uptake of the tracer, the radiation-absorbed dose to the thyroid would be approximately 600 rad (6 Gy). The second example is a patient who has a 1-g remnant and 2% uptake and received a diagnostic dose of 10 mCi (370 MBq), and treatment was delayed for 1 wk. The thyroid could receive 8000 rad (80 Gy), assuming an effective half-life of 100 h. Neither of these doses would be enough to cause ablation. Obviously, larger diagnostic doses and longer delays between diagnosis and therapy result in more radiation to thyroid tissue. Thus, it is prudent to use 2–3 mCi (74–111 MBq) of ^{131}I, and be prepared to treat quickly.

In summary, several studies that involve large patient populations do not support the concept of stunning, whether this means absent uptake on the posttherapy scan or reduced efficacy of ^{131}I treatment. Consequently, this author does not consider stunning to be a clinically significant phenomenon.

REFERENCES

1. Park HM, Perkins OW, Edmondson JW, et al. Influence of diagnostic radioiodines on the uptake of ablative dose of iodine-131. Thyroid 1994; 4:49–54.
2. Park HM, Park YH, Zhou XH. Detection of thyroid remnant/metastasis without stunning: an ongoing dilemma. Thyroid 1997; 7:277–280.
3. Mandel SJ, Shankar LK, Benard F, et al. Superiority of iodine-123 compared with iodine-131 scanning for thyroid remnants in patients with differentiated thyroid cancer. Clin Nucl Med 2001; 26:6–9.
4. Gerard SK. Whole-body thyroid tumor 123I scintigraphy. J Nucl Med 2003; 44:852.
5. Allman KC. Thyroid stunning revisited. J Nucl Med 2003; 44:1194.
6. Coakley A. Thyroid stunning. Eur J Nucl Med 1998; 25:203–204.
7. Brenner W. Is thyroid stunning a real phenomenon or just fiction? J Nucl Med 2002; 43:835–836.
8. Hurley JR. Management of thyroid cancer: radioiodine ablation, "stunning," and treatment of thyroglobulin-positive, (131)I scan-negative patients. Endocr Pract 2000; 6:401–406.
9. Medvedec M. Thyroid stunning. J Nucl Med 2001; 42:1129–1131.
10. Diehl M, Grunwald F. Stunning after tracer dosimetry. J Nucl Med 2001; 42:1129.
11. Mazzaferri EL, Jhiang SM. Long-term impact of initial surgical and medical therapy on papillary and follicular thyroid cancer. Am J Med 1994; 97:418–428.
12. Nemec J, Röhling S, Zamrazil V, Pohunková D. Comparison of the distribution of diagnostic and thyroablative I-131 in the evaluation of differentiated thyroid cancers. J Nucl Med 1979; 20:92–97.
13. Waxman A, Ramana L, Chapman N, et al. The significance of I-131 scan dose in patients with thyroid cancer: Determination of ablation: Concise communication. J Nucl Med 1981; 22:861–865.
14. Spies W, Wojtowicz CH, Spies SH, et al. Value of post-therapy whole-body I-131 imaging in the evaluation of patients with thyroid carcinoma having undergone high-dose I-131 therapy. Clin Nucl Med 1989; 14:793–800.
15. Pacini F, Lippi L, Formica M, et al. Therapeutic doses of iodine-131 reveal undiagnosed metastases in thyroid cancer patients with detectable serum-thyroglobulin levels. J Nucl Med 1987; 28:1888–1891.
16. Schlumberger M, Mancusi F, Baudin E, Pacini F. 131I therapy for elevated thyroglobulin levels. 1997; 7:273–276.
17. Pineda J, Lee T, Ain K, et al. Iodine-131 therapy for thyroid cancer patients with elevated thyroglobulin and negative diagnostic scan. J Clin Endocrinol Metab 1995; 80:1488–1492.
18. Rawson R, Rall JE, Peacock W. Limitations and indications in the treatment of thyroid cancer with radioactive iodine. J Clin Endocrinol Metab 1951; 11:1128–1142.
19. Cholewinski SP, Yoo KS, Klieger PS, O'Mara RE. Absence of thyroid stunning after diagnostic whole-body scanning with 185 MBq 131I. J Nucl Med 2000; 41:1198–1202.
20. Fatourechi V, Hay ID, Mullan BP, et al. Are posttherapy radioiodine scans informative and do they influence subsequent therapy of patients with differentiated thyroid cancer? Thyroid 2000; 10:573–577.
21. Bajen M, Mane S, Munoz A, Garcia JR. Effect of a diagnostic dose of 185 MBq 131I on postsurgical thyroid remnants. J Nucl Med 2000; 41:2038–2042.
22. Yeung H, Humm JL, Larson SM. Thyroid stunning. J Nucl Med 2001; 42:1130–1131.
23. McDougall IR. 74 MBq radioiodine 131I does not prevent uptake of therapeutic doses of 131I (i.e., it does not cause stunning) in differentiated thyroid cancer. Nucl Med Commun 1997; 18:505–512.
24. Cohen J, Kalinyak JE, McDougall IR. Clinical implications of the differences between diagnostic 123I and post-therapy 131I scans. Nucl Med Commun 2004; 25:129–134.
25. Hu YH, Wang PW, Wang ST, et al. Influence of 131I diagnostic dose on subsequent ablation in patients with differentiated thyroid carcinoma: discrepancy between the presence of visually apparent stunning and the impairment of successful ablation. Nucl Med Commun 2004; 25:793–797.
26. Morris LF, Waxman AD, Braunstein GD. The nonimpact of thyroid stunning: remnant ablation rates in 131I-scanned and nonscanned individuals. J Clin Endocrinol Metab 2001; 86:3507–3511.
27. Karam M, Gianoukas A, Feustel PJ, et al. Influence of diagnostic and therapeutic doses on thyroid remnant ablation rates. Nucl Med Commun 2003; 24:489–495.
28. Maxon HR, Thomas SR, Hertzberg VS, et al. Relation between effective radiation dose and outcome of radioiodine therapy for thyroid cancer. N Engl J Med 1983; 309:937–941.
29. Maxon HR. Quantitative radioiodine therapy in the treatment of differentiated thyroid cancer. Q J Nucl Med 1999; 43:313–323.

36 PART C

Stunning: Does it Exist? A Commentary

Douglas Van Nostrand

Do diagnostic prescribed activities (dosages) of ^{131}I cause stunning or not? In the first part of this section, Drs. Park and Gerard present arguments supporting the presence of stunning secondary to the administration of diagnostic dosages of ^{131}I, and in the second section, Dr. McDougall presents arguments against the presence of stunning as a significant issue. In the end, each physician will most likely select the information that one believes makes the stronger argument or best supports one's prior viewpoint. However, a third viewpoint exists to either a "yes" or "no" answer. It is a compromised viewpoint that holds: "Diagnostic doses of ^{131}I result in a spectrum ranging from no stunning to significant stunning and even treatment."

This author submits that the authors of the above two sections, as well as the authors of the references cited and not cited [1-5], are good physicians, observers, and researchers. Consequently, although one particular study may be flawed, it would be statistically unlikely that all the authors, their data, and their arguments on the positive or negative side were all wrong. Notably, all the authors appear to agree that the radiation-absorbed dose of ^{131}I to thyroid tissue and metastases depends on many factors (see Table 1). Although the specific factors that may account for the discordant observations between the various articles cannot be identified, more likely, such uncontrolled factors as those listed in Table 1 produced these discordant results, rather than the belief that all the data on a particular side were wrong. Accordingly, to answer the question, "Does stunning exist?," the author's response is: "It is a spectrum ranging from no stunning to significant stunning and even treatment."

Of course, some readers may still want to continue the debate, taking one of the two extreme positions on the stunning issue. However, to do so provides little chance of any further progress. Would it not be more productive to redirect our energy to try to identify those patients who may or may not have a high risk of clinically significant stunning? Another approach might be to change the original question regarding stunning and ask instead: "Regardless of the frequency or severity of stunning or treatment, are there reasonable alternatives for the management of patients that would eliminate, or at least minimize, the real or theoretical effects of stunning by diagnostic amounts of ^{131}I?" These alternatives might include: (1) ablation or treatment using empiric dosages of radioiodine without radioiodine scanning; (2) ^{123}I for whole body scanning; or (3) if ^{131}I is needed for dosimetry, then use the smallest amount of ^{131}I possible to achieve the desired objective. Perhaps our energy should be redirected to:

1. Evaluating and refining these alternatives.
2. Comparing the sensitivity of rhTSH-stimulated ^{123}I to ^{131}I whole-body scans.
3. Determining the feasibility of higher amounts of ^{123}I for dosimetry.
4. Encouraging commercial companies to increase the amount of ^{123}I available in a single dose at a reasonable cost.
5. Evaluating the utility of ^{124}I.

With that matter resolved, one might next wonder whether ^{124}I causes stunning?

Table 1
Factors Influencing Radiation-Absorbed Dose to Thyroid Tissue

Amount of diagnostic prescribed activity (dosage) of radioiodine administered
Uptake of radioiodine by the thyroid tissue or metastasis
Variability of residence time of radioiodine in the thyroid tissue or thyroid metastasis
Volume of thyroid tissue or metastasis
Whether the tissue consistes of normal thyroid cells or metastatic cells
Whether the metastatic cells are well-differentiated or more dedifferentiated
Interval of time from the diagnostic prescribed activity (dosage) to the time of treatment
Investigator compulsiveness in looking for "stunning"
Method to confirm or disprove stunning

REFERENCES

1. Dam HQ, Kim SM, Lin HC, Intenzo CM. 131-I therapeutic efficacy is not influenced by stunning after diagnostic whole body scanning. Radiology 2004; 232:527–533.

2. Bajen MT, Mane S, Munoz A, Garcia JR. Effect of diagnostic dose of 185 MBq 131-I on postsurgical thyroid remnants. J Nucl Med 2000; 41:2038–2042.
3. Dam HQ, Kim SM, Lin HC, Intenzo CM. ^{131}I therapeutic efficacy is not influenced by stunning after diagnostic whole body scanning. Radiology 2004; 232:527–533.
4. Gerard SK. Stunning with ^{131}I diagnostic whole-body imaging of patients with thyroid cancer. Radiology 2004; 232:972–973.
5. Dam HQ. Stunning with ^{131}I diagnostic whole-body imaging of patients with thyroid cancer. Radiology 2004; 232:973–974.

37
Ultrasonic Imaging and Identification of Metastases in Cervical Lymph Nodes

Manfred Blum

INTRODUCTION

Ultrasonography may offer diagnostic insights that improve the management of patients who have lymphadenopathy and are suspected to have thyroid cancer or who have had a thyroidectomy for cancer. This examination is valuable to assess the nature of palpable lymph nodes, detect and characterize impalpable lymphadenopathy, and also to facilitate their percutaneous aspiration biopsy. Benign nodes are common. They tend to be elliptical and have a narrow central hilum. The sonographic features of a cervical lymph node that should be regarded with high suspicion for malignancy include a plump round shape, narrowing of the hilum that is associated with widening of the cortex, inability to identify a hilum, and chaotic blood vessels, especially if they do not emanate solely from the hilum.

LYMPH NODE ANATOMY

In brief, the lymph nodes in the neck are generally divided to include: superficial cervical, anterior cervical, submental, submaxillary, and deep cervical nodes. The latter are retropharengeal, superior and inferior jugular, spinal accessory, and transverse cervical. An anatomic standard has evolved, particularly among surgeons and oncologists to communicate the location of lymphadenopathy. The system establishes seven levels according to easily recognized landmarks by dividing the neck into triangles or regions:

I: Submandibular and submental regions
II: Nodes from the skull base to the bottom of the hyoid bone (upper internal jugular or digastric nodes)
III: Nodes from the bottom of the hyoid to the bottom level of the cricoid cartilage (middle internal jugular or supraomohyoid nodes)
IV: Nodes from the bottom of the cricoid to the clavicle level (low internal jugular or infraomohyoid nodes)
V: Nodes from the skull base to the clavicle posterior to the sternocleidomastoid muscle (spinal accessory and transverse cervical nodes)
VI: Nodes between the carotid arteries from the bottom of the hyoid bone to the top of the mamubrium
VII: Nodes in the superior mediastinum below the top of the manubrium and above the innominate vein, as well as between the carotid arteries

The cervical lymph nodes are positioned to interact with antigens that are drained through afferent lymphatic channels from regional glands and other tissues. Each lymph node is surrounded by a capsule, has a distinct cortex, and a medulla that is permeated by sinusoidal channels. The subcortical region is particularly rich in sinuses. Efferent lymphatic vessels from superficial lymph nodes drain into one or more central lymph node groups before joining the thoracic duct in the left side of the neck or the lymphatic duct on the right side of the neck.

There are lymphatic capillary plexus in and around the thyroid gland that drain into lymphatic vessels and then enter lymph nodes. The internal jugular group of nodes is the main collecting system and contains 10–20 nodes on each side that are adjacent to the internal jugular vein, deep to the sternocleidomastoid muscle.

LYMPH NODES IN THYROID CANCER

In patients with thyroid cancer, as in other malignancies, we search for early manifestations of recurrent cancer. We practice with the expectation that early detection will result in successful intervention, improved outcome, and cost-effectiveness. For differentiated thyroid cancer, these hopes are unproven and difficult to substantiate because after a total thyroidectomy has been done, there is usually long survival and minimal mortality. Even patients who have recurrent thyroid cancer typically die but of other causes, and often not directly from their thyroid cancer. Some have questioned the rationale of early detection of recurrent differentiated thyroid cancer with ultrasonography. Recurrence of thyroid cancer does occur, can invade vital structures (e.g., the trachea, larynx, bone, blood vessels, and the recurrent laryngeal nerves), and can adversely affect the quality of life.

From: *Thyroid Cancer: A Comprehensive Guide to Clinical Management, 2/e*
Edited by: L. Wartofsky and D. Van Nostrand © Humana Press Inc., Totowa, NJ

These tumor deposits must be detected to initiate treatment, and it seems prudent to make the discovery as early as possible before invasion has occurred to prevent or ameliorate morbidity and, in a few cases, to forestall death. Ultrasonography makes this possible with complete safety, less cost, and with greater sensitivity than other imaging methods. Therefore, we engage in early detection with the unproven but logical expectation that early intervention will improve palliation and health.

How common are metastases to nodes in patients with differentiated thyroid cancer? The incidence of nodal metastases for differentiated thyroid cancer is greater with papillary cancer (33–61%) than with follicular cancer (5–20%), which is a relatively rare tumor (1). Based on a review of 13 large series of patients with thyroid cancer, it has been calculated that metastasis to lymph nodes will occur in 36% of 8029 adults with papillary carcinoma (2). In children, metastasis to lymph nodes may occur twice as much (3). Pathologists have shown undetected microscopic nodal metastasis with greater frequency than is perceptible during surgery or pathologic gross examination. The clinical corollary of that assertion is the demonstration that an elevated thyroglobulin concentration in the blood after a total thyroidectomy has been done is usually linked to undetected micrometastases, even if there is no ^{131}I uptake in the thyroid bed (4).

There is diverse evidence about the importance to prognosis to detect nodal recurrence after thyroidectomy for differentiated thyroid cancer. In one series, 15% of patients who had cervical lymph node metastasis died of thyroid cancer, compared with no deaths among the thyroid cancer patients with no evidence of lymph node involvement (5). Several publications have reported a higher cancer death rate when there are mediastinal or bilateral cervical lymphadenopathy (5–8). Furthermore, the 30-year cancer-specific mortality rate is threefold higher in patients who had bilateral cervical or mediastinal lymph node metastasis than in patients without lymph node disease (9). Yet, some investigations have found that lymph node metastases are of little prognostic importance in patients with thyroid cancer (10–12).

PALPATING THYROID ADENOPATHY

Several factors influence the chance that even the most experienced examiner can palpate abnormal lymph nodes. Among these are the size and consistency of the node and the habitus of the patient. Successful palpation increases with the skill and experience of the examiner and is generally limited to lymph nodes at least 1 cm in diameter and are of hard consistency. Even larger lymph nodes that are soft or are located deep in the neck, behind the carotid artery, in the tracheoesophageal groove, under the sternocleidomastoid muscle, and low in the thoracic inlet are particularly difficult to palpate, as are nodes in a very muscular or obese patient.

Table 1
Role of Thyroid Ultrasonography of Lymphadenopathy

Detect and characterize impalpable lymphadenopathy
Assess the nature of palpable lymph nodes
Ascertain the anatomic relationship of nodes to surrounding structures
Enhance the accuracy of aspiration biopsy of nodes
Provide clues that can facilitate diagnosis and treatment

Table 2
Characteristics of Benign Nodes

Elliptical or lima bean–shaped
Sharply margined
Uniform echo pattern except for hyperechogenic, narrow central hilum
L:T ratio is greater than 2
Vascular pattern is orderly and not intense
RI below 0.6
Size is not a reliable criterion

ULTRASONOGRAPHY OF CERVICAL LYMPH NODES

Cervical ultrasonography is valuable to detect impalpable lymphadenopathy, review palpable lymph nodes, ascertain the anatomic relationship of nodes to surrounding structures, enhance the accuracy of aspiration biopsy, and provide clues that can facilitate diagnosis and treatment (Table 1).

Ultrasonography of the neck can reveal normal and pathologic structures, such as cervical lymph nodes that are larger than 2–3 mm in size (13), whereas the most skilled palpation can only detect nodes that have grown to at least 1–1.5 cm. Although neither palpation nor cervical ultrsonography can reliably differentiate malignant and benign nodes, sonographic examination can offer diagnostic insights for patients suspected with thyroid cancer or who had a thyroidectomy.

ULTRASONOGRAPHY OF BENIGN LYMPH NODES

Normal nodes are commonly impalpable but detectable by ultrasonic examination (Table 2). A normal lymph node tends to be elliptical or the shape of a narrow lima bean and is sharply margined. The ratio of the longitudinal to the transverse diameter of a noncancerous lymph node (L:T ratio) is less than 1.5 (14). It has a uniform ground-glass appearance, except for a hyperechogenic, narrow but not "slit-like," central hilum (Fig. 1). On Doppler examination, the vascular pattern is orderly and not intense (15). The ratio of systolic to diastolic blood flow within a lymph node, which is the resistive index (RI), has been reported below 0.6 in benign reactive nodes (Fig. 2; 16).

Ultrasonic Imaging

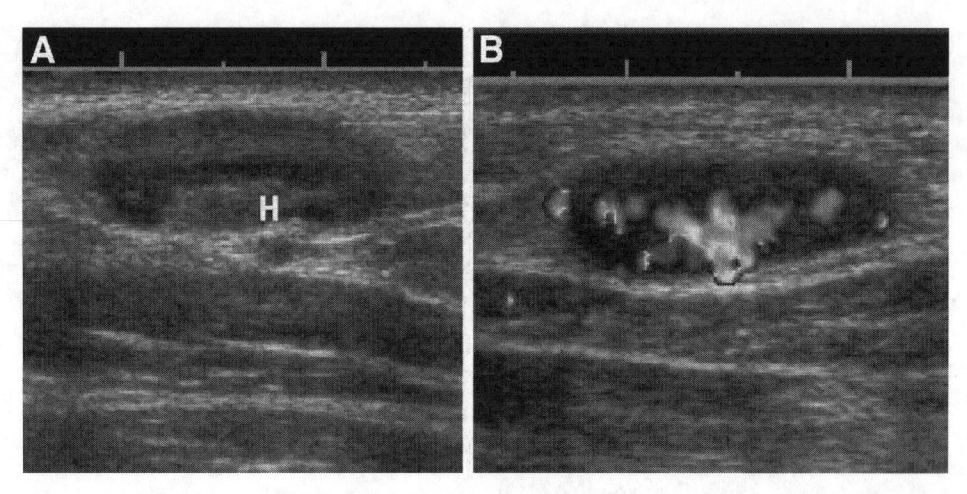

Fig. 1. Longitudinal projections of a normal lymph node on sonographic examination. **(A)** A hyperechogenic hilum. **(B)** The sonogram with Doppler, demonstrating the vascularity of the hilum. H, hilum. (Color illustration appears in insert following p. 198.)

Table 3
Characteristics That Suggest Cancerous Nodes

Plump, round shape
L:T ratio is less than 1.5
Indistinct margins
Nonhomogeneous echo pattern (sometimes cystic)
Pinhead size calcifications (psammoma bodies; coarse
 calcifications in medullary cancer)
Narrowing of the hilum associated with widening of the cortex
 or lack of a hilum
Hypervascular and with chaotic vessels on Doppler examination
RI significantly above 0.6 (mean 0.92)
Malignant nodes may cluster (like a small bunch of grapes)
Nodes are especially suggestive of metastases in the drainage
 area of the primary cancer
Size is not a reliable criterion

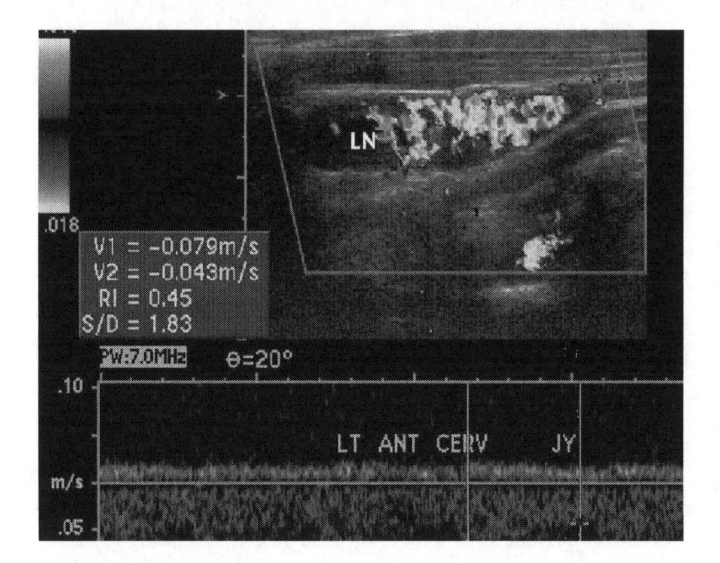

Fig. 2. Longitudinal view of a narrow, oval normal lymph node with Doppler showing physiologic vasculature. The RI is normal (0.45). LN, lymph node. (Color illustration appears in insert following p. 198.)

Size is not a reliable criterion; benign nodes may be large. In infants, children, and adolescents, nodes are more abundant and larger than in adults. Nodes may be bulky and can confuse the ultrasonic diagnosis, especially during and after regional infections and for 1–3 mo after head and neck surgery.

ULTRASONOGRAPHY OF METASTATIC THYROID CANCER LYMPH NODES

The sonographic features of a cervical lymph node that may suggest malignancy are presented in Table 3. Characteristics of nodes associated with cancer include a plump round shape, indistinct margins, narrowing of the hilum associated with widening of the cortex, lack of an identifiable hilum, a heterogeneous echo pattern that may contain cystic spaces, and changes in blood flow on Doppler examination (Fig. 3).

It is essential to have state-of-the-art ultrasound equipment and employ 12–14-MHz transducers to obtain useful information about lymphadenopathy, except that lower energy transducers are adequate to ascertain if a lymph node is elliptical or round.

Several studies have investigated the efficacy of these ultrasonic features of lymph nodes in differentiating benign and malignant processes *(14,17–20)*. Ultrasound has been reported to be able to detect thyroid cancer that is metastatic to cervical lymph nodes with a sensitivity of 92.6% *(19)*. The most useful diagnostic characteristic may be the L:T ratio, which reflects a plump shape and the presence of a central

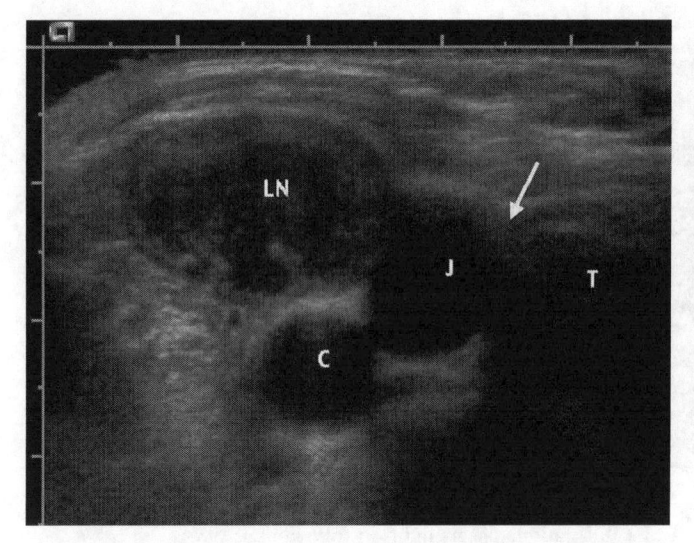

Fig. 3. Sonogram of the neck from a patient who had a total thyroidectomy for papillary cancer of thyroid. This is a transverse projection of a rounded, heterogeneous lymph node without Doppler. The node is involved with papillary thyroid cancer. The thyroidectomy bed (→) is free of thyroid tissue. LN, pathologic lymph node; J, jugular vein; C, carotid artery; T, air in the trachea. (Color illustration appears in insert following p. 198.)

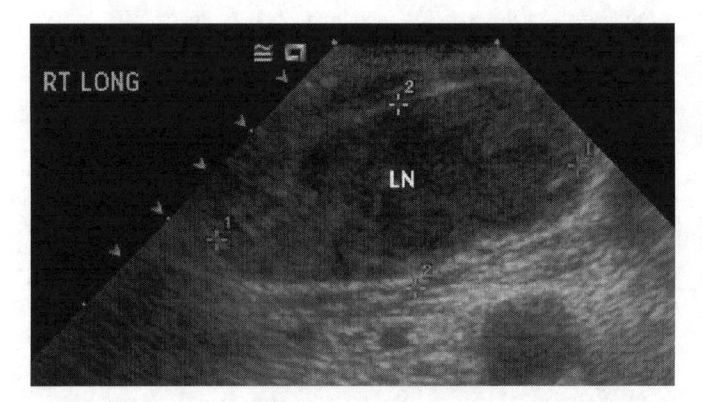

Fig. 4. Longitudinal projection of a sonogram of a plump, heterogeneous lymph node involved with metastatic papillary thyroid cancer. The L:T ratio was 2.5. Note the absence of a hilum. LN, lymph node. (Color illustration appears in insert following p. 198.)

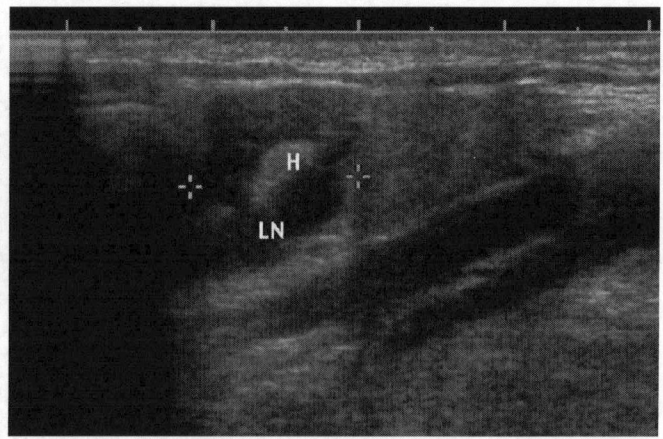

Fig. 5. Longitudinal view of a sonogram of a lymph node that was plump and was therefore deemed suspicious by the fatty hilum, suggesting benign disease. Biopsy revealed a reactive node, not cancer. LN, lymph node; H, hilum. (Color illustration appears in insert following p. 198.)

echogenic hilum (14,18,19). Vassallo and associates found that the L:T ratio was less than 1.5 in 62% of metastatic nodes and greater than 2 in 79% of reactive nodes (14; Fig. 4). Furthermore, using rotation of the scanning plane to identify the largest diameter of a node, they provided fairly convincing evidence that benign lymph nodes tend to be narrowly oval in shape; those malignant are usually round. Solbaiti and associates (18) evaluating 291 lymph nodes in 143 patients before surgical dissection of the neck because of thyroid cancer reported on the significance of a central echogenic hilum and a peripheral hypoechogenic cortex. The combination of the narrowing hilum and cortex widening was seen in 90% of malignant nodes but in only 54% of benign nodes. In contrast, an elliptical or wide hilum was a useful criterion for identifying low likelihood of malignancy, as confirmed by Vassallo et al. (14) in 15 of 26 (58%) of benign reactive nodes and in only 5 of 68 (8%) of malignant nodes. In the same publication, they reported that the inability to identify a hilum with high-resolution equipment was uncommon in benign nodes (Fig. 5) but not a good indicator of malignancy. In their series, only 2 of 26 (8%) reactive nodes lacked a hilum, but a hilum was not observed in only 36 of 68 (44%) nodes that were occupied by malignancy. Finding a "slit-like" narrow hilum was also not that useful to identify a cancerous node in their series, observed in 33 of 68 (49%) benign nodules and 9 of 26 (35%) malignant nodules.

The margin of a lymph node has been reported as offering insight into the risk of malignancy but has poor sensitivity. However, special wariness is appropriate when a node exhibits focal loss of a distinct interface between the nodes and its surroundings, a bulge, or indentation or displacement of an adjacent structure.

Certain characteristics of nodal vascularity on Doppler examination may be diagnostically useful to identify cancer, but the results are controversial. The blood vessel flow in cancerous nodes has been described as enhanced and chaotic. One study found that malignant nodes demonstrate enhanced color flow signals more often (29 of 32) than benign (6 of 16; 20). Prominent hilar vascularity has been reported in metastatic nodes from papillary carcinoma, but this may also be observed in reactive nodes (21). Indeed, another investigation suggested that these abundant color flow signals are not at all useful for identifying cancer in lymph nodes (16; Fig. 6). Perhaps, more diagnostically important than the

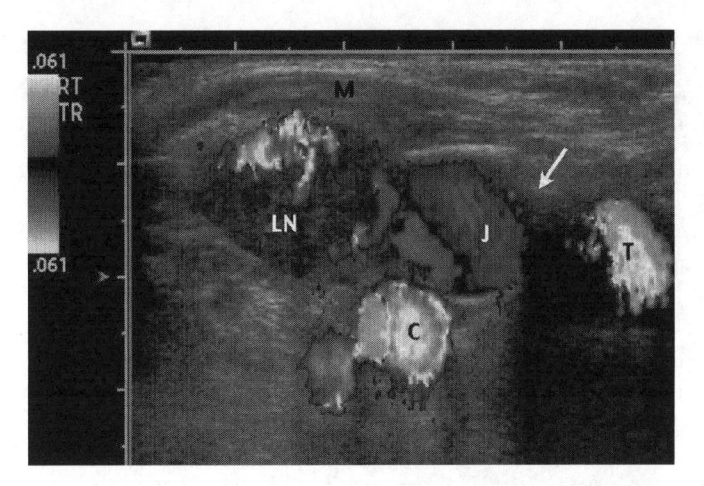

Fig. 6. Transverse projection of a sonogram of a rounded lymph node in the right jugular chain after thyroidectomy for papillary cancer of thyroid. The RI was 7.7, which is abnormally high. (→), Note absence of thyroid lobe; LN, pathologic lymph node with prominent heterogeneous vascular channels in its superficial and medial regions. J, jugular vein; C, carotid artery; T, artifact created by air in the trachea; M, muscle. (Color illustration appears in insert following p. 198.)

magnitude of enhanced blood flow from the hilum will be establishing that the chaotic blood vessels emanate from the periphery of the node (signifying the neovascularity of cancer), rather than from the hilum. Another useful feature appears to be the RI. It has been reported that cancerous lymph nodes have a RI above 0.6 (mean 0.92), whereas reactive nodes have a considerably lower index (<0.6; *16*).

There may be calcifications in cancerous nodes. Pinhead size specks of calcium may represent the psammoma bodies of papillary cancer (Figs. 7 and 8), but coarse deposits are not specific; however, in medullary thyroid cancer, large accretions of calcium are a typical finding.

Malignant nodes may cluster like a small bunch of grapes, and nodes are particularly suggestive of metastases if they occur in the drainage area of the cancer. However, isolated nodes even when they are contralateral to the primary lesion may be cancerous.

To reiterate an important point, size is not a reliable criterion; benign nodes may be large, and those that are cancerous can be quite small and nonpalpable (Fig. 7). Sutton and colleagues *(17)* reported that size, shape, and gross internal architecture of lymph nodes did not reliably segregate benign and malignant lesions.

Kessler et al. reported that cystic changes in enlarged nodes should suggest papillary thyroid cancer *(22)*. A total of 63 patients with enlarged cervical lymph nodes, all of whom had ultrasound-guided aspiration biopsy and 27 had surgical excision, were analyzed retrospectively. Of 20 patients who had papillary thyroid cancer, 14 (70%) had cystic changes in the nodes. Intranodal cystic changes were not observed among

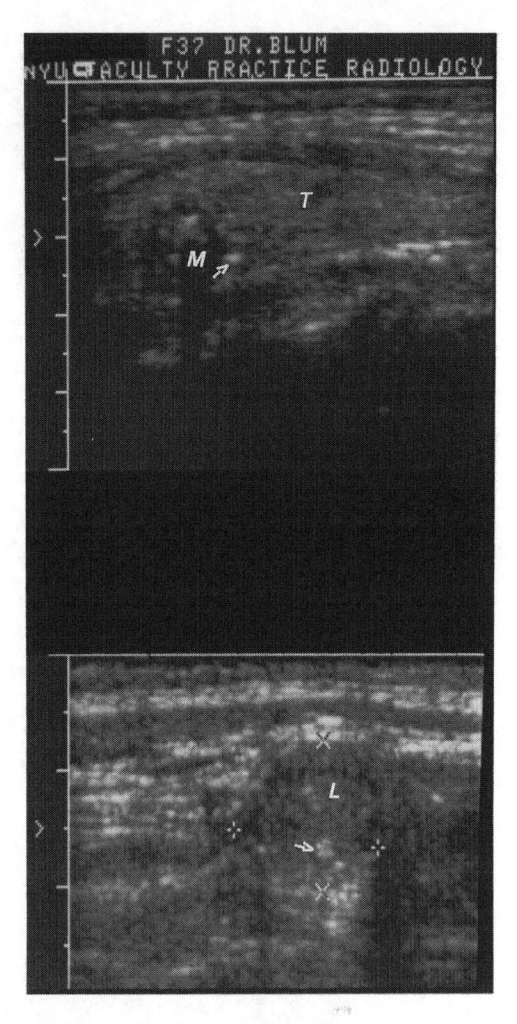

Fig. 7. The images demonstrate the use of sonography to detect a nonpalpable primary thyroid when adenopathy is palpated. A 37-yr-old obese female had a palpable, firm, 2-cm lymph node in the right jugular chain of nodes. The thyroid region was not abnormal on palpation. Sonograms of the neck in the longitudinal plane are shown. **(Top)** A 1-cm hypoechoic mass is seen in the upper posterior portion of the right thyroid lobe. Minute bright spots are calcifications (possibly psammoma bodies). **(Bottom)** The lymph node that was palpated is 1.8 cm in diameter, rounded, and also has calcifications. Surgery revealed papillary thyroid cancer with psammoma bodies and adenopathy. T, thyroid lobe; L, lymph node; arrow, calcification.

the patients with other cancers that were metastatic to nodes or in benign reactive lymphadenopathy. Although the data yielded a 70% sensitivity, 100% specificity, 100% positive predictive value, 88% negative predictive value, and 90% overall accuracy for cystic spaces in enlarged pathologic nodes, caution is advised with this criterion because cystic degeneration of tuberculous nodes has been seen. Therefore, certain chronic infections could lead to confusion. Examination of a larger series is needed to validate the reported perfect specificity and positive predictive value of this observation.

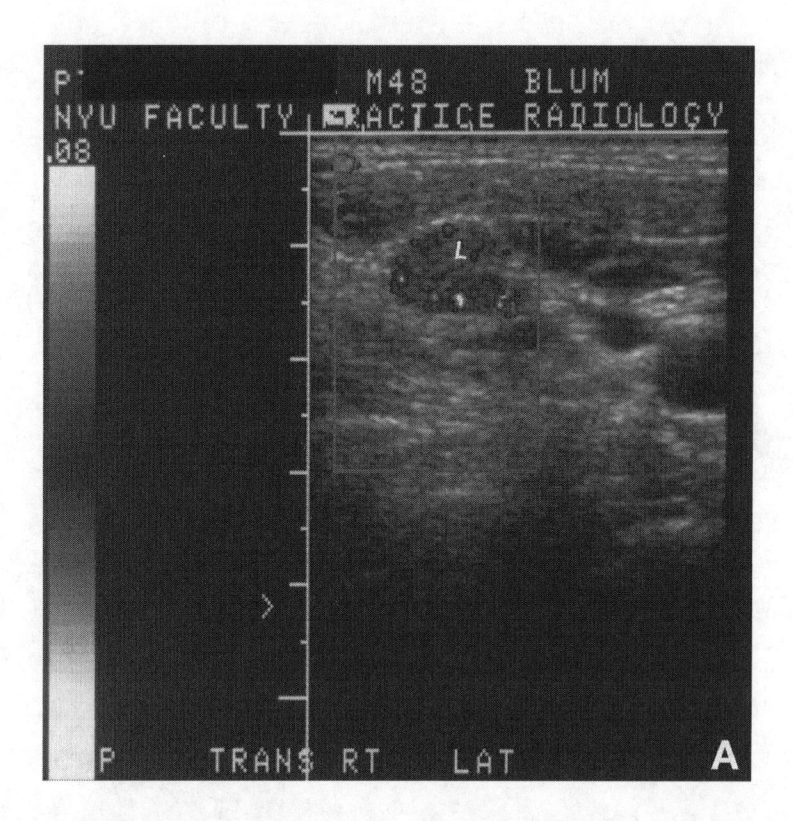

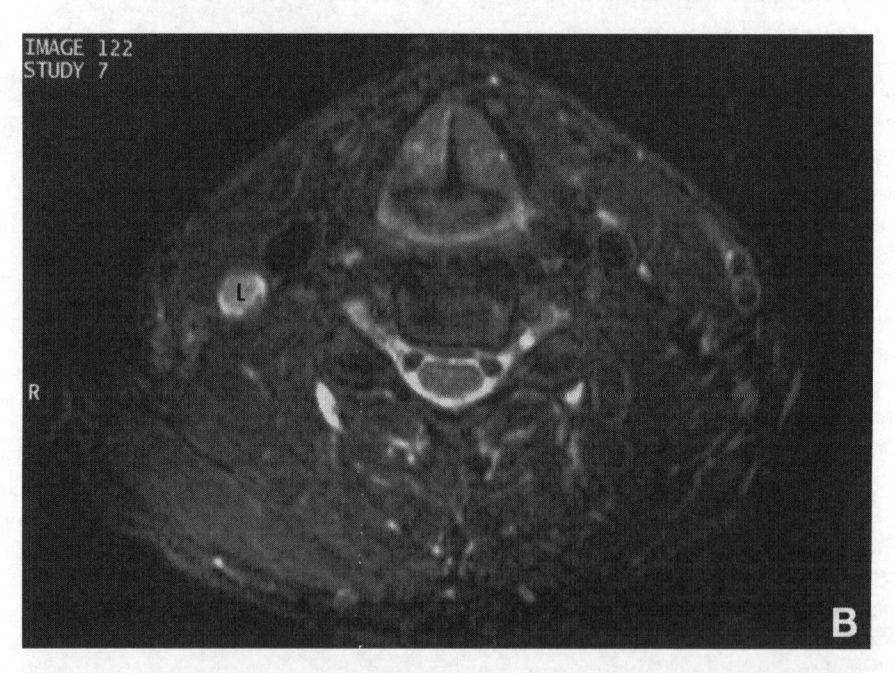

Fig. 8. Use of sonography in routine follow-up; nonpalpable adenopathy was found. Magnetic resonance imaging confirmed the abnormality. The node was malignant. The images are from a 48-yr-old muscular male who had a total thyroidectomy 5 yr previously for papillary thyroid cancer. The examination was physiologic, thyrotropin was 0.2 µIU/mL, and thyroglobulin was less than 0.5 ng/dL while he was taking 200 µg of L-thyroxine daily. A sonogram of the neck was done as part of routine reevaluation. **(A)** One film of the sonogram demonstrating a rounded pathologic lymph node with loss of the fatty hilum. The rectangle denotes a Doppler examination. The bright spots indicate blood vessels. The patient and referring physician were unwilling to accept the need for treatment until magnetic resonance imaging was done, as shown in **B**. The lesion was confirmed as a bright mass on the T-2 image, consistent with cancer. Subsequently, the suppressive therapy was discontinued, thyrotropin and thyroglobulin rose, a whole-body ^{131}I scan was found positive, and he was treated with [131]I. L, pathologic lymph node.

CLINICAL PERSPECTIVE ON ULTRASONOGRAPHY OF ADENOPATHY

A useful working concept is that the sonographic anatomic and vascular features of nodes provide useful hints in clinical problem-solving, but ultrasound correlates imperfectly with histology. State-of-the-art equipment with Doppler capability and an experienced examiner aware of the medical question and willing to devote the time required for a thorough evaluation, performed in multiple planes, are necessary to evaluate lymphadenopathy properly. Primitive apparatus with transducers below 10 MHz and routine scanning by the average technician with subsequent image interpretation by a radiologist or clinician who lacks specific education and experience cannot be expected to yield optimal diagnostic information. With those cautions, one may conclude that a reasonably accurate clinical diagnosis of nodal metastatic disease is possible using multiple criteria described but not one feature alone. Also, malignancy is highly unlikely when a node is narrow with an L:T ratio that is significantly greater than 2, especially if the node has a central echogenic hilum. Unfortunately, the sensitivity and specificity for detecting cancer in a lymph node with any of the ultrasonographic features are not that high unless the node is quite plump and impinges on or invades adjacent structures. Furthermore, prudence is warranted in interpreting sonographic images of adenopathy in children.

ULTRASOUND SURVEILLANCE AFTER THYROIDECTOMY

Although relapses from thyroid cancer most often occur in the first decade after the cancer has been discovered (23), cancer may recur many years after apparent complete remission (24,25). Therefore it is reasonable to repeat cervical ultrasonography annually for 10 yr after thyroidectomy for differentiated thyroid cancer, then at infrequent intervals, perhaps every 5–10 yr.

ULTRASOUND-GUIDED PERCUTANEOUS ASPIRATION BIOPSY OF CERVICAL LYMPH NODES

Percutaneous biopsy of thyroid nodules and adenopathy with and without ultrasound guidance is discussed in Chapters 17, 18, 25. Several investigators have studied the utility of aspiration biopsy of lymph nodes that are involved with metastatic thyroid cancer. Takashima reported correlation with the surgical findings in 62 patients who had impalpable cervical lymph nodes (mean diameter, 0.8 cm), with 95% sensitivity, 94% specificity, and 94% accuracy (26). Lee and colleagues (27) reported on 36 cervical lymph node biopsies in 29 patients with cervical lymphadenopathy and suspected recurrent differentiated thyroid cancer. They found 91% sensitivity and 100% specificity. Furthermore, the presence of a high concentration of thyroglobulin in the biopsy aspirate of a lymph node should strongly suggest the diagnosis of metastasis from thyroid carcinoma (4). The combined diagnostic sensitivity and specificity of tissue marker analysis (thyroglobulin or calcitonin) and cytopathological examination has been extimated as 100% (27).

INTRAOPERATIVE ULTRASONOGRAPHY AND LYMPHADENOPATHY

Intraoperative ultrasonic examination performed by the surgeon has been reported to enhance the detection of nonpalpable adenopathy, as well as to alter the surgical management. However, there is no information on the benefit of surgically removing small (or larger) pathologic nodes; however, in the past, radical dissection of the neck did not enhance the outcome of patients with differentiated thyroid cancer when compared to more limited surgery. Yet, in selected patients, when a tumor deposit is located in a vital area, and therapy with ^{131}I is not possible, surgery may be palliative or conceivably curative. In that case, intraoperative ultrasonic identification of nonpalpable tumor may be important. After the surgeon has completed a thyroidectomy, intraoperative ultrasonography could become standard to assess for adequacy of dissection, looking for and removing undetected nodes before "closing."

The feasibility of intraoperative ultrasonography in the surgical management of patients with recurrent thyroid cancer is under investigation. In one study, ultrasound was required to identify nonpalpable deposits of tumor in 7 of 13 patients with recurrent, scan-negative papillary thyroid cancer, 11 of whom had elevated thyroglobulin levels. In these 11 patients, the preoperative thyroglobulin level declined in 10 patients and became undetectable in 7 (28). They also reported that ultrasonography was the most useful in patients with a history of external-beam radiotherapy. Another investigation focused on surgeon-controlled real-time ultrasound (29). Sonography was performed intraoperatively when nonpalpable, cancerous cervical lymph nodes were suspected and was reported to significantly influence surgical management.

ULTRASONOGRAPHY WITH OTHER IMAGING

It is necessary at times to augment sonography selectively to elucidate distorted anatomy, resolve conflicting medical opinions, or expose the origin of tumor markers, such as elevation of calcitonin or thyroglobulin when sonography does not reveal the responsible site (Fig. 8). In such circumstances, scintiscanning, computed tomography, or magnetic resonance imaging should be employed, as discussed in Chapter 38.

REFERENCES

1. Simpson WJ, McKinney SE, Carruthers JS, et al. Papillary and follicular thyroid cancer: prognostic factors in 1,578 patient. Am J Med 1987; 83:479–488.
2. Mazzaferri EL. Thyroid carcinoma: Papillary and follicular. In Mazzaferri EL, Samaan N, editors. Endocrine Tumors. Cambridge, MA: Blackwell Scientific Publications, 1993.
3. De Keyser LFM, Van Herle AJ. Differentiated thyroid cancer in children. Head and Neck Surg 1985; 8:100–114.
4. Pacini F, Fugazzola L, Lippi F, et al. Detection of thyroglobulin in fine needle aspirates of non-thyroidal neck masses: a clue to the diagnosis of metastatic differentiated thyroid cancer. J Clin Endocrinol Metab 1992; 74:1401–1404.
5. Sellers M, Beenken S, Blankenship A, et al. Prognostic significance of cervical lymph nodes metastasis in differentiated thyroid cancer. Am J Surg 1992; 164:578–581.
6. Akslen LA, Haldorsen T, Thoresen SO, Glattre E. Survival and causes of death in thyroid cancer. A population-based study of 2,479 cases from Norway. Cancer Res 1991; 51:1234–1241.
7. De Groot LJ, Kaplan EL, McCormick M, Straus FH. Natural history, and course of papillary thyroid carcinoma. J Clin Endocrinol Metabol 1990; 71:414–424.
8. Scheumann GSW, Gimm O, Wegener G, et al. Prognostic significance and surgical management of locoregional lymph node metastasis in papillary thyroid cancer. World J Surg 1994; 18:559–568.
9. Mazzaferri EL, Jhiang SM. Long term impact of initial surgical and medical therapy on papillary and follicular thyroid cancer. Am J Med 1994; 97:418.
10. al-Saleh MS, al-Kattan TM. Incidence of carcinoma in multinodular goiter in Saudi Arabia. J R Coll Surg Edimb 1994; 39:106.
11. Carcangiu ML. Papillary carcinoma of the thyroid: a clinical pathologic study of 241 cases treated at the University of Florence, Italy. Cancer 1985; 55:805.
12. Hay ID, Bergstralh EJ, Goellner JR, Ebersold JR, Grant CS. Predicting outcome in papillary thyroid carcinoma: development of a reliable prognostic scoring system in a cohort of 1,779 patients surgically treated at one institution during 1940-1989. Surgery 1993; 114:1050.
13. Blum M. Evaluation of thyroid function; sonography, computed tomography and magnetic resonance imaging. In Becker KL, editor. Principles and Practice of Endocrinology and Metabolism. Philadelphia, PA: Lippincott Co., 1990: 289–293.
14. Vassallo P, Wernecke K, Roos N, Peters PE. Differentiation of benign from malignant superficial lymphadenopathy: the role of high-resolution US. Radiology 1992; 183:215–220.
15. Kakkos SK, Scopa CD, Chalmoukis AK, et al. Relative risk of cancer in sonographically dectected thyroid nodules with calcifications. J Clin Ultrasound 2000; 28:347.
16. Choi M, Lee JW, Jang KJ. Distinction between benign and malignant causes of cervical, axillary, and inguinal adenopathy: value of Doppler spectral waveform analysis. Am J Roentg 1995; 165:981–984.
17. Sutton RT, Reading CC, Charboneau JW, et al. US-guided biopsy of neck masses in preoperative management of patients with thyroid cancer. Radiology 1988; 168:769–772.
18. Solbiati L, Arsizio B, Rizzatto G, et al. High resolution sonography of cervical lymph nodes in head and neck cancer: criteria for differentiation of reactive versus malignant nodes. Radiology 1988; 169:113.
19. Bruneton JN, Roux P, Caramella E, et al. Ear, nose, and throat cancer: Ultrasound diagnosis of metastasis to cervical lymph nodes. Radiology 1984; 152:771–773.
20. Chang DB, Yuan A, Yu CJ, et al. Differentiation of benign and malignant cervical lymph nodes with color Doppler sonography. Am J Roentg 1994; 162:965–968.
21. Ahuja AT, Ying M, Yuen HY, Metreweli C. Power Doppler sonography of metastatic nodes from papillary carcinoma of the thyroid. Clin Radiol 2001; 56:284–288.
22. Kessler A, Rappaport Y, Blank A, et al. Cystic appearance of cervical lymph nodes is characteristic of metastatic papillary thyroid carcinoma. J Clin Ultrasound 2003; 31:21–25.
23. Mazzaferri EL, et al. Papillary thyroid carcinoma: the impact of therapy in 576 patients. Medicine 1997; 56:171.
24. Schlumberger, et al. Follow-up of patients with differentiated thyroid carcinoma. Eur J Cancer Calan Oncol 1988; 24:345.
25. Blum M, Perlman S. Reducing suppressive therapy in patients with a history of thyroid cancer. Ann Int Med 1995; 123:807–809.
26. Takashima S, Yoshida J, Kishimoto H, et al. Nonpalpable lymph nodes of the neck: assessment with US and US-guided fine-needle aspiration biopsy. Radiology 1995; 197(Suppl):270.
27. Lee MJ, Ross DS, Mueller PR, et al. Fine-needle biopsy of cervical lymph nodes in patients with thyroid cancer: a prospective comparison of cytopathologic and tissue marker analysis. Radiology 1993; 187:851–854.
28. Karwowski JK, Jeffrey RB, McDougall IR, Weigel RJ. Intraoperative ultrasonography improves identification of recurrent thyroid cancer. Surgery 2002; 132:924–928.
29. Solorzano CC, Carneiro DM, Ramirez M, et al. Surgeon-performed ultrasound in the management of thyroid malignancy. Am Surg 2004; 70:576–580.

38
Magnetic Resonance Imaging and Computed Tomography of Thyroid Cancer

James J. Jelinek, Kenneth D. Burman, Richard S. Young, and Alexander S. Mark

INTRODUCTION

This chapter discusses the role of magnetic resonance imaging (MRI) and computed tomography (CT) in the evaluation of patients with thyroid cancer. Traditionally, patients with thyroid cancer have been diagnosed based on an evaluation initiated by clinical examination of a palpable thyroid nodule, accounting for about 60% of ultimate diagnoses of thyroid cancer. An additional 20% or more patients are found to have thyroid cancer based on a clinical presentation with findings of adjacent cervical and/or supraclavicular lymph nodes. However, the increased utilization of both MRI and CT of the head and neck has led to the "incidental" discovery of thyroid lesions that may comprise as many as 20% of patients who are diagnosed with thyroid cancer. For example, there is widespread use of CT in the evaluation of the cervical spine in trauma, evaluation of the neck for any type of neck mass or hoarseness, and significantly increased use in the evaluation of patients with lung disease and/or suspected pulmonary embolism. Similarly, MRI is increasingly utilized, particularly in the examination of pathology related to the cervical spine (e.g., disc herniation and stenosis). MRI angiography is also more frequently used for the analysis of stroke to assess possible stenosis of the carotid and vertebral arteries. Furthermore, these techniques demonstrate and image abnormalities of the thyroid gland and, when a suspected mass is seen, lead to a work-up of potential thyroid tumor. With the growing utilization of both MRI and CT, the rate of discovery of thyroid cancer is expected to increase.

INCIDENTALOMAS

The incidental finding of thyroid masses is becoming more common. Although less than 1% of all cancers are present in the thyroid gland, thyroid nodules are found in at least 4–10% of the adult population [1]. However, in the routine interpretation of neck and chest CT and MRI, a higher percentage of the adult population have only small lesions or "incidentalomas" detected on CT, MRI, or ultrasound. These could be present in as many as 40% of the adult population. The decision when incidental lesions should be evaluated further for possible thyroid cancer is extremely controversial and difficult given the high prevalence of thyroid lesions detected by both CT and MRI (see Chapters 17 and 23). However, when a nodule is greater than 1–1.5 cm in size, it may be more prudent to seek consultation regarding potential thyroid aspiration and biopsy. Even smaller lesions may be biopsied in special circumstances, such as a history of neck radiation exposure or a family history of thyroid cancer. Clearly, the major role of clinical history and careful physical examination of the neck remains paramount. Ultrasound guidance for fine-needle aspiration (FNA) is commonplace today (see Chapter 21), and MRI and CT do not have an impact in the guidance of biopsy for most thyroid nodules [1,2]. Only rare incidentally diagnosed masses of the thyroid gland that are not reachable by traditional ultrasound methods (e.g., substernal mass) should be biopsied by CT. Even small thyroid nodules that are immediately adjacent to the carotid artery and jugular veins do not preclude biopsy with ultrasound. In fact, such location may make FNA under ultrasound guidance even more strongly warranted. In our institution, the overwhelming majority of FNAs are performed with no imaging guidance. However, of those FNAs performed with radiologic guidance, 99% are performed with ultrasound with biopsy under CT, accounting for only an unusual subset of patients, specifically for deep cervical or infraclavicular postoperative recurrences. When needle aspirations should be performed with radiology guidance is a controversial issue. In the past, the vast majority of aspirations were of palpable nodules, and the aspirations were performed by palpation. More recently, as techniques have evolved, a greater percentage of all aspirations are performed under radiological guidance. Obviously, all nonpalpable nodules must be treated with imaging guidance.

ANATOMY OF THE NECK

The primary role of MRI and CT in the evaluation of thyroid cancer is in the follow-up of recurrent thyroid cancer. To

From: *Thyroid Cancer: A Comprehensive Guide to Clinical Management, 2/e*
Edited by: L. Wartofsky and D. Van Nostrand © Humana Press Inc., Totowa, NJ

appreciate the value of MRI and CT of the neck, a brief review of the anatomy of the neck is required. The thyroid gland is present in the lowest part of the neck, just above the sternal notch. The thyroid gland lies deep to the anterior neck muscles: the sternocleidomastoid muscle, omohyoid muscle, sternothyroid muscles, and sternohyoid muscles (3). The thyroid gland sits like a saddle over the trachea with the thinnest portion of the thyroid gland (isthmus) lying directly anterior to the trachea. The vital structures of the neck adjacent to the thyroid gland are all posterior. Moving from lateral to medial, the largest vital structure posterior and lateral is the internal jugular vein. The carotid artery, with its adjacent vagus nerve, typically resides directly medial to the jugular vein (3). Resulting from normal variations of anatomy in patients, the internal carotid artery and jugular vein can reside relatively more lateral or even quite close to midline. The recurrent laryngeal nerve resides immediately between each lateral lobe of the thyroid gland and the trachea. The esophagus is directly posterior to the trachea but may be slightly to the left and posterior to the trachea.

Other important structures include the phrenic nerve, which is typically more posterior to the jugular vein. The muscles of the longus colli and scalenus muscles are posterior to these vital structures. Notably, the roots of the brachial plexus reside between the anterior and middle scalene muscles. The important structures of the larynx, including the cricoid cartilage, thyroid cartilage, cartilage of the arytenoids, cuniculate, and cuneiforms are just cephalad to the thyroid gland.

CLASSIFICATION OF LYMPH NODES

Lymph nodes have been classified by the American Joint Committee on Cancer (4). Classification systems typically refer to the size and character of the lymph nodes. Nodes larger than 1 cm are considered more at risk of harboring cancer, and benign nodes are typically oval-shaped and comprise a discernable hilum (see Chapter 37 on Ultrasound of Lymph Nodes). Unfortunately, it is becoming clear that thyroid cancer may be found in lymph nodes smaller than 1 cm, which lack classic suspicious characteristics (5). The typical staging describes *level I* lymph nodes as those that are present directly below the myohyoid tongue muscles and anterior to the submandibular glands. Typically, level I lymph nodes have been described as submental lymph nodes; however, particularly in the newer classification (6), lymph nodes that are lateral to the medial edge of the anterior belly of the gastric muscle are also considered level I. These have also been previously referred to as "submandbular lymph nodes." *Level II* are lymph nodes above the level of the hyoid bone, along the carotid artery and jugular veins, typically referred to as "upper jugular lymph nodes." *Level III* are middle level jugular nodes that are present at the level of the hyoid bone. *Level IV* are lower jugular nodes and are below the level of the hyoid bone, extending down to the level of the clavicle. *Level V* are lymph nodes anterior to the trapezius muscle but posterior to the sternocleidomastoid muscle. *Level VI* (anterior compartment) are midline anterior nodes between the manubrium and hyoid bone anteriorly (4).

COMPUTED TOMOGRAPHY

CT generates images using a series of X-ray beams and detectors. As in other areas of medicine, there have been huge strides in the technological advances of CT. Older CT studies were typically performed with slice thickness ranging from 5 to 10 mm. Today, slice thickness is usually 3 mm. In many advanced centers, 1–2-mm thickness is obtained, and the set of images are not just presented in the axial plane. Using 1 mm or less slice thickness allows the performance of isotropic images to enable the neck to be imaged in any plane, most commonly in the axial, sagittal, and coronal planes. Images can also be easily presented as a full three-dimensional color image.

CT scanners today are considerably faster than any other imaging modality; in most cases, the total time of the imaging is less than 60 s. Specifically for the evaluation of the neck, almost all radiologists strongly prefer X-ray contrast, which contains a high-iodine content. Contrast is ideal to show a marked difference between the arteries and veins against their adjacent structures. With the infusion of iodinated contrast, there is a more striking contrast in the soft-tissue appearance of lymph nodes vs muscle and other adjacent tissues, e.g., the salivary glands. Unfortunately, in patients with thyroid cancer, the ability to use iodinated contrast is restricted because of the effect of iodine excess on potential radioiodine scanning and/or therapy. Noncontrast CTs of the neck are much more difficult to interpret and have a lower sensitivity and specificity. The use of iodine may interfere with diagnostic evaluation by ^{123}I or ^{131}I, as well as the treatment of many thyroid cancers with ^{131}I. For some thyroid cancers, such as the anaplastic form, this may not be an issue. Nonetheless, as a standard default, it is prudent for all thyroid cancer patients imaged by CT to not be given iodinated contrast unless it is explicitly stated by the managing physician that it is permissible. It is unpredictable how long it may take the radioiodinated contrast to be dissipated in a given individual, as this may be influenced by thyroid or metabolic status, renal function, and so on. Iodine uptake may be blunted for 3–8 wk.

The typical advantages of CT are the widespread availability of CT scanners, the quick scan times, the increasing ability to achieve slice thickness of 1–3 mm, and the easy generation of reformatted images in any plane, including axial, sagittal, and oblique images. The major drawback is that the CT of the soft-tissue neck is markedly limited by the inability to use iodinated contrast in many thyroid cancer patients. For this reason, most centers do not use CT in the early evaluation and subsequent follow-up of patients with thyroid cancer.

MAGNETIC RESONANCE IMAGING

Unlike CT, MRI does not require the use of X-rays; hence, there is no radiation to the patient. Nonetheless, MRI does generate electromagnetic waves and images primarily the hydrogen atoms within the body. Different pulse sequences are performed by applying radiofrequency pulses to the body. Typically, MRI has employed T1- and T2-weighted images. These two properties of T1 and T2 would be difficult to explain without some degree of physics explanation of radiofrequency-generated pulses and the effect on H protons, which is beyond the scope of this book. The T1-weighted images typically show excellent anatomic boundaries between tissues. T2-weighted images are more useful in the evaluation of pathologic processes, particularly local lymph nodes and tumors. T2-weighted images often demonstrate tumors, adenopathy, fluid, and inflammation as being "bright" *(7)*. In addition to the typical T1- and T2-weighted sequences, newer MRI sequences are usually used in other parts of the body, specifically short T1 inversion recovery (STIR) sequences that are used as a fat-suppressing, water/edema/tumor–enhancing modality. This is frequently utilized in neuroimaging, as well as the detection of bone lesions. STIR imaging is not frequently involved in neck imaging. Other sequences, such as gradient-echo images, are quite sensitive to the detection of hemorrhage. Similar to STIR imaging, most centers do not use gradient sequences in neck evaluation.

Benefits and Disadvantages

When performing oncology imaging, many centers currently give MRI contrast. Most MRI contrast gadolinium, which is an inert element. Several features make the MRI contrast agent significantly better than CT contrast agents. Unlike CT contrast agents, there is no iodine and consequently no contraindication for the routine imaging of patients with thyroid cancer. Other significant advantages of the MRI contrast agent are the incredibly low incidence of minor contrast reactions. With iodine-related CT contrast agents, 5% of patients will experience hives, extreme warmth, or nausea. These side effects are extremely rare with the gadolinium MRI contrast agent. Furthermore, the rare incidence of major anaphylactic reactions associated with CT contrast is almost nonexistent with MRI. Nonetheless, there are rare cases of MRI contrast reactions. Typically, these reactions are minor and include headaches. Only extremely rare reports of severe reactions to gadolinium have been documented in the worldwide literature over the last two decades. The volume of gadolinium contrast is typically 15 mL, as opposed to over 100 mL used for contrast CT.

The disadvantages to MRI are that the overall examination time is significantly longer than that of CT. However, today's MRI scanners are much faster than older equipment, and examinations can be frequently completed in 30–40 min, whereas previous examinations performed in the 1980s and 90s often took over 1 h. With modern equipment today, imaging techniques have now also changed. Imaging slice thickness used to vary between 5 and 10 mm; on current examination scanners, even with reduced scan time, a typical image sequence can be obtained using 3-mm slice thickness. As has always been the case, an advantage of MRI is that it can be obtained in the axial, sagittal, and coronal planes.

The most significant factors that would preclude a patient from getting an MRI are the interference with metallic devices. The devices that cause potential problems include pacemakers, some implanted cochlear (ear) devices, and older aneurysm clips. (Most modern intracranial aneurysm clips are now made of material that is MRI-compatible.) Before any patient with an intracranial aneurysm clip has an MRI, it should be confirmed that the clip is MRI-compatible. Regardless, all patients should be carefully screened before entering the MRI to make sure there are no metallic substances on their body. An additional problem is that there is an increasing problem of claustrophobia associated with CT. For some patients, it may be beneficial to provide medication to decrease the anxiety of being within a closed space. Valium is typically used for this condition. Newer MRI units are available in an "open" configuration. However, the "open" MRI units do not have the same resolution capacity as the high-field closed units. Particularly with thyroid imaging, it is not uncommon to try to detect 3–4-mm lymph nodes. The "open" MRI units are simply not able to image to this detail. Generally, the cost of CT imaging is 20–30% less than MRI. Ultrasound is significantly less expensive, but its image quality varies greatly depending on the skill of the ultrasonographer *(8)*.

MRI VS CT

In the follow-up of patients with thyroid cancer, the older literature seems to indicate a preference for contrast CT over MRI *(9,10)*. Most of these studies were performed in the evaluation of cervical lymph nodes in patients with primary head and neck (squamous) carcinoma *(11)*. No study has been performed that directly compares MRI vs CT in the evaluation of thyroid cancer; however, patients with thyroid cancer are not typically recommended for iodinated contrast. There is little benefit of imaging by noncontrast CT over an MRI. Furthermore, with the newer equipment, higher soft-tissue contrast and spatial resolution, along with the use of MRI contrast agents, newer literature shows a preference for contrast MRI over contrast CT *(8,12)*. Thus, most radiologists evaluating the extent of recurrent adenopathy in the neck or chest prefer MRI both without and with contrast, which has become the mainstay when advanced cross-sectional imaging is required, especially for the evaluation of recurrence in patients with thyroid cancer.

APPROPRIATE MRI AND CT USE IN FOLLOW-UP OF PATIENTS WITH THYROID CANCER

Physicians reviewing patients with thyroid cancer have a number of different physiologic and anatomic studies at their disposal (13). Typically, follow-up imaging has been performed with ^{123}I and ^{131}I but in most cases, ^{123}I is preferable. In addition, a standard of practice is to follow serum thyroglobulin levels in appropriate individuals. Large recurrences are easily detected by clinical examination and ultrasound; however, it is not uncommon for patients to have abnormal ^{123}I uptake or increasing thyroglobulin levels, with no abnormal findings on clinical exam or ultrasound. Therefore, MRI has a more important role in the detection of small lesions. The sensitivity and specificity of MRI varies based on the criteria utilized. Traditional imaging with CT and MRI has often used a short-axis diameter dimension of 1 cm for determining if an individual lymph node is either benign or malignant. However, in the evaluation of thyroid cancer, this method is no longer valid. Many small local recurrent lymph nodes detected by ^{123}I, rising thyroglobulin levels, or positron emission tomography (PET) scanning, have short-axis diameters of 4–5 mm. A 3-mm slice thickness is required to detect these small recurrences.

The use of PET using fluorodeoxyglucose (FDG) has had a significant impact on the follow-up of patients with thyroid cancer (14,14a). PET imaging may be more sensitive and specific in the detection of early thyroid cancer (14,15; see Chapters 34, 61, 71, 76, and 79). The major drawbacks of PET imaging, however, are that it is not universally approved by various payers, it is significantly more expensive, and it is not widely available. Two new exciting technologies that combine the value of PET with CT or with MRI are now available (14,14a). The combination of PET imaging with MRI using fusion software is extremely helpful to physically fuse the physiologic images of the FDG uptake with the cross-sectional images of MRI in the axial, coronal, or sagittal planes. This fusion allows a higher sensitivity and specificity. The second exciting technology is PET-CT images, where a combined PET-CT study is done in one setting. The major drawback of PET-CT for patients with thyroid cancer, however, is that CT has limited diagnostic utility in evaluating small neck nodes when no intravenous contrast can be given. Contrast-enhanced CT in a combined PET-CT scanner is extremely useful in the evaluation of lymphomas, lung cancer, breast cancer, and colon cancer. This is not the case when using noncontrast CT in the evaluation of neck small lesions, particularly when there is little body fat within the neck or there are complicating factors, such as postsurgical changes or postradiation changes. The evolving appropriate strategies for patient follow-up using PET with either CT or MRI is evolving (14,15).

MRI AND CT FINDINGS IN PATIENTS WITH THYROID CANCER

The appearance of thyroid masses or recurrent thyroid nodules can be variable. In some cases, the thyroid cancer recurrences can be cystic, and in other cases, especially for papillary carcinoma, the lesions may contain focal areas of calcification (5). In most instances, on CT or MRI, abnormal lymph nodes will have a more rounded, bulbous, or spherical appearance, rather than a typical "kidney bean" shape with a narrow waist. On MRI, all lymph nodes are mostly similar to muscle on T1-weighted images and bright on T2-weighted images but usually not as bright as water. A pathologically enlarged MRI lymph node often has a more rounded appearance and is larger in size. A lymph node is most likely malignant if the short-axis diameter is greater than 1 cm. However, it can be inferred that even smaller 4–5-mm nodes may be pathologic when they appear together with rising thyroglobulin levels or positive uptake on PET scan, correlating with MRI by fusion software. Thus, any size lesion can be a recurrent malignant lymph node, but the traditional usage of MRI and CT has been to designate a lymph node less than 1 cm in size as benign.

Because papillary lymph nodes typically have a more rounded appearance when pathologic, the accuracy and positive predictive value of evaluating patients with recurrent papillary carcinoma is better than that of follicular carcinoma, with a positive predictive value and accuracy of 86% and 85% for papillary cancer and 63% positive predictive value and 67% accuracy for follicular carcinoma, respectively (7). However, there is no specific imaging appearance on either CT or MRI that would define nodes as malignant. Abnormal uptake by ^{123}I or PET, combined with growing size, are the key predictors that signify a lymph node is malignant, regardless of size or appearance (whether cystic or with calcification).

Common tumor characteristics should be considered in regard to imaging and follow-up of the specific types of thyroid cancers. Papillary cancers are the most common, accounting for approx 60–80% of thyroid cancers. Papillary carcinoma is multifocal in 15–30% of cases and most often spreads by intraglandular metastasis and presents with local adenopathy. A specific feature of papillary cancer is the presence of psammoma bodies, which can give the appearance of calcification (3). Furthermore, a mixed papillary-follicular carcinoma might also have evidence of psammomatous calcifications. The calcifications are easily detected by CT but would not be visible on MRI. Some papillary carcinomas may also have a "cystic" appearance on both CT and MRI. (5,16). Although lymph node involvement from papillary carcinoma mostly occurs at levels IV and VI, more distant metastatic lymph adenopathy can occur into the chest or up to level II or III lymph nodes *(16)*. Because papillary cancer typically uptakes iodine, the radioiodine scintigrams are usually positive *(13)*.

The second most common type of thyroid cancer, follicular carcinoma, comprises less than 20% of all thyroid cancers. Because follicular carcinoma is more likely to spread by hematogenous processes, regional lymph node metastases are less likely to occur. In the follow-up of follicular carcinoma, it may be more important to obtain CT scans to evaluate for lung nodules. (MRI is not significantly useful in the evaluation of small pulmonary nodules.) The detection of pulmonary nodules by CT does not require iodinated contrast. Notably, there is wide variability in the clinical manifestations of papillary and follicular thyroid cancer, and individual considerations should be made for each patient. For example, papillary thyroid cancer can metastasize to the lungs with or without detectable cervical lymph node involvement.

Anaplastic carcinoma of the thyroid gland accounts for less than 10% of thyroid cancers and is the least common, consisting of 1–4% of thyroid cancers. Because these are more poorly differentiated tumors, they are more likely to attain a larger size (see Chapters 77–83). In addition, because of their rapid growth, they are frequently associated with areas of hemorrhage and internal necrosis. Many cases of anaplastic carcinoma arise within a preexisting multinodular goiter or arise rarely within a more well-differentiated type of thyroid cancer.

The last common primary type of thyroid cancer is the medullary carcinoma, accounting for 2–6% of thyroid cancers (see Chapters 67–73). Medullary thyroid cancers may be associated with multiple endocrine neoplasias and are associated with elevated levels of calcitonin. The MRI and CT features are not specific. Similarly to papillary carcinoma, the CT appearance may show the presence of psammomatous calcification, but it is typically denser than that seen with papillary cancer. Peripheral metastatic lesions to the lung and liver may also show calcification. When medullary thyroid cancer is familial, it may also be associated with hyperparathyroidism and pheochromocytomas.

MRI AND CT IN THE PREOPERATIVE STAGING OF THYROID CANCER

Although MRI and CT are not routinely used in the preoperative staging of a small thyroid nodule, some large thyroid cancers may require more careful preoperative planning. Specifically, large tumors that have invaded the thyroid cartilage, esophagus, or adjacent local structures need a more careful preoperative plan to determine what type of resection may be required or whether the tumor is, in fact, inoperable. For the extent and invasion of tumor into critical structures, MRI is the ideal study that is most sensitive and specific for detection of invasion. MRI has been assessed for its accuracy in the identification of invasion of the tracheal cartilage, involvement of the current laryngeal nerve, and esophagus involvement. MRI is often 80–95% sensitive in detecting invasion of these critical structures, with a slightly higher specificity *(16–18)*. In contrast to therapeutic approaches for other types of carcinoma, papillary cancer remains the most radiosensitive. The intent of most surgical resections is to obtain a clear margin. However, a significant debulking of the papillary thyroid tumor allows a potentially greater response to radioactive iodine. The criticality of negative surgical margins is not as stringent for the radioactive iodine–sensitive thyroid carcinomas.

POSTOPERATIVE AND POSTRADIATION IMAGING OF THYROID CANCER

The postoperative and postradiation imaging of thyroid cancer is best achieved with MRI. CT, in most cases, is again limited by the inability to use iodinated contrast. With the follow-up findings of scarring, thickening, and loss of fascial planes, CT becomes even more difficult to assess for recurrent tumor *(19)*. The abnormal changes on MRI become easier to interpret after a latency period of 4–6 wk in which postoperative edema subsides. For those patients receiving whole-neck external-beam radiation, there is a latency period of 4–6 mo in which residual edema may be present. Because the normal anatomic planes that are usually clearly outlined by fat between the fascia delineate the structures, loss of these normal fascial planes makes interpretation of recurrence significantly more difficult *(19)*. However, as time lengthens from the patient's initial surgery and from postoperative radiation, any new findings in the surgical bed or in the upper neck or mediastinum are more likely to represent recurrence. This is particularly true when correlated with positive findings seen on PET or radioactive iodine scanning. In many cases, early studies can serve as a valuable baseline for comparison on follow-up study, thereby allowing newly developing interval processes to be detected sooner.

MULTIDISCIPLINARY APPROACH TO THE INTERPRETATION OF RECURRENT THYROID CANCER

There are likely not as many diverse disciplines and tools available to detect recurrence of a specific cancer in any other area of oncology imaging. A close working relationship between radiologists, nuclear medicine physicians, pathologists, surgeons, and endocrinologists is optimal. Correlating PET scan findings with abnormalities detected on MRI (or less likely, CT), in combination with changing thyroglobulin levels, can become challenging, particularly if each physician works within a vacuum. A multidisciplinary approach enables a much more sensitive and significant detection of

Jellinek et al.

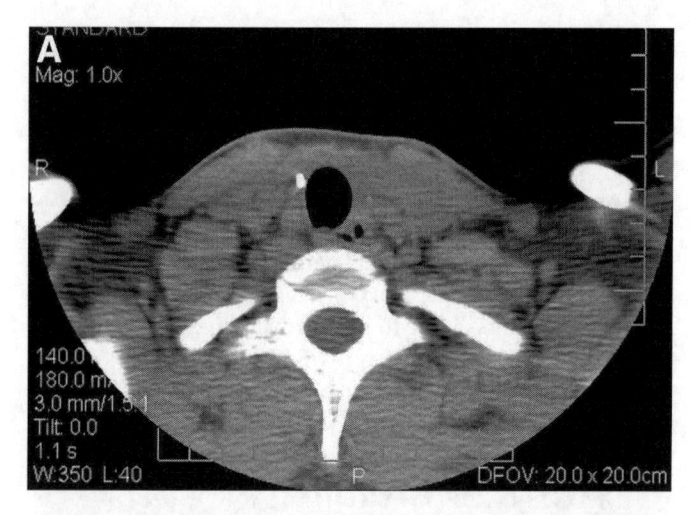

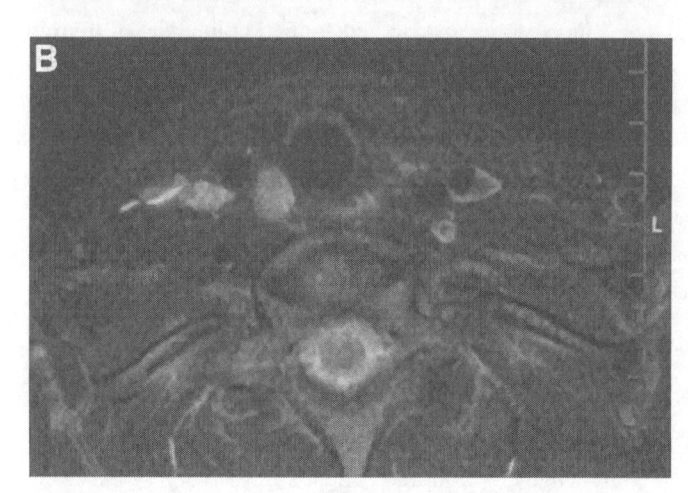

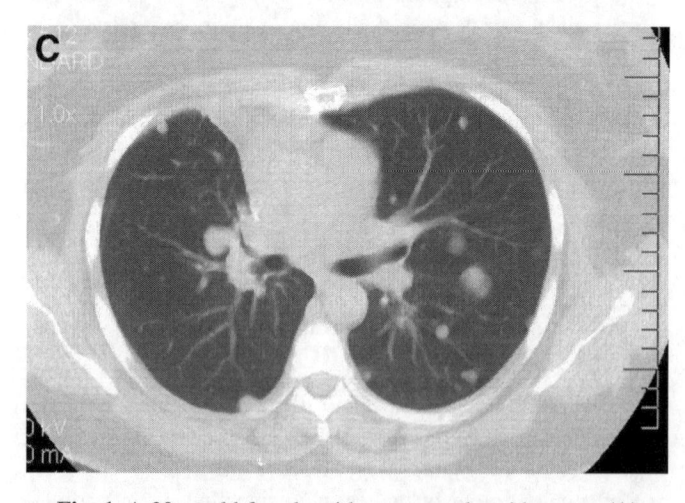

Fig. 1. A 39-yr-old female with recurrent thyroid cancer. (**A**) Recurrent adenopathy is hard to assess on this noncontrast CT. (**B**) The recurrent adenopathy of the right neck is more obvious on this axial T2-weighted image. (**C**) Noncontrast CT of the lungs show multiple pulmonary nodules from metastatic disease.

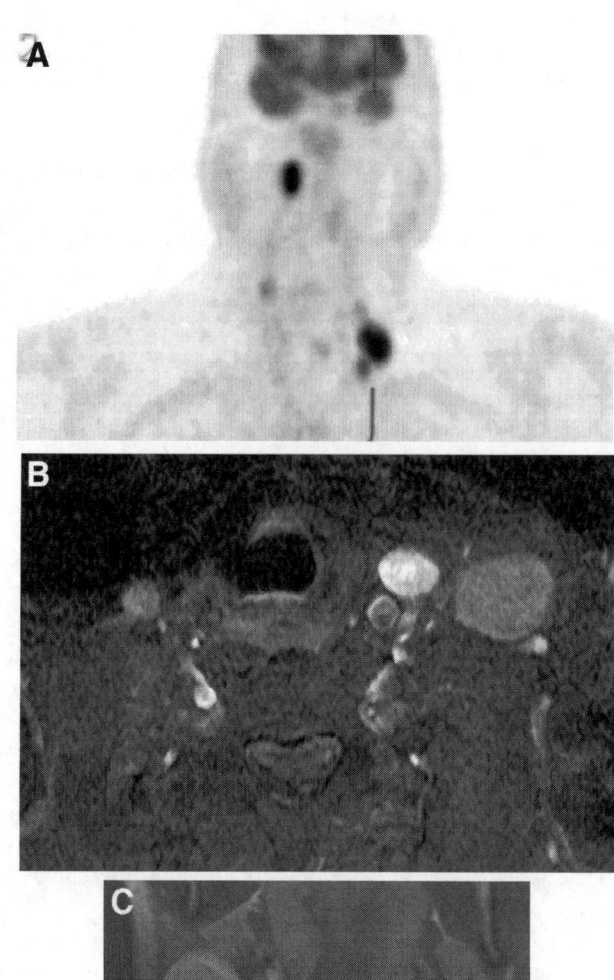

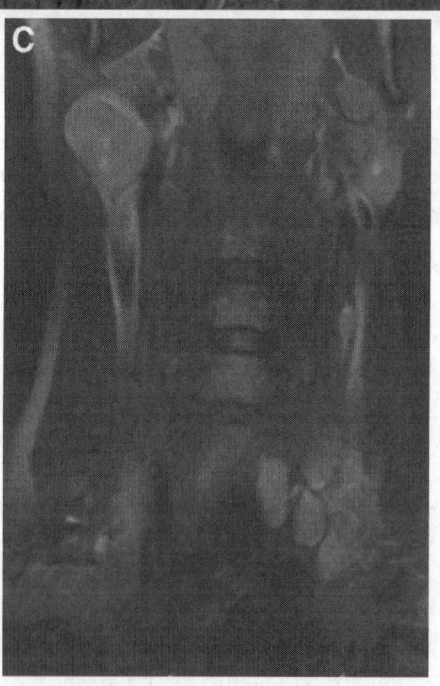

Fig. 2. A 38-yr-old male with recurrent thyroid cancer. Comparison of PET and MRI. (**A**) PET image of the neck showing left lower neck lymph nodes and a single, large, right, level II lymph node. (**B**) Axial postcontrast-enhanced fat-saturated T1-weighted MRI shows recurrent left lower neck lymph nodes corresponding to the PET study. (**C**) Coronal T2-weighted MRI correlates well with the PET findings that show both left lower neck adenopathy and a single, enlarged, right level II lymph node.

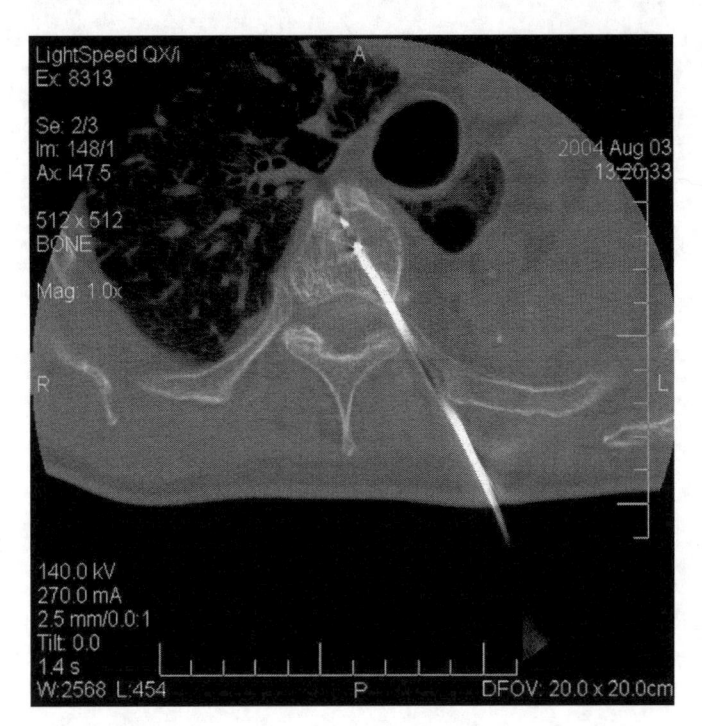

Fig. 3. A 75-yr-old male with metastatic disease to thoracic spine. Axial CT image shows a biopsy needle with radiofrequency (RF) prongs deployed into the thoracic vertebral body metastasis for treatment.

recurrent tumors. A traditional imager using MRI or CT would be looking for lymph nodes with a short axial diameter of 1 cm. However, when combining endocrine findings of a rising thyroglobulin level with associated positive findings on either PET or ^{123}I or ^{131}I, small (4 mm) lymph nodes can be identified as reflecting recurrence and (in some cases with an experienced ultrasonographer) then undergo FNA biopsy. In other cases, positive findings by MRI or PET may have other anatomic or physiologic causes unrelated to recurrence of thyroid cancer. Each single modality can be nonspecific or insensitive. Deciphering these different possibilities is greatly facilitated by a multidisciplinary approach with combined conferences.

CT GUIDANCE FOR ABLATION OF PERIPHERAL METASTATIC THYROID CANCER

The newest weapon in the oncologist armamentarium against cancer is local ablative therapy (see Chapter 54). Radiofrequency ablation and cryotherapy can be used to ablate both neck recurrence and distal metastasis (20,21). Using CT guidance (as used for CT-guided biopsies), a large needle (e.g., a 14-gauge needle) can be placed into the center of tumor recurrence. A "hot"-tip radiofrequency wire or a cryotherapy probe can be guided through the needle, and then the lesion is either "heated" or "frozen." The ablative therapy can be palliative or helpful in "debulking" tumor to make radioactive iodine more effective (Figs. 1–3).

REFERENCES

1. Weiss RE, Lado-Abeal J. Thyroid nodules: diagnosis and therapy. Curr Opin Oncol 2002; 14:46–52.
2. Blum M. Nonisotopic imaging of the neck in patients with thyroid nodules or cancer. In Wartofsky L, editor. Thyroid Cancer; A Comprehensive Guide to Clinical Management. Totowa, NJ: Humana, 2000:9–34.
3. Smoker WRK, Harnsberger HR, Reede DL, et al. The neck. In Som PM, Bergeron RT, editors. Head and Neck Imaging, 2nd ed. St. Louis, MO: Mosby Yearbook, 1991:497–592.
4. Becker M. Other infrahyoid neck lesions. In Mafer MF, Valvassori GE, Becker M, editors. Imaging of the Head and Neck, 2nd ed. Stuttgart, Germany: Thieme, 2005:780–845.
5. Som PM, Brandwein M, Lidov M, et al. The varied presentations of papillary thyroid cervical nodal disease: CT and MR findings. Am J Neuroradiol 1994; 15:1123–1128.
6. Som PM, Curtin HD, Mancuso AA. Imaging-based nodal classification for evaluation of neck metastatic adenopathy. Am J Roentgenol 2000; 174:837–844.
7. Gross ND, Weissman JL, Talbot JM, et al. MRI detection of cervical metastases from differentiated thyroid carcinoma. Laryngoscope 2001; 111:1905–1909.
8. Schroder RJ, Rost B, Hidajat N, et al. Value of contrast-enhanced ultrasound vs. CT and MR in palpable enlarged lymph node of the head and neck. Rofo 2002; 174:1099–1106.
9. Curtin HD, Ishwaran H, Mancuso AA, et al. Comparison of CT and MR imaging in staging of neck metastases. Radiology 1998; 207:123–130.
10. Yousem DM, Som PM, Hackney DB, et al. Central necrosis and extracapsular neoplastic spread in cervical lymph nodes: MR imaging versus CT. Radiology 1992; 182:753–759.
11. Von den Brekel MWM. Lymph node metastasis: CT and MRI. Eur J Radiol 2000; 22:230–238.
12. King AD, Tse GM, Yuen EH, et al. Comparison of CT and MR imaging for the detection of extranodal neoplastic spread in metastatic neck nodes. Eur J Radiol 2004; 52:264–270.
13. James C, Starks M, MacGillroy DC, White J. The use of imaging studies in the diagnosis and management of thyroid cancer and hyperparathyroidism. Surg Oncol Clin N Am 1999; 8:145–169.
14. Benchaou M, Lehmann W, Slosmann DO, et al. The role of FDG-PET in the preoperative assessment of N-staging in head and neck cancer. Acta Otolaryngol 1996; 116:332–335.
14a. Nahas Z, Goldenberg D, Fakhry C, et al. The role of positron emission tomography/computed tomography in the management of recurrent papillary thyroid carcinoma. Laryngoscope 2005; 115:237–243.
15. Popperl G, Lang S, Dogdelen O. Correlation of FDG-PET and MRI/CT with histopathology in primary diagnosis, lymph node staging and diagnosis of recurrency of head and neck cancer. Rofo 2002; 174: 714–720.
16. Takashima S, Matsushita T, Takayama F, et al. Prognostic significance of magnetic resonance findings in advanced papillary thyroid cancer. Thyroid 2001; 11:1153–1159.
17. Takashima S, Takayama F, Wong J, et al. Using MR imaging to predict invasion of the recurrent laryngeal nerve by thyroid cancer. Am J Roentgenol 2003; 180:837–842.

18. Wang JC, Takashima S, Takayama F, et al. Tracheal invasion by thyroid carcinoma: prediction using MR imaging. Am J Roentgenol 2001; 177:926–936.
19. Becker M, Schroth G, Zbaren P, et al. Long-term changes induced by high-dose irradiation of the head and neck region: image findings. Radiographics 1997; 17:5–26.
20. Dupuy DE, Monchick JM, Decrea C, Pisharodi L. Radio-frequency ablation of regional recurrence from well-differentiated thyroid malignancy. Surgery 2001; 130:971–977.
21. Lee JM, Jin GY, Goldberg SN, et al. Percutaneous radio-frequency ablation for inoperable non-small cell lung cancer and metastases: preliminary report. Radiology 2004; 230:125–134.

39
Management of the Patients with Negative Radioiodine Scan and Elevated Serum Thyroglobulin

Leonard Wartofsky

In the past two decades, significant improvements in the assays for serum thyroglobulin (Tg) have revolutionized the standard follow-up and surveillance for recurrence in patients with thyroid carcinoma (1–5). Not infrequently, we are faced with the management dilemma presented by patients with differentiated thyroid cancer (DTC) in whom measurable or high serum Tg levels suggest residual or metastatic disease, but their radioiodine diagnostic survey scans are negative.

Some workers have advocated empiric high-dose radioiodine therapy in these patients, based on the Tg levels indicating disease, even when the negative scan suggests there will be little to no uptake. However, this approach has been somewhat controversial (6–12a). The National Comprehensive Cancer Network guidelines (12) are far from definitive on this issue but point out that no studies have yet demonstrated significantly reduced morbidity and mortality from radioiodine therapy given strictly for elevated serum Tg levels. The British Thyroid Association guidelines (13) are completely silent on the dilemma. Pacini and Schlumberger (14) were the first investigators to advocate this empiric high-dose ^{131}I therapy for patients who are "scan-negative, Tg-positive," whereas Sherman and Gopal (15) advised caution in the absence of data confirming efficacy and an acceptable risk:benefit ratio.

When initially faced with this perplexing pairing of diagnostic data—positive Tg and negative scan—it is essential to first attempt to uncover a cause for a possibly false-negative scan or a false-positive elevation of serum Tg before even considering empiric radioiodine therapy. For example, a falsely positive serum Tg level could occur because of interfering anti-Tg antibodies (16). Explanations for a false-negative radioiodine scan include inadequate thyrotropin (TSH) elevation, stable iodine contamination (e.g., history of recent iodine contrast radiography), dispersed microscopic metastases too small to visualize, or such dedifferentiation of the tumor that it can still produce Tg but has lost its iodide-trapping ability. To rule out iodine contamination, serum or urinary iodide can be measured and a repeat total-body scan (TBS) 4–6 wk after an iodide depletion regimen can be considered (17). In some series of patients (18), a significant number of subjects had both negative serum Tg and a negative scan, presumably representing dedifferentiation of these tumors.

In managing the patient who presents with a negative scan and positive thyroglobulin, clinical aspects should be taken into account before definitive action is taken to prescribe radioiodine therapy. Important matters to consider include risk factors, evidence of prior metastatic or aggressive disease, and any arguments for employing other imaging tools, such as magnetic resonance imaging (MRI) or ultrasound to visualize potential occult disease. How the clinical context can alter the approach is illustrated by two hypothetical cases. First, in a 60-yr-old man with a history of a stage III 4-cm papillary or 2-cm follicular lesion, the author would consider the Pacini-Schlumberger approach of empiric treatment with high-dose radioiodine. Alternatively, in a 25-yr-old woman with a history of a 2-cm stage I papillary cancer with negative nodes and only marginally measurable or slightly elevated Tg (e.g., <4 ng/mL), the author might favor a more conservative approach, at least for a period of time.

Whether serum Tg levels are stable or rising is significantly useful in the decision-making process regarding radioiodine therapy. Of course, the patient must be brought into the decision-making process and informed fully of the extent of collective knowledge, experience, and biases pertaining to that patient's specific situation. We would like to avoid treatment with aggressive high-dose radioiodine for uncertain indications and treatment that might result in harmful sequelae, such as neutropenia, xerostomia, and/or azoospermia.

As pointed out by Sherman and Gopal (15), the risks of aggressive radioiodine therapy may not be warranted given the ill-defined goals, unless there is evidence of progressive disease. Pacini et al. (14) and Schlumberger et al. (19) are not the only investigators to describe a salutary result from empiric treatment of the Tg-positive/scan-negative patient. Pineda et al. (20) reported their results in

17 Tg-positive/scan-negative patients who all had prior total thyroidectomy and radioiodine ablation. After empiric treatment with 150–300 mCi of ^{131}I, 16 of 17 had visualization of metastases on their posttreatment scan. Tg levels decreased in 81% of patients after their first treatment dose and decreased in 90% and 100% of those who received second and third doses, respectively. Although these results sound impressive (20,21), examination of the individual patient's Tg level response is less so. Mean Tg decreased from 74 to 62 to 32 over 1–2 yr of follow-up, and only 6 of 29 positive scans became negative.

A definite tilt toward empiric radioiodine therapy in 16 scan-negative/Tg-positive patients was evident in the report by de Keizer et al. (22) who described a decreased Tg level in 88% of patients. The period of follow-up was too short to indicate any improvement in survival or disease-free interval; however, the authors proposed treatment of such patients with at least one dose when scans were negative. As with the Pineda and Robbins studies (20), serum Tg did decline in the majority of patients but not dramatically.

The cogent issues raised by Sherman and Gopal, and previously by McDougall (23) and Mazzaferri (24), reflect the fact that many patients treated by Schlumberger et al. and Pineda and Robbins had minimal, if any, disease that would affect their life expectancy. The empiric therapy would expose them to unwarranted doses of radiation exposure, unwarranted at least until sufficient data is obtained from well-controlled studies that confirm efficacy of therapy. Based on their own experience in 24 patients (25) and their analysis of the literature (26), Fatourechi and Hay suggested two general patient categories. The first group has a higher risk of demonstrating uptake on the scan after high-dose therapy, representing younger patients with diffuse micrometastases and negative whole-body scan and conventional imaging but moderately elevated Tg levels. Patients in the second group are likely to be older, higher risk patients with known metastases that release Tg and do not take up radioiodine but are identified by other imaging. In their experience, this latter group will not demonstrate uptake on a posttreatment scan and therefore do not require therapy.

Arguably, the most useful experience reported to date is that of Pacini et al. (27) who compared the outcomes in 42 scan-negative/Tg-positive patients (group 1) treated with radioiodine to 28 patients (group 2) followed without treatment, where the average follow-up was 6.7 and 11.9 yr, respectively. The first posttherapy scan was positive in 30 of 42 treated patients, negative in 12, and only the patients with positive scans were given additional ^{131}I therapy. Complete remission was seen in 10 of 30 (normalized Tg levels), partial remission (still detectable Tg) in 9 of 30, and evidence of persistent disease in 11 of 30 (measurable Tg and scans became positive). Among these 30 patients with positive posttherapy scans, when radioiodine uptake was seen in the lungs (metastatic disease) on the posttherapy scan, it resolved in 8 of 9 (89%) cases but in only 11 of 18 cases with cervical lymph node involvement. In the remaining 12 of the 42 group 1 patients who did not have positive scans after treatment doses, two entered remission, 7 had persistent Tg elevations, 2 had mediastinal lymph node involvement, and only 1 died of disease during the follow-up period. The changes in Tg were not directly compared to the changes in the no-treatment group. Significantly, of these 28 patients (group 2) who were followed with no treatment, 19 of 28 (68%) became Tg-negative, another 6 of 28 (21.4%) were unchanged, and only 3 (11%) had an increase in Tg levels. Pacini et al. concluded that there may be a role for empiric ^{131}I therapy in patients with pulmonary metastases, but that their data supporting empiric therapy in patients with cervical lymph nodes was far from compelling. In view of the remarkable stability in those who were not treated, they did not advocate further radioiodine therapy in those patients whose first posttherapy scan remains negative—an approach that seems to be quite balanced.

It was possible to compare the change in Tg levels in 28 treated vs 32 nonradioiodine-treated patients in the study by Koh et al. (28). Significantly greater reductions in Tg were seen with ^{131}I therapy, with four patients actually becoming undetectable. Posttherapy scans became positive in 12 of 28 (43%) of the scan-negative/Tg-positive patients. Like deKeizer et al. (22), the authors encouraged consideration of empiric radioiodine therapy, both for palliation and potential localization of lesions on the posttreatment scan.

In their review of the literature, Ma et al. (28a) concluded that the decision to treat should be individualized on the basis of the extent of disease as indicated by serum thyroglobulin levels. Thus, individuals with thyroglobulin levels >10 ng/mL or patients stratified at high risk for recurrence should be treated with radioiodine with the expectation that approximately two thirds will show both a fall in thyroglobulin and a positive post-treatment scan.

It may seem easy to recommend empiric therapy based on these data of declines in serum Tg, but it should be noted that improvement in survival is yet to be shown. In addition to the potential untoward complications of high-dose radioiodine therapy mentioned above (and enumerated in Chapter 50), another important aspect of empiric therapy is the cost to the patient regarding morbidity of hypothyroidism and its negative impact on productivity, as well as the cost in health care related to hospitalization and the associated expensive technological procedures.

In the author's approach to the scan-negative/Tg-positive patient, it is important to turn at an early stage in evaluation to alternative imaging procedures. Although radioiodine therapy may not be feasible because of the lack of visible uptake on diagnostic scanning, alternative therapeutic approaches to metastatic deposits of thyroid cancer may be available. These might include surgical excision, localized ablation by ethanol instillation or radiofrequency ablation (see Chapter 54), or localized external-radiation therapy *(29,30;* see Chapter 51), but the location of the metastases should first be identified and assessed before one of these approaches is taken. Imaging with computed tomography (CT) MRI, and ultrasound have been employed for this purpose, and alternative scanning agents may have a role in identifying lesions that are not visualized with traditional ^{131}I whole-body scan (see Chapter 35).

ALTERNATIVE SCANNING AGENTS

Two early scanning agents used as alternatives to radioiodine were ^{201}Tl *(31)* and ^{99m}Tc sestamibi *(32)*. In one study of patients with bone metastases documented with positive ^{131}I scans, ^{201}Tl was compared to the bone agent, ^{99m}Tc hydroxymethylene diphosphonate (^{99m}Tc-HMDP; *31*). The two agents had a combined sensitivity of 93.5%. In a group of 14 patients with negative ^{131}I scans and other evidence of thyroid malignancy, ^{201}Tl was positive in 10 of 14, and ^{99m}Tc-HMDP was positive in all 14. Carril et al. *(33)* found that ^{201}Tl showed a sensitivity and specificity higher than that associated with ^{131}I for recurrent or persistent disease. Lesions were detected in 31 of 116 patients by ^{201}Tl but not by ^{131}I TBS. In patients who have been ablated and show no further ^{131}I uptake, the authors proposed continuing management with no additional ^{131}I scans. Because ^{201}Tl scanning does not require levothyroxine withdrawal, follow-up would be guided only by ^{201}Tl scanning and monitoring serum Tg. Dadparvar et al. *(34)* compared ^{201}Tl and scanning with ^{99m}Tc-methoxyisobutyl isonitrile (^{99m}Tc-MIBI). They found that a ^{131}I TBS alone was satisfactory as a preablation diagnostic study, but the addition of either alternative agent increased the diagnostic yield postablation, particularly when the ^{131}I TBS was negative. However, these results have not been universal because Lorberboym et al. *(35)* found ^{131}I TBS to be more sensitive and specific than ^{201}Tl, with the latter giving several false-positive scans. Ugur et al. *(36)* noted a 70% overall concordance between ^{201}Tl, ^{99m}Tc-MIBI, and ^{131}I TBS but observed false-negatives with both alternative agents, concluding that they should not be used in lieu of ^{131}I TBS. In one reported case, ^{201}Tl scanning was positive and useful in a patient with metastatic disease with *both* negative ^{131}I TBS and negative serum Tg levels *(37)*.

Employing the agent, ^{99m}Tc sestamibi, Elser et al. *(38)* noted a 94% sensitivity for the detection of positive lymph nodes and local recurrence; they detected 32 of 40 metastases with sestamibi vs only 18 of 40 with an ^{131}I TBS. Another cationic scanning agent, ^{99m}Tc tetrafosmin, which has been used previously for myocardial perfusion imaging, was assessed for the detection of thyroid cancer *(39–41)*. For 12 patients with elevated serum Tg (4 with negative ^{131}I TBS), tetrafosmin was slightly superior to ^{201}Tl and ^{99m}Tc-MIBI. This same group of workers *(41)* reported that tetrafosmin successfully identified all of 21 lesions that were positive by ^{131}I TBS, as well as an additional 17 of 23 lesions that were negative by ^{131}I TBS. The agent had 86% sensitivity for distant metastases, and was positive in four patients with ^{131}I-negative proven pulmonary metastases. The findings correlated with other imaging modalities for tumor identification, e.g., CT or ultrasound.

It is also significant that these alternative agents are logistically both more convenient and expedient than scanning with ^{131}I. Along with the ability to scan patients while euthyroid and still on TSH-suppressive levothyroxine therapy, the time required for evaluation is much reduced. Instead of scanning 48–72 h after a dose of ^{131}I, the ^{99m}Tc tetrafosmin planar scan is performed 20 min after injection of the isotope, with additional images taken by single-photon emission computed tomography of any suspicious lesions. ^{99m}Tc tetrafosmin scans were negative in all 68 patients studied by Lind et al. *(41)*, who were free of disease on the basis of ^{131}I TBS and serum Tg.

FLUORODEOXYGLUCOSE-POSITRON EMISSION TOMOGRAPHY (Chapters 34, 61)

Another agent, 18-fluorine fluorodeoxyglucose (FDG) has been employed with positron emission tomography (PET) for detection of thyroid cancer with uptake of the agent related to glucose utilization by tumor tissue *(42–45)*. Indeed, PET scanning is rapidly becoming a part of the routine armamentarium of diagnostic imaging procedures for thyroid cancer and may be the optimal imaging modality for medullary thyroid cancer *(46)*. Its more widespread adoption has been limited by its relatively high cost and the reluctance of insurers to provide coverage for all but selected patient populations. In fact, one of those populations in which PET scanning has been found useful is the scan-negative/Tg-positive patients. Numerous publications testify to its utility in both individual patient case reports and small patient series *(47–51)*.

The greatest uptake sensitivity for FDG-PET scanning has been noted with the fastest growing undifferentiated tumors. Grunwald et al. *(52)* compared FDG-PET to ^{99m}Tc sestamibi and ^{131}I TBS. Of 29 studies, 11 of 29 had disease detected only with FDG-PET, 8 of 29 were detected only with ^{131}I TBS, and 10 of 29 were detected by both. Five sites were found by FDG-PET and not by ^{99m}Tc sestamibi. FDG-PET may be useful in patients in whom ^{131}I TBS is not feasible owing to a history of iodine exposure; similarly, its use would not preclude CT scanning (with contrast if desired) as an additional means to image tumors.

A more recent, larger study by Schluter et al. *(53)* described 118 PET scans in 64 scan-negative/Tg-positive patients. Of 64 patients, 44 had positive PET studies, 34 of whom were proven to be true positives, leading to an altered therapeutic approach in 19 of 34 (surgery and/or external irradiation), whereas 20 patients had negative scans. Their results indicated a positive predictive value (PPV) for PET of 83% but a negative predictive value (NPV) of only 25%. In seven patients, there was so much metastatic disease identified that a palliative, rather than curative, approach was taken. Yet, for the most part, they found PET to be a valuable adjunct to identify patients who could benefit from further therapy. Wang and coworkers (54) reported good results with PET scanning in 37 patients with negative ^{131}I scans. PET identified occult lesions in 71%, with a 92% PPV in patients with high serum Tg and a 93% NPV in patients with lower Tg levels. Chung et al. (55) reported excellent utility of FDG-PET scanning in 54 patients with negative ^{131}I scans after thyroxine withdrawal, and they demonstrated a 94% PPV and a 93% NPV. FDG-PET may be particularly useful when both the iodine scan and serum Tg are false-negatives, and this often applies when the low-serum Tg is a result of interfering antithyroglobulin antibodies. Chung et al. noted that this often implied regional lymph node involvement. Although Wang et al. (54) found that FDG-PET was not that useful in detecting small degrees of residual papillary tumor in the neck, Chung et al. showed PET to be positive more often with neck disease and conventional scanning than in detecting pulmonary metastases. Comparably encouraging results have been reported by Helal et al. (56) in a series of 37 scan-negative/Tg-positive patients with DTC. In a group of 10 patients with known metastases via conventional imaging, PET confirmed tumor at 17 of 18 sites and identified tumors at 11 additional sites. PET was positive in 19 of 27 patients in a second group with negative imaging by other methods. These findings led to a change in treatment management in 29 of 37 patients, with 23 receiving further surgery and 14 of 23 achieving disease-free status. These authors proposed PET as the "first-line investigation" in scan-negative/Tg-positive patients. A more pessimistic view was expounded by van Tol and colleagues in a letter to the editor (57) in which they described an extraordinary high rate of false-positives (64%) with PET, and that the findings led to a significant change in management in only 1 of 11 (9%) patients. A drawback is the lack of widespread availability of PET scanners because of their high cost and, most importantly, these scans are currently not reimbursed by most insurers in the United States except for specific indications. (This situation is likely to improve in the future.)

Fridrich et al. (58) compared FDG-PET to ^{99m}Tc-MIBI and ^{131}I TBS and found both to be more sensitive than ^{131}I TBS, with a slight edge in favor of ^{99m}Tc-MIBI. In addition to the benefit of good uptake, independent of the patients, serum TSH level, FDG-PET, or MIBI did not have the propensity for high background in the neck, mediastinum, and chest, as with ^{131}I, and could be used more effectively to detect small metastases in these areas. In contrast, liver and brain demonstrate high FDG uptake, and the ability to detect metastases in these areas is limited with this agent. Indeed, Feine et al. (59) were able to localize and identify positive neck metastases with FDG-PET in six patients with elevated serum Tg levels. Dietlein et al. proposed a more conservative perspective regarding the utility of FDG-PET scanning (60). They observed positive FDG-PET images in 7 of 21 patients with positive lymph node metastases but negative ^{131}I TBS; sensitivity was 82% in patients with high-serum Tg but negative TBS. They concluded that FDG-PET should not be used in lieu of ^{131}I-TBS but would serve as a useful adjunct or complement to evaluation, particularly when the ^{131}I TBS was negative in conflict with a rising or elevated level of serum Tg. Altenvoerde et al. (61) performed PET studies in 12 of 32 patients with scan-negative/Tg-positive findings, and the PET scans were positive in 6 of 12. Interestingly, the mean Tg level in the six positive patients was 147 ± 90, whereas the PET-negative patients had a mean Tg of only 9 ± 7.6, suggesting that PET is most useful in those patients with more aggressive and/or larger metastases. Similar conclusions were reached by Grunwald et al. (62) and Wang et al. (63). In this regard, PET-positive patients with larger volume disease have a worse prognosis (54).

Clearly, PET scanning may miss some types of metastases. In the report of Hung et al. (64), 20 scan-negative/Tg-positive patients underwent FDG-PET scanning, with lesions detected in 17 of 20, but PET scans were negative in two patients proven to have miliary distribution of pulmonary metastases. The authors suggest chest CT scans in such cases. Most valuable has been the newest technology that combines PET scanning with CT or MRI by either fusion software, or preferably within one dedicated PET/CT scanner (64a). An overlay of high SUV on a CT or MR image provides much greater specificity that the imaged finding is cancer. As with many diagnostic modalities, negative findings would not preclude disease, but positive findings on PET/CT would dictate CT-guided or ultrasound-guided FNA cytology and then surgery if tumor is confirmed.

TSH STIMULATION OF FDG-PET

Whether FDG uptake might be enhanced by either endogenous TSH after levothyroxine withdrawal or by recombinant human TSH (rhTSH) remains somewhat controversial. Relating to in vitro thyroid cell cultures, TSH will increase uptake of both FDG (65) and ^{201}Tl (66), but that does not prove that thyroid cancer cells will respond in the same way in vivo. TSH could probably improve imaging because TSH stimulates glucose transport into the cells and cellular metabolism. The best proof of this concept is derived from several clinical studies. For example, Chin et al. (67) evaluated seven patients who were scan-negative/Tg-positive and compared PET scans of those patients on thyroxine suppression to PET scans after rhTSH. The scans after rhTSH disclosed more lesions, and the average tumor-to-background (T:B) ratio values were higher. Similar results were seen by Petrich et al. (68) in 30 patients with largely negative radioiodine scans. rhTSH stimulation provided higher T:B ratios and uncovered more lesions in more patients. Comparing PET scans after thyroxine withdrawal (not rhTSH) to PET scans of patients on suppressive therapy, both Moog et al. (69)

and van Tol et al. *(70)* concluded that TSH stimulation detected more lesions. Rational patient selection is needed, and clinicians and payors have to determine whether the additional cost burden of rhTSH to an already expensive PET scan will constitute a favorable cost–benefit ratio.

Unrelated to PET scanning but relevant to rhTSH, there is a case report of a scan-negative/Tg-positive patient in whom radioiodine trapping was restored after a period of levothyroxine withdrawal and rhTSH stimulation *(71)*. Occasionally, radioiodine trapping may also be restored after chemotherapy *(72)*, and the matter of redifferentiation is discussed in Chapter 86.

SOMATOSTATIN IMAGING

DTC imaging by somatostatin receptor scintigraphy (SRS) with octreotide has been reported *(73,74)*. Of 25 patients with DTC and elevated serum Tg levels studied by Baudin *(73)*, 16 of 25 had negative ^{131}I TBS, and SRS was positive in 12 of these patients as well as in 8 of 9 patients with positive ^{131}I TBS. Stokkel et al. *(75)* studied 10 Tg-positive/^{131}I scan-negative patients with octreotide scanning and described multiple metastases in 9 of 10. Based on octreotide uptake, the authors speculate that ^{111}In-labeled octreotide or its analogs might be useful for therapy of such patients. Sarlis et al. *(76)* compared octreotide scanning to PET and conventional imaging in 21 patients with aggressive disease, finding that octreotide had only moderate sensitivity yet detected disease in five patients who were negative by PET and other imaging. Confirmatory studies are required, but SRS with labeled octreotide may represent another useful alternative to ^{131}I TBS, with the advantage of lacking the need to withdraw TSH-suppressive levothyroxine therapy.

SURGERY

As mentioned above, ultrasonography of the neck is extremely useful to identify occult metastases of papillary thyroid cancer *(77)* and deserves to be an almost routine imaging tool for this purpose (see Chapters 21, 37), particularly if used in conjunction with rhTSH-stimulated thyroglobulin levels *(78)*. Another approach has been to proceed with cervical exploration and node dissection in the case of papillary carcinoma, even when all additional imaging studies are unrevealing. In one such series of 21 patients, Alzahrani et al. *(79)* performed neck dissections after confirming the presence of tumor by ultrasound-guided fine-needle aspiration cytology. Postoperatively, serum Tg fell from a mean of 185 ± 79 to 127 ± 59, with 4 patients who achieved remission, 13 had persistent disease, and 4 showed progression. They concluded that the additional surgery offered benefit in a minority of patients and that most remained stable. Moreover, the intraoperative use of ultrasound can readily improve the detection of residual or recurrent thyroid cancer *(80)*, and there has been greater success with positive node dissections since its use by our surgeons.

CONCLUSIONS

In conclusion, how should the scan-negative/Tg-positive patient be managed with no underlying reason to suspect either false-negative scan or false-positive serum Tg level? Schlumberger *(81,82)* would empirically administer 100 mCi ^{131}I to any patient with a Tg level more than 10 ng/mL while off of levothyroxine and only repeat the ^{131}I whole-body scan every 2–5 yr when the Tg level is in the range of 1–10 ng/mL. As mentioned above, no studies show improved survival with this approach. On the contrary, the follow-up study of van Tol et al. *(83)* indicates little support for empiric therapy based on an average follow-up period of 4.2 yr. Of 56 patients given a "blind" dose of 150 mCi of ^{131}I, uptake was revealed on the posttreatment scan in 28 of 56 (50%) of the patients with no difference in serum Tg levels. They concluded that therapy had no salutary effect on survival or reduction of tumor burden. There may be many factors that could differentiate those patients who seem to respond to empiric therapy from those who do not. One factor could be the size of the lesions as micrometastases may be more readily ablated than macrometastases *(84)*. At this point in our knowledge, I am attracted to the concept of individualization of empiric therapy as proposed by Ma et al. *(28a)* based upon the height of the thyroglobulin levels and whether or not they are seen to be increasing during follow-up. Indeed, although controversial as discussed above and elsewhere *(12a)*, empiric radioiodine therapy should probably be attempted at least one more time in selected patients with thyroglobulin levels >10 ng/mL or rising. Post-therapy thyroglobulin levels and the post-therapy scan should be examined to assess potential benefit. In an attempt to maximize the efficacy of the radioiodine, I employ a low iodine diet for 4 wk prior to therapy supplemented by low dose diuretic (20 mg/day furoseamide) and confirm the patient's adherence to the diet by measurement of urinary iodine 1 wk prior to the planned therapy. We proceed with therapy if the urinary iodide is less than 50 μg/L, and most patients can achieve levels of less than 20 μg/L. In addition, radioiodine retention and presumed therapeutic benefit can be augmented by lithium carbonate therapy as discussed in Chapter 49. The growing number of reports *(22, 27–28a,84,85)* indicating benefit of empiric therapy appear to justify this approach.

If radioiodine therapy is not to be given in the face of clearly measurable Tg levels, alternative imaging procedures should be encouraged. For papillary thyroid carcinoma with a propensity to regional recurrence, that could include ultrasound, CT, MRI, ^{99m}Tc-MIBI, or FDG-PET, with fine needle aspiration cytology when feasible to confirm the diagnosis. For follicular thyroid cancer with its propensity for distant metastases (especially to bone and lung), imaging with ^{99m}Tc tetrafosmin, ^{99m}Tc-HMDP, or ^{201}Tl could be attempted. Identification of isolated distant lesions by these methods would allow earlier intervention by surgical excision, a local ablative technique, or external radiotherapy instead of delaying further treatment until a subsequent ^{131}I TBS might become positive or serum Tg levels might increase further because of further tumor growth. In patients with higher risk disease following early total thyroidectomy and high-dose radioiodine ablation, this approach should permit effective management until more target-specific tumoricidal therapies become available.

REFERENCES

1. Spencer CA. New insights for using serum thyroglobulin (Tg) measurement for managing patients with differentiated thyroid carcinomas. Thyroid International 2003; 4:1–14.
2. Spencer CA, LoPresti JS, Fatemi S, Nicoloff JT. Detection of residual and recurrent differentiated thyroid carcinoma by serum thyroglobulin measurement. Thyroid 1999; 9:435–441.
3. Torrens JI, Burch HB. Serum thyroglobulin measurement. Utility in clinical practice. Endocrinol Metab Clin N Amer 2001; 30:429–467.
4. Whitley RJ, Ain KB. Thyroglobulin: a specific serum marker for the management of thyroid carcinoma. Clinics Lab Med 2004; 24:29–47.
5. Toubeau M, Touzery C, Arveux P, et al. Predictive value for disease progression of serum thyroglobulin levels measured in the postoperative period and after (131)I ablation therapy in patients with differentiated thyroid cancer. J Nucl Med 2004; 45:988–994.
6. Robbins J. Management of thyroglobulin-positive, body scan-negative thyroid cancer patients: evidence for the utility of I-131 therapy. J Endocrinol Investig 1999; 22:808–810.
7. Clark OH, Hoelting T. Management of patients with differentiated thyroid cancer who have positive serum thyroglobulin levels and negative radioiodine scans. Thyroid 1994; 4:501–505.
8. McDougall IR. Management of thyroglobulin positive/whole-body scan negative: is 131-I therapy useful? J Endocrinol Invest 2001; 24: 194–198.
9. Levy EG, Fatourechi V, Robbins R, Ringel MD. Thyroglobulin-positive, radioiodine-negative thyroid cancer. Thyroid 2001; 11:599–602.
10. Gemsenjager E. Thyroglobulin-positive, radioiodine-negative thyroid cancer (Letter to Editor). Thyroid 2003; 13:833–834.
11. Hurley JR. Management of thyroid cancer: radioiodine ablation, "stunning," and treatment of thyroglobulin-positive, (131)I scan-negative patients. Endocr Pract 2000; 6:401–406.
12. National Comprehensive Cancer Network (NCCN) Thyroid Carcinoma Guidelines 2003, March 20, 2004. Available at: www.nccn.org/professionals/physician_gls/f_guidelines.asp#site.
12a. Mazzaferri EL. Empirically treating high serum thyroglobulin levels. J Nucl Med 2005; 46:1079–1088.
13. British Thyroid Association. Guidelines for the management of differentiated thyroid cancer in adults. Available at: www.british-thyroid-association.org/guidelines.htm. 2002.
14. Pacini F, Lippi F, Formica N, et al. Therapeutic doses of iodine-131 reveal undiagnosed metastases in thyroid cancer patients with detectable serum thyroglobulin levels. J Nucl Med 1987; 28:1888–1891.
15. Wartofsky L, Sherman SI, Gopal J, et al. The use of radioactive iodine in patients with papillary and follicular thyroid cancer. J Clin Endocrinol Metab 1998; 83:4195–4203.
16. Spencer CA, Takeuchi M, Kazaroxyan M, et al. Serum thyroglobulin autoantibodies: prevalence, influence on serum thyroglobulin measurement, and prognostic significance in patients with differentiated thyroid carcinoma. J Clin Endocrinol Metab 1998; 83:1121–1127.
17. Maxon HR, Thomas SR, Boehringer A, et al. Low iodine diet in I-131 ablation of thyroid remnants. Clin Nucl Med 1983; 8:123–126.
18. Klutmann S, Jenicke L, Geiss-Tonshoff M, et al. Prevalence of iodine- and thyroglobulin-negative findings in differentiated thyroid cancer. A retrospective analysis of patients treated from 1951 to 1998 in university hospital. Nuklearmedizin 2001; 40:143–147.
19. Schlumberger M, Mancusi F, Baudin E, Pacini F. 131-I therapy for elevated thyroglobulin levels. Thyroid 1997; 7:273–276.
20. Pineda JD, Lee T, Ain K, et al. Iodine-131 therapy for thyroid cancer patients with elevated thyroglobulin and negative diagnostic scan. J Clin Endocrinol Metab 1995; 80:1488–1492.
21. Robbins J. Management of thyroglobulin-positive, body scan-negative thyroid cancer patients: evidence for the utility of I-131 therapy. J Endocrinol Investig 1999; 22:808–810.
22. De Keizer B, Koppeschaar HP, Zelissen PM, et al. Efficacy of high therapeutic doses of iodine-131 in patients with differentiated thyroid cancer and detectable serum thyroglobulin. Eur J Nucl Med 2001; 28:198–202.
23. McDougall IR. 131-I treatment of 131-I negative whole body scan, and positive thyroglobulin in differentiated thyroid carcinoma: what is being treated? Thyroid 1997; 7:669–672.
24. Mazzaferri EL. Editorial: Treating high thyroglobulin with radioiodine: A magic bullet or a shot in the dark? J Clin Endocrinol Metab 1995; 80:1485–1487.
25. Fatourechi V, Hay ID, Javedan H, et al. Lack of impact of radioiodine therapy in Tg-positive, diagnostic whole-body scan-negative patients with follicular cell-derived thyroid cancer. J Clin Endocrinol Metab 2002; 87:1521–1526.
26. Fatourechi V, Hay ID. Treating the patient with differentiated thyroid cancer with thyroglobulin-positive iodine-131 diagnostic scan-negative metastases: including comments on the role of serum thyroglobulin monitoring in tumor surveillance. Seminars Nucl Med 2000; 30:107–114.
27. Pacini F, Agate L, Elisei R, et al. Outcome of differentiated thyroid cancer with detectable serum Tg and negative diagnostic (131)I whole body scan: comparison of patients treated with high (131)I activities versus untreated patients. J Clin Endocrinol Metab 2001; 86:4092–4097.
28. Koh JM, Kim ES, Ryu JS, et al. Effects of therapeutic doses of 131-I in thyroid papillary carcinoma patients with elevated thyroglobulin level and negative 131-I whole-body scan: comparative study. Clin Endocrinol 2003; 58:421–427.
28a. Ma C, Xie J, Kuang A. Is empiric 131-I therapy justified for patients with positive thyroglobulin and negative 131-K whole-body scanning results? J Nucl Med 2005; 46:1164–1170.
29. Ford D, Giridharan S, McConkey C, et al. External beam radiotherapy in the managment of differentiated thyroid cancer. Clin Oncol 2003; 15:337–341.
30. Brierley JD, Tsang RW. External-beam radiation therapy in the treatment of differentiated thyroid cancer. Semin Surg Oncol 1999; 16: 42–49.
31. Alam MS, Takeuchi R, Kasagi K, et al. Value of combined technetium-99m hydroxy methylene diphosphonate and Thallium-201 imaging in detecting bone metastases from thyroid carcinoma. Thyroid 1997; 7:705–712.
32. Almeida-Filho P, Ravizzini GC, Almeida C, et al. Whole-body Tc-99m sestamibi scintigraphy in the follow-up of differentiated thyroid carcinoma. Clin Nucl Med 2000; 25:443–446.
33. Carril JM, Quirce R, Serrano J, et al. Total body scintigraphy with thallium-201 and iodine-131 in the follow-up of differentiated thyroid cancer. J Nucl Med 1997; 38:686–692.
34. Dadparvar S, Chevres A, Tulchinsky M, et al. Clinical utility of technetium-99m methoxisobutylisonitrile imaging in differentiated thyroid carcinoma: comparison with thallium-201 and iodine-131 scintigraphy and serum thyroglobulin quantitation. Eur J Nucl Med 1995; 22:1330–1338.
35. Lorberboym M, Murthy S, Mechanick JI, et al. Thallium-201 and iodine-131 scintigraphy in differentiated thyroid carcinoma. J Nucl Med 1996; 37:1487–1491.
36. Ugur O, Kostakoglu L, Caner B, et al. Comparison of 201-Tl, 99mTc-MIBI and 131-I imaging in the follow-up of patients with well differentiated thyroid carcinoma. Nucl Med Commun 1996; 17:373–377.

37. Harder W, Lind P, Molnar M, et al. Thallium-201 uptake with negative iodine-131 scintigraphy and serum thyroglobulin in metastatic oxyphilic papillary thyroid carcinoma. J Nucl Med 1998; 39:236–238.
38. Elser H, Henze M, Hermann C, et al. 99m-Tc-MIBI for recurrent and metastatic differentiated thyroid carcinoma. Nuklearmedizin 1997; 36:7–12.
39. Lind P, Gallowitsch HJ. The use of non-specific tracers in the follow up of differentiated thyroid cancer: results with Tc-99m tetrofosmin whole body scintigraphy. Acta Med Austr 1996; 23:69–75.
40. Gallowitsch HJ, Kresnik E, Mikosch P, et al. Tc-99m-tetrafosmin scintigraphy: an alternative scintigraphic method for following up differentiated thyroid carcinoma—preliminary results. Nuklearmedizin 1996; 35:230–235.
41. Lind P, Gallowitsch HJ, Langsteger W, et al. Technetium-99m-tetrafosmin whole-body scintigraphy in the follow-up of differentiated thyroid carcinoma. J Nucl Med 1997; 38:348–352.
42. Macapinlac HA. Clinical usefulness of FDG PET in differentiated thyroid cancer. J Nucl Med 2001; 42:77–78.
43. Adler LP, Bloom AD. Positron emission tomography of thyroid masses. Thyroid 1993; 3:195–200.
44. McDougall IR, Davidson J, Segall GM. Positron emission tomography of the thyroid, with an emphasis on thyroid cancer. Nucl Med Commun 2001; 22:485–492.
45. Schoder H, Yeung HWD. Positiron emission imaging of head and neck cancer, including thyroid carcinoma. Semin Nucl Med 2004; 34:180–197.
46. deGroot JW, Links TP, Jager PL, et al. Impact of 18F-fluoro-2-D-glucose positron emission tomograph (FDG-PET) in patients with biochemical evidence of recurrent or residual medullary thyroid cancer. Ann Surg Oncol 2004; 11:786–794.
47. Ortega F, Maldonado A, Maranes P, et al. PET-FDG in thyroid cancer with high thyroglobulin levels and negative 131-I scan. A case report. Revista Espanola de Medicina Nuclear 1999; 18:50–54.
48. Muros MA, Llamas-Elvira JM, Ramirez-Navarro A, et al. Utility of fluorine-18-fluorodeoxyglucose positron emission tomography in differentiated thyroid carcinoma with negative radioiodine scans and elevated serum thyroglobulin levels. Am J Surg 2000; 179:457–461.
49. Laking GR, Price PM. Clinical impact of (18)F-FDG PET in thyroid carcinoma patients with elevated thyroglobulin levels and negative (131)I scanning results after therapy. J Nucl Med 2002; 43:1728–1729.
50. Frilling A, Tecklenborg K, Gorges R, et al. Preoperative diagnostic value of [(18)F] fluorodeoxyglucose positron emission tomography in patients with radioiodine-negative recurrent well-differentiated thyroid carcinoma. Ann Surg 2001; 234:804–811.
51. Alnafisi NS, Driedger A, Coates G, et al. FDG-PET of recurrent or metastatic 131I-negative papillary thyroid carcinoma. J Nucl Med 2000; 41:1010–1015.
52. Grunwald F, Menzel C, Bender H, et al. Comparison of 18FDG-PET with 131-Iodine and 99m-Tc-sestamibi scintigraphy in differentiated thyroid cancer. Thyroid 1997; 7:327–335.
53. Schluter B, Bohuslavizki KH, Beyer W, et al. Impact of FDG PET on patients with differentiated thyroid cancer who present with elevated thyroglobulin and negative 131I scan. J Nucl Med 2001; 42:71–76.
54. Wang W, Macapinlac H, Larson SM, et al. [18F]-2-fluoro-2-deoxy-D-glucose positron emission tomography localizes residual thyroid cancer in patients with negative diagnostic (131)I whole body scans and elevated serum thyroglobulin levels. J Clin Endocrinol Metab 1999; 84:2291–2302.
55. Chung JK, So Y, Lee JS, et al. Value of FDG-PET in papillary thyroid carcinoma with negative 131-I whole body scan. J Nucl Med 1999; 40:986–992.
56. Helal BO, Merlet P, Toubert ME, et al. Clinical impact of (18)F-FDG PET in thyroid carcinoma patients with elevated thyroglobulin levels and negative (131)I scanning results after therapy. J Nucl Med 2001; 42:1464–1469.
57. van Tol KM, Jager PL, Dullaart RP. Links TP. Follow-up in patients with differentiated thyroid carcinoma with positive 18F-fluoro-2-deoxy-D-glucose-positron emission tomography results, elevated thyroglobulin levels, and negative high-dose 131I posttreatment whole body scans. J Clin Endocrinol Metab 2000; 85:2082–2083.
58. Fridrich L, Messa C, Landoni C, et al. Whole-body scintigraphy with 99m-TC-MIBI, 18F-FDG and 131-I in patients with metastatic thyroid carcinoma. Nucl Med Commun 1997; 18:3–9.
59. Feine U, Lietzenmayer R, Hanke JP, et al. Fluorine-18-FDG and iodine-131 uptake in thyroid cancer. J Nucl Med 1996; 37:1468–1472.
60. Dietlein M, Scheidhauer K, Voth E, et al. Fluorine-18 fluorodeoxyglucose positron emission tomography and iodine-131 whole-body scintigraphy in the follow-up of differentiated thyroid cancer. Eur J Nucl Med 1997; 24:1342–1348.
61. Altenvoerde G, Lerch H, Kuwert T, et al. Positron emission tomography with F-18-deoxyglucose in patients with differentiated thyroid carcinoma, elevated thyroglobulin levels, and negative iodine scans. Langenbecks Arch Surg 1998; 383:160–163.
62. Grunwald F, Kalicke T, Feine U, et al. (18)F-FDG PET scanning in patients with thyroid cancer: results of a multicentre study. Eur J Nucl Med 1999; 26:1547–1552.
63. Wang W, Larson SM, Fazzari M, et al. Prognostic value of (18)F-FDG PET scanning in patients with thyroid cancer. J Clin Endocrinol Metab 2000; 85:1107–1113.
64. Hung MC, Wu HS, Kao Ch, et al. F18-fluorodeoxyglucose positron emission tomography in detecting metastatic papillary thyroid carcinoma with elevated human serum thyroglobulin levels but negative I-131 whole body scan. Endocr Res 2003; 29:169–175.
65. Deichen JT, Schmidt C, Prante O, et al. Influence of TSH on uptake of [18F]fluorodeoxyglucose in human thyroid cells in vitro. Eur J Nucl Med Mol Imaging 2004; 31:507–512.
66. Mruck S, Pfahlberg A, Papadopoulos T, et al. Uptake of ^{201}TI in primary cell cultures from human thyroid tissue is multiplied by TSH. J Nucl Med 2002; 43:145–152.
67. Chin BB, Patel P, Chhade C, et al. Recombinant human thyrotropin stimulation of fluoro-d-glucose positron emission tomography uptake in well-differentiated thyroid carcinoma. J Clin Endocrinol Metab 2004; 89:91–95.
68. Petrich T, Borner AR, Otto D, et al. Influence of rhTSH on [18-F] fluorodeoxyglucose uptake by differentiated thyroid carcinoma. Eur J Nucl Med Molec Imaging 2002; 29:641–647.
69. Moog F, Linke R, Manthey N, et al. Influence of thyroid-stimulating hormone levels on uptake of FDG in recurrent and metastatic differentiated thyroid carcinoma. J Nucl Med 2000; 41:1989–1995.
70. van Tol KM, Jager PL, Piers DA, et al. Better yield of 18-fluorodeoxyglucose-positron emission tomography in patiens with metastatic differentiated thyroid carcinoma during thyrotropin stimulation. Thyroid 2002; 12:381–387.
71. Kasner DL, Spieth ME, Starkman ME, Zdor-North D. Iodine-131-negative whole body scan reverses to positive after a combination thyrogen stimulation and withdrawal. Clin Nucl Med 2002; 27:772–780.
72. Morris JC, Kim CK, Padilla MLK, et al. Conversion of non-iodine-concentrating differentiated thyroid carcinoma metastases into iodine-concentrating foci after anticancer chemotherapy. Thyroid 1997; 7:63–66.
73. Baudin E, Schlumberger M, Lumbroso J, et al. Octreotide scintigraphy in patients with differentiated thyroid carcinoma: contribution for patients with negative radioiodine scan. J Clin Endocrinol Metab 1996; 81:2541–2544.

74. Haslinghuis LM, Krenning EP, De Herder WW, et al. Somatostatin receptor scintigraphy in the follow-up of patients with differentiated thyroid cancer. J Endocrinol Invest 2001; 24:415–422.
75. Stokkel MP, Reigman HI, Verkooijen RB, Smit JW. Indium-11-Octreotide scintigraphy in differentiated thyroid carcinoma metastases that do not respond to treatment with high-dose I-131. J Cancer Res Clin Oncol 2003; 129:287–294.
76. Sarlis NJ, Gourgiotis L, Guthrie LC, et al. In-111 DTPA-Octreotide scintigraphy for disease detection in metastatic thyroid cancer: Comparison with F-18 FDG PET and extensive conventional radiographic imaging. Clin Nucl Med 2003; 28:208–217.
77. Antonelli A, Miccoli P, Ferdeghini M, et al. Role of neck ultrasonography in the follow-up of patients operated on for thyroid cancer. Thyroid 1995; 5:25–28.
78. Pacini F, Molinaro E, Castagna MG, et al. Recombinant human thyrotropin-stimulated serum thyroglobulin combined with neck ultrasonography has the highest sensitivity in monitoring differentiated thyroid carcinoma. J Clin Endocrinol Metab 2003; 88:3668–3673.
79. Alzahrani AS, Raef H, Sultan A, et al. Impact of cervical lymph node dissection on serum TG and the course of disease in TG-positive, radioactive iodine whole body scan-negative recurrent/persistent papillary thyroid cancer. J Endocrinol Invest 2002; 25:526–531.
80. Karwowski JK, Jeffrey B, McDougall IR, Weigel RJ. Intraoperative ultrasonography improves identification of recurrent thyroid cancer. Surgery 2002; 132:924–929.
81. Schlumberger MJ. Papillary and follicular thyroid carcinoma. N Engl J Med 1998; 338:297–306.
82. Schlumberger M, Hay ID. Use of radioactive iodine in patients with papillary and follicular thyroid cancer. J Clin Endocrinol Metab 1998; 83:4195–4203.
83. van Tol KM, Jager PL, deVries EG, et al. Outcome in patients with differentiated thyroid cancer with negative diagnostic whole-body scanning and detectable stimulated thyrglobulin. Eur J Endocrinol 2003; 148:589–596.
84. Kabasakal L, Selcuk NA, Shafipour H, et al. Treatment of iodine-negative thyroglobulin-positive thyroid cancer; differences in outcome in patients with macrometastases and patients with micrometastases. Europ J Nucl Med Molec Imaging 2004; 31:1500–1504.
85. Kamel N, Corapcioglu D, Sahin M, et al. I-131 therapy for thyroglobulin positive patients without anatomical evidence of persistent disease. J Endocrinol Invest 2004; 27:949–953.

40
Determinants of Prognosis in Papillary Thyroid Cancer

Henry B. Burch

INTRODUCTION

What features distinguish the rare patient with rapidly progressive and ultimately fatal papillary thyroid cancer from the more typical patient with an essentially normal survival? Prognostication in papillary thyroid cancer has been facilitated by the recognition of clinical and pathological features that correlate with the risk of recurrence and death from disease (Table 1). Numerous retrospective analyses have identified several factors that contribute to a negative impact on survival. These include patient age older than 40–50 yr, tumor size larger than 4 cm, advanced tumor grade, male sex, local tumor invasion beyond the thyroid capsule, and distant metastatic disease (1–5).

The Mayo Clinic provided a detailed account of 1500 consecutive cases of papillary thyroid cancer over a 40-yr period (2). The 20-yr cancer-specific mortality in this cohort was 0.8% for patients less than 50 yr of age, 7% for patients 50–59 yr of age, 20% for patients 60–69 yr of age, and 47% for patients ages 70 or higher. Similarly, mortality from thyroid cancer increased with tumor size, with a 20-yr mortality of 0.8% for patients with tumors less than 2.0 cm in diameter, 6% for tumors 2.0–3.9 cm, 16% for tumors 4.0–6.9 cm, and 50% for tumors greater than 7 cm. Patients with tumors extending through the thyroid capsule had a 20-yr mortality rate of 28%, compared to only 1.9% of patients with tumor confined to the thyroid. The worst outcome occurred in patients with distant metastases at presentation, for whom the 10-yr cancer mortality was 69% vs 3% in those patients with tumors confined to the neck. Overall mortality from thyroid cancer was 9% for men and 4% for women.

Mazzaferri has reported long-term follow-up on a large cohort of differentiated thyroid cancer patients, with the longest follow-up at 40 yr (1,3). Although the cohort analysis included patients with follicular thyroid cancer (21% of patients in 1994), a great deal of useful information has been gathered from this series and recently updated (1). For the patients with papillary thyroid cancer, the overall recurrence rate at 30 yr was 31%, and the disease-specific death rate was 6% (3). Age at diagnosis was an important determinant of disease-specific mortality, with a 1.8% death rate for patients less than 40 yr old, 12% for patients greater than age 40, and 21% for patients older than 50 at diagnosis (3). Tumor size was also predictive of recurrence and death. Size less than 1.5 cm in diameter yielded a recurrence rate of 11% and a tumor-specific death rate of 0.4%, compared to 33% and 7%, respectively, for patients with tumors more than 1.5 cm at diagnosis.

A series of 810 patients with papillary thyroid cancer seen at Memorial Sloan-Kettering Cancer Center from 1930 to 1985 was examined for prognostic factors and reported the results in 1996 after a median follow-up duration of 20 yr (5). Patients younger than 45 yr old had a 4% disease-specific death rate at 20 yr, compared to 27% in those ages 45 yr old or older. Local tumor extension into the surrounding neck structures was associated with a 61% cancer death rate at 20 yr vs only 5% in patients with no local extension. Patients with distant metastases had a 54% cancer death rate at 20 yr. Other significant predictors of mortality by multivariate analysis were tumor size (greater than 4 cm) and male gender but not multifocality or positive lymph nodes. A unique feature of this report involved the description of an intermediate-risk group, defined as either an age older than 45 but tumor 4 cm, or older than 45 but tumor smaller than 4 cm and without local invasion or distant metastases. These two patient groups together comprised 39% of all patients and appeared to have an intermediate risk of death (8% at 20 yr vs 1% for the lowest-risk patients and 57% for high-risk patients) that was independent of patient age.

Lastly, a study of 269 patients with papillary thyroid cancer, who were followed an average of 12 yr after diagnosis at the University of Chicago, found an overall recurrence rate of 25% and a cancer death rate of 8.2% (4). Regarding the risk of death from thyroid cancer, age more than 45 yr was associated with a 32-fold increased risk, a tumor larger than 3.0 cm with a 5.8-fold increased risk, extrathyroidal extension with a 7.7-fold increased risk, and distant metastases with a 47-fold increased risk.

Although this discussion has focused on cause-specific *mortality* from thyroid cancer, many of the same prognostic

From: *Thyroid Cancer: A Comprehensive Guide to Clinical Management, 2/e*
Edited by: L. Wartofsky and D. Van Nostrand © Humana Press Inc., Totowa, NJ

Table 1
Consistently Poor Prognostic Factors for Papillary Thyroid Cancer

Patient age >40 at diagnosis
Large tumors (>4.0 cm)
Male gender
Advanced tumor grade
Tumors with local extension
Distant metastases

indicators cited in this section are also predictive of local recurrences and distant metastases *(2,6)*.

EFFECT OF TREATMENT ON OUTCOME

The extent of initial therapy for papillary thyroid cancer has value for predicting tumor recurrence and cancer-related death. In a study consisting of 1077 patients with papillary thyroid cancer and 278 with follicular thyroid cancer, patients with tumors greater than 1.5 cm and no distant metastases had a 30-yr recurrence rate of 26%. They also had a cancer-related mortality rate of 6% when treated with total or near-total thyroidectomy, compared to rates of 40% and 9%, respectively, for patients treated with less-complete surgery *(3)*. These same authors found that despite experiencing more advanced disease, patients treated with postoperative radioiodine ablation for tumors greater than 1.5 cm, as well as no distant metastases (stages II and III), had significantly lower rates of tumor recurrence (16% vs 38%, $p < 0.001$) and cause-specific mortality (3% vs 9%, $p = 0.03$) than patients not taking radioiodine ablation *(3)*. Another study that involved 269 patients with papillary thyroid cancer for an average follow-up of 12 yr found that patients with tumors larger than 1 cm in diameter had a lower incidence of recurrence and death when a total or near-total thyroidectomy was performed *(4)*. Similarly, this study determined that postoperative radioiodine ablation resulted in lower rates of recurrence and death from thyroid cancer. However, this result had marginal statistical significance and was limited to patients with tumors larger than 1 cm and confined to the thyroid or tumors metastatic only to cervical lymph nodes *(4)*.

Not all studies have supported the use of prophylactic radioiodine ablation following surgery for papillary thyroid cancer. In the Mayo Clinic review of 1500 patients with papillary thyroid cancer, no difference in recurrence or cause-specific mortality was found between 946 patients treated with surgery alone and 220 patients treated with surgery and radioiodine ablation *(2)*. This disparity likely reflects the restraints imposed by the application of retrospective data to judge treatment efficacy for thyroid cancer. Patients treated more aggressively are likely to have been at a higher risk for recurrence and death from disease. This confounding effect tends to underestimate the benefit of therapy. Conversely, the inclusion of patients administered radioiodine therapy for known residual disease in an analysis of remnant ablation tends to overestimate the benefit of the latter practice.

EFFECT OF TUMOR SUBTYPE

Although papillary thyroid cancer in its entirety has an excellent prognosis, it is evident that certain rare subtypes of this disease have a distinctly poor prognosis (see Chapters 65, 66). These subtypes include the tall-cell variant, columnar variant, and insular-pattern thyroid carcinomas, as has been recently reviewed *(7,8)*. The follicular variant of papillary thyroid cancer is a subtype with a microfollicular histological pattern but nuclear features and biological behavior similar to typical papillary thyroid cancer *(9)*.

REFERENCES

1. Mazzaferri EL, Kloos RT. Clinical review 128: Current approaches to primary therapy for papillary and follicular thyroid cancer. J Clin Endocrinol Metab 2001; 86:1447–1463.
2. Hay ID. Papillary thyroid carcinoma. Endocrinol Metab Clin North Am 1990; 19:545–576.
3. Mazzaferri EL, Jhiang SM. Long-term impact of initial surgical and medical therapy on papillary and follicular thyroid cancer. Am J Med 1994; 97:418–428.
4. DeGroot LJ, Kaplan EL, McCormick M, Straus FH. Natural history, treatment, and course of papillary thyroid carcinoma. J Clin Endocrinol Metab 1990; 71:414–424.
5. Shaha AR, Shah JP, Loree TR. Risk group stratification and prognostic factors in papillary carcinoma of thyroid. Ann Surg Oncol 1996; 3:534 538.
6. Ain KB. Papillary thyroid carcinoma. Etiology, assessment, and therapy. Endocrinol Metab Clin North Am 1995; 24:711–760.
7. Prendiville S, Burman KD, Ringel MD, et al. Tall cell variant: an aggressive form of papillary thyroid carcinoma. Otolaryngol Head Neck Surg 2000; 122:352–357.
8. Burman KD, Ringel MD, Wartofsky L. Unusual types of thyroid neoplasms. Endocrinol Metab Clin North Am 1996; 25:49–68.
9. Zidan J, Karen D, Stein M, et al. Pure versus follicular variant of papillary thyroid carcinoma: clinical features, prognostic factors, treatment, and survival. Cancer 2003; 97:1181–1185.

41
Papillary Cancer
Special Aspects in Children

Andrew J. Bauer and Merrily Poth

INTRODUCTION

Similarly to adults, the most common form of thyroid malignancy in children is papillary thyroid cancer (PTC), accounting for approx 70–80% of newly diagnosed pediatric thyroid cancers *(1–3)*. In contrast to adults, however, pediatric patients with PTC have more locally invasive disease and more pulmonary metastases at presentation, as well as a higher incidence of recurrent or persistent disease after initial treatment. Despite these apparently ominous features, 5- and 10-yr survival rates and disease-specific mortality for children with PTC remains favorable *(1–9c)*.

Our current approach to evaluation and treatment of PTC in children and adolescents has been extrapolated from the old treatment of PTC in adults. Although the cancer's histology is the same, its clinical behavior in children is much different, with pediatric PTC showing even much faster growth, often presenting with extensive regional disease and pulmonary metastases. Even after treatment, 15–35% of cases recur or persist and need to be retreated. As the medical community continues to search for the safest, most effective treatment options for children, the fact remains that much of our knowledge is based on retrospective chart reviews. These reviews often cover decades of time, with great variations in length of time to diagnosis, patient age, degree of iodine sufficiency, and details of surgical and medical management. The last decade has witnessed a marked increase in the number of reports on pediatric thyroid cancer, but information on 30–40-yr post-treatment follow-up remains quite limited. Because of this lack of controlled and definitive data, the ability to individualize treatment plans to ensure optimum outcome with the least risk of therapy remains limited *(1–3,5,10)*.

The low incidence of PTC mitigates against any single center or physician group accumulating enough patients to conduct a long-term study with treatment and survival data. Thus, disparities and unknowns continue to create controversy in treatment as we strive to balance the use of intense treatment for cancer that, on presentation, appears aggressive with regional and pulmonary metastases but contrary to adults, seems to have a more indolent, long-term natural history.

PRESENTATION AND EVALUATION

As stated in the overview on thyroid cancer in children (Chapter 10), the most typical presentation for thyroid cancer in children and adolescents is an asymptomatic, solitary thyroid nodule, either noted in a patient followed for autoimmune thyroid disease or during routine physical exam *(11–16)*. Thyroid nodules are thought to be relatively uncommon in children, historically reported at a prevalence of less than 2% *(17)*; the true incidence may be higher because not all children have careful routine thyroid exams. Unlike nodular thyroid disease in adults, up to 50% of pediatric thyroid nodules may be malignant *(18,19)*.

Importantly, as many as 50% of children with thyroid cancer present with persistent cervical adenopathy as their initial symptom *(13,15,16)*. Because palpable cervical lymphadenopathy from benign causes is common in children, deciphering which lymph nodes are potentially malignant may present a significant challenge for clinicians *(12–16)*.

In our experience, several of the worst cases relating to the extent of disease at diagnosis and treatment difficulty were referred only after relatively extended evaluations for what was believed to be cervical adenitis. In each case, this evaluation included several courses of antibiotic therapy and repeated examinations. It was only when eventual biopsy of the lymph node revealed thyroid cancer that the thyroid was carefully examined and the primary lesion identified. Thus, education must be provided and emphasized to primary care providers and surgeons regarding the need for thorough examination of the thyroid gland as part of the evaluation of persistent cervical adenopathy.

The opinions and assertions contained herein are the private views of the authors and are not to be construed as official or as reflecting the opinions of the Uniformed Services University of the Health Sciences, the Department of the Army or the Department of Defense.

From: *Thyroid Cancer: A Comprehensive Guide to Clinical Management, 2/e*
Edited by: L. Wartofsky and D. Van Nostrand © Humana Press Inc., Totowa, NJ

PTC in children has a high rate of metastasis, often showing regional and distant metastasis at the time of diagnosis. At the time of diagnosis, 30–70% of these patients have palpable lymph nodes, and up to 90% of PTC lesions are already locally invasive at initial surgery, most commonly metastasizing to regional lymph nodes (1–5,7,8,12–16, 20–22). Lung metastases are reported in 6–20% of children (2–4,7,9,23,24), depending on the technique used to determine their presence. Chest radiographs and chest computed tomography (CT) scans are relatively insensitive in detecting lung metastases, with normal chest X-rays quite common in the presence of diffuse pulmonary disease (13,21,23). Whole-body scanning (WBS), whether postsurgical, postablation, or posttherapy, is more sensitive, but this is positively correlated to the amount of ^{131}I administered and negatively correlated with the amount of thyroid tissue present in the thyroid bed or cervical region. In a study of 122 patients under 20 yr of age, of which 28 had pulmonary metastasis, only 7 had metastatic disease seen on chest X-ray (23). Pulmonary disease was diagnosed in eight patients on first postsurgery WBS (2–3 mCi of ^{131}I), seven patients on first postablation scan, and six on later posttherapy scans (23). Of these patients, 85% had near-total thyroidectomies as their initial treatment (23).

Therefore, in patients found to have regional lymph node metastases at diagnosis, underlying lung metastases may be present but only detected on scan after complete surgical resection of cervical disease. In some cases, it may be first noted on later WBS performed during long-term follow-up, reflecting progression of disease (13–16,20–22). One argument supporting aggressive initial surgery is based on improved sensitivity for early detection of pulmonary disease, which may stimulate the clinician to employ a higher initial ^{131}I ablative dose to be used. The use of large quantities of ^{131}I must be balanced with the realization that less than 10% of children and adolescents with thyroid cancer die of their disease, even with extensive, locally invasive, or recurrent disease (12–16,20–22).

Although local invasion of tumor and metastases to the lungs are common (and long-term prognosis remains good even with this extensive disease), bone metastases are rare in children, occurring in less than 1% in all reported series. When bone metastases do occur in children, they carry a poor prognosis.

The recommended process to evaluate a child or adolescent with a thyroid nodule has changed with the use of fine-needle aspiration (FNA) and the availability of this technique for children. Proven to be effective in selecting patients for surgery in adult populations, FNA has now been instituted as a primary tool for younger patients (25–27). In a recent report of 42 pediatric patients with thyroid nodules that ultimately had surgical resection, the sensitivity, specificity, and accuracy of FNA was reported to be 95%, 86.3%, and 90.4%, respectively (27). There are well-developed guidelines for this procedure, the most stringent and perhaps appropriate were those detailed by Hamburger (28). He clearly articulated the need to acquire sufficient material and recommended the use of six separate aspirates in a given biopsy procedure as a technique for ensuring sufficient clinical material. The use of local anesthesia before aspiration, and even the use of sedation in younger or more anxious patients, enable this process. He and others have emphasized the critical need for experienced and competent cytopathologists to ensure that the pathological interpretation of material is accurate (see Chapters 18, 25). With the use of FNA, the finding of clearly malignant cells allows the opportunity for appropriate preoperative planning of a "cancer" operation and thoughtful counseling between parents and child before the operation (29). Presence of the molecular marker, galectin-3, has been assessed in cells obtained by FNA in adults as an indicator of malignancy (see Chapter 19) but studies in children have not found this marker to be useful (29a).

Notably, in adults with a lower incidence of malignant thyroid nodules, it may be easier to follow a nodule after a negative or even an equivocal FNA cytology result. In younger children and adolescents, the much higher incidence of malignancy (up to 50% vs 10–14% reported in adults) means that only the most benign and definitive FNA results will allow the endocrinologist to follow the patient expectantly (27). Diagnostic data from preoperative FNA in a child with a thyroid nodule may obviate the need for frozen-section tissue examination during the surgical removal of the mass (lobectomy). Many surgeons feel that frozen-section examination adds little to the data obtained with a preoperative FNA (30). If the FNA yields cells consistent with "follicular neoplasm," the frozen-section evaluation will rarely give more definitive results. Most pediatric surgeons would rather remove the affected lobe and possibly the isthmus, then await the final pathology report before deciding whether to proceed with a completion subtotal thyroidectomy. However, this issue remains under debate (31).

In contrast to the increasing use of FNA in the evaluation of childhood thyroid nodules, the routine use of scintigraphic procedures to characterize a nodule as "hot," "warm," or "cold" is decreasing. Numerous reports describe malignant lesions in warm or hot nodules; thus, these distinctions do not clearly define the ultimate risk of malignancy (27, 32–34). The thyroid scan was once a standard part of the initial evaluation of a thyroid nodule, now most practitioners no longer use thyroid scans as a routine examination of thyroid lesions (27). However, thyroid scans may be useful to rule out the entity of hemiagenesis of the thyroid in which the apparent mass is an enlarged single lobe of the thyroid gland, although this can be determined by ultrasound as well. In our view, a reasonable plan for evaluation of thyroid nodules or persistent cervical adenopathy in children would include thyroid ultrasound to assess the size, number, centricity (bilateral, multicentric, or focal), and characteristics (cystic, solid, mixed) of the nodule, followed by FNA *(35a)*.

Although the ultrasound findings do not predict whether a lesion is benign or malignant, the information is useful to decide where to attempt FNA (especially in the case of more than one nodule) and whether drainage of the nodule would be effective with cystic lesions. The ultrasound results may also be helpful in planning surgical intervention. Routine use of cervical CT scans or magnetic resonance imaging (MRI) to assess local or regional disease has not been formally assessed but may be considered on an individual basis. If CT is used for this evaluation, it is extremely important to avoid the use of iodine-rich contrast in the study.

A subgroup of children with thyroid nodules are those with a history of exposure to radiation, whether from environmental accidents (Chernobyl) or as survivors of childhood nonthyroid cancer who received external-beam irradiation during treatment *(36–42)*. In these children, there are often multiple thyroid lesions that may be benign adenomas, multicentric cancers, or a mixture of these *(43–45)*. The overall risk of thyroid nodules has been reported to be as high as 27 times above sibling controls *(37)*, and the increased risk of malignancy, most often PTC, is 18–53-fold higher *(37,38)*. Based on these data, it may be argued that the appearance of a thyroid nodule in a child with a history of significant radiation exposure is sufficient to indicate the need for surgery without any additional preoperative evaluation.

In addition to annual physical examinations in following children with previous radiation exposure, the issue of if and when to perform regular thyroid ultrasound is debated. It is our belief that an ultrasound should be performed at least once within 5 yr of radiation treatment. Scheduled repeat exams are then individualized according to the results, physical exam, radiation dose, and age at time of radiation therapy. Patients younger than 10 yr old at the time of initial radiation therapy, as well as patients with Hodgkin's disease, are more closely followed.

APPROACH TO TREATMENT

As in adults, the initial therapy of childhood thyroid cancer involves surgical resection. However, the extent of surgery recommended does remain somewhat controversial. In PTC, which comprises the vast majority of childhood thyroid cancer cases, the general recommendation for surgery includes a near-total or total thyroidectomy, along with the removal of local lymph nodes *(1,2,4,5,9,10,24,46–54)*. The safety of this procedure is dependent on the extent of disease found at surgery and the surgeon's experience. With an inexperienced surgeon, there may be a high morbidity, including hypoparathyroidism and recurrent laryngeal nerve (RLN) damage. However, if the procedure is performed by a surgeon experienced with this operation in children, there is a low incidence of complications and essentially no mortality *(46,47,54a)*.

Regarding the complications of permanent hypoparathyroidism and RLN damage, a review documents the most recent pediatric thyroid cancer case reports over a period of 40 yr. It indicated a 0–15% incidence of permanent hypoparathyroidism and a 0–9% incidence of permanent RLN damage *(1–3,9,10,24)*. One outlier is a report by Brink et al. who reviewed a group of 14 patients with pulmonary metastases, showing 30% and 38% incidences, respectively *(4)*. The importance of surgical experience is illustrated by the fact that even this study did not find any cases of hypoparathyroidism after 1980 *(4)*. Analysis of the reports from the mid-1970s to the present show a lower incidence: 0–4% for hypoparathyroidism and 0% for RLN damage ($n = 69$, combined). Again, this is likely a reflection of improved surgical techniques and experience *(2,24)*. Thus, it cannot be overemphasized that thyroid surgery, particularly in children and adolescents, is a procedure that should be performed only by a professional with extensive, successful experience relating to this disease. Autotransplantation of a parathyroid is occasionally performed to preserve parathyroid function.

Previous controversy existed regarding the need to remove the contralateral lobe of the thyroid. Those that advocated a more limited procedure than a near-total or total thyroidectomy argued that it was not worth the additional risk because: (1) the more extreme operation carried a higher risk of complications, and (2) thyroid cancer in children had a good prognosis, and a simple lobectomy was therefore sufficient for the initial operation *(55)*. Those in favor of total thyroidectomy base their argument on the observation that up to 65% of pediatric PTC is multifocal *(4,8,20,32)* and often bilateral *(2)*, with an even higher incidence of multicentricity in patient's postradiation exposure.

In the absence of a prospective study, deciding which surgical approach is the most appropriate requires balancing the desire to improve disease-free survival with the risk of surgical complications. Several other arguments favor the use of more aggressive surgical intervention, the primary one being improved disease-free survival *(5,7,9)*. A multivariate analysis by Jarzab et al. of 109 children (71% PTC; 29% follicular thyroid cancer) reported on radical surgery. (Radical is designated as total thyroidectomy with central lymph node dissection and bilateral node biopsy with radical-modified dissection if positive nodes were found.) This type of surgery was the most significant factor in predicting disease-free survival *(9)*. In this study, children who received less than a "radical" surgery had a 10-fold increase in the relative risk of recurrence *(9)*. Similar results supporting the utility of radical surgery have been described by both Chow et al. and Landau et al. A decrease was shown from 38% to 3% in local and from 17% to 0% in distant relapse rates, along with a decline from 60% to 30% in local recurrence rates, respectively *(5,7)*.

In addition to improving disease-free survival, surgical removal of the entire thyroid and any regional disease allows for the most efficient use of adjunctive ^{131}I therapy and improves the sensitivity of WBS for detecting persistent or recurrent disease. Most would agree that pediatric PTC patients experience long-term survival, but this good prognosis is applicable only with the use of ^{131}I to treat residual or recurrent disease *(5,7,9,51,52)*. With less than a near-total thyroidectomy, the presence of large amounts of normal thyroid tissue makes the effective use of ^{131}I to eradicate thyroid cancer cells, with their less efficient iodine-uptake mechanism, difficult, if not impossible. For the same reasons, scanning with ^{131}I to search for the presence of residual or recurrent tumor is impeded by the presence of normal thyroid tissue. Finally, the use of serum thyroglobulin measurements to search for recurrent or persistent malignant disease is problematic in the presence of normal thyroid tissue.

In summary, despite the obvious potential for increased surgical complications with more extensive surgery in children, the authors believe that either total thyroidectomy or removal of the affected lobe and the isthmus, with a subtotal resection of the contralateral lobe, is the preferred operation for PTC in children and adolescents. Surgery should also encompass central-compartment dissection with biopsy of all suspicious lymph nodes and extension to unilateral-modified radical neck dissection if positive lymph nodes are found.

Ensuring that this surgery is only performed by surgeons with extensive experience with this procedure in children results in a drastically decreased rate of both minor and major complications. Currently, at most centers with this standard of practice, the incidence of complications is well below 5%; the most common is mild temporary hypocalcemia *(46–52)*. The incidence of significant RLN damage (not from compression of the nerve by tumor before surgery) is low, and bilateral damage during surgery is very rare. Even authors who argue against the routine use of near-total thyroidectomy note excellent results and low rates of problems in initial operations performed by more experienced surgeons *(55)*.

^{131}I ABLATION

The incorporation of ^{131}I ablation into the postsurgical therapeutic modality for PTC has become common. In fact, it has been suggested that greater reliance on radioiodine in combination with less aggressive surgery may decrease the surgical complication rate without compromising long-term outcome *(56)*. However, this approach has not been formally studied. Regardless, there are clear advantages to the use of ^{131}I ablation that, in addition to the destruction of malignant cells, include the destruction of all residual normal thyroid tissue, allowing for the more effective use of surveillance methods. These include ^{131}I scanning and serum thyroglobulin measurements (see Chapter 33).

A current recommendation is to administer an ablative dose of ^{131}I to patients with differentiated thyroid cancer, usually 4–6 wk after surgery. Thyroid hormone replacement is usually withheld during this time. The patient is placed on a reduced iodine diet for at least the last 2 wk before receiving ^{131}I. A serum thyrotropin (TSH) should be performed before the administration of ^{131}I. If sufficient thyroid was removed at surgery, it should be more than 30 μU/mL. This will ensure effective uptake of iodine into both residual normal residual tissue and malignant cells. Some centers are using recombinant TSH to prepare adult patients for this ablation. Although we do use this therapy for follow-up scanning in some patients, we would not recommend its use for ablation in children or adolescents considering the need for a significantly increased ^{131}I dose with recombinant TSH to achieve successful ablation vs that obtained with the standard hypothyroid regimen.

There is some debate about how much ^{131}I should be given for this initial ablative dose. A relatively small dose of 30 mCi can be administered as an outpatient procedure. This dosage results in ablation of residual thyroid tissue in 93% of patients who, at the time of this dose, have an uptake of less than 0.3% on follow-up scan, where this uptake is only in the thyroid bed *(57)*. Unfortunately, in patients with higher estimates of uptake and/or with metastatic disease, this low dose leads to successful ablation in only 59%. In one study where four patients under age 20 were initially treated with this low dose, only two were effectively ablated. Additionally, some patients initially thought to be successfully ablated had later recurrences *(57)*.

Therefore, it is probably preferable to give a larger dose of ^{131}I, usually 80–150 mCi, which is sufficient to ablate normal tissue in almost all patients. The higher dose would be linked to the stage of disease. In stage III or IV patients, this dosage also serves as an initial treatment for metastatic disease and allows identification and localization of metastatic disease in a postablation WBS (performed 7–10 d postablation; *58, 58a*). Very limited data are available on the use of recombinant human TSH to facilitate radioiodine therapy *(58b)*.

Follow-Up ^{131}I Treatment

As is typically done in adults, children should be reevaluated for residual disease 6 mo after initial RAI ablation. Currently, thyroid hormone withdrawal is instituted 4–6 wk before, and the patient is placed on triiodothyronine. Triiodothyronine is withdrawn, and a low-iodine diet is instituted 2 wk prior to RIA. As previously addressed, concerns over compliance and safety continue, and changes to this regimen may be forthcoming over the next several years. While hypothyroid, a TSH-stimulated serum thyroglobulin level is sent at the time of the scan. Therapy is dictated based on clinical suspicion of disease, radiologic evidence of disease, and proof of disease found on ^{131}I or ^{123}I scan. If available, dosimetry should be employed to provide the safest, most effective RAI dose. Reasonable doses to consider in the absence of dosimetry are 100–125 mCi for thyroid bed and/or lymph node involvement and 125–150 mCi if pulmonary metastases are present.

Efficacy of ^{131}I has been established in several recent studies, showing decreased recurrence (2–4,7,9). ^{131}I treatment reduced the relative risk factor for relapse by a factor of 5 in a study of 109 children, ages 6–17 yr, 74% of whom received total thyroidectomy with lymph node dissection, 55% who received ^{131}I ablation (60–80 mCi), and 78% of whom received ^{131}I treatment (cumulative dose of 60–580 mCi; 9–9c). In addition, after 5 yr of observation, 97% of children treated with ^{131}I were disease-free, whereas 40% and 60% of children without ^{131}I therapy relapsed after 5 and 10 yr, respectively (9–9c). Of note, all the children ($n = 14$) in the 6–10 yr age group relapsed within 5 yr, supporting the observation that younger age may portend a reduced disease-free survival (9–9c).

Overall, ^{131}I therapy, in cumulative doses of less than 600 mCi, have been associated with a twofold decrease in relapse and improved disease-free survival. However, follow-up data extending beyond 20 yr is extremely limited, and an eventual recurrence rate of 15–25% may be seen on a cumulative basis, despite aggressive surgical and RAI therapy (1,3–5,7–9c,24).

There are multiple areas of concern regarding potential long-term toxicity of ^{131}I in children. Because of the relatively smaller total-body mass in most children and adolescents in comparison to adults, there has been some hesitancy to use ^{131}I for the treatment of pediatric thyroid disease, both benign and malignant. This reluctance is based on the increased sensitivity of young individuals to the effects of radiation and their relatively longer life expectancy. Overall, most published data are relatively reassuring about toxicity. However, it is important to be familiar with potential long-term effects of RAI therapy and to address them with patients and family members in the context of the risks and benefits.

Issues of particular concern include effects on bone marrow, effects on reproductive function in both boys and girls, and potential carcinogenic effects (see Chapters 7, 50). In addition, there are the relatively acute toxic effects of ^{131}I of thyroiditis and inflammation of salivary glands, as well as acute nausea and vomiting (58,59). Salivary gland effects may be reduced with careful attention to hydration and measures to increase salivary flow during the exposure.

Effects of acute suppression of bone marrow can be monitored, and hematologic parameters are usually normalized by 60 d. Untoward long-term consequences of this level of acute bone marrow suppression are extremely rare and should therefore not be a cause of concern. However, it is important to allow recovery of bone marrow before retreatment with ^{131}I to ensure that full recovery will occur. Current recommendations are to space treatments at least 6 mo apart. Leukemia has been reported after multiple high doses of ^{131}I were given over a short period of time (58).

Gonadal toxicity is another potential long-term effect of ^{131}I and should be discussed with the patient and parents prior to therapy. In postpubertal males, a transient rise in follicular-stimulating hormone is common and may persist for up to 9 mo, but decreased fertility has not been reported (59,60). After a single dose of ^{131}I therapy, the estimated radiation dose to each testis appears to be lower than the dose associated with permanent damage to the germinal epithelium. However, with repeated doses of ^{131}I, along with decreased renal clearance of iodine secondary to hypothyroidism, there is still some concern. Current recommendations state that males should avoid impregnation for at least 4 mo after treatment, and that counseling for sperm banking should be given and documented for postpubertal male patients receiving cumulative doses in excess of 400 mCi (61). Data on the association of testicular function with the toxic effects of radiation, relative to the process of sexual maturation, seem to indicate that more mature testicles are more vulnerable to toxic effects. Thus, testicular effects may not be a major source of concern when treating prepubertal children.

Transient amenorrhea and menstrual irregularities have been reported in up to 17% of females younger than 40 yr, 65% of whom were treated with a single ablative dose of 81 mCi (62). Although permanent ovarian failure was not reported, and the incidence of congenital abnormalities was not increased, 14 miscarriages in 441 pregnancies occurred. The increase in miscarriage rate within the year after large ^{131}I doses led to the recommendation for conception to be avoided during the year after ^{131}I (63).

The potential for an elevated risk of secondary malignancy is also an issue of concern. There are reports of young women diagnosed with breast cancer who were treated during adolescence with ^{131}I for thyroid cancer (64,64a). Other malignancies have been reported after high-dose ^{131}I therapy, including bladder cancer, leukemia, and colorectal cancer (58,65). Vigorous hydration, frequent urination, and emptying of the bowel are recommended after high doses of ^{131}I to decrease colon, bladder, and total-body exposure. A recent study comparing the risk of second malignancy in 875 patients treated with ^{131}I for thyroid cancer did not indicate any relationship to radioiodine treatment or dosage (64a). Although the patient population included both adults and children, the implication for children being treated with ^{131}I is reassuring.

There is an increased risk of subsequent development of thyroid nodules in patients treated with small doses of ^{131}I for toxic nodules or Graves' disease. This risk generally does not apply to the amount used for the treatment of malignant disease (>20 mCi). Obviously, this is particularly true when there is complete or near-complete thyroidectomy before treatment with ^{131}I. Thus, there is no evidence of subsequent increases in thyroid disease after ^{131}I treatment for thyroid cancer.

THYROID HORMONE REPLACEMENT

Irrespective of the extent of surgical resection or whether ^{131}I ablation was performed, all children with thyroid cancer ultimately need to be treated with thyroid hormone therapy. Physiologic replacement dosing in children and adolescents is 1–3 μg/kg/d or 75–100 μg/m^2/d, and a dose of 2.1–4.5 μg/kg/d is usually sufficient to suppress the TSH to a goal of 0.01–0.02 μU/mL *(66)*. With the above dosing guideline, the goal is to suppress TSH to a level below assay detection. The individual patient may require a dose greater than that determined by calculation.

Although all patients will require lifelong thyroid hormone therapy, release from near-total suppression to physiologic replacement doses may be considered when the patient appears to be in remission. The time at which to decrease the dose is debatable and must be individualized on the basis of negative scans and undetectable serum thyroglobulin after a number of years postthyroidectomy. When free of demonstrable disease, the goal of this phase of replacement therapy dosage is to keep the TSH just above the detection limit of the assay, typically at 0.1–0.4 μU/mL *(66)*. This is particularly important in children, as the hyperthyroidism from the relatively high levels of free T_4 needed for TSH suppression may result in potential negative long-term effects on bone density *(67,68)* and behavioral symptoms similar to attention deficit disorder *(66)*. Any effect on bone density is especially problematic in children and adolescents treated for thyroid cancer who will be administered these suppressive doses of thyroxine during the critical time of peak bone mass acquisition. Long-term studies are needed to assess the impact of suppressive thyroid hormone therapy on peak bone mass acquisition and to determine whether clinically detrimental bone loss results.

PROGNOSTIC FACTORS

Review of the literature available generally shows that children with PTC, despite their high incidence of local spread at diagnosis and high rates of recurrence, experience low disease-related mortality. However, as previously stated, all studies on the effects of therapy, including the extent of surgery and the use of ^{131}I, are retrospective and therefore not conclusive in regard to determining the effects of specific treatment modalities on long-term outcomes. It may be appropriate to state that children diagnosed with PTC have good prognosis, but large studies separating patient age groups (prepubertal vs pubertal vs postpubertal), extent of surgery, and extent of ^{131}I therapy do not exist. Also, there are no studies of large groups of children followed for 20+ yr after treatment of thyroid cancer; yet, it is conceivable that a significant risk of recurrence may exist during this time span.

The search for reliable prognostic factors useful for individualizing treatment has involved interrogation of epidemiologic data (e.g., gender, age at presentation, tumor size, and presence of local and/or regional disease). Assessment of treatment is also important, including total thyroidectomy vs lobectomy, extent of lymph node dissection, ^{131}I ablation, and suppressive thyroid hormone replacement therapy.

Age, sex, and tumor size at presentation have shown inconsistent results relating to prognosis *(5,6,9)*. Intuitively, one might suspect that children under the age of 10 yr may have more aggressive PTC because the disease is often invasive at diagnosis. In fact, several reports have suggested this possibility *(5,6,9)*, with one study showing a 100% recurrence rate within 5 yr of initial therapy in 6–10-yr-old patients *(9)*. These recurrences occurred despite that patients received aggressive therapy: 74% had total thyroidectomy and 87% had received ^{131}I ablative therapy *(9)*. Male sex, previously associated with worse prognosis *(6)*, was not associated with a worse outcome *(9)*. To settle the question of whether young age and male gender really portend a worse prognosis, larger numbers of carefully studied patients are needed.

A recent study examining 47 patients with PTC reported that tumor size at presentation was linked with more advanced disease (distant metastasis) and was associated with a lower chance of response to initial therapy *(8)*. Overall, although 88% of these patients had aggressive initial therapy (88% had total thyroidectomy and all had ^{131}I ablation), patients with larger tumor size (4.2 vs 2.0 cm) required a greater number of doses of ^{131}I and a greater cumulative dose (333 vs 104 mCi) to achieve first remission *(8)*. Despite intense initial therapy, repeated ^{131}I treatment, and suppressive thyroid hormone therapy, 62.5% of these patients had persistent disease at last follow-up *(8)*. Other studies have not shown size to have prognostic significance *(3,7)*. More importantly, smaller tumor size may predict remission, as one study found a recurrence rate of 32% (11 of 34) in tumors with an average size of 2.7 cm (range 0.9–4.0 cm; *3*). Based on these data, tumor size should probably not be used to guide the extent of surgery or medical management in children.

The extent of surgery, ^{131}I ablative therapy, and suppressive thyroid hormone replacement has also been examined in regard to predicting prognosis of long-term disease outcome. Those clinicians against aggressive surgery (total or near-total thyroidectomy with modified radical neck dissection) report an undue risk of complications for disease with low mortality. Proponents of aggressive surgery argue that PTC in children is more often multifocal, bilateral, and has more frequently progressed to regional and distal metastasis at the time of initial evaluation *(1,2,4,7–9c,24)*. In several recent studies, total thyroidectomy with ablation has clearly been shown to improve 10-yr disease-free survival and decrease the incidence of recurrence *(1,2,4,7,9,24)*. One study demonstrated a 10-fold reduction in the risk of recurrence with total vs nontotal thyroidectomy and a fivefold reduction in the recurrence risk with the use of ^{131}I ablation *(9)*.

With the present state of our knowledge, it is recommended that all papillary thyroid tumors in children and adolescents be treated and followed aggressively. Because the disease-free survival of children with PTC is reported to be 80–90%, and the long-term mortality from PTC is less than 10% *(12–16,20–22,69–72)*, controversies relating to the appropriateness of aggressive therapy still exist. With the advent of improved surgical techniques and potential use of parathyroid autotransplantation, the risk of more intense surgery seems to be justified by a decreased risk of recurrence when led by a surgeon with extensive pediatric thyroid surgery experience. In addition, as previously stated, aggressive surgery enables the optimum benefit of ^{131}I therapy, allows for more accurate assessment of pulmonary disease, and provides clinicians with the ability to use serum thyroglobulin levels effectively to monitor disease over the long term.

Optimism is clearly justified, as the vast majority of patients attain long-term disease-free survival; however, the current treatment modalities are nonetheless onerous and include some morbidity. In addition, good long-term outcomes are predicated on both careful monitoring for recurrent disease and appropriate treatment. The possibility of recurrent disease many years after apparently negative evaluations mandates that patients once diagnosed with thyroid cancer should be followed expectantly for at least 20 yr, with the transition from pediatric to adult care being a critical time to avoid the lack of follow-up. In addition, reports of disease recurrence in some patients during pregnancy after many years of negative evaluations *(73)* suggests that pregnancy is also a period of time with a higher rate of recurrence. Patient education concerning lifelong risk is of outmost importance.

SUMMARY

Despite that the long-term excellent prognosis for children and adolescents with PTC, it is important to ensure that all patients continue to be followed closely for an extended length of time, perhaps for life. Recurrences may occur years after the initial diagnosis and treatment, even when appropriately treated and after a patient appears to be disease-free. Although aggressive initial management and suppressive thyroid hormone therapy appear to improve prognosis, these encouraging findings must be tempered with the realization that up to 15–35% of patients who receive aggressive initial therapy still experience recurrence of their disease *(1,2,4,7,9,24)*.

More specific recommendations regarding prognosis and the need for more or less aggressive treatment may evolve as studies to characterize tumors using molecular techniques are available. Currently, the recommendation for therapy includes at least subtotal thyroidectomy with modified neck dissection, followed by ^{131}I ablation and suppressive doses of thyroxine. Serum thyroglobulin measurements *(74)* and follow-up ^{131}I scans to monitor for recurrent or persistent disease and repeat treatment of disease with ^{131}I should result in an excellent long-term prognosis in the vast majority of cases.

REFERENCES

1. Kumar A, Bal CS. Differentiated thyroid cancer. Indian J Pediatr 2003; 70:707–713.
2. Giuffrida D, Scollo C, Pellegriti G, et al. Differentiated thyroid cancer in children and adolescents. J Endocrinol Invest 2002; 25:18–24.
3. Lee YM, Lo CY, Lam KY, et al. Well-differentiated thyroid carcinoma in Hong Kong Chinese patients under 21 years of age: A 35-year experience. J Am Coll Surg 2002; 194:711–716.
4. Brink JS, van Heerden JA, McIver B, et al. Papillary thyroid cancer with pulmonary metastases in children: Long-term prognosis. Surgery 2000; 128:881–887.
5. Landau D, Vini L, A'Hern R, Harmer C. Thyroid cancer in children: the Royal Marsden Hospital experience. Eur J Cancer 2000; 36:214–220.
6. Welch-Dinauer C, Tuttle RM, Robie D, et al. Clinical features associated with metastasis and recurrence of differentiated thyroid cancer in children, adolescents, and young adults. Clin Endocrinol 1997; 49:619–628.
7. Chow SM, Law S, Mendenhall WM, et al. Differentiated thyroid carcinoma in childhood and adolescence—clinical course and role of radioiodine. Pediatr Blood Cancer 2004; 42:176–183.
8. Powers PA, Dinauer CA, Tuttle RM, et al. Tumor size and extent of disease at diagnosis predict the response to initial therapy for papillary thyroid carcinoma in children and adolescents. J Pediatr Endocrinol Metab 2003; 16:693–702.
9. Jarzab B, Junak D, Wloch J, et al. Multivariate analysis of prognostic factors for differentiated thyroid carcinoma in children. Eur J Nucl Med 2000; 27:833–841.
9a. Borson-Chazot F, Causeret S, Lifante JC, et al. Predictive factors for recurrence from a series of 74 children and adolescents with differentiated thyroid cancer. World J Surg 2004; 28:1088–1092.
9b. Shapiro NL, Bhattacharyya N. Population-based outcomes for pediatric thyroid carcinoma. Laryngoscope 2005; 115:337–340.
9c. Leboulleux S, Baudin E, Hartl DW, Travagli JP, Schlumberger M. Follicular cell-derived thyroid cancer in children. Hormone Res. 2005; 63:145–151.
10. Kowalski LP, Filho JG, Pinto CA, et al. Long-term survival rates in young patients with thyroid carcinoma. Arch Otolaryngol Head Neck Surg 2003; 129:746–749.
11. Jocham A, Joppich I, Hecker W, et al. Thyroid carcinoma in childhood: Management and follow up of 11 cases. Eur J Pediatr 1994; 153:17–22.
12. Samuel AM, Sharma SM. Differentiated thyroid carcinomas in children and adolescents. Cancer 1991; 67:2186–2190.
13. Ceccarelli C, Pacini F, Lippi F, et al. Thyroid cancer in children and adolescents. Surgery 1988; 104:1143–1148.
14. Viswanathan K, Gierlowski TC, Schneider AB. Childhood thyroid cancer: characteristics and long-term outcome in children irradiated for benign conditions of the head and neck. Arch Pediatr Adolesc Med 1994; 148:260–263.
15. Harness JK, Thompson NW, McLeod MK, et al. Differentiated thyroid carcinoma in children and adolescents. World J Surg 1992; 16:47–54.
16. Schlumberger M, De Vathaire F, Travagli JP, et al. Differentiated thyroid carcinoma in childhood: long term follow-up of 72 patients. J Clin Endocr Metab 1987; 65:1088–1094.
17. Bentley AA, Gillespie C, Malis D. Evaluation and management of a solitary thyroid nodule in a child. Otolaryngol Clin N Am 2003; 36:117–128.
18. Hopwood NJ, Kelch RP. Thyroid masses: approach to diagnosis and management in childhood and adolescence. Pediatr Rev 1993; 14:481–487.

19. Hung W, Anderson KD, Chandra RS, et al. Solitary thyroid nodules in 71 children and adolescents. J Pediatr Surg 1992; 27:1407–1409.
20. Welch-Dinauer CA, Tuttle RM, Robie DK, et al. Clinical features associated with metastasis and recurrence of differentiated thyroid cancer in children, adolescents and young adults. Clin Endocrinol 1998; 49: 619–628.
21. Fassina AS, Rupolo M, Pelizzo MR, Casara D. Thyroid cancer in children and adolescents. Tumori 1994; 80:257–262.
22. Lamberg BA, Karkinen-Jaaskelainen M, Franssila KO. Differentiated follicle-derived thyroid carcinoma in children. Acta Pediatr Scand 1989; 78:419–425.
23. Bal CS, Kumar A, Chandra P, et al. Is chest x-ray or high-resolution computed tomography scan of the chest sufficient investigation to detect pulmonary metastasis in pediatric differentiated thyroid cancer? Thyroid 2004; 14:217–224.
24. Haveman JW, Van Tol KM, Rouwe CW, et al. Surgical experience in children with differentiated thyroid carcinoma. Ann Surg Oncol 2003; 10:15–20.
25. Degnan BM, McClellan DR, Francis GL. An analysis of fine-needle aspiration biopsy of the thyroid in children and adolescents. J Pediatr Surg 1996; 31:903–907.
26. Raab SS, Silverman JF, Elsheikh TM, et al. Pediatric thyroid nodules: disease demographics and clinical management as determined by fine needle aspiration biopsy. Pediatrics 1995; 95:46–49.
27. Corrias A, Einaudi S, Chiorboli E, et al. Accuracy of fine needle aspiration biopsy of thyroid nodules in detecting malignancy in childhood: Comparison with conventional clinical, laboratory, and imaging approaches. J Clin Endocrinol Metab 2001; 86:4644–4648.
28. Hamburger JL Diagnosis of thyroid nodules by fine needle biopsy: use and abuse. J Clin Endocrinol Metab 1994; 79:335–338.
29. De Keyser LF, Van Herle AJ. Differentiated thyroid cancer in children. Head Neck Surg 1985; 8:100–114.
29a. Niedziela M, Maceluch J, Korman E. Galectin-3 is not an universal marker of malignancy in thyroid nodular disease in children and adolescents. J Clin Endocrinol Metab 2002; 87:4411–4415.
30. Rodriguez JM, Parrilla P, Sola J, et al. Comparison between preoperative cytology and intraoperative frozen-section biopsy in the diagnosis of thyroid nodules. Br J Surg 1994; 81:1151–1154.
31. Gibb GK, Pasiek JL. Assessing the need for frozen sections: still a valuable tool in thyroid surgery. Surgery 1995; 118:1005–1010.
32. Croom RD III, Thomas CG Jr, Reddick RL, Tawil MT. Autonomously functioning thyroid nodules in childhood and adolescence. Surgery 1987; 102:1101–1108.
33. Hopwood NJ, Carroll RG, Kenny FM, Foley TP Jr. Functioning thyroid masses in childhood and adolescence. J Pediatr 1976; 89: 710–718.
34. Smith M, McHenry C, Jarosz H, et al. Carcinoma of the thyroid in patients with autonomous nodules. Am Surg 1988; 54:448–449.
35. De Roy van Zuidewijn DB, Songun I, Hamming J, et al. Preoperative diagnostic tests for operable thyroid disease. World J Surg 1994; 18: 506–510.
35a. Lyshchik A, Drozd V, Demidchik Y, Reiners C. Diagnosis of thyroid cancer in children: value of gray-scale and power Doppler ultrasound. Radiology 2005; 235:604–613.
36. Bhatia s, Yasui Y, Robison LL, et al. High risk of subsequent neoplasms continues with extended follow-up for the late effects study group. J Clin Oncol 2003; 21:4386–4394.
36a. Willams ED, Abrosimov A, Boghdanova T, et al. Thyroid carcinoma after Chernobyl: latent period, morphology and aggressiveness. Brit J Cancer 2004; 90:2219–2224.
36b. Cardis E, Kesminiene A, Ivanov V, et al. Risk of thyroid cancer after exposure to ^{131}I in childhood. J Natl Cancer Inst 2005; 97:724–732.
37. Sklar C, Whitton J, Mertens A, et al. Abnormalities of the thyroid in survivors of Hodgkin's Disease: data from the Childhood Cancer Survivor Study. J Clin Endocrinol Metab 2000; 85:3227–3232.
38. Tucker MA, Morris Jones PH, Boice JD, et al. Therapeutic radiation at a young age is linked to secondary thyroid cancer. Cancer Res 1991; 51:2885–2888.
39. Farahati J, Demidchik EP, BIko J, Reiner C. Inverse association between age at the time of radiation exposure and extent of disease in cases of radiation-induced thyroid carcinoma in Belarus. Cancer 2000; 88:1470–1476.
40. Acharya S, Sarafoglou K, LaQuaglia M, et al. Thyroid neoplasms after therapeutic radiation for malignancies during childhood and adolescence. Cancer 2003; 97:2397–2403.
41. Niedziela M, Korman E, Breborowicz D, et al. A prospective study of thyroid nodular disease in children and adolescents in western Poland from 1996 to 2000 and the incidence of thyroid carcinoma relative to iodine deficiency and the Chernobyl disaster. Pediatr Blood Cancer 2004; 42:84–92.
42. Jacob P, Goulko G, Heidenreich WF, et al. Thyroid cancer risk to children calculated. Nature 1998; 392: 31–32.
43. Shore RE, Hildreth N, Dvoretsky P, et al. Thyroid cancer among persons given x-ray treatment in infancy for an enlarged thymus gland. Am J Epidemiol 1993; 137:1068–1080.
44. Nikiforov YE, Gnepp DR, Fagin JA. Thyroid lesions in children and adolescents after the Chernobyl disaster: implications for the study of radiation tumorigenesis. J Clin Endocrinol Metab 1996; 81: 9–14.
45. Nikiforov YE, Gnepp DR. Pediatric thyroid cancer after the Chernobyl disaster: pathomorphologic study of 84 cases (1991–1992) from the Republic of Belarus. Cancer 1994; 74:748–766.
46. Farahati J, Bucsky P, Parlowsky T, et al. Characteristics of differentiated thyroid carcinoma in children and adolescents with respect to age, gender, and histology. Cancer 1997; 80:2156–2162.
47. Stael AP, Plukker JT, Piers DA, et al. Total thyroidectomy in the treatment of thyroid carcinoma in childhood. Br J Surg 1995; 82: 1083–1085.
48. Patwardhan N, Cataldo T, Braverman LE. Surgical management of the patient with papillary cancer. Surg Clin North Am 1995; 75: 449–464.
49. Shindo ML. Considerations in surgery of the thyroid gland. Otolaryn Clin North Am 1996; 29:629–635.
50. Vassilopoulou-Sellin R, Goepfert H, Raney B, Schultz PN. Differentiated thyroid cancer in children and adolescents: clinical outcome and mortality after long-term follow-up. Head Neck 1998; 20: 549–555.
51. Frankenthaler RA, Sellin RV, Cangir A, Goepfert H. Lymph node metastasis from papillary-follicular thyroid carcinoma in young patients. Am J Surg 1990; 160:341–343.
52. Massimino M, Gasparini M, Ballerini E, Del Bo R. Primary thyroid carcinoma in children: a retrospective study of 20 patients. Med Pediatr Oncol 1995; 24:13–17.
53. Robie DK, Welch-Dinauer C, Tuttle RM, et al. The impact of initial surgical management on outcome in young patients with differentiated thyroid cancer. J Pediatr Surg 1999; 33:1134–1140.
54. Welch-Dinauer CA, Tuttle MR, Robie DK, et al. Extensive surgery improves recurrence-free survival for children and young patients with class I papillary thyroid carcinoma. J Pediatr Surg 1999; 34: 1799–1804.
54a. Thompson GB, Hay ID. Current strategies for surgical management and adjuvant treatment of childhood papillary thyroid carcinoma. World J Surg 2004; 28:1187–1198.
55. Cohn KH, Bäckdahl M, Forsslund G, et al. Biologic considerations and operative strategy in papillary thyroid carcinoma: arguments against the routine performance of total thyroidectomy. Surgery 1984; 96:957–971.
56. Ringel MD, Levine MA. Current therapy for childhood thyroid cancer: Optimal surgery and the legacy of King Pyrrhus. Ann Surg Oncol 2003; 10:4–6.

57. Van Wyngaarden M, McDougall IR. What is the role of 1100 MBq (<30 mCi) radioiodine 131-I in the treatment of patients with differentiated thyroid cancer? Nucl Med Commun 1996; 17: 199–207.
58. Maxon HR III, Smith HS. Radioiodine-131 in the diagnosis and treatment of metastatic well differentiated thyroid cancer. Endocrinol Metab Clin North Am 1990; 19:685–715.
58a. Bal CS, Chandra P, Swivedi SM, Mukhopadhyaya S. Is chest x-ray or high-resolution computerized tomography of the chest sufficient investigation to detect pulmonary metastasis in pediatric differentiated thyroid cancer? Thyroid 2004; 14:217–225.
58b. Ralli M, Cohan P, Lee K. Successful use of recombinant human thyrotropin in the therapy of pediatric well-differentiated thyroid cancer. J Endocrinol Invst 2006; 28:270–273.
59. Edmonds CJ, Smith T. The long-term hazards of the treatment of thyroid cancer with radioiodine. Br J Radiol 1986; 59:45–51.
59a. Van Santen HM, Aronson FC, Vulsma T, et al. Frequent adverse events after treatment for childhood-onset differentiated carcinoma: a single institute experience. Europ J Cancer 2004; 40:1743–1751.
60. Hyer S, Vini L, O'Connell M, Pratt B, Harmer C. Testicular dose and fertility in men following I131 therapy for thyroid cancer. Clin Endocrinol 2002; 56:755–758.
61. Pacini F, Gasperi M, Fugazzola L, et al. Testicular function in patients with differentiated thyroid carcinoma treated with radioiodine. J Nucl Med 1994; 35:1418–1422.
62. Vini L, Hyer S, Al-Saadi A, et al. Prognosis for fertility and ovarian function after treatment with radioiodine for thyroid cancer. Postgrad Med J 2002; 78:92–93.
63. Casara D, Rubello D, Piotto A, et al. Pregnancy after high therapeutic doses of iodone-131 in differentiated thyroid cancer: potential risks and recommendations. Eur J Nucl Med 1993; 20:192–194.
64. Green DM, Edge SB, Penetrante RB, et al. In situ breast carcinoma treatment during adolescence for thyroid cancer with radioiodine. Med Pediatr Oncol 1995; 24:82–86.
64a. Berthe E, Henry-Amar M, Michels JJ, et al. Risk of second primary cancer following differentiated thyroid cancer. Eur J Nucl Med 2004; 31:685–691.
65. Rubino C, de Vathaire F, Dottorini ME, et al. Second primary malignancies in thyroid cancer patients. Br J Cancer 2003; 89:1638–1644.
66. Hung W, Sarlis NJ. Current controversies in the management of pediatric patients with well-differentiated nonmedulllary thyroid cancer: a review. Thyroid 2002; 12:683–702.
67. Solomon BL, Wartofsky L, Burman KD. Prevalence of fractures in postmenopausal women with thyroid disease. Thyroid 1993; 3:17–23.
68. Radetti G, Castellan C, Tato L, et al. Bone mineral density in children and adolescent females treated with high doses of L-thyroxine. Horm Res 1993; 39:127–131.
69. Feinmesser R, Lubin E, Segal K, Noyek A. Carcinoma of the thyroid in children—a review. Pediatr Endocrinol Metab 1997; 10:561–568.
70. Zimmerman D, Jay ID, Gough IR, et al. Papillary thyroid carcinoma in children and adults: long-term follow-up of 1039 patients conservatively treated at one institution during three decades. Surgery 1988; 104:1157–1166.
71. Samaan NA, Schultz PN, Hickey RC, et al. The results of various modalities of treatment of well differentiated thyroid carcinoma: a retrospective review of 1599 patients. J Clin Endocrinol Metab 1992; 75:714–720.
72. Travagli JP, Schlumberger M, De Vatharie F, et al. Differentiated thyroid carcinoma in childhood. J Endocrinol Invest 1995; 18:161–164.
73. Merrick Y, Hansen HS. Thyroid cancer in children and adolescents in Denmark. Eur J Surg Oncol 1989; 15:49–53.
74. Kirk JMW, Mort C, Grant DB, et al. The usefulness of serum thyroglobulin in the follow-up of differentiated thyroid carcinoma in children. Med Pediatr Oncol 1992; 20:201–208.

42
Special Presentations of Thyroid Cancer in Pregnancy, Renal Failure, Thyrotoxicosis, and Struma Ovarii

Kenneth D. Burman

INTRODUCTION

Differentiated thyroid cancer most commonly exists in euthyroid individuals, who present with a thyroid mass or who have a structural thyroidal abnormality detected on a radiologic study. In contrast to this typical presentation, there are several groups of patients who have thyroid cancer associated with other clinical circumstances and therefore require special attention. This chapter discusses these special situations and includes patients with thyroid cancer and (1) concomitant thyrotoxicosis, (2) renal failure on dialysis, (3) pregnancy, and (4) tumor origin in an ectopic site. (Patients with thyroglossal duct thyroid cancer are discussed in Chapter 43.) The general principles underlying the diagnosis and treatment of thyroid cancer in these subgroups are comparable to cancer presenting in the more typical cases, but these special circumstances require additional considerations.

CONCOMITANT THYROTOXICOSIS

The association between thyroid cancer and hyperthyroidism can occur in several different forms. Thyroid cancer, for instance, can occur in a patient with known or suspected Graves' disease. Often, this occurs when a thyroid nodule or "hypofunctioning area" is detected by sonogram, isotope scan, and/or palpation. Occasionally, a cervical lymph node is detected in combination with the thyroid nodule or as a separate and distinct finding. This topic has been recently reviewed by Stocker and Burch (1). Thyroid cancer has been estimated to range between 1% and 9% of Graves' disease patients. Of course, this detection rate depends on how assiduous the search is for nodules and thyroid cancer. Although controversial, it has been speculated that thyroid cancer is more aggressive when it occurs in conjunction with Graves' disease, possibly from the presence of thyrotropin (TSH) receptor–stimulating antibodies that may directly stimulate growth and differentiation of the malignant thyroid cells (1,2). It is a relatively rare occurrence; however, it may prove prudent to perform both a careful thyroid and neck examination and a thyroid sonogram in patients with Graves' disease.

If there is a distinct thyroid nodule (generally ≥1 cm), then fine-needle aspiration (FNA) cytology should be performed. If the lesion has suspicious or malignant cytology, then a thyroidectomy becomes the preferred therapy for both the suspicious nodule and the thyrotoxicosis. Of course, the patient's hyperthyroidism should be controlled prior to surgery, usually with the use of an antithyroid agent (methimazole or propylthiouracil) and β blockers. The patient should be rendered clinically and biochemically euthyroid as rapidly as possible to not delay definitive therapy.

After restoring euthyroidism, it is also optimal to deplete thyroidal stores of thyroid hormone by continuing the thiourea treatment for several weeks prior to surgery. Some clinicians will utilize preoperative treatment with iodine (SSKI or Lugol's) for about 7–10 d before surgery to help reduce thyroid function quickly, possibly reduce gland vascularity, and hopefully decrease the risk of acute thyroid hormonal release at surgery or shortly thereafter. Particularly when used for more than many weeks, iodine preparations can actually enhance thyroid hormone release (escape from the Wolff-Chaikoff effect); thus, care must be taken when employing these agents. Radiocontrast agents, e.g., ipodate, had been utilized effectively in the preoperative treatment of thyrotoxic patients, but these agents are not presently available in the United States. Following thyroidectomy, the treatment and monitoring plans for a patient with concomitant Graves' hyperthyroidism and differentiated thyroid cancer is basically the same as if thyrotoxicosis had not been present.

METASTATIC THYROID CANCER AND THYROTOXICOSIS

A separate and also unusual presentation is the occurrence of thyrotoxicosis in the setting of widespread metastatic thyroid cancer. The occurrence of this rare syndrome is related to the volume of functioning differentiated thyroid cancer cells in the patient. It occurs when there is extensive thyroidal tissue in metastatic foci that can trap iodine, synthesize iodothyronines, and then secrete sufficient thyroxine (T4) and triiodothyronine (T3) to render the patient biochemically (and usually clinically) hyperthyroid, despite a previous thyroidectomy and likely radioactive iodine ablative therapy. Generally, it is easily recognized that these patients have widespread metastases, but the appearance of hyperthyroidism may initially be thought as associated with excessive exogenous L-thyroxine administration. When the patient remains hyperthyroid, even when the dosage of levothyroxine gradually tapers, the mechanism for the hyperthyroidism becomes clear. Occasionally, this condition is recognized when a patient is prepared for a withdrawal ^{131}I scan. The clue is that the serum TSH fails to sufficiently rise after the withdrawal of levothyroxine therapy to perform radioisotopic scanning or therapy. The pituitary thyrotropic cells are suppressed by the high circulating levels of thyroid hormone from the metastases. This circumstance can be differentiated from a patient who has not discontinued exogenous L-T4 as scheduled because of elevated serum thyroglobulin and the presence of metastatic lesions when a radioiodine scan is ultimately performed. Scanning and therapy when TSH fails to rise can be achieved with the use of recombinant human TSH (Thyrogen®). The treatment of these patients is directed at the malignant lesions using ^{131}I therapy (or other direct modalities, such as surgery or external radiation as appropriate). However, attention may also have to be directed at treating the hyperthyroidism with antithyroid agents, e.g., methimazole or propylthiouracil and β blockers.

Although this syndrome is usually because of widespread metastatic disease, it may be rarely related to minimal residual disease that is stimulated by thyroid-stimulating immunoglobulins (TSH-R-AB) in a patient with underlying Graves' disease *(3,4)*. Metastatic thyroid cancer–causing hyperthyroidism is seen most frequently with follicular cancer, but it has also been described with other types, including papillary and anaplastic cancer *(5,6)*.

RENAL FAILURE

The presence of thyroid cancer in a patient with end-stage renal disease (ESRD) requiring hemodialysis needs special consideration resulting from the issue of radioactive iodine therapy *(7–9)*. This circumstance should be managed by an experienced multidisciplinary approach, involving endocrinologists, nuclear medicine specialists, radiation safety officers, and nurses. This discussion focuses on the use of radioactive iodine, but general medical and surgical principles should be used in the diagnosis and management.

Regarding ^{131}I therapy, there are specific considerations because iodine clearance is usually primarily via the kidneys; therefore, the clearance of radioiodine in a patient taking ^{131}I therapy is controlled with the use of hemodialysis. In general, our approach is to perform hemodialysis immediately prior to ^{131}I treatment, and then dialyze the patient again about 24 h after the ^{131}I dose. Some articles in the literature review these issues, and we have recently reviewed the topic *(7–9)*. We conclude that it is preferable, if possible, to perform dosimetry—a process that provides a quantitative estimate of the isotope retention and exposure in the individual patient. If this technique is not available, it seems appropriate to administer approximately 30–40% of the usual empiric ^{131}I dose that would be given to the patient if they did not have ESRD. Based on the literature and our experience, hemodialysis can be safely performed after radioiodine therapy using the standard precautions but with some caveats. Because there is significant radioiodine removal by dialysis initially, special precautions should include using adequate distance and shielding between the dialysis technician and patient. The dialysate should be disposed into the sewer system, preferably via a closed system. Following the first three or four dialysis procedures, a large fraction of the radioiodine should have been cleared from the blood, and the patient can then continue on dialysis in the usual manner. All medical health personnel involved in the patient's care should be advised of the radiation safety issues and should wear a radiation badge for exposure to be monitored and documented.

PREGNANCY

The normal pregnancy is associated with physiologic alterations in thyroid hormone levels and overall thyroidal economy *(10–12)*. In some patients during the first trimester of pregnancy, particularly when hyperemesis occurs human choriogonadotropin (hCG) in high concentrations binds to and stimulates the TSH receptor, resulting in enhanced thyroidal secretion. As a result, free T4 and T3 levels are increased, and TSH is suppressed. Symptoms of hyperthyroidism may be present but can be difficult to differentiate from symptoms of a normal pregnancy. The elevations in iodothyronine levels are transient in the vast majority of patients, as thyroid secretion returns to normal when the marked elevations in hCG begin to decline. In addition to these changes, thyroid hormone–binding proteins increase with the influence of estrogens, mediating an elevation of total T4 and T3. In the absence of hCG elevations, free T4 and T3 are unchanged by the increases in binding proteins during pregnancy. However, depending on the type of free T4 assay employed, the normal range of free T4 may decrease *(11)*. Following pregnancy, postpartum thyroiditis may occur, especially in patients with elevated antithyroperoxidase antibodies. A further discussion of the functional thyroidal changes during or after pregnancy is beyond the scope of this chapter.

Thyroid volume increases normally during pregnancy *(11)*. However, the finding of a specific nodule needs to be pursued in a comparable fashion as in a nonpregnant individual. There is controversy whether the risk of thyroid cancer increases during pregnancy. To assess the effects of pregnancy on the risk of thyroid cancer, Rossing et al. *(13)* performed a population-based case-control study comparing the presentation of thyroid cancer in 410 women 18–64 yr old at time of diagnosis with papillary thyroid cancer vs 574 controls. Their results suggested that both pregnancy and lactation may result in a transient increase in risk of papillary thyroid cancer. Mack et al. *(14)*, however, noted there was no elevated risk of thyroid cancer with the use of oral contraceptives or other exogenous estrogens. Yet, the risk of thyroid cancer increased with the number of pregnancies in women who used lactation suppressants and decreased with duration of breastfeeding. They concluded that their data provided only limited support of a possible link between reproductive history and increased risk of thyroid cancer in women.

Moosa and Mazzaferri *(15)* studied the outcome of thyroid cancer in 61 pregnant women in comparison to outcomes in 528 female age-matched controls who also had thyroid cancer discovered but not when they were pregnant. Median follow-up was approx 20 yr. The thyroid nodule was asymptomatic and was found on routine examination more often in the pregnant women (74%) than in controls (43%, $p < 0.001$).

Thyroidectomy was conducted in the postpartum period in 77% of the women and in 20% during their second trimester of pregnancy. Near-total thyroidectomy was performed in 43 (73%) of the pregnant women and 265 (59%) of the controls ($p = NS$). Nearly the same proportion of both groups (30% and 25%, respectively) were treated with ^{131}I postoperatively. Cancer recurrences, distant recurrences, and cancer deaths were comparable in each group. Outcomes were similar whether surgery was performed during or after pregnancy, despite a longer delay in treatment of the latter (1.1 ± 1.0 vs 16.1 ± 19.7 mo, $p < 0.001$). They concluded that the prognosis of differentiated thyroid cancer is comparable in pregnant women to that in nonpregnant women of the same age, and that further diagnostic procedures and surgical treatment of FNA-proven thyroid cancer that occurs during pregnancy can be delayed until after delivery.

Our opinion is similar to that of Moosa and Mazzaferri, with emphasis on individualized management according to the tumor characteristics of a given patient. If the nodule is diagnosed in the first trimester of pregnancy as differentiated thyroid cancer, and the decision is to wait until after delivery to perform a thyroidectomy, it does seem prudent to repeat the neck exam and thyroid sonogram periodically during the pregnancy to help ensure that the lesion is not growing rapidly. Serum thyroglobulin levels may be monitored during pregnancy and appear to be valid, not inordinately influenced by this condition. The obstetrician should be advised to avoid using topical iodine solutions as antisepsis at delivery, if possible, because of their potential deleterious effect on ^{131}I treatments.

Sometimes a definitive diagnosis of thyroid cancer is not made during pregnancy, and the patient has either FNA cytology suggestive of follicular neoplasm or a clinical context that is worrisome (e.g., rapid growth of nodules or lymph nodes). These circumstances are complex, and there are no evidence-based studies available to use as guidelines for action. To confirm the diagnosis of follicular neoplasm, it may help to have several experienced cytologists review the material. The cytologic criteria for thyroid lesions do not change during pregnancy *(16)*.

Once the diagnosis is confirmed, then the options of either following until after delivery or having the thyroidectomy during the mid-trimester of pregnancy are discussed and decided on by a multidisciplinary team with full involvement of the patient. A FNA cytology indicating follicular neoplasm represents thyroid cancer only about 20% of the time. For that percentage of lesions ultimately diagnosed as cancer, they could be a follicular variant of papillary thyroid cancer or follicular cancer, with the latter cancer being less common, potentially more aggressive, and its course less well-defined during pregnancy. These issues have to be considered carefully in deciding whether to operate during pregnancy or wait until after delivery.

The type of surgery to perform during pregnancy is also controversial. When the FNA cytology illustrates papillary thyroid cancer in a nonpregnant individual, the recommended surgery is typically a near-total thyroidectomy. If the aspiration suggests a follicular neoplasm, the sonogram shows no evidence of disease on the contralateral side, and there is no history of radiation, either an isthmusectomy and lobectomy or a near-total thyroidectomy may be conducted. Ensuring intact parathyroid function is even more important in pregnant than in nonpregnant women. The risk of hypocalcemia and hoarseness is slightly higher even with an experienced surgeon performing a near-total thyroidectomy. Normal fetal and neonatal calcium homeostasis relies on an appropriate supply of calcium from the mother *(17)*. Both maternal hypercalcemia and hypocalcemia can cause metabolic bone disease or disorders of calcium homeostasis in neonates. Maternal hypercalcemia can suppress fetal parathyroid function and cause neonatal hypocalcemia. Conversely, maternal hypocalcemia can stimulate fetal parathyroid tissue, resulting in bone demineralization. On rare occasions, administration of large calcium doses to pregnant women may be associated with neonatal hypocalcemia *(18)*. Thus, the potential effect of hypocalcemia on the pregnant woman and fetus is concerning and has to be taken into account. In any case, parathyroid function should be carefully assessed postoperatively in the pregnant patient, with serial measurements of both total and ionized calcium and parathyroid hormone.

Whether to administer levothyroxine to a patient who has had only a lobectomy and isthmusectomy with a final diagnosis of a benign lesion is controversial. Clearly, replacement exogenous L-T4 is required with the development of an elevated TSH level. L-T4 replacement is slightly more difficult to manage during pregnancy because requirements increase *(10)*. Although the need for increased dosage depends on the integrity of any remaining endogenous thyroid hormone production, the precise percentage increase varies; some patients require a significant increase in their L-T4 therapy *(10,19)*. Dosage is determined by monitoring TSH levels and return to the prepregnant level soon after delivery.

The effect of radioactive iodine treatments for thyroid cancer on the integrity of future conception and delivery is an important issue. Lin et al. *(20)* sought to ascertain the outcome of pregnancy in women with differentiated thyroid carcinoma who became pregnant after radioactive iodine treatment. They analyzed the medical records of 779 patients, 37 of whom had received radioiodine therapy prior to conception. There were 58 pregnancies recorded by these women during the study, and 47 babies were delivered. Three artificial and eight spontaneous abortions were documented. Seven patients conceived within 6 mo after the last administration of radioiodine, including two cases within 1 mo, and one of these seven patients had a spontaneous abortion. The authors concluded that previous administration of ^{131}I in women with well-differentiated thyroid cancer does not result in demonstrable adverse effects on subsequent pregnancies.

However, this experience has not been uniform. In apparent contrast, Ayala et al. *(21)* reached a different conclusion after reviewing the medical history of 26 women with differentiated thyroid cancer who became pregnant after receiving a therapeutic dose of radioactive iodine. There were 39 pregnancies, and 6 occurred during the first year after therapy. Anomalies were noted in three cases: a male suffering from Trisomy 18, a girl with constitutional aplastic anemia, and a boy with a congenital hip dysplasia. Of the 33 pregnancies that occurred after the first-year posttherapy, there were two spontaneous abortions, and one boy was affected by ureteral stenosis. It cannot be confirmed or concluded that these congenital disorders were from the ^{131}I therapy, but these authors recommend that pregnancy should be avoided for the first year after radioiodine therapy.

Chou et al. *(22)* recently examined the gestational history of 104 patients who previously had differentiated thyroid cancer and then became pregnant. The prior use of ^{131}I for scanning or therapeutic purposes (in 153 patients, 263 pregnancies) did not adversely affect the pregnancy outcome, the chance of congenital malformations, or first-year neonatal mortality. There were 116 pregnancies in 68 patients administered an ablative dose of radioiodine. Their children (ages 1 mo to 30.8 yr) had no evidence of any detectable abnormalities. The incidence of preterm deliveries was higher in those with a history of radioactive iodine exposure, but this estimate was not correlated with a higher ablative dose or a shorter time interval between therapy and conception. The miscarriage rate was not increased.

Vini et al. *(23)* studied the possible effect of radioiodine therapy on fertility and ovarian function. A total of 322 patients with differentiated thyroid cancer received a 3-GBq ablation dose, and 174 subjects received total cumulative doses ranging from 8.5 to 59 GBq for residual, recurrent, or metastatic thyroid cancer. During the first 10 mo following therapy, 17% ($n = 83$) of women noted menstrual irregularities, but no case of permanent ovarian failure was reported. Of 276 women who had 427 children, there were no congenital abnormalities, 4 premature births, and 14 miscarriages.

This literature is difficult to interpret given the relatively small number of cases and because specific information is lacking related to doses of ^{131}I and subsequent dosimetric analyses. In addition, matched case-controlled studies have not been performed in the same geographical and epidemiologic area. Nonetheless, it does seem prudent to request that women delay becoming pregnant for at least 6–12 mo following radioactive iodine therapy.

ECTOPIC SITES OF THYROID CANCER

Thyroid tissue can arise in ectopic locations, presumably from variant embryologic migration. Such ectopic thyroid tissue is thought to have the same risk of developing thyroid cancer as thyroid tissue in its eutopic location. However, the identification of this ectopic tissue and the ability to diagnose thyroid cancer may be often difficult. Perhaps the most commonly discussed location for ectopic thyroid tissue is in the ovary (i.e., struma ovarii). Most ectopic thyroid tissue in the ovary is benign, but there are numerous case reports of thyroid cancer that originates in the ovarian location *(24)*. When metastases occur, they typically manifest as peritoneal studding; however, distant metastases to the lung and other sites (e.g., bone, brain, and liver) may also occur. Whether the struma ovarii is benign or malignant, it can produce sufficient thyroid hormone to cause biochemical or clinical thyrotoxicosis. Radioactive iodine scans may show uptake in the ovary, as well as in the normal thyroid location in the neck.

Malignant struma ovarii is typically diagnosed incidentally in the evaluation of an ovarian mass *(24–37)*. Occasionally, the first presentation is metastases, perhaps in the peritoneal or pulmonary area. Given the rarity of the condition, there are no evidence-based studies to direct what may be optimal evaluation and treatment. The general approach is to remove the ectopic cancer tissue by an oophorectomy with related surgery for local disease, such as taking multiple peritoneal and omental biopsies with common iliac and paracaval node sampling as appropriate. Tumor staging with radiologic studies of the neck, chest, abdomen, pelvis, and possibly brain and bone are needed, with special attention to the thyroid gland. A thyroid sonogram might yield a thyroid nodule that requires FNA.

It is possible, albeit rare, that eutopic thyroid cancer will metastasize to the ovary *(31)* and there is a histologic variant of ovarian cancer that is papillary in nature *(38–40)* making identification of the site of origin of the primary tumor problematic. Papillary thyroid cancer will stain histochemically for thyroglobulin *(37)*. Ascites may occur and, surprisingly, thyroid cancer can also elevate the ovarian marker CA 125 *(29)*. Primary thyroid cancer that originates within the ovary is usually papillary in nature, with a few cases of follicular and anaplastic cancer reported *(28,30,35,37)*.

In addition to appropriate surgery and staging in conjunction with radiologic assessment, ^{131}I scans, ^{131}I treatment and monitoring via ultrasound, computed tomography or magnetic resonance imaging and serum thyroglobulin determinations seem to be valuable in patients with primary ovarian thyroid cancer *(34)*. Most authorities also recommend that a near-total thyroidectomy be performed when ovarian thyroid cancer is detected, which allows more accurate utilization of radioiodine treatment and monitoring. Because the ability of ectopic thyroid tissue to trap iodine is relatively limited, recombinant TSH has been used to enhance radioiodine uptake and treatment *(34)*.

Thyroid tissue and cancer can also occur at ectopic sites closer to the thyroid bed *(41)*. Such tissue, either benign or harboring cancer, has been identified in the tongue *(42)*, within the tracheal lumen *(41)*, or in the thyroglossal duct *(43;* see Chapter 43*)*. Thyroid cancer that arises in ectopic locations represents an unusual clinical circumstance. We believe that the same general principles guiding our approach to eutopic thyroid cancer apply to ectopic thyroid cancer, but individual variation based on the specific tumor site and other aspects is warranted.

In conclusion, thyroid cancer linked to special circumstances, such as in conjunction with hyperthyroidism or ESRD, during pregnancy, or in anatomically ectopic locations, should be treated similarly to eutopic thyroid cancer in euthyroid, otherwise "normal" subjects. These specific conditions are unusual but should be considered when assessing thyroid cancer patients.

REFERENCES

1. Stocker DJ, Burch HB. Thyroid cancer yield in patients with Graves' disease. Minerva Endocrinol 2003; 28:205–212.
2. Filetti S, Belfiore A, Amir SM, et al. The role of thyroid-stimulating antibodies of Graves' disease in differentiated thyroid cancer. N Engl J Med 1988; 318:753–759.
3. Basaria S, Salvatori R. Thyrotoxicosis due to metastatic papillary thyroid cancer in a patient with Graves' disease. J Endocrinol Invest 2002; 25:639–642.
4. Guglielmi R, Pacella CM, Dottorini ME, et al. Severe thyrotoxicosis due to hyperfunctioning liver metastasis from follicular carcinoma: treatment with (131)I and interstitial laser ablation. Thyroid 1999; 9:173–177.
5. Alagol F, Tanakol R, Boztepe H, et al. Anaplastic thyroid cancer with transient thyrotoxicosis: case report and literature review. Thyroid 1999; 9:1029–1032.
6. Salvatori M, Saletnich I, Rufini V, et al. Severe thyrotoxicosis due to functioning pulmonary metastases of well-differentiated thyroid cancer. J Nucl Med 1998; 39:1202–1207.
7. Holst J, Jonklaas J, Atkins F, et al. Dosimetric analysis of radioiodine therapy for thyroid cancer and hyperthyroidism in patients with end stage renal disease on hemodialysis; Thyroid, in press.
8. Jimenez RG, Moreno AS, Gonzalez EN, et al. Iodine-131 treatment of thyroid papillary carcinoma in patients undergoing dialysis for chronic renal failure: a dosimetric method. Thyroid 2001; 11:1031–1034.
9. Mello A, Isaacs R, Petersen J, et al. Management of papillary thyroid carcinoma with radioiodine in a patient with end stage renal disease on hemodialysis. Clin Nuc Med 1992; 19:776–781.
10. Alexander EK, Marqusee E, Lawrence J, et al. Timing and magnitude of increases in levothyroxine requirements during pregnancy in women with hypothyroidism. N Engl J Med 2004; 351:241–249.
11. Glinoer D. What happens to the normal thyroid during pregnancy? Thyroid 1999; 9:631–635.
12. Toft A. Increased levothyroxine requirements in pregnancy—why, when, and how much? N Engl J Med 2004; 351:292–294.
13. Rossing MA, Voigt LF, Wicklund KG, Daling JR. Reproductive factors and risk of papillary thyroid cancer in women. Am J Epidemiol 2000; 151:765–772.
14. Mack WJ, Preston-Martin S, Bernstein L, et al. Reproductive and hormonal risk factors for thyroid cancer in Los Angeles County females. Cancer Epidemiol Biomarkers Prev 1999; 8:991–997.
15. Moosa M, Mazzaferri EL. Outcome of differentiated thyroid cancer diagnosed in pregnant women. J Clin Endocrinol Metab 1997; 82:2862–2866.
16. Marley EF, Oertel YC. Fine-needle aspiration of thyroid lesions in 57 pregnant and postpartum women. Diagn Cytopathol 1997; 16:122–125.
17. Thomas AK, McVie R, Levine SN. Disorders of maternal calcium metabolism implicated by abnormal calcium metabolism in the neonate. Am J Perinatol 1999; 16:515–520.
18. Robertson WC, Jr. Calcium carbonate consumption during pregnancy: an unusual cause of neonatal hypocalcemia. J Child Neurol 2002; 17:853–855.
19. Chopra IJ, Baber K. Treatment of primary hypothyroidism during pregnancy: is there an increase in thyroxine dose requirement in pregnancy? Metabolism 2003; 52:122–128.
20. Lin JD, Wang HS, Weng HF, Kao PF. Outcome of pregnancy after radioactive iodine treatment for well differentiated thyroid carcinomas. J Endocrinol Invest 1998; 21:662–667.
21. Ayala C, Navarro E, Rodriguez JR, et al. Conception after iodine-131 therapy for differentiated thyroid cancer. Thyroid 1998; 8:1009–1011.
22. Chow SM, Yau S, Lee SH, et al. Pregnancy outcome after diagnosis of differentiated thyroid carcinoma: no deleterious effect after radioactive iodine treatment. Int J Radiat Oncol Biol Phys 2004; 59:992–1000.
23. Vini L, Hyer S, Al-Saadi A, et al. Prognosis for fertility and ovarian function after treatment with radioiodine for thyroid cancer. Postgrad Med J 2002; 78:92–93.
24. Takeuchi K, Murata K, Fujita I. "Malignant struma ovarii" with peritoneal metastasis: report of two cases. Eur J Gynaecol Oncol 2000; 21:260–261.
25. Chan SW, Farrell KE. Metastatic thyroid carcinoma in the presence of struma ovarii. Med J Aust 2001; 175:373–374.
26. Checrallah A, Medlej R, Saade C, et al. Malignant struma ovarii: an unusual presentation. Thyroid 2001; 11:889–892.
27. Dardik RB, Dardik M, Westra W, Montz FJ. Malignant struma ovarii: two case reports and a review of the literature. Gynecol Oncol 1999; 73:447–451.
28. Griffiths AN, Jain B, Vine SJ. Papillary thyroid carcinoma of struma ovarii. J Obstet Gynaecol 2004; 24:92–93.
29. Huh JJ, Montz FJ, Bristow RE. Struma ovarii associated with pseudo-Meigs' syndrome and elevated serum CA 125. Gynecol Oncol 2002; 86:231–234.
30. Hemli JM, Barakate MS, Appleberg M, Delbridge LW. Papillary carcinoma of the thyroid arising in struma ovarii—report of a case

30. and review of management guidelines. Gynecol Endocrinol 2001; 15: 243–247.
31. Logani S, Baloch ZW, Snyder PJ, et al. Cystic ovarian metastasis from papillary thyroid carcinoma: a case report. Thyroid 2001; 11: 1073–1075.
32. Nahn PA, Robinson E, Strassman M. Conservative therapy for malignant struma ovarii. A case report. J Reprod Med 2002; 47: 943–945.
33. Ribeiro-Silva A, Bezerra AM, Serafini LN. Malignant struma ovarii: an autopsy report of a clinically unsuspected tumor. Gynecol Oncol 2002; 87:213–215.
34. Rotman-Pikielny P, Reynolds JC, Barker WC, et al. Recombinant human thyrotropin for the diagnosis and treatment of a highly functional metastatic struma ovarii. J Clin Endocrinol Metab 2000; 85: 237–244.
35. Soto Moreno A, Venegas EM, Rodriguez JR, et al. Thyroid carcinoma on an ovarian teratoma: a case report and review of the literature. Gynecol Endocrinol 2002; 16:207–211.
36. Utsunomiya D, Shiraishi S, Kawanaka K, et al. Struma ovarii coexisting with mucinous cystadenoma detected by radioactive iodine. Clin Nucl Med 2003; 28:725–727.
37. Volpi E, Ferrero A, Nasi PG, Sismondi P. Malignant struma ovarii: a case report of laparoscopic management. Gynecol Oncol 2003; 90: 191–194.
38. Santin AD, Zhan F, Bellone S, et al. Discrimination between uterine serous papillary carcinomas and ovarian serous papillary tumours by gene expression profiling. Br J Cancer 2004; 90:1814–1824.
39. Soliman PT, Slomovitz BM, Broaddus RR, et al. Synchronous primary cancers of the endometrium and ovary: a single institution review of 84 cases. Gynecol Oncol 2004; 94:456–462.
40. Ryu DR, Yoo TH, Kim YT, et al. Minimal change disease in a patient with ovarian papillary serous carcinoma. Gynecol Oncol 2004; 93: 554–556.
41. Byrd MC, Thompson LD, Wieneke JA. Intratracheal ectopic thyroid tissue: a case report and literature review. Ear Nose Throat J 2003; 82:514–518.
42. Kao SY, Tu H, Chang RC, et al. Primary ectopic thyroid papillary carcinoma in the floor of the mouth and tongue: a case report. Br J Oral Maxillofac Surg 2002; 40:213–215.
43. LiVolsi VA, Perzin KH, Savetsky L. Carcinoma arising in median ectopic thyroid (including thyroglossal duct tissue). Cancer 1974; 34: 1303–1315.

43
Thyroglossal Duct Carcinoma

Leonard Wartofsky and Nikolaos Stathatos

Papillary thyroid cancer is the most common endocrine malignancy. In the vast majority of cases, it presents initially as a nodule within the thyroid gland, with or without metastatic disease (local or distal). Rarely, extrathyroidal or ectopic origin of this malignancy has been documented, typically in embryologic rests of thyroid cells. One common site is the thyroglossal duct. Although a cystic nodule within a remnant of this duct is the most typical neck mass detected during childhood, such nodules are almost always histologically benign.

During embryologic development, the thyroid gland descends in a caudal direction from the foramen cecum, initially forming the thyroglossal duct. In most individuals, this structure disappears completely by week 10 of gestation. In some cases, however, it fails to completely atrophy and persists, often forming a cyst of varying size and histology. These cystic remnants most often contain a lining of follicular thyroid tissue (60% of cases; *1*). Other epithelial types have been described, such as squamous, cuboidal, columnar *(2,3)*, intestinal, and gastric *(4)*. As much as 7% of the healthy population may have some remnant of the thyroglossal duct at postmortem *(5)*.

Thyroglossal duct remnants are the most common neck masses diagnosed during childhood and account for about 70% of all neck masses in children *(6)*. Most remain asymptomatic into adulthood, but in a few rare cases, these remnants have been the site of malignant tumors. Brentano *(7)* may have reported the first case of carcinoma derived in a thyroglossal duct cyst in 1911; since then, there have been about 300–350 published cases. The reported prevalence of cancer is approx 1% of all diagnosed thyroglossal duct remnants *(8,9)*. Thyroid cancer may present at any age and has been reported to affect patients between 6 and 81 yr of age. The most frequent presentation occurs in the fourth decade of life, with a female predominance (2:1 ratio; *10*).

The origin of these cancers has brought much debate: do they arise *de novo* or represent metastatic disease from a primary lesion inside the thyroid gland itself? Criteria have been proposed to help with this distinction *(11)* and include the presence of a thyroglossal duct remnant lined with epithelial cells and the documentation of a normal thyroid gland. The majority of these tumors are papillary thyroid carcinomas (80%), followed by squamous cell carcinomas (6%), and mixed follicular tumors (4%; *10*). Even Hürthle cell and anaplastic carcinoma *(12)* have been reported, but our review of the literature failed to find any cases of medullary thyroid cancer in a thyroglossal duct remnant. This latter finding is probably because of the different embryologic origin of the C cells from which medullary thyroid tumors originate.

For the evaluation of these lesions, a physical exam can provide important clues. A neck mass that moves with swallowing and tongue movement is characteristic. The possibility of metastatic papillary carcinoma to a Delphian lymph node in the same midline location must be considered. Some authors advocate obtaining a thyroid nuclear scan *(10)* to detect ectopic thyroid tissue and to determine if there is actually a fully functioning thyroid gland prior to removing the cyst. Although this may provide such evidence, results may be difficult to interpret because of the adjacent presence of a normal thyroid gland. It may not be possible to distinguish a small ectopic focus from the thyroid gland itself. Other imaging techniques can be used to make this diagnosis, including ultrasound and magnetic resonance image (MRI). These methods are not able to give clues to the histologic composition of the masses, but they can be helpful preoperatively for anatomic localization and evaluation of possible metastatic disease.

A more widely accepted method of testing for the presence of thyroid tissue is fine-needle aspiration (FNA) cytology of the mass *(13)*. Although significantly less than 100% sensitive, it is one of the most reliable preoperative diagnostic tools, not only for detecting thyroid tissue but also for diagnosing malignancy, if present. In our view, a tissue diagnosis prior to the definitive surgical procedure should be considered mandatory. If the initial FNA is nondiagnostic, a repeated attempt with ultrasound guidance should be done with multiple aspirates. If still nondiagnostic, frozen-section analysis of the excised duct at surgery before closure has been recommended, along with careful intraoperative digital examination of the thyroid gland *(14)*.

The most frequently used surgical therapeutic approach for these tumors is the Sistrunk procedure *(13a,15)*, which involves dissection of the thyroglossal cyst. Prior to FNA, carcinoma of the thyroglossal duct would be typically identified during the pathologic analysis of a thyroglossal duct cyst removed during a Sistrunk operation. Lymph node dissection is then performed, as needed, with lymph node metastases reported in 7–12% of thyroglossal duct carcinomas *(8,16)*. The operation involves the hyoid bone because of the embryologic development of the hyoid from the second branchial arch through which the thyroglossal duct passes. Invasion into the hyoid bone has been described in as many as 30% of malignant cases—an estimate that some authors believe necessitates the Sistrunk procedure *(17)*. In this procedure, the tract is dissected down to the hyoid bone, and the middle or median portion of the hyoid bone is also removed.

A recent review of thyroglossal duct carcinoma cases in children *(18)* provides similar data to that summarized above for adults. Of 21 cases, 12 were present in girls at a mean age of 13 yr old. All cases were the papillary type, except for three that were mixed papillary and follicular. The tumor was confined to the thyroglossal duct in all the patients with the thyroid gland found negative for carcinoma, but there was invasion of the duct capsule in 10 of 21 (45%) and local invasion in 5 of 21 (23%), one of whom had pulmonary metastases. All patients generally had surgery for a nontender, painless, asymptomatic mass with carcinoma diagnosed by pathology; no patients had FNA cytology. One patient died 8 h postoperatively, and all the others had a relatively uneventful follow-up period. The same positive and negative arguments for thyroidectomy appear to apply in children as in adults, and these authors favored management by near-total thyroidectomy, radioiodine ablation, and levothyroxine suppressive therapy.

The controversy regarding whether adult patients should have a total thyroidectomy if thyroid cancer is identified in a thyroglossal duct remnant is ongoing *(13a)*. For tumors originating in the thyroid gland, an incidental malignant focus in the opposite lobe of the gland is not an uncommon finding. Thus, it is recommended that patients with intrathyroidal cancer have a total thyroidectomy and is considered by some as the standard of care today (see Chapters 22, 24). Although these data could suggest that the same management should apply for a tumor originating in a thyroglossal duct remnant, there has not been a sufficient number of these cases to draw a more definite conclusion. There remain cogent arguments against routine-associated thyroidectomy for papillary cancer *(1)*, given the excellent prognosis for the overwhelming majority of small stage I lesions, particularly in young patients. However, the case for thyroidectomy is more compelling when the tumor is follicular, considering the propensity for angioinvasion and a more aggressive course of the latter cancer. Depending on the histology and extent of the primary tumor, and the need for further therapy with radioactive iodine, a total thyroidectomy may be a necessary step to ensure a cure. Incidence may be as high as 25% for associated carcinoma within the thyroid gland *(19)*. On the contrary, because many of these carcinomas have been detected in the duct without any evidence of tumor within the thyroid gland, thyroidectomy might be avoided if the thyroid has no demonstrable nodules by ultrasound, and the primary tumor is small without proof of metastasis to cervical nodes. Proponents of concomitant thyroidectomy *(20)* point out that there may be a high incidence of local spread of these tumors not detected at a Sistrunk procedure. The full procedure with thyroidectomy allows appropriate staging and subsequent monitoring by isotopic scans and serum thyroglobulin measurements. Moreover, a patient was reported to develop lung metastases and die following treatment with only cyst removal and without thyroidectomy *(13)*.

If the tumor histology is that of squamous cell carcinoma, a more extensive surgical excision is usually required. These tumors generally have a much worse prognosis, whereas papillary thyroid carcinomas have the same excellent prognosis as those originating from the thyroid gland, depending (as always) on the stage of the disease at diagnosis. With squamous cell carcinoma, adjunctive postoperative external radiation therapy may also be warranted. In the final analysis, whether to perform thyroidectomy at the same time as the Sistrunk procedure is a highly complex issue. As summarized by Mazzaferri *(21)*, we may not be in a position to always make a fully rational judgment based on the data available on these tumors. However, the presence of characteristics associated with a more aggressive cancer course will make the decision easier in many cases.

REFERENCES

1. LiVolsi V, Perzen K, Savetsky L. Carcinoma arising in median ectopic thyroid. Cancer 1974; 34:1303–1313.
2. Akbari Y, Richter P, Papadakis L. Thyroid carcinoma arising in thyroglossal duct remnants. Arch Surg 1967; 94:235–239.
3. Magsalin R, Diener C, Jawadi H. Thyroglossal cyst carcinoma. J Kans Med Soc 1982; 83:426–427.
4. Chandrasoma P, Janssen M. A thyroglossal cyst lined by gastric epithelium. JAMA 1982; 247:1406.
5. Hilger AW, Thompson SD, Smallman LA. Papillary carcinoma arising in a thyroglossal cyst: A case report and literature review. J Laryngol Otol 1995; 109:1124–1127.
6. Gardner D. Unusual appearance of a thyroglossal duct cyst carcinoma. J Oto-Laryngol 1989; 18:258–259.
7. Brentano H. Struma aberrata lingual mit drusen metastasen. Deutsch Med Wschr 1911; 37:665.
8. Weiss SD, Orlich CC. Primary papillary carcinoma of a thyroglossal duct cyst: report of a case and literature review. Brit J Surg 1991; 78: 87–89.
9. Boswell W, Zoller M, Williams J. Thyroglossal duct carcinoma. Am Surg 1994; 60:650–655.
10. Renard T, Choucair R, Stevenson W, et al. Carcinoma of the thyroglossal duct. Surg Gyn Obst 1990; 171:305–308.
11. Komorowski R, Joseph T. Thyroglossal duct carcinoma. Hum Pathol 1975; 6:717–729.

12. Woods RH, Saunders JR Jr, Pearlman S, et al. Anaplastic carcinoma arising in a thyroglossal duct tract. Otolaryngol Head Neck Surg 1993; 109:945–949.
13. Bardales RH, Suhrland MJ, Korourian S, et al. Cytologic findings in thyroglossal duct carcinoma. Am J Clin Pathol 1996; 106:615–619.
14. Luna-Ortiz K, Hurtado-Lopez LM, Valderrama-Landaeta JL, Ruiz-Vega A. Thyroglossal duct cyst with papillary carcinoma: what must be done? Thyroid 2004; 14:363–366.
15. Sistrunk W. The surgical treatment of cysts of the thyroglossal tract. Ann Surg 1920; 71:121–122.
16. Patel SG, Escrig M, Shaha AR, et al. Management of well-differentiated thyroid carcinoma presenting within thyroglossal duct cyst. J Surg Oncol 2002; 79:134–139.
17. Stephenson B, Wheeler M. Carcinoma of the thyroglossal duct. Surg 1994; 64:212.
18. Peretz A, Leiberman E, Kapelushnik J, Hershkovitz E. Thyroglossal duct carcinoma in children: Case presentation and review of the literature. Thyroid 2004; 14:777–785.
19. Stephenson B, Wheeler M. Carcinoma of the thyroglossal duct. Aust N Z J Surg 1994; 64:212.
20. Miccoli P, Minuto MN, Galleri D, et al. Extent of surgery in thyroglossal duct carcinoma: Reflections on a series of eighteen cases. Thyroid 2004; 14:121–123.
21. Mazzaferri EL. Editorial: Thyroid cancer in thyroglossal duct remnants: a diagnostic and therapeutic dilemma. Thyroid 2004; 14:335–336.

Part IV
Well-Differentiated Thyroid Cancer
Treatment

44
Radiation and Radioactivity

John E. Glenn

INTRODUCTION

Radioiodine therapy has a unique effect: the patient may become a hazard to other people. Thus, special governmental regulations affect the management of patients who are treated with radioiodine, and the physician administering the radioiodine must comply with these governmental policies. In addition, the treating physician has to understand and communicate the risk of radiation from the radioiodine treatment to the patient, as well as to the patient's family, friends, and caretakers. However, this is not an easy task. A balance must be achieved in convincing the patient to agree with these specific instructions, and at the same time, dispel unnecessary fear. For this balance, the physician should be able to adopt different strategies with different patients, requiring a good working knowledge of radiation and radioactivity, ionizing and nonionizing radiation, and units of radioactivity and radiation dosage. The physician must also know the regulations for hospitalization, conditions for earlier release, radiation safety precautions during hospital stay and upon release, and the myths and fears about radioactivity. This chapter presents an overview of these topics.

RADIATION AND RADIOACTIVITY

The physician and patient should have a clear understanding of the difference between radiation and radioactivity. Both are closely related concepts, but the distinction is important to determine methods to protect patients and their loved ones.

Radiation

Radiation is a means of transporting small bundles of energy from one place to another. Light from a flashlight is radiation. The microwaves that cook food are radiation. The heat that warms our faces in front of the fireplace is radiation. The atomic particles released by the sun as solar wind are radiation. The waves (X-rays or γ waves) or particles (α or β) released from radioactivity are radiation. People who come into close proximity with a patient treated with radioactivity are exposed to radiation but not contaminated with radiation. Simply, radiation exposure is an event, not a substance.

Radioactivity

Alternatively, radioactivity is "stuff" made up of atoms, just like people, houses, food, and everything else that we can see, feel, taste, smell, or touch. Radioactive atoms are different from other atoms because they can release energy in the form of radiation as discussed above. People can get radioactivity in or on themselves, and unwanted radioactivity on a person or thing is contamination. In other words, radioactivity is a substance that emits radiation and is not an event.

Types of Radiation From Radioactivity

The most important types of radiation emitted from radioactivity are α, β, positron, and γ waves.

α *radiation* is a rapidly moving nucleus of the helium atom (two protons and two neutrons). The α particle is massive (heavy) and energetic. Because it is heavy, it loses energy very rapidly. This property means that it gives high-radiation doses when ingested, injected, or otherwise inserted into tissue. However, because an α particle quickly loses energy, it almost never penetrates the skin. Thus, patients receiving radioactive material emitting only α radiation will receive high doses but are not a hazard to people in their vicinity.

β *radiation* is an atomic electron. The β particle is created when a neutron in the nucleus is converted into a proton, plus an electron (β) and an antineutrino. The β particle has a small mass, which is about 2000 times less than the smallest atom and has a negative electric charge. The β particle loses energy less rapidly than an α particle and can penetrate tissue for a short distance of 1 or 2 cm. Thus, patients receiving radioactive material emitting only β radiation will receive moderately high doses; however, as a source of radiation, they are not normally a hazard to people in their vicinity. The antineutrino carries off energy but does not interact with either the patient or nearby objects.

Positron is another form of radiation that nuclear medicine has recently harnessed for diagnostic purposes. In nuclear and radioactive decay processes, a particle not normally found in nature is created that has exactly the same mass as a β particle or electron. This particle is the positron, termed so because it carries a positive electric charge, rather the negative charge of the β particle. The positron is classified as the antimatter twin of the electron. An amazing property of antimatter/matter twins is that when they collide, they annihilate each other. All the mass is converted into pure energy, according to Einstein's famous equation ($E = mc^2$). This energy always shows up as two γ rays of identical energy, traveling in exactly opposite directions. This property allows precise spatial imaging. The imaging process is referred to as *positron emission tomography* (PET). With PET, the radiation exposure always includes positron and γ radiation.

γ *radiation* is electromagnetic energy. γ radiation has no resting mass but a relativistic mass given by the equation, $E = mc^2$. γ rays only give up energy when colliding with atomic electrons. Thus, individual γ rays release energy less rapidly than α or β particles and may pass through the human body without giving any radiation dose. Patients who receive radioactive material emitting only γ radiation will receive moderately low doses but may be a hazard to people in their vicinity.

^{131}I emits both β and γ radiation. The β radiation is the major source of radiation to any remaining normal thyroid tissue and functioning metastatic thyroid cancer cells. Yet, a significant portion of the γ radiation "escapes" the patient. Although this energy can be harnessed to obtain images, γ waves can result in the radiation dose affecting family and friends. Accordingly, the γ radiation emitted from the patient is one of the forms of radioiodine therapy that must be monitored and controlled to minimize its effect to family, friends, and caretakers.

Ionizing and Nonionizing Radiation

Some forms of radiation are ionizing and emitted from radioactivity, such as α, β, and γ, and other forms are non-ionizing radiation, e.g., light and microwaves.

Unlike nonionizing radiation, ionizing radiation alters the number of electrons within the atoms of matter that the ionizing radiation has penetrated. Those affected atoms are called *ions* because they have either lost or gained one or more electrons. The number of ions created within matter, including the human tissue, depends on the amount of energy given off by the ionizing radiation. This amount is the *radiation dose*. A high radiation dose entails a large number of ions.

The creation of ions (free radicals with changed oxidation states) inside the cell can interact with other molecules and cause the cell's chemical properties to change. Particularly, changes may cause damage to the molecules that control the body's ability to replace or regulate cells. For example, DNA may undergo breaks, and the repair process may lead to errors in the sequences or faulty joining of the broken helical strands. These errors may result in cell death or propagation of the error (mutation) to the daughter cells after division.

Nonionizing radiation does not create ions; however, it can cause damage through other mechanisms, such as heat.

DETERMINISTIC AND STOCHASTIC EFFECTS

The effects of ionizing radiation may be either deterministic or stochastic. Death of the residual thyroid cells or thyroid cancer cells is the objective of radioiodine therapy, and death (and consequential inflammation) of nonthyroid tissue causes untoward effects. These effects are *deterministic* and have a radiation-dose threshold beyond which the effect is almost always seen. For deterministic effects, severity increases with radiation dose. The suppression of bone marrow stem cells in the ^{131}I patient is a deterministic effect.

Cancer induction is a *stochastic* process—the cancer mutation is dependent on the probability of the effect occurring, rather than the severity of the effect. Further details on the patient risk from medical procedures are published by The International Commission on Radiological Protection *(1)*.

UNITS OF RADIOACTIVITY AND RADIATION DOSE

Science needs to precisely define the units of measurement. A problem in the United States is our reluctance to adopt international systems, including the metric system. Thus, the physician will encounter two different systems for measuring radioactivity and radiation dose.

International System

In the international system, named units are based on the three fundamental metric units: the meter, kilogram, and second. Radiation dose is defined as the energy deposited in tissue per unit mass. Thus, the unit of absorbed radiation dose, *Gray* (Gy), is calculated as:

$$1 \text{ Gy} = 1 \text{ J/kg} = 1 \text{ m}^2/\text{s}^2$$

Radioactivity is the measure of the number of atomic nuclei disintegrating per unit of time. The fundamental unit has been named the *Becquerel* (Bq) and is estimated as:

$$1 \text{ Bq} = 1 \text{ disintegration/s}$$

Special Units System

The "special units" is a hybrid system widely used in the United States. Radiation dose is still absorbed energy per unit mass. However, the unit of energy is a much smaller metric unit, *erg*, and the unit of mass is *gram*, rather than the kilogram. The unit of absorbed dose is the *rad*.

$$1 \text{ rad} = 100 \text{ erg/g} = 100 \text{ cm}^2/\text{s}^2 = 0.01 \text{ Gy}$$

or

$$1 \text{ Gy} = 100 \text{ rad}$$

Radioactivity is still the measure of the number of atomic nuclei disintegrating per unit of time. The unit is the *Curie* (Ci) and equals the number of disintegrations in 1 g of ^{226}Ra in 1 s. A Curie turns out to be 37 billion disintegrations per second.

$$1 \text{ Ci} = 37 \text{ billion Bq}$$
$$1 \text{ mCi} = 37 \text{ million Bq}$$
$$1 \text{ disintegration/min} = 1 \text{ disintegration}/(60 \text{ s}) = 0.0167 \text{ Bq}$$

In this discussion, the international units will be used with the special units in parentheses.

U.S. REGULATORY FRAMEWORK

The establishment of radiation standards in the United States is a federal function. The Environmental Protection Agency is the lead agency, but several agencies participate in the standards-setting process. The Nuclear Regulatory Commission (NRC) is the federal agency with statutory responsibility for all radioactive material produced by the nuclear fuel cycle. These radioactive materials include thorium and uranium processed from ore, radioactive materials enriched in fissionable materials by physical processes, and materials that are made radioactive by fission or exposure to radiation from fission. The Atomic Energy Act allows the NRC to relinquish regulatory authority to states that establish a compatible regulatory program by written agreement (i.e., Agreement States). The NRC Agreement States regulate ^{131}I, and possession requires a license from the appropriate group or agency. To determine if your state is an Agreement State, the following Internet address displays a map showing NRC and Agreement States: www.hsrd.ornl.gov/nrc/rulemaking.htm.

The Occupational Health and Safety Administration (OSHA) has the responsibility to protect occupationally exposed individuals but avoids dual regulation with the NRC. OSHA and the Agreement States regulate nonfuel cycle radioactive materials like radium or radioactivity produced in a cyclotron. The NRC does not have the authority to regulate nonfuel cycle radioactivity. ^{123}I is cyclotron-produced, and not regulated by the NRC. Most states that are not part of the Agreement States either license cyclotron-produced radioactive material or require facility registration.

Before the mid-1990s, the Atomic Energy Commission, and later the NRC, had required that all patients receiving more than 1.11 billion Bq (1.11 GBq or 30 mCi) of radioactive material for therapy remain in the hospital until the radioactivity dropped below 1.11 GBq (30 mCi). Patients could also leave if the radiation dose, measured at 1 m from their bodies, dropped below 0.00005 Gy (50 µGy/h or 5 mrad/h). These criteria were intended to make sure family and friends would not be exposed to more than 0.005 Gy (0.5 rad) from any patient receiving ^{131}I. The criteria were derived from some cautious assumptions:

- None of the radioactive material would be eliminated except by natural decay. (This assumption is contrary to real experience in cancer patients, where 80–90% of the radioiodine may be excreted in the first 24 h.)
- The patient's body would not absorb any radiation emitted. (In practice, the patient's tissues reduce external-radiation doses from ^{131}I by a measurable, albeit not large, amount.)
- The most exposed individual family member or friend would spend no more than 25% of their time within 3 ft of the patient until all the radioactive material was gone from natural decay. (This is not a cautious assumption unless the patient has been advised to sleep in a separated bed for a few days.)

Based on comments from physicians treating patients with radioactive materials, the NRC changed its patient-release criteria in 1997 *(5)*. The Agreement States had 3 yr to adopt "compatible" regulations. Thus, the description of the NRC's requirements presented here may vary slightly (but not significantly) from state to state.

Instead of a specified level of radioactivity or radiation dose rate of 1 m from the patient, the physician as a NRC or Agreement State licensee are now required to demonstrate that family and friends will not receive a radiation dose in excess of 0.005 Gy (0.5 rad) from the patient if the patient is released from the hospital. The physician has two choices:

1. Base the estimated radiation dose on the administered dose and the same cautious assumptions the NRC had previously used.
2. Base the estimated dose on the activity at the time of release and more realistic assumptions according to the actual circumstances of the patient.

Of note, the earlier numerical radioactivity and dose-rate values used for patient release involved rounding down calculated values. The NRC has adjusted its guidance for default release limit for ^{131}I based on only the radioactivity remaining in the body and its cautious assumptions to be slightly more accurate. The revised default values are:

- Radioactivity less than or equal to 1.221 GBq (33 mCi), or
- Measured dose rate less than or equal to 70 µGy/h (7 mrad/h).

If the radiation dose to family and friends could exceed 0.001 Gy (0.1 rad), the regulations also require that the patient is given written instructions. These instructions, if followed, should be adequate to keep actual radiation doses below 0.001 Gy (0.1 rad).

INTERNET RESOURCES

The Internet offers the opportunity to access current regulations and guidance of the NRC and many Agreement

States. The NRC has a toolkit with many links to help review licensing, procedures, and inspections. The address is: www.nrc.gov/materials/miau/med-use-toolkit.html.

Extensive guidance for the release of patients on ^{131}I therapy is provided in Appendix U, "Model Procedure for Release of Patients or Human Research Subjects Administered Radioactive Materials" in the NRC's *Consolidated Guidance About Materials Licenses Program—Specific Guidance About Medical Use Licenses, vol. 9*. The address for a copy of volume 9 is: www.nrc.gov/reading-rm/doc-collections/nuregs/ staff/sr1556/v9. An earlier version of only the patient release information can be found at: www.nrc.gov/reading-rm/doc-collections/reg-guides/occupational-health/active/8-39/08-039.pdf. The Conference of Radiation Control Program Directors. Inc. has posted free documents for downloading at: www.crcpd.org. In addition, you may find more information and links at the Society of Nuclear Medicine website: interactive.snm.org.

PROTECTION OF PEOPLE OTHER THAN PATIENTS

Immediately after cancer treatment, anyone in contact with or near the patient is at risk of receiving a radiation dose from the radioactive iodine within the patient. This can occur directly from the radiation emitted from the patient's body or by ingesting or inhaling radioactive iodine that the patient sheds through breath or body fluids. The current scientific consensus about the risks from exposure to radiation has been published by the National Academy of Sciences *(2)*.

To maintain the cancer risk to friends and family members As Low As Reasonably Achievable—a concept radiation health experts refer to as ALARA—some patients may require hospitalization, and all patients must receive specific radiation safety instructions whether released after hospitalization or immediately after treatment. Both of these circumstances are discussed below; however, the instructions are based on radiation protection standards set by the NRC or similar regulations *(3)* adopted by many state agencies *(4)*. These instructions are intended to establish a level of risk comparable to activities normally considered "safe," like office work. Thus, the most exposed individual in contact with the patient should receive a radiation dose and has an estimated risk of less than 0.04% of developing a fatal cancer from radiation in the next 10–60 yr. Simply, fewer than 4 of every 100,000 people in close contact with the patient may develop a fatal cancer later in life because of radiation from the patient. Internet resources regarding radiation protection in the United States have already been listed above. An example of an instruction is included (see Example 1).

Hospitalization

Hospitalization was required for all isotope administrations above 1.11 GBq (30 mCi) before the NRC made changes to its regulations. With these changes, hospitalization may not be necessary under certain restrictions. The physician as a licensee of the NRC or Agreement State is responsible for the assessment as to when a patient requires initial hospitalization and when the patient can be released. Training of hospital staff is required for success and necessary by regulation. A sample handout for alerting patients to hospital restrictions is included as Example 2.

As time passes after the radioactive iodine is administered, the risk of exposing anyone else to radiation decreases. Table 1 shows how the dose rate drops off with time for measurements made at 1 m from the patient's body. This table is calculated from the ^{131}I retention assumptions for a cancer patient in the NRC's Regulatory Guide 8.39 *(6)*.

Generally, the physician does not have to hospitalize the patient or keep them any longer if the *measured* dose rate is less than 70 µGy/h (7 mrad/h). However, the physician is required to provide written instructions for:

- Guidance on the interruption or discontinuation of breast-feeding.
- Guidance on practices to reduce the radiation dose to others.
- Information on the consequences of failure to follow the guidance.

For the release of a patient at higher measured dose rates, the physician must ask the patient questions to document that he or she is a suitable candidate for release. The physician must also ascertain that the patient does not plan any extended travel time in public transportation. A sample questionnaire is shown in Example 3, which is discussed further below.

Even if the patient can maintain isolation, concern may still persist regarding the patient's potential to contaminate the living space during the first 24–36 h. However, after 2 d, the patient usually will not emit any radioactive contamination that is seriously consequential (see Table 2). During the first 24 h, urine, saliva, breath, and blood contain concentrations of radioactive iodine that could harm another person's thyroid. Again, the physician must seriously evaluate both the probability and consequences of an accident that could result in another person's uptake of radioactive iodine. Keeping the patient for an 18-h hospital stay or longer significantly reduces the risks associated with any accidental exposure to bodily fluids.

Radiation Safety Precautions

The medical staff, support staff, other patients, visitors and the next patient to occupy the room must be protected from unnecessary exposure to radiation and radioactive material. The methods of achieving protection are: (1) isolation of the patient, (2) containment of radioactive material to the assigned room, (3) measurement and release of anything leaving the room, and (4) good hygiene by anyone entering and leaving the room.

> **Example 1**
>
> **Written Instructions for The Patient At Home**
>
> The main protection for family and friends is for you to avoid close contact for about 3 days after coming home.
>
> **There is one critical person who is at potential great risk of harm.** Nursing an infant or small child after receiving radioactive iodine will transfer the radioactive iodine from the mother to the child in the milk. Radioactive iodine ingested by the child will expose the thyroid of the child to potentially harmful levels of radiation. Lifelong medication may be required to prevent serious effects both mentally and physically if the child's thyroid receives a high dose of radiation.
>
> Although there is no evidence that the amount of radiation received by those people coming close to you will do detectable harm, it is reasonable to take certain precautions for at least three days following release.
>
> Once you get home:
>
> 1. Keep a safe distance from other people –
>   - Sleep alone for three nights.
>   - Avoid kissing and sexual intercourse for seven days.
>   - Minimize time in public places including public transportation, theaters, sporting events for 3 days. You can eat meals with your family during this time.
>   - Stay at least three feet away from people if you will be involved with them for more than an hour in the first three days.
> 2. You may care for children during this time, but time spent holding a child on a lap or lying next to you should be minimized.
> 3. Breast-feeding must be avoided because it could seriously harm the infant.
> 4. Wash hands frequently for several days. Sweat contains some minuscule amount of radioactive iodine.
> 5. Wash bed linens and clothes separately for three days. After three days, resume normal care.
> 6. Use a separate bathroom for three days, if possible. Urine contains excreted radioactive iodine. Flush twice when using the toilet. If separate facilities are not available, good hygiene habits are adequate to minimize exposure.
>
> These guidelines will limit exposure to others far below acceptable levels. Radioactive iodine will disappear completely through your own body excretions

Isolation

The patient is isolated from all but a few hospital staff. Hospital staff are instructed to have as little contact as possible, consistent with the standard of care. Isolation is not required because of immediate danger to people coming in close contact with the patient, but it is to ensure the ALARA principle. In an emergency, the medical staff should provide all the necessary medical attention that the patient needs regardless of the radiation exposure to themselves. The maximum radiation dose likely during a 1-h emergency is about equal to the radiation dose from nature in 1 yr: 0.003 Gy (0.3 rad).

If radiation doses to medical staff are likely to exceed 0.005 Gy (0.5 rad), personal dosimetry must be provided. Proximity to the patient, even right after treatment, should not expose staff to more radiation than a member of the public receives in 1 yr from natural background radiation. However, that kind of radiation exposure for 20–40 times a year would result in unreasonably high radiation exposure and an unnecessary but small risk of cancer later in life.

Visitors are not permitted unless the physician managing the radioiodine administration believes certain family members or close friends are needed to provide unique care or support. If visitors are allowed, they must be monitored for

> **Example 2**
>
> **Information concerning your hospitalization**
>
> 1. There will be restrictions on visitors during your hospitalization. Minors (under age 18) and pregnant women will not be permitted to visit. All visits will be restricted to a few minutes and persons must remain a marked distance away. You are encouraged to tell friends and family not to visit.
>
> 2. Any personal belongings you bring with you will be checked for radioactive iodine before you leave. Belongings that can not be cleaned to acceptable release levels such as radios, magazines, books, etc. may have to be held for you until the radioactive iodine has decayed. Therefore, you should not bring with you any belongings that you can not afford to be without for possibly a few weeks.
>
> 3. Nurses will be able to provide medical care but will use gloves and shoe covers when entering your room.
>
> 4. Housekeeping will be limited in your room. Housekeeping personnel are not permitted to enter the room and all items must be measured using radiation detection instruments before leaving the room.
>
> 5. You may use the toilet without concern about the radioactive iodine. One should sit while using the toilet. All other normal sanitary practices should be followed. The toilet should be flushed three times with the lid down.

Table 1
Predicted Dose Rate at 1 m µGy/h and mrad/h

Time	*Dosage*		
	3.7 GBq (100 mCi)	5.55 GBq (150 mCi)	7.4 GBq (200 mCi)
0 d	500 µGy/h (50 mrad/h)	750 µGy/h (75 mrad/h)	1000 µGy/h (100 mrad/h)
0.25 d	300 µGy/h (30 mrad/h)	450 µGy/h (45 mrad/h)	600 µGy/h (60 mrad/h)
0.5 d	180 µGy/h (18 mrad/h)	270 µGy/h (27 mrad/h)	360 µGy/h (36 mrad/h)
0.75 d	110 µGy/h (11 mrad/h)	165 µGy/h (16.5 mrad/h)	220 µGy/h (22 mrad/h)
1 d	70 µGy/h (7 mrad/h)	105 µGy/h (10.5 mrad/h)	140 µGy/h (14 mrad/h)
2 d	25 µGy/h (2.5 mrad/h)	38 µGy/h (3.8 mrad/h)	50 µGy/h (5 mrad/h)
3 d	16 µGy/h (1.6 mrad/h)	24 µGy/h (2.4 mrad/h)	32 µGy/h (3.2 mrad/h)
4 d	15 µGy/h (1.5 mrad/h)	18 µGy/h (1.8 mrad/h)	30 µGy/h (3.0 mrad/h)
5 d	13 µGy/h (1.3 mrad/h)	19.5 µGy/h (1.95 mrad/h)	26 µGy/h (2.6 mrad/h)
6 d	12 µGy/h (1.2 mrad/h)	18 µGy/h (1.8 mrad/h)	24 µGy/h (2.4 mrad/h)
7 d	11 µGy/h (1.1 mrad/h)	17 µGy/h (1.7 mrad/h)	22 µGy/h (2.2 mrad/h)
14 d	6 µGy/h (0.6 mrad/h)	9 µGy/h (0.9 mrad/h)	12 µGy/h (1.2 mrad/h)
21 d	3 µGy/h (0.3 mrad/h)	4.5 µGy/h (0.45 mrad/h)	6 µGy/h (0.6 mrad/h)

radiation dose and precautions must be taken to keep doses below 0.005 Gy (0.5 rad).

Containment

Everything that enters the room should be left in the room unless cleared by radiation safety personnel. The hospital population is not exposed to radioactive material as long as it stays in the room. Personal belongings should be limited to clothes, disposable materials, or items that can be cleaned easily. Personal possessions that cannot be cleaned and are contaminated with ^{131}I above a certain limit should be disposed of by the hospital or kept until the radioactivity decays.

Measurement and Release

All contents in the room, along with the patient, should be measured for radiation before leaving. There are three possibilities: (1) release, if not contaminated above the release limit, (2) held for later release after radioactive decay,

Example 3

Questionnaire Concerning Hospitalization For Patients Administered Radioactive Iodine

By answering the following questions and agreeing to follow the guidelines, you may be able to be released earlier because of your limited contact with other people.

1. Are you a woman nursing a small child or infant?

    Yes ____   No ____

    NOTE: Nursing an infant or small child after receiving radioactive iodine will transfer the radioactive iodine from the mother to the child through the milk. Radioactive iodine ingested by the child will expose the thyroid of the child to potentially harmful levels of radiation. Lifelong medication may be required to prevent serious effects both mentally and physically if the child's thyroid receives a high dose of radiation. **If you are nursing a child, inform Nuclear Medicine personnel and we must reschedule your administration at a later date after you have permanently ceased nursing this child.**

2. Can you take care of yourself except for brief visits and not be in the same room with another person for more than three hours total during each of the first two days?

    Yes ____   No ____

    If no, briefly explain circumstances: _____
    _____

3. Will you be able to maintain distance from other people, including:

    – Sleeping alone for at least one night (recommend 3 nights)?

 – Avoiding kissing and sexual intercourse for at least 3 days?

 – Staying at least 3 feet away from people if you will be involved with them for more than an hour a day in the first 3 days?

    Yes ____   No ____

    If no, briefly explain circumstances: _____
    _____

4. Will you avoid travel by airplane or mass transit for the first day?

    Yes ____   No ____

    If no, briefly explain circumstances: _____
    _____

5. Will you avoid prolonged travel in an automobile with others for the at least first two days?

    Yes ____   No ____

    If no, briefly explain circumstances: _____
    _____

6. Will you have sole use of a bathroom for at least two days?

    Yes ____   No ____

    If no, briefly explain circumstances: _____
    _____

I have read these guidelines, understand the instructions and agree to avoid contacts in accordance with my answers to items 2 through 6. [Note: If you can not manage at home and avoid close contact, it may be necessary for you to remain in the hospital up to an additional 24 hours.]

Signature: _____   Date: _____

(Patient or other person in accordance with hospital informed consent policy.)

Table 2
Radioactive Iodine Excreted by Various Pathways During Days Following Dosage

Day	Perspiration (activity on whole body)	Saliva (per cubic centimeter)	Breath	Urine
1	925,000 Bq	1,702,000 Bq	1,665,000 Bq	2,960,000,000 Bq
	25 µCi	46 µCi	45 µCi	80,000 µCi
2	481,000 Bq	296,000 Bq	407,000 Bq	318,200,000 Bq
	13 µCi	8 µCi	11 µCi	8600 µCi
3	74,000 Bq	33,300 Bq	48,100 Bq	37,000,000 Bq
	2 µCi	0.9 µCi	1.3 µCi	1000 µCi
4	7400 Bq	3700 Bq	7400 Bq	3,700,000 Bq
	0.2 µCi	0.11 µCi	0.2 µCi	100 µCi
5	740 Bq	370 Bq	740 Bq	481,000 Bq
	0.02 µCi	0.01 µCi	0.02 µCi	13 µCi
6	74 Bq	37 Bq	74 Bq	74,000 Bq
	0.002 µCi	0.001 µCi	0.002 µCi	2 µCi
7	Minimal	Minimal	Minimal	7400 Bq
	Minimal	Minimal	Minimal	0.2 µCi

The excreted activity is Becquerel (mCi) per 3.7 GBq (100 mCi) administered.

and (3) disposal as radioactive waste. Preparing the room before the patient is admitted enables more rapid cleanup of the room and quicker release. Floors, door handles, telephones, and other items likely to be touched should be covered with paper or plastic to help the prevention of radioactive contamination.

Hygiene

Everyone who enters the patient's room should wear gloves and shoe covers and remove their gloves and shoe covers as they leave the room. Washing their hands promptly provides additional benefit against contamination.

Conditions for Earlier Release

A patient's agreement to limit close contact, within arms length with family and friends, to 3 h a day for the first few days is often enough for a licensee to justify earlier release. Under certain circumstances, an NRC licensee may immediately release a patient who has been given hundreds of millicuries of radioactive material based on that patient's ability to be isolated from other people. Most hospitals release all but a few patients within 18–30 h after the administration of radioactive iodine.

Considerations for release earlier than 18 h should include:

- Almost total isolation at home for the first day.
- Separate eating, bathing, and toilet facilities for the first few days.
- No use of public facilities or transportation for the first few days.
- No trips longer than 1 h in a private automobile or sitting in contact with another passenger during the first day after administration.
- The ability of the patient to provide self-care without assistance.
- No medical need to observe the patient for the first day.

A worksheet for documenting patient release above the default values, based on the questionnaire (Example 3), is included as Example 4. Note that the sample includes the derivation of a release criterion based only on the occupancy factor (E). Based on this derivation, the maximum acceptable dose rate at release is:

$$dD/dt = 1.79/E \text{ mrad/h}$$

Other Considerations

There is a potential risk of injury to another individual's thyroid if more than 1.1 million Bq (0.030 mCi) is ingested or inhaled as a result of exposure to radioactive iodine from the thyroid cancer patient. Washing hands and staying at least 1 m away from other people will prevent an unhealthy dose of radiation. Certain intimate contacts could transfer more than 1.1 million Bq (0.030 mCi) in the very early days after administering radioactive iodine. Breast milk and pregnancy are particularly concerning. Women of childbearing age must avoid pregnancy during their treatment, and mothers must not nurse infants.

The amount of radioactivity shed through breath, saliva, urine, and perspiration drops rapidly. Intimate contact should be avoided only for days, rather than weeks. As noted, Table 2 shows estimates of the amount of radioactivity the patient will release through perspiration, saliva, breath, and urine during each day following dosage. Other than radioactivity excreted in urine, by day 4, the levels are much smaller than

Example 4

Worksheet For Determining Acceptable Dose Rates For Release Of Patients Administered Radioactive Iodine

I. Regulatory Limit

10 CFR 35.75 permits release of patients if the total effective dose equivalent to any other individual from exposure to the released individual is not likely to exceed 0.5 rad.

II. Acceptable methods

Acceptable methods are described in Regulatory Guide 8.39 *"Release Of Patients Administered Radioactive Materials."*

III. Calculations

Calculations will be based on Equation B-1 from Regulatory Guide 8.39.

$$D(t) = \frac{34.6 \, \Gamma \, Q_0 \, T_p \, E \, (1 - e^{-0.693t/T_p})}{r^2}$$

where

$D(t)$ = Accumulated dose to time t, in rad

34.6 = Conversion factor of 24 hrs/day times the total integration of decay (1.44)

Γ = Exposure rate constant for a point source, rad/mCi x hour at 1 cm

Q_O = Initial activity at the start of the time interval
T_p = Physical half-life in days

E = Occupancy factor that accounts for different occupancy times and distances when an individual is around a patient

r = Distance in centimeters. This value is typically 100 cm

t = exposure time in days

The dose rate in rad/hour for the effective remaining activity Q_m at time t_m (when a measurement is made) is by the definition of Γ:

$$\frac{dD(t)}{dt} = \frac{\Gamma Q_m}{r^2} \quad \text{or} \quad Q_m = \frac{dD(t)}{dt} \times \frac{r^2}{\Gamma}$$

and since the dose to infinity after the dose rate measurement at time t_m is:

$$D_\infty = \frac{34.6 \, \Gamma \, Q_m \, T_p \, E \, (1 - 0)}{r^2}$$

Then $D_\infty = (dD/dt) * 34.6 * T_p * E$

(continued)

Example 4 (*continues*)

For the purposes of this worksheet:

Dmax = 500 millirad
T_p = 8.08 days

And the acceptable dose rate is therefore

dD/dt = 500/(34.6*8.08*E) = 1.79/E mrad/hour

E = .25 or 0.125 depending on the patient circumstances.

IV. **Evaluation** (Sign for the appropriate dose rate for this administration)

1. If the patient has not submitted information about possible contacts with other people, we can assume without further justification the occupancy factor is 0.25. [Reference: Regulatory Guide 8.39 "Release Of Patients Administered Radioactive Materials" and 10 CFR 35.75]

   E = 0.25. The measured dose rate at 1 meter must be equal to or less than 1.79/0.25 = 7.1 millirad/hour

   Signature of person making evaluation_____

2. If the patient has submitted information about possible contacts with other people and has answered yes to all questions 2 – 6 of the questionnaire, we can assume the occupancy factor is 0.125. [Reference: Section B.1.2, "Occupancy Factors To Consider for Patient-Specific Calculations," Regulatory Guide 8.39 *"Release Of Patients Administered Radioactive Materials"*.

   E =0.125. The measured dose rate at 1 meter must be equal to or less than 1.79/0.125 = 14.3 mrad/hour.

   Signature of person making evaluation_____

3. If the patient has submitted information about possible contacts with other people but has answered no to any of the questions 2 – 6 of the questionnaire, the Radiation Safety Officer will make the determination of acceptable dose rate.

   [Reference: Section B.1.2, Regulatory Guide 8.39 *"Release Of Patients Administered Radioactive Materials"*.

   The measured dose rate at 1 meter must be equal to or less than ___ millirad/hour
   Basis:
   _____
   _____
   _____

   Signature of Radiation Safety Officer_____

1.1 million Bq (0.030 mCi), and by day 7, are extremely small. Table 2 was calculated using an average of measurements made at 24 and 48 h by the Medical College of Wisconsin *(7)*, with the assumption that the measured levels after 48 h would drop as predicted using the NRC Regulatory Guide 8.39 retention model. These measurements indicated that the levels (except for urine) are greatest at 24 h.

MYTHS AND FEARS ABOUT RADIOACTIVITY

1. *Radiation exposure will make a person radioactive.* This statement is false. A patient who has received radioiodine is radioactive and is a source of radiation exposure only as long as radioactive iodine remains in the body. More than 99% of the radioactive iodine is eliminated in the first few days.

Table 3
Natural and Manmade Sources of Radiation

Natural sources
- Radon gas (55%)
- Natural radioactivity in your body (11%)
- Natural radioactivity in the earth (8%)
- Radiation from outer space (8%)

Manmade sources
- Medical therapy and diagnosis (15%)
- Consumer products (3%)
- Nuclear power (<1%)

2. *Radiation exposure is unusual and is very dangerous.* In fact, most radiation exposure comes from nature, whereas the minority is manmade (see Table 3). A large radiation dose can cause injury or death. Large doses during pregnancy can cause developmental deficiencies. Small doses may increase the risk for cancer.
3. *If I avoid manmade sources of radiation, I will not get any extra radiation dose.* Compare flying in a high-altitude airplane with living near a nuclear power plant: nuclear power plant at plant boundary (0.6 mrad/yr) vs coast-to-coast airplane roundtrip (5 mrad).

CONCLUSION

This chapter has discussed the differentiation of radiation and radioactivity, ionizing and nonionizing radiation, units of radioactivity and radiation dose, hospitalization regulations, conditions for earlier release, radiation safety precautions during the hospital stay and upon release, and myths and fears about radioactivity. Protection of the public to prevent unnecessary exposure from patients taking radioiodine therapy requires knowledge, planning, procedures, and education. Advance communication with the patient about radiation, radioactivity, risks, regulations, hospitalization, and appropriate precautions at home will help ensure good compliance, resulting in reduced radiation exposure to family, friends, caretakers, and the general public.

REFERENCES

1. Radiation and your patient: a guide for medical practitioners. Ann ICRP 2001; 2001:1–52.
2. Health Effects of Exposure to Low Levels of Ionizing Radiation: BEIR V. The National Academies Press, 1990.
3. Part 35, Medical Use of Byproduct Material. Title 10, Code of Federal Regulations, Section 35.75.
4. Part G, Use of Radionuclides in the Healing Arts. Suggested State Regulations for Control of Radiation, vol. I, Ionizing Radiation. Conference of Radiation Control Program Directors. Inc.
5. Federal Register, 62 FR 4120, Jan. 29, 1997.
6. Release of Patients Administered Radioactive Materials. Division 8, Occupational Health, Regulatory Guide 8.39, U.S. Nuclear Regulatory Commission, 1997.
7. Ibis E, Wilson CR, Collier BD, et al. Iodine-131 contamination from thyroid cancer patients. Nucl Med 1992; 33:2110–2115.

45
Radioiodine Treatment of Distant Metastases

Douglas Van Nostrand

INTRODUCTION

Radioiodine has been used for many years for the treatment of patients who have distant metastases derived from well-differentiated thyroid cancer (1). This chapter presents an overview of the literature regarding the efficacy of radioiodine therapy in the treatment of distant metastases and discusses the approaches to select the prescribed activity (dosage) of radioiodine for these treatments.

Efficacy of Radioiodine Treatment in Distant Metastases

The major difficulty in assessing this efficacy is that no prospective study has been performed, and the likelihood of such is remote. However, multiple retrospective studies are available (2–29). Selected research for radioiodine treatment for lung metastases is listed in Table 1; pulmonary and bone metastases, Table 2; bone, Table 3; and distant metastases not separated by site, Table 4. The numerous limitations associated with retrospective studies are listed in Table 5. Metastases to bone are also discussed in Chapter 53.

Pulmonary Metastases

As applicable to many areas of thyroid cancer management, controversy exists regarding whether radioiodine therapy increases survival, reduces recurrence, and/or palliates metastasis in patients with pulmonary metastases. Data from Ruegemer (9), Dinneen (16), and Sisson (21) show little or no evidence to suggest a therapeutically beneficial effect of radioiodine, whereas data from Casara (14), Schlumberger (8,18), Samaan (7), Pacini (15), Ronga (29), and others support a therapeutic impact from radioiodine in pulmonary metastases.

Ruegemer et al. (9) from the Mayo Clinic reported that, "By univariate analysis, patient age, tumor extent ($p = 0.0002$), pattern of lung involvement ($p = 0.0001$), radioiodine uptake of the metastases, and radioiodine treatment were significant prognostic factors." Naturally, potential benefit from radioiodine therapy must depend on the presence of radioiodine uptake; in their series, mortality was lower in 19 patients with radioiodine uptake than in the 33 patients with no evidence of radioiodine uptake on scan ($p = 0.016$). In addition, a higher proportion of micronodular lung involvement was present in the 19 patients (58%) vs the 33 patients who had no radioiodine uptake (12%; $p = 0.0005$). However, Ruegemer stated, "By multivariate analysis, only age at the time of first diagnosis of distant metastases and involvement of multiple organ sites were independently associated with cancer mortality." The Cox regression model suggested that after adjustment for age and extent of metastatic involvement, radioiodine administration did not have a significant influence on survival.

Another Mayo Clinic series, reported by Dinneen et al. (16), described 100 patients with pulmonary metastases, as well as other various distant metastases. The favorable prognostic factors by univariate analysis included the use of radioiodine therapy ($p < 0.001$), age at diagnosis of distant metastases, complete resection of the primary tumor, histological grade 1, diploid nuclear DNA, and lung as the first site of metastases. However, again, radioiodine treatment was not identified as a favorable prognostic factor by multivariate analysis. The other favorable prognostic factors by multivariate analysis were age, site of distant metastasis, and degree of extrathyroidal invasion of the primary tumor. In contrast to the observations of Schlumberger et al. (18), Dinneen et al. noted no difference in survival for the time periods of 1940–1954, 1955–1969, and 1970–1989. He concluded that this indirect evidence suggested that recent advances in the diagnosis and management of distant metastasis, such as radioiodine treatment, had no effect on survival.

Maheshwari et al. (4) from the University of Texas/MD Anderson Hospital and Tumor Institute reviewed 53 patients with pulmonary metastases and 31 patients with metastases to the bone. Although specific data on these patients were not presented, Maheshwari stated, "Repeated therapy with ^{131}I did not appear to improve the patients' survival rate."

In an analysis of 12 patients, Sisson et al. (21) reported that it was uncommon to achieve complete remission of distant metastases with radioiodine. Their administered activity ranged from 60 to 350 mCi (2.2–13 GBq), with total accumulative prescribed activity ranging from 140 to 800 mCi

Table 1
Pulmonary Metastases

Author		No. of Patients	1-yr Survival	5-yr Survival	10-yr Survival	15-yr Survival	Remission	Comments
Brown (5)	Normal chest X-ray, positive ^{131}I scan	20		63%	54%		65%	
Casara (14)		42	100%	100%	96%		Complete remission 78%	
	Abnormal chest X-ray, positive ^{131}I scan	54	~92%	~55%	36%		Complete remission 3.7%	
	Abnormal chest X-ray, negative ^{131}I scan	38	~75%	~18%	11%		None	
Massin (6)	Overall	58	68%	44%	14%			
	Radioiodine-treated group	24		74%	42% (8 yr)			
	Micronodular	11			77% (8 yr)		9/11 considered cured	
	Macronodular	13					3/13 considered cured	Macronodular disease, low or no ^{131}I uptake
	Untreated	29	50%	10%				
Schlumberger (18)	Lung only	214			61%		50%	Survival following diagnosis of thyroid cancer
Nemec (3)	All pulmonary metastases	78		29%	12%	36%		4 Patients had bone metastases
	Fine pattern	25		76%	59%	39		19 Patients had bone metastases
	Coarse pattern	33		41%	14%	4%		
	^{131}I uptake	66		92%	70%	35%		
	No ^{131}I uptake or not treated	12		32%	6%	3%		
Hindié (28)	Positive ^{131}I scans	20		90%	84%			Average follow-up for the 17 survivors was 12.7 yr
	Negative chest X-ray, positive ^{131}I scan	11			90%		73%	
	Abnormal chest X-ray, positive ^{131}I scan	9			78%		22%	
	Negative ^{131}I scan	12		33%	0%			

Dorn (32)		13			Lung without bone metastases. But patient may have had other nonskeletal metastases. Follow-up was an average of 4.1 yr (range of 1.1 to 9.5 yr). 62% survival yr to date with 3 deaths attributable to thyroid cancer and 2 to other causes
Samaan (7)	Overall	101	69%	44%	26 Patients had other sites of metastases
	Radioiodine +	59	61%	31%	Concluded that radioiodine increased survival
Ronga (29)	Radioiodine −	42	29%	7%	
	Overall	96	78%	59%	43%
	Miliary	49	86%	75%	61%
	Nodular	46	68%	47%	26%
	Radioiodine +	65	87%	76%	58%
	Radioiodine −	30	53%	25%	0%
Vassilopoulou-Sellin (20)		16			Little data available, but the only patient free of disease is a 6-yr-old female with radioiodine-positive, X-ray-negative lung metastases

413

Table 2
Pulmonary and Bone Metastases

Author		No. of Patients	1-yr Survival	5-yr Survival	10-yr Survival	Remission	Comments
Brown (5)		11				9%	Improvement in only 1 patient. See Table 3
Schlumberger (18)		72			13%	7%	
Petrich (26)	Radioiodine +	41					Mean survival of 7.3 yr
Dorn (32)		6					Follow-up was an average of 3.7 yr (range of 1.2–7.2 yr). 85% Survival to date, with 1 death attributable to thyroid cancer

(5.2–29.6 GBq). In a subsequent report, Sisson et al. *(30)* questioned whether radioiodine could deliver enough of a radiation-absorbed dose to small pulmonary metastases less than 1 mm in diameter. Their concern was based on the fact that as a tumor becomes smaller and smaller, the β and γ energy deposited within the actual tumor decreases; for a sphere of 0.5-mm diameter, less than 40% of radioiodine energy is deposited within that sphere *(30)*. In addition, even if a 1-mm focus of pulmonary metastases could receive enough rads to be treated successfully, that focus may have small 100–500 μ papillary projections that may not receive sufficient rads.

In a multivariate analysis of 134 patients who had pulmonary metastases, Casara et al. *(14)*, from the University of Padua and the Institute of Semeiotica Medica in Italy, showed that only radioiodine uptake ($p < 0.0001$), chest X-ray ($p = 0.0014$), and multiple distant metastases ($p = 0.01$) were significant independent variables. Univariate analysis identified radioiodine uptake ($p < 000.1$), patient age ($p < 0.0001$), histology ($p = 0.04$), chest X-ray, and the presence of multiple distant metastases ($p < 0.0001$) as prognostic factors. Casara concluded that early scintigraphic diagnosis and radioiodine therapy of lung metastases appeared to be the most important factors to obtain a significant improvement in survival rate and a prolonged disease-free time interval. Regarding the different results of Casara and Ruemeger, Casara raised the possibility that the lack of radioiodine influence in the Mayo Clinic data may have been partly a result of the performance of only partial thyroidectomies. Casara *(14)* further commented that:

"When the pulmonary metastases were <5 mm in diameter with a negative chest X-ray, complete disease remission following ^{131}I therapy almost always occurred. When metastases were >5 mm in diameter (positive chest X-ray), the survival rate is still considered fairly good, but the probability of obtaining complete disease remission was very low despite ^{131}I uptake. Moreover, when the macronodular metastases lose the capability of radioiodine uptake, a fatal outcome was almost always observed."

In 1996, Schlumberger et al. *(18)*, from Institut Gustave-Roussy in Villejuif, France, reported the therapeutic benefit of ^{131}I in 394 patients with distant metastases. Positive prognostic factors for survival by multivariate analysis were (1) radioiodine uptake, (2) a younger age, (3) the time of metastases detection, (4) histological type, and (5) small extent of disease. Schlumberger summarized that radioiodine treatment was one of the factors that increased survival. Schlumberger also noted that patients who had their distant metastases discovered after 1976 had a 140% increase in survival, relative to those patients who had their distant metastases discovered before 1960. For patients who had their distant metastases discovered between 1960 and 1977, the increase in survival was 30%. He proposed that these improvements might have been because of the introduction of radioiodine in 1960 and serum thyroglobulin measurements in 1977. As Ruegemer noted, the discordance between the results of Ruegemer and Schlumberger may be relating to a difference in patient population. Only one of Ruegemer's patients had a positive radioiodine scan and negative chest X-ray, whereas 18% (51 of 281) of patients evaluated by Schlumberger had a positive radioiodine scan and negative chest and bone X-ray.

Samaan et al. *(7)* reviewed 101 patients with pulmonary metastases, who were also studied at the University of Texas/MD Anderson Hospital and Tumor Institute. Samaan concluded that patients treated with radioactive iodine had a longer survival than those not treated ($p < 0.002$), and uptake of radioactive iodine by lung metastasis was a favorable prognostic factor, especially in patients with negative chest X-rays. However, he also observed the link between age and radioactive iodine uptake.

Hindié et al. *(28)*, from Hôpital Saint-Antoine, stated that ^{131}I had a beneficial impact on pulmonary functioning metastases. However, he questioned that the "beneficial impact" of

Table 3
Bone Metastases

Author		No. of Patients	1-yr Survival*	5-yr Survival*	10-yr Survival*	20-yr Survival*	Remission	Comments
Brown (5)		21		7%	0%		0%	11 Patients also had lung metastases
Schlumberger (18)		108			21%		10%	
Marcocci (11)		30	98%	65%	18%		10%	3 Patients with complete remission had both surgery and radioiodine treatment
Petrich (26)	Radioiodine +	60						Mean survival of 8.9 yr (survival longer in those with uptake. $p<0.0005$)
	Radioiodine −	6						Mean survival of 1.2 yr
Proye (13)		28	53%				36% Responded 7% (2) cured	Combination of treatments. 7 Patients alive with follow-up of 8 mo to 8 yr
	Radioiodine + Radiographically −	12					2/12 cured	
Bernier (27)		109	41%	15%		7%		Median survival of 3.9 yr
Pittas (25)		146		25%	13%			1% Patients had anaplastic carcinoma, 6 had medullary, and 3 had lymphoma
Fanchiang (34)		39		64.9%				16 Patients had other organ involvement. 25 Patients had surgical treatment, and 18 patients received external radiotherapy
Woods (12)		37		47%	34% Projected			Only 1 patient received just radioiodine intra-arterially
Zettinig (33)		41		59%	39%			
Dorn (32)		9					Follow-up was an average of 6.7 yr (range of 1.3–10.9) 88% survival to date, with 2 deaths not attributed to thyroid cancer	Patients may have had other non-lung metastases

*Time is from diagnosis of initial bone metastasis to death.

Table 4
Distant Metastases Not Separated by Location

Author		No. of Patients	1-yr Survival	5-yr Survival	10-yr Survival	15-yr Survival	Remission	Comments
Petrich (26)	<45 yr old	8					63% Total or partial remission	
	>45 yr old	99					50% Total or partial remission	Lung metastases present in 44. No difference in survival of patients with or without lung metastases
Schlumberger (18)	Complete response	124		96%	93%	89%		
	No complete response	270		37%	14%	8%		
	<40 yr old with neg X-rays	56			96%			
	>40 yr old with macronodular lung or multiple bone metastases	156			7%			
Pacini (15)		118					36% cured	76% Survival at end of follow-up, with a mean survival of 5.8 yr (86 lung only, 13 lung and bone, 16 bone only, and 3 other sites)
Høi (10)		91	58%	20%	Approx 6% (9 yr)		8%	
Ruegemer (9)		85	76%	42%	33%			
Dineen (16)		100	40%	27%	24%			
Menzel (19)		26					35% Complete or partial remission	Mean follow-up of 52 mo

Table 5
Variables Limiting Retrospective Studies on the Efficacy of Radioiodine in Distant Metastases

Method and depth of review
Small patient populations
Histopathology
Extent of initial surgery
Use of radioiodine ablation
Amount of radioiodine used for ablation
Extent of metastases
Sites of metastases
Use of radioiodine for treatment
Amount of radioiodine used for treatment
Length and frequency of follow-up
Definition of clinical remission

radioiodine in patients who had negative chest X-rays and positive radioiodine scans, compared to patients with positive chest X-rays and negative radioiodine scans, may not be the result of the radioiodine. Rather, this impact may represent two distinct entities, or two stages, of the same disease but with different prognoses, regardless of the radioiodine.

Relating to the different results that Hindié observed in comparision to Ruegemer's findings at Mayo Clinic, Hindié suggested this might be partly explained by different stages of metastatic disease at the time of diagnosis, as well as the intensity of radioiodine therapy. The group of 85 patients in Ruegemer's series (Mayo Clinic) did not receive radioiodine ablation after thyroid surgery, and distant metastases were detected by chest or bone X-ray in 99% (84 of 85) of patients. Furthermore, only 37% of patients who subsequently received radioiodine therapy in the Mayo Clinic series had ^{131}I uptake. In Hindié's series, 63% of patients had radioiodine uptake. Again, these discordances may be owing to either a difference in the stage of disease at diagnosis and/or intensity of therapy.

Ronga et al. (29), from La Sapienza University in Rome, Italy, evaluated 96 patients with pulmonary metastases from 1958 until 2000, concluding that the most important factors increasing survival rates were a young age at diagnosis and radioiodine uptake by metastases. The multivariate analysis demonstrated that the risk of death was 5.4 times higher in patients over age 45 yr and was reduced by radioiodine treatment to nearly 1/6. Although Ronga's data indicated that improved survival also appeared associated with a miliary vs a nodular pattern, Ronga thought this link was related to radioiodine uptake and possibly a more favorable prognosis for patients with a miliary pattern.

Nemec et al. (3), from the Research Institute of Endocrinology in Prague, reviewed 78 patients with pulmonary metastases. Nemec implied survival was improved in patients who were younger and had a pattern of radioiodine uptake in the lung that was considered "fine" (<10 mm). The survival rate was worse with abnormalities on chest X-rays and bone metastases. He stated that the most important factor for survival was radioiodine uptake; however, he did not correct his data to include the impact of age.

Massin et al. (6), from Groupe Hospitalier Pitié-Salpétriére, evaluated 58 cases of pulmonary metastases, of which 24 were treated with radioiodine and 29 were untreated. The survival for the radioiodine-treated group at 5 and 8 yr was 74% and 42%, respectively, whereas the untreated survival at the same follow-up was 50% and 10%, respectively. Massin proposed that radioiodine uptake, age, and tumor invasion were favorable prognostic factors. He further suggested that the favorable prognostic aspect of the radioiodine uptake had a direct relationship to therapy with radioiodine. However, this was not a multivariate analysis, and he stated radioiodine uptake was more likely in patients 30 yr of age or younger and less likely in patients more than 80 yr old.

Brown et al. (5) examined 42 patients with distant metastases at the Royal Marsden Hospital Thyroid Unit. In patients with only lung metastases, 54% were alive and free of disease 10 yr after radioiodine treatment. The average total prescribed activity of radioiodine administered in the entire series was 680 mCi (25.2 GBq), and 7 patients received more than 1000 mCi (37 GBq). There were 13 patients (65%) who had only pulmonary metastases that showed complete remission, which were all achieved with a total cumulative amount of radioiodine of 800 mCi (29.6 GBq) or less. In 11 patients with lung (and bone metastases), complete resolution of the lung "deposits" were seen in 1 patient, with definite improvement in the chest X-ray in 3 patients.

Menzel et al. (19), from the University of Bonn, treated 26 patients with various combinations of distant metastases and empiric activity of 300 mCi (1.11 GBq) at approx 3-mo intervals. Menzel reported complete or partial remission in 35%, stable disease in 23%, and progressive disease in 42%. The mean overall follow-up after the onset of metastatic spread was 52 mo (range 9–157 mo). He concluded that high prescribed activity with repetitive treatments of 300 mCi (11.1 GBq), and cumulative activities of up to 2000 mCi (74 GBq) of radioiodine, were beneficial in the treatment of advanced differentiated thyroid carcinoma.

Pacini et al. (15), from the Institute of Endocrinology of the University of Pisa, reported on 118 patients with metastatic disease—the majority of whom had lung metastases. Specifically, 86 patients had only lung metastases; 16 had only bone metastases; 13 had lung and bone metastases; and 3 had other metastases. Although the results were not separated and analyzed by site of distant metastases, the overall "cure" rate for distant metastases was 36% (43 of 118). They observed that the efficacy of radioiodine therapy depended predominately on the size, location, and number of distant metastatic lesions. The best chance for a favorable response was in patients with radioiodine-positive, radiograph-negative, micronodular diffuse lung metastases. Radioiodine's

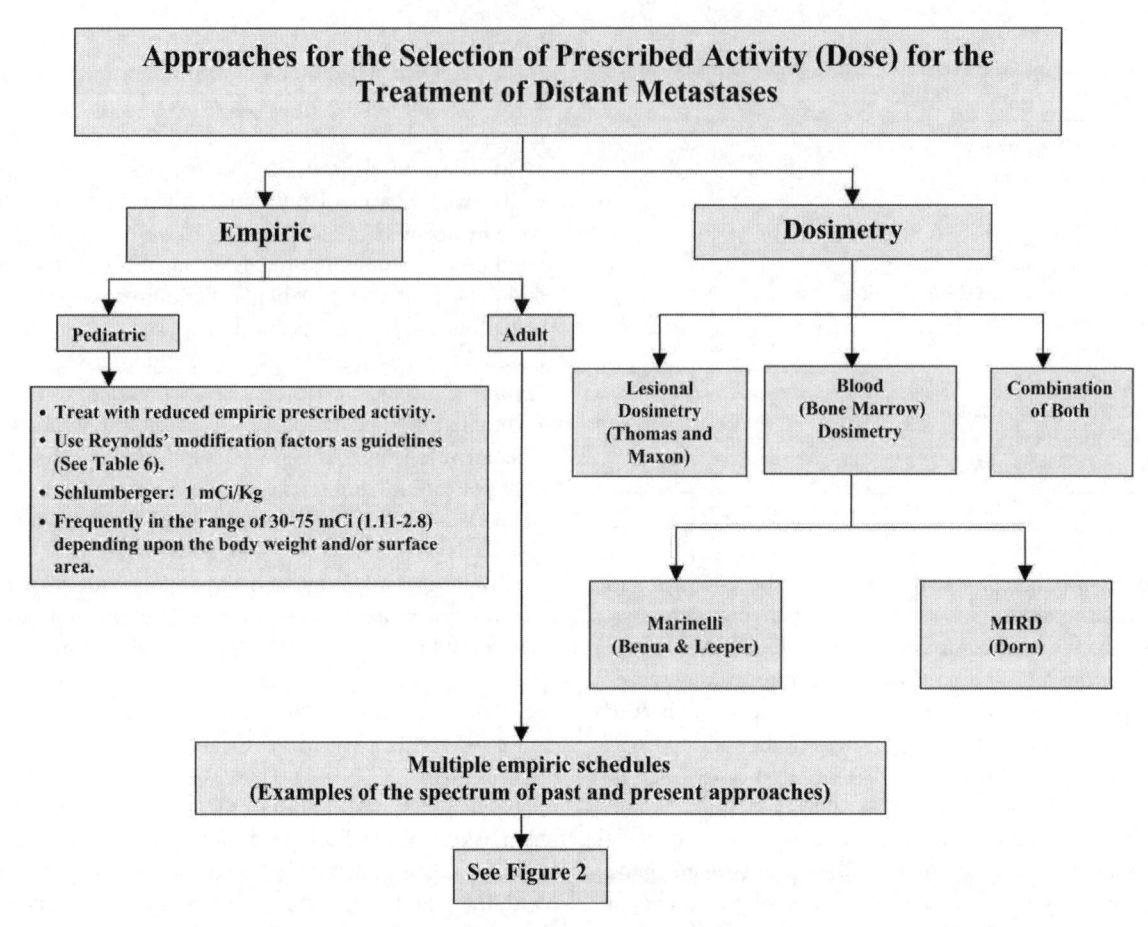

```
Approaches for the Selection of Prescribed Activity (Dose) for the
              Treatment of Distant Metastases
                              │
                ┌─────────────┴─────────────┐
            Empiric                     Dosimetry
        ┌──────┴──────┐        ┌───────────┼───────────┐
    Pediatric       Adult   Lesional     Blood      Combination
                            Dosimetry  (Bone Marrow)  of Both
                            (Thomas and  Dosimetry
                             Maxon)
    • Treat with reduced empiric prescribed activity.
    • Use Reynolds' modification factors as guidelines
      (See Table 6).                              ┌────┴────┐
    • Schlumberger: 1 mCi/Kg                   Marinelli   MIRD
    • Frequently in the range of 30-75 mCi    (Benua &    (Dorn)
      (1.11-2.8) depending upon the body       Leeper)
      weight and/or surface area.

              Multiple empiric schedules
      (Examples of the spectrum of past and present approaches)
                         │
                    See Figure 2
```

Fig. 1. Approaches for the selection of prescribed activity (dosage) for the treatment of distant metastases.

Table 6
Modification Factors of Prescribed Activity for Treatment for Children

Factor	Body Weight (kg)	Body Surface Area (m²)
0.2	10	0.4
0.4	25	0.8
0.6	40	1.2
0.8	55	1.4
1.0	77	1.7

Body surface area = $0.1 \times$ (weight in kg)$^{0.67}$. Source: refs. 48,49.

effects appeared even more favorable in children. Furthermore, they commented that early recognition and treatment of pulmonary metastases might improve the effectiveness of radioiodine therapy.

Vassilopoulou-Sellin et al. (20), from the University of Texas MD Anderson Cancer Center, reviewed 18 patients who developed distant metastases, of whom 16 had pulmonary metastases with and without other sites of metastases. Although few data are available, the one patient free of disease after 9 yr of follow-up was a 6-yr-old female child with radioiodine-positive, radiograph-negative lung metastases.

Høie et al. (10), from the Norwegian Radium Hospital in Norway, reported on 91 patients with distant metastases, and the overall survival data after 1 yr was 50%. Of the 91 patients, 73 had intrathoracic metastases, and two types of radioiodine accumulation patterns were described. One pattern had miliary or multiple parenchymal lesions, with either granular or nodular X-ray changes, and was observed in 48 patients. A second pattern of pulmonary infiltrations was observed in 25 patients and was associated with hilar or mediastinal enlargement and pleural effusions. However, they did not separate the survival data for patients who had only lung metastases, lung and other metastases, or nonlung metastases. Additionally, the authors did not distinguish between the results of the patients treated and not treated with radioiodine. Postoperative radioiodine ablation was not routine.

Leeper (2), from Memorial Sloan Kettering Cancer Center, reported that 11 of 18 older patients with distant metastases from follicular carcinoma were treated with radioiodine, and 6 patients demonstrated tumor regression. He concluded that the survival time of patients was enhanced

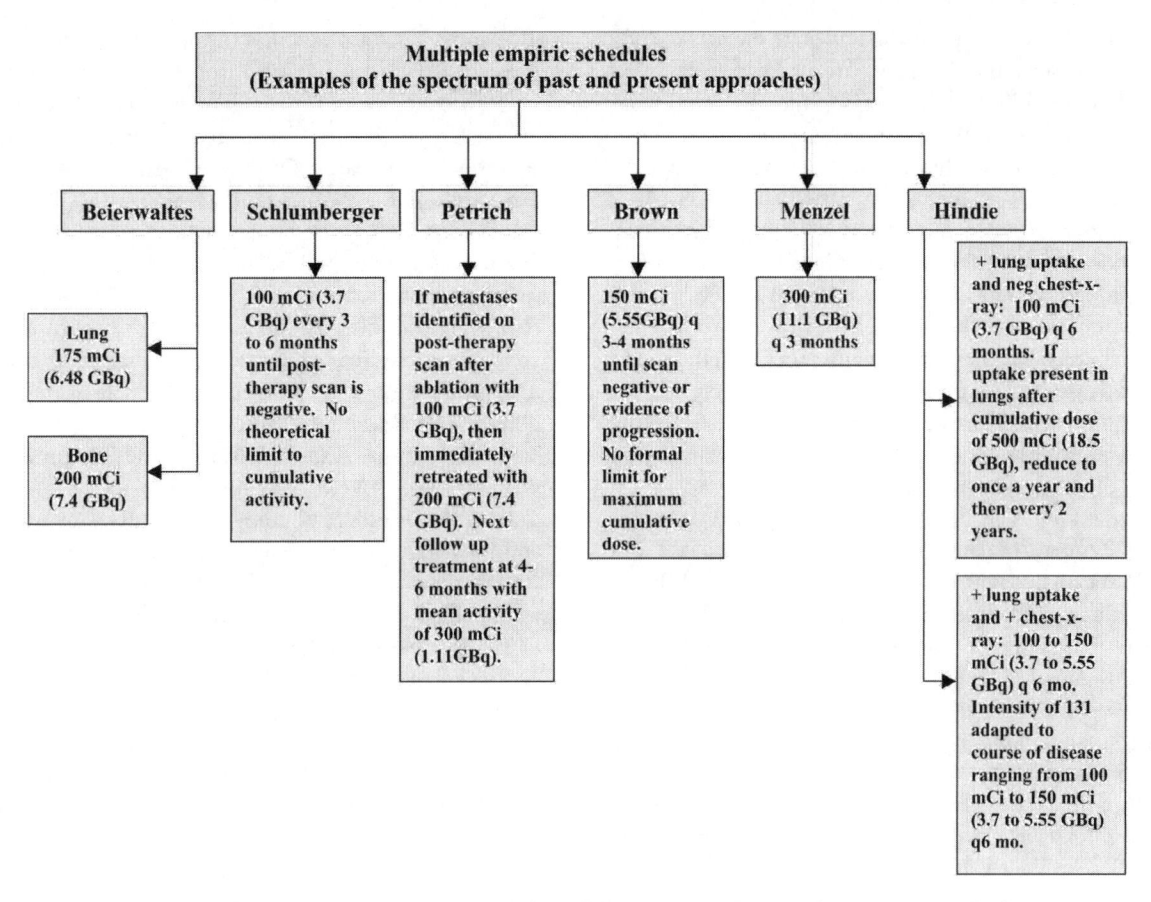

Fig. 2. Multiple empiric schedules (examples of the spectrum of past and present approaches).

Beierwaltes	Schlumberger	Petrich	Brown	Menzel	Hindie
Lung 175 mCi (6.48 GBq); Bone 200 mCi (7.4 GBq)	100 mCi (3.7 GBq) every 3 to 6 months until post-therapy scan is negative. No theoretical limit to cumulative activity.	If metastases identified on post-therapy scan after ablation with 100 mCi (3.7 GBq), then immediately retreated with 200 mCi (7.4 GBq). Next follow up treatment at 4–6 months with mean activity of 300 mCi (1.11 GBq).	150 mCi (5.55 GBq) q 3–4 months until scan negative or evidence of progression. No formal limit for maximum cumulative dose.	300 mCi (11.1 GBq) q 3 months	+ lung uptake and neg chest-x-ray: 100 mCi (3.7 GBq) q 6 months. If uptake present in lungs after cumulative dose of 500 mCi (18.5 GBq), reduce to once a year and then every 2 years. + lung uptake and + chest-x-ray: 100 to 150 mCi (3.7 to 5.55 GBq) q 6 mo. Intensity of 131 adapted to course of disease ranging from 100 mCi to 150 mCi (3.7 to 5.55 GBq) q6 mo.

significantly by radioiodine therapy. Also from Memorial Sloan Kettering Cancer Center, Robbins et al. *(31)* reported that after one high-dose treatment of radioiodine, complete resolution of radioiodine uptake was achieved in 33% of patients with pulmonary metastases.

Although the debate continues regarding the effect on survival, recurrence, and palliation of patients treated with radioiodine for lung metastases, this author believes that the data support the use in selected patients, as discussed below in the summary and illustrated in Figs. 1 and 2.

Bone Metastases

Many studies advocate radioiodine as valuable in the management of bone metastases *(15,18,20,25–27,32)*, although several others do not *(9–11,13,15,16,24,33;* see also Chapter 53).

Bernier et al. *(27)*, evaluated 109 patients with bone metastases at the Groupe Hospitalier Pitié-Salpétriér. The survival rates after 5 and 10 yr were 41% and 15%, respectively. Factors associated with an improved survival by univariate analysis were (1) radioiodine therapy, (2) younger age at discovery of bone metastases, (3) bone metastases as the revealing symptom for well-differentiated thyroid cancer, and (4) surgery for bone metastasis. Prognostic features associated with an improved survival by multivariate analysis included (1) the cumulative dose of radioiodine therapy, (2) absence of metastases in other organs, and (3) complete surgical removal of bone metastases in patients younger than 45 yr old.

Pittas et al. *(25)* at Memorial Sloan Kettering Cancer Center analyzed 146 patients with bone metastases from thyroid carcinoma. These results did include 13 (1%) patients with anaplastic thyroid carcinoma, 6 with medullary carcinoma, and 3 with lymphoma. The significant prognostic factors by univariate analysis of their data were (1) radioiodine uptake, (2) treatment with radioiodine ($p = 0.001$), (3) time from initial bone metastasis, and (4) absence of nonosseous metastases. Neither surgery nor external radiotherapy was a significant factor. The major prognostic factors for improved survival by multivariate analysis were radioiodine uptake and absence of nonosseous metastases—these were independent variables. However, after adjusting for all variables, radioiodine treatment was not identified to affect survival. Pittas concluded that the "overall survival is best in those whose lesions concentrate radioactive iodine and those who have no nonosseous metastases."

Petrich et al. *(26)*, from Hannover University Medical School in Germany, evaluated 107 patients with bone metastases. There were 60 patients who had bone metastases with radioiodine uptake, and the mean survival time was 8.9 yr. In patients with both bone metastases and lung metastases without radioiodine uptake, the mean survival was 1.2 yr. As other authors have noted, the data of Petrich et al. suggested that age was important, and 4 of 8 patients who were 45 yr old or younger achieved complete remission, whereas only 21 of 99 patients older than 45 yr achieved complete remission. Complete remission was also twice as likely to be achieved in patients with three or less sites of bone metastases, compared to those patients with more than three sites of bone metastases. Notably, no statistical difference was found in the mean survival in patients with radioiodine uptake in only bone metastases vs patients who had both bone and lung metastases (7.3 yr).

In the data reported by Dorn et al. *(32)*, from Augsburg Clinic in Germany, 15 patients who had bone metastases were selected to be treated with dosimetrically determined amounts of radioiodine. At the time of publication, 87% (13 of 15) of the patients had survived, with an average follow-up of 5.1 yr, mean follow-up of 5.0 yr, and range of 0.6–10.9 yr. The two deaths at 3.2 and 10.9 yr were attributed to thyroid cancer. The largest single amount of radioiodine administered was 1040 mCi (38.5 GBq).

In 28 patients with bone metastases, evaluated at the Surgical Professorial Unit at Lille University in France, Proye et al. *(13)* described a 1-yr survival rate of 53%; 43% of patients with bone metastases had positive radioiodine scans. Two patients were reported to have been "cured," and six patients had a partial remission. Both patients with "normal" X-rays and the diagnosis of bone metastasis on radioiodine scans alone had a response. Bone metastases with an X-ray abnormality never disappeared with radioiodine therapy alone. Of patients with positive radioiodine scans with or without an X-ray abnormality, the response rate was 50% (6 of 12). Regardless of whether there was radioiodine uptake, the response rate was 36% (8 of 22). Most patients received a combination of treatments, including radioiodine, surgery, and external radiotherapy. Patients who had bone metastases at the time of their initial diagnosis of well-differentiated thyroid carcinoma had a worse prognosis than those patients who subsequently developed bone metastases. These data of Proye et al. suggests that overall bone metastases respond poorly to radioiodine, and bone metastases that do respond to radioiodine were radioiodine-positive and radiographically-negative. Finally, they stated that surgical excision should be considered for isolated radiographically positive bone metastasis.

Zettinig et al. *(33)*, from the University of Vienna, analyzed 41 consecutive patients with bone metastases. By univariate analysis, total thyroidectomy, lymph node surgery, radioiodine therapy, and the absence of extraskeletal distant metastases were significant predictors of survival. However, no major prognostic factors were identified by multivariate analysis. In patients with only bone metastasis, univariate analysis determined that surgical expiration of the bone metastases was a prognostic factor for improved survival.

Marcocci et al. *(11)*, from the Instituto di Endocrinologia at the University of Pisa, Italy, reported on 30 patients with bone metastases. Of these patients, 25 were administered radioiodine with cumulative doses of 50–1810 mCi (1.85–6.7 GBq). Eleven bone metastases were radioiodine-positive and radiograph-negative; in 6 of these patients, the radioiodine uptake resolved. None of the 27 bone metastases that were radioiodine-positive and radiograph-positive showed a complete response. Marcocci et al. stated that apparently only surgical treatment can lead to a cure for bone metastases and is the preferred treatment for resectable bone metastases. Although Marcocci et al. suggested this was especially true for a single-bone lesion, Pittas et al. *(25)* indicated that other subclinical bone metastases are likely, and metastatic bone disease is virtually always a multicentric process.

Fanchiang et al. *(24)*, from Chang Gung Memorial Hospital in Taipei, reported on 39 patients, of whom 32 patients had bone metastases at the time of diagnosis. Using the Kaplan-Meier method of analysis, the 5-yr survival rate was estimated to be 64.9%. A total of 31 patients had multiple bone metastases, and the radiographs were abnormal in 33 of the 39 patients. There were 25 patients who received surgical intervention, and 18 received external radiotherapy. Although 28 patients had radioiodine uptake on scan, the number of patients treated with radioiodine was not indicated in the article, and no data were presented regarding the overall utility of radioiodine treatment. Fanchiang et al. concluded that surgery was the recommended treatment for surgically resectable and radiographically positive bone metastases because radioiodine could not eradicate the metastases completely.

As noted above, Pacini et al. *(15)* reported on 118 patients with metastatic disease, of whom 16 patients had bone metastases. However, the data of these patients was not separated from that of the patients with other sites of metastases. The authors did comment that some complete remissions were obtained in single radioiodine-positive, radiograph-negative bone metastases, but the overall response rate was poor. He proposed that, "Surgical removal of accessible bone metastases should be considered whenever possible *(15)*."

Woods et al. *(12)*, from the University of Texas/MD Anderson Cancer Center, could not assess the effect of radioactive iodine, as only one patient received radioiodine alone, and this was given as an intra-arterial injection into the axillary artery.

In summary, the role of radioiodine therapy in bone metastases continues to remain controversial. However, as more studies are reported, we may become more adept in identifying which patients with bone metastases will or will not benefit from radioiodine treatment. A patient who may benefit from radioiodine is one whose bone metastasis is (1) radioiodine-positive, (2) radiographically negative (3) not associated with other organ involvement, and (4) not potentially curable from surgery or other treatment modalities. Further studies are needed to determine if radioiodine is more effective in bone metastases with dosimetry-determined amounts of radioiodine, rather than empiric amounts. As noted elsewhere, the amounts of radioiodine that may be given based on dosimetry are typically higher than most empiric-prescribed activities. With higher quantities of prescribed activity, radioiodine may be significantly more effective because of higher radiation-absorbed doses, higher radiation-absorbed dose rates, and less fractionation of treatments. Finally, combination treatments, e.g., surgery and radioiodine with dosimetrically-determined prescribed activity followed immediately by external radiotherapy, deserve further studies.

Other Sites of Distant Metastases

Although less common, metastases to other distant sites do occur, such as to the mediastinum, brain, liver, adrenal gland, skin, kidney, and pancreas. However, little information is available relating to the efficacy of radioiodine treatment for these sites.

Metastases to the mediastinum are probably the third most frequent site for distant metastases *(16)*; however, no specific data exists pertaining to radioiodine's effect on mediastinal metastases. Of note, Massin et al. *(6)* suggested that mediastinal metastases are secondary from pulmonary metastases, rather than representing spread from cervical node metastases. This theory was based on their observations that (1) there was no statistical correlation between cervical and mediastinal lymph node metastases, (2) the main histological patterns were different at both sites (follicular was the most frequent histology in the mediastinal nodes, whereas papillary histology predominated in the cervical nodes), and (3) isolated mediastinal nodes were rare. Høie et al. *(10)* also implied that the source of mediastinal metastases was pulmonary metastases. Irrespective of the pattern of metastatic spread, further study is needed regarding the utility of radioiodine treatment on mediastinal metastases.

Chiu et al. *(34)*, from the University of Texas/MD Anderson Cancer Center, analyzed 32 patients with brain metastases from well-differentiated thyroid carcinoma. No evidence of survival benefit was found from radioiodine therapy. However, resection of one or more foci of brain metastases significantly improved survival. Surgical excision improved the median disease-specific survival since diagnosis of brain metastases from 3.4 to 16.7 mo ($p < 0.05$).

McWilliams et al. *(35)* of the Mayo Clinic reported on 16 patients with brain metastases. Four received radioiodine treatment. Of these, one patient had uptake on the radioiodine scan, and two patients had no uptake. No scan results were available for the fourth patient. None of the patients had an objective response to radioiodine treatment. Surgical excision appeared to improve the average survival after diagnosis of brain metastases from 2.7 to 20.8 mo.

Brown et al. *(5)* reported a single patient whose only site of metastatic disease was in the liver. The patient's condition was stable for 12 yr after radioiodine therapy but then developed gross hepatomegaly and died within several weeks.

SELECTION OF PRESCRIBED ACTIVITY FOR RADIOIODINE TREATMENT OF DISTANT METASTASES

The selection of a prescribed radioiodine activity for treatment of distant metastases of well-differentiated thyroid cancer has been based on either empiric recommendations or dosimetric calculations (see Fig. 1). As discussed in Chapter 26 on radioiodine ablation, the term "empiric" is defined by Webster's New World Dictionary as: "relying or based on practical experience without reference to scientific principles." Beierwaltes proposed empiric-prescribed activities for radioiodine treatment of recurrent and metastatic disease *(36)*, and empiric prescribed activities for radioiodine treatment of patients with recurrent or metastatic disease may range from 150 to 300 mCi (5.55–11.1 GBq) using multiple schedules (see Fig. 2; *2,5,18,19,21,26,28*). The determination of prescribed activity for these treatments has also been based on dosimetric calculations of either the lesion(s), blood (bone marrow), or both *(32,37–41)*. A detailed discussion of dosimetry, along with the advantages and disadvantages of empiric and dosimetrically determined prescribed activity, are presented in Chapters 46 and 47.

Beierwaltes *(36)* proposed treatment with prescribed activities of 150–175 mCi (5.55–6.48 GBq) for cervical lymph nodes metastases, 175–200 mCi (6.48–7.4 GBq) for pulmonary metastases, and 200 mCi (7.4 GBq) for bone metastases. Schlumberger et al. *(18)* typically treated patients with 100 mCi (3.7 GBq) every 3–6 mo until the posttherapy scan was negative, with no theoretical limit for cumulative prescribed activity. If metastasis was identified on a posttherapy scan, Petrich et al. *(26)* would then immediately retreat with 200 mCi (7.4 GBq), and their next follow-up treatment was typically at 4–6 mo, with mean activity of 300 mCi (11.1 GBq). Their prescribed activity for ablation was 100 mCi (3.7 GBq). Brown et al. *(5)* treated patients with 150 mCi (5.55 GBq) every 3–4 mo until the scan was negative or there was evidence of progression. They also had no formal limit for maximum cumulative prescribed activity. Menzel et al. *(19)* used 300 mCi (11.1 GBq) at 3-mo intervals after the diagnosis of metastatic disease. The maximum total activity administered in 1 yr was 1200 mCi (44.4 GBq), which was given to 7 patients, and the range of total cumulative activity was 400 mCi to 2.7 Ci (14.80–99.90 GBq) in 26 patients treated for advanced thyroid cancer. Hindié et al. *(28)* treated patients with 100 mCi (3.7 GBq) of ^{131}I every 6 mo until no uptake was present. If

Proposed Algorithm for Radioiodine Treatment of Distant Metastases

```
                        Preferred
           ┌───────────────┴───────────────┐
        Empiric                          Dosimetry
      ┌────┴────┐                            │
  Pediatric   Adult                   Blood Dosimetry
      │         │                      (Bone Marrow)
      │         │                      (Benua & Leeper)
```

Pediatric: Refer the patient to a facility that performs blood (bone marrow) dosimetry

Adult: Follow one of the approaches listed in Figure 2.

Perform 48-hour whole body retention such as described by Sisson (see text)

- **Diffuse Pulmonary Metastases:** Reduce empiric prescribed activity such that the 48-hour whole body retention will not exceed 80 mCi (2.96 GBq)
- **Macronodular Pulmonary Metastases:** Reduce empiric prescribed activity such that the 48-hour whole body retention will not exceed 120 mCi (4.44 GBq). Depending upon the number and extent of the macronodular metastases, this may be reduced further.
- **Bone, Liver, Kidney, Brain, Pancreas, etc. Metastases:** Reduce empiric prescribed activity such that the 48-hour whole body retention will not exceed 120 mCi (4.44 GBq).

Dosimetry (Blood Dosimetry):
1. Do not exceed maximal dosimetric-determined prescribed activity.
2. Do not exceed 120 mCi (4.44 GBq) whole body retention at 48-hours, and if diffuse pulmonary metastases, then do not exceed 80 mCi (2.96 GBq) whole body retention at 48-hours.
3. Modify the prescribed activity based upon factors such as listed in Table 7.
4. As possible, extend the time between treatments (e.g. at least one year).
5. No maximum cumulative prescribed activity. This should also be individualized with an assessment of risk versus benefit.

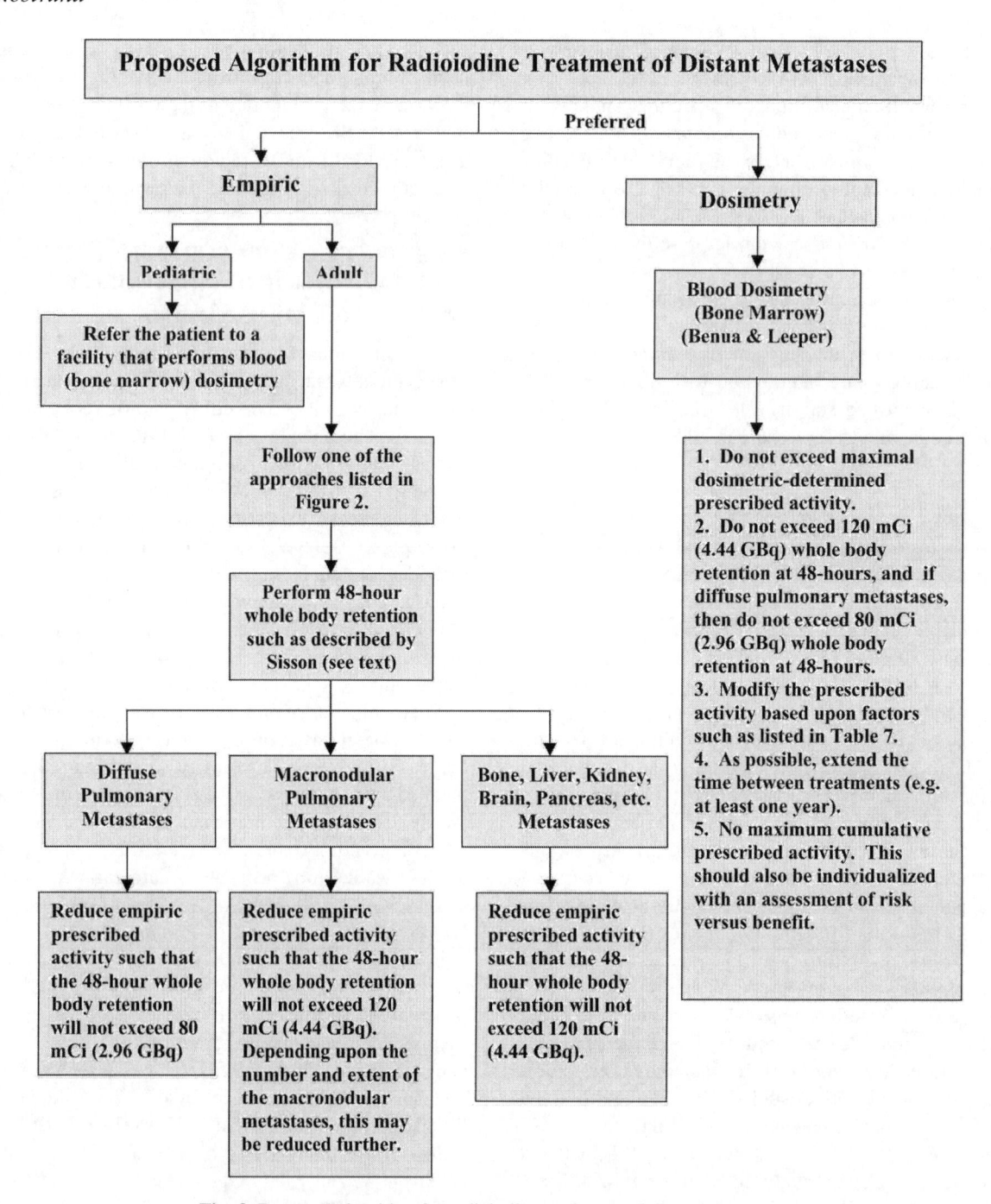

Fig. 3. Proposed algorithm for radioiodine treatment of distant metastases.

pulmonary uptake was still visible on the post-^{131}I therapy scan after a cumulative activity of 500 mCi (18.5 GBq), then the frequency of radioiodine therapy was reduced to once a year, then to once every 2 yr. For patients with positive findings on chest X-ray, Hindié administered 100–150 mCi (3.7–5.55 GBq) of radioiodine every 6 mo and altered the prescribed activity and frequency according to the course of the disease. This dosage ranged from 100 mCi (3.7 GBq) once a year to 150 mCi (5.55 GBq) every 6 mo.

SUMMARY

In summary, no prospective study is available to prove whether radioiodine treatment for distant metastases increases survival, reduces recurrences, and/or has significant palliative effects. The retrospective studies also do not resolve this issue. Thus, the debate continues. Similarly, when radioiodine is used for treatment, decisions will be made with incomplete information about what is the appropriate amount of radioiodine to administer and the method to determine that amount.

Based on the data noted above and in other chapters, such as Chapters 26, 39, 46, 49, and 53, this author submits the following conclusions and opinions. From these conclusions, guidelines are illustrated in Fig. 3.

1. The prognosis of patients with distant metastases may be reduced by many interrelated factors. Such factors are increasing age of patient, increasing size of metastasis(es), increasing number of metastases, location of metastases (e.g., lung, bone, or brain), increasing number of organs involved, pattern of metastases (e.g., macronodular vs micronodular, focal vs diffuse), radiological evidence of metastasis, and absence of radioiodine uptake.
2. Radioiodine treatment can be curative in selected patients who have distant metastases.
3. Radioiodine therapy can be palliative in certain patients with distant metastases.
4. A large proportion of patients who have distant metastases are not cured and may receive only minimal to no palliation from radioiodine.
5. The selection of patients for radioiodine treatment is important.
    a. Patients with diffuse pulmonary metastases that are not visualized on chest X-ray and computed tomography (CT) ("X-ray-negative") but are seen on radioiodine scan ("radioiodine-positive") are good candidates for radioiodine treatments. The potential benefit from radioiodine appears to decrease when the pulmonary metastases are visualized with chest X-ray/CT or F-18 fluorodeoxyglucose positron emission tomography, are more focal, and/or do not take up radioiodine.
    b. Early diagnosis and treatment of selected pulmonary metastases are important to maximize the efficacy of radioiodine therapy, to increase the probability of achieving a complete remission, and/or to increase survival. Notably, this may also be a result, at least in part, of the metastases being more radiosensitive at this stage.
    c. Children who have diffuse pulmonary metastases that are X-ray-negative and radioiodine-positive may have an excellent prognosis, and this prognosis typically is many years. However, these patients are still good candidates for treatment with radioiodine. Considering their excellent prognosis, it is particularly important that every effort be made to select the appropriate amount of radioiodine to maximize the chance for cure or to increase survival, while minimizing significant bone marrow suppression, radiation pneumonitis, and pulmonary fibrosis (Table 6). In addition, aggressive efforts should be made at the time of treatment to reduce the radiation-absorbed dose to the salivary glands, gastrointestinal system, urinary bladder, and so on.
    d. Radioiodine alone does not significantly increase survival or achieve significant palliation for patients who have pulmonary metastases that are macronodular in size (>1 cm) on X-ray and are radioiodine-negative.
    e. A single-bone metastasis that is X-ray-negative and radioiodine-positive may respond well to radioiodine and may be especially true for metastases at the base of the skull (42). However, alternative therapy, e.g., complete surgical excision, external radiotherapy, radiofrequency ablation, or arterial embolization, should be considered first (see Chapters 50, 51, 53, and 54). Radioiodine may be used as adjunctive therapy, or if the above treatments are not options, then as an alternative therapy.
    f. For patients with multiple, extensive, radioiodine-negative bone metastases, radioiodine treatments do not appear to significantly increase survival or achieve significant palliation.
    g. For patients who have brain metastases, surgical excision of the brain metastases, external radiotherapy (e.g., γ knife radiosurgery), and so forth, should be considered first. Radioiodine may be used as adjunctive or palliative treatment, but the probability of any significant effect is low.
    h. A "blind treatment" is an option in patients with negative radioiodine whole body scans and elevated thyroglobulin levels* (see Chapter 39).
    i. Patients who have a negative posttherapy scan should not receive any further radioiodine treatment unless redifferentiation—reestablishment of radioiodine uptake—is achieved and/or a significant reduction in a tumor marker (e.g., size of masses or serum thyroglobulin levels) has occurred. However, with a negative posttherapy scan, a major decrease in a tumor marker is highly unlikely.
6. The method to select the amount of radioiodine depends on the medical practice and capabilities of the specific facility.
    a. The first treatment ("first strike") of distant metastases has the highest chance of being curative (32).
    b. Tumor destruction is not linearly related to radiation-absorbed dose (rad, Gy), but the radiation-absorbed dose delivered to the tumor must exceed a minimum level to have a notable effect (39).
    c. The difference between a significant effect and a minimal effect from radioiodine treatment may be a very small difference in regard to the amount of radiation-absorbed dose delivered and, thus, the amount of millicuries (Bq) administered (39).
    d. Higher dose *rates* (rad/h and Gy/h) are more effective (43,44).
    e. For radioiodine-positive distant metastases, radioiodine administered in a single treatment is more likely to have a greater effect on the tumor than when the same amount of radioiodine is administered in fractionated treatments over 3 mo to several years. The lower response from fractionated treatments is a result of (1) low radiation-absorbed dose *rates* and (2) reduced radiation-absorbed doses deliv-

---

*A "blind treatment" is the medical slang for the treatment of a patient whose serum thyroglobulin level is positive but radioiodine scan is negative. Like many other factors, this circumstance is very controversial. Even if a blind treatment is considered, the level of serum thyroglobulin above which a blind-treatment is indicated is also controversial.

Table 7
Factors That Individualize Treatments of Patients With Distant Metastases

Age
Histology
Location of metastases (e.g., lung, bone, or brain)
Number of metastases
Size of metastasis(s)
Number of organs involved
Signs and symptoms secondary to metastases
Uptake of radioiodine
Radiological evidence of disease
Potential for surgical excision
Response of metastases to any previous radioiodine treatment (e.g., indicated by physical exam, radioiodine scan, chest X-ray, computed tomography, magnetic resonance, ultrasound, serum thyroglobulin levels)
Baseline CBC and differential pretreatment, with special attention to granulocytes, lymphocytes, and platelets
Response of CBC and differential during the 3–6 wk after previous treatment
Change in baseline CBC and differential after previous treatment
Pulmonary function tests pretreatment
Change in pulmonary function tests since previous treatment
Bone marrow biopsy for assessment, not of metastases, but percent cellularity and adipose tissue in the bone marrow
Concomitant disease(s)
Facilities available
Patient desire(s)

CBC, complete blood count.

ered from the second and subsequent treatments because of decreased radioiodine uptake from the first or preceding treatments.

f. As radiation-absorbed doses and dose rates are increased, the frequency and severity of side effects also increase (see Chapter 49).

g. As medical treatment plans are individualized for each patient, the amount of radioiodine to treat distant metastases should also be individualized. The purpose of this individualization is to maximize the potential radiation-absorbed dose and dose rate to the tumor without exceeding the maximal tolerated radiation-absorbed dose to the bone marrow or lungs.

h. Dosimetrically-determined amounts of radioiodine, as determined by the Benua-Leeper or the MIRD methods (see Chapters 47 and 48 on Dosimetry), allow more patients to receive higher radiation-absorbed doses and higher dose rates to the metastases than empiric amounts of radioiodine.

i. Dosimetrically-determined amounts of radioiodine can identify as many as 11–19% *(45,46)* of patients who would have received more than 200 rad to the bone marrow if treated with an empiric-prescribed activity of 200 mCi (7.4 GBq) of radioiodine. This percentage is even higher if the empiric-prescribed activity is 300 mCi (11.1 GBq).

j. Patients who (1) have distant metastases, (2) are going to be treated with radioiodine, and (3) may receive multiple subsequent radioiodine treatments should be managed *early* and *aggressively* to reduce the radiation-absorbed dose to nontarget organs, such as salivary glands, gastrointestinal tract, and urinary bladder. In addition, this management should be regardless of the amount of radioiodine administered for the initial treatment (see Chapter 50 on side effects).

k. If dosimetry cannot be performed, than the measurement of a 48-h whole-body retention, as described by Sisson et al. *(47)*, may help identify patients who may be eligible for higher empiric amounts of radioiodine or should have their empiric-prescribed activity reduced.

Based on the above conclusions and opinions, this author proposes an algorithm for the selection of the amount of radioiodine to be administered to patients with distant metastases (Fig. 3). However, there are two caveats. The algorithm in Fig. 3 is not for the selection of patients for radioiodine treatment but for the selection of the activity to be administered. In addition, this algorithm is not absolute. Rather, the algorithm is one physician's guidelines. The decision whether to treat and the amount of radioiodine to administer must be individualized according to many factors; a few are listed in Table 7. Thus, the "practice" of medicine continues.

REFERENCES

1. Seidlin SM, Marinelli LD, Oshry E. Radioactive iodine therapy: effect on functioning metastases of adenocarcinoma of the thyroid. JAMA 1946; 132:838–847.
2. Leeper RD. The effect of I-131 therapy on survival of patients with metastatic papillary or follicular thyroid carcinoma. J Clin Endocrinol Metab 1973; 36:1143–1152.
3. Nemec J, Zamrazil V, Pohunkova D, Rohling S. Radioiodide treatment of pulmonary metastases of differentiated thyroid cancer: results and prognostic factors. Nucl Med 1979; 18:86–90.
4. Maheshwari YK, Strattton Hill C, Haynie TP, et al. Iodine-131 therapy in differentiated thyroid carcinoma: M.D. Anderson Hospital experience. Cancer 1981; 47:664–671.
5. Brown AP, Greening WP, McCready VR, et al. Radioiodine treatment of Metastatic thyroid carcinoma: the Royal Marsden hospital experience: Br J Radiol 1984; 57:323–327.
6. Massin JP, Savoie JC, Garnier H, et al. Pulmonary metastases in differentiated thyroid carcinoma: study of 58 cases with implications for the primary tumor treatment. Cancer 1984; 53:982–992.
7. Samaan, NA, Schultz PN, Haynie TP, Ordonez NG. Pulmonary metastasis of differentiated thyroid carcinoma: treatment results in 101 patients. J Clin Endocrinol Metab 1985; 65:376–380.
8. Schlumberger M, Arcangioli O, Piekarski JD, et al. Detection of and treatment of lung metastases of differentiated thyroid carcinoma in patients with normal chest x-rays. J Nucl Med 1988; 29:1790–1794.
9. Ruegemer JJ, Hay ID, Bergstralh EJ, et al. Distant metastases in differentiated thyroid carcinoma: a multivariate analysis of prognostic variables. J Clin Endocrinol Metab 1988; 67:501–508.
10. Hoie J, Stenwig AE, Kullman G, Lindegaard M. Distant metastases in papillary thyroid cancer: a review of 91 patients. Cancer 1988; 61:1–6.

11. Marcocci C, Pacini F, Elisi R, et al. Clinical and biological behavior of bone metastases from differentiated thyroid carcinoma. Surgery 1989; 106:960–966.
12. Woods WJ, Singletary SE, Hickey RC. Current results of treatment for distant metastatic well-differentiated thyroid carcinoma. Arch Surg 1989; 124:1374–1377.
13. Proye CAG, Dromer DHR, Carnaille BM, et al. Is it still worthwhile to treat bone metastases from differentiated thyroid carcinoma with radioactive iodine? World J Surg 1992; 16:640–646.
14. Casara D, Rubello D, Saladini G, et al. Different features of pulmonary metastases in differentiated thyroid cancer: natural history and multivariate statistical analysis of prognostic variables. J Nucl Med 1993; 34:1626–1631.
15. Pacini F, Cetani F, Miccoli P, et al. Outcome of 309 patients with metastatic thyroid carcinoma treated with radioiodine. World J Surg 1994; 18:600–604.
16. Dinneen SF, Valimaki MJ, Bergstralh, EJ, et al. Distant metastases in papillary thyroid carcinoma: 100 cases observed at one institution during 5 decades. J Clin Endocrinol Metab 1995; 80:2041–2045.
17. Vassilopoulou-Sellin R, Libshitz HI, Haynie TP. Papillary thyroid cancer with pulmonary metastases beginning in childhood. Clinical course over three decades. Med Pediatr Oncol 1995; 24:119–122.
18. Schlumberger M, Challeton C, De Vathaire F, et al. Radioactive iodine treatment and external radiotherapy for lung and bone metastases from thyroid carcinoma. J Nucl Med 1996; 37:598–605.
19. Menzel C, Grunwald F, Schomburg A, et al. "High-dose" radioiodine therapy in advanced differentiated thyroid carcinoma. J Nucl Med 1996; 37:1496–1503.
20. Vassilopoulou-Sellin R, Schultz P, Haynie TP. Clinical outcome of patients with papillary thyroid carcinoma who have recurrence after initial radioactive iodine therapy. Cancer 1996; 78:494–501.
21. Sisson JC, Giordano TJ, Jamadar DA, et al. Treatment of micronodular pulmonary metastases from papillary thyroid cancer with I-131. Cancer 1996; 78:2184–2192.
22. Shaha AR, Shah JP, Loree TR. Patterns of nodal and distant metastasis based on histologic varieties in differentiated thyroid carcinoma of the thyroid. Am J Surg 1996; 172:692–694.
23. Samuel AM, Rajashekharrao B, Shah DH. Pulmonary metastases in children and adolescents with well-differentiated thyroid cancer. J Nucl Med 1998; 30:1531–1536.
24. Fanchiang JK, Lin JD, Huang MJ, Shih NW. Papillary and follicular thyroid carcinomas with bone metastases: A series of 39 cases during a period of 18 years. Chang Gung Med J 1998; 21:377–382.
25. Pittas AG, Adler M, Fazzari M, et al. Bone metastases from thyroid carcinoma; clinical characteristics and prognostic variables in one hundred forty six patients. Thyroid 2000; 10:261–268.
26. Petrich T, Widjaja A, Musholt TJ, et al. Outcome after radioiodine therapy in 107 patients with differentiated thyroid carcinoma and initial bone metastases: side effects and influence of age. Eur J Nucl Med 2001; 28:203–208.
27. Bernier MO, Leenhardt L, Hoang C, et al. Survival and therapeutic modalities in patients with bone metastases of differentiated thyroid carcinomas. J Clin Endocrinol Metab 2001; 86:1568–1473.
28. Hindié E, Melliere D, Lange F, et al. Functioning pulmonary metastases of thyroid cancer: does radioiodine influence the prognosis? Eur J Nucl Med 2003; 30:974–981.
29. Ronga G, Filesi M, Montesano T, et al. Lung metastases from differentiated thyroid carcinoma. A 40 years' experience. Q J Nucl Med Mol Imaging 2004; 48:12–19.
30. Sisson JC, Jamadar DDA, Kazerooni EA, et al. Treatment of micronodular lung metastases of papillary thyroid cancer: are the tumors too small for effective irradiation from radioiodine? Thyroid 1998; 8:215–221.
31. Robbins RJ, Larson SM, Pentlow KS, Tuttle RM. Treatment of thyroid cancer metastases with I-131 following thyroid hormone withdrawal or recombinant human TSH. Thyroid 2003; 13:702.
32. Dorn R, Kopp J, Vogt H, et al. Dosimetry-guided radioactive iodine treatment in patients with metastatic differentiated thyroid cancer: largest safe dose using a risk—adapted approach. J Nucl Med 2003; 44:451–456.
33. Zettinig G, Fueger B, Passier C, et al. Long-term follow-up of patients with bone metastases from differentiated thyroid carcinoma—surgery or conventional therapy? Clin Endocrinol 2002; 56:377–382.
34. Chiu AC, Delpassand ES, Sherman SI. Prognosis and treatment of brain metastases in thyroid carcinoma. J Clin Endocrinol Metab 1997; 82:3637–3642.
35. McWilliams RR, Giannini C, Hay ID, et al. Management of brain metastases from thyroid carcinoma: a study of 16 pathologically confirmed cases over 25 years. Cancer 2003; 98:356–362.
36. Beierwaltes WH. The treatment of thyroid carcinoma with radioactive iodine. Semin Nucl Med 1978; 8:79–94.
37. Thomas SR, Maxon HR, Kereiakes JG. In vivo quantitation of lesion radioactivity using external counting methods. Med Phys 1976; 3:253–255.
38. Thomas SR, Maxon HR, Kereiakes JG, Saenger EL. Quantitative external counting techniques enabling improved diagnostic and therapeutic decisions in patients with well-differentiated thyroid cancer. Radiology 1977; 122:731–737.
39. Maxon HR, Thomas SR, Hertzbert VS, et al. Relation between effective radiation dose and outcome of radioiodine therapy for thyroid cancer. N Engl J Med 1983; 309:937–941.
40. Benua RS, Cicale NR, Sonenberg M, Rawson RW. The relation of radioiodine dosimetry to results and complications in the treatment of metastatic thyroid cancer. Am J Roentgenol Radium Ther Nucl Med 1962; 87:171–182.
41. Leeper RD. Thyroid cancer. Med Clin North Am 1985; 69:1079–1096.
42. Schlumberger J, Tubiana M, De Vathaire F, et al. Long term results of treatment of 283 patients with lung and bone metastases from differentiated thyroid carcinoma. J Clin Endocrinol Metab 1998; 63:960–967.
43. Samuel AM, Rajashekharrao B. Radioiodine therapy for well-differentiated thyroid cancer: A quantitative dosimetric evaluation for remnant thyroid ablation after surgery. J Nucl Med 1994; 35:1944–1950.
44. Kassis AI, Adelstein SJ. Radiobiologic principles of radionuclide therapy. J Nucl Med 2005; 46:4S–12S.
45. Atkins FB, Van Nostrand D, Kulkarni K, et al. The frequency with which empiric amounts of radioiodine "over-" or "under-" treat patients with metastatic well-differentiated thyroid cancer. J Nucl Med 2005; 46:129P.
46. Leeper R. Controversies in the treatment of thyroid cancer: the New York Memorial Hospital Approach. Thyroid Today 1982; 5:1–4.
47. Sisson JC, Shulkin BL, Lawson S. Increasing efficacy and safety of treatments of patients with well-differentiated thyroid carcinoma by measuring body retentions of I-131. J Nucl Med 2003; 44:898–903.
48. Reynolds JC. Comparison of I-131 absorbed radiation doses in children and adults; a tool for estimating therapeutic I-131 doses in children. In Robbins J, editor. Treatment of thyroid cancer in children. Springfield, VA: US Department of Commerce Technology Administration, National Technical Information Service, 1994:127–135.
49. Maxon HR. Quantitative radioiodine therapy in the treatment of differentiated thyroid cancer. Q J Nucl Med 1999; 43:313–323.

46
^{131}I Treatment of Metastatic Thyroid Carcinoma Following Preparation by Recombinant Human Thyrotropin

Richard J. Robbins and R. Michael Tuttle

INTRODUCTION

Eradication of metastatic thyroid carcinoma is a challenge. This challenge is attributed to the marked reduction in iodine uptake and organification in thyroid cancer cells, the relatively slow and unpredictable rate of progression, and the generally high quality of life (QOL), even in those patients with widely metastatic lesions. Furthermore, relatively few studies have identified reliable predictors of the progression rate, the pattern of metastatic spread, or the sensitivity to ^{131}I therapy. Patients and their physicians often continue to administer large amounts of ^{131}I to lesions that appear iodine-avid, even in the absence of previous tumor responses. A common rationalization for this approach is that the subsequent progression would have been worse if another dose of ^{131}I had not been administered.

To compound this dilemma, evidence suggests that thyrotropin (TSH) is a progression factor for the growth of metastatic thyroid carcinoma. Therefore, the standard management approach employs constant suppression of this hormone. Unfortunately, TSH is the only known activator of the sodium-iodide symporter (NIS), which must be maximally stimulated to deliver the optimal amount of administered ^{131}I. Thus, it has become routine to withdraw patients from thyroid hormone replacement to produce elevated endogenous TSH production, allowing TSH stimulation and possible cancer cell proliferation for 6–8 wk. In vitro, in vivo, and clinical studies all support this contention, and examples of tumor expansion and progression have been documented in this setting *(1–3)*.

Numerous leading thyroid cancer authorities have tried to attenuate the clinical symptoms of hypothyroidism by reducing the time of thyroid hormone withdrawal or by using triiodothyronine (T3) for a few weeks to minimize the hypothyroid state. These strategies all rely on the assumption that maximum radioiodine uptake by malignant thyroid tissues occurs when the serum TSH has risen above the 25–30-mU/mL range. There is remarkably little evidence that indicates this assumption is true, despite its widespread acceptance within the community of thyroid specialists.

The advent of clinical-grade recombinant human TSH (rhTSH) provided an opportunity to examine the possibility that short-term elevations in serum TSH (3–4 d) might enable a comparable activation of the NIS *(4)* in thyroid cancer tissue, without the need for hypothyroidism associated with prolonged TSH stimulation, which might result in disease progression. rhTSH-assisted treatment is usually given when patients are taking full therapeutic doses of thyroxine (T4) and a low-iodine diet. A reduced whole-body radiation load is an additional theoretical advantage, considering the known reduced renal iodine clearance that exists in hypothyroidism, which would lead to longer radioiodine retention and greater radiation exposure with the regimen of T4 withdrawal *(5)*. Finally, in our experience with thousands of patients, thyroid cancer survivors are generally reluctant to withdraw from T4 because of its negative effect on their QOL, as shown by Cohen et al. *(6)*. Many patients simply choose to forgo the possible benefit of radioiodine therapy simply because they want to avoid hypothyroidism.

Immediately after the preliminary results from the phase II testing of rhTSH were announced, clinicians began requesting access to rhTSH for "unusual" patients who could not produce TSH endogenously or who were too unstable to undergo thyroid hormone withdrawal. Through a compassionate need program supported by the Genzyme Corporation and sanctioned by federal agencies, rhTSH (Thyrogen) was made available to physicians on a case-by-case basis in April 1995.

CASE REPORTS (TABLE 1)

The first evidence that rhTSH could be used to stimulate ^{131}I uptake in metastatic lesions was presented at the annual meeting of the American Thyroid Association in November 1996 *(7)*. All four patients in this preliminary report remained on TSH suppressive doses of T4 throughout testing and

Table 1
Individual Case Reports of rhTSH as Preparation for Radioiodine Therapy

Author	Metastatic Sites	^{131}I (mCi)	Side Effects	Outcome
Rudavsky (8)	Lung, bone	515	Vomiting	PR
Chiu (1)	Brain	200	NA	NA
Adler (2)	Brain, lung, bone	434–506	Bone pain	PR
Colleran (9)	Neck	150	NA	NA
Perros (3)	Neck	135, 141	None	PR
Risse (11)	Pituitary	0	None	Not treated
Masiukiewicz (12)	Pituitary	200	NA	NA
Vargas (13)	Brain	304	Hemiplegia	PR
Mazzaferri (14)	Lung	100–140	NA	PR
Robbins (15)	Brain	154	Papilledema	PR
Rotman (10)	Liver	65	Nausea	PR
Aslam (16)	C-spine, neck, mediastinum	209	NA	NA
Serafini (17)	Orbit	207	NA	NA
Goffman (18)	Lung, neck	157	Vomiting, dyspnea	PR

PR, partial response; NA, not available.

therapy. Uptake of ^{131}I into metastatic lesions was demonstrated on posttherapy scans in all four patients.

The initial published report on rhTSH-assisted ^{131}I therapy of metastatic thyroid carcinoma was by Rudavsky and Freedman (8). These physicians also showed that rhTSH could substitute for endogenously produced TSH and stimulate the uptake of ^{131}I into lung and bone metastases in one patient. Their patient received 515 mCi of ^{131}I 24 h after the second of two daily 0.9-mg injections of rhTSH. Within 2 wk, the patient had a substantial reduction in bone pain related to his metastases. His serum thyroglobulin (Tg) level fell from 7800 ng/mL to 1924 ng/mL over a 4-mo interval. Subsequent to this report, many clinicians and investigators began to apply this approach to selected patients.

Chiu et al. (1) administered 200 mCi of ^{131}I following two 0.9-mg doses of rhTSH to treat brain metastases in a patient with a tall-cell variant of papillary thyroid carcinoma and demonstrated uptake of the isotope into the lesions.

Adler et al. (2) reported that rhTSH could stimulate uptake of a therapeutic dose of ^{131}I into the brain, spine, and lung metastases. One patient had central TSH deficiency. Improvement in the lung metastases was observed in one patient.

Colleran and Burge (9) reported on the use of rhTSH for a patient whose TSH level did not elevate following 7 wk of thyroxine withdrawal, despite being clinically hypothyroid. Magnetic resonance imaging (MRI) of the pituitary revealed an empty sella. rhTSH was then used to stimulate ^{131}I uptake.

Rotman-Pikielny et al. (10) used rhTSH to assist ^{131}I therapy in a patient with functioning hepatic metastases, which prevented an elevation of TSH after thyroid hormone withdrawal. A partial reduction in liver metastases was found 6 mo after therapy.

Perros (3) reported on a patient with unstable angina who sustained a myocardial infarction following thyroid hormone withdrawal in preparation for radioiodine therapy for follicular thyroid carcinoma. rhTSH was then used to prepare the patient for ^{131}I administration, without any adverse cardiovascular events, on two different occasions.

Risse et al. and Masiukiewicz et al. (11,12) both reported on the use of rhTSH to assist in ^{131}I therapy of patients with hypopituitarism from thyroid cancer involvement of the pituitary gland. Vargas et al. (13) also reviewed a patient with thyroid cancer involving the pituitary region. Unfortunately, in this case, rapid expansion of the lesion following rhTSH was associated with the onset of hemiplegia. After 4 d, the patient received 304 mCi of ^{131}I. A follow-up MRI scan 2 yr later documented a reduction in the size of the pituitary mass.

Mazzaferri and Kloos (14) described a patient with papillary thyroid cancer and end-stage renal failure who could not tolerate hypothyroidism. Following two doses of rhTSH, the patient was treated with ^{131}I, and the posttherapy scan revealed uptake in lung metastases that was not seen on chest X-ray.

Robbins et al. (15) examined a patient with follicular thyroid cancer who developed rapid expansion of a previously undiagnosed brain metastasis associated with hemiplegia after two rhTSH injections. The patient demonstrated good uptake of ^{131}I in lung, bone, and central nervous system lesions. This patient was treated on two subsequent occasions with the assistance of rhTSH and glucocorticoids and had no neurologic complications.

Aslam and Daly (16) reported on a 62-yr-old man treated with radioactive iodine for widely metastatic papillary thyroid cancer that was enabled by rhTSH.

Serafini et al. (17) reported on a woman with papillary thyroid cancer who was unable to tolerate hypothyroidism

Table 2
Reports of Larger Series of Patients Who Received rhTSH-Assisted Therapy

Author	rhTSH Schedule	^{131}I Administered	Side Effects	Outcomes
Luster (19)	0.9 mg IM 48 and 24 h prior	27–200 mCi	Headache, bone pain	PR: 5 POD: 5
Mariani (20)	0.9 mg IM 48 and 24 h prior	NA	Mild nausea, malaise	NA
Lippi (21)	0.9 mg IM four doses prior	100 MBq/kg	Bone pain, nausea, fever	PR: 4 Stable: 2 POD: 4
Berg (22)	0.9 mg IM 48 and 24 h prior	108 mCi	Nausea, bone pain	PR: 5 NR: 2
De Keizer (23)	0.9 mg IM 48 and 24 h prior	200 mCi	None	PR: 3 Stable: 2 POD: 6
Jarzab (24)	0.9 mg IM 48 and 24 h prior	100–200 mCi	Bone pain, lesion edema, paresthesiae, rash	CR: 1 PR: 12 Stable: 19 POD: 15

CR, complete response; PR, partial response; stable, stable disease; POD, progression of disease; NR, no response; IM, intramuscular.

because of severe generalized malaise. On multiple occasions, she refused to be withdrawn from thyroid hormone, and rhTSH was used to prepare her for a therapeutic dose of ^{131}I. The posttherapy scan revealed radioiodine uptake in the thyroid bed region and disclosed a new metastatic lesion in her left orbit.

Finally, Goffman et al. (18) analyzed a patient with diffuse lung metastases who was considered too ill to undergo thyroid hormone withdrawal as preparation for ^{131}I treatment. After two rhTSH injections, she developed moderate swelling of her neck lesions and dyspnea. She then received 157 mCi of ^{131}I; 2 d later, she developed severe respiratory failure, necessitating oxygen, steroids, and antibiotics. She gradually improved, and her serum Tg level declined. The sudden deterioration in pulmonary function was thought to be most likely the result of lesional edema, partly owing to the direct effect of rhTSH.

Although these reports describe a diverse set of patients and circumstances, they have established that:

1. Serum TSH is reliably elevated considerably higher than 30 mU/L, which is often considered the standard of care after T4 withdrawal.
2. Uptake of radioiodine is routinely demonstrated on posttherapy scans.
3. Although rhTSH is generally well-tolerated, large metastatic lesions can rapidly swell, causing neurological, respiratory, or painful events.
4. The vast majority of patients experience no symptoms of hypothyroidism.
5. Evidence of partial response or stabilization of disease is often realized.

However, individual case reports do not provide the full perspective of the possible risks and benefits of this approach that become evident in larger standardized trials.

LARGER SERIES (TABLE 2)

From Wurzburg, Germany, Luster et al. (19) reported their observations in 10 patients with advanced metastatic thyroid carcinoma who were treated with ^{131}I after rhTSH preparation, according to a standard protocol. Patients were offered this option because of the inability to produce sufficient TSH or because of a medical contraindication to hypothyroidism. Each patient received two daily 0.9-mg rhTSH injections, and the therapeutic administration of ^{131}I was given on the third day. T4 therapy was continued throughout the procedure. Those with brain or spinal cord metastases received high-dose steroids to prevent lesion edema. At follow-up (a mean of 4.3 mo), three patients had died of progressive disease. Six of the eight surviving patients had evidence of partial responses, as indicated by reductions (at least 30% lower than baseline) in serum Tg, and the other two were stable. No major adverse events occurred; however, headache ($n = 2$), bone pain ($n = 1$), fever ($n = 1$), and rash ($n = 1$) were reported. The authors concluded that this approach was a reasonable alternative to thyroid hormone withdrawal in selected patients.

Mariani et al. (20) administered ^{131}I to eight thyroid cancer survivors after preparation with rhTSH, which was administered as two 0.9-mg injections per day, and the ^{131}I was administered on day 3. Posttherapy scans showed considerable radioiodine uptake in residual disease in seven of the eight patients, but no long-term follow-up data was available to analyze its efficacy.

Lippi et al. from Pisa, Italy, (21) used rhTSH-assisted ^{131}I therapy for 12 patients who had differentiated thyroid carcinoma and residual metastatic disease. They used two 0.9-mg injections of rhTSH for a 4-mCi diagnostic whole-body scan (WBS), then two more injections of rhTSH within 1 wk to prepare for ^{131}I therapy, which was given 24 h following the last rhTSH injection. Based on published data suggesting that blood clearance rates of iodine were 50% slower in hypothyroid patients, they doubled their usual activity administered to compensate. Serum TSH levels rose to over 100 mU/L in all patients. The posttherapy WBS showed radioiodine uptake into metastatic lesions in all as well. Despite relatively advanced disease and previous high doses of ^{131}I, 4 of 10 evaluable patients had a reduction in their serum Tg. Although this approach was well-tolerated, two patients had swelling and pain in bone lesions, similar to their past experience when withdrawn from T4. As in other reports, nausea and fever in low levels were also present. The authors concluded that rhTSH-assisted treatment of metastatic thyroid carcinoma was a safe method to administer ^{131}I, preventing the debilitating effects of hypothyroidism.

Berg et al. (22) from Sweden also investigated the safety and efficacy of rhTSH-treated ^{131}I in 11 frail thyroid cancer patients. Patients remained on T4 and were placed on a low-iodine diet for the 2 wk prior to therapy. After two daily 0.9-mg injections of rhTSH, the patients each received approx 108 mCi of ^{131}I. Of the 11 patients, 8 were being treated for metastatic disease. Five of the eight patients showed partial response to the therapy, two showed no response, and one is under surveillance. The rhTSH was well-tolerated, with the exception of two patients who developed lesional swelling, one with nausea and the other with bone pain. No serious adverse events occurred. The authors concluded that rhTSH-assisted ^{131}I was safe and feasible in frail elderly patients, and that it offered a means to reasonable palliative therapy for those with widely metastatic disease.

De Keizer et al. (23) applied this same strategy in 16 patients who underwent 19 rhTSH-administered ^{131}I treatments for metastatic disease. All patients had total thyroidectomy with radioiodine remnant ablation and were being treated for residual cancer. Patients were on a low-iodine diet and received two daily 0.9-mg injections of rhTSH, then ^{131}I on day 3. The radiation to individual lesions was estimated by posttherapy scanning techniques. Tumor response was solely based on changes in serum Tg. In 11 evaluable treatments, a partial Tg response occurred in 27%, stable disease in 18%, and progression of disease was seen in 55%. None of those whose disease progressed received a lesion dose of more than 30 Gy. The treatments were well-tolerated, with only one patient showing spinal cord compression that responded to corticosteroid administration. The authors thought that this approach was reasonable for those with advanced disease who were not good candidates for thyroid hormone withdrawal.

The largest report yet on this strategy is from Jarzab et al. (24) in Poland. They used rhTSH-assisted ^{131}I therapy in 54 patients who, with a few exceptions, had a total thyroidectomy and radioiodine remnant ablation. All the patients had clear evidence of residual thyroid carcinoma. There were 31 patients who had radioiodine-avid metastases, whereas the rest had nonfunctional metastases. Those with nonfunctional metastases were given retinoic acid prior to the rhTSH to determine if they could reinduce radioiodine avidity. All patients received twice-daily 0.9-mg rhTSH injections, followed by ^{131}I on day 3 (median, 100 mCi; range, 100–250 mCi). They were not placed on low-iodine diets. The patients who qualified for this trial had a large amount of residual cancer that was considered at risk for growth during a prolonged thyroid hormone withdrawal preparation. A total of 18 patients were considered to have insufficient endogenous TSH production. In 49 patients, the serum TSH at the time of treatment was significantly higher after rhTSH than in previous thyroid hormone withdrawal treatments (mean, 190 mU/L vs 70 mU/L). Bone pain occurred in 25% of those with known bone metastases. Tumor edema in the neck was seen in three patients, tachycardia in five, and a rash occurred in two. Of 47 evaluable patients at follow-up, these investigators found 1 who had a complete response to ^{131}I treatment; 12 (26%) had partial responses; 19 (40%) had stable disease; 15 (32%) had progression of disease; and 5 patients died. Of the subset ($n = 20$) with nonradioiodine-avid disease following retinoids, 2 had partial responses, 11 had stable disease, and 7 had progression. In 34 patients, there was a 46% reduction in the median serum Tg; however, this did not have statistical significance. There were 44 patients who had a previous withdrawal assisted ^{131}I therapy, allowing outcomes to be compared between the two methods of preparation, where patients served as their own controls. The early outcomes were found to be identical in 52%, better after rhTSH in 32%, and inferior following rhTSH in 16%, compared to preparation by thyroid hormone withdrawal. The authors concluded that rhTSH-administered ^{131}I therapy of metastatic thyroid cancer was safe and as equally effective as T4 withdrawal.

These larger series provide a better sense that this approach can stimulate radioiodine uptake in metastatic lesions, that the approach is generally safe, and that steroid pretreatment should be considered in any lesions of the bone, pleura, or near the central nervous system. These series also show that partial responses and/or disease stabilization is the most common short-term outcome. The main issues that remain unresolved are how rhTSH preparation compares to T4 withdrawal preparation regarding: (1) comparisons of long-term survival and progression-free survival; (2) measurements of whole-body radiation exposure; and (3) estimates of ^{131}I-associated side effects.

Other issues that need to be carefully addressed include:

1. What are the optimum rhTSH doses and schedules for rhTSH-assisted 131I therapy? Some studies utilize four 0.9-mg injections just prior to therapy, whereas others use only two.
2. Should strict low-iodine diets be routinely employed, and should patients continue taking T4 immediately preceding the

administration of ^{131}I? However, in fairness, the precise value of such an approach has never been rigorously evaluated.

3. Uniform criteria should be established to define complete and partial responses, stability, and progression of disease. A consensus on this point among the leaders in the field would be valuable, as research on this approach moves forward.

4. It is clear that radioiodine clearance from blood and bodily tissues is not the same in the hypothyroid state when compared to the slightly hyperthyroid state. The differences in blood and lesional clearance should be more carefully defined so that investigators can agree whether to adjust the therapeutic-administered activity of ^{131}I.

5. Most studies published thus far use short follow-up periods. Much longer monitoring periods (5–10 yr) will be necessary before this approach can be considered comparable to preparation by thyroid hormone withdrawal.

6. The incidence of adverse effects should be prospectively studied in a randomized controlled trial of rhTSH preparation vs T4 withdrawal. The evidence that repeated episodes of prolonged serum TSH elevations may foster tumor progression is only referred to anecdotally by thyroid cancer experts.

SUMMARY

The international use of rhTSH to prepare thyroid cancer patients for high-dose ^{131}I therapy of metastatic disease is growing. Given the small number of patients who die each year of thyroid cancer, it is unlikely that any federal agencies will support research analyzing the rhTSH preparation vs withdrawal preparation. Second, it is unlikely that any single center has sufficient patients to answer the many questions that have been raised. Therefore, it is time for leaders in the field to develop a set of guidelines regarding the appropriate use of this approach and design multicentered trials to quantify the safety and efficacy of rhTSH preparation in comparison to the traditional method of thyroid hormone withdrawal.

ACKNOWLEDGMENTS

We thank Anne Robbins, MLS for valuable bibliographic searching and critical review of the manuscript.

REFERENCES

1. Chiu AC, Delpassand ES, Sherman SI. Prognosis and treatment of brain metastases in thyroid carcinoma. J Clin Endocrinol Metab 1997; 82:3637–3642.
2. Adler M, Macapinlac HA, Robbins RJ. Radioiodine treatment of thyroid cancer with the aid of recombinant human thyrotropin. Endocr Pract 1998; 4:282–286.
3. Perros P. Recombinant human thyroid-stimulating hormone (rhTSH) in the radioablation of well-differentiated thyroid cancer: preliminary therapeutic experience. J Endocrinol Invest 1999; 22:30–34.
4. Dai G, Levy O, Carrasco N. Cloning and characterization of the thyroid iodide transporter. Nature 1996; 379:458–460.
5. Villabona C, Sahun M, Roca M, et al. Blood volumes and renal function in overt and subclinical primary hypothyroidism. Am J Med Sci 1999; 318:277–280.
6. Cohen O, Dabhi S, Karasik A, Zila Zwas S. Compliance with follow-up and the informative value of diagnostic whole-body scan in patients with differentiated thyroid carcinoma given recombinant human TSH. Eur J Endocrinol 2004; 150:285–290.
7. Robbins R, Macapinlac H, Yeung H, Larson S. 131-Iodine therapy of metastatic thyroid cancer with the aid of human recombinant TSH. Thyroid 1996; 6:S1–S6.
8. Rudavsky AZ, Freeman LM. Treatment of scan-negative, thyroglobulin-positive metastatic thyroid cancer using radioiodine 131I and recombinant human thyroid stimulating hormone. J Clin Endocrinol Metab 1997; 82:11–14.
9. Colleran KM, Burge MR. Isolated thyrotropin deficiency secondary to primary empty sella in a patient with differentiated thyroid carcinoma: an indication for recombinant thyrotropin. Thyroid 1999; 9:1249–1252.
10. Rotman-Pikielny P, Reynolds JC, Barker WC, et al. Recombinant human thyrotropin for the diagnosis and treatment of a highly functional metastatic struma ovarii. J Clin Endocrinol Metab 2000; 85:237–244.
11. Risse JH, Grunwald F, Bender H, et al. Recombinant human thyrotropin in thyroid cancer and hypopituitarism due to sella metastasis. Thyroid 1999; 9:1253–1256.
12. Masiukiewicz US, Nakchbandi IA, Stewart AF, Inzucchi SE. Papillary thyroid carcinoma metastatic to the pituitary gland. Thyroid 1999; 9:1023–1027.
13. Vargas GE, Uy H, Bazan C, et al. Hemiplegia after thyrotropin alfa in a hypothyroid patient with thyroid carcinoma metastatic to the brain. J Clin Endocrinol Metab 1999; 84:3867–3871.
14. Mazzaferri EL, Kloos RT. Using recombinant human TSH in the management of well-differentiated thyroid cancer: current strategies and future directions. Thyroid 2000; 10:767–778.
15. Robbins RJ, Voelker E, Wang W, et al. Compassionate use of recombinant human thyrotropin to facilitate radioiodine therapy: case report and review of literature. Endocr Pract 2000; 6:460–464.
16. Aslam SN, Daly RG. Use of recombinant human thyrotropin in a complicated case of metastatic papillary thyroid carcinoma. Endocr Pract 2001; 7:99–101.
17. Serafini AN, Clauss RP, Levis-Dusseau S. Protocol for the combined diagnostic and therapeutic use of recombinant human thyroid-stimulating hormone. Clin Nucl Med 2003; 28:14–17.
18. Goffman T, Ioffe V, Tuttle M, et al. Near-lethal respiratory failure after recombinant human thyroid-stimulating hormone use in a patient with metastatic thyroid carcinoma. Thyroid 2003; 13:827–830.
19. Luster M, Lassmann M, Haenscheid H, et al. Use of recombinant human thyrotropin before radioiodine therapy in patients with advanced differentiated thyroid carcinoma. J Clin Endocrinol Metab 2000; 85:3640–3645.
20. Mariani G, Ferdeghini M, Augeri C, et al. Clinical experience with recombinant human thyrotrophin (rhTSH) in the management of patients with differentiated thyroid cancer. Cancer Biother Radiopharm 2000; 15:211–217.
21. Lippi F, Capezzone M, Angelini F, et al. Radioiodine treatment of metastatic differentiated thyroid cancer in patients on L-thyroxine, using recombinant human TSH. Eur J Endocrinol 2001; 144:5–11.
22. Berg G, Lindstedt G, Suurkula M, Jansson S. Radioiodine ablation and therapy in differentiated thyroid cancer under stimulation with recombinant human thyroid-stimulating hormone. J Endocrinol Invest 2002; 25:44–52.
23. de Keizer B, Brans B, Hoekstra A, et al. Tumour dosimetry and response in patients with metastatic differentiated thyroid cancer using recombinant human thyrotropin before radioiodine therapy. Eur J Nucl Med Mol Imaging 2003; 30:367–373.
24. Jarzab B, Handkiewicz-Junak D, Roskosz J, et al. Recombinant human TSH-aided radioiodine treatment of advanced differentiated thyroid carcinoma: a single-centre study of 54 patients. Eur J Nucl Med Mol Imaging 2003; 30:1077–1086.

47

Dosimetry

*Dosimetrically-Determined Prescribed Activity of Radioiodine for the Treatment of Metastatic Thyroid Carcinoma**

Frank B. Atkins, Douglas Van Nostrand, and Leonard Wartofsky

OVERVIEW

In the absence of definitive studies relating radioiodine-prescribed activity (dosage**) to outcomes, selection of a specific prescribed activity of radioiodine to treat metastatic thyroid carcinoma is problematic, and several approaches have been used. These include empiric fixed prescribed activity and prescribed activity based on dosimetric approaches specific for each patient. This chapter reviews the rationale and technique for "dosimetrically-determined" prescribed activity of radioiodine for the treatment of metastatic thyroid carcinoma. The chapter includes discussion of (1) the alternatives for selection of a prescribed activity, (2) the two major approaches for determining radioiodine prescribed activity dosimetrically, (3) the several modifications of these approaches, (4) the literature regarding the results, and then concludes with (5) recommendations for patient management and future research. This review does not address use of dosimetrically-determined prescribed activity of radioiodine for the initial (postoperative) ablation of thyroid tissue.

INTRODUCTION

Although a favorable prognosis is typically associated with well-differentiated thyroid carcinoma, that is not necessarily the case for metastatic well-differentiated thyroid carcinoma (1). Consequently, modifications in therapeutic approach, particularly with radioiodine, may be required to achieve good outcomes in patients with metastatic disease. Radioiodine was first shown to localize in metastatic thyroid carcinoma over half a century ago (2) and has been used extensively since then in the management of these patients (1,3–5).

However, there is no consensus among clinicians managing these patients regarding what constitutes an appropriate radioiodine dosage for the treatment of metastatic thyroid carcinoma. Several approaches to select a therapeutic dosage of radioiodine have been advocated. These can be broadly classified into two groups: (1) "empiric fixed prescribed activity" or (2) "dosimetrically determined" prescribed activity. Given the heterogeneity of thyroid cancer patients, empiric dosing may not be associated with optimal results in all patients. This chapter reviews the principles and methodologies of "dosimetrically-determined" prescribed activity of radioiodine for the treatment of metastatic thyroid carcinoma.

EMPIRIC FIXED PRESCRIBED ACTIVITY

Many excellent reviews of empiric fixed prescribed activity have been previously published (1,4,6–10). One of the most frequently used sets of empiric fixed prescribed activities was proposed by Beierwaltes (3) and is summarized in Table 1. With this approach, the fixed prescribed activities are typically in the range of 5.55–7.4 GBq (150–200 mCi). However, both smaller and larger prescribed activities have been proposed and used (11,12). Other methods have used intermittent moderate dosage. For example, Schlumberger et al. used an initial dosage of 3.7 GBq (100 mCi) of ^{131}I to treat metastasis of the lung and bone, which might be repeated every 3–6 mo. The cumulative radioiodine dosage in this group of patients ranged from 2 to 55.5 GBq (54–1500 mCi), with a mean of 12.5 GBq (339 mCi [±281 mCi]; 11). Menzel adopted a more aggressive approach, employing empiric fixed prescribed activity of 11.1 GBq (300 mCi), with intervals as short as 3 mo (12).

---

*A large portion of this chapter was reproduced from: Van Nostrand D, Atkins F, Yeganeh F, et al. Dosimetrically determined doses of radioiodine for the treatment of metastatic thyroid carcinoma. Thyroid 2002; 12:121–134, with the permission of the journal, *Thyroid*, published by Mary Ann Liebert Publishers, Inc.

**The word "dose" can be used to refer either to the amount of a radiopharmaceutical for a diagnostic scan, ablation, and treatment (mCi and Bq) or to the amount of radiation exposure to an organ or patient (rad or Gy). Because this may result in confusion, authors frequently use the word "dosage" to refer to the amount of a radiopharmaceutical for diagnostic scan, ablation, and treatment and reserve "dose" for the radiation exposure. Others have suggested "prescribed activity" to refer to the amount of a radiopharmaceutical for scan or treatment; in this chapter, dosage will be used.

Table 1
Empiric Fixed Prescribed Activity

Regional nodes that could not be removed by surgery	5.55–6.2 GBq (150–175 mCi)
Pulmonary metastasis	6.2–7.4 GBq (175–200 mCi)
Bone metastasis	7.4 GBq (200 mCi)

Source: ref. 3.

"DOSIMETRICALLY-DETERMINED" PRESCRIBED ACTIVITY

Although the simplicity of a set of empiric fixed prescribed activities is appealing and convenient, the persistence of disease in a significant proportion of patients has led to attempts to improve the empiric approach to therapy. We adhere to the proposition that the ideal treatment dose would be based on the minimum amount of radioiodine needed to successfully treat the patient's metastases without exceeding a dosage to the patient that would result in unacceptable side effects or risks. Efforts to meet this goal have led to two major approaches, each of which addresses a different aspect of this problem. Benua et al. developed an approach to help determine the maximum amount of radioiodine that could be administered without significant bone marrow suppression *(13)*. Thomas and Maxon developed a method to evaluate the amount of radioiodine needed to adequately treat metastatic lymph nodes *(14)*. This section discusses the two basic approaches of dosimetrically-determined prescribed activity and begins with a brief review of the principles involved to better understand the rationale for and the potential greater efficacy of the dosimetric approaches.

Background

Dosimetry

The term *dosimetry* has been used in a variety of contexts. It has been most commonly employed in the area of radiation oncology to describe the methodology and analysis used to calculate a treatment plan designed to deliver a prescribed radiation dose to the patient's tumor using external radiation. Within radiation safety programs and services, it has been used to describe the *monitoring* of the exposure of individuals from internal and external radiation hazards within a working environment. Finally, regarding thyroid cancer therapy with radionuclides, this terminology has been used in two contexts: (1) the calculation of a maximally safe dosage of ^{131}I that can be administered to a given patient, which would not exceed some empirical-limiting radiation dose to the blood or blood-forming components; and (2) the calculation of the radiation dose that would (or has been) delivered to individually identifiable and quantifiable thyroid tissue, remnants, or metastatic lesions. The latter conforms more closely with the traditional usage of this term within the radiation oncology community, as it applies to the calculation of the dose specifically for the cancer being treated. However, just as in the case of external radiation therapy, it is the radiation dose delivered to the patient's normal tissues that frequently limits the maximum tumor dose. With radioiodine therapy, the most radiosensitive organ of greatest concern is the patient's bone marrow.

Internal Radiation Dosimetry

When ionizing radiation is absorbed in living tissues, it can cause cellular damage because of the energy that is deposited. Different cell types will respond differently to the same amount of absorbed radiation. Nevertheless, one of the most important parameters used in the assessment of the radiation effects on any particular organ is the amount of energy deposited by the radionuclide in that organ. This calculation is the subject of what has become termed as *internal radiation dosimetry*. When radionuclides were first used for medical purposes, at best, this type of information was fragmented. Consequently, conservative estimates were used to estimate the order of magnitude of the radiation dose to the body and other critical organs that resulted from the administration of a radionuclide. This radiation dose is expressed in units of centigray (rad), which is a measure of the total amount of energy deposited per gram of tissue by all the radiation types emitted by the radionuclide. To perform this calculation, we need to know detailed information about (1) the types of radiation emitted in each disintegration (i.e., charged particles or photons), their relative abundance, and their energy; (2) how many disintegrations occur in each organ; and (3) what fraction of the energy of each radiation type that is released in any given organ is absorbed in another organ (including itself). The nuclear decay data required for the first issue can be found in the physics literature *(15)* based on experimental measurements performed in the laboratory. The second issue requires detailed knowledge about the uptake and clearance of the radionuclide in various organs within the patient. The third issue requires knowledge not only of the absorption and penetration characteristics of the various radiations emitted, but also the size, shape, volume, and geometrical arrangements of the various organs within the patient. Ideally, direct measurements of the absorbed dose at relevant locations within each patient would be best, but this is nearly impossible. Thus, we are instead restricted to theoretical estimates according to models and measurements performed in standardized humanoid phantoms.

CLASSICAL DOSIMETRY

The so-called classical dosimetry method was first published in 1948 by Marinelli et al. *(16)*. This was refined in 1956 by Loevinger et al. *(17)* and soon became the standard method *(18)* for calculating the radiation dose from internal sources. Because charged particles (i.e., β radiation) typically only travel a few millimeters in tissue, it is generally assumed that all the energy carried by this radiation is locally absorbed in the organ in which the radioactive decay occurs. In the case of ^{131}I, the maximum range of β particles in tissue *(19)* is 2.4 mm. The model developed by Loevinger addressed the more penetrating radiation: the γ emissions. Therefore, the radiation dose from the two components (penetrating and nonpenetrating) can be expressed as:

$$D_\beta = 73.8C <E_\beta> T_e$$
$$D_\gamma = 0.0346C\Gamma g T_e$$

where C is the initial concentration of the radionuclide in the organ (μCi/g); $<E_\beta>$ is the mean energy of the β radiation; Γ is the exposure rate constant specific to ^{131}I, T_e is the effective half-life in days, and g is a geometric factor to account for variations in the organ's size, shape, and volume. The constants that appear in these equations are conversion factors, such that the dose is expressed in units of centigray (rad).

MEDICAL INTERNAL RADIATION DOSE SCHEMA

The medical internal radiation dose (MIRD) methodology was developed by a committee within the Society of Nuclear Medicine to provide a more sophisticated approach to calculate the radiation dose to various organs from radionuclides that are internally deposited and accumulate in other organs. The initial models were released in the mid-1970s *(20)* and continue to be expanded and refined with the publication of new pamphlets. A review of the basic concepts and recent developments in internal radionuclide radiation dosimetry has been published *(21)*. This formulation simplified the calculation of radiation dose to varying organs within the patient by separating biological parameters that describe the uptake and clearance, along with physical decay from the details of energy absorption of the radiation released in each decay. All the absorption characteristics have been lumped into a single quantity: the "S" factor. These "S" factors incorporate (1) the details of the types and energies of the radiations emitted (e.g., how many, how much energy, what type); (2) the size and shape of the organ in which the radionuclide is distributed; (3) the size, shape, and geometrical relationship of any other organ within the patient; and (4) the energy fraction of each possible emission absorbed in any given organ from radiation that originated in any organ. Consequently, this single factor depends on the radionuclide, the organ containing the radionuclide (source), and the organ for which the dose is calculated (target). We can then express the dose to the target organ, D_t, as follows:

$$D_t = \sum_s \tilde{A}_s S(t \rightarrow s)$$

where $\tilde{A}_s$ represents the total number of decays that occur for the radionuclide in a given source organ, s. Finally, we sum the dose contributions from all the possible source organs to the target organ, indicated by Σ in this equation, which can include the target organ as one of the source organs.

Dosimetry Approaches

Based on the principles outlined above, Benua *(13)* developed an approach that set an upper limit of the radiation dose to the patient's blood, whereas Maxon *(14)* calculated the radiation dose that could be delivered to the lesion.

Limited Bone Marrow (Benua Approach)

It has been noted *(22)* that even with relatively conservative fixed prescribed activity of ^{131}I, bone marrow depression can still occur in about one quarter of all patients treated for metastatic thyroid cancer. Unfortunately, the empiric methods do not provide any information to help predict in which patients this would occur. However, the method reported by Benua et al. *(13,23)* allows an estimate to be calculated for the radiation dose that will be delivered to the hematopoietic system from each gigabecquerel (mCi) administered to a given patient. This is possible because it involves data collection over the course of 4 d or more following the administration of a tracer dosage of ^{131}I to the patient. Considering the time period when this methodology was developed, the dosimetry calculations were based on the classical formulations, rather than on MIRD. Furthermore, it should be emphasized that these calculations yield the radiation dose to the whole-blood compartment, not to the bone marrow directly. In their study, a total of 122 administrations in 59 patients were reviewed. However, adequate data were only available to calculate a dose in 85 of these treatments. For this group, the whole-blood dose ranged from 45 to 740 cGy (rad), with a mean of 267 cGy (rad), whereas the largest single dosage of ^{131}I was 22.2 GBq (600 mCi). As might be expected, several serious complications and side effects occurred in this group. However, within a patient subgroup, i.e., those that received 200 cGy (rad) or less to the blood, the side effects were not as serious. Based on these observations, a protocol was implemented by Benua and Leeper at the Memorial Sloan-Kettering Cancer Center (MSKCC), in which a treatment dosage was selected that would restrict delivery to no more than 200 cGy (rad) to the blood *(24)*.

DESCRIPTION OF THE BENUA PROTOCOL

Regardless of the dosimetric methodology employed, a common feature is the incorporation of the radioiodine pharmacokinetics in a given patient. Consequently, a tracer dosage of ^{131}I is first administered to the patient, and then the clearance is followed for a specified period. The form of ^{131}I (e.g., liquid or capsule) should be the same as the form of ^{131}I used for therapy. In this classical approach, the blood is considered the critical organ, which is irradiated either from the particles emitted from activity in the blood or from the emissions originating from activity dispersed throughout the remainder of the body. Therefore, only two compartments need to be monitored for radioactivity: the blood and whole body. The activity in the blood is determined from periodic 5-mL heparinized blood samples. The activity in the whole body (i.e., the activity remaining in the patient) is monitored redundantly using two independent techniques: 24-h urine collections and whole-body counting using a single uncollimated probe with a fixed geometry. The patient-to-detector distance should be sufficiently large to allow the activity from the entire patient to be detected while standing, with nearly the same sensitivity from head to foot. Typically, this would require distances greater than 3 m. A 12.7-cm diameter NaI (Tl) detector was used originally, but smaller diameter probes could be used with a corresponding increase in the acquisition time to offset the reduction in sensitivity. Benua employed an energy window of ±50 keV centered on the 364-keV γ emission. Although their original investigation followed patients for at least 6 d after the tracer-prescribed activity, their protocol was modified to end after 4 d; thus, a study beginning on Monday would be completed by Friday.

Data Collection:
- Blood samples (5 mL, heparinized) at 2, 4, 24, 48, 72, and 96 h
- Whole-body counts at 0, 2, 4, 24, 48, 72, and 96 h
- Total urine collection at 24, 48, 72, and 96 h
- Activity administered to patient as tracer dosage (approx 37 MBq [1 mCi])

In addition, a standard was prepared at the study onset of 37 MBq (1 mCi) of ^{131}I to normalize the whole-body counts. This was counted at a distance comparable to that of the patient in a reproducible geometry and was used throughout the 4-d monitoring period. During the initial 4-h period following the ^{131}I administration, the patient is not allowed to urinate or defecate. Under these circumstances, essentially 100% of the dosage will be contained within the patient at any time during the initial 4 h. The maximum value at 0, 2, or 4 h is then defined to represent the 100% value, and subsequent daily measurements are normalized to this value using this formula.

$$Retention(t) = \frac{Patient\ counts(t)}{Standard\ counts(t)} \times \frac{Standard\ counts\ @\ MaxTime}{Patient\ counts\ @\ MaxTime} \times 100\%$$

When used in this way, the standard will correct for variations in detector sensitivity from measurement to measurement, as well as for physical decay. Absolute calibrations are not necessary, as the patient is used as his or her reference. The blood and urine samples are counted using scintillation well-detector systems. Because the activity must be established in these samples, it is necessary to make up a calibration standard that can be counted at the same time. This involves the addition of a carefully assayed quantity of ^{131}I (approx 3.7–7.4 MBq [100–200 µCi]) to a total volume of 500–1000 mL. Such a small concentration is necessary to avoid saturating the detector. An alternative might be to use a ^{133}Ba rod source that has been cross-calibrated against the ^{131}I standard. With its relatively long half-life (10.5 yr) and similar γ emissions, ^{133}Ba could serve as a suitable replacement for the prepared ^{131}I standard, which simplifies the protocol. At the conclusion of the data acquisition, 2-mL aliquots of whole blood, diluted or undiluted urine, and the in vitro standard are counted. Using this information, it is possible to calculate the percent of administered dose per liter of whole blood at each timed sample. A zero time point is calculated by dividing the total dosage by the patient's total blood volume. However, a patient-specific blood volume is not determined but is assumed to equal 20% of the body weight. As indicated in the section on internal radiation dosimetry, one of the factors needed in the dose calculation is the total number of disintegrations that occur in the organ over time. This is reflected in the effective half-life T_e that appears in the first two equations. This formulation assumes that the radionuclide clearance from the organ of interest follows a single exponential curve that can be characterized by the effective half-life. Alternatively, knowing the organ activity as a function of time, and because activity is a measure of disintegrations per second, then the integral (i.e., area under this curve) is a measure of the total number of disintegrations. Therefore, based on his *classical* dosimetry approach, the formula to calculate the radiation dose to the whole blood follows.

The calculation of the area under these two curves is based on a mathematical fit to the data points using a multiple exponential function. Because the data collection is terminated after 4 d, these curves must then be extrapolated to infinity. A conservative estimate is employed by assuming that the clearance following the final measured data point is based simply on the physical decay:

$$\gamma(cGy/MBq) = 0.0000141g \times \left[\frac{1}{weight\ (kg)}\right] \times [area\ under\ body\ curve]$$

in cGy (rad) per MBq ^{131}I administered are given as:

$$\beta(cGy/MBq) = 0.00259 \times [area\ under\ blood\ curve]$$

This estimate ignores any biological clearance and results in an overestimate of the area of these tails and, hence, in the radiation dose. Examples of two patient studies are shown in Fig. 1; one demonstrates rapid clearance, and the other shows relatively slow clearance. The *maximum treatment prescribed activity* is then calculated as the activity of ^{131}I that would deliver a combined β and γ dose to the blood component of 200 cGy (200 rad) and is given by:

$$Treatment\ dose\ (MBq) = 200\ cGy/(\beta[cGy/MBq] + \gamma[cGy/MBq])$$

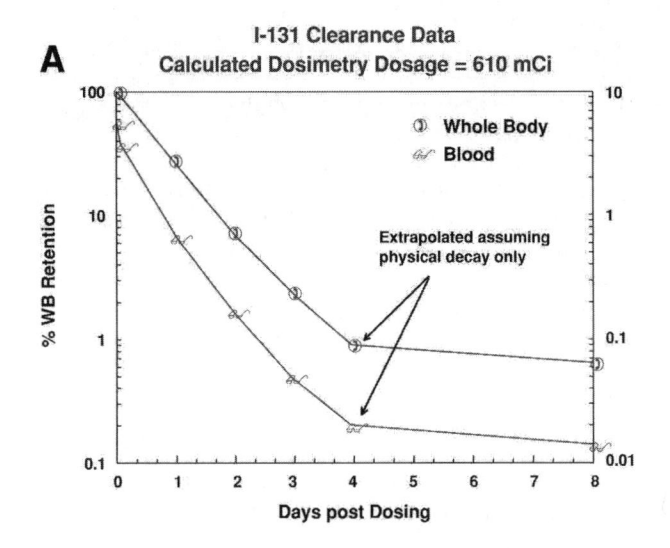

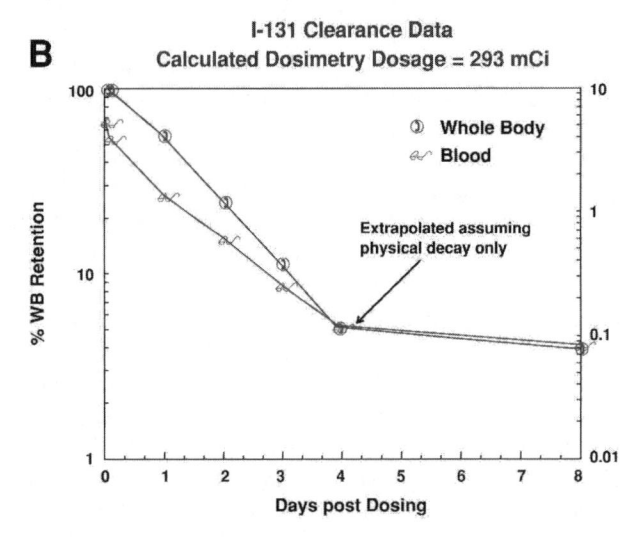

Fig. 1. Whole-body and blood clearance curves of ^{131}I for two dosimetry patients. In both cases, the final measured data point was determined at 4-d postdosing. The classical dosimetry model then uses a conservative assumption of only physical decay, which can be seen as the abrupt change in the slope of the curves at this time point. The patient in **A** has rapid clearance, and there is little additional area under the extrapolated segment, which results in a calculated dosage of 610 mCi to deliver 200 cGy to the blood. In contrast, in a patient with slower clearance, such as in **B**, there is a greater contribution to the total area under these curves, which leads to a lower calculated value for the maximum treatment dosage of 293 mCi.

ADJUSTMENTS TO ORIGINAL PROTOCOL

To improve reliability and simplify the original dosimetry protocol, several groups have introduced a number of modifications and enhancements; the more significant are outlined below.

Elimination of the Urine Collection. As previously mentioned, the urine data was used as a redundant method to determine the whole body activity as a function of time and served as a check of the probe data. The whole body retention was inferred from the difference between the administered activity and accumulated urine activity. Consequently, there is an inherent problem with this method: any error that may have occurred at one time point is propagated throughout *all* of the following data points as well. Particularly, some potential problems are associated with this measurement, including:

- Incomplete urine collection.
- Loss of iodine through alternative pathways, principally fecal, but also sweat, saliva, respiration, and so on.
- The high concentration of activity in the first 2 d can frequently saturate a well-counter detector, such that an additional 10:1 dilution might be required to avoid deadtime-counting errors.
- Errors in measuring the volume for each 24-h collection.
- Pipetting errors.

Removing the urine collection step, which is a burden for many patients, substantially reduces the complexity of this protocol by eliminating all the problems linked with the transport, storage, and handling of large volumes of radioactive body fluids. The net effect is that cumulative errors as high as factors of 2–5 in specific cases *(25)* can occur. By eliminating the urine assay from the protocol, the possible risk to personnel is also eliminated from accidental spills and radiation exposure from handling the radioactive urine. Most importantly, this can be accomplished without compromising the objective.

Geometric Mean for Whole Body Counting. A method of organ and body activity quantitation that has been widely adopted in nuclear medicine incorporates a geometric mean approach. Because the γ rays from ^{131}I are absorbed by varying amounts, depending on the depth of the source in the patient, neither an anterior nor a posterior orientation alone is appropriate. This is especially the case as the radionuclide redistributes over time after the absorption from the stomach. However, the geometric mean ($\sqrt{ant \times post}$) has been shown to be less sensitive to these variations *(26)*.

Timing and Number of Data Points. Whole body counting immediately following the ^{131}I tracer dose is generally neither practical nor useful. This is more true today when capsules are used instead of liquids for the isotope administration. The activity at this point in time is essentially confined to the stomach in a geometry that does not match the more diffuse body distribution at later times. In addition, a delayed sample at 4 h is inconvenient and may be difficult for the patient to avoid urinating before this measurement can be performed, which would invalidate this sample for normalization purposes. By this point, there can also be significant accumulation of activity in the bladder that can bias this data point. Therefore, a single data point at approx 2 h postadministration is sufficient for the normalization operation. Although this might seem to be an insufficient number of data points, it has been shown *(27)* that a sampling scheme, such as the one outlined above, provides basically the same accuracy as more extensive sampling, at least in the case of radioimmunotherapy. The last data point is also collected at approx 96-h postadministration of the tracer dose, provided that the whole-body retention at this time is 4% or less. If not, then an additional measurement may be performed on the following Monday, i.e., day 7.

Whole Body Counting Using the γ Camera. As an alternative to using an external probe to measure whole body retention, a dual detector γ camera system can be used. In this case, the patient is scanned in the whole body mode in a reproducible geometry while lying supine on the imaging table. This method has been generally accepted for patient-specific whole body dosimetry of ^{131}I-radiolabeled antibodies *(28)*. Furthermore, it has been shown to yield comparable results with the external probe data *(29)*. This technique has the following features:

- Simultaneous anterior and posterior images using a high-energy collimator.
- Table height, detector radii, scan length, scan speed, and energy window are standardized and reproduced for each data point.
- Scan speed can be relatively rapid (typically 30 cm/min) to complete the data acquisition in approx 8 min and is comparable to the time required using an external probe.
- Additional scans are performed each day for background and a counting standard (vial containing about 37 MBq [1 mCi] of ^{131}I).
- Total counts in the image or fixed regions of interest encompassing the entire body are used for the calculation of whole-body retention.

Although the images are not used for diagnostic purposes, this approach has the added advantage that if for some reason there is delayed absorption of the tracer dosage in the stomach, then the measurement could be repeated after 4 h. There are many other advantages when using this technique in the dosimetry protocol. This method is easier for patients who are unable to stand for the 5–10 min needed when using a probe, but the patient can be counted in a seated position. More importantly, it utilizes space and equipment normally found in a nuclear medicine laboratory. In most centers, a radiation probe that can be dedicated to this purpose is not available; hence, a standard thyroid uptake probe is used. These detectors typically have only a 1-in. diameter, and their geometric efficiency is therefore only one twenty-fifth of that of the 5-in. detector used by Benua and Leeper. It is also frequently difficult to locate space where there is an unobstructed area that the probe and patient can be positioned with the required minimum separation of about 3 m. A revised classical blood dosimetry protocol, incorporating the changes discussed above, is summarized in Table 2.

OTHER MODIFICATIONS

Other modifications and refinements to this dosimetry protocol have also been proposed. Furhang et al. *(30)* suggested

Table 2
Modified Classical Dosimetry Protocol

Whole body counting (conjugate counting)
2, 24, 48, 72, and 96 h
Count standard and background
Normalize data points to 100% using 2-h value
Calculate γ component of dose (Gy/MBq) using classical approach

Blood sample (5-mL heparinized)
2, 24, 48, 72, and 96 h
At conclusion of data collection, make counting standard 0.1–0.2 µCi/mL
Pipet 1 mL of whole blood from each collection and from standard
Count duplicate samples in well counter in same run
Convert blood data into units of % ingested dose/l
Calculate β component of dose (Gy/MBq) using classical approach

an analytical curve-fitting technique to generate a more realistic extrapolation of the clearance curve beyond the final data point. Another attempt at simplifying this dosimetry protocol *(31)* suggested the elimination of blood samples. Their investigation examined the accuracy with which the total dose to the blood could be predicted using only the whole body data. Although there is a strong correlation between these two components, this method assumes that the β and γ doses are in a fixed ratio to each other. Unfortunately, there is a wide range in this value among patients, as shown in the data of Thomas et al. *(31)*, as well as in the study by Robeson et al. *(32)*. Our own data from a group of 18 patients demonstrated a mean β:γ ratio of 3.68 and a broad range of 2.75–5.12. Given the inaccuracy that can be introduced in the calculation for any individual patient, and the fact that the β dose (i.e., blood compartment) is the major contributor to the radiation dose to the blood, we would strongly argue for the continued use of blood samples.

Another area involves the transition from the *classical* model to the MIRD schema. For example, all the β energy released in the blood is assumed to be absorbed in the blood. Because these particles can travel several millimeters, this is likely an overestimate. More sophisticated models that account for the vascular space and geometrical configurations have suggested a value of 0.82 for the absorbed fraction *(33)*. The recent successes in the use of ^{131}I radioimmunotherapy for B-cell lymphoma have focused considerable attention on patient-specific dosimetry. Again, the radiation dose to the bone marrow is the limiting factor *(34)*.

Hermanska *(35)* has suggested using a biphasic model, not a monoexponential model. The objective is to approximate the more accurate results of complex multicompartmental models. This biphasic model considers the uptake phase and attempts to better predict the long-term clearance phase. However, Hermanska's biphasic model requires more data points than a monoexponential model. Also, the evaluation of the biphasic model was performed in patients who were receiving their first radioiodine treatment.

Finally, Sisson *(36)* has suggested additional empiric modifications of dosimetrically determined prescribed activity in patients who have functioning metastasis with measurable serum thyroxine. For these atypical patients, he has recommended reduction in their therapy dosage.

OTHER RADIOIODINES FOR DOSIMETRY

Although all the discussions in this chapter involved the use of ^{131}I for conducting dosimetry, it is feasible that other radioiodines (e.g., ^{124}I and ^{123}I) could also be used for this purpose. The primary reasons that ^{131}I is used are that (1) it is readily available and relatively inexpensive; (2) it has a physical half-life suited for the required 4–8 d monitoring period; and (3) the γ emission, although somewhat high in energy, is appropriate for imaging with conventional scintillation cameras. Unfortunately, for the radionuclide ^{123}I, the first two requirements are unfavorable. A potentially significant advantage of ^{123}I over ^{131}I is that on a per millicurie basis, the radiation dose delivered to a thyroid remnant or metastatic lesion is about 100-fold less. Consequently, potential "stunning" because of the dosimetry procedure prior to treatment would be less concerning. However, the relatively short 13-h half-life of this radionuclide makes it impractical for a prolonged biokinetic study. It might be feasible to use ^{123}I in a patient for whom it is known that 4 d would be an adequate observation period, but even in this case, the tracer dosage would have to increase to about 20 mCi. Given the current pricing for ^{123}I, this would not be practical, even though the radiation dose would still be a fraction of that from a typical 2-mCi ^{131}I tracer dosage, along with the added benefit of improved image quality for the 24- and 48-h metastatic surveys.

The other potential candidate, ^{124}I, a positron emitter, could quite possibly become the preferred radioiodine not only for dosimetry, but for all thyroid cancer imaging. Unfortunately, it is currently not widely available and requires a positron emission tomography (PET)-imaging system; however, both of these limitations are changing. As this radionuclide emits charged particles during the decay (i.e., the positrons), the dose advantage over ^{131}I, if any, is not as great. In a study by Eschmann et al. *(37)*, it was concluded that ^{124}I, despite its complicated decay scheme, is suitable for the dosimetry of radioiodine therapy in both benign and malignant thyroid diseases.

Lesion-Based Dosimetry (Maxon Approach)

Calculating a treatment plan based on delivering a prescribed radiation dose to the tumor is the fundamental tenet of radiotherapy, whereas the classical dosimetry approach of Benua was based on giving the maximum dosage of ^{131}I that was safe and therefore more in line with thermotherapeutic strategies. The implicit assumption in the lesion-based dosimetry is that a treatment dosage derived in this manner would achieve the maximum therapeutic effect to any metastatic disease while minimizing the risk to the patient. Numerous investigations have been performed to determine the radiation dose that would be delivered to residual thyroid and metastatic tissue, with the objective to correlate the radiation dose with the therapeutic effect. However, to perform these calculations, it is necessary to measure the uptake and clearance of ^{131}I from identifiable thyroid remnants and/or metastatic lesions. This calculation of lesion dose *(38)* is generally based on a classical model, which for ^{131}I is given by:

$$Dose\ (cGy) = 0.63\ C_0 T_{1/2\ lesion}$$

where C_0 is the initial concentration (µCi/g) of ^{131}I in the lesion, and $T_{1/2\ lesion}$ is the effective half-life of the lesion activity in hours. To determine the concentration of ^{131}I, how much activity (in absolute units) is contained in the lesion must be known. One way to ascertain this is based on an analysis of selected regions of interest on conjugate view γ camera images. These images are obtained at several time points, measured from the time of administration of the tracer dosage. Typically, these images would be acquired at 24, 48, and 72 h, but later time samples might be necessary if the uptake and clearance are delayed. In addition, transmission images to correct for attenuation in the lesion area, as well as images of a standard for calibration purposes, are necessary. A curve-fitting procedure is then used to establish the assumed single-exponential half-life value and to extrapolate the curve-to-zero time to determine the lesion's initial activity. Another parameter needed to calculate the activity concentration is the lesion mass. Various approaches have been suggested for this determination. For example, Maxon *(50)* used nonmagnified anterior images from a rectilinear scanner to determine the lesion dimensions and assumed a spherical or elliptical shape; Koral *(40)* used both anterior and lateral pinhole camera images with corrections for magnification and an ellipsoidal shape. Others *(39)* have used alternative, higher spatial resolution images, such as computed tomography (CT) or ultrasound, to determine the mass.

Many investigators have reported the effective half-life of ^{131}I in thyroid metastatic lesions as within a range of about 1–5 d. Thus, a limited number of temporal samples may not accurately predict this curve. Furthermore, in a small sampling of patients studied posttherapy *(40)*, the uptake in the lesion did not achieve its maximum value until 1–3 d postadministration. An assumption of instantaneous uptake therefore results in an overestimate of the radiation dose. Determining the lesion dimensions on a γ camera image has inherent problems. If the projected dimensions of the lesion are small compared to the spatial resolution of the imaging system, then partial volume errors are introduced. In addition, only distances (e.g., the major and minor axes) are measured, and the volume is calculated from a presumed three-dimensional (3D) shape. Furthermore, if the dimensions are smaller than about 5 mm (assuming that this could be accurately determined), then the range of the β particles can no longer be neglected in the dose calculation. For example, small spherical tissues of 0.1 or 1.0 mm in diameter receive relative doses of 8.6% or 56% *(41)*, respectively, compared to a 5-mm diameter lesion. Consequently, if the concentration of ^{131}I is a constant, then the absorbed dose rate initially increases as the radius of a spherical lesion increases. This curve begins to flatten off at a radius of about 7 mm and is essentially constant for lesions with radii more than 10 mm. Over the range of radii from 1 to 10 mm, there is approximately a threefold increase *(42)* in the dose rate. In fact, the dose rate is a factor that has been generally ignored in radioiodine therapy. It is well known in external radiation treatment that the dose rate, as well as the total dose, has an impact on cell survival. As the dose rate is reduced, more and more of the sublethal cell damage may be repaired during the exposure. Below about 0.6 Gy/h (60 rad/h), there is only a little dose rate effect *(43)*, with the residual cell killing effect from nonrepairable injury associated with the total cumulative radiation dose. However, these are realistic dose rates for radioiodine therapy. For example, Schlesinger et al. *(44)* calculated that for a treatment dosage of 5.5 GBq (150 mCi) and a lesion uptake of 0.3% per gram, the initial dose rate would be 1.83 Gy/h. Assuming an effective half-life of 3 d, their data showed that it would take about 5 d to reduce the dose rate to this critical value.

MIRD Dosimetry

Dosimetric approaches have improved significantly over the past 40 yr and continue to evolve into more sophisticated methodologies to characterize the transport and absorption of radiation in complex biological systems. Patient-specific models employing Monte Carlo simulations have even been proposed. Indeed, it is generally believed that the MIRD methodology is a more accurate approach to dosimetry than the classical models employed in the Benua and Leeper approach. Using the MIRD methodology, it is possible to estimate the radiation dose that would be delivered not only to critical organs, such as the bone marrow and lung, but also to the lesion(s) to be treated. However, the latter is considerably more complicated and often not technically feasible if the lesion cannot be visualized with a small tracer dosage of ^{131}I. Nevertheless, dosimetry-guided radioiodine therapy for metastatic thyroid cancer has also been reported, based on the MIRD methodology by Dorn et al. *(45)*. This group used the red marrow as the critical target organ, rather than the whole blood, which is used as a surrogate for the bone marrow. Furthermore, for the bone marrow 3 Gy (300 rad) was selected as their upper limit for safety purposes or 30 Gy (3000 rad) for the lungs. Out of all their treatments with a curative intent ($n = 41$), only 19 treatments resulted in the maximum of 3 Gy (300 rad) to the bone marrow. Based on this approach and the higher safety limit chosen, a single treatment dosage of ^{131}I as high as 38.5 GBq (1040 mCi) could be given. Although these workers claimed that such a dose limit (i.e., 3 Gy [300 rad]) to the bone marrow is safe and does not result in permanent marrow suppression, the evidence is still somewhat limited to support this conclusion. Note also that the Benua and Leeper model uses 2 Gy (200 rad) to the whole blood, not the bone marrow, as the limit. The actual radiation dose to the bone marrow is less than that delivered to the whole blood and, at most, is probably about 60–70% of this value.

RESULTS

Patient outcomes of ^{131}I treatment for metastatic thyroid carcinoma have been previously reported for (1) empiric fixed prescribed activity *(1,5,46–49)*, (2) the Maxon dosimetric approach *(14,50–52)* and (3) the Benua dosimetric approach *(24,53,54)*. Outcomes of radioiodine treatments are also discussed in Chapters 45, 46, 59. The following is an overview of outcomes related to empiric fixed prescribed activity, the Maxon dosimetric approach, and the Benua dosimetric approach.

Maxon and Smith reviewed the literature for the effects of radioiodine on functioning metastatic disease, where the radioiodine-prescribed activities used were predominantly empiric fixed prescribed activity similar to those in Table 1 *(5)*. Complete resolution was typically defined as no evidence of disease by scan, X-ray, and clinical examination. For metastasis to the lymph nodes, complete resolution of disease was seen in 68.2% (58 of 85), "improvement but still evident" disease in 18.8%, and no apparent effect was seen in 12.5%. For metastasis to the lung, complete resolution of disease was seen in 45.9% (134 of 292), "improvement but still evident" disease in 27.7%, and no apparent effect in 24.5%. For metastasis to the bone, complete resolution of disease was seen in 6.8% (16 of 233), "improvement but still evident" disease in 35.6%, and no apparent effect in 54.2%. Examining results after empiric prescribed activity, Schlumberger reported survival rates measured from the time of metastases discovery of 53% at 5 yr, 38% at 10 yr, and 30% at 15 yr. Remission was achieved in only 79 of 283 patients (28%) once metastases were discovered *(11)*. Subsequently, Schlumberger indicated (1) a remission rate of 50% with a 10-yr survival rate of 61% for lung metastasis; (2) a remission rate of 10% with a 10-yr survival rate of 21% for bone metastasis, and (3) a remission rate of 7% with a 10-yr survival rate of 13% for lung and bone metastasis *(55)*. Also using empiric fixed prescribed activity, Menzel reported clinical remission in 14 patients, partial remission in 3, stable disease in 16, and progressive disease in 37 *(12)*. Dinneen found overall survival rates (for all causes) for distant metastasis to be 37% at 5 yr, 24% at 10 yr, and 20% at 15 yr *(56)*.

Table 3
Memorial Sloan-Kettering Cancer Center 1974–1981 Experience

Status	Number of Patients	Number of ^{131}I Treatments						Average Total Dose (mCi ^{131}I)
		1	2	3	4	5	6	
Cured	21	13	6	1	0	0	1	463
Died of disease	17	9	3	3	0	1	1	630
Died of other causes	4	2	2	0	0	0	0	568
Under treatment	19	10	6	1	2	0	0	514
Living with disease; no further treatment	6	5	1	0	0	0	0	466
Lost to follow-up	3	2	1	0	0	0	0	379
Total	70	41	19	5	2	1	2	520

After implementation of restriction of maximum (a) 200 rads total-blood radiation, (b) 120 mCi of ^{131}I whole-body retention at 48 h, and (c) 80 mCi of ^{131}I whole-body retention at 48 h if pulmonary metastases are present. *Source:* ref. *54*.

With the Benua approach, Leeper described the status and treatment for metastatic differentiated thyroid cancer of 70 patients treated at MSKCC from 1974 to 1981 (*54*; see Table 3) and from 1974 to 1984 (*23*; see Table 4). This occured after Benua had implemented several restrictions (see footnotes, Tables 3 and 4). Benua and Leeper administered an average single therapeutic dose of 11.4 GBq (308 mCi ^{131}I [range 70–654 mCi]). Total radioiodine-prescribed activity exceeded 37 GBq (1 Ci) in six patients. The largest cumulative dose was 77.7 GBq (2.1 Ci). Of Leeper's patients, 19% were treated with prescribed activity lower than 7.4 GBq (200 mCi). In most cases, each treatment delivered a calculated radiation exposure of 200 cGy (200 rads) to the blood. "Cures" were defined as negative roentgenograms, clinical examination, and radioiodine scan. Thyroglobulin assays, albeit relatively insensitive by today's standards, were only used near the end of the above time period. Treatments were repeated, if necessary, at annual intervals. In 1984, Leeper reported that 58% of the patients receiving one dose were "cured." Patients younger than age 40 had a higher "cure" rate (30 of 33, 90%) than those over age 40 (10 of 23, 43%).

Using his quantitative approach, Maxon (*50*) treated 26 patients with over 67 metastatic lesions. There were 63 lesions in the neck, 1 in the lung, and 2 in the mediastinum. One patient had numerous abnormalities in the neck, chest, and abdomen, which were not detailed in the report. Of the 67 lesions in 25 patients, 59 responded to ^{131}I. None of the numerous lesions in the 26th patient responded. Based on the location of the abnormalities, the response was 58 of 63 (92%) in the neck, 1 of 2 in the mediastinum, 0 of 1 in lung, and 0 of 1 in bone. Maxon reported that the response rate significantly increased in those lesions that received over 8000 cGy (rads), as determined by his dosimetric approach. Little chance of a response was seen if the radiation dose was less than 3500 cGy (rads). In a subsequent article, Maxon

Table 4
Memorial Sloan-Kettering Cancer Center 1974–1984 Experience

Status	Number of Patients
Cured	45
Died of all causes	28
Under treatment	29
Living with disease	9
Status unknown	5
Total	116

After implementation of restriction of maximum (a) 200 rads total-blood radiation, (b) 120 mCi of ^{131}I whole-body retention at 48 h, and (c) 80 mCi of ^{131}I whole-body retention at 24 h if pulmonary metastases are present. *Source:* ref. *23*.

(*51*) reported successful treatment in 81% (63 of 78) of lymph node metastases and in 74% (17 of 23) of overall patients. Notably, some of these patients had residual thyroid tissue in the thyroid bed. The results were achieved after a single radioiodine administration calculated to deliver a radiation exposure of at least 8500 cGy (rads). The mean dose of ^{131}I in this group was 5.8 ± 1.9 GBq (156.7 ± 51.7 mCi), with a range of 1.8–9.1 GBq (48.6–246.3 mCi). When no residual thyroid tissue was present in the thyroid bed, and no distant metastasis was noted, Maxon's success with treatment increased to 90% (26 of 29) of lymph node metastases and 86% (6 of 7) of patients. This success was seen after a single administration of radioiodine delivered radiation exposures of at least 14,000 cGy (rads). The definition of "success" in this case was absence of evident lymph node metastasis on physical examination and on a 37-MBq (2-mCi) radio-iodine scan.

Despite the published outcomes for empiric fixed prescribed activity or prescribed activity determined by the Maxon and Benua approach, a comparison of those results is difficult and unreliable. The difficulty lies in differences in the (1) definition of successful treatment, (2) changing definition of successful treatment, (3) duration of follow-up, and (4) variability in data collection. In addition, no prospective study comparing the outcomes of empiric dosages to dosimetrically-determined dosages has been published. Obtaining adequate statistical samples with reliable follow-up over long time periods is very difficult. However, regardless of these limitations, we believe that reasonable inferences may be drawn from the data to allow development of guidelines for the use of dosimetry (see Recommendations section).

STRENGTHS AND LIMITATIONS OF THE VARIOUS APPROACHES

Empiric Fixed Prescribed Activity

The strengths of using the empiric fixed prescribed activity, such as those of Beierwaltes, are convenience, a long history of use, and a reasonably acceptable rate and severity of complications. A theoretical strength of the higher empiric fixed-dose approach, e.g., protocols using 7.4 GBq (300 mCi) of radioiodine at 3–6 mo intervals, is improved outcome, but a limitation is the lack of significant data confirming outcomes, as well as the rate and severity of complications. In additional, empiric fixed prescribed activity permit the option of treating recurrent disease as detected by ^{123}I scans, thyroglobulin blood levels, and/or other imaging modalities without using ^{131}I diagnostically. Avoiding the use of diagnostic ^{131}I eliminates potential reduction of therapeutic ^{131}I uptake because of "stunning" by the diagnostic dosage.

In our view, a major limitation of empiric fixed prescribed activity is the failure to consider the individual status of the patient. The ideal radioiodine dosage to treat metastatic thyroid carcinoma is the lowest possible amount of radioiodine that delivers a lethal dose of radiation to the entire metastasis while minimizing side effects. Empiric fixed prescribed activity dosages, by their very nature, do not permit determination of either the minimal radioiodine that will deliver a lethal dose or the reasonably safe maximum allowable dosage. An additional limitation is that multiple empiric fixed prescribed activities (fractionated radiotherapy) may not be equivalent to the same total radioiodine dosage calculated by dosimetry given at one time. Dose rate is important; thus, multiple smaller dosages may have less therapeutic benefit than the same total dosage given at one time. Moreover, previous nontumoricidal doses may reduce the efficacy of subsequent doses.

The Benua Approach

The strengths of the Benua approach are the (1) determination in each patient of the maximal allowable "safe" dosage of radioiodine, (2) identification of as many as one in five patients whose maximal allowable "safe" dosage of radioiodine is less than the empiric fixed prescribed activity, (3) potential to give higher radiation doses to metastasis at one time, rather than multiple lower empiric prescribed activity with potentially lower total effective radiation doses, (4) experience of a long history of use by Benua, Leeper, and Larson at MSKCC, (5) empiric modifications of the original protocol based on observed initial complications, and (6) reasonable complications rates relative to the disease severity after the implementation of empiric modifications.

There are several limitations of the Benua approach. First, the approach results in increased cost and inconvenience. However, we believe this is reasonable and not unlike treatment programs for metastatic disease from other cancers. Second, the approach does not estimate the radiation dose to the metastasis, and the "maximal allowable safe dosage" may be given without any therapeutic effect. Third, the program requires a commited medical staff. Like any treatment program for metastatic disease, the institution must see a reasonable number of patients to establish efficiency and assure quality. Fourth, present dosimetric approaches use ^{131}I diagnostically, which may reduce uptake of the therapeutic dosage and therefore reduce the radiation dose delivered to the metastasis (stunning).

The Maxon Approach

The strength of the Maxon approach, as originally discussed by Maxon, is "[a] more selective exposure to individual patients based upon their individual needs without an increase in radiation exposure to the total patient population and lower overall costs." This could improve the outcome in some patients and avoid complications in those patients who receive no benefit or no significant benefit from the radioiodine treatment. The proposed lower overall costs may be offset by either the new Nuclear Research Commission guidelines, which allow earlier release from hospitals, or more expensive imaging methods to evaluate volume of metastases.

Some technical limitations of the Maxon approach are noted in Table 5. Other limitations include (1) increased cost and inconvenience, albeit, we again believe that this is also modest and reasonable; (2) no significant data regarding its use in distant metastasis; and (3) potentially difficult implementation of the approach in distant metastasis.

Another potential disadvantage of the Maxon approach is whether nonvisualization of a lymph node or any distant metastasis on a 74-Bq (2-mCi) radioiodine scan implies that the metastasis is not treatable with radioiodine. Again, Maxon indicated that delivery of 8000 cGy (rads) to the lymph node metastasis was associated with an excellent chance of successful treatment, and doses of less than 3500 cGy (rads) reduce the chance of effective treatment. However, does this suggest that the necessary centigray (rads) cannot be delivered to a functioning metastasis that is not visualized on a 2-mCi radioiodine scan? Arnstein (57) has suggested that significant centigray (rads) can be delivered to lesions not

Table 5
Potential Problems and Limitations of Lesion-Based Dosimetry

A single-exponential model may not accurately reflect the kinetics of the radioiodine in the lesion
Assumption of instantaneous uptake and maximum at time zero
Estimation of the lesion mass
Assumption of uniform distribution of ^{131}I in lesion
Statistical errors in the measurements
Therapeutic response relative to dose rate
Dosage reduction for lesions <5 mm in diameter

seen on scans performed with 74 Bq (2 mCi) and even as high as 1.11 GBq (30 mCi). This issue is one of the arguments for a treatment when serum thyroglobulin is elevated, and the pretherapy radioiodine scan is negative, but no further subsequent radioiodine prescribed activity if the posttherapy radioiodine scan is negative. Clearly, further study is warranted.

All Approaches

A major downfall of all the approaches is the less than optimal definition of "success." This includes not only the criteria for complete remission (no evidence of disease) and partial remission, but also the length of follow-up. For example, the criteria for "success" could be merely a normal physical exam and negative radioiodine whole-body survey within less than 3 yr of follow-up. These criteria may have been reasonable at the time of original studies, but it is arguable whether these criteria and the short length of follow-up provide much information about patient outcomes, e.g., the rate of complete remission, partial remission, and length of remission. For example, diagnostic modalities other than physical exam, such as ultrasound of the neck and CT of the chest, were available and have been used since the 1970s. Additional modalities to detect residual disease became available and were used in the 1980s and 90s, such as serum thyroglobulin assays and magnetic resonance imaging (MRI). By today's standards, the results of radioiodine whole body surveys may be poor criteria for success. For example, we now know that the lack of uptake on a 7.4-MBq (2-mCi) radioiodine scan is not necessarily evidence of successful treatment. The size and/or uptake of the metastasis after treatment may be too little to be visualized on the radioiodine scan, and/or the metastasis may have dedifferentiated and lost its functional ability to trap iodide. To simply rely on physical exam and a negative radioiodine scan is a less than optimal definition of success. In addition, the described follow-up periods of only several years to assess altered outcomes in a disease that may take significant longer time periods to recur is problematic. Accordingly, the less than optimally rigorous definitions of success and the frequently short follow-up periods may overestimate "success" as defined by earlier reports. In addition, the variability of the definitions makes meaningful comparisons unreliable.

However, this should not devalue these approaches but rather encourage us to reevaluate the approaches with more specific definitions of complete and partial remissions that encompass the longer term follow-up and are more appropriate for the current time.

In summary, many problems exist regarding any dosimetric approach, but physicians and patients should not see these problems as deterrents in using the Maxon and/or Benua approach when appropriate. In addition, third-party insurance payers should not interpret these problematic issues with dosimetric approaches to therapy as rationale to declare them experimental and thereby justify denial of reimbursement. Rather, any additional costs of these improved approaches over empiric fixed prescribed activity is warranted by the greater expectation of remission or cure. The remaining questions or issues regarding dosimetric approaches to therapy must be studied, resolved, and then we can move forward and achieve greater future benefit for our patients.

RECOMMENDATIONS AND SUMMARY

Recommendations

The selection of radioiodine prescribed activity is discussed in multiple other chapters of this book (see Chapters 45, 46, 48, 59). Our recommendations for the use of dosimetry to help select radioiodine prescribed activity for the treatment of metastatic thyroid carcinoma are noted in Tables 6–8. Although this chapter did not summarize all the literature that supports our recommendations, we believe the recommendations are sufficiently reasonable for our current knowledge. We also recognize that other factors related to the clinical status of the patient, and the patient's own desires, may influence the selection of the radioiodine dosage. In addition, we encourage the development and use of adjunctive methods to enhance the potential dose of radiation delivered to the metastasis. For example, we believe that all patients with metastatic disease should be prepared for diagnostic dosimetric studies and therapy by strict adherence to a low-iodine diet for 4 wk prior to evaluation (an interval that usually coincides with the thyroid hormone withdrawal period; see Chapter 88). The compliance with the diet should be assessed by iodide measurement in one 24-h urine collection prior to therapy. In contrast to the average normal daily excretion of 300–400 µg in the United States, urinary iodine should be less than 50 µg after 4 wk of a low-iodine diet and no levothyroxine therapy. One should also consider adjuvant lithium carbonate, which has been reported to prolong ^{131}I retention in metastasis *(58,59)*.

In patients whose serum thyroglobulin levels are elevated and radioiodine scans are negative, it is even more problem-

Table 6
General Recommendations of Radioiodine Therapy for Well-Differentiated Metastatic Thyroid Carcinoma

Recommend referral of patient to a site that performs dosimetry.
If referral to a site that performs dosimetry is not possible, use empiric fixed prescribed activity as noted in previous tables.
Empirical fixed prescribed activity of radioiodine above 200 mCi (7.4 GBq) is not recommended.
Recommend retreatment preferably no sooner than 1 yr from previous treatment.
For patients treated with 200 mCi (7.4 GBq) or more, recommend antiemetics, laxatives, and aggressive sialogogues (e.g., lemons) during the day and night.
For prescribed activity of 200 mCi (7.4 GBq) or more, obtain baseline CBC and monitor CBCs for 6 wk posttherapy. (If future radioiodine is used, the CBC response may be helpful.)
If baseline blood counts are reduced, creatinine and BUN are elevated, or patient had a significant drop of blood counts after previous radiotherapy, consider reducing any subsequent dosage.

CBC, complete blood count; BUN, blood urea nitrogen.

Table 7
Recommendations for Treatment of Functioning Lung Metastasis of Well-Differentiated Thyroid Carcinoma

In the absence of dosimetry availability, we recommend empiric fixed prescribed activity of 175–200 mCi (6.2–7.4 GBq)
With availability of the Benua dosimetry protocols or an equivalent approach, we recommend selection of a dosage that does not exceed 200 rads (cGy) to the blood, and the whole body retained dosage of radioiodine at 48 h does not exceed 80 mCi (2.96 GBq)

Table 8
Recommendations for Functioning Nonpulmonary Distant Metastasis

For bone or brain metastasis, recommend consideration of surgical excision prior to radioiodine therapy.
In the absence of dosimetry availability, we recommend empiric fixed prescribed activity of 200 mCi (7.4 GBq).
With availability of Benua dosimetry or an equivalent approach, we recommend selection of a dosage that does not exceed 200 rads (cGy) to the blood, and the whole body retained dosage of radioiodine at 48 h does not exceed 120 mCi (4.44 GBq).
Recommend consideration of additional external-beam radiotherapy or radiofrequency ablation for focal and/or symptomatic bone metastasis and "γ knife" radiotherapy for brain metastasis.
Recommend pretreatment of brain metastasis (e.g., steroids) and recommend reduction of dosimetrically-determined dose.

atic if they should be treated with radioiodine and/or further evaluated with other imaging modalities. The latter include F-18 fluorodeoxyglucose-PET, ^{99m}Tc sestamibi, ^{201}Tl, computer axial tomography, ultrasonography, and MRI; these approaches are reviewed in Chapters 35 and 39. Identification of one or several foci of tumor on these imaging modalities may allow surgical excision, thus avoiding radiation exposure. If this is not the case, then empiric radioiodine therapy is an option and can result in clinical improvement and reduction in serum thyroglobulin levels in many, but clearly not all, patients *(60–63)*. We would concur with this approach and are reassured by the appearance of uptake seen in lesions on the posttreatment scan.

Summary

Radioiodine is an important option in the therapeutic armamentarium for metastatic thyroid carcinoma, and a significant amount of information has been published regarding the dosage selection of radioiodine for the treatment of metastatic well-differentiated thyroid carcinoma. From these data, we believe the following. First, empiric fixed prescribed activity, as suggested by Dr. Beierwaltes, appears to be a reasonable alternative for the selection of prescribed activity because of convenience, a long history of use, and a reasonably acceptable rate and severity of complications. Second, less outcome data are available with other empiric fixed dosage schedules, e.g., 300 mCi every 3–6 mo, and further evaluation of such approaches are needed. Third, "dosimetrically determined" prescribed activity of radioiodine seems to be intuitively an improvement over empiric fixed prescribed activity. An empiric fixed dosage does not consider any detailed information relating to the individual, including the size, uptake, retention, and delivery of radiation to a metastasis or the individual's whole body clearance and radiation dose to the blood. Fourth, the Maxon approach appears to allow more selective exposure to individual patients based on their specific needs for metastatic lymph nodes without increased radiation exposure to the total patient population, in addition to potentially lower overall costs. Fifth, the Benua approach is a reasonable approach for the selection of the "maximum-allowable" radioiodine dosage for the treatment of metastatic disease. Finally, more research is needed to compare the long-term outcome, benefits, and risks of these approaches, as well as to evaluate new approaches, such as patient-specific dosimetry with ^{124}I PET and the 3D-internal dosimetry software developed by Sgouros and colleagues *(64)*.

REFERENCES

1. Beierwaltes WH, Nishiyama RH, Thompson NW, et al. Survival time and "cure" in papillary and follicular thyroid carcinoma with distant metastases: statistics following University of Michigan therapy. J Nucl Med 1982; 23:561–568.

2. Seidlin SM, Marinelli LD, Oshry E. Radioactive iodine therapy effect on functioning metastases of adenocarcinoma of the thyroid. JAMA 1946; 132:838–847.
3. Beierwaltes WH. The treatment of thyroid carcinoma with radioactive iodine. Semin Nucl Med 1978; 8:79–94.
4. Freitas JE, Gross MD, Ripley S, Shapiro B. Radionuclide diagnosis and therapy of thyroid cancer: current status report. Sem Nucl Med 1985; 15:106–131.
5. Maxon HR, Smith HS. Radioiodine-131 in the diagnosis and treatment of metastatic well differentiated thyroid cancer. Endocrinol Metab Clin North Am 1990; 19:685–718.
6. Krishnamurthy GT, Blahd W. Radioiodine I-131 therapy in the management of thyroid cancer. Cancer 1977; 40:195–202.
7. Maheshwari YK, Hill CS Jr, Haynie TP III, et al. I-131 therapy in differentiated thyroid carcinoma. Cancer 1981; 47:664–671.
8. Edmonds CJ. Treatment of thyroid cancer. Clin Endocrinol Metab 1979; 8:223–243.
9. Tubiana M. Thyroid cancer. In Beckers C, editor. Thyroid Disease. France: Pergamon, 1982: 187–227.
10. Robbins J. The role of TRH and lithium in the management of thyroid cancer. In Andreoli M, Monaco F, Robbins J, editors. Advances in Thyroid Neoplasia. Rome: Field Educational Italia, 1981: 233–244.
11. Schlumberger M, Tubiana M, DeVathaire F, et al. Long-term results of treatment of 283 patients with lung and bone metastases from differentiated thyroid carcinoma. J Clin Endocrinol Metab 1986; 63: 960–967.
12. Menzel C, Grunwald A, Palmedo H, et al. "High-dose" radioiodine therapy in advanced differentiated thyroid carcinoma. J Nucl Med 1996; 37:1496–1503.
13. Benua RS, Cicale NR, Sonenberg M, Rawson RW. The relation of radioiodine dosimetry to results and complications in the treatment of metastatic thyroid cancer. Am J Roentgenol Radium Ther Nucl Med 1962; 87:171–182.
14. Thomas SR, Maxon HR, Kereiakes JG. In vivo quantitation of lesion radioactivity using external counting methods. Med Phys 1976; 3: 253–255.
15. International Commission on Radiological Protection. Radionuclide transformations. Energy and intensity of emissions. ICRP Publication 38. Ann ICRP 1983 Vol.11–13.
16. Marinelli LD, Quimby EH, Hine GJ. Dosage determination with radioactive isotopes. II. Practical considerations in therapy and protection. Am J Roentgenol 1948; 59:260–281.
17. Loevinger R, Holt JG, Hine JG. Internally administered radioisotopes. In Attix F, Roesch W, and Tochlin E, editors. Radiation Dosimetry. New York: Academic Press, 1956: 803–875.
18. Quimby EH. In Radionuclides in Medicine and Biology. Philadelphia, PA: Lea & Febiger, 1970.
19. Howell RW, Dandamudi VR, Sastry KS. Macroscopic dosimetry for radioimmunotherapy: nonuniform activity distribution in solid tumors. Med Phys 1989; 16:66–74.
20. Snyder WS, Ford MR, Warner GG, et al. "S" absorbed dose per unit cumulated activity for selected radionuclides and organs. In MIRD Pamphlet, no. 11. Reston, VA: Society of Nuclear Medicine, 1975.
21. Zanzonico PB. Internal radionuclide radiation dosimetry: a review of basic concepts and recent developments. J Nucl Med 2000; 41: 297–308.
22. Keldsen N, Mortensen BT, Hansen HS. Bone marrow depression due to I131 treatment of thyroid cancer. Ugeskr Laeger 1988; 150: 2817–2819.
23. Benua RS, Leeper RD. A method and rationale for treating metastatic thyroid carcinoma with the largest safe dose of I-131. In Medeiros-Neto G, Gaitan E, editors. Frontiers in Thyroidology, vol. 2. New York: Plenum Medical Book Co., 1986: 1317–1321.
24. Leeper RD, Shimaoka K. Treatment of metastatic thyroid cancer. Clin Endocrinol Metab 1980; 9:383–404.
25. Thomas SR, Maxon HR, Fritz KM, et al. A comparison of methods for assessing patient body burden following I-131 therapy for thyroid cancer. Radiology 1980; 137:839–842.
26. Thomas SR, Maxon HR, Kereiakes JG, Saenger EL. Quantitative external counting techniques enabling improved diagnostic and therapeutic decisions in patients with well-differentiated thyroid cancer. Radiology 1977; 122:731–737.
27. Erwin W, Groch M. Quantitative radioimmunoimaging for radioimmunotherapy treatment planning: effect of reduction in data sampling on dosimetric estimates. Cancer Biother Radiopharm 2002; 17: 699–711.
28. Wahl RL, Kroll S, Zasadny KR. Patient-specific whole-body dosimetry: principles and a simplified method for clinical implementation. J Nucl Med 1998; 39(Suppl):14S–20S.
29. Zasadny KR, Gates VL, Moon S, et al. Comparison of total body dosimetry predicted with gamma-camera whole-body scans versus collimated probe for patients receiving I-131 anti-B1 antibody. Radiology 1996; 201:300P.
30. Furhang EE, Larson SM, Buranapong P, Humm JL. Thyroid cancer dosimetry using clearance fitting. J Nucl Med 1999; 40:131–136.
31. Thomas SR, Samaratunga RS, Sperling M, Maxon HR. Predictive estimate of blood dose from external counting data preceding radioioine therapy for thyroid cancer. Nucl Med Biol 1993; 20: 157–162.
32. Robeson W, Zanzi I, Yoshida M, et al. Validation study to determine if accurate dosimetry for radioiodine therapy for thyroid cancer can be performed using only external counting data. J Nucl Med 1994; 15S:112P.
33. McEwan AC. Absorbed doses in the marrow during I-131 therapy. Br J Radiol 1997; 50:329–331.
34. Sgouros G. Bone marrow dosimetry for radioimmunotherapy: theoretical considerations. J Nucl Med 1993; 34:689–694.
35. Hermanska J, Karny M, Zimak J, et al. Improved prediction of therapeutic absorbed doses of radioiodine in the treatment of thyroid carcinoma. J Nucl Med 2001; 42:1084–1090.
36. Sisson JC, Carey JE. Thyroid carcinoma with high levels of function: treatment with I-131. J Nucl Med 2001; 42:975–983.
37. Eschmann S, Reischl G, Bilger K, et al. Evaluation of dosimetry of radioiodine therapy in benign and malignant thyroid disorders by means of I-124 and PET. Eur J Nucl Med 2002; 29:760–767.
38. Maxon, HR. Quantitative radioiodine therapy in the treatment of differentiated thyroid cancer. Q J Nucl Med 1999; 43:313–323.
39. Kimmig B, Hermann HJ. Measurement of dose during radioiodine treatment of thyroid cancer. Acta Endocrinol 1983;S252:72.
40. Koral KF, Adler RS, Carey JE, Beierwaltes WH. Iodine-131 treatment of thyroid cancer: absorbed dose calculated from post-therapy scans. J Nucl Med 1986; 27:1207–1211.
41. Schlesinger T, Flower MA, McCready VR. Radiation dose assessments in radioiodine (I-131) therapy. The necessity for in vivo quantitation and dosimetry in the treatment of carcinoma of the thyroid. Radiother Oncol 1989; 14:35–41.
42. Leichner PK. A unified approach to photon and beta particle dosimetry. J Nucl Med 1994; 35:1721–1729.
43. Hall JH. Radiation dose rate: a factor of importance in radiobiology and radiotherapy. Br J Radiol 1972; 45:81–97.
44. Schlesinger T, Flower M, McCready V. Radiation dose assessments in radioiodine (I-131) therapy. The necessity for in-vivo quantitation and dosimetry in the treatment of carcinoma of the thyroid. Radiother Oncol 1989; 14:35–41.
45. Dorn R, Kopp J, Vogt H, et al. Dosimetry-guided radioactive iodine treatment in patients with metastatic differentiated thyroid cancer: largest safe dose using a risk-based approach. J Nucl Med 2003; 44:451–456.
46. Pochin EE. Radioiodine therapy of thyroid cancer. Semin Nucl Med 1971; 1:503–515.

47. Varma VM, Beierwaltes WH, Nofal MM, et al. Treatment of thyroid cancer: death rates after surgery and after surgery followed by sodium iodides I-131. JAMA 1970; 214:1437–1442.
48. Nemec J, Zamrazil V, Pohunkova D, et al. Bone metastases of thyroid cancer, biological behavior and therapeutic possibilities. Acta Univ Carol Med Monogr 1978; 83:1–106.
49. Pochin EE. Prospects from the treatment of thyroid carcinoma with radioiodine. Clin Radiol 1967; 18:113–135.
50. Maxon HR, Thomas SR, Hertzbert VS, et al. Relation between effective radiation dose and outcome of radioiodine therapy for thyroid cancer. N Engl J Med 1983; 309:937–941.
51. Maxon HR, Englaro EE, Thomas SR, et al. Radioiodine-131 therapy for well differentiated thyroid cancer—a quantitative radiation dosimetric approach: outcome and validation in 85 patients. J Nucl Med 1992; 33:1132–1136.
52. Thomas SR, Maxon HR, Kereiakes JG, Saenger EL. Quantitative external counting techniques enabling improved diagnostic and therapeutic decisions in patients with well differentiated thyroid cancer. Radiology 1997; 122:731–737.
53. Benua RS, Cicale NR, Sonenberg M, Rawson RW. The relation of radioiodine dosimetry to results and complications in the treatment of metastatic thyroid cancer. Am J Roentgenol Radium Ther Nucl Med 1962; 87:171–182.
54. Leeper RR. Thyroid cancer. Med Clin North Am 1985; 69:1079–1096.
55. Schlumberger M, Challeton C, De Vathaire F, et al. Radioactive iodine treatment and external radiotherapy for lung and bone metastases from thyroid carcinoma. J Nucl Med 1996; 37:598–605.
56. Dinneen SF, Valimaki MJ, Bergstralh EJ, et al. Distant metastases in papillary thyroid carcinoma: 100 cases observed at one institution during 5 decades. J Clin Endocrinol Metab 1995; 80:2041–2045.
57. Arnstein NB, Carey JE, Spaulding SA, et al. Determination of iodine-131 diagnostic dose for imaging metastatic thyroid cancer. J Nucl Med 1986; 27:1764–1769.
58. Koong SS, Reynolds JC, Movius EG, et al. Lithium as a potential adjuvant to I-131 therapy of metastatic, well-differentiated thyroid carcinoma. J Clin Endocrinol Metab 1999; 84:912–916.
59. Reynolds JC, Robbins J. The changing role of radioiodine in the management of differentiated thyroid cancer. Semin Nucl Med 1997; 27:152–164.
60. Pacini F, Lippi F, Formica N, et al. Therapeutic doses of iodine-131 reveal undiagnosed metastases in thyroid cancer patients with detectable serum thyroglobulin levels. J Nucl Med 1987; 28:1888–1891.
61. Pineda JD, Lee T, Ain K, et al. Iodine-131 therapy for thyroid cancer patients with elevated thyroglobulin and negative diagnostic scan. J Clin Endocrinol Metab 1995; 80:1488–1492.
62. Schlumberger M, Mancusi F, Baudin E, et al. I-131 therapy for elevated thyroglobulin levels. Thyroid 1997; 7:273–276.
63. Schlumberger M, Baudin E. Serum thyroglobulin determination in the follow-up of patients with differentiated thyroid carcinoma. Eur J Endocrinol 1998; 138:249–252.
64. Sgouros G, Kolbert KS, Sheikh A, et al. Patient-specific dosimetry for I-131 thyroid cancer therapy using I-124 PET and 3-dimensional-internal dosimetry (3D-ID) software. J Nucl Med 2004; 45:1366–1372.

48
Radioiodine Dosimetry with Recombinant Human Thyrotropin

R. Michael Tuttle and Richard J. Robbins

INTRODUCTION

Although radioactive iodine (RAI) has been an essential tool in the management of thyroid cancer for more than 50 yr, there continues to be a lack of scientific rigor regarding the optimal choice of administered activity for individual patients. Often, activities of 30–150 mCi are administered for RAI remnant ablation, whereas activities ranging from 150–250 mCi are usually reserved for treatment of metastatic disease. In most cases, the activity selected is based on an empiric regimen without knowledge of the rate of RAI clearance for that individual patient.

In the 1950s, methods were established to calculate the maximal tolerable activity (MTA) of RAI, based principally on the rate of clearance of "tracer" doses of ^{131}I from the blood and entire body in patients undergoing traditional thyroid hormone withdrawal preparation (1–4). In these early studies, administered activities that resulted in more than 2 Gy to the blood were associated with significant bone marrow depression. Additionally, whole-body retention of more than 80 mCi of ^{131}I at 48 h in patients with diffuse lung metastases was linked with subsequent pulmonary fibrosis (2,5). Using these parameters, it is often possible to safely administer activities of 500–600 mCi in selected patients with metastatic thyroid carcinoma.

The advent of recombinant human thyrotropin (rhTSH) has sparked a reevaluation of the approach to RAI scanning, remnant ablation, and therapy (6). rhTSH is now widely used as preparation for diagnostic whole-body scanning and is increasingly employed as a preparation for RAI remnant ablation (1,7). However, whole-body RAI clearance is significantly faster in patients prepared for RAI studies using rhTSH. Because iodine is principally excreted by the kidney, and hypothyroidism is associated with a significant decrease in renal glomerular filtration rate, thyroid hormone withdrawal is associated with a marked increase in whole-body RAI retention times. Patients prepared with rhTSH are either euthyroid or mildly thyrotoxic and would be expected to have a more rapid renal clearance of RAI, shorter RAI retention times and, hence, lower whole-body radiation exposure for a given administered activity of RAI.

This chapter reviews the available data on whole-body RAI clearance and lesional dosimetry to determine the magnitude and clinical significance of the enhanced clearance of RAI in patients prepared for RAI studies with rhTSH.

WHOLE-BODY AND BLOOD CLEARANCE OF RAI

Whole-body retention was established in both the hypothyroid state and rhTSH preparation in seven patients studied at the National Cancer Institute, part of the phase I/II multicenter study examining the diagnostic use of rhTSH in thyroid cancer (8). In these patients, thyroid hormone withdrawal resulted in a 24-h whole-body retention of 16.8 ± 7% of the administered activity compared to 7.4 ± 5% in those prepared with rhTSH.

These findings are consistent with our initial observations, which determined RAI clearance based on multiple blood and whole-body measurements over 72 h following a tracer dose of ^{131}I (1) in patients undergoing rhTSH stimulation. In most patients, the radioactive iodine clearance is faster after rhTSH than when the RAI clearance was determined in the same patient during thyroid hormone withdrawal (see Fig. 1). As part of our routine clinical care, we performed standard RAI clearance studies in our first 97 patients following rhTSH preparation and a comparison group of 52 patients during thyroid hormone withdrawal. In these cohorts, traditional thyroid hormone withdrawal was associated with a MTA of 462 ± 33 mCi. Preparation with rhTSH was linked with a significantly higher MTA (640 ± 26 mCi), consistent with more rapid RAI clearance and decreased whole-body retention. Our studies suggest that whole-body RAI clearance is approx 30% faster after rhTSH preparation vs traditional thyroid hormone withdrawal.

Luster et al. studied RAI blood and whole-body clearance in 9 subjects during both thyroid hormone withdrawal and

From: *Thyroid Cancer: A Comprehensive Guide to Clinical Management, 2/e*
Edited by: L. Wartofsky and D. Van Nostrand © Humana Press Inc., Totowa, NJ

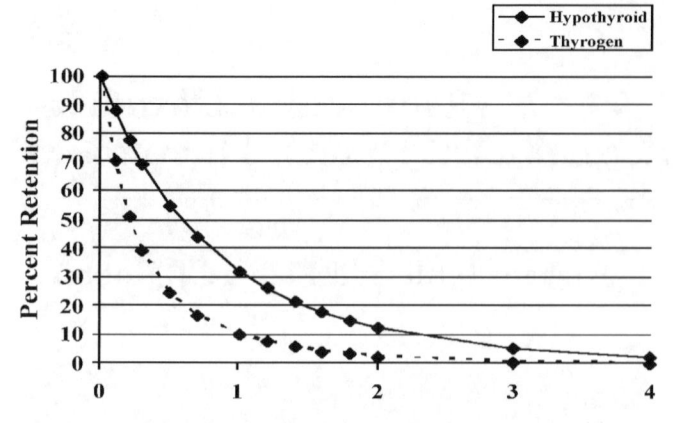

Fig. 1. RAI clearance curves in a representative patient studied during hypothyroid withdrawal and following rhTSH stimulation.

Table 1
Associations of Thyroid Withdrawal to Uptake Value and IDR vs rhTSH Preparation

Preparation	24-h Uptake in Remnant (%)	IDR (Gy/h)
Thyroid hormone withdrawal	5.8 ± 5.7	27.1 ± 42.5
Thyroid hormone withdrawal and rhTSH	9.4 ± 9.5	48.5 ± 43
rhTSH	2.5 ± 4.3	10.7 ± 12.6

Data is mean ± standard deviation.

rhTSH preparation using multiple blood and whole-body counts at several time points over 48 h (9). The effective half-time of RAI in the blood was 9.7 ± 2 h following rhTSH preparation in comparison to 11.7 ± 2 h after thyroid hormone withdrawal. The effective half-time of RAI in the remaining whole body (not counting the thyroid remnant) was also shorter following rhTSH preparation (9.4 ± 1.5 h) than thyroid hormone withdrawal (12.4 ± 2.5 h). Therefore, the same administered activity would result in lower whole-body radiation exposure in rhTSH-prepared patients when compared to hypothyroid patients after thyroid hormone withdrawal.

From the information above, radioactive iodine clearance from the blood and whole body can be estimated as about 25–30% faster in euthyroid patients prepared with rhTSH than with thyroid hormone withdrawal (Fig. 1). The apparent benefit of lower total-body radiation exposure for a specific administered RAI activity needs to be balanced by the risk that RAI clearance is too rapid to allow adequate uptake of RAI for effective treatment of thyroid remnants or metastatic lesions.

DOSIMETRY IN THYROID REMNANTS

RAI uptake in thyroid remnants (after total thyroidectomy) was carefully examined in a phase I/II multicenter study in patients prepared with either thyroid hormone withdrawal or a wide range of rhTSH doses (8). When all rhTSH-dosing regimens were analyzed together, the uptake in the thyroid remnant was higher after thyroid hormone withdrawal in 72% (13 of 18) of patients (2% uptake following thyroid hormone withdrawal and 1.2% uptake following rhTSH; $p < 0.05$). However, rhTSH in doses of 10 U/d for two consecutive days (similar to 0.9 mg intramuscularly for 2 d as currently used for diagnostic scanning preparation), or 20 of U rhTSH as a single dose, resulted in uptake in the thyroid remnant that was not significantly different than thyroid hormone withdrawal. As described above, the effective half-time of RAI was significantly shortened with rhTSH preparation; thus, that part of the decreased uptake by the thyroid remnant could be likely explained by the more rapid clearance of RAI from the blood. Indeed, in a subgroup analysis of the seven subjects that had both thyroid remnant dosimetry and whole-body/blood dosimetry, no difference was seen in RAI uptake into the thyroid remnant when uptake values were corrected for RAI whole-body retention. Therefore, the percentage uptake into thyroid remnants appears to be very comparable between the preparation methods, but hypothyroidism was associated with a greater radiation delivered to the thyroid because of the slower RAI clearance from the blood.

Pacini et al. examined 24-h RAI uptake in thyroid remnants and the initial dose rate (IDR) (amount of radiation delivered to the thyroid remnant in the first hour after dosing) in three patient cohorts undergoing RAI remnant ablation (7). Thyroid hormone withdrawal was related to a significantly higher 24-h uptake value and IDR, compared to rhTSH preparation (see Table 1). Interestingly, the highest uptake values and IDR were seen in patients prepared with traditional thyroid hormone withdrawal who then received rhTSH injections just prior to RAI dosing. The 24-h thyroid remnant uptake was higher in this group of Italian patients vs the patients studied by Meier et al. within the United States (8). This difference may be because of the difference in dietary iodine intake between the two countries. As would be expected, the lower RAI uptake in the thyroid remnants, combined with an administered activity of only 30 mCi given 48 h after the second rhTSH dose, led to successful remnant ablation in only 54% of the patients prepared with rhTSH, compared to an 84% success rate when 30 mCi was used after thyroid hormone withdrawal. (For additional information on rhTSH in remnant ablation, see Chapter 27.)

In addition to evaluating whole-body and blood RAI clearance, Luster et al. also carefully examined 24-h uptake, effective half-life, and residence times within the thyroid remnants (9). In eight of nine patients, rhTSH preparation was associated with a higher 24-h uptake, a longer effective half-life, and a longer residence time in the thyroid remnant, compared with the same values determined while hypothyroid. These findings vary with the reports above. The authors hypothesized that stunning could have had a major role in the findings, as all patients served as their own controls, with the rhTSH preparation evaluations conducted before the hypothyroid withdrawal studies. This sequential effect could have artificially decreased the RAI uptakes in the second scans (all done while hypothyroid), causing the uptake measured during thyroid hormone withdrawal to appear lower than it would have been if studied without the prior rhTSH scan. In support of this hypothesis, Lassmann et al. reported that thyroid remnant dosimetry with rhTSH stimulation following a thyroid hormone withdrawal scan was associated with a decrease in 24-h uptake, a reduction in effective half-life, and shorter residency time *(10)*.

Because of the potential effect of stunning, it is difficult to compare uptake of RAI into thyroid remnants in individual patients. For practical and logistical reasons, it would be challenging to enroll patients into a study in which the order of the rhTSH scan and thyroid hormone withdrawal scan are randomized. Therefore, the current published literature cannot accurately determine the differences in RAI uptake into thyroid remnants. However, the reported clinical success of rhTSH-assisted RAI remnant ablation certainly verifies that adequate doses of radiation are being delivered to the thyroid remnants of most patients.

TUMOR DOSIMETRY

Although the data presented above provides much information on whole-body and blood clearance rates, as well as effective half-times and residency rates within presumably "normal" thyroid remnants following total thyroidectomy, much less is known about radiation doses that can be achieved within metastatic deposits of thyroid cancer cells (lesional dosimetry). Several small series and anecdotal cases have been reported in which rhTSH stimulation prior to RAI therapy has resulted in tumoricidal effects in metastatic lesions, as evidenced in follow-up RAI imaging and cross-section imaging studies (see Chapter 46 on the use of rhTSH in RAI therapy).

A precise estimate of lesional dosimetry can be obtained when images are acquired with positron emission tomography (PET) scanners following tracer doses of the positron emitter ^{124}I *(11)*. Figure 2 demonstrates RAI-avid distant metastatic disease on a 2-mCi ^{131}I rhTSH-stimulated diagnostic scan in an elderly male with recurrent, widespread metastatic follicular thyroid cancer *(12)*. The results of whole-body and blood ^{131}I dosimetry and ^{124}I PET lesional imaging after rhTSH stimulation are shown in Fig. 3. Despite what appears to be a markedly positive diagnostic whole-body scan, the lesion dosimetry analysis shows that the individual metastatic lesions are receiving far less than adequate tumoricidal doses (see Fig. 4).

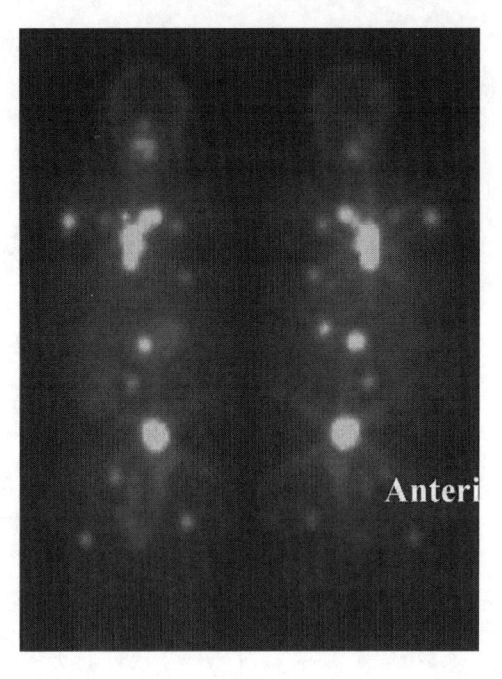

Fig. 2. A 2-mCi diagnostic ^{131}I scan in an elderly male with widespread RAI-avid metastatic follicular cancer.

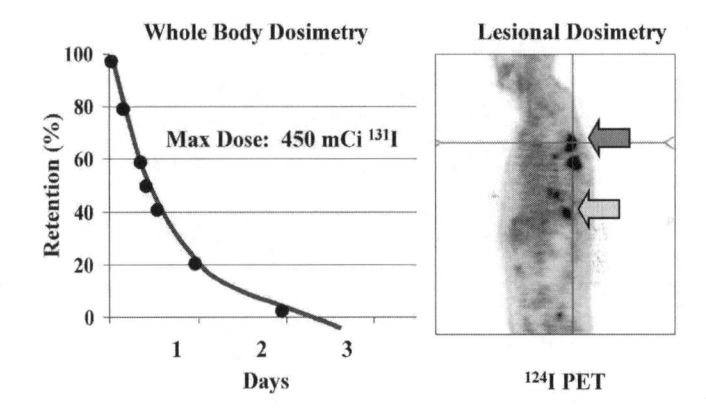

Fig. 3. Results of whole-body dosimetry (RAI clearance) presented on the left panel and a ^{124}I PET scan image in the right panel, showing spinal and paraspinal metastatic lesions. (Color illustration appears in insert following p. 198.)

In other cases, rhTSH stimulation leads to more than adequate lesional, dosimetry and documented regression of metastatic lesions, as demonstrated in an elderly female with recurrent papillary thyroid cancer (see Figs. 5 and 6). In this patient, serial structural imaging after two rhTSH-assisted RAI therapies 6 mo apart confirmed that tumoricidal doses were achieved by showing a marked decrease in the size of her mediastinal recurrence and pulmonary metastases. These anecdotal cases suggest that rhTSH stimulation can achieve tumoricidal doses of RAI within metastatic lesions in some patients.

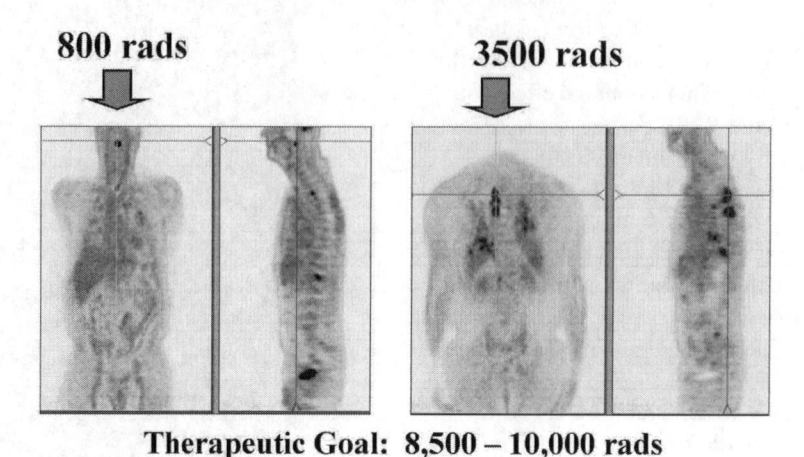

Fig. 4. Lesional dosimetry calculations based on a 400-mCi administered activity. Predicted lesional dosimetry is far below expected tumoricidal doses in most of his lesions. (Color illustration appears in insert following p. 198.)

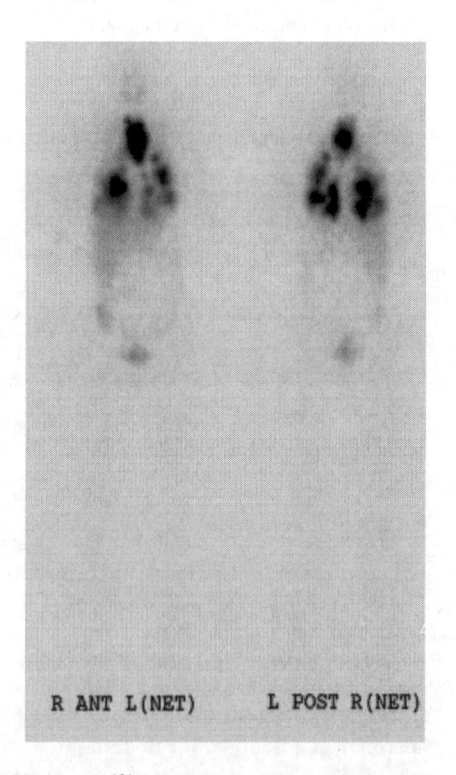

Fig. 5. A 2-mCi ^{131}I scan in an elderly female with recurrent metastatic papillary thyroid cancer, showing RAI-avid disease in the mediastinum and lungs.

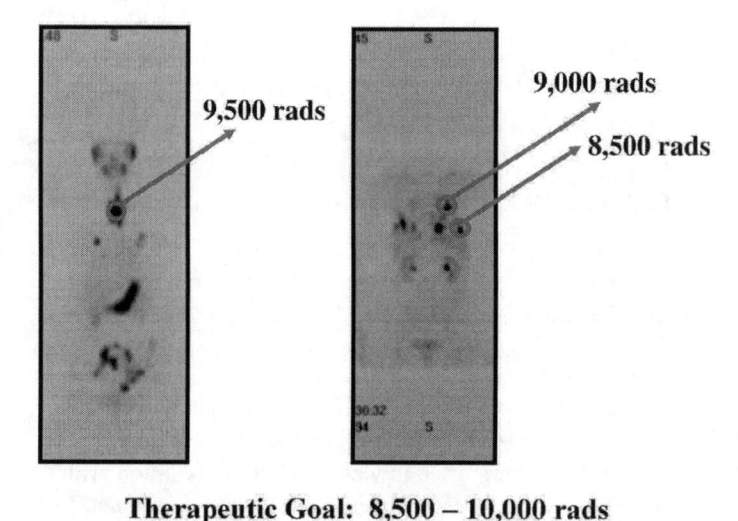

Fig. 6. ^{124}I PET lesional dosimetry that shows predicted lesional doses following administration of 120 mCi of ^{131}I. (Color illustration appears in insert following p. 198.)

Keizer et al. reported the results of classical lesional dosimetry studies using rhTSH-assisted ^{131}I tumor uptake measurements from posttherapy RAI scans and tumor volume estimates from structural imaging studies in 16 patients with recurrent or metastatic differentiated thyroid cancer *(13)*. The median lesional radiation dose was 26.3 Gy (range 1.3–368 Gy), with a median effective half-time of 2.7 d (range 0.5–6.4 d). Even within the multiple pulmonary metastatic lesions studied in a individual patient, estimated radiation doses to individual lesions ranged from 19.5 to 87.1 Gy. Although similar data on thyroid hormone withdrawal patients was not available in this study, the authors did note that the iodine kinetics within metastatic lesions was quite similar to that reported by Maxon et al. in previously published detailed lesional dosimetry studies in hypothyroid patients *(14)*.

Based on the data above, it is clear that rhTSH preparation can induce sufficient ^{131}I uptake to result in tumoricidal doses of RAI in many patients with metastatic thyroid cancer. These dosimetry data are consistent with the previous series of patients with metastatic thyroid cancer treated with RAI following rhTSH preparation, as reviewed in Chapter 46.

IMPACT OF IODINE CONTAMINATION ON DOSIMETRY STUDIES

When comparing radioiodine kinetics in patients prepared with rhTSH to those prepared with traditional thyroid hormone withdrawal, it is important to consider the impact of the stable iodine contamination at the time of each study. As approx 65% of the molecular weight of levothyroxine derives from iodine, continued thyroid hormone replacement therapy during rhTSH, by necessity, adds unwanted iodine to the diet. Loffler et al. examined urinary iodine excretion in 85 patients undergoing thyroid hormone withdrawal and 61 patients undergoing rhTSH while continuing levothyroxine replacement before diagnostic RAI scanning *(15)*. Whereas the urinary iodine excretion was quite low in both groups of patients, the median iodine excretion rate was lower in hypothyroid withdrawal (50 µg/L) than in the rhTSH stimulation group (75 µg/L). However, the range of urinary iodine excretion rates was identical in both groups (25–600 µg/L).

From these data, it is clear that adequate levels of iodine depletion can be achieved with either preparation method following an adequate low-iodine diet; very similar remnant ablation rates and lesional radiation doses can be expected. It seems unlikely that the small amount of obligatory iodine contained with levothyroxine preparation would significantly impact the results of diagnostic whole-body scans or RAI therapies as used in clinical practice. However, a small effect on the precise measures of lesional dosimetry studies cannot be ruled out and needs to be considered when rhTSH dosimetry is compared with thyroid hormone withdrawal dosimetry studies.

REFERENCES

1. Robbins, RJ, Larson SM, Sinha N, et al. A retrospective review of the effectiveness of recombinant human TSH as a preparation for radioiodine thyroid remnant ablation. J Nucl Med 2002; 43:1482–1488.
2. Furhang EE, Larson SM, Buranapong P, Humm JL. Thyroid cancer dosimetry using clearance fitting. J Nucl Med 1999; 40:131–136.
3. Leeper RD. The effect of 131 I therapy on survival of patients with metastatic papillary or follicular thyroid carcinoma. J Clin Endocrinol Metab 1973; 36:1143–1152.
4. Benua RS, Cicale NR, Sonenberg M, Rawson RW. The relation of radioiodine dosimetry to results and complications in the treatment of metastatic thyroid cancer. Am J Roentgenol Radium Ther Nucl Med 1962; 87:171–182.
5. Rall JE, Alpers JB, Lewallen CG, et al. Radiation pneumonitis and fibrosis: a complication of radioiodine treatment of pulmonary metastases from cancer of the thyroid. J Clin Endocrinol Metab 1957; 17:1263–1276.
6. Robbins RJ, Robbins AK. Clinical review 156: Recombinant human thyrotropin and thyroid cancer management. J Clin Endocrinol Metab 2003; 88:1933–1938.
7. Pacini F, Molinaro E, Castagna MG, et al. Ablation of thyroid residues with 30 mCi (131)I: a comparison in thyroid cancer patients prepared with recombinant human TSH or thyroid hormone withdrawal. J Clin Endocrinol Metab 2002; 87:4063–4068.
8. Meier CA, Braverman LE, Ebner SA, et al. Diagnostic use of recombinant human thyrotropin in patients with thyroid carcinoma (phase I/II study). J Clin Endocrinol Metab 1994; 78:188–196.
9. Luster M, Sherman SI, Skarulis MC, et al. Comparison of radioiodine biokinetics following the administration of recombinant human thyroid stimulating hormone and after thyroid hormone withdrawal in thyroid carcinoma. Eur J Nucl Med Mol Imaging 2003; 30:1371–1377.
10. Lassmann M, Luster M, Hanscheid H, Reiners C. Impact of 131 I diagnostic activities on the biokinetics of thyroid remnants. J Nucl Med 2004; 45:619–625.
11. Erdi YE, Macapinlac H, Larson SM, et al. Radiation dose assessment for I-131 therapy of thyroid cancer using I-124 PET Imaging. Clin Positron Imaging 1999; 2:41–46.
12. Tuttle M, Robbins R, Larson SM, Strauss HW. Challenging cases in thyroid cancer: a multidisciplinary approach. Eur J Nucl Med Mol Imaging 2004; 31:605–612.
13. de Keizer B, Brans B, Hoekstra A, et al. Tumour dosimetry and response in patients with metastatic differentiated thyroid cancer using recombinant human thyrotropin before radioiodine therapy. Eur J Nucl Med Mol Imaging 2003; 30:367–373.
14. Maxon HR, Thomas SR, Hertzberg VS, et al. Relation between effective radiation dose and outcome of radioiodine therapy for thyroid cancer. N Engl J Med 1983; 309:937–941.
15. Loffler M, Weckesser M, Franzius C, et al. Iodine excretion during stimulation with rhTSH in differentiated thyroid carcinoma. Nuklearmedizin 2003; 42:240–243.

49
Use of Lithium as an Adjuvant to Radioiodine in the Treatment of Thyroid Cancer

Monica C. Skarulis, Marina S. Zemskova, and Jacob Robbins

INTRODUCTION

Radioactive iodine (^{131}I) is the most effective medical therapy for metastatic thyroid cancer. Eradication of persistent or recurrent cancer with radioiodine is dependent on successful uptake and adequate retention of ^{131}I in tumor deposits. To optimize radionuclide uptake, dietary depletion of iodide and thyrotropin-secreting hormone (TSH)-induced sodium-iodide symporter activity are required. Methods to enhance the half-time of ^{131}I in the tumor tissue are limited. Iodine clearance is prolonged by alterations of renal function that occur in the hypothyroid state or by chronic administration of diuretics. Hydrochlorothiazide, furosemide, and salt loading increase renal sodium excretion, leading to iodide depletion. Unfortunately, the reduced blood volume from the associated loss of water ultimately diminishes iodine clearance, thereby increasing radiation to tumor and whole-body proportionately (1). High-iodide concentrations can also inhibit proteolytic enzymes and release of ^{131}I incorporated into thyroid hormone; however, this effect cannot be exploited as an advantage in the treatment of thyroid cancer because it also diminishes uptake.

Lithium ion, administered as the carbonate salt, blocks thyrocyte release of ^{131}I incorporated in thyroid hormone. Unlike iodide, lithium does not affect ^{131}I uptake and is the most promising method to enhance the radiation dose to tumors and improve the therapeutic efficacy of radioiodine.

LITHIUM'S EFFECT ON THE THYROID

In the mid-19th century, the alkaline properties of lithium salts were widely used to treat various uric acid diatheses, which involved the many manifestations of "brain gout," including headache, epilepsy, mania, and depression (2). The modern use of lithium in the management of mania and bipolar disease was established during the 1950s, and the association of lithium use with goiter and thyroid dysfunction was reported by several investigators (3–5). Subsequently, investigations commenced to discover the full effects of lithium on thyroid function (6,7).

Early human studies by Sedvall demonstrated that lithium decreased serum protein–bound iodine (PBI) and increased thyroidal radioiodine uptake after 7–20 d of lithium treatment (8). The effect was transient, and both PBI and uptake returned to baseline after several months of continued lithium therapy (9,10). Although a direct lithium effect on the hypothalamus and/or pituitary has been proposed, observed elevations in basal TSH (11) and enhanced response to thyrotropin-releasing hormone (12) during lithium treatment are most likely compensatory and secondary to the sometimes subtle, diminished thyroid hormone feedback that occurs.

Lithium interferes with thyroid hormone synthesis and secretion, and its perturbations are dose-dependent. Lithium is concentrated in the thyroid, achieving levels three to four times that of the serum (5). Iodide enters the thyrocyte through an active sodium-dependent iodide transport system known as the Na$^+$/I$^-$ symporter (NIS). NIS activity occurs in a 2 Na$^+$: 1 anion stoichiometry and is not restricted to sodium as the driving cation (13,14) Lithium can drive iodide transport at approx 10–20% of the level achieved by sodium (14). The exact role that NIS has in achieving the high thyrocyte concentrations has yet to be examined. Studies of the inhibitory effect of lithium on rat thyroid demonstrated that doses above 2 mEq per liter interfered with multiple steps in iodine metabolism, including iodide trapping (15). However, at therapeutic concentrations, TSH-induced iodine accumulation persisted, whereas TSH-induced endocytosis of colloid and release of thyroid hormone was reduced (16). Lithium reduces TSH-induced adenyl cylase activity through competition with magnesium at binding sites essential for enzyme activity and cyclic adenosine monophosphate (cAMP) generation (16,17). Additional data suggest that lithium may also act in steps subsequent to cAMP formation (16,18). Lithium effects on colloid droplet formation, microtubule function (19), and thyroglobulin hydrolysis (20) have been observed.

From: *Thyroid Cancer: A Comprehensive Guide to Clinical Management, 2/e*
Edited by: L. Wartofsky and D. Van Nostrand © Humana Press Inc., Totowa, NJ

The least understood effect of lithium is on peripheral thyroxine (T4) degradation, which appears to be decreased in both euthyroid and hyperthyroid subjects *(21,22)*.

LITHIUM IN HYPERTHYROIDISM

Recognition of lithium's ability to inhibit thyroid hormone release *(15,23)* inspired several small clinical studies in the early 1970s to study its efficacy either alone or in combination with thionamides or radioiodine in the management of hyperthyroid patients *(24)*. Used as a single agent, lithium quickly decreased serum thyroxine levels by approx 30% *(24–26)* and achieved a euthyroid state after 2–6 wk of therapy in 11 of 12 patients in an observational intervention trial *(27)*. Several studies using lithium in combination with a thionamide resulted in greater reductions of T4 and triiodothyronine levels when compared to thionamide alone *(28–30)*. Boehm et al. *(31)* studied the combination of lithium and iodide, noting an additive inhibition on thyroid hormone release only when lithium preceded the administration of iodide.

Importantly, several studies demonstrated that lithium prolonged the half-life of radioiodine within the thyroid gland *(15,23,32)*. It is proposed that retention of iodine within the thyroid gland maximizes the local radiation effect and minimizes total-body exposure *(28,33)*, particularly in patients with rapid thyroidal turnover *(28)*; however, no studies have shown improved cure rates with adjuvant lithium *(33–35)*. Lithium is rarely used to treat hyperthyroidism and is generally restricted to patients in whom the conventional therapeutic options are associated with dose-limiting adverse effects.

DEMONSTRATION OF LITHIUM ACTION IN THYROID CANCER

Malignant thyroid cells are less efficient in transporting and retaining ^{131}I than normal thyroid cells. The biological half-time of ^{131}I is shorter in malignant thyroid tumors (<10 d) than in the normal thyroid gland (approx 60 d, *36*), which limits the efficacy of therapeutic radioiodine. Using quantitative radiation dosimetry, Maxon and coworkers showed that among metastatic deposits, variability in iodine turnover modifies the effect of therapy *(37)*. Comparing the iodine kinetics in metastases that were successfully eradicated with radioactive iodine to those that were not, the effective half-time and thus the radiation dose (rad) were significantly lower in unresponsive tumors (2.5 d) vs responsive tumors (5.5 d). However, the percent uptake of radiation was similar between the groups. The estimated lethal dose for metastases was greater than 8000 rad, and subsequent studies found that a quantitative dosimetry strategy to achieve this dose was associated with a high cure rate *(38)*. In addition to the total amount of radioiodine given, the duration of its residence in metastatic lesions is a critically important factor to reach a successful therapeutic outcome, thus providing the rationale for adjuvant lithium therapy.

The first published research on the effect of lithium in thyroid cancer patients was a small case series by Briere *(39)* and a case study by Gershengorn *(40)*. In both studies, lithium increased the dose of radiation delivered to well-differentiated thyroid cancer, as shown by measuring the rate of radioiodine release after a tracer dose of ^{131}I. The prelithium half-time ranged from 3 to 11 d (mean 6.6 d). Lithium slowed the release of radioiodine in each case but was most effective when the prelithium half-time of ^{131}I was less than 6 d.

Movius and coworkers showed that in the majority of metastases examined before and after lithium in a small series of patients with well-differentiated thyroid cancer, the biological half-time of ^{131}I in the individual lesions was increased 20–770% over baseline *(41)*. Whole-body radiation was not significantly altered, except in a single patient with highly functional, bulky metastases *(40,41)*. Lithium appeared to have its greatest effect in tumors with rapid turnover; on average, the calculated radiation dose to all tumors was increased by 30%, and those that had at least a 25% increase in tumor radiation dose had prelithium biological half-times less than 6 d *(41)*.

Additional studies at the National Institutes of Health by Koong *(42)* further confirmed the inverse relationship between the beneficial lithium impact and baseline half-time values. Lithium prolonged the effective half-time in 77% of metastases studied, and an increase of more than 50% was observed when the control biological half-time was less than 3 d. As lithium treatment also increased ^{131}I accumulation in the tumor, the average tumor radiation dose increased twofold. No significant lithium effect could be seen if the half-time was greater than 6 d. In six of seven thyroid remnants studied, a similar positive effect was noted.

PATIENT SELECTION

Although the ability of lithium to enhance radioiodine retention in metastatic lesions has been known for several decades, there are no well-designed clinical studies demonstrating improved outcomes, such as survival or disease-free survival, associated with its use as an adjuvant. Factors that have curtailed its use include lack of practice guidelines derived from clinical trials, limited availability of ^{131}I dosimetry to identify patients likely to benefit from lithium therapy, and inexperience prescribing this psychotherapeutic agent, which has a narrow therapeutic range, to hypothyroid patients. Despite these concerns, lithium therapy should be considered in high-risk patients with demonstrated radioiodine uptake in metastatic deposits to augment the radiation dose, particularly if there has been a minimal response to prior therapy. Even when lesion dosimetry cannot be performed to identify those with rapid turnover and potential benefit, lithium can be used as an adjunct to optimize the radiation dose delivered by standard fixed quantities of ^{131}I typically given in practice.

PROTOCOL FOR LITHIUM USE

Patients who receive adjuvant lithium should be rigorously prepared for radioiodine therapy to assure adequate TSH levels and iodine deficiency, achieved by dietary restriction. Lithium is administered as lithium carbonate 2–5 d prior to the tracer dose for dosimetry and before ^{131}I therapy. All studies in the literature have been performed with the short-acting lithium carbonate preparation. No experience with the long-acting lithium salt has been reported, but it should be avoided because of the short therapy duration. Blockade of thyroidal iodine release occurs at serum lithium levels between 0.6 and 1.2 mEq/L, which is the same therapeutic target range for manic depressive disorder (32). The target concentration of lithium is generally achieved in 2–3 d if a loading dose of 600 mg is given followed by 300 mg three times daily (42). Lithium is measured by atomic absorption spectrophotometry in serum obtained 8–12 h after the previous dose, and the administered dose is adjusted accordingly. The total daily dose required is generally 900–1600 mg/d. Lithium carbonate is continued for 5–7 d after the therapeutic radioiodine dose is administered. During this period, toxicity must be assessed clinically, as serum levels cannot be measured because of the specimen's radioactivity, and lithium should be stopped if toxicity is suspected.

RISKS OF THERAPY

Although lithium carbonate is associated with many side effects (Table 1), short-term therapy is well-tolerated by most individuals. No serious toxicity has been observed with lithium in any patients with thyroid cancer reported in the literature. Mild gastrointestinal disturbances, e.g., nausea, vomiting, or diarrhea, were indicated in 10–20% (43) of patients. In all cases that symptoms occurred, none were severe enough to require discontinuation of the drug.

To avoid toxicity, patients must be closely monitored at the initiation of therapy. Blood levels are measured daily in the morning, and the dosage is adjusted to achieve the desired therapeutic range. Gastrointestinal side effects generally arise when serum concentrations are greater than 1.5 mEq/L, and central nervous system effects (confusion, somnolence, and seizures) occur when levels approach 2.0 mEq/L. Lethal toxicity is linked with levels greater than 2.5 mEq/L.

Lithium is excreted almost entirely in the urine and is associated with diminished renal-concentrating ability and nephrogenic diabetes insipidus that improves when lithium is discontinued. Patients should be counseled to avoid

Table 1
Adverse Effects and Toxicities of Lithium Administration

Mild	Dry mouth, polyuria, polydipsia, and mild nausea
Moderate	Drowsiness, muscular weakness, diarrhea, and vomiting
Severe	Vomiting, dehydration, high-urine output, tinnitus, blurred vision, pseudotumor cerebri, ataxia, seizure, coma, bradycardia, and hypotension

volume depletion while on lithium. Reversible mild elevations in serum creatinine concentrations are frequently observed in hypothyroid patients as a result of the reduced glomerular filtration rate. These expected changes in renal function should not preclude the use of lithium. However, extreme caution should be taken in patients with renal impairment. A 25–50% reduction of lithium dose is recommended if the creatinine clearance is 10–50 mL/min, and a 50–75% reduction is advised if the creatinine clearance is less than 10 mL/min.

The mean whole-body radiation dose is usually not significantly altered by lithium, despite its ability to increase the retention in tumor deposits (41–43). However, in a study of a single patient treated with lithium, an unexpected increase in whole-body radiation was attributed to ^{131}I-labeled thyroglobulin release from bulky metastases (40). Transient leukopenia and thrombocytopenia was noted. Quantitative whole-body dosimetry is recommended in all patients taking radioiodine therapy doses of 200 mCi or greater, regardless if adjuvant lithium carbonate is used. Close monitoring of blood counts for 6–10 wk after high-dose ^{131}I therapy is advised to determine the effect on hematopoiesis.

FUTURE DIRECTIONS

Although ample scientific evidence supporting the use of lithium as an adjuvant to radioiodine is available, there have been no controlled clinical trials to establish its effectiveness. Empiric use of lithium with standard fixed doses of radioiodine is acceptable; however, quantitative lesion dosimetry studies are required to calculate the lowest effective amount of radioiodine needed to eradicate metastatic disease. Assessment of the long-term outcomes associated with the use of such tailored therapy is warranted. Adjuvant lithium may also be useful in patients receiving radioiodine to ablate remnant thyroid. Clinical trials are needed to determine if lithium administration can improve the success rate of low-dose ^{131}I. Studies designed to simplify the methodology of lesional dosimetry, allowing easy tumor identification with rapid radioiodine turnover and calculation of the radiation dose associated with a given quantity of ^{131}I administered, would facilitate the conduct of such studies.

SUMMARY

Sufficient scientific evidence demonstrates that the effects of lithium carbonate on thyrocyte function result in an increased dose of radiation delivered to thyroid cancer from a given amount of ^{131}I. The patients most likely to benefit from adjuvant lithium are those who have tumors unresponsive to previous therapy and whose tumors have a short biological half-time. Lithium can be administered safely to hypothyroid patients during preparation for ^{131}I therapy but must be monitored carefully to achieve therapeutic levels and avoid toxicity. If quantitative lesional dosimetry is employed, lithium can achieve effective therapy with a lower administered dose of radioiodine and lower whole-body radiation. Studies of adjuvant lithium for both the eradication of metastatic disease and remnant ablation are needed to evaluate its ability to reduce the cumulative dose of radioiodine required to successfully treat thyroid cancer and to examine its impact on the ultimate outcome: disease-free survival.

REFERENCES

1. Maruca J, Santner S, Miller K, Santen RJ. Prolonged iodine clearance with a depletion regimen for thyroid carcinoma: concise communication. J Nucl Med 1984; 25:1089–1093.
2. Amdisen A, Hildebrandt J. Use of lithium in the medically ill. Psychother Psychosom 1988; 49:103–119.
3. Fieve RR, Platman S. Lithium and thyroid function in manic-depressive psychosis. Am J Psychiatry 1968; 125:527–530.
4. Gonzales R, Lauter H. On the therapy of manic-depressive psychoses with lithium salts. Nervenarzt 1968; 39:11–16.
5. Schou M, Amdisen A, Jensen S, Olsen T. Occurrence of goitre during lithium treatment. Br Med J 1968; 3:710–713.
6. Robbins J. Perturbations of iodine metabolism by lithium. Mathematical Biosciences 1984; 72:337–347.
7. Kushner J, Wartofsky L. Lithium-thyroid interactions. In Johnson L, editor. Lithium Therapy Monographs, vol. 2. Basel, Switzerland: S. Karger, 1988:74–98.
8. Sedvall G, Jonsson B, Pettersson U, Levin K. Effects of lithium salts on plasma protein bound iodine and uptake of 131I in thyroid gland of man and rat. Life Sciences 1968; 7:1257–1264.
9. Cooper TB, Simpson GM. Preliminary report of a longitudinal study of the effects of lithium on iodine metabolism. Curr Ther Res Clin Exp 1969; 11:603–608.
10. Fyro B, Petterson U, Sedvall G. Time course for the effect of lithium on thyroid function in men and women. Acta Psychiatr Scand 1973; 49:230–236.
11. Emerson CH, Dysno WL, Utiger RD. Serum thyrotropin and thyroxine concentrations in patients recieving lithium carbonate. J Clin Endocrinol Metab 1973; 36:338–346.
12. Lauridsen UB, Kirkegaard C, Nerup J. Lithium and the pituitary-thyroid axis in normal subjects. J Clin Endocrinol Metab 1974; 39: 383–385.
13. O'Neill B, Magnolato D, Semenza G. The electrogenic, Na+-dependent I-transport system in plasma membrane vesicles from thyroid glands. Biochim Biophys Acta 1987; 896:263–274.
14. Eskandari S, Loo DD, Dai G, et al. Thyroid Na+/I– symporter. Mechanism, stoichiometry, and specificity. J Biol Chem 1997; 272: 27,230–27,238.
15. Berens SC, Bernstein RS, Robbins J, Wolff J. Antithyroid effects of lithium. J Clin Invest 1970; 49:1357–1367.
16. Williams JA, Berens SC, Wolff J. Thyroid secretion in vitro: inhibition of TSH and dibutyryl cyclic-AMP stimulated 131-I release by Li+1. Endocrinology 1971; 88:1385–1388.
17. Burke G. Effects of cations and ouabain on thyroid adenyl cyclase. Biochim Biophys Acta 1970; 220:30–41.
18. Mori M, Tajima K, Oda Y, et al. Inhibitory effect of lithium on the release of thyroid hormones from thyrotropin-stimulated mouse thyroids in a perifusion system. Endocrinology 1989; 124: 1365–1369.
19. Bhattacharyya B, Wolff J. Stabilization of microtubules by lithium ion. Biochem Biophys Res Commun 1976; 73:383–390.
20. Bagchi N, Brown T, Mack R. Studies on the mechanism of inhibition of thyroid function by lithium. Biochim Biophys Acta 1978; 542: 163–169.
21. Spaulding SW, Burrow GN, Bermudez F, Himmelhoch JM. The inhibitory effect of lithium on thyroid hormone release in both euthyroid and thyrotoxic patients. J Clin Endocrinol Metab 1972; 35: 905–911.
22. Carlson HE, Tample R, Robbins J. Effect of lithium on thyroxine disappearance in man. J Clin Endocrinol Metab 1973; 36:1251–1254.
23. Sedvall G, Jonsson B, Pettersson V. Evidence of an altered thyroid function in man during treatment with lithium carbonate. Acta Psychiat Scand 1969; (Suppl):59–67.
24. Temple R, Berman M, Wolff J. Reduction of thyroid hormone release by lithium in thyrotoxicosis. J Clin Invest 1971; 50.
25. Gerdes H, Littmann KP, Joseph K, et al. Successful treatment of thyrotoxicosis by lithium. Acta Endocrinol Suppl (Copenh) 1973; 173:23.
26. Kristensen O, Andersen HH, Pallisgaard G. Lithium carbonate in the treatment of thyrotoxicosis. A controlled trial. Lancet 1976; 1: 603–605.
27. Lazarus JH, Richards AR, Addison GM, Owen GM. Treatment of thyrotoxicosis with lithium carbonate. Lancet 1974; 2:1160–1163.
28. Turner JG, Brownlie BE, Rogers TG. Lithium as an adjunct to radioiodine therapy for thyrotoxicosis. Lancet 1976; 1:614–615.
29. Hedley JM, Turner JG, Brownlie BE, Sadler WA. Low dose lithium-carbimazole in the treatment of thyrotoxicosis. Aust N Z J Med 1978; 8:628–630.
30. Turner JBB. Use of lithium in the treatment of thyrotoxicosis. Aust N Z J Med 1978; 8:628–630.
31. Boehm TM, Burman KD, Barnes S, Wartofsky L. Lithium and iodine combination therapy for thyrotoxicosis. Acta Endocrinol (Copenh) 1980; 94:174–183.
32. Temple R, Berman M, Robbins J, Wolff J. The use of lithium in the treatment of thyrotoxicosis. J Clin Invest 1972; 51:2746–2756.
33. Bogazzi F, Bartalena L, Brogioni S, et al. Comparison of radioiodine with radioiodine plus lithium in the treatment of Graves' hyperthyroidism. J Clin Endocrinol Metab 1999; 84:499–503.
34. Brownlie BE, Turner JG, Millner GM, et al. Lithium associated thyroid cancer. Aust N Z J Med 1980; 10:62–63.
35. Bal CS, Kumar A, Pandey RM. A randomized controlled trial to evaluate the adjuvant effect of lithium on radioiodine treatment of hyperthyroidism. Thyroid 2002; 12:399–405.
36. Berman M, Hoff E, Barandes M, et al. Iodine kinetics in man—a model. J Clin Endocrinol Metab 1968; 28:1–14.
37. Maxon HR, Thomas SR, Hertzberg VS, et al. Relation between effective radiation dose and outcome of radioiodine therapy for thyroid cancer. N Engl J Med 1983; 309:937–941.
38. Maxon HR, III, Englaro EE, Thomas SR, et al. Radioiodine-131 therapy for well-differentiated thyroid cancer—a quantitative radiation dosimetric approach: outcome and validation in 85 patients. J Nucl Med 1992; 33:1132–1136.

39. Briere J, Pousset G, Darsy P, Guinet. The advantage of lithium in association with iodine 131 in the treatment of functioning metastasis of the thyroid cancer (author's transl). Ann Endocrinol (Paris) 1974; 35:281–282.
40. Gershengorn MC, Izumi M, Robbins J. Use of lithium as an adjunct to radioiodine therapy of thyroid carcinoma. J Clin Endocrinol Metab 1976; 42:105–111.
41. Movius EG, Robbins J, Pierce LR, et al. The value of lithium in radioiodine therapy of thyroid carcinoma. In Medeiros-Neto G, Gaitan E, editors. Frontiers in Thyroidology. New York: Plenum, 1986: 1269–1272.
42. Koong SS, Reynolds JC, Movius EG, et al. Lithium as a potential adjuvant to 131I therapy of metastatic, well differentiated thyroid carcinoma. J Clin Endocrinol Metab 1999; 84:912–916.
43. Pons F, Carrio I, Estorch M, et al. Lithium as an adjuvant of iodine-131 uptake when treating patients with well-differentiated thyroid carcinoma. Clin Nucl Med 1987; 12:644–647.

50
Side Effects of ^{131}I for Ablation and Treatment of Well-Differentiated Thyroid Carcinoma

Douglas Van Nostrand and John Freitas

INTRODUCTION

The use of radioactive iodine (^{131}I) in the ablation and treatment of well-differentiated thyroid carcinoma may be associated with side effects in numerous organ systems (Table 1). Although many articles address the side effects of radioiodine, the characterizations of these effects vary widely because of a host of different factors (Table 2). This chapter attempts to consolidate the literature by presenting, where appropriate, (1) the spectrum of signs and symptoms, as well as the frequency and severity of side effects, (2) a review of selected articles, (3) a discussion of preventive measures to lessen the frequency and severity of side effects, and/or (4) a discussion of the medical management when the side effect occurs.

HAIR

The loss of hair secondary to radioiodine treatment is an infrequent complication and has been reported in a patient with an underlying skull metastasis (1). Although Alexander et al. (2) found transient episodes of more generalized alopecia in 28% (57 of 203) of patients that occurred one to several weeks after discharge from radioiodine treatment, this side effect was not dependent on the radioiodine dosage administered. Because hypothyroid patients suffer hair loss, and cancer patients have been traditionally hypothyroid when radioiodine is administered, the hair loss has been generally considered due to the hypothyroidism, not the radioiodine *per se*. As more radioiodine treatments may be used with recombinant human thyrotropin (rhTSH) while patients are euthyroid, it will be of interest to determine whether there is any associated hair loss.

BRAIN

Brain metastases diagnosed premortem are rare in patients with thyroid cancer and, when present, are usually linked with other sites of distant metastases. Most thyroid cancer brain metastases are not iodine-avid (17% in one series), as shown on diagnostic whole body scans (3). Patients with ^{131}I-avid brain metastases can experience abrupt marked deterioration or death if metastases swell or hemorrhage, or if cerebral edema develops in response to ^{131}I therapy (4–6). Prior to ^{131}I treatment, the possibility of surgical resection to debulk tumor mass of isolated brain lesions (even if iodine-avid) should be considered, because survival is improved significantly for those treated with surgical extirpation (3). If metastasectomy is not feasible for iodine-avid metastases, such patients should be pretreated for several hours orally with 16–32 mg of oral dexamethasone daily in divided dosages to prevent developing or worsening peritumoral edema. Steroids should be continued for 5–7 d following ^{131}I therapy (3). Although glucocorticoids have been identified as a cause of reduced radioiodine uptake in benign thyroid tissue in euthyroid patients, the rapidity at which this effect occurs is probably over several days (not hours) and may not be as marked in hypothyroid individuals (7). If an alternative to glucocorticoids is required, 50% oral glycerol (1.2–2.0 g/kg) daily has been shown as effective to reduce cerebral edema in patients undergoing external-beam therapy of brain metastases and may have similar efficacy in ^{131}I-treated patients (8).

SPINAL CORD

Simpson (9) reported two deaths from spinal cord necrosis, but these patients had been treated with external-beam radiotherapy. In general, the same precautions for spinal cord metastases apply for the brain. Acute swelling of cord lesions has been seen after rhTSH-stimulated ^{131}I therapy, but it is difficult to distinguish whether the etiologic factor was the TSH or the radioiodine.

EYE

The three most important side effects involving the eye area are inflammation of the lacrimal gland, obstruction of the lacrimal duct, and conjunctivitis. Although these side effects have not been well-characterized, some data are available.

Table 1
Sites of Side Effects Associated With Radioiodine Treatment

Hair
Brain
Spinal cord
Eye
Salivary glands
Taste and smell
Nose
Facial nerve
Vocal cord
Thyroid
Parathyroid
Pulmonary
Gastrointestinal system
Urinary bladder
Bone marrow
Fertility
Neoplasms

Table 2
Factors Causing Variability of Characterizations of Radioiodine Side Effects

Criteria for the presence of side effects
Thoroughness in the search for signs and symptoms of side effects
Length of follow-up
Grading of side effects
Prescribed activities of radioiodine for ablation or treatment
Total cumulative prescribed activities of radioiodine
Time intervals between treatments
Methods implemented or not implemented to prevent side effects

The mechanism for lacrimal gland inflammation is similar to sialadenitis of the salivary glands (see below). Radioiodine is known to accumulate within the lacrimal gland and, in sufficient concentration, may deliver enough radiation exposure to result in local inflammation and subsequent reduced production of tears. The reduced function has been well-studied by Zettinig *(10)* and appears to occur frequently after radioiodine therapy. In the evaluation of 88 patients, 81 patients had at least one abnormal result out of a set of three tests used to assess the quality and quantity of tears. The Schirmer tear test, which measures the quantity of aqueous tear production, was positive (decreased tears) in 40% of patients in one eye and 20% in both eyes. The tear film break-up time, which measures the tear film's stability, was abnormal in 71% of patients in at least one eye and in 57% of patients in both eyes. The lacrimal lipid layer that thickens, stabilizes, and retards evaporation of the aqueous layer underneath was abnormal in 49% of patients in at least one eye and in 34% of patients in both eyes. The lipid layer is produced by the sebaceous Meibomian glands in the lids, as well as by the Zeis and Moll glands along the eyelid margin and lashes.

The mechanism of the obstruction of the lacrimal duct, which drains the tears to the nasal cavity, is hypothesized to be the effects of radiation exposure to the duct lining from the radioiodine in the tears and/or possibly in the cells of the duct lining, leading to subsequent inflammation, fibrosis, and narrowing. Radioiodine activity in the tears has been well-described, with as much as 0.01% of the administered radioiodine dosage secreted in tears in each eye during the first 4 h after radioiodine administration *(11)*.

The mechanism of conjunctivitis is not well-understood but is most likely the result, at least in part, of documented changes in the tear quality and quantity. Zettinig *(10)* showed changes in the external eye morphology, demonstrating corneal staining with fluorescein in 42% (37 of 88) of patients, and 35% of patients had abnormal conjunctival findings on visual inspection.

The clinical presentation of lacrimal inflammation is xerophthalmia (dry eye). Typically, the patient has no initial symptoms of pain or swelling but subsequently develops reduced production of tears, resulting in dry eyes (xerophthalmia). The frequency of xerophthalmia was 16% (14 of 88) in patients studied. Seven patients had xerophthalmia and xerostomia, and seven had only xerophthalmia *(10)*. Solans *(12)* reported xerophthalmia in 33% (26 of 79), which persisted for 1 yr in 25%, for 2 yr in 17%, and into the third year in 14% of patients. Keratoconjunctivitis sicca persisted in 14% (11 of 88) of patients into the second year and in 8% (6 of 88) after the third year. No significant relationship of xerophthalmia was found with cumulative prescribed activity of radioiodine.

The clinical presentation of nasolacrimal duct obstruction is epiphora (excessive tearing). Zettinig *(10)* reported epiphora in 11% (10 of 88) and epiphora with photophobia in 1% of patients. The mechanism of photophobia was not discussed. The exact mechanism of epiphora was also not discussed but must relate to the failure of normal tear drainage to the nasal cavity. Kloos *(13)* reported a 2.6% incidence of epiphora (10 of 390), with symptoms appearing a mean of 6.5 mo after the last radioiodine dose (range of 3–16 months). Subsequently, Burns et al. *(13a)* described a highly documented and suspected incidence of obstructed nasolacrimal drainage of 3.4% and 4.6%, respectively.

Conjunctivitis typically presents with pain and erythema. Alexander *(2)* indicated a frequency of chronic or recurrent conjunctivitis in 23% (46 of 203) of patients.

Currently, no proven recommendations to reduce the radiation exposure to the lacrimal glands and ducts are available. Further research is warranted to evaluate methods that may reduce the radiation dose to the lacrimal gland and nasolacrimal duct. Regarding the management of xerophthalmia, obstruction of the nasolacrimal duct, or conjunctivitis, the first and most important aspect is for the physician and patient to be aware of potential side effects and their presenting signs and symptoms. Thus, when they do occur, the physician can implement treatment and/or refer the patient to an ophthalmologist. Depending on the severity, the patient may be simply observed without treatment, treated with artificial tears, or possibly referred to an ophthalmologist for additional treatments, such as a dacryocystorhinostomy (surgical creation of communication between the lacrimal sac and nasal cavity) for patients with severe epiphora. Alexander (2) found that 4 of 46 patients underwent dacryocystorhinostomy.

In summary, side effects of the lacrimal gland, lacrimal duct, and conjunctiva occur frequently, are often overlooked, may require referral to an ophthalmologist, and need further study.

SALIVARY GLAND

Significant radioiodine can accumulate in and pass through the salivary glands; therefore, radioiodine ablation and therapy can also result in a major radiation dose to the salivary glands that is manifested by both early and late untoward effects. These untoward effects include sialoadenitis, xerostomia, salivary duct obstruction, and possibly tumors of the salivary gland. (The latter is discussed in the Neoplasms section.) The terms "sialoadenitis" and "sialadenitis" have been used interchangeably in the medical literature, and both mean inflammation of the salivary gland. For this chapter, "sialoadenitis" will be used.

Anatomy and Physiology

To discuss the anatomy and physiology of the salivary glands in depth is beyond the scope of this book. However, the major pairs of salivary glands—the parotid, submandibular, and sublingual glands—can concentrate iodine as high as 7–700 times the plasma levels (14–17). The salivary glands are composed of serous cells and mucous cells. The parotid glands have predominately serous cells, and its saliva is predominately serous secretion. The submandibular glands have a mixture of serous and mucinous cells, and its saliva is predominately mucinous secretion. The sublingual glands also have a mixture of cells and make only a small contribution in volume but affect the viscosity of saliva. The parotid glands demonstrate a higher frequency of radiation sialoadenitis than submandibular and sublingual salivary glands, the hypothetical basis for which is that the serous cells have a greater ability to concentrate radioiodine than the mucous cells (18). An important mechanism of salivary iodide transport is (as in the thyroid gland itself) the sodium-iodide symporter (NIS) in salivary ductal cells. However, despite the presence of NIS, the salivary accumulation of radioiodine does not appear to be affected by the TSH level or the state of thyroid function (16,17,19). Relating to this,

Table 3
Incidence of Sialoadenitis

Author (Ref.)	Incidence (No. of Patients)
Alexander (2)	33% (67/203)
Albrecht (26)	59% (30/51) (parotid)
Alweiss (28)	12% (10/87)
Benua (23)	2% (3/122)
Edmonds (25)	10% (26/258)
Kahn (23)	34% (17/50)
Maier (29)	8% (3/37)
Pan (29)	4.6% (16/342)
Van Nostrand (22)	67% (9/15)

Table 4
Multiple Factors Affecting the Frequency and Severity of Sialoadenitis and Xerostomia

Diligence in looking for signs and symptoms of sialoadenitis or xerostomia
Individual prescribed activity of radioiodine
Cumulative dosage of radioiodine
Interval and frequency of treatment
Amount of radioiodine uptake in the salivary glands
Previous history of other salivary gland disease
Administration of drugs that cause xerostomia
Diligence of the patient and physician in reducing the radiation exposure to the salivary gland prior to and during radioiodine therapy

Rice's histopathologic studies indicate that the parotid acini and serous cells are severely injured after external radiotherapy, with little discernible change in the mucous cells (20). The salivary glands are controlled by the autonomic nervous system. The parasympathetic system apparently has a more significant impact on saliva production than the sympathetic system, but the latter still has a role (21).

Salivary Side Effects

Frequency

The most frequently reported side effect is acute radiation sialoadenitis, which has an incidence ranging from 10% to 67% (2,22–28; see Table 3). As noted earlier, the variability in frequency and severity is multifactorial (see Table 4), and correlations with both individual prescribed activity (27,31) and cumulative prescribed activity of radioiodine have been reported (26).

Signs and Symptoms

EARLY PRESENTATIONS

The spectrum of the signs and symptoms of sialoadenitis range from an asymptomatic sialoadenitis to a very

Table 5
Incidence of Xerostomia

Author (Ref.)	Incidence (No. of Patients)
Albrecht (26)	22% (11/51)
Alexander (2)	43% (87/203)
Alweiss (28)	30% (3/10)
Benua (23)	2% (3/122)
Edmonds (25)	10% (26*/258)
Kahn (23)	18% (10/55)
Leeper (91)	Common
Lin (32)	5.4% (3/56)
Solans (12)	33% (26/79)
Van Nostrand (22)	13% (2/15)

*Calculated.

painful, tender, and swollen salivary gland that may persist for many months. After employing the usual salivary gland–protective precautions, the glands of a patient treated for the first time with a prescribed activity of 5.55 GBq (150 mCi) or less of ^{131}I will most likely be asymptomatic, but this does not negate the presence of sialoadenitis. Although an asymptomatic form of sialoadenitis is difficult to confirm histopathologically, a "silent" sialoadenitis is indirectly or retrospectively implicated if there is subsequent development of xerostomia. Alexander reported that 56% of patients with xerostomia had no prior symptoms of sialoadenitis (2). However, many patients do develop symptoms. As many as one third of the patients will report at least mild pain, with or without tenderness and swelling of the salivary glands. This pain may begin as early as 6 h or as late as several days to even several weeks after radioiodine treatment. The pain, tenderness, swelling, or all three symptoms may be unilateral or bilateral and are more common in the parotid glands. However, the submandibular and lingual glands are still often involved. Alexander (2) found that in the group of patients with sialoadenitis (67 of 203), 80.6% (54 of 67) involved the parotids, and 14 of these were unilateral, and 40 were bilateral. Signs and symptoms of sialoadenitis in the submandibular glands were seen in 46% (31 of 67); 8 were unilateral and 23 bilateral. Albrecht (26) found 59% (30 of 51) of the patients had parotid gland involvement, with 25 bilateral and 5 unilateral, whereas 16% (8 of 51) had involvement of the submandibular glands. The signs and symptoms may last several weeks and occasionally as long as 1 yr, but most resolved spontaneously within several hours to several days with no specific treatment. If treatment was necessary, symptoms were usually easily controlled with hydration, anti-inflammatory agents (e.g., aspirin and ibuprofen), or an analgesic (e.g., acetaminophen; see discussion below for more detail). Sometimes, the symptoms may be more severe and chronic, and steroids may be required. If there is a suppurative parotitis, antibiotics may be required. In three patients, Allweiss reported a suppurative sialoadenitis that needed antibiotics (28).

LATE PRESENTATIONS

Obstruction. Although patients may present with the early signs and symptoms of an acute radiation sialoadenitis, some patients may initially present 1–12 mo after radioiodine ablation or treatment or secondarily after initial signs of an acute radiation sialoadenitis with new and different pain, tenderness, and swelling. The process of eating or just the sight of appetizing foods often invokes these symptoms, which may resolve within minutes to hours and are typically recurrent. The pathogenesis is different from those of the initial acute radiation sialoadenitis and is most likely a combination of (1) narrowing of the salivary ducts secondary to scarring and (2) altered quality and/or quantity of saliva. With normal saliva, there may be ductal narrowing with acute partial obstruction upon salivation. With reduced flow and thicker saliva, there may be stagnation and mucus precipitation, resulting in a plug (or calculus) with obstruction. Nevertheless, the pathogenesis is probably a combination of both reduced flow and narrowing of the duct to varying degrees. Although the natural history of this side effect has not been well-described, in the experience of one of the authors, these symptoms usually, but not always, slowly resolve over several months, but the signs and symptoms can be persistent.

XEROSTOMIA

Xerostomia is an important complication of radiation sialoadenitis. In addition to dry mouth, it may also present as burning oral discomfort, difficulty in eating dry foods, decreased taste sensitivity, increased production of viscous mucus or morning expectoration, and mucosal ulcerations. The reported frequency of xerostomia ranges from 2% to 55% (2,22,26,33; see Table 5), and the frequency and severity is again multifactorial. If xerostomia occurs, it may begin within several weeks after radioiodine treatment and usually resolves within 3 mo (2,22,33). For the condition to last greater than 1 yr is infrequent but does occur in 4.4–7% of patients (2,22,28,31). Xerostomia may even be permanent (34,35). Interestingly, Alexander (2) reported one patient whose xerostomia resolved 7 yr after the last radioiodine treatment.

Currently, there does not appear to be a demonstrable relationship of xerostomia to an earlier clinically evident presentation of sialoadenitis. As noted above, Alexander (2) showed that more than half the patients (56.1%; 63 of 96) who were diagnosed with xerostomia did not have clinically evident sialoadenitis, and Malpani (36) also found no link between significant reduction in the function of the salivary glands and the symptoms of sialoadenitis.

Regarding the prescribed activity of radioiodine, Spiegel (37) evaluated 20 patients with thyroid cancer and reported a dose-dependent decrease in salivary gland function. The same group specifically described a 40% reduction of parotid gland function after prescribed activities of 9.99 GBq (270 mCi; 38). Solans (12) demonstrated no association between xerostomia and cumulative prescribed activity.

Complications of Xerostomia. Salivary gland dysfunction after radioiodine therapy was the focus of a recent excellent review (39). Complications of xerostomia include dental caries and candidiasis. Although xerostomia has been suggested to significantly increase dental caries (39,40), this complication may be less frequent than suspected. Laupa (40) found that despite the lower salivary flow rates after radioiodine treatment, the frequency of widespread dental caries and demineralization, similar to that observed in externally irradiated patients, was not evident. Candidiasis is a rare but possible side effect of xerostomia, which may be severe enough to require treatment (e.g., with nystatin and clotrimazole; 41). Recommendations for xerostomia management and preventive care to minimize dental caries are noted in Table 6.

Although xerostomia is a major complication of radiation sialoadenitis, it is important to note that xerostomia is a reported side effect of over 500 medications (46), and the temporal relationship of radioiodine ablation or treatment to xerostomia does not prove that the condition is because of prior radiation. Similarly, in a study of 65-yr-old residents in Maryland, an epidemiological study indicated a 17% prevalence of dry mouth (47). Radiation sialoadenitis may be the most likely cause, but an evaluation by an otolaryngologist is recommended.

STOMATITIS

Stomatitis is rare, but if it occurs, it may be very painful (35). Its mechanism has not been clarified. If severe, stomatitis may require treatment with dexamethasone elixir mouthwash or mouthwash containing viscous lidocaine, diphenhydramine and aluminum, and magnesium hydroxides (35). Referral to an otolaryngologist is advised.

Radiation Dose

The radiation exposure to the salivary glands has not been well-studied. Donachi (48) reported approximately 250 rads (250 cGy) to the salivary gland from a 185-MBq (5-mCi) dose, and Goolden (49) demonstrated 700 rads (700 cGy) during the first 24 h.

Preventive Treatment

The most important aspect of treatment to prevent or minimize sialoadenitis is to begin with the first ablation. However, three factors often undermine efforts to aggressively reduce radiation exposure to the salivary glands on the initial ablation. First, the initial signs or symptoms of radiation sialoadenitis are either silent or mild and transient. Second, most patients will never require another radioiodine ablation or treatment. Third, staging helps predict which

Table 6
Recommendations for the Management of Xerostomia and Dental Caries

Referral to an otolaryngologist and dentist
Treatment of causes other than radiation sialoadenitis, such as changing a drug or drug dosage that is causing xerostomia
Adequate hydration
Impeccable dental hygiene
Artificial saliva swirled in the mouth and swallowed every 3–4 h
Repeated massages of the gland as necessary
Avoidance of anticholinergics
Administration of sialogogues (42)
    Pilocarpine (Salagen), 5–10 mg postoperatively TID. Oral tablet may need to be taken for 6–12 wk before full benefit is realized
    Cevimeline (43; Evoxac), cholinesterase inhibitor, 30 mg postoperatively TID
    Anethole trithione (Hepasulfol, Mucinol, Sialor, Sonicur, and Sufralem). The standard dose is 37.5–75 mg typically in divided doses before meals. Doses of up to 150 mg daily have been used.
    Chewing gum
    Trial of saliva-stimulating tablets (44), including such potential agents as disaccharides and low-dose interferon-α lozenges
    Acupuncture (45)
Fluoride therapy in the form of topical fluoride applications, fluoride mouthwashes, and fluoride toothpastes
Hydrogen peroxide mouthwash diluted with mouthwash, e.g., Listerine®
Antibiotics for suppurative sialoadenitis

group of patients are at risk for metastasis and thus additional radioiodine treatments. However, neither the relative minor initial signs and symptoms, the likelihood of not needing another treatment, nor the implication of staging, helps the individual patient who does need additional treatments and is at risk for sialoadenitis and its associated consequences. Thus, because the patient still has the potential of additional radioiodine ablations or treatments and to reduce the severity and frequency of subsequent sialoadenitis and its associated consequences, we strongly recommend aggressive measures to minimize the radiation dose to the salivary gland beginning with the *first* radioiodine treatment. This will serve to reduce the severity and frequency of subsequent sialoadenitis and its associated consequences (see Table 7).

Preablation

ASSESSMENT OF SALIVARY GLANDS

Kulkarni (50) demonstrated that although there was no significantly statistical difference, the incidence of salivary gland dysfunction was higher in patients who showed moderate and marked salivary uptake of radioiodine on the diagnostic scans than those patients who had none or mild salivary gland uptake. This preliminary data should not alter

Table 7
Approaches to Minimize Radiation Sialoadenitis and its Consequences

Preablation
    Assessment of salivary glands on preablation or pretreatment radioiodine whole body scans
    Patient education about prevention
    Patient participation in implementing the preventive measures
    Hydration
    Suspension of anticholinergic medications
    Amifostine
    Reserpine
Immediately postablation
    Hydration
    Sour candies
    Lemon juice
    Massage
    Waking up multiple times during the first night to implement candies, hydration, and message
Postablation
    Anti-inflammatory agents
    Steroids

the aggressive management to minimize radiation dose to the salivary glands; however, assessment of the uptake in the salivary glands on such scans still may be useful. For example, asymmetric, persistent, relatively increased uptake in one parotid gland may forewarn of a problem in that gland. Alternatively, minimal or no radioactivity in any of the salivary glands may suggest a lower radiation dose to the salivary glands from radioiodine and thus a lower chance of radiation sialoadenitis in that patient. In patients considered for high empiric or dosimetrically-determined radioiodine-prescribed activities, marked salivary gland uptake may indicate the need to consider a reduction in prescribed activity to minimize sialoadenitis. Further research is warranted to evaluate the utility of the salivary gland uptake on pretreatment radioiodine scans; yet, until that data is available, a general assessment of salivary gland uptake may be useful.

PATIENT EDUCATION

Two crucial factors to lessen radiation to the salivary gland are (1) educating the patient about the importance of minimizing the radiation dose to the salivary gland, along with the techniques to do so, and (2) encouraging the patient to be part of the treatment team, allowing potentially beneficial tasks to be performed.

HYDRATION

Although there is no direct evidence to demonstrate the value of hydration to reduce the radiation dose to the salivary glands, hydration is recommended on a purely empiric basis. Dehydration is known to lower saliva production, thereby increasing stasis of saliva, stasis of radioiodine in the salivary glands, and the radiation dose to the salivary glands. Hydration is also important for renal clearance of the radioiodine circulating in the blood, thus reducing the amount and duration of radioiodine available in the blood for the salivary gland to take up.

CHOLINERGIC AND ANTICHOLINERGIC MEDICATIONS

Although anticholinergic drugs may decrease the initial radioiodine uptake in the salivary glands in some patients, as a general rule, all anticholinergic medications should be discontinued.

Cholinergics (e.g., pilocarpine, cevimeline, anetholetrithione, and bromhexine) may be useful to stimulate salivation and hopefully increase radioiodine turnover or throughput in the salivary gland. An empiric treatment plan based on a 5-d regimen, beginning 2 d prior to radioiodine treatment, has been proposed (35). However, the utility of cholinergic drugs remains controversial. Alexander (2) showed no difference in the frequency and severity of sialoadenitis in those who received pilocarpine compared to those who did not.

AMIFOSTINE

Amifostine (WR–2721, Ethyol) has been shown to protect the salivary gland from the damaging effects of ionizing radiation of external radiotherapy for head and neck tumors (51–53). Amifostine is an organic thiophosphate and is dephosphorylated to its active metabolite WR-1065. The latter is a scavenger of oxygen-free radicals, which are the primary cause of radiation-induced tissue damage. Amifostine concentration can be 100 times greater in normal tissue than tumor tissue (54), and the conversion of amifostine to WR-1065 is more effective in an alkaline environment. Normal tissue is more alkaline than tumor tissue. One side effect of amifostine was a temporary drop in blood pressure that required temporary suspension of the infusion. However, this is usually not a problem; if it occurs, it is manageable.

Because of its value for external radiotherapy for head and neck tumors, amifostine has been proposed for use in patients with thyroid cancer. With salivary gland scintigraphy, Bohuslavizki assessed the influence of amifostine on the adverse effects of radioiodine treatments on salivary gland function and demonstrated that parotid and submandibular function was reduced by approximately 40% in the placebo group and remained unchanged in the amifostine group (55). Despite these data, amifostine is presently not widely used in patients receiving radioiodine treatment, as no data are available to show whether amifostine also protects the thyroid cancer from the desired radiation effect. More research is needed.

RESERPINE

In addition to the innervation of the salivary glands by the parasympathetic system, the salivary glands are also innervated by the sympathetic system. Therefore, antisympathomimetic agents may have utility. Levy (56) evaluated

12 patients: 9 received reserpine and 3 did not. Based on radioiodine uptake on whole body images relative to patients not given reserpine, his data suggested that the patients taking reserpine had a significant decrease in the ratio of parotid-to-background counts. However, it is uncertain whether the reduced salivary gland uptake was secondary either to the reserpine or stunning from a 370-MBq (10-mCi) diagnostic prescribed activity of ^{131}I or partial treatment of the salivary gland from the 3.7–5.55-GBq (100–150 mCi) ablative prescribed activities of radioiodine.

Immediate Postablation

On the day of ablation and immediately afterward, hydration is again thought to be indicated and valuable. Also the administration of sialogogues is routinely recommended shortly after ablation or treatment (57). This includes sour candies, lemon juice, lemon drops, or other candies or foods that make the patient salivate. Although oral hydration and the use of sialogogues cease while the patient is asleep, the radiation exposure from radioiodine in the salivary gland does not, and it is proposed that the greatest radiation exposure to the salivary gland from radioiodine occurs during sleep. Accordingly, one of the authors recommends that the patient be encouraged to wake up several times (i.e., four or five) during the first night to use sialogogues, drink fluids, and void. This additional fluid intake is valuable to increase urine flow and reduce radiation dose to the urinary bladder (see below). An alternative to oral intake of fluid would be continuous intravenous hydration; however, if the intravenous line is placed after therapy, this may raise radiation safety issues for the phlebotomist. Massage of the parotid glands may also be beneficial, especially if there is initial partial-flow obstruction (35; see Fig. 1).

Despite their generally accepted use, some authors have questioned the utility of empiric sialogogues. Nakada (58) reported that postponing the use of sialogogues until 24 h after the administration of the radioiodine therapeutic dose reduced sialoadenitis from 63.8% (67 of 105) to 36.8% (46 of 125), hypogeusia (abnormally diminished acuteness of the sense of taste) or taste loss from 39% to 25.6%, and dry mouth from 23.8% to 11.2%. Permanent xerostomia decreased from 14.3% to 5.6%. However, in their study, the sialogogues were administered every 2–3 h during the daytime, which may not be frequent enough or of sufficient duration to be beneficial. Moreover, there was no documentation of sialogogue type or of patient adherence to the regimen. Further research is needed to identify methods to reduce the radiation exposure to the salivary glands.

Postablation

Whether patients should prophylactically take anti-inflammatory agents, such as nonsteroidal drugs, to reduce the inflammation and/or the signs and symptoms of sialoadenitis is not known. However, once the patient develops clinical

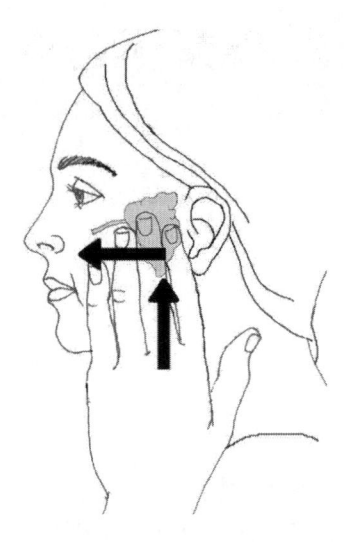

Fig. 1. For antegrade massage, push with the fingers mildly on the parotid gland cephalad and then anteriorly. (Reproduced with permission from Keystone Press from the book entitled "Thyroid Cancer: A Guide for Patients.")

symptoms of acute radiation sialoadenitis, anti-inflammatory agents should be used. Steroids are not routinely recommended but may be considered for more severe acute radiation sialoadenitis.

Management of Long-Term Complications

If sialoadenitis persists for longer than several days, then administration of anti-inflammatory agents and referral to an otolaryngologist should be considered.

The symptoms of obstruction (as described earlier) should neither be mistaken as chronic sialoadenitis nor treated as chronic sialoadenitis. Although a component of chronic sialoadenitis may be present and warrant treatment, ductal obstruction should also be considered because the management is different. If the pain and swelling is mild, owing to obstruction from a soft plug or radiation fibrosis, then occasional increased retrograde or antegrade pressure with massage may resolve the symptoms by helping the normal or thickened saliva pass the ductal narrowing or help spontaneously extrude a plug (see Fig. 1). If the symptoms are not mild or transient, then referral to otolaryngologist is strongly recommended. The otolaryngologist can then evaluate for other, albeit unlikely, etiologies of obstruction, consider periodic ductal dilation of Stenson's duct, and, in rare cases, consider tympanic neurectomy or ligation of the duct. Although excision of the gland should be avoided, Allweiss (28) reported one patient who required a parotidectomy because of intractable salivary gland pain and discomfort. Finally, a secondary infection can occur that may require antibiotics.

In summary, sialoadenitis is an important side effect of radioiodine therapy. Awareness of this side effect and appropriate preventive care and treatment can help its prevention.

Table 8
Incidence of Change in Taste and/or Smell

Author (Ref.)	Incidence (No. of Patients)
Albrecht (36)	58% (30/51)
Alexander (3)	27% (55/203)
Benua (23)	2% (3/122)
Kahn (23)	16% (8/50)
Lin (32)	1.8% (1/56)
Van Nostrand (22)	33% (5/15)
Varma (59)	48% (41/85)

TASTE AND SMELL

Alteration of taste and smell is well-documented after radioiodine (2,22,23,59) and may be described as simply a loss of taste, loss of smell (2), metallic taste, or chemical taste (59). Occasionally, these patients may describe a salty taste that may be secondary to inadequately absorbed sodium and chloride ions in the saliva (60). The frequency varies from 2% to 58% of patients, as noted in Table 8. The loss or change in taste or smell may occur as early as 24 h after radioiodine ablation and was reported to occur within 168 h (59). Although transient, the change persisted from 4 to as long as 52 wk in 37% of those patients who had changes in taste (60). Alexander (2) found that it occurred up to several weeks after discharge and persisted for 1–12 wk. The mechanism is most likely ^{131}I uptake in von Ebner's serous gland, located in the vicinity of the taste bud–containing circumvallate papilla (35,59). Albrecht (26) demonstrated a dependence or direct relationship on administered activity. Preventive care parallels that for sialoadenitis.

NASAL EFFECTS

Pain in the tip of the nose and epistaxis is a rare but real side effect of radioiodine. Van Nostrand et al. (22) described 2 of 15 patients who had received prescribed radioiodine activities greater than 7.4 GBq (200 mCi) and had nasal complaints. One patient had dry nasal mucosa at 1 wk, followed by easily controlled epistaxis and a tender nose with clots and scabs during the second week. The lining of the nose has mucous cells that can accumulate radioiodine; this accumulation can be the most prominent in the tip of the nose, which is frequently seen and confirmed on radioiodine whole body scans (61) (see Chapter 15 entitled "Atlas of Radioiodine Whole-Body Scans"). At the present time, little is known regarding methods to reduce this infrequent side effect of radioiodine. However, if performing dosimetry and planning to administer prescribed radioiodine activity higher than 7.4 GBq (200 mCi), the pretherapy scan for nasal uptake can be assessed to anticipate this potential complication. If there is facial activity with focal uptake in the nose area, consider a lateral view with appropriate markers. If there is marked uptake in the nose and if a high-prescribed activity of radioiodine is being considered, then the prescribed activity can be reduced. Further research is warranted relating to drugs that may reduce this uptake.

FACIAL NERVE

Radioiodine has been associated as a rare cause of transient facial nerve paralysis. Levinson (62) reported two patients who rapidly developed transient facial paralysis after ^{131}I. The proposed mechanism was the passage of the affected nerve through the parotid gland, and the paralysis was attributed to the gland swelling secondary to radiation sialoadenitis with ischemia of the nerve. After resolution of the sialoadenitis, the facial nerve palsies resolved.

THYROID TISSUE

Radiation Thyroiditis

The most recent analysis of United States surgical procedures demonstrated that 77.4% of thyroid cancer patients underwent a total thyroidectomy independent of stage or tumor histology (63). The surgical removal of most benign or malignant thyroid tissue facilitates subsequent ^{131}I therapy. However, many patients are still referred for ^{131}I therapy, who harbor up to a lobe of residual thyroid tissue either by design or following a complicated, less than satisfactory surgical procedure.

Radiation thyroiditis postablation is commonly seen in patients with large benign thyroid remnants (≥10% neck uptake), especially when treated with >2.8–3.7 GBq (≥75–100 mCi) or more of ^{131}I, delivering radiation doses more than 50,000 rads (cGy). In 10 patients studied retrospectively after lobectomy only, 60% demonstrated neck pain or tenderness with ^{131}I ablation of the residual lobe (24). Neck and ear pain, dysphagia, painful swallowing, thyroid tenderness, and even airway compromise requiring intubation can be seen beginning 2-4-d postablation. With more extensive surgery, such as total or near-total thyroidectomy (<5% neck uptake), radiation thyroiditis is rarely seen. However, extensive neck metastases with avid radioiodine uptake can also demonstrate marked pain and swelling and even hemorrhage following ^{131}I therapy, particularly if radiation doses exceed 40,000 cGy (rads). Strong consideration should be given to surgical removal of all palpable neck metastatic disease to prevent such sequelae. A less common phenomenon is painless neck swelling that is manifested by edematous and firm induration of the neck, typically seen within 1–2 d of ^{131}I treatment of more than 10–15 g of thyroid tissue (64). This is frequently associated with a neck-tightening or strangling sensation that can be very alarming to some patients. Although mild symptoms often recede with just analgesics, an oral prednisone burst and taper is both necessary and beneficial in some patients with painful radiation thyroiditis and most patients with painless neck edema, using 30–60 mg daily for 3–5 d initially, followed by a gradual taper over 7–10 d.

Thyrotoxicosis

Thyrotoxicosis has been well-documented in patients with functioning well-differentiated thyroid carcinoma after radioiodine treatment *(61,65–68)*. Trunnel *(68)* reported that the signs and symptoms of hyperthyroidism appeared within 2 wk of treatment. Cerletty *(69)* described two cases in which the failure to control the thyrotoxic state led to thyroid storm and death.

HYPOPARATHYROIDISM

Therapeutic prescribed activity of ^{131}I can easily deliver greater than 10,000 rads (cGy) to the thyroid bed with lesser radiation to adjacent parathyroid tissue at 5–6 wk postthyroidectomy when surgically induced parathyroid injury may still be present. However, ^{131}I β particles (negatrons) have a range of only 2.05 mm in soft tissue, and parathyroid irradiation would only be significant for intrathyroidal or closely adherent parathyroid glands. Only two cases of permanent hypoparathyroidism after ^{131}I therapy of thyroid cancer have been reported in patients known to be normocalcemic prior to treatment. One case occurred within 4 mo of ^{131}I following transient well-documented hyocalcemia postthyroidectomy but returned to a eucalcemic state before ^{131}I therapy *(70,71)*. Glazebrook has postulated that many thyroid cancer patients treated with ^{131}I exhibit diminished parathyroid reserve, as shown by stress testing in 53 patients postthyroidectomy. When salt and water loaded prior to forced diuresis, 58% of the 53 patients treated with 2.96–5.55 GBq (80–150 mCi) demonstrated transient hypocalcemia. In this prospective study, affected patients were more likely to have lower prestress serum calcium levels than the unaffected patients. In the absence of symptoms, routine monitoring of calcemic status does not appear to be warranted.

VOCAL CORDS

Recurrent laryngeal nerve injury or direct trauma from endotracheal tube placement during thyroidectomy can induce transient or permanent vocal cord paralysis, manifested by stridor or hoarseness. In symptomatic patients seen prior to anticipated ^{131}I therapy, direct laryngoscopy can document vocal cord dysfunction and should be performed. ^{131}I treatment of residual thyroid bed tissue can cause significant thyroid tissue swelling that is associated with laryngeal nerve compression and dysfunction *(72,73)*. As reported by Lee et al. *(72)*, 5.55 GBq (150 mCi) prescribed activity of ^{131}I given to treat residual right-thyroid bed tissue in a patient with papillary thyroid cancer was followed by the gradual development of bilateral vocal cord paresis within 72 h. As only right-thyroid bed irradiation occurred (no significant left-lobe uptake present), it was believed that a partial left recurrent laryngeal nerve injury had been present since the surgery, necessitating an emergent tracheostomy. Fortunately, the bilateral vocal cord dysfunction resolved after 8 wk.

PULMONARY EFFECTS

Acute radiation pneumonitis (ARP) and pulmonary fibrosis (PF) are potentially serious complications of radioiodine treatment in patients who have pulmonary metastasis from well-differentiated thyroid carcinoma. Fortunately, this is very rare; however, because it is rare, most of the information regarding ARP and PF secondary to radioiodine comes from (1) radiation pathology from external radiotherapy *(74)*, (2) two important case reports described in 1957 by Rall *(75)*, and (3) several additional reports in the literature *(23,25,31–33,76,77)*. Occurrence of ARP, PF, or both is directly related to the extent of pulmonary metastasis, the prescribed activity of radioiodine, and its uptake and retention in the lung lesions. However, based on the information derived from these resources, radiation pneumonitis and pulmonary fibrosis is expected to be an infrequent and manageable complication of radioiodine treatment.

Presentation

Based upon radiation pathology from external radiotherapy *(74)*, the time of ARP onset is usually 1–20 wk after initial treatment. Its clinical presentation includes dyspnea, nonproductive cough, possible pleuritic pain, fever, and rales. Radiographic changes are similar to other pneumonitis secondary to other causes. Although these changes are typically confined to the field of irradiation, they may occur outside the field, known as *abscopal effects (78–80)*. Morgan suggested that these changes outside the irradiation field are from other mechanisms, such as generalized immunologically mediated lung damage *(81)*.

The pathologic changes include congestion and intra-alveolar edema with alveolar macrophages, and the initial lesions probably occur in the endothelial cells of alveolar wall capillaries. Protein-rich fluid then leaks through the damaged capillary wall into the interstitium and alveolar lumen, with resultant edema in the alveolar septa and hyperplasia of the alveolar-lining cells. A hyaline membrane may occur, comparable to the pathogenesis of other etiologies of acute respiratory distress syndromes (ARDS); however, if formed, the hyaline membrane is more prominent in ARP. This description is similar to the autopsy reports of the two patients with ARP and PF, as reported by Rall *(75)*.

PF is a late clinical sequela of ARP. Although PF is typically present in most individuals who recover from ARP, PF can develop in patients who never had an initial acute illness. Most patients who develop PF are symptomatic 1 yr later. If PF does occur, it is usually established and stable by 1 yr after exposure and is irreversible. However, PF can also be chronic and progressive.

The pathophysiology of PF involves progressive fibrosis of the alveolar septa. The laboratory changes include mildly reduced pulmonary functions, such as decreased vital capacity, decreased forced expiratory volume (FEV_1), decreased carbon monoxide diffusing capacity (DLCO), mild arterial hypoxia, decreased compliance, and reduced alveolar-capillary membrane integrity. Radiographically, computed tomography (CT) is a more sensitive test than chest radiography and can demonstrate a progressive decrease in lung volumes, a reduction of pulmonary blood flow, and the fibrotic changes associated with PF.

Risk factors for clinical radiation pneumonitis are controversial. Monson (80) demonstrated an increase in clinical radiation pneumonitis in patients with a low Karnofsky performance status, a history of smoking, comorbid lung disease, or low pulmonary function tests (PFTs). In those patients with an FEV_1 of 2 or less, 24% (16 of 66) developed clinical radiation pneumonitis, whereas in patients with an FEV_1 above 2, only 6% (1 of 17) developed clinical radiation pneumonitis. In those patients with a forced vital capacity (FVC) of 3 or less, 31% (17 of 54) developed clinical radiation pneumonitis, but no patient with an FVC more than 3 developed clinical radiation pneumonitis. These patients had received external radiotherapy for lung carcinoma (80). However, there is a diversity of opinions regarding risk factors such as pulmonary function (82).

As noted previously, limited reports exist in the literature regarding ARP and PF secondary to radioiodine treatment in patients who have well-differentiated thyroid carcinoma with pulmonary metastasis. One of the most detailed reports (75) provides valuable descriptions of two patients with documented fatal ARP and PF. Several salient features about these two patients are summarized here. First, the initial respiratory symptoms occurred approximately 60 and 61 d after their radioiodine treatments, respectively. For one patient, the presenting symptoms were shortness of breath and substernal pressure during exertion. For the other patient, symptoms were coldness, fatigue, shortness of breath, and a slightly nonproductive cough. The time interval from the initially reported respiratory symptoms to death from respiratory failure was 48 and 49 d, respectively. Rapid deterioration appeared to occur over the last 23 and 38 d. Steroids were used in one patient, which produced a significant but only transient improvement. Although other reports of ARP and PF are noted, no other significant information is available regarding time until symptoms, course of respiratory failure, use of steroids, and so on.

Although these are only two cases and little additional information is available in the literature, several warnings appear to be appropriate and prudent. First, the signs or symptoms of ARP and/or its sequela do not necessarily occur immediately after treatment but can be delayed as long as 8 wk, and possibly longer. Second, the initial symptoms may appear to be minor and nonspecific but should not be dismissed as unimportant or owing to other causes. Third, there may be an initial symptomatic period where *early* treatment with steroids could alter the patient's course before progressive, irreversible respiratory failure begins.

Radiation Dose to the Lung

Estimating the radiation dose to the lung from radioiodine treatment is problematic on several counts. There are challenges in estimating the radioiodine uptake in a pulmonary lesion, effects of inhomogeneous radioiodine uptake within the lesion, lesion depth, attenuation of the radioactivity, radioactivity clearance from the lesion, lesion volume, and the radiation exposure to adjacent normal pulmonary tissue. Consequently, the radiation exposure to the lungs, or even a portion of the lungs, from radioiodine is difficult to accurately determine. However, more specific data are available from external radiotherapy on the relationship between radiation dose and side effects of the lung (see Tables 9–11). The data from external radiotherapy are useful for an overall perspective, but extrapolation of the data to radioiodine therapy is again difficult. Similarly, although dosimetric analysis of radiation exposure to the lungs from radioiodine with phantoms has been reported (98), the information is limited.

In the literature on ARP and PF secondary to radioiodine treatment, the most valuable data are from Rall (75) and Benua (23). Rall observed 15 patients with pulmonary metastasis from well-differentiated thyroid carcinoma who were treated with radioiodine. Four of these patients developed pulmonary changes, and two subsequently died from the pulmonary changes. Figure 2 demonstrates the relationship between prescribed ^{131}I activity deposited in the chest and the pulmonary assessment. When the study was reported in 1957, the pulmonary assessment was made by X-ray and evaluation of symptoms. No patient that retained less than 4.63 GBq (125 mCi) in the chest at 24 h developed radiographic changes or symptoms to suggest pulmonary changes secondary to radiation effects. In Fig. 3, Rall's data demonstrate an association between pulmonary assessment and the quantity of ^{131}I deposited in the chest over the first 20 d following treatment. The quantity of ^{131}I deposited was expressed in units of "curie-day," which represents the sum for each of the 20 d of the ^{131}I estimated quantity deposited in the lungs. Both fatalities had the highest estimates of ^{131}I exposure to the chest with over 1 Ci-d. Furthermore, no patient with approximately 0.75 Ci-d of ^{131}I deposited in the chest developed radiographic changes or symptoms to suggest any pulmonary changes secondary to radiation. In 1961, Benua (23) reported on an expanded group of patients at Memorial Sloan Kettering Cancer Institution (MSKCI), which included Rall's patients; 59 patients were treated with 122 doses of ^{131}I. Radiation pneumonitis occurred in five of these patients. However, radiation pneumonitis did not occur when the calculated radiation dose to the blood was less than or equal to 200 cGy (rads) and the whole-body reten-

**Table 9
Fractionated Radiation Dose and Side Effects of the Lung**

34.9 Gy (3490 rads), 15 fractions over 19 d = 50% developed radiographic evidence of lung damage *(83)*
40 Gy (4000 rads), 20–30 fractions = 8–15% severe ARP clinically *(78,84)*
54 Gy (5400 rads; fractionation N/A) = 20% developed clinical ARP *(80)*
Occasionally severe lesions have occurred with lower doses
Of 377 patients treated to the mantle for Hodgkin's disease, 20 developed ARP; three died with less than 600 cGy (600 rads) to one whole lung. Five died after 600–1500 cGy (600–1500 rads; *85)*

N/A, not available.

**Table 10
Single Radiation Dose (SD) and Side Effects of the Lung**

After 600–1000 cGy (rads) single dose, 17.5% developed ARP 100 d later and 15% died of ARP within 2 wk *(86)*
820 cGy (rads) for 5% incidence of ARP
930 cGy (rads) for 50% incidence of ARP
1100 cGy (rads) for 90% incidence of ARP *(87)*
700 cGy (rads) for SD to both lungs is current proposed limit *(87–89)*

**Table 11
Pulmonary Fibrosis**

Difficult to establish because it is typically asymptomatic but probably very frequent *(90)*
After 3000 cGy over 10–15 d, 30% had radiographic changes *(83,87)*
After 5000 cGy (rads) over 25 d, 90% had radiographic changes *(83,87)*

tion of radioiodine at 48 h was less than or equal to 2.96 GBq (80 mCi). (See Chapter 47 for additional information regarding the Benua and Leeper's dosimetry protocol).

Based on their early experience, Benua and Leeper proposed and implemented the above restrictions for patients with pulmonary metastasis. In 1982, Leeper *(91)* reported that no subsequent radiation pneumonitis had been observed at MSKCI over approximately 20 yr since the original group of five patients. In the intervening years, other institutions have adopted the Benua and Leeper (MSKCC) dosimetry protocol with the above restrictions. A review of the literature of those patients who have had pulmonary metastases and were treated with a prescribed activity of radioiodine, according to dosimetry and the above restrictions or an empiric formula, is noted in Table 12. The frequency of observed radiation pneumonitis in the pooled group of patients was 2%, PF was approximately 3%, and death secondary to radiation effects to the lung was 2%.

Thus, despite the absence of prospective data in the literature and the inability to extrapolate the data from external radiation therapy, significant empirical data has been accumulated over the last 50 yr. These data allow at least one approach that has a reasonably acceptable risk of ARP and PF complications.

Appropriate Time Interval Between Radioiodine Treatments

It is also problematic to determine the appropriate time interval between radioiodine treatments to minimize the patient's chance of developing ARP and PF. Schlumberger *(94)* found no ARP or PF in a patient group with pulmonary metastases who were treated with radioiodine every 4–6 mo, but the prescribed activity used was only 3.7 GBq (100 mCi). Hindié et al. *(95)* also reported no ARP or PF with treatments every 6 mo until a cumulative prescribed activity of 18.5 GBq (500 mCi), at which time the interval was increased to 1 or 2 yr. However, Hindié *(95)* also treated patients with prescribed activities of 3.7–5.55 GBq (100–150 mCi). Rall suggested that the recovery from ARP was exponential, and that multiple doses should be separated by intervals of 6 mo or more *(75)*. Leeper, who administered much higher prescribed activities of radioiodine, empirically recommended extending the time between treatments to approximately 1 yr *(91)*. Although further study is needed, these studies will be difficult to perform.

Existence of Prior Pulmonary Disease

Aldrich *(76)* evaluated pulmonary function in 12 of 35 patients with well-differentiated thyroid carcinoma metastatic to the lung. Five patients had other known causes for lung disease, but no distinctive type of abnormal pulmonary function (e.g., obstructive, restrictive, or mixed) was identified with pulmonary metastases. Interestingly, no patient died from pulmonary complications of radioiodine treatment if the pretreatment pulmonary functions tests were normal.

Recommended Pretreatment Management of Pulmonary Metastases

If a patient has known pulmonary metastases secondary to well-differentiated thyroid carcinoma, we recommend the following approach.

1. Obtain the history of pulmonary disease and the results of all previous PFTs, if any.
2. Assess extent of pulmonary metastases based on chest X-ray and chest CT without contrast.
3. Examine present pulmonary function using PFTs and DLCO.
4. Assess the pattern of metastases on the chest X-ray, the chest CT without contrast, and the radioiodine scan. According to the limited literature (and intuitively), the risk of ARP and PF appears to be lower when:
   a. The radioactive uptake in the lungs is lower.
   b. The radioactivity in the lungs clears faster.

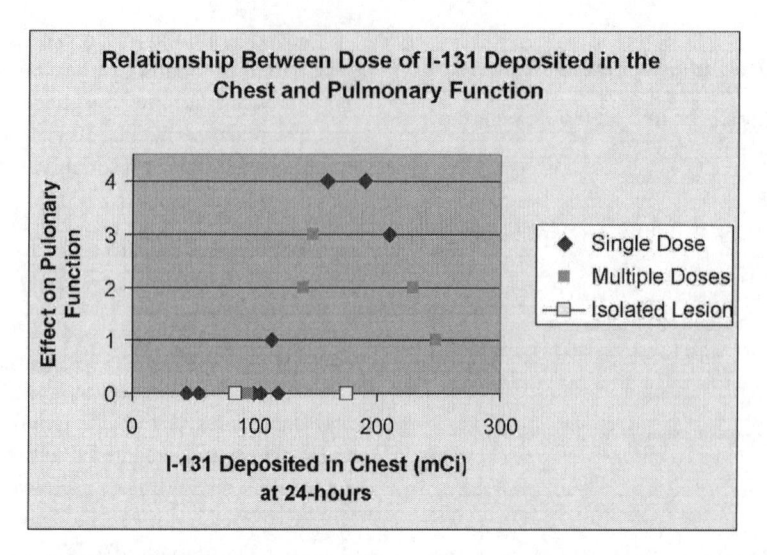

Fig. 2. This data was compiled from Rall's original article. Changes in pulmonary function begin to appear after the ^{131}I deposited in the chest at 24 h exceeded 125 mCi. The effect of pulmonary function was graded as following: 0 = none; 1 = minimal X-ray reaction; 2 = moderate X-ray reaction; 3 = moderate X-ray reaction + symptoms; 4 = death from pulmonary insufficiency.

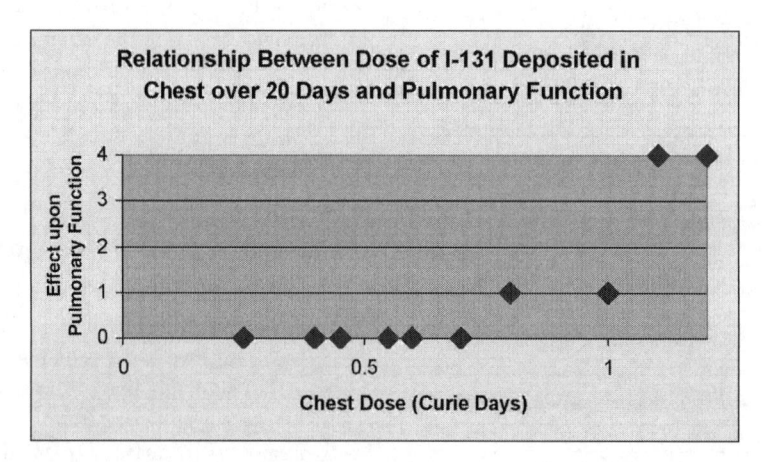

Fig. 3. The two fatalities from radiation pneumonitis reported by Rall each had over 1 Ci-d of radioiodine retention in the lung. This was calculated by summing the calculated lung retention for each day over 20 d. The effect of pulmonary function was graded as following: 0 = none; 1 = minimal X-ray reaction; 2 = moderate X-ray reaction; 3 = moderate X-ray reaction + symptoms; 4 = death from pulmonary insufficiency.

   c. The disease is a single focus, rather than multiple foci.
   d. The disease pattern is more regional than diffuse, such as one or two macronodular areas of disease instead of diffuse micronodular or miliary disease. (However, note that patients with a micronodular or miliary pattern of metastases with good radioiodine uptake may have an improved response and prognosis after treatment with radioiodine *(96–98)*.
5. Determine the response on clinical exam, chest X-ray, CT without contrast, PFT with DLCOs, radioiodine scans, and blood thyroglobulin levels after previous treatments.
6. Recommend dosimetry, and follow the restrictions for pulmonary metastases, as described by Benua and Leeper.
   a. Do not exceed a radioiodine-prescribed activity that would result in whole-body retention at 48 h of more than 2.96 GBq (80 mCi).
   b. Do not exceed a radioiodine-prescribed activity that would result in greater than 200 cGy (rads) to the blood (bone marrow).
7. If an empiric prescribed activity of 7.4 GBq (200 mCi) or more is going to be used, and the patient has a diffuse micronodular or miliary pattern of metastases in the lung, we strongly recommend that a reliable effort be made to estimate the whole-body retention at 48 h or the whole lung retention at 24 h, and adjust the prescribed activity accordingly. Of note, Leeper *(99)* reported that 19% of the radioiodine-prescribed activities that delivered 200 cGy (rads) to the blood were below 7.4 GBq (200 mCi). Tuttle et al. *(139)* reported that 5% of patients receiving 200 mCi (7.5 GBq) of ^{131}I would have received 200 rads (cGy) or more to the blood. Atkins et al. *(140)* reported 11% (14 of 127) of the radioiodine prescribed activities administering 200 cGy (rads) to the blood were less than 7.4 GBq (200 mCi).

Table 12
Review of the Literature

Author (Ref.)	Pneumonitis	Pulmonary Fibrosis or Impairment	Fatal	Dosimetry	Comments
Aldrich (76)		7/35	2/35	No	Impairment may have been part of thyroid cancer or concomitant lung disease
Benua (23)	5/59	1/59	2/59	Yes	
Brown (33)	0/31	0/31	0/31	No	1. Dose typically 150 mCi 2. Average dose 680 mCi
Edmonds (25)	0/5	1/5	0/5	No	1. Dose typically 150 mCi 2. Range 378–973 mCi 3. Follow-up 8–17 yr 4. Progressive impairment, which may have been part of disease itself
Leeper (92)	0/70*	0/70*	0/70*	Yes	1. Average dose of 309 mCi 2. Range 70–654 mCi
Maheshwari (30)	0/53	1/53	0/53	No	Dose typically 50–200 mCi
Menzel (77)	0/23	0/23	0/23	No	Used empiric dose as high as 300 mCi
Pacini (138)		1/86	1/86	No	Respiratory failure from thyroid cancer, ^{131}I, or both could not be differentiated
Samuel (93)	1/35	1/35	0/35	No	1. Highest dose 270 mCi 2. Highest total dose 1194 mCi 3. Data based on ^{99m}Tc-DTPA clearance
Schlumberger (94)	0/23	0/23	0/23	No	Administer repeated prescribed activities of 100 mCi
Van Nostrand (22)	0/6*	0/6*	0/6*	Yes	Highest dose 450 mCi
Total	6/305	12/426	5/426		

*After restriction imposed of not exceeding 80 mCi of ^{131}I whole body retention at 48 h.

8. Reduce prescribed activity of radioiodine in the presence of impaired pretreatment PFTs.
9. With higher empiric or dosimetrically determined doses, retreat with radioiodine no sooner than 1 yr from the last treatment.
10. For patients with changes indicating PF from previous radioiodine therapy, consider pulmonary biopsy to assess the degree of PF.

Recommended Posttreatment Management

In follow-up for the radioiodine treatment of patients who have functioning pulmonary metastases from well-differentiated thyroid carcinoma, we recommend the following:

- Educate the patient regarding the signs and symptoms to carefully monitor, including any cough or shortness of breath, which may be the initial warning of pulmonary complications.
- Encourage the patient to seek *early* evaluation for any respiratory symptoms.
- Schedule routine follow-up evaluations at 1- and 2-mo post-therapy.
- Recommend PFTs at 1 and 2 mo. (Until data is available to demonstrate that there is no value of PFTs at these time points, we believe these should be performed as part of the assessment for early pulmonary changes that may benefit from early treatment.)
- Repeat PFTs at 4, 6, and 12 mo.
- Schedule follow-up visits with the patient at monthly intervals for a minimum of 1 yr.

For those patients with possible ARP and PF, we recommend the following:

- Begin treatment as soon as possible.
- Consider initial therapy with nonsteroidal anti-inflammatory agents or inhaled steroids, and
- Consider the *early* use of oral or intravenous steroids and antibiotics.

Summary

In summary, ARP and PF can be serious conditions of radioiodine treatment in patients who have functioning pulmonary metastases from well-differentiated thyroid cancer. Although scientific data are still limited, evidence is available based on approximately 50 yr of clinical experience that suggests empiric and dosimetric approaches for the radioiodine treatment of pulmonary metastases, with a minimal risk of complications. Nevertheless, additional research is needed in this area. If ARP does occur, early detection and treatment is strongly recommended.

GASTROINTESTINAL EFFECTS

^{131}I ingestion is followed by rapid absorption through the stomach and small-bowel wall into the systemic circulation, with subsequent active gastric mucosa concentration and secretion. This direct stomach irradiation engenders no symptoms in most patients at ingested dosage below 1.11 GBq (30 mCi). As the administered ^{131}I dosage escalates, nausea is experienced by more patients; 5.35% of patients complain of this side effect at a standard dose of 1.48 GBq (40 mCi; 32). In 78 patients treated with a standard ablation-prescribed activity of 2.78 GBq (75 mCi) for residual thyroid bed activity, nausea was reported in 12% of patients when questioned at 4–5 d postablation (J. Freitas, unpublished data). The majority of patients (50–67%) treated with prescribed activity of 5.55 GBq (150 mCi) of ^{131}I will complain of nausea that usually develops after 18–24 h, but can be seen within 2–4 h of therapy and persists for 24–48 h (22,23). Whether the frequency of ^{131}I associated nausea in these studies and seen in our practice is accentuated by the concomitant use of sialogogues (e.g., tart candies) is not known. Vomiting with or without preceding nausea is rarely seen (probably <1%) at a prescribed activity less than 3.7 GBq (<100 mCi) but does occur at higher ^{131}I prescribed activity (8%) with 5.55 GBq (150 mCi) and 15% with an average dose of 11.7 GBq (316 mCi; 2,3). Prior to May 29, 1997, Nuclear Regulatory Commission (NRC) guidelines mandated in-patient hospitalization for any patient whose whole-body retention exceeded 1.11 GBq (30 mCi) of ^{131}I (equivalent to ≥5 mR at 1 m). If vomiting occurred in the in-patient setting, radioiodine in gastric contents was contained within a controlled area (100). New NRC guidelines, the so-called "Patient Discharge Rules," are "exposure"-based, rather than patient activity–based. Patients receiving up to 7.4 GBq (200 mCi) of ^{131}I are now routinely released by many licensees when the total effective dose equivalent of a member of the public exposed to the patient is not likely to exceed 5 mSv (0.5 rem; 101). Patients treated with more than 3.7 GBq (>100 mCi) of ^{131}I have returned to a medical facility after vomiting unknown quantities of ^{131}I in an uncontrolled location. The possibility of an outpatient vomiting over 1.85 GBq (>50 mCi) of ^{131}I in the home environment (or local motel), significantly contaminating family members or the general public, has greatly heightened the awareness of this issue. Patients with a multiplicity of disease processes are at increased risk of vomiting ingested ^{131}I, including anxiety disorder, cerebral palsy, any pharyngeal or esophageal motility disorder, gastroesophageal reflux disease, gastroparesis, gastric outlet obstruction, and other similar entities. To lessen the chance of dealing with a large quantity of vomited radioiodine, one patient with a prior vomiting history shortly after a diagnostic ^{131}I ingestion and another patient with marked diabetic gastroparesis received their therapy with the commercially available oral formulation (after sterilization) intravenously with no subsequent nausea, vomiting, or other sequelae. However, intravenous ^{131}I does not eliminate the possibility of vomiting ^{131}I entirely because blood clearance curves of oral and intravenous ^{131}I are similar. Additionally, a significant percentage of the intravenously administered radioiodine will be secreted into the stomach within the next 24 h, as noted above.

For most patients, nausea and vomiting can usually be averted or ameliorated by premedication with antiemetic preparations, such as ondansetron (Zofran), prochlorperazine (Compazine), or triethylperazine (Torecan). Emphasizing the possible side effects of nausea and vomiting seems to help precipitate their occurrence, especially in anxious patients. Our current practice is to provide the patient with a prescription for six ondansetron 8-mg tablets, taking one tablet three times daily beginning 30 min prior to ^{131}I therapy. If necessary, the first 8-mg dose of ondansetron can be administered intravenously if the patient neglects to take the medication as prescribed. With ^{131}I-prescribed activity more than 7.4 GBq (>200 mCi), total-body radiation dose can exceed 50 rem, and fatigue, headache, nausea, and vomiting attributable to acute radiation sickness can occur within 12 h but usually dissipate within 24–36 h as retained ^{131}I decreases with diuresis and catharsis. Fatalities at a threshold of approximately 100 Sv (rem) of whole-body exposure can occur. Such exposures can be seen even with prescribed activity of less than 7.4 GBq (<200 mCi) if renal failure ensues before excretion of the majority of administered ^{131}I (102). Such sequelae as acute radiation sickness are less frequently seen now than (36%) when much larger prescribed activities were more commonly given (23). We now administer ^{131}I-prescribed activity in a narrower range and optimize the environment surrounding the procedure to maximize results and minimize complications.

Finally, Kinuya (103) reported a Mallory-Weiss syndrome caused by ^{131}I therapy for metastatic thyroid carcinoma. The patient had massive hematemesis secondary to a tear at the gastroesophageal junction, with only mild nausea and no initial vomiting.

RADIATION CYSTITIS

Balan (104) reported one case of cystitis, as did Dobyns (105).

BONE MARROW

Bone marrow suppression, aplastic anemia, and leukemia are some of the most serious potential untoward affects of radioiodine therapy. This section discusses bone marrow suppression and aplastic anemia. Leukemia is discussed separately in this chapter.

Review of the Literature

Like all side effects of radioiodine ablation and treatment, the variability in the reported frequency and severity of bone marrow suppression is also multifactorial, and some of these factors are noted in Table 13. A summary of the frequency occurrence of bone marrow suppression based on a review of the literature is presented in Table 14. To demonstrate examples of the severity of bone marrow suppression according to National Cancer Institute (NCI) criteria and the typical time courses, two hypothetical cases are shown in Figs. 4 and 5. The Common Terminology Criteria for Adverse Events for hematologic toxicities are noted in Table 15. A review of the literature on the frequency of reported aplastic anemia is noted in Table 16. The specifics of selected articles are subsequently discussed.

Alexander et al. *(2)* reported that 9 out of 203 patients treated with between 3.7 and 7.4 GBq (100–200 mCi) of radioiodine demonstrated hematological abnormalities involving moderate reduction of their leukocytes that ranged from 3200 to 4200 per µL (normal range: 4300–10,000/µL). They also reported no signs of thrombocytopenia or aplastic anemia, and the total cumulative prescribed activity ranged from 0.1 to 1.9 Ci (3.7–70.3 GBq).

Benua et al. *(23)* reported bone marrow suppression in 38 of 59 patients who received 122 treatments. Serious bone marrow depression was observed following these treatments in eight patients; two patients subsequently died of bone marrow suppression. Benua has suggested a relationship of significant bone marrow suppression when the total radiation dose to the blood exceeded 200 cGy (rads). Serious complications, including bone marrow suppression, were observed in 21% when total radiation to the blood exceeded 200 cGy (rads) but in only 3% when the total radiation to the blood was less than 200 cGy (rads). Furthermore, bone marrow suppression was also increased when the whole-body retention at 48 h exceeded 4.44 GBq (120 mCi). Although Benua reported severe and permanent bone marrow suppression in 8 of 59 patients, after Benua imposed the restrictions of (1) a maximum of 200 cGy (rads) to the blood and (2) 4.44 GBq (120 mCi) whole-body retention at 48 h, no subsequent cases of permanent bone marrow suppression have occurred as reported by Leeper *(91)*.

Benua further reported that the mean whole-blood radiation dose from the ^{131}I treatments in the 59 patients was 267 rads (2.67 Gy), with a range of 45–740 rads (0.45–7.4 Gy). For the eight patients with severe bone marrow suppression, the calculated total radiation dose to the blood from the last radioiodine treatment ranged from 170 rads (1.7 Gy) to 582 rads (5.8 Gy). However, all had been previously treated. For six of the eight patients with severe bone marrow sup-

Table 13
Variability of Frequency and Severity of Bone Marrow Suppression

Individual prescribed activity of radioiodine
Patient's rate of radioiodine clearance
Frequency of treatments
Interval between treatments
Total cumulative prescribed activities of radioiodine
Frequency of prescribed activities delivering greater than 200 or 300 cGy (rads) to the bone marrow
Performance of Benua and Leeper dosimetry
Variability in the definition of bone marrow suppression
Variability in the diligence in evaluating bone marrow suppression
Patient bone marrow reserve
Extensive bone metastases
Prior or concomitant radiation therapy to the bone

pression in whom total-blood radiation dose could be calculated for the cumulative radioiodine administered, the total radiation dose to the blood ranged from 300 to 1100 rads (3–11 Gy). Severe bone marrow suppression was not observed if the total cumulative radiation dose to the blood was less than 300 cGy (rads).

Dobyns et al. *(105)* noted that the most likely change in the blood is a decline in the lymphocytes.

Dorn et al. *(106)* performed 104 treatments with prescribed activities determined by a dosimetric MIRD methodology (see Chapter 47 on dosimetry). In 100% (25 of 25) of patients who received absorbed doses of lower than 300 cGy (rads) to the bone marrow, transient bone marrow suppression was present. However, no permanent bone marrow suppression was observed. The maximum single administered dose was 38.5 GBq (1040 mCi).

Edmonds and Smith *(25)* found that 3 patients from a group of 258 developed aplastic anemia and died within 4 yr; they had extensive metastases and were treated multiple times. The total radioactivity was 63 GBq (1700 mCi), 40 GBq (1080 mCi), and 31 GBq (850 mCi). In this study, patients were initially treated with 2.9 GBq (80 mCi) for ablation and, when necessary, with additional treatments of 5.5 GBq (150 mCi) every few months.

Grunwald et al. *(107)* indicated that 1% (7 of 567) of patients who had radioiodine treatments had persistent changes in blood counts. In patients who received prescribed cumulative activities of less than 18.5 GBq (500 mCi), only 5 of 469 had a hemoglobin less than or equal to 9.0, white blood cell count (WBC) 2500 or less, and/or platelets 50,000 or less. For prescribed activities of 18.5 GBq (500 mCi) to less than 37 GBq (<1000 mCi), 1 of 77 patients had changes, and with prescribed activities of 37 GBq (≥1000 mCi), 6 of 21 patients had blood changes, and four of these patients had pancyotpenia.

Table 14
Summary of Bone Marrow Suppression

Author (Ref.)	Year	Total	Any Hematological Abnormality	Hemoglobin	WBC	Platelets
Alexander (26)	1998	203	4.4% (9)	0% (0)	4.4% (9)	No evidence
Benua (23)	1962 1980	122	31% (38)[a]	–	–	–
Dorn (106)	2003	25	100% (25)	–	–	–
Leeper (91)	1982		No permanent bone marrow suppression	–	–	–
Edmonds (25)	1986	258	1.1% (3)[b]	–	–	–
Grunwald (107)	1994	567	1.4% (8)	–	–	–
Haynie (108)	1963	159	–	34% (54)	10%	8.4% (5)
Keldsen (109)	1988	27	26% (15)	–	33% in female (and increased in male)	30% in female and 17 in male
Matthies (110)	2004	68			22% (15)	12% (8)
Menzel (77) (low prescribed activity, see text)	1996	84	3.6% (3)[c]	0% (0)	3.6% (3)	0% (0)
Menzel (77) (high prescribed activity, see text)	1996	78	50% (34)[d]	–	–	–
Pan (29)	2004	–	–	–	4.0%	10.4%
Petrich (111)	2001	107	37.4% (40/107)	–	–	–
Robeson (112)	2002	12	42% (5/12)	25% (3/12)	42% (5/12)	17% (2)
Schober (113)	1987	296		24% (71)	11% (33)	35% (104)
Trunnell (68)	1949	9	100% (9)	–	–	–
Van Nostrand (22)	1986	10	90% (9)	–	–	–

[a]Total of 59 patients and 122 doses. Six of the 122 treatments produced severe bone marrow suppression, with two resulting in death.
[b]It is unclear from the article if the author looked for bone marrow suppression other than when it was fatal.
[c]Prescribed activities of radioiodine were 1.8–5.5 GBq (49–200 mCi).
[d]Prescribed activities of radioiodine were greater than 7.4 GBq (200 mCi). Bone marrow suppression was mild in thirty, grade II in three patients and severe in one patient. The data was not fully described.

Haynie and Beierwaltes (108) reported their observations in 159 patients who received ^{131}I for treatment of thyroid cancer at 3-mo intervals (if needed) between 1947 and 1960. Evaluation of these patients included a baseline and at least one posttreatment complete blood count (CBC). The patients received prescribed activities of usually 3.7–11.1 GBq (100–300 mCi) of ^{131}I with follow-up CBC at 3 mo and 1-yr intervals for 10 yr after completion of therapy. The most frequently observed abnormality was a subnormal hemoglobin concentration, which occurred in 34% (54 of 159). However, only 5 of 159 developed a significant anemia less than 10 gram percent. The hemoglobin concentration returned to the normal range in all but eight patients by 1 yr. Subnormal WBC was observed in about 10% of these patients, and the lowest value was 2000 per mm^3. No leukopenia persisted beyond 1 yr. Thrombocytopenia was seen in only five (3%) patients, whose levels were only slightly decreased below the normal limits. If it did occur, thrombocytopenia was always transient and returned to normal by 1 yr. The degree of suppressed blood counts did appear to correlate with several factors: total ^{131}I dosage, prior radiation therapy, and the presence of widely disseminated metastases. Nevertheless, the authors reported that the suppressed blood count duration was brief and not associated with symptoms. They also reported no incidence of aplastic anemia.

Keldsen et al. (109) reported that 26% (15 of 27) of their patients' WBC count dropped below 2500 and/or platelet count fell less than 150,000 at some point after treatment. The drop in platelet count was 30% (305,000–212,000) in females and 17% (271,000–224,000) in males. The WBC lowered 33% (6000 to 4400) in women and increased in men.

In a group of 70 patients treated from 1973 through 1982, Leeper (91) observed no permanent bone marrow suppression. As previously noted, the average single therapeutic dose was

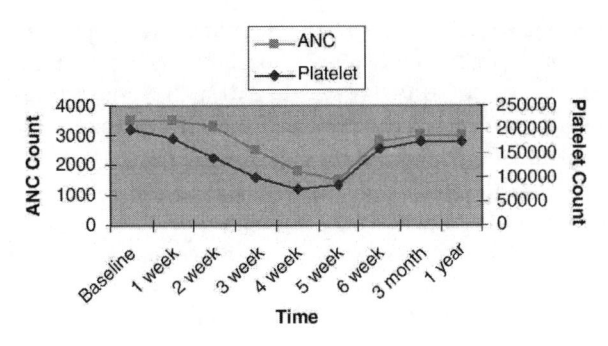

Fig. 4. Hypothetical course NCI grade 1 mild to moderate bone marrow suppression.

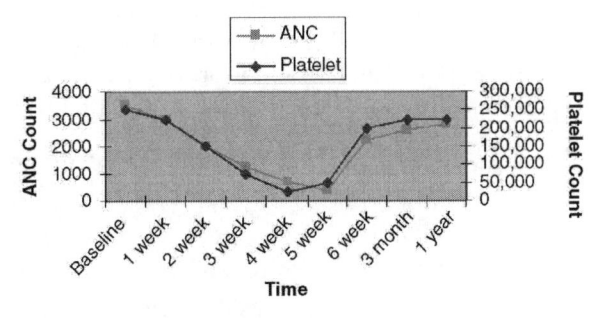

Fig. 5. Hypothetical course NCI grade 4 severe bone marrow suppression.

Table 15
The NCI Common Terminology Criteria for Adverse Events

Adverse Event	Grade 1	Grade 2	Grade 3	Grade 4	Grade 5
Hemoglobin	<LLN–10.0 g/dL	<10.0–8.0 g/dL	<8.0–6.5 g/dL	<6.5 g/dL	Death
Leukocytes (total WBCs)	<LLN–3000 mm^3	<3000–2000 mm^3	<2000–1000 mm^3	<1000 mm^3	Death
Neutrophils/granulocytes	<LLN–1500 mm^3	<1500–1000 mm^3	<1000–500 mm^3	<500 mm^3	Death
Platelets	<LLN–75,000 mm^3	<75,000–50,000 mm^3	<50,000–25,000 mm^3	<25,000 mm^3	Death

<LLN, less than the lower limits of normal for that particular laboratory. Criteria is from December 12, 2003.

Table 16
Aplastic Anemia or Death Attributed to Bone Marrow Suppression

Author (Ref.)	Year	Aplastic Anemia
Alexander (2)	1998	0% (0/203)
Benua (23)	1962	1.6% (2/122)
Dorn (106)	2003	0% (25/25)
Edmonds (25)	1986	1.2% (3/258)
Haynie (108)	1963	0% (0/159)
Leeper (92)	1982	0% (0/70)
Menzel (77)	1996	0.5% (1/167)[a]
Petrich (111)	2001	3.7% (4/107)
Schober (113)	1987	1.0% (3/296)
Schumichen (114)	1983	0.75% (3/400)
Tollefson (31)	1964	0% (0/70)[b]
Van Nostrand (22)	1986	0% (0/10)

[a]Patient rejected for additional treatments because of persistent severe bone marrow suppression.

[b]In the evaluation of 70 fatalities in patients with thyroid cancer, none were because of bone marrow suppression.

11.4 GBq (309 mCi), with a range of 70 to 2.59–24.2 GBq (654 mCi). No additional data was reported pertaining to the extent of reversible bone marrow suppression.

Matthias et al. (110) reported on the hematologic toxicity in 68 patients who received cumulative radioiodine prescribed activities that ranged from 18.5 to 153.5 GBq (500–4150 mCi.) Thrombocytopenia occurred in five patients with grade I or II and in three patients with grade III or IV. Grade I comprises anemia of 9.5–10.0 g Hb/100/mL, thrombocytopenia of 75,000–99,000/mm^3 or leukopenia of 3000–3900 mm^3. Grade II is anemia of 8.0–9.4 g Hb/100 mL, thrombocytopenia of 50,000–74,000/mm^3, or leukopenia of 2000–2900/mm^3. Grade III is classified as persistent and distinct anemia of less than 7.9 g Hb/100 mL, thrombocytopenia of less than 49,000/mm^3 or leukopenia below 1900/mm^3. Leukopenia was observed in 14 patients with grade I or II and 1 patient with grade IV. The specific-grading scale used was not noted.

Menzel et al. *(77)* evaluated a group of 26 patients with 167 treatments. He reported that only 3 of 84 treatments with a low-radioiodine dose of less than 1.8–5.55 GBq (<49–200 mCi) resulted in mild hematological toxicity (leukocytes <3000/nL and/or thrombocytes <75,000/nL. For patients who received high-prescribed activities (11.1 GBq [300 mCi] or higher), 38% (30 of 78) of treatments caused a mild decline of leukocyte count. Three patients developed World Health Organization (WHO) grade II hematotoxicity. One patient had four therapies totaling 44.4 GBq (1200 mCi); one had two therapies that totaled 22.2 GBq (600 mCi), and one patient developed severe leucopenia and thrombocytopenia (WHO grade III) after three high-activity therapies. The patients in this study were typically treated at 3-mo intervals.

Pan et al. *(29)* evaluated 342 patients over approximately 10 yr. Transient platelet reduction was noted in 10.4%, and transient leukopenia was found in 4% of patients. The frequency of abnormalities was higher with cumulative radioiodine doses greater than 18.5 GBq (500 mCi).

Petrich et al. *(111)* described the side effects of radioiodine in the treatment of 107 patients who had bone metastases secondary to well-differentiated thyroid carcinoma. Of 107 patients, 40 (37.4%) had a change in their blood counts. Most of the changes were WHO grade I or grade II. A total of 10 patients had grade III and 4 patients had bone marrow aplasia.

With prescribed activities of radioiodine equal to or exceeding 80% of the dosimetrically-determined dosage, Robeson et al. *(112)* found that 42% (5 of 12) of patients had mild leukopenia, 17% (2 of 12) had mild thrombocytopenia, and 25% (3 of 12) had anemia. Hypocellular bone marrow biopsy was noted in one patient. He reported no difference in the average cumulative prescribed activity in patients with and without bone marrow suppression.

Schober et al. *(113)* reported on 296 patients who were treated with an average cumulative prescribed activity of 19.8 GBq (536 mCi). The observation period was a median of 65 mo. The most frequently observed hematologic change was thrombocytopenia, occurring in 35% of patients. Erythrocytopenia occurred in 24%, and the leukocytes decreased in 11% but increased in 23%, with a median decrease of 7%. The most severe decreased counts occurred after a high dose of 37 GBq or more (≥1000 mCi). Pancytopenia was present in 4.4% of all patients and was probably a contributing cause of death in three patients.

Tollefsen et al. *(31)* examined the cause of fatalities in 70 patients who had thyroid carcinoma. None of these deaths were attributed to bone marrow suppression. Notably, some of these patients were included in earlier reports from MSKCI *(119)*.

Trunnell et al. *(68)* reported that all patients (9 of 9) treated for metastatic thyroid cancer had depression of one or more peripheral blood elements. The greatest drop occurred in lymphocytes from a level of one third to one fourth of baseline. They reported one fatality from pancytopenia that occurred 1 mo after the last treatment, which was 9.25 GBq (250 mCi), and a total prescribed activity of 638 mCi (23.6 GBq). Bone marrow aspiration biopsies were performed in seven patients, demonstrating a uniform drop in total cell count and reversal of the erythroid myeloid ratio. With the exception of the fatality noted above, peripheral bloods counts recovered in 4–6 mo.

Van Nostrand et al. *(22)* described 9 of 10 patients who had bone marrow suppression that was transient and never required any transfusions. The most severe bone marrow suppression was <NCI grade I for hemoglobin, NCI grade II for leukocytes, and NCI grade I for platelets. Radioiodine-prescribed activities ranged from 1.9 to 16.7 GBq (51–450 mCi), and the total previous cumulative prescribed activity was 0–25 GBq (0–665 mCi).

Recommendations for Pretreatment and Posttherapy Management

The difficulty with suggesting recommendations for the pre- and posttreatment management of possible bone marrow suppression secondary to radioiodine therapy is that there are no good studies that have evaluated the efficacy of any specific pre- or posttreatment plan. However, the physician must still act. In the absence of good prospective data, the recommendations must be made upon incomplete retrospective data. Various suggestions have been proposed by different workers in the field, but a discussion of all these approaches is beyond the scope of this chapter. Instead, one proposed set of recommendations is presented below. These recommendations should be appropriately modified according to the specific clinical situation unique to each patient, the objectives of the physician, and the potential clinical benefit vs the risk of irreversible bone marrow suppression.

General Recommendations for all Patients

Several key methods are proposed for all patients regarding the pretreatment and posttherapy management of potential bone marrow suppression.

1. Obtain baseline CBC. Importantly, all other recommendations are based on a CBC with differential that was obtained when the patient was in a euthyroid state. Because the absolute neutrophil count (ANC) may be reduced in the hypothyroid state *(115,116)*, a baseline CBC obtained under this condition may not be appropriate to use for long-term follow-up. However, an additional baseline CBC when the patient is hypothyroid just before ablation may be useful for the short-term follow-up. This information might help identify any initial decline in blood counts relative to the baseline euthyroid CBC as secondary to the hypothyroidism, not the radioiodine.
2. For any reduction of the baseline CBC values, evaluate and correct any other cause for the reduced baseline CBC.
3. If the pretherapy scan demonstrates significant radioiodine uptake in bone or lung metastases, consider dosimetric modification of the prescribed radioiodine activity.

4. Recommend CBC with differential at 3, 4, 5, and 6 wk after radioiodine ablation. If the patient has no decrease in any blood counts after ablation or treatment, then discontinue CBCs after 6 wk. If the patient has a significant drop in blood counts within the first 6 wk, then continue weekly blood counts until the patient clearly has a rising ANC and platelet count and is no longer at risk for infection or bleeding.
5. For significant bone marrow suppression, administer colony-stimulating factor(s) or transfusion as may be clinically warranted. An oncologist should be part of the treating team.
6. Finally, obtain CBC with differential at 3 mo and 1 yr after ablation.

Sequential CBCs after initial ablation will most likely not affect the clinical management of these patients; however, we believe that this data could be important if a subsequent treatment is required. Most patients will not require retreatment, and although staging can help predict which groups of patients are more likely to need retreatment, the physician can never be certain of this for any specific patient. Sequential CBCs obtained after initial ablation may be the only information regarding the response of the patient's bone marrow to previous therapeutic prescribed activities of radioiodine. Because of the potential value of this information, and because four to six CBCs are relatively inexpensive and usually associated with minor inconvenience, this author recommends that this be obtained in every patient.

Specific Recommendations for Selected Patients

For initial ablations with an empiric dose of up to 5.55 GBq (150 mCi) in patients whose CBC and differential is abnormal and cannot be corrected, reduction of the ablative prescribed activity of radioiodine should be considered. Unfortunately, no data are available regarding how much the empiric ablative prescribed activity should be reduced, if at all, and this also depends on what the original planned empiric ablative prescribed activity would have been. However, despite the lack of information, the physician must again still make a decision. Accordingly, we propose that if the euthyroid baseline CBC is reduced to NCI grade I (see above), and the planned prescribed activity was 5.55 GBq (150 mCi), then the prescribed activity should be lowered by 20–30%. For NCI grade II or higher, dosimetry can be used to derive a maximum prescribed activity, then reducing this value can account for the patient's compromised hematological status.

Subsequent treatments for metastases in patients who have normal baseline CBC, ANC, and platelet count should not exceed an empiric prescribed activity greater than 7.4 GBq (200 mCi). If the prescribed activity is based instead on dosimetry, then as much as one's facility allows up to the dosimetrically-determined prescribed activity should be administered. A minimum of 6 mo and preferably 1 yr is recommended between treatments of dosimetrically-determined prescribed activities. At the present time, there is no evidence whether the total cumulative estimated radiation dose to the blood (not the total cumulative radioiodine prescribed activity) should influence any reduction in dosimetrically-determined prescribed activity.

For subsequent treatments of metastases in patients who had previous radioiodine treatments with an uncorrectable abnormal CBC, then the suggestions in Table 18 should be considered.

Summary

Bone marrow suppression is an important untoward effect of radioiodine treatment. Clinically significant bone marrow suppression because of the first radioiodine ablation is unlikely. However, the overall data indicates that the frequency and severity of bone marrow suppression increases as (1) the individual prescribed activity of radioiodine increases, (2) the individual radiation dose to the blood exceeds 200 or 300 cGy (rads), (3) the frequency of treatments increases, (4) the interval between treatments decreases, (5) the total cumulative prescribed activity of radioiodine rises, (6) the total cumulative radiation dose to the blood increases, and (7) extensive bone marrow metastases occurs.

Sequential routine CBCs after *all* ablations and treatments may be helpful in those patients who develop subsequent metastases and require repeated, higher prescribed activities of radioiodine. With a carefully considered plan, the availability of colony-stimulating factors, and good follow-up, bone marrow suppression should be manageable.

FERTILITY

Gonadal irradiation from ^{131}I therapy is derived from multiple sources (blood, bladder, gut, and local metastases) and leads to concerns about subsequent infertility and genetic change. Transient ovarian failure manifested by menses cessation and elevated levels of serum follicle-stimulating hormone (FSH) and luteinizing hormone during the first-year posttherapy was seen in 27% (18 of 66) of a group of older women (median age 34 yr) treated with an average single ^{131}I dose of 9.99 GBq (270 mCi; *117*). The estimated mean ovarian dose in the amenorrheic women was 176 vs 158 cGy (rads; $p > 0.5$) in the menstruating women, but the amenorrheic group was significantly older (median 40 vs 32 yr; $p < 0.001$). The onset of amenorrhea was delayed for at least one menstrual cycle following ^{131}I therapy in all effected women and persisted for less than 6 mo in 14 of 18 patients, despite a usually prompt return to a euthyroid status after ^{131}I therapy. In another study, transient ovarian failure was less frequent, occurring in 8% of 409 younger women (median age 31 yr), but again, the amenorrheic women were older (mean age 36) than their normal menstruating cohort (mean age 31; *118*). The delay in onset of the amenorrhea suggests a radiation effect on developing oocytes, rather than on a maturing follicle.

Table 17
Recommendations for Evaluation and Treatment of Patients With Bone Marrow Suppression

Obtain unilateral or bilateral bone marrow biopsy to assess the bone marrow cellularity and degree of adipose tissue.
    Unless the purpose of the bone marrow biopsy is to assess a specific area for the presence of metastatic well-differentiated thyroid carcinoma, the bone marrow biopsy should not be obtained from a bone that is suspected to have metastasis or has had previous external radiotherapy.
    Fibrosis of the marrow is not a manifestation of delayed radiation injury of the bone marrow.
Assess for the presence and extent of bone metastases such as with bone scan, radiographic bone survey, magnetic resonance, and/or positron emission tomography scan.
Review the baseline and subsequent CBCs after previous treatments.
Review the history for extent of any external radiation therapy to the bone marrow.
Review the response to previous radioiodine therapy, such as change in scan, change in thyroglobulin level, or size of masses clinically or on other radiographic studies.
Recommend blood and whole body dosimetry:
    Do not exceed the prescribed activity calculated by dosimetry.
    Do not exceed 4.44 GBq (120 mCi) of ^{131}I whole-body retention at 48 h (In the presence of pulmonary metastases whole body retention at 48 h should not exceed 2.96 GBq [80 mCi]. See the Acute Radiation Pneumonitis and the Pulmonary Fibrosis section in this chapter and Chapter 47 on dosimetry).
If the bone marrow aspiration/biopsy is normal:
    Weigh the potential benefit of radioiodine vs other treatments, which will depend on such factors as the degree of radioiodine uptake, size of tumor, patient desires, and so on.
    Consider reduction of the prescribed activity below the maximum calculated dosimetry prescribed activity. In the absence of data, suggest a 20–25% reduction of prescribed activity for patients who have a NCI grade I or II reduction of leukocytes, absolute neutrophil count, and/or platelets.
    Consider pretreatment with the appropriate colony-stimulating factor(s).
If bone marrow biopsy is abnormal:
    Weigh the potential benefit of radioiodine vs other treatments, which will depend on such factors as the bone marrow cellularity and degree of fat on the bone marrow biopsy, degree of radioiodine uptake in the metastases, tumor size, patient desires, and so forth. "Blind treatments" (treatment when no uptake is seen on radioiodine scan) are not recommended in these patients.
    Reduce the administered prescribed activity below the maximum calculated dosimetric-determined prescribed activity.
    Prophylactically treat with granulocyte- or platelet-stimulating factor.
    Consider stem cell harvest for rescue bone marrow transplantation. No data is available regarding this option.
    If possible, avoid treating within 1 yr from previous treatment.
    Consider amifostine treatment. Amifostine has been proposed to help protect the bone marrow; however, no data is available regarding whether the amifostine also protects thyroid cancer. Amifostine has been discussed elsewhere (see section on salivary gland side effects).

However, no decrease in fertility in women treated with ^{131}I has been shown, but the miscarriage rate appears higher in the first year following ^{131}I therapy. Whether this is secondary to radioiodine irradiation or simply reflects insufficient thyroid hormone control during this time remains to be established, but it should be standard practice to strongly discourage conception in the first year following ^{131}I treatment (118–120). No significant increase in congenital anomalies has been seen in subsequent pregnancies of ^{131}I treated thyroid cancer patients, despite cumulative radiation exposures to ovaries of more than 100 cGy (rads) (122). Such ovarian radiation exposure can be reduced by forced hydration for 24–48 h after ^{131}I administration, frequent micturition during the day and night, and laxatives to prevent constipation and retention of isotope in the colon.

Similarly, transient testicular failure manifested by elevated serum FSH concentrations and depressed inhibin B levels, the best markers of germinal cell injury, was seen by 6 mo in men (100%) following their initial ^{131}I therapy but returned to normal by 18 mo (121). Employing thermoluminescence dosimetry in 14 patients, the testicular radiation dose was shown prospectively to approximate 2.3 cGy/GBq/testes (0.085 rad/mCi/testes) (not higher postulated levels) that should be insufficient to induce infertility with typical single therapies of prescribed activity of 2.8–5.55 GBq (75–150 mCi), delivering 6.3–12.6 cGy (rads; 122). However, each subsequent ^{131}I therapy magnifies the initial germinal cell insult and leads to a gradual elevation of baseline FSH levels (measured prior to subsequent ^{131}I therapy), with the degree of baseline FSH elevation directly related to the cumulative prescribed activity of ^{131}I received (123). This rise in FSH was associated with a fall in sperm count and motility in eight of nine patients tested. Thus, permanent germinal cell damage may be more common in males than in females, leading to a significant risk of infertility in those patients with locally extensive or metastatic disease who are likely to receive large cumulative ^{131}I-prescribed activity.

In males with extensive or resistant thyroid cancer likely to receive cumulative ^{131}I-prescribed activity more than 14.8 GBq (400 mCi), family planning should be discussed. The possibility of storage of sperm or fertilized ova of these patients should be discussed if future offspring are desired. In addition, it should be noted that the testicular radiation exposure from each ^{131}I treatment can be reduced by forced hydration, frequent urination, and prevention of constipation (as discussed above), and such practices should be strongly encouraged. In several follow-up studies of male thyroid cancer patients treated with ^{131}I (123,124), fertility was not reduced, compared to the general population. There are no data to suggest an increase in congenital anomalies or in the miscarriage rate of sexual partners impregnated by male patients in the first year after ^{131}I treatment. Nevertheless, it would seem prudent to discourage impregnation during the first year following such therapy. In the past, male patients have not been typically discouraged from impregnating their sexual partners in the first year after ^{131}I treatment, but this perspective is changing.

OTHER CANCERS

Long-term follow-up studies have indicated an increased incidence in comparison to the general population of one or more second primary cancers following an initial thyroid cancer diagnosis (25,120,125–131). In one large follow-up study involving 6941 thyroid cancer patients, there was a 27% significantly increased risk, expressed as standardized incidence ratio (SIR), of developing a second malignancy, compared to the general population (130). Excess second primary cancers were seen with increasing SIRs (1.2–5.9) in the digestive tract, female breast cancer, male genital cancer, leukemias, skin melanoma, central nervous system, kidney, endocrine gland other than thyroid, and bone and soft tissue. When the ^{131}I-treated thyroid cancer patient group was compared to thyroid cancer patients not treated with ^{131}I, the overall SIRs for the two groups were identical (SIR = 1.3), suggesting that prior thyroid cancer predisposes patients to the development of other second malignancies, perhaps because of polygenic factors. However, in such studies, some secondary malignancies have been shown to be more frequent (a greater relative risk) in ^{131}I-treated patients than patients not receiving ^{131}I in their postoperative care.

Typically, hematological malignances exhibit a shorter latency period (time interval from the therapy to the second malignancy) than solid tumors. As a complication of ^{131}I therapy, leukemia has been reported in the literature with an incidence below 0.3%, and the majority of leukemia patients over age 50 received a cumulative dose of 29.6 GBq (>800 mCi; 25,120,125–131). Those patients who received the largest ^{131}I cumulative dose in the shortest time interval were most susceptible to this complication, and acute myeloid leukemia was seen most often within 10 yr of initial ^{131}I therapy (25,119). In several series, a linear dose–response relationship was exhibited. For this reason, repeated ^{131}I therapies should be ideally spaced at least at 1-yr intervals, with each therapy giving less than 200 rads (cGy) to the blood. However, patients with progressive ^{131}I-avid disease should not be denied potentially effective or curative therapy because of possible leukemia concerns when they otherwise could be treated (prescribed activity <200 rads to the blood) at 6–9 mo after the previous therapy.

Colorectal cancer has been shown to have an increased relative risk in one series of 846 thyroid cancer patients treated with ^{131}I (without concomitant external-beam therapy) and followed for a mean of 10 yr, and this result has been supported in a larger pooled study of 4225 ^{131}I-treated patients (including the initial 846 patients; 127,130). The risk of colorectal cancer was related to the cumulative ^{131}I dose administered 5 years or more prior to the diagnosis of colorectal cancer as the second primary malignancy (127,130). This increased colorectal cancer incidence is probably related to ^{131}I accumulation (typically 1–3% of treatment dose) in the colonic lumen, which is potentiated or prolonged by the hypothyroid state. To reduce colonic radiation exposure, some therapists routinely prescribe laxatives, and this appears reasonable, especially in patients with infrequent (<2 daily) bowel movements (125).

Although the bladder is exposed to large quantities of excreted ^{131}I, an increased rate of bladder cancer deaths was shown in only one study of 258 patients, but not in other long-term follow-up studies (25,120,127,128,130). As the administered dose of ^{131}I increases, and the ^{131}I uptake by benign or malignant thyroid tissue decreases, the more ^{131}I will be excreted into the urinary bladder. The two bladder cancer deaths reported by Edmonds occurred in patients receiving 48.1 GBq (≥1300 mCi) of ^{131}I, with an estimated radiation dose to the urinary bladder of 29,000 rads (cGy) or more (25). For any administered ^{131}I quantity, the radiation dose to the bladder can be reduced by aggressive hydration within the first 48 h and frequent micturition, especially during the first 24 h, to lower the urinary ^{131}I concentration and bladder residence time of excreted ^{131}I.

As noted previously, the salivary glands receive a significant radiation dose even from a single ^{131}I administration. Salivary gland tumors have been noted in various follow-up studies and case reports (120,128,130–133). The latency period in the three case reports were 3, 3, and 10 yr and 3, 5, and 11 yr in one large follow-up study (120). Rubino et al. demonstrated a significant increase in salivary gland tumors in the 4225 patients receiving ^{131}I therapy, compared to 2616 non-^{131}I-treated patients with a relative risk of 7.5 (130). To lessen this risk, special attention should be paid to maximize hydration and the use of sialogogues, as detailed previously.

Breast duct epithelium is capable of transporting radioiodine into the breast and faint-to-moderate ^{131}I uptake is seen in nonlactating breast tissue after ^{131}I therapy *(134,135)*. The lactating breast can demonstrate intense radioiodine uptake that persists with decreasing intensity for many weeks to months after lactation ceases. Although breast cancer has been noted in several follow-up studies of secondary primary neoplasms, it has not attained statistical significance in association to ^{131}I treatment *(25,130,132,136)*. It remains to be seen whether a group of lactating women treated with ^{131}I while exhibiting much higher breast ^{131}I uptake and radiation dose would reveal an excess number of breast cancers with long-term monitoring. There appears to be a higher incidence of breast cancer in patients with Hashimoto's disease, and the latter may underlie up to 20% of patients with thyroid cancer.

Anaplastic thyroid cancer can occur late in the natural history of differentiated thyroid cancer, and a literature review reveals that more than half of patients developing anaplastic transformation have no antecedent history of ^{131}I therapy *(137)*. Using pooled data from Swedish, Italian, and French long-term follow-up data, Rubino et al. have shown a previously unreported significant increase in incidence of bone and soft-tissue cancers (4.0 relative risk), with a strong relationship to cumulative ^{131}I dosage. Most likely, this has not been demonstrated in other smaller long-term studies because of the relative rarity of these tumors. Many of these second primary malignancies developed in patients with thyroid cancer bone metastases who were treated with large prescribed activity of ^{131}I with concomitant external-beam therapy. However, even when adjusted for concomitant therapy, the increased association of bone and soft-tissue cancers with ^{131}I therapy persisted.

REFERENCES

1. Benua RS, Cicale NR, Sonenberg M, Rawson RW. The relation of radioiodine dosimetry to results and complications in the treatment of metastatic thyroid cancer. Am J Roentgenol Radium Ther Nucl Med 1962; 87:171–182.
2. Alexander C, Bader JB, Schaefer A, et al. Intermediate and long-term side effects of high-dose radioiodine therapy for thyroid carcinoma. J Nucl Med 1998; 39:1551–1554.
3. Chiu AC, Delpassand ES, Sherman SI. Prognosis and treatment of brain metastases in thyroid carcinoma. J Clin Endocrinol Metab 1997; 82:3637–3642.
4. Holmquest DL, Lake P. Sudden hemorrhage in metastatic thyroid carcinoma of the brain during treatment with iodine-I31. J Nucl Med 1976; 17:307–309.
5. Datz FL. Cerebral edema following iodine-131 therapy for thyroid carcinoma metastatic to the brain. J Nucl Med 1986; 27:637–640.
6. Hurley JR, Becker DV. The use of radioiodine in the management of thyroid cancer. In Freeman LM, Weissman HS, editors. Nuclear Medicine Annual 1983. New York: Raven Press, 1983:329–384.
7. Grayson RR. Factors which influence the radioactive iodine thyroidal uptake test. Am J Med 1960; 24:397–415.
8. Bedikian AY, Valdivieso M, Heilbrun LK, et al. Glycerol: a successful alternative to dexamethasone for patients receiving brain irradiation for metastatic disease. Cancer Treat Rep 1978; 62:1081–1083.
9. Simpson WJ, Panzarella T, Carruthers JS, et al. Papillary and follicular thyroid cancer: Impact of treatment in 1578 patients. Int J Radiat Oncol Biol Phys 1988; 14:1063–1075.
10. Zettinig G, Hanselmayer G, Fueger B, et al. Long-term impairment of the lacrimal glands after radioiodine therapy: a cross-sectional study. Eur J Nucl Med 2002; 29:1428–1432.
11. Bakheet SMB, Hammami MM, Hemidan A, et al. Radioiodine secretion in tears. J Nucl Med 1998; 39:1452–1454.
12. Solans R, Bosch JA, Galofre P, et al. Salivary and lacrimal gland dysfunction (sicca syndrome) after radioiodine therapy. J Nucl Med 2001; 42:738–743.
13. Kloos RT, Duvuuri V, Jhiang SM, et al. Nasolacrimal drainage system obstruction from radioactive iodine therapy for thyroid carcinoma. J Clin Endocrinol Metab 2002; 87:5817–5820.
13a. Burns JA, Morgenstern KE, Cahill KV, et al. Nasolacrimal obstruction secondary to I-131 therapy. Ophthal Plast Reconstr Surg 2004; 20:126–129.
14. Schiff L, Stevens CD, Molle WE, et al. Gastric (and salivary) excretion of radioiodine in man (preliminary report). J Natl Cancer Inst 1947; 7:349–354.
15. Rice DH. Advances in diagnosis and management of salivary gland diseases. West J Med 1984; 140:238–249.
16. Myant NB. Iodine metabolism of salivary glands. Ann NY Acad Sci 1960; 85:208.
17. Freinkel N, Ingbar SH. Concentration gradients for inorganic I-131 and chloride in mixed human saliva. J Clin Invest 1953; 32:1077–1084.
18. Honour AJ, Myant NB, Rowlands EN. Secretion of radioiodine in digestive juices and milk in man. Clin Sc 1952; 11:449–462.
19. Jhiang SM, Cho JY, Ryu KY, et al. An immunohistochemical study of Na+/I–symporter in human thyroid tissues and salivary gland tissues. Endocrinology 1998; 139:4416–4419.
20. Rice DH. Advances in diagnosis and management of salivary gland diseases. West J Med 1984; 140:238–249.
21. Batsakis JG. Physiology. In Cummings CW, Schuller DE, editors. Otolaryngology-Head and Neck surgery, vol. 2. St. Louis, MO: Mosby-Year Book, 1998; 1210–1222.
22. Van Nostrand DV, Neutze J, Atkins F. Side effects of "rational dose" iodine-131 therapy for metastatic well differentiated thyroid carcinoma. J Nucl Med 1986; 27:1519–1527.
23. Kahn S, Waxman A, Ramanna L, et al. Transient radiation effects following high dose I-131 therapy for differentiated thyroid cancer (DTC). J Nucl Med 1994; 35:15P.
24. Burmeister LA, du Cret RP, Mariash CN. Local reaction to radioiodine in the treatment of thyroid cancer. Am J Med 1991; 90: 217–222.
25. Edmonds CJ, Smith T. The long-term hazards of the treatment of thyroid cancer with radioiodine. Br J Radiol 1986; 59:45–51.
26. Albrecht HH, Creutzig H. Salivary gland scintigraphy after radioiodine therapy. Functional scintigraphy of the salivary gland after high dose radioiodine therapy. Fortschr Rontgenstr 1976; 125: 546–551.
27. Tubiana M, Lacour J, Monnier JP, et al. External radiotherapy and radioiodine in the treatment of 359 thyroid cancers. Br J Radiol 1975; 48:894–907.
28. Allweiss P, Braunstein GD, Katz A, Waxman A. Sialadenitis following I-131 therapy for thyroid carcinoma: Concise communication. J Nucl Med 1984; 25:755–758.
29. Pan MS. Follow-up study of side effects for iodine-131 treatment in patients with differentiated thyroid cancer. J Nucl Med 2004; 5S: 386P.

30. Maheshwari YK, Strattton Hill C, Haynie TP, et al. Iodine-131 therapy in differentiated thyroid carcinoma: M.D. Anderson Hospital experience. Cancer 1981; 47:664–671.
31. Tollefsen HR, DeCosse JJ, Hutter RVP. Papillary carcinoma of the thyroid. A clinical and pathological study of 70 fatal cases. Cancer 1964; 17:1035–1043.
32. Lin WY, Shen YY, Wang SJ. Short-term hazards of low-dose radioiodine ablation therapy in postsurgical thyroid cancer patients. Clin Nucl Med 1996; 21:780–782.
33. Brown AP, Greening WP, McCready VR, et al. Radioiodine treatment of metastatic thyroid carcinoma: the Royal Marsden hospital experience. Br J Radiol 1984; 57:323–327.
34. Schneyer LH, Tanchester D. Some oral aspects of radioactive iodine therapy for thyroid disease. NYJ Dent 1954; 24:308–309.
35. Mandel S, Mandel L. Persistent sialadenitis after radioactive iodine therapy: report of two cases. J Oral Maxillofac Surg 1999; 57:738–741.
36. Malpani BL, Samuel AM, Ray S. Quantification of salivary gland function in thyroid cancer patients treated with radioiodine. Int J Radiat Oncol Biol Phys 1996; 35:535–540.
37. Spiegel W, Reiners C, Borner W. Sialadenitis following iodine-131 therapy for thyroid carcinoma. J Nucl Med 1985; 26:816.
38. Reiners C, Eichner R, Eilles C, et al. Kamera-funktionsszintigraphie der kopfspeicheldrusen nach hoch-dosierter radiojodtherapie bei schilddrusenkarzinoma patienten. In Nuklearmedizin, Schmidt HAE, Riccabona G, editors. Stuttgart, New York: Schattauer 1980; 477–481.
39. Mandel SJ, Mandel L. Radioactive iodine and the salivary glands. Thyroid 2003; 13:265–271.
40. Laupa MS, Toth BB, Keene HJ. Effect of radioactive iodine therapy on salivary flow rates and oral streptococcus mutants prevalence in patients with thyroid cancer. Oral Surg Oral Med Oral Pathol 1993; 75:312–317.
41. Busnell DL, Boles MA, Kaufman GE, et al. Complications, sequela and dosimetry of iodine-131 therapy for thyroid carcinoma. J Nucl Med 1992; 33:2214–2221.
42. Davies AN. The management of xerostomia: a review. Eur J Cancer Care 1997; 6:209–214.
43. Nakada K, Hirata K, Ishibashi T, et al. Cevimeline hydrochloride hydate in treating salivary gland dysfunction following radioiodine therapy for thyroid cancer. J Nucl Med 2004; 45S: 17P.
44. Ericson T, Lindberg A. Clinical trial of a saliva stimulating tablet SST. Tandjakartidningen 1982; 74:713–716.
45. Blom M, Lunderberg T. Long term follow up of patients treated with acupuncture for xerostomia and the influence of additional treatment. Oral Diseases 2000; 6:15–24.
46. Sreebny LM, Schwartz SS. A reference guide to drugs and dry mouth. Gerodontology 1986; 5:75–99.
47. Hochberg MC, Tielsch J, Munoz B, et al. Prevalence of symptoms of dry mouth and their relationship to saliva production in community dwelling elderly; the SEE project. J Rheumatol 1998; 25: 486–491.
48. Donachi I. Biologic effects of radiation on the thyroid. In Werner SC, Ingbar SH, editors. The Thyroid New York: Harper & Row, 1978; 274–283.
49. Goolden AWG, Mallard JR, Farran HEA. Radiation sialitis following radioiodine therapy. Br J Radiol 1957; 30:210–212.
50. Kulkarni K, Kim SM, Intenzo C. Can salivary gland uptakes on a diagnostic I-131 scan predict acute salivary gland dysfunction in patients receiving radioiodine therapy for thyroid cancer? J Nucl Med 2004; 5S:291P.
51. Shaw LM, Bonner HS, Schuchter L, et al. Pharmacokinetics of amifostine: effects of dose and method of administration. Semin Oncol 1999; 26:34–36.
52. Werner-Wasik M. Future development of amifostine as a radioprotectant. Semin Oncol 1999; 26:129–1234.
53. Dorr RT, Holmes BC. Dosing considerations with amifostine: a review of the literature and clinical experience. Semin Oncol 1999; 26: 108–119.
54. Hall P, Holm LE, Lundell G, Ruden BI. Tumors after radiotherapy for thyroid cancer. Acta Oncol 1992; 31:403–407.
55. Bohuslavizki KH, Klutmann S, Jenicke L, et al. Salivary gland protection by S-2-(3-amiopropylamino)-ethylphosphorothioic acid (amifostine) in high-dose radioiodine treatment: results obtained in a rabbit animal model and in a double blind multi-arm trial. Cancer Biother Radiopharm 1999; 13:337–347.
56. Levy HA, Park CH. Effect of reserpine on salivary gland radioiodine uptake in thyroid cancer. Clin Nucl Med 1987; 12:303–307.
57. Freitas JE, Gross MD, Ripley S, Shapiro B. Radionuclide diagnosis and therapy of thyroid cancer; current status report. Semin Nucl Med 1985; 15:106–131.
58. Nakada K, Ishibashi T, Takei K, et al. Does lemon candy decrease salivary gland damage following radioiodine therapy for thyroid cancer? J Nucl Med 2005; 46:261–266.
59. Varma VM, Dai WL, Henkin RI. Taste dysfunction in patients with thyroid cancer following treat with I-131. J Nucl Med 1992; 33:996.
60. Maier H, Bihl H. Effect of radioactive iodine therapy on parotid gland function. Acta Otolaryngol 1987; 103:318–324.
61. Norby EH, Neutze JH, Van Nostrand D, et al. Nasal radioactive iodine uptake: a prospective study of frequency, intensity and pattern. J Nucl Med 1990; 31:52–54.
62. Levenson D, Coulec S, Sonnenberg M, et al. Peripheral facial nerve palsy after high-dose radioiodine therapy in patients with papillary thyroid carcinoma. Ann Intern Med 1994; 120:576–578.
63. Hundahl SA, Cady B, Cunningham MP, et al. Initial results from a prospective cohort study of 5583 cases of thyroid carcinoma treated in the United States in 1996. U.S. and German Thyroid Cancer Study Group. An American College of Surgeons Commission on Cancer Patient Care Evaluation Study. Cancer 2000; 89:202–217.
64. Goolden AWG, Kam KC, Fitzpatrick ML, Munro AJ. Oedema of the neck after ablation of the thyroid with radioactive iodine. Br J Radiol 1986; 59:583–586.
65. Cooper DS, Ridgway EC, Maloof F. Unusual types of hyperthyroidism. Clin Endocrinol Metab 1978; 7:199–220.
66. Smith R, Blum C, Benua RS, Fawwaz R. Radioactive iodine treatment of metastatic thyroid carcinoma with clinical thyrotoxicosis. Clin Nucl Med 1985; 10:874–875.
67. Ikejiri K, Furuyama M, Muranaka T, et al. Carcinoma of the thyroid manifested as hyperthyroidism caused by functional bone metastasis. Clin Nucl Med 1997; 22:227–230.
68. Trunnell JB, Marinelli LD, Duffy BJ Jr., et al. The treatment of metastatic thyroid cancer with radioactive iodine: credits and debits. J Clin Endocrinol 1949; 9:1138–1152.
69. Cerletty JM, Listwan WJ. Hyperthyroidism due to functioning metastatic thyroid carcinoma. Precipitation of thyroid storm with therapeutic radioactive iodine. JAMA 1979; 242:269–270.
70. Winslow CP, Meyers AD. Hypocalcemia as a complication of radioiodine therapy. Am J Otolaryngol 1998; 19:401–403.
71. Glazebrook GA. Effect of decicurie prescribed activity of radioactive I-131 on parathyroid function. Am J Surg 1987; 154:368–373.
72. Lee TC, Harbert JC, Dejter SW, et al. Vocal cord paralysis following I-131 ablation of a postthyroidectomy remnant. J Nucl Med 1985; 26: 49–50.
73. Pochin EE. Radioiodine treatment of thyroid cancer. In Hahn PF, editor. Therapeutic Use of Artificial Radioisotopes. New York: John Wiley & Sons, 1956; 195.
74. Fajardo L. G LF, Berthrong M, Anderson, editors. Radiation Pathology. Oxford: University Press, 2001.
75. Rall JE, Alpers JB, Lewallen CG, et al. Radiation pneumonitis and fibrosis: a complication of radioiodine treatment of pulmonary metas-

tases from cancer of the thyroid. J Clin Endocrinol Metab 1957; 17: 1263–1276.
76. Aldrich LB, Sisson JC, Grum CM. Pulmonary function in thyroid carcinoma metastatic to the lung. J Endocrinol Invest 1987; 10:111–116.
77. Menzel C, Grunwald F, Schomburg A, et al. "High-dose" radioiodine therapy in advanced differentiated thyroid carcinoma. J Nucl Med 1996; 37:1496–1503.
78. Bennett DE, Million RR, Ackerman IV. Bilateral radiation pneumonitis. A complication of the radiotherapy of bronchogenic carcinoma. Cancer 1969; 23:1001–1018.
79. Fulkerson WJ, McLendon RE, Prosnitz LR. Adult respiratory distress syndrome after limited radiotherapy. Cancer 1986; 57:1941–1946.
80. Monson JM, Stark P, Reily JJ, et al. Clinical radiation pneumonitis and radiographic changes after thoracic radiation therapy for lung carcinoma. Cancer 1998; 82:842–850.
81. Morgan GW, Pharm B, Breit SN. Radiation and the lung. Int J Radiat Oncol Biol Phys 1995; 31:361–369.
82. Choi NC, Kanarek DJ, Kazemi H. Physiologic changes in pulmonary function after thoracic radiotherapy for patients with lung cancer and role of regional pulmonary function studies predicting postradiotherapy pulmonary function before radiotherapy. Cancer Treat Symp 1985; 2:119–130.
83. Mah K, Van Dyk J, Keane T, Poon PY. Acute radiation-induced pulmonary damage: a clinical study on the response to fractionated radiation therapy. Int J Radiat Oncol Biol Phys 1987; 13:179–188.
84. Smith JC. Radiation pneumonitis. A review. Am Rev Respir Dis 1963; 87:647–665.
85. Carmel RJ, Kaplan HS. Mantle irradiation for Hodgkin's disease. An analysis of technique, tumor eradication and complications. Cancer 1976; 37:2813–2825.
86. Fryer CJH, Fitzpatrick PJ, Rider WD, et al. Radiation pneumonitis: experience following a large single dose of radiation. Int J Radiat Oncol Biol Phys 1978; 4:931–936.
87. McDonald S, Rubin P, Philips TL, Marks LB. Injury to the lung from cancer therapy: clinical syndromes, measurable endpoints, and potential scoring systems. Int J Radiat Oncol Biol Phys 1995; 31: 1187–1203.
88. Fowler JF, Travis EL. The radiation pneumonitis syndrome in half-body radiation therapy. Int J Radiat Oncol Biol Phys 1978; 4: 1111–1113.
89. Keane T, Van Dyk J, Rider WD. Idiopathic interstitial pneumonia following bone marrow transplantation. The relationship with total body irradiation. Int J Radiat Oncol Biol Phys 1981; 7:1365–1370.
90. Gross NJ. Pulmonary effects of radiation therapy. Ann Intern Med 1977; 86:81–92.
91. Leeper R. Controversies in the treatment of thyroid carcinoma: the New York Memorial Hospital approach. Thyroid Today 1982; 4:1–6.
92. Leeper RD. The effect of I-131 therapy on survival of patients with metastatic papillary or follicular thyroid carcinoma. J Clin Endocrinol Metab 1973; 36:1143–1152.
93. Samuel AM, Unnikrishnan TP, Baghel NS, Rajashekharrao B. Effect of radioiodine therapy on pulmonary alveolar-capillary membrane integrity. J Nucl Med 1995; 36:783–787.
94. Schlumberger M, Arcangioli O, Piekarski JD, et al. Detection of and treatment of lung metastases of differentiated thyroid carcinoma in patients with normal chest X-rays. J Nucl Med 1988; 29: 1790–1794.
95. Hindié E, Melliere D, Lange F, et al. Functioning pulmonary metastases of thyroid cancer: does radioiodine influence the prognosis? J Nucl Med 2003; 30; 974–981.
96. Nemec J, Zamrazil V, Pohunkova D, Roohling S. Radioiodide treatment of pulmonary metastases of differentiated thyroid cancer; results and prognostic factors. Nuklearmedizin 1979; 18:86–90.
97. Massin JP, Savoie JC, Garnier H, et al. Pulmonary metastases in differentiated thyroid carcinoma: study of 58 cases with implications for the primary tumor treatment. Cancer 1984; 53:982–992.
98. Samaan NA, Schultz PN, Haynie TP, Ordonez NG. Pulmonary metastasis of differentiated thyroid carcinoma: treatment results in 101 patients. J Clin Endocrinol Metab 1985; 60:376–380.
99. Leeper RD, Shimaoka K. Treatment of metastatic thyroid cancer. Clin Endocrinol Metab 1980; 9:383–404.
100. Quimby ES, Feitelberg S, Laughlin JS, et al. NCRP Report 37: Precautions in the management of patients who have received therapeutic amounts of radionuclides. Washington, DC: National Council on Radiation Protection, 1970.
101. US Nuclear Regulatory Commission 1997 Criteria for release of individuals administered radioactive materials. Federal Reg 1997; 62: 4120.
102. Marcus CS, Siegel JA. NRC absorbed dose reconstruction for family members of I-131 therapy patient: case study and commentary. J Nucl Med 2004; 45:13N–16N.
103. Kinuya S, Hwang E, Ikeda E, et al. Mallory-Weiss Syndrome caused by iodine-131 therapy for metastatic thyroid carcinoma. J Nucl Med 1997; 38:1831–1832.
104. Balan KK, Raouf AH, Critchley M. Outcome of 249 patients attending a nuclear medicine department with well-differentiated thyroid cancer; a 23 year review. Br J Radiol 1994; 67:283–291.
105. Dobyns BM, Maloof F. The study and treatment of 119 cases of carcinoma of the thyroid with radioactive iodine. J Clin Endocrinol 1951; 11:1323–1360.
106. Dorn R, Kopp J, Vogt H, et al. Dosimetry-guided radioactive iodine treatment in patients with metastatic differentiated thyroid cancer: largest safe dose using a risk—adapted approach. J Nucl Med 2003; 44:451–456.
107. Grunwald F, Schomburg A, Menzel C, et al. Blood count changes after radioiodine treatment in thyroid carcinoma. Med Klin 1994; 89: 522–528.
108. Haynie T, Beierwaltes W. Hematologic changes observed following therapy for thyroid carcinoma. J Nucl Med 1963; 4:85–91.
109. Keldsen N, Mortensen BT, Hansen HS. Bone marrow depression due to I-131 treat of thyroid cancer. Ugeskr Laeger 1988; 50: 2817–2819.
110. Matthies A, Bender H, Distelmaier M, et al. Efficacy and side effects of high dose iodine-131 therapy in metastatic thyroid carcinoma. J Nucl Med 2004; 45S:189P.
111. Petrich T, Widjaja A, Musholt TJ, et al. Outcome after radioiodine therapy in 107 patients with differentiated thyroid carcinoma and initial bone metastases: side effects and influence of age. Eur J Nucl Med 2001; 28:203–208.
112. Robeson WR, Ellwood JE, Margulies P, Margouleff D. Outcome and toxicity associated with maximum safe dose radioiodine treatment of metastatic thyroid cancer. Clin Nucl Med 2002; 27:556–666.
113. Schober O, Gunter HH, Schwarzrock R, Hundeshagen H. Hamatologische langzeitveranderungen bei der Radiojodtherapie des Schilddrusenkarzinoms. Strahlenther Onkol 1987; 163; 464–474.
114. Schumichen C, Schmitt E, Scheuffele C. Influence of the therapy concept onto the prognosis of thyroid carcinoma. Nuklearmedizin 1983; 22:97–105.
115. Kuhn JM, Rieu M, Wolf LM, et al. Hematologic repercussions of disorders of thyroid secretion. Presse Med 1984; 13:421–425.
116. Donate RM, Gallagher NI. Hematologic alteration associated with endocrine disease. Med Clin N Am 1968; 52; 231–241.
117. Raymond JP, Izembart M, Marliac V, et al. Temporary ovarian failure in thyroid cancer patients after thyroid remnant ablation with radioactive iodine. J Clin Endocrinol Metab 1989; 69:186–190.
118. Vini L, Hyer S, Al-Saadi A, et al. Prognosis for fertility and ovarian function after treatment with radioiodine for thyroid cancer. Postgrad Med J 2002; 78:92–93.
119. Schlumberger M, De Vathaire F, Ceccarelli C, et al. Exposure to radioactive iodine-131 for scintigraphy or therapy does not preclude pregnancy in thyroid cancer patients. J Nucl Med 1996; 37:606–612.

120. Dottorini ME, Lomuscio G, Mazzucchelli L, et al. Assessment of female fertility and carcinogenesis after iodine-131 therapy for differentiated thyroid carcinoma. J Nucl Med1995; 36:21–27.
121. Wichers M, Benz E, Palmedo H, et al. Testicular function after radiodiodine therapy for thyroid carcinoma. Eur J Nucl Med 2000; 27: 503–507.
122. Hyer S, Vini L, O'Connell M, et al. Testicular dose and fertility in men following I (131). therapy for thyroid cancer. Clin Endocrinol 2002; 56:755–758.
123. Pacini F, Gasperi M, Fugazzola L, et al. Testicular function in patients with differentiated thyroid carcinoma treated with radioiodine. J Nucl Med 1994; 35:1418–1422.
124. Sarkar SD, Beierwaltes WH, Gill SP, Cowley BJ. Subsequent fertility and birth histories of children and adolescents treated with I-131 for thyroid cancer. J Nucl Med 1976; 17:460–464.
125. Maxon HR III, Smith HD. Radioiodine-131 in the diagnosis and treatment of metastatic well differentiated thyroid cancer. Endocrinol Metab Clinics North Am 1990; 19:685–718.
126. Bitton R, Sachmechi I, Benegalrao Y, Schneider BS. Leukemia after a small dose of radioiodine for metastatic thyroid cancer. J Clin Endocrinol Metab 1993; 77:1423–1426.
127. de Vathaire F, Schlumberger M, Delisle MJ, et al. Leukaemias and cancers following iodine-131administration from thyroid cancer. Br J Cancer 1997; 75:734–739.
128. Hall P, Holm LE, Lundell G, et al. Cancer risks in thyroid cancer patients. Br J Cancer 1991; 64:159–163.
129. Pochin EE. Radioiodine therapy of thyroid cancer. Semin Nucl Med 1971; 1:503–515.
130. Rubino C, de Vathaire F, Dottorini ME, et al. Second primary malignancies in thyroid cancer patients. Br J Cancer 2003; 89:1638–1644.
131. Berthe E, Henry-Amar M, Michels JJ, et al. Risk of second primary cancer following differentiated thyroid cancer. Eur J Nucl Med Mol Imaging 2004; 31:685–691.
132. Wiseman JC, Hales IB, Joasoo A. Two cases of lymphoma of the parotid gland following ablative radioiodine therapy for thyroid carcinoma. Clin Endocrinol 1982; 17:85–89.
133. Rodriguez-Cuevas S, Ocampo LB. A case report of mucoepidermoid carcinoma of the parotid gland developing after radioiodine therapy for thyroid carcinoma. Eur J Surg Oncol 1995; 21:692.
134. Spitzberg C, Joba W, Eisenmenger W, Heufelder AE. Analysis of human sodium iodide symporter gene expression in extrathyroidal tissues and cloning of its complementary deoxyribonucleic acids from salivary gland, mammary gland, and gastric mucosa. J Clin Endocrinol Metab 1998; 83:1746–1751.
135. Hammami MM, Bakheet S. Radioiodine breast uptake in non-breast feeding women. Clinical and scintigraphic characteristics. J Nucl Med 1996; 37:26–31.
136. Adjadj E, Rubino C, Shamsaldim A, et al. The risk of multiple primary breast and thyroid carcinomas. Cancer 2003; 98: 1309–1317.
137. Mazzaferri EL, Young RL, Oertel JE, et al. Papillary thyroid carcinoma: the impact of therapy in 576 patients. Medicine 1977; 56: 171–196.
138. Pacini F, Cetani F, Miccoli P, et al. Outcome of 309 patients with metastatic thyroid carcinoma treated with radioiodine. World J Surg 1994; 18:600–604.
139. Tuttle RM, Pentlow K, Qualey R, et al. Empiric radioactive iodine (RAI) dosing regimens frequently exceed maximum tolerated activity levels in elderly patients with metastatic thyroid cancer. (abstract #177). 74th Annual meeting, American Thyroid Association, Los Angeles CA, October 10–13, 2002, p 198.
140. Atkins FB, Van Nostrand D, Kulkarni K, et al. The frequency with which empiric amounts of radioiodine "over-" or "under-" treat patients with metastatic well-differentiated thyroid cancer. J Nucl Med 2005; 46:129P.

51
External Radiation Therapy of Papillary Cancer

James D. Brierley and Richard W. Tsang

INTRODUCTION

External-beam radiotherapy (RT) in the management of papillary thyroid cancer can be subdivided regarding its purpose into adjuvant, radical, and palliative. The intent of adjuvant therapy is to improve the results of standard therapy that consists of surgery and radioactive iodine; however, its exact role is controversial. Unlike radioactive iodine, external-beam RT is a local therapy, which confines its impact to cases where a local treatment is required to maximize local regional control of the disease beyond what can be achieved with optimal surgery and radioactive iodine. Therefore, RT is generally limited to patients considered to have a high risk of locoregional recurrence, e.g., older patients with significant extrathyroidal extension of disease, residual disease following surgery, or extensive lymphatic spread.

RADICAL EXTERNAL-BEAM RT FOR GROSS DISEASE

For patients with residual tumor following attempted surgical resection, ^{131}I is unlikely to eradicate such disease unless a highly absorbed radiation dose is achieved. O'Connell et al. *(1)* suggested that an absorbed dose of 100 Gy is required to destroy small remnants of tumor. However, Maxon et al. *(2)* have shown that a single radioiodine administration of an absorbed dose greater than 80 Gy eliminated neck nodes in only 74% of patients with small-volume disease less than 2 g. Thus, in the presence of gross residual disease after excision, ^{131}I therapy is likely insufficient to achieve local tumor control.

The efficacy of external-beam radiation in controlling gross residual papillary cancer has been known since at least 1966, when Sheline et al. *(3)* reported their RT experience in 58 patients treated between 1935 and 1964. Although the radiation given would no longer be considered adequate in many current cases, they reported a good response rate. There were 15 patients with papillary cancer who had gross residual disease or inoperable recurrence in the surgical bed. After follow-up from 1 to 25 yr, eight patients with papillary tumors were alive with no evidence of disease; for patients with palpable disease, the complete response (CR) rate was 78%.

More recently, Chow et al. *(4)* reported their experience from Hong Kong. They identified 124 patients with gross residual locoregional disease after surgery for papillary thyroid cancer. Patients were stratified by whether they also received RT after surgery. Those patients who received radiation had a significantly greater local regional control rate at 5 yr follow up (67% vs 38%, $p = 0.001$).

Other studies have reported a similar result, with an approx 40% CR of gross disease after RT *(5,6)* and local control rates of about 60% at 5 yr *(7,8)*. Some retrospective series have reported good local control of gross disease with RT *(4,9,10)*. However, most of these studies did not separate the results of treatment between follicular and papillary tumors.

These reports suggest that long-term control is possible in patients with thyroid cancer with gross residual disease after attempted resection or when no resection is possible. Not all attempts to resect gross disease should be dissuaded, but circumstances still exist where surgery is not possible. These include invasion of prevertebral fascia or carotid artery and situations where resection would result in loss of function, e.g., if laryngectomy is required. In adddition, if the patient is elderly or has a poor performance status, and extensive surgery is not deemed appropriate or possible, leaving residual disease may be appropriate. Such scenarios that result in gross disease after resection should be followed by ^{131}I and radical external-beam RT and may lead to improved long-term local control.

EXTERNAL-BEAM RT AS ADJUVANT THERAPY

One reason that the adjuvant role of external RT remains uncertain and controversial is that studies reporting its use are generally all retrospective. They have included many patients who either have not been adequately treated with standard therapy (total/near total thyroidectomy and radioactive iodine) or who would not be expected to benefit from

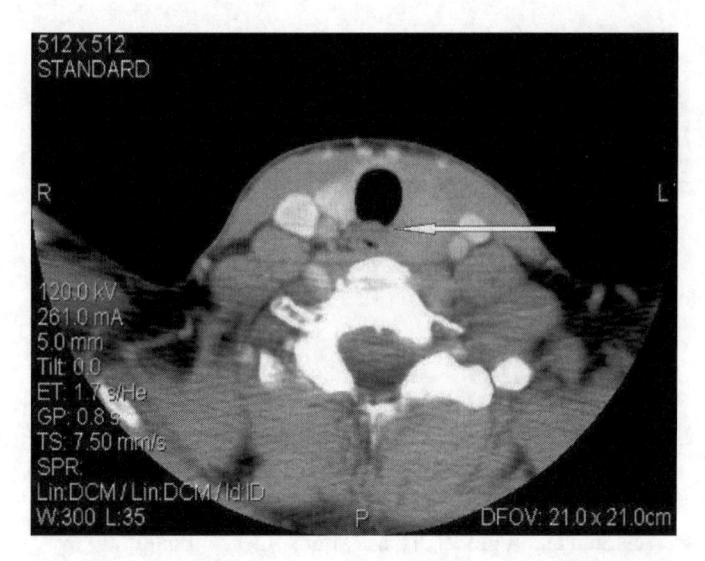

Fig. 1. A computed tomography scan slice showing ETE and invasion into the tracheoesophageal groove. The scan is from a 64-yr-old woman who presented with an asymptomatic 3-cm mass in the left thyroid lobe. Fiberoptic laryngoscopy was normal; fine-needle aspiration was consistent with papillary thyroid cancer. At surgery, there was gross ETE into strap muscles, the tracheoesophageal groove, and recurrent laryngeal nerve. Tumor was resected off of the recurrent laryngeal nerve. There was no evidence of gross residual disease. Bilateral paratracheal nodes were resected. The final pathology confirmed a 4-cm papillary thyroid carcinoma with ETE, a positive surgical margin, and two nodes containing metastatic tumor. Radioactive iodine was given, and the posttherapy scan demonstrated minimal uptake in the thyroid bed with thyrotropin (147) and thyroglobulin (5.7). External-beam radiation (50 Gy in 20 fractions) was given to the thyroid bed.

external-beam RT because they were not at high risk from local recurrence. Hence, for patient selection, it is important to identify patients who are at high risk of local recurrence and who may therefore benefit from adjuvant radiation, as well as radioactive iodine. The prognostic factors for poor outcome have been described in detail in Chapter 40, but both extrathyroidal extension and age are major factors predicting the risk of recurrence.

Mazzaferri and Jhiang *(11)* reported on 1355 patients with differentiated thyroid cancer, of whom 1077 had papillary cancer; 8% proved to have extrathyroidal extension (ETE). The local recurrence rate was 38% in patients with ETE, compared to 25% in patients without ETE ($p = 0.001$). Similarly, these patients were at higher risk of death from their cancer (20% vs 9% if there was no ETE; $p = 0.001$).

Further evidence, that these patients are at high risk was reported by Vassilopoulou-Selin et al., who studied 65 patients with recurrent papillary thyroid cancer. All patients had prior surgery and radioactive iodine *(12)*. Subjects with recurrence in lymph nodes were far more likely to respond to further radioactive iodine and far less likely to die from their disease. In contrast, the patients with the greatest degree of recurrence in the thyroid bed (14 of 15 patients) failed to take up radioactive iodine. This deleterious effect is more marked in older patients, as demonstrated in a study from Memorial Sloan Kettering. A 30-yr disease-free survival was indicated for patients without ETE of 87% but only 29% with ETE ($p < 0.0001$). This negative effect of ETE on outcome was seen only in patients over the age of 45 *(13)*.

It may be concluded that specifically older patients with ETE, as shown in Fig. 1, are at higher risk of local recurrence and are more likely to die from their disease. This group of patients may benefit from intensifying their local regional therapy with the addition of external-beam RT, surgery, and radioactive iodine to reduce the risk of recurrence in the thyroid bed.

An analysis from Princess Margaret Hospital examined patients with papillary histology and microscopic residual disease after surgical resection (defined as tumor at or within 2 mm from the resection margin). Those who received additional adjuvant external RT to the neck benefited from this treatment with an increased cause-specific survival (CSS) and local relapse-free rate (LRFR; *14*). This analysis has recently been updated with more follow-up. There were 154 patients: 90 received RT and 64 did not. The CSS was 100% at 10 yr in patients given RT, compared to 95.3% if RT was not prescribed ($p = 0.01$). Similarly, the LRFR was greater in patients given RT (94.2%) vs those who did not receive RT (83.9%, $p = 0.02$; *15*). For patients 60 yr old or younger, a benefit in LRFR was shown but not survival (CSS 98.2% no RT vs 100% RT, $p = 0.09$; LRFR 85.4% no RT vs 95.9% RT, $p = 0.03$; Fig. 2).

A different study was also performed in patients with papillary or follicular carcinoma. A subgroup was considered to be at high risk of relapse in the thyroid bed. These were older patients over age 60 yr with ETE and no gross residual disease. There were 70 patients identified who fell into this high-risk group, of whom 47 received RT and 23 did not. There was a higher CSS (81.0% vs 64.6%, $p = 0.04$) and LRFR (86.4% vs 65.7%, $p = 0.01$) in patients who received RT *(15)*.

These data suggest that external-beam RT improves both local control and survival in patients at high risk of recurrence in the thyroid bed. Unfortunately, like all studies reviewing the role of external RT, these data have limitations because the studies are retrospective. Unknown selection factors may have influenced the results by introducing bias in how patients were chosen for external-beam radiation. In addition, although these patients were considered at high risk, not all received what would now be considered standard therapy with total thyroidectomy and radioactive iodine, especially those in the earlier time period of the study.

However, there are two important studies that also suggest an adjuvant role for external-beam radiation where all patients had total thyroidectomy and radioactive iodine. Phlips et al. *(16)* reported a small series of 94 patients with differentiated thyroid cancer. All patients received radioiodine after surgical

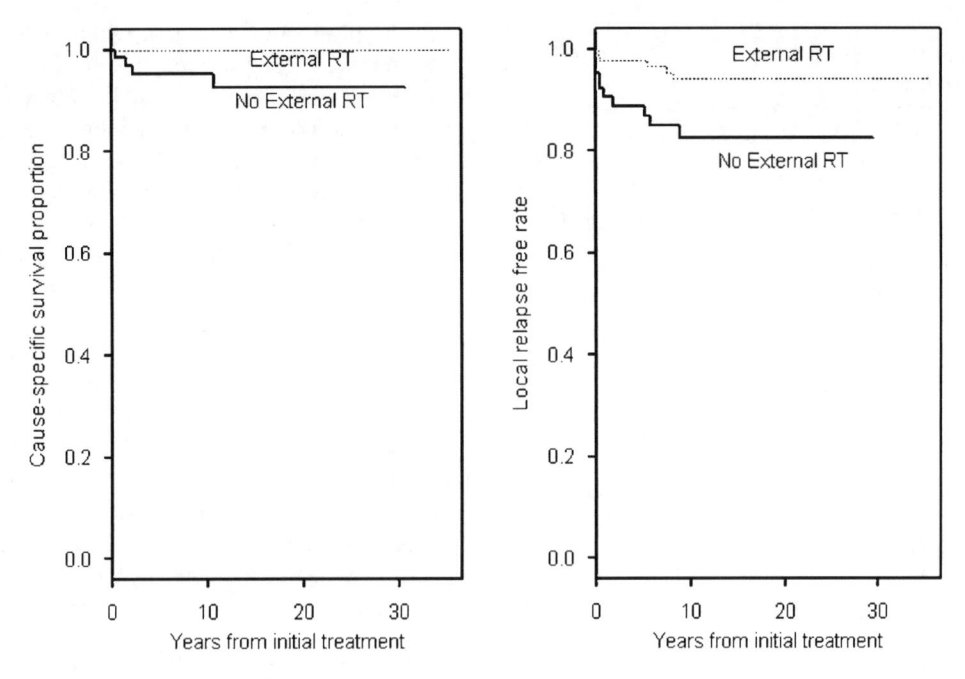

Fig. 2. Effect of external-beam RT on CSS and LRFR in patients with papillary thyroid cancer and microscopic residual disease (defined as tumor at or within 2 mm of the resection margin; *15*).

resection and 38 also had RT. The overall survival was identical for the two groups, but the LRFR was 21% for those who received only radioiodine and 3% for those who received RT. Patients who received RT were considered to have either microscopic or minimal residual disease or positive lymph node involvement with ETE. These adverse features were less frequent in the group treated with ^{131}I alone, who would therefore be expected to have a lower LRFR. The numbers are small, and the study was retrospective, but it does suggest a role for RT, in addition to ^{131}I in improving local control in a selected group of high-risk patients.

There have been two reports on the use of RT in differentiated thyroid cancer from Germany. In the first, Benker et al. *(17)* reviewed 932 patients, of whom 346 had been given RT prior to ^{131}I. Survival was not prolonged following postoperative RT; in patients older than 40 with T3 or T4 tumors, the 10-yr survival rate was 48% for those treated without RT and 58% for those who received XRT ($p = 0.09$). Subsequently, the same group *(18)* reported that adjuvant RT was associated with reduced locoregional and distant recurrence in patients over age 40 with differentiated thyroid cancer with ETE and lymph node involvement. All patients had standard therapy of total thyroidectomy, ^{131}I ablation, and thyrotropin suppression, in addition to RT. RT was a predictive factor for improvement in both the time to locoregional recurrence ($p = 0.004$) and time to distant failure ($p = 0.0003$). This benefit, however, was seen only with papillary thyroid cancer ($p = 0.0001$), not follicular thyroid cancer ($p = 0.38$).

Although all the above studies suggest a role for external-beam RT in patients at high risk of recurrence in the thyroid bed and neck, other research suggests that external-beam RT may not be beneficial *(19,20)* (Table 1). Although the former studies have been criticized *(21)*, the only way to definitively determine if external-beam RT has a role would be by a randomized controlled study. Such a study was started in Germany, but it has ended because of poor accrual *(22)*. Nevertheless, In the absence of randomized data, we believe there is still sufficient evidence from all the retrospective data to recommend external-beam RT, in addition to standard therapy, in high-risk patients (defined as older than age 45 with clinical ETE (i.e., cT4) and gross or microscopic residual disease after resection). At Princess Margaret Hospital, we currently recommend external-beam RT in patients over age 45 who have gross ETE at the time of resection (i.e., cT4) with presumed microscopic disease (i.e., gross tumor "shaved" off the larynx). However, there is nothing absolute about the age of 45, as prognosis does not change dramatically at that age *(11)*. Older patients may have a similar therapeutic gain from adjuvant RT with less extensive ETE compared to younger patients with extensive ETE or poor prognostic features, such as insular variant histology.

Once it is decided to recommend external radiation, another controversial issue arises. Should the cervical nodes be included in the treated volume, or should only the thyroid bed and adjacent soft tissues be irradiated? The advantage of irradiating only the thyroid bed is the volume irradiated is smaller, and the side effects are consequently less. This is especially true, because the salivary glands, which may already have reduced function following radioactive iodine, can be spared.

Table 1
Adjuvant External RT in High-Risk Papillary Thyroid Cancer

	10-yr Local Recurrence	
	Surgery (With and Without ^{131}I)	Surgery and RT (With and Without ^{131}I)
Esik (35)	80%[a]	37%[a]
Farahati (18)	56%[b]	10%[b]
Ford (36)	63%[a]	18%[a]
Kim (23)[c]	37.5%	4.8%
Phlips (16)	21%	3%
Simpson (9)	18%	14%
Tsang (7)	22%	7%
Tubiana (8)	21%	14%

[a] Compares low dose vs higher dose.
[b] Local and distant failures.
[c] 5-yr LRFR.

The study by Farahati et al. previously mentioned had included the cervical nodes and cervical node involvement as criterion for recommending external-beam RT (18). More recently, Kim et al. examined 91 patients with locally advanced papillary thyroid cancer (defined as pathological T4 or N1 disease; 23). A total of 68 received radioiodine alone, and 23 received external-beam RT with or without iodine. Although there was no difference in survival, there was a significantly better LRFR in patients who received external-beam RT (95.2% vs 67.5% respectively; $p = 0.04$). However, the vast majority of patients with nodal disease can be adequately treated with surgery and radioactive iodine alone (11). Nevertheless, patients who have lymph node metastases with extra nodal capsular extension and local invasion of adjacent soft tissues are at high risk of disease recurrence and poorer prognosis (24).

At Princess Margaret Hospital, we reserve cervical irradiation for patients with extensive nodal involvement, including gross ETE and local invasion. It is also considered in patients who have relapsed with tumor in cervical nodes, despite previous nodal resection and high-dose radioactive iodine, and whose disease is resistant to radioactive iodine. In younger patients, RT is usually considered after the second cervical or superior mediastinal lymph node recurrence.

EXTERNAL-BEAM RT

The thyroid bed is a technically challenging volume to treat, as it curves around the vertebral body and includes the air column in the trachea. It can be difficult to adequately treat the thyroid bed and also spare the spinal cord to a tolerable dose. A variety of techniques have been described that produce sufficient dose distribution (25). Advances in radiation techniques that result in better dose distribution to the areas at risk and reduce the volume of normal tissues to a minimum are described in Chapter 84. Well-planned external-beam RT has acceptable acute toxicity and rarely causes serious complications. In patients assigned to the radiation arm of the German randomized control study that ended because of poor accrual, it was noted that most patients experience mild-to-moderate side effects from adjuvant external-beam RT (22). At the first follow-up, most side effects had subsided, and acute toxicity was tolerable in these patients. Late toxicity is infrequent; the most common problems were skin telangiectasia, increased skin pigmentation, soft-tissue fibrosis, and mild lymphedema, predominantly in the submental area. Esophageal and tracheal stenosis are extremely rare. Neither Tsang et al. (26) nor Farahati et al. (27) reported any Radiation Therapy Oncology Group grade IV late toxicity. If the external-beam radiation dose does not result in local control, and the patient relapses in the thyroid bed area, salvage surgery may still be possible with an experienced surgeon conducting postradiation surgery in the head and neck region.

EXTERNAL-BEAM RT FOR METASTASES

The effectiveness of ^{131}I for metastatic disease greatly depends on the metastasis site. It is well known that lung metastases generally respond well to radioactive iodine. In a series of patients with distant metastases, Casara et al. found that those over age 40 or with bone metastases were much less likely to concentrate radioactive iodine (28). Only 3% of bone metastases were considered to have achieved a CR following radioactive iodine. Similar poor control of bone metastases has been indicated by others (29–31); therefore, an aggressive surgical approach has been recommended (31,32). Not all bone secondaries, however, are amenable to surgical resection, and high-dose external-beam radiation (e.g., 50 Gy in 25 fractions), as well as radioactive iodine, is thus appropriate and may result in long-term control (33). External-beam radiation also has an important role in palliating symptomatic bone metastases and cord compression.

Brain metastases from papillary thyroid cancer are unusual. In a study of metastases from the brain of all histologies (32 were differentiated cancers), surgical resection resulted in improved survival, but there was no benefit from external-beam radiation. In another series, external-beam radiation led to a CR in three out of four patients with measurable disease (34). External-beam RT should probably be provided if surgical resection is not possible. Yet, it is uncertain if it has any benefit if complete excision of brain metastases was performed. Single large lung metastases causing hemoptysis or obstruction may also respond to RT.

The role of RT in controlling gross residual disease after surgery and in unresectable disease has been discussed. In patients with symptomatic recurrent disease with poor performance status or widespread incurable disease, in whom high-dose RT for long-term control is not thought appropriate, shorter course RT may be effective to control local symptoms, such as pain, skin ulceration, and obstruction.

REFERENCES

1. O'Connell M, Flower MA, Hinton PJ, et al. Radiation dose assessment in radioiodine therapy. Dose-response relationships in differentiated thyroid carcinoma using quantitative scanning and PET. Radiother Oncol 1993; 28:16–26.
2. Maxon HR, Englaro EE, Thomas SR, et al. Radioiodine-131 therapy for well-differentiated thyroid cancer—a quantitative radiation dosimetric approach: outcome and validation in 85 patients. J Nucl Med 1992; 33:1132–1136.
3. Sheline GE, Galante M, Lindsay S. Radiation therapy in the control of persistent thyroid cancer. Am J Roentgenol Radium Ther Nucl Med 1966; 97:923–930.
4. Chow S-M, Law SCK, Mendenhall WM, et al. Papillary thyroid carcinoma: prognostic factors and the role of radioiodine and external radiotherapy. Int J Radiat Oncol Biol Phys 2002; 52:784–795.
5. Glanzmann C, Lutolf UM. Long-term follow-up of 92 patients with locally advanced follicular or papillary thyroid cancer after combined treatment. Strahlenther Onkol 1992; 168:260–269.
6. O'Connell M, A'Hern RP, Harmer CL. Results of external beam radiotherapy in differentiated thyroid carcinoma: a retrospective study from the Royal Marsden Hospital. Eur J Cancer 1994; 30A:733–739.
7. Tsang RW, Brierley JD, Simpson WJ, et al. The effects of surgery, radioiodine and external radiation therapy on the clinical outcome of patients with differentiated thyroid cancer. Cancer 1998; 82:375–388.
8. Tubiana M, Haddad E, Schlumberger M, et al. External radiotherapy in thyroid cancers. Cancer 1985; 55:2062–2071.
9. Simpson WJ, Panzarella T, Carruthers JS, et al. Papillary and follicular thyroid cancer: impact of treatment in 1578 patients. Int J Radiat Oncol Biol Phys 1988; 14:1063–1075.
10. Wu LT, Averbuch SD, Ball DW, et al. Treatment of advanced medullary thyroid carcinoma with a combination of cyclophosphamide, vincristine, and dacarbazine. Cancer 1994; 73:432–436.
11. Mazzaferri EL, Jhiang SM. Long-term impact of initial surgical and medical therapy on papillary and follicular thyroid cancer. Am J Med 1994; 97:418–428.
12. Vassilopoulou-Sellin R, Schultz PN, Haynie TP. Clinical outcome of patients with papillary thyroid carcinoma who have recurrence after initial radioactive iodine therapy. Cancer 1996; 78:493–501.
13. Coburn MC, Wanebo HJ. Age correlates with increased frequency of high risk factors in elderly patients with thyroid cancer. Am J Surg 1995; 170:471–475.
14. Tsang RW, Brierley JD, Simpson WJ, et al. The effects of surgery, radioiodine and external radiation therapy on the clinical outcome of patients with differentiated thyroid cancer. Cancer 1998; 82:375–388.
15. Brierley JD, Tsang RW, Panzarella T. Analysis of prognostic factors and effect of treatment from a single institution on patients treated over forty years. Thyroid 2003; 13.
16. Phlips P, Hanzen C, Andry G, et al. Postoperative irradiation for thyroid cancer. Eur J Surg Oncol 1993; 19:399–404.
17. Benker G, Olbricht T, Reinwein D, et al. Survival rates in patients with differentiated thyroid carcinoma. Influence of postoperative external radiotherapy. Cancer 1990; 65:1517–1520.
18. Farahati J, Reiners C, Stuschke M, et al. Differentiated thyroid cancer. Impact of adjuvant external radiotherapy in patients with perithyroidal tumor infiltration (stage pT4). Cancer 1996; 77:172–180.
19. Samaan NA, Schultz PN, Hickey RC, et al. The results of various modalities of treatment of well differentiated thyroid carcinomas: a retrospective review of 1599 patients. J Clin Endocrinol Metab 1992; 75:714–720.
20. Mazzaferri EL, Young RL. Papillary thyroid carcinoma: a 10 year follow-up report of the impact of therapy in 576 patients. Am J Med 1981; 70:511–518.
21. Brierley JD, Tsang RW. External radiation therapy in the treatment of differentiated cancer. Semin Surg Oncol 1999; 16:42–49.
22. Schuck A, Biermann M, Pixberg MK, et al. Acute toxicity of adjuvant radiotherapy in locally advanced differentiated thyroid carcinoma. First results of the multicenter study differentiated thyroid carcinoma (MSDS). Strahlenther Onkol 2003; 179:832–839.
23. Kim TH, Yang DS, Jung KY, et al. Value of external irradiation for locally advanced papillary thyroid cancer. Int J Radiat Oncol Biol Phys 2003; 55:1006–1012.
24. Yamashita H, Noguchi S, Murakami N, et al. Extracapsular invasion of lymph node metastasis. A good indicator of disease recurrence and poor prognosis in patients with thyroid microcarcinoma. Cancer 1999; 86:842–849.
25. Tsang RW, Brierley JD. The thyroid. In Kian Ang K, editor. Radiation Oncology. St. Louis, MO: Mosby, 2003.
26. Tsang RW, Brierley JD, Simpson WJ, et al. The effects of surgery, radioiodine and external radiation therapy on the clinical outcome of patients with differentiated thyroid cancer. Cancer. 1998; 82:375–388.
27. Farahati J, Reiners C, Stuschke M, et al. Differentiated thyroid cancer. Impact of adjuvant external radiotherapy in patients with perithyroidal tumor infiltration (stage pT4). Cancer 1996; 77:172–180.
28. Casara D, Rubello D, Saladini G, et al. Distant metastases in diffentiated thyroid cancer: longterm results of radioiodine treatment. Tumori 1991; 77:432–436.
29. Brown AP, Greening WP, McCready VR, et al. Radioiodine treatment of metastatic thyroid carcinoma: the Royal Marsden Hospital experience. Br J Radiol 1984; 57:323–327.
30. Schlumberger M, Challeton C, De Vathaire F, et al. Radioactive iodine treatment and external radiotherapy for lung and bone metastases from thyroid carcinoma. J Nucl Med 1996; 37:598–605.
31. Proye CA, Dromer DH, Carnaille BM, et al. Is it still worthwhile to treat bone metastases from differentiated thyroid carcinoma with radioactive iodine? World J Surg 1992; 16:640–645; discussion 645–646.
32. Niederle B, Roka R, Schemper M, et al. Surgical treatment of distant metastases in differentiated thyroid cancer: indication and results. Surgery 1986; 100:1088–1097.
33. Brierley JD, Tsang RW. External-beam radiation therapy in the treatment of differentiated thyroid cancer. Semin Surg Oncol 1999; 16:42–49.
34. Chiu AC, Delpassand ES, Sherman SI. Prognosis and treatment of brain metastases in thyroid carcinoma. J Clin Endocrinol Metab 1997; 82:3637–3642.
35. Esik O, Nemeth G, Eller J. Prophylactic external irradiation in differentiated thyroid cancer: a retrospective study over a 30-year observation period. Oncology 1994; 51:372–379.
36. Ford D, Giridharan S, McConkey C, et al. External beam radiotherapy in the management of differentiated thyroid cancer. Clin Oncol (R Coll Radiol) 2003; 15:337–341.

52 PART A
Chemotherapy for Thyroid Cancer
General Principles

Lawrence S. Lessin

INTRODUCTION

Chemotherapy has been used as a single modality treatment or as part of combined modality therapy in metastatic or locally advanced thyroid cancer when other conventional treatments (e.g., surgery and radiation therapy) have failed. Cytotoxic chemotherapy is predominantly employed in anaplastic carcinomas and may be used in the 20% of differentiated (papillary, follicular, and mixed) thyroid carcinomas that do not concentrate iodine. Although chemotherapy may induce a tumor response and provide palliation of troublesome symptoms, no established evidence shows it prolongs survival. Numerous reports on the use of chemotherapy in a variety of thyroid cancers have been published, but only a few controlled clinical trials compare the efficacy of different drug regimens. Generally, the response to chemotherapy is modest, but some investigators have stated that patients who respond to the first chemotherapeutic agent are more likely to respond to a second agent when relapse occurs (1).

CHEMOTHERAPEUTIC AGENTS USED IN THYROID CANCER

Individual chemotherapeutic agents with known (or proposed) antitumor activity against thyroid cancer are listed in Table 1.

Doxorubicin

Doxorubicin is an anthracycline derivative that has been the most widely used and studied chemotherapeutic agent in thyroid cancer. In 1974, one of the earliest studies on doxorubicin was reported by Gottlieb and Hill (2), who treated 30 patients with different types of refractory thyroid carcinoma. Of 30 patients, 11 (37%) achieved a partial response. Median survival was found to be significantly better in responders compared to nonresponders (11 mo vs 4 mo). Since then, many reports on the use of doxorubicin in advanced thyroid cancer have been published, with response rates varying from 30% to 45%. Currently, doxorubicin is considered the most effective single agent at a dose of 60 mg/m^2 every 3 wk (1). Lower doxorubicin doses at 45 mg/m^2 were found by Gottlieb and Hill (2) to be inferior to 60 mg/m^2, with no responses in three patients. In contrast, 3 of 13 patients responded to 60 mg/m^2, three additional responses were seen when the dose was escalated to 75 mg/m^2, and two more responses were seen with a further increase to 90 mg/m^2. Doxorubicin-induced cardiomyopathy was found to be the limiting toxicity. Droz and colleagues also found a lack of response to low-dose doxorubicin (3). The patient's nutritional and performance status also seemed to influence the response to doxorubicin. O'Bryan and coworkers (4), as well as Benker and Reinwein (5), noted that poorer response to doxorubicin occurred in patients with low performance status. In the only randomized trial published, Shimaoka and associates (6) also described performance status as a significant predictor of response. Doxorubicin has been used in combination with other agents, including cisplatinum, bleomycin, vincristine, and vindesine, without clear advantage.

Epirubicin

Epirubicin is an anthracycline analog of doxorubicin, with dose-limiting myelosuppression and less cardiotoxicity. In 2002, Santini and colleagues treated 14 patients with metastatic poorly differentiated thyroid cancer, utilizing a combination of epirubicin and carboplatin at 4–6 wk intervals for 4–6 wk (7). Thyrotropin (TSH) stimulation was achieved by either levothyroxine withdrawal or recombinant human TSH. A single complete remission was observed, five patients had partial remissions, and seven had stable disease. Half of patients showed a decline in thyroglobulin levels.

Mitoxantrone

Mitoxantrone, an anthracenedicine DNA intercalator, is related to doxorubicin but is much less cardiotoxic.

From: *Thyroid Cancer: A Comprehensive Guide to Clinical Management, 2/e*
Edited by: L. Wartofsky and D. Van Nostrand © Humana Press Inc., Totowa, NJ

Table 1
Chemotherapeutic Agents Used in Thyroid Cancer

Drug	Class	Major Toxicity
Doxorubicin	Anthracycline	Cardiac, limit to 550 mg/m^2, mucositis
Epirubicin	Anthracycine	Less cardiotoxic than doxorubicin, myelosuppression
Mitoxantrone	Anthracenedione, DNA intercalator	Myelosuppression, less cardiotoxic than anthracyclines
Bleomycin	Antitumor antibiotic	Pulmonary toxicity, follow pulmonary diffusion capacity
Cisplatin	Heavy metal, binds directly to DNA	Nephrotoxicity, follow electrolytes closely
Carboplatinum	Heavy metal, analog of cisplatin	Myelotoxicity
Etoposide	Epipodophyllotoxin, topoisomerase II inhibitor	Myelosuppression
Topotecan	Topoisomerase I inhibitor, analog of etoposide	Myelosuppression, mucositis
Irinotecan	Topoisomerase I inhibitor, analog of etoposide	Myelosuppression, diarrhea
Dacarbazine	Alkylating-like activity	Myelosuppression, gastrointestinal toxicity
Cyclophosphamide	Alkylating agent	Myelosuppression, hemorrhagic cystitis
Paclitaxel	Taxane	Myelosuppression, neuropathy
Vincristine	Vinca alkyloid	Peripheral neuropathy
Methotrexate	Antimetabolite	Gastrointestinal toxicity, liver fibrosis
Capecitabine	Oral fluoropyrimidine prodrug of 5-FU	Hand–foot syndrome, diarrhea
Gemcitabine	Antimetabolie	Myelosuppression

Myelosuppression is the principal limiting toxicity. It has been substituted for doxorubicin as a radiation sensitizer in patients whose poor cardiac function precludes the use of an anthracycline. A phase II study with this agent by Schlumberger et al. showed a 6.3% response rate in 16 patients with nonanaplastic thyroid cancer (8).

Bleomycin

Bleomycin was the first chemotherapeutic agent to be used in metastatic differentiated thyroid cancer. Although relatively ineffective as a single agent, when used in combination with doxorubicin and vincristine or with doxorubicin and cisplatin, response rates up to 30% were reported (9).

Cisplatin

Cisplatin has been used as monotherapy in heavily pretreated patients with a variety of thyroid cancers. Hoskin and Harmer (1) indicated 5 responded of 13 patients (38%) treated. Droz and colleagues (10) treated 18 patients with medullary thyroid carcinoma and reported 3 responses (21%), including 1 with a complete response that lasted 9 mo. Along with doxorubicin, cisplatin is commonly used as part of a combination chemotherapy regimen. Droz and colleagues (10) also conducted a phase II study of 44 cases with both differentiated and anaplastic thyroid cancer, utilizing doxorubicin and cisplatin as either monotherapy or in combination. No objective responses were seen in the 19 patients treated with single-agent cisplatin, 13 of whom had previously failed doxorubicin therapy. Therefore, in patients refractory to doxorubicin, cisplatin may produce responses in patients with medullary carcinoma but not in differentiated and anaplastic carcinoma.

Etoposide

Hoskin and Harmer (1) described their experience with etoposide, a topoisomerase II inhibitor, as a single agent in 22 heavily pretreated patients, with 4 responses in various thyroid cancers. Etoposide was used as monotherapy by Kelsen and coworkers (11) in medullary thyroid carcinoma and had a response rate of 14%. Related neuroendocrine tumors, such as small-cell lung cancer and peripheral neuroectodermal tumors, are highly responsive to etoposide used singly or in combination.

Topotecan and Irinotecan

These analogs of camptothecin are topoisomerase I inhibitors, and both have shown in vitro activity against medullary and poorly differentiated thyroid cancers and are currently employed in clinical trials *(12)*. Camptothecin is an inhibitor of topoisomerase I—the parent substance of irinotecan and the taxane, paclitaxel—and has displayed some promise in vitro against medullary thyroid cancer cells *(13)*.

Carboplatin

Hoskin and Harmer *(1)* had limited experience with single-agent carboplatin in nine heavily pretreated patients; two of nine showed partial responses.

Methotrexate

Methotrexate, the antifolate antimetabolite, was used in the early 1980s in combination with doxorubicin and lomustine (a nitrosourea). Because of poor response rates, little usage of methotrexate has been recently reported in the treatment of thyroid cancer.

Capecitabine

Capecitabine, an oral prodrug of 5-fluorouracil (5-FU), is activated within tumor cells and has minimal systemic toxicity. It is active as a single agent or in combination against colon and breast cancers. The hand–foot syndrome (erythema and scaling of hands and feet) and diarrhea are dose-limiting. The drug is converted to 5-FU within tumor cells by thymidine phosphorylase (TP). 5-FU blocks thymidylate synthase and is inactivated by dihydropyrimidine dehydrogenase (DPD). In 2004, Patel et al. showed that the majority of differentiated thyroid cancers express TP with low levels of DPD, which suggests potential clinical activity of capecitabine in thyroid cancer *(14)*.

Gemcitabine

Gemcitabine, a fluorinated nucleoside analog, is used clinically to treat pancreas, lung, and breast cancer. In vitro studies of this agent in both solution and liposomal-encapsulated forms against three poorly differentialed and anaplastic thyroid cancer cell lines have shown significant cytotoxic effect at clinically achievable concentrations *(15,16)*. These observations indicate potential efficacy in poorly differentiated thyroid cancer and warrant further testing in clinical trials.

Application of the various chemotherapeutic agents to specific thyroid cancers is discussed for differentiated, papillary, and follicular thyroid cancer, medullary thyroid cancer, and anaplastic thyroid carcinoma in Chapters 52B, 73, 82, and 87.

REFERENCES

1. Hoskin PJ, Harmer C. Chemotherapy for thyroid cancer. Radiother Oncol 1987; 10:187–194.
2. Gottlieb JA, Hill CS. Chemotherapy of thyroid cancer with Adriamycin: experience with 30 patients. N Engl J Med 1974; 290:193–197.
3. Droz JP, Charbord P, Rougier P, Parmentier C. Echec de la chimiotherapie des cancers de la thyroide. Bull Cancer 1981; 68:350–352.
4. O'Bryan RM, Baker LH, Gottlieb JE, et al. Dose response evaluation of Adriamycin in human neoplasia. Cancer 1977; 39:1940–1948.
5. Benker G, Reinwein D. Ergegnisse der chemotherapie des schilddrusenkarzinoms. Dtsch Med Wochenschr 1983; 11:403–406.
6. Shimaoka K, Schoenfeld D, DeWys W, et al. A randomized trial of doxorubicin vs doxorubicin plus cisplatin in patients with advanced thyroid carcinoma. Cancer 1985; 56:2155–2160.
7. Santini F, Bottici V, Elisei R, et al. Cytotoxic effects of carboplatinum and epirubicin in the setting of an elevated serum thyrotropin for advanced poorly differentiated thyroid cancer. J Clin Endocrinol Metab 2002; 87:4160–4165.
8. Schlumberger M, Parmentier C. Phase II evaluation of mitoxantrone in advanced non anaplastic thyroid cancer. Bull Cancer 1989; 76:403–406.
9. Harada T, Nishikawa Y, Suzuki T, et al. Bleomycin treatment for cancer of the thyroid. Am J Surg 1971; 22:53–57.
10. Droz JP, Schlumberger M, Rougier P, et al. Phase II trials of chemotherapy with adriamycin, cisplatin and their combination in thyroid cancers: a review of 44 cases. Int Congr Ser 1985; 684:203–208.
11. Kelsen D, Fiore J, Heelan R, et al. Phase II trial of etoposide in APUD tumors. Cancer Treat Rep 1987; 71:305–307.
12. Kuefer MU, Moinuddin M, Heideman RL, et al. Papillary thyroid carcinoma: demographics, treatment, and outcome in eleven pediatric patients treated at a single institution. Med Pediatr Oncol 1997; 28:433–440.
13. Kaczirek K, Schindl M, Weinhausel A, et al. Cytotoxic activity of camptothecin and paclitaxel in newly established continuous human medullary thyroid carcinoma cell lines. J Clin Endocrinol Metab 2004; 89:2397–2401.
14. Patel A, Pluim T, Helms A, et al. Enzyme expression profiles suggest the novel tumor-activated fluoropyrimidine carbamate capecitabine (Xeloda) might be effective against papillary thyroid cancers of children and young adults. Cancer Chemother Pharmacol 2004; 53:409–414.
15. Celano M, Calvagno MG, Bulotta S, et al. Cytotoxic effects of gemcitabine-loaded liposomes in human anaplastic thyroid carcinoma cells. BMC Cancer 2004; 4:63.
16. Ringel MD, Greenberg J, Chen X, et al. Cytotoxic activity of 2′ 2′-difluorodeoxycytidine (gemcitabine) in poorly differentiated thyroid carcinoma cells. Thyroid 2000; 10:865–869.

52 PART B
Chemotherapy of Differentiated Papillary or Follicular Thyroid Carcinoma

Lawrence S. Lessin

SINGLE MODALITY TREATMENT WITH CHEMOTHERAPY

Chemotherapy is used as a palliative measure in 25% of recurrent inoperable or metastatic papillary, follicular, or mixed thyroid cancers that do not concentrate ^{131}I. Doxorubicin, bleomycin, and cisplatin have been the principal agents employed. As advanced thyroid cancer is rare, there are few meaningful clinical trials that compare single- and multi-agent chemotherapy for differences in efficacy and toxicity. The Eastern Cooperative Oncology Group (ECOG) designed and completed the only randomized study of doxorubicin vs doxorubicin plus cisplatin in inoperable, radioiodine-resistant advanced thyroid cancer in chemotherapy-naive patients. In this study reported in 1985 (1), 41 patients received doxorubicin alone, and 43 patients received the combination. There were 16 patients with differentiated thyroid cancers who received single-agent doxorubicin, given at a dose of 60 mg/m^2 intravenously every 3 wk. A total of 19 comparable patients received the combination of doxorubicin at 60 mg/m^2 and cisplatin at 40 mg/m^2 every 3 wk. Treatment was discontinued when stable disease was achieved after three cycles of therapy, when disease progressed after two treatment cycles, or when the total dose of doxorubicin exceeded 550 mg/m^2. Suppressive thyroid hormone administration was continued throughout the treatment duration in both groups of patients. The overall response rate for all patients was 21%. In the doxorubicin-alone arm, the response rate was 17% vs 26% in the combination arm; however, because of the small number of patients, this difference was not statistically significant. Moreover, neither the time to relapse nor overall survival was found to be statistically different between the two groups. Weight loss of more than 10%, presence of lung metastases, and poor performance status were found to be significant prognostic indicators. Treatment-related toxicity, predominantly hematological and gastrointestinal effects, was worse in the combination group, but no treatment-related fatalities were reported in either treatment arm. Although the combination regimen was not statistically superior to doxorubicin alone regarding response rate and survival, all five complete responders received the combination regimen. Two of the five complete responders had differentiated thyroid cancers.

In contrast, a similar combination treatment tested in a phase II study by the Southeastern Cancer Study Group in 22 patients produced only two partial responses with serious toxic reactions (2). In 1997, the St. Jude's group reported unsustained complete response of childhood papillary cancer to both doxorubicin and a combination of topotecan and carboplatin (3). In 2002, Leaf and colleagues (4) published an ECOG phase II study of single-agent etoposide at 140 mg/m^2 for 3 d every 3 wk until progression. No responses were seen among the 10 patients accrued, and the study was closed after 18 mo. In 2002, Santini et al. conducted a study of 14 patients with poorly differentiated thyroid cancer, who were treated with carboplatin and epirubicin at 4–6 wk intervals for six courses (5). TSH stimulation was accomplished by either reduction of L-thyroxine dosage (eight patients) or administration of recombinant human TSH (six patients). Hematologic toxicity was the dose-limiting factor. One patient had complete remission, five patients had partial remission, and eight had stable disease. Overall response rate was 37%. Serum thyroglobulin levels decreased by more than 50% in six patients. Endogenous vs exogenous TSH stimulation had no statistically significant effect on response rates, but the authors believed that TSH stimulation generally improved response. Median survival was 21 mo from the start of chemotherapy, and six patients showed no progression of lung metastases.

CHEMOTHERAPY COMBINED WITH EXTERNAL-BEAM RADIATION THERAPY

The combined modality approach for locally advanced, ^{131}I refractory, differentiated thyroid cancer using low-dose doxorubicin combined with external-beam radiation was prospectively studied by Kim and Leeper (5). In their series, 22 patients with histologically confirmed, well-differentiated papillary, follicular, or mixed thyroid cancer were given doxorubicin at a dose of 10 mg/m^2 per week by bolus injection with concomitant radiation therapy. Radiation was administered at doses of 200 cGy/d for 5 d each week to total a tumor dose of 5600 cGy. A 91% com-

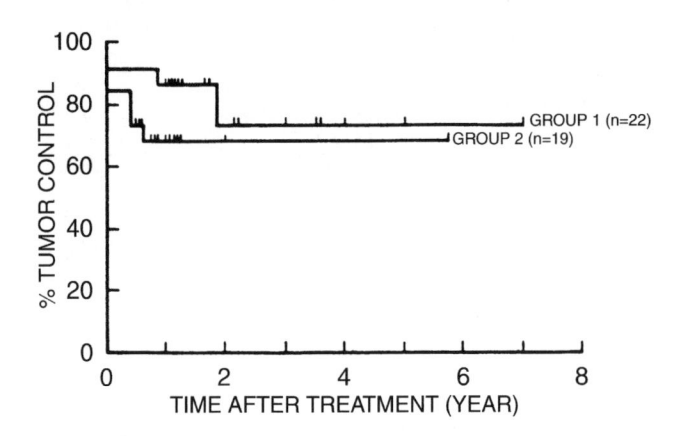

Fig. 1. Local tumor control rate as a function of time after combined treatment for patients with differentiated (group 1) vs anaplastic (group 2) thyroid cancers. (From Kim JH, Leeper RD, Cancer 1987; 60:2372–2375, with permission.)

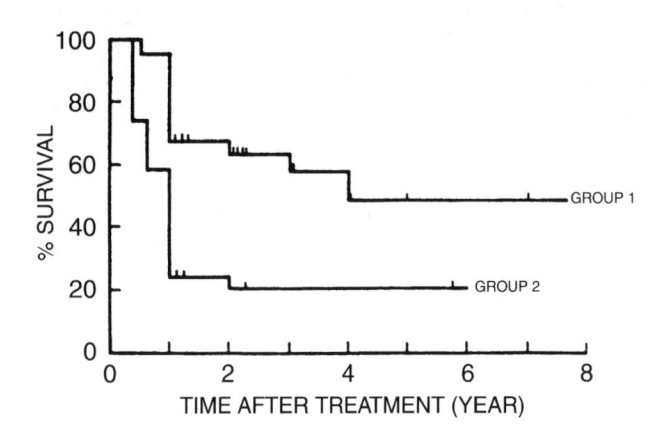

Fig. 2. The actuarial survival curves of the two groups of patients after combined therapy. (From Kim JH, Leeper RD, Cancer 1987; 60:2372–2375, with permission.)

plete response rate was observed with 77% long-term local control (see Fig. 1). In patients with differentiated thyroid cancers, the overall survival was 50% at 5 yr (Fig. 2). In this study, deaths of patients with differentiated thyroid cancers were due to distant metastases, rather than local tumor invasion. All patients developed moderate, treatment-related pharyngoesophagitis and tracheitis within 3–4 wk after initiation of combined chemoradiotherapy, but none required cessation of treatment. Before this study, combined modality treatments for locally advanced thyroid cancer with higher doses of doxorubicin were plagued by increased local tissue toxicity and increased systemic morbidity (6). This approach provides a fairly effective and well-tolerated treatment option for locally advanced refractory differenatiated (and anaplastic) thyroid cancer.

In summary, single-agent or combination chemotherapy containing doxorubicin is beneficial in metastatic, refractory differentiated thyroid cancer, with improved survival in responders. For locally advanced cancer, combined low-dose chemoradiotherapy offers an effective means of palliation. Differentiated thyroid cancers are relatively resistant to chemotherapeutic agents, and some investigators are testing the effect of endogenous or exogenous TSH stimulation on response enhancement to antitumor agents. This chapter has summarized data from clinical trials of chemotherapeutics for well-differentiated thyroid cancer for which radioiodine or surgery are no longer options. Some promising new agents are being investigated with data confined to in vitro cell culture studies, which are provided in Chapters 86 and 87. In addition, there are exciting new molecular approaches to chemotherapy that employ either gene or redifferentiation therapy, and these have been reviewed by Braga-Basaria and Ringel (8) and Park and Clark (9), as well as in Chapter 86. The primary application of the latter approaches has been to address undifferentiated or anaplastic thyroid cancer.

However, some studies have related to follicular thyroid cancer as well, including the potential use of endogenous inhibitors of angiogenesis and tumor growth, such as endostatin (10), a peptide derived from proteolysis of collagen XVIII, and other gene therapy approaches (11).

REFERENCES

1. Shimaoka K, Shoenfeld D, De Wys W, et al. A randomized trial of doxorubicin vs. doxorubicin plus cisplatin in patients with advanced thyroid carcinoma. Cancer 1985; 56:2155–2160.
2. Williams SD, Birch R, Einhorn LH. Phase II evaluation of doxorubicin plus cisplatin in advanced thyroid cancer: a Southeastern Cancer Study Group Trial. Cancer Treat Rep 1986; 70:405–407.
3. Kuefer MU, Moinuddin M, Heideman RL, et al. Papillary thyroid carcinoma: demographics, treatment and outcome in eleven pediatrics treated at a single institution. Med Pediatr Oncol 1997; 28:433–440.
4. Kim JH, Leeper RD. Treatment of locally advanced thyroid carcinoma: with combination doxorubicin and radiation therapy. Cancer 1987; 60:2372–2375.
5. Santini F, Bottici V, Elisei R, et al. Cytotoxic effects of carboplatinum and epirubicin in the setting of an elevated serum thyrotropin for advanced poorly differentiated thyroid cancer. J Clin Endocrinol Metab 2002; 87:4150–4165.
6. Tallroth E, Lundell G, Tennvall J, Wallin G. Chemotherapy and multimodality treatment in thyroid carcinoma: disorders of the thyroid and parathyroid II. Otolaryngol Clin North Am 1990; 23:523–527.
7. Leaf AN, Wolf BC, Kirkwood JM, Haselow RE. Phase II study of etoposide (VP-16) in patients with thyroid cancer with no prior chemotherapy: an Eastern Cooperative Oncology Group Study (E1385); Med Oncol 2000; 17:47–51.
8. Braga-Basaria M, Ringel MD. Beyond radioiodine: a review of potential new therapeutic approaches for thyroid cancer. J Clin Endocrinol Metab 2003; 88:1947–1960.
9. Park JW, Clark OH. Redifferentiation therapy for thyroid cancer. Surg Clin N Am 2004; 84:921–943.
10. Ye C, Feng C, Wang S, et al. Antiangiogenic and antitumor effects of endostatin on follicular thyroid cancer. Endocrinology 2002; 143:3522–3528.
11. Ye C, Feng C, Wang S, et al. sFlt-1 gene therapy of follicular thyroid carcinoma. Endocrinology 2004; 145:817–822.

53
Thyroid Carcinoma
Metastases to Bone

Steven P. Hodak and Kenneth D. Burman

Bone metastases occur in 10%–30% of all cancer patients *(1)*. Although thyroid carcinoma accounts for only 1% of all reported malignancies *(2)*, it is one of the top five cancers that most frequently produce bone metastases. Manifestations of thyroid cancer generally vary because of the different types of thyroid malignancies. Papillary and follicular thyroid cancers are frequently referred to as "differentiated," because they trap iodine, respond to radioiodine therapy, and synthesize and secrete thyroglobulin. However, within this group, some tumors become poorly differentiated and may lose or not exhibit one or more of these features. Poorly differentiated, undifferentiated, and medullary thyroid cancers tend to behave aggressively and often produce distant metastases. Medullary thyroid cancer is not iodine-avid and cannot be identified with radioiodine scans or treated with radioactive iodine. Similarly, poorly differentiated and undifferentiated thyroid cancers may exhibit reduced or no iodine avidity.

Fortunately, however, medullary and poorly differentiated thyroid cancers are uncommon. Despite the aggressive behavior of poorly and undifferentiated thyroid cancer, their relative rarity makes the overall incidence of bone metastases from these cancers similarly rare. Additionally, because these cancers show poor-iodine avidity, limited options exist for successful treatment when there are distant metastases in bone. Most protocols used in such cases are adapted from approaches for the treatment of other solid or neuroendocrine tumors. Prognosis is generally poor. Because of these facts, careful distinctions should be made when considering the complications of bone metastases from this latter group of thyroid malignancies. As a result of the significant differences in tumor biology and response to radioiodine, metastatic complications of medullary thyroid cancer and poorly and undifferentiated thyroid cancer are discussed in Chapter 67. This chapter largely focuses on bone metastases of differentiated thyroid cancer.

FREQUENCY AND SURVIVAL

Because of the greater frequency of papillary and follicular cancer when compared to poorly differentiated cancer, most osseous metastases arise in patients with differentiated thyroid cancer. Papillary cancer is the most common type of thyroid malignancy, accounting for up to 80% of all thyroid malignancies *(2)*. Bone metastases from papillary thyroid cancer are rare, with an estimated incidence less than 2%. However, papillary thyroid cancer is so prevalent, it is still responsible for the majority of thyroid cancer bone metastases. Follicular thyroid cancer is far less common than papillary carcinoma, representing less than 15% of all differentiated thyroid cancers *(2)*. Yet, it is much more metastatic to bone and has a reported incidence from 7% to 20% (Fig. 1). Despite an almost 10-fold increase in the risk of follicular thyroid carcinoma (vs papillary) to metastasize to bone, its relative infrequency results in bone metastases of follicular thyroid cancer that are far less common than those of papillary thyroid cancer.

The overall incidence of bone metastases varies partly by the histologic type of cancer, but usually has a range of 2.3–12.7% *(8)* and has been reported as high as 60% in some reviews *(9)*. Clinical series that attempt to define the frequency and behavior of bone metastases often contain methodologic limitations that account for widely discrepant results. These studies are almost exclusively retrospective and typically include the populations of highly specialized centers, thereby resulting in referral bias. Patients within these referral populations are likely to have more advanced and atypical disease in comparison to the general population. This results in additional bias, and limited ability to generalize from such data *(2)*.

Studies are often constrained by insufficient institutional records that do not contain adequate documentation of the metastases histopathology and their ^{131}I avidity. Consequently,

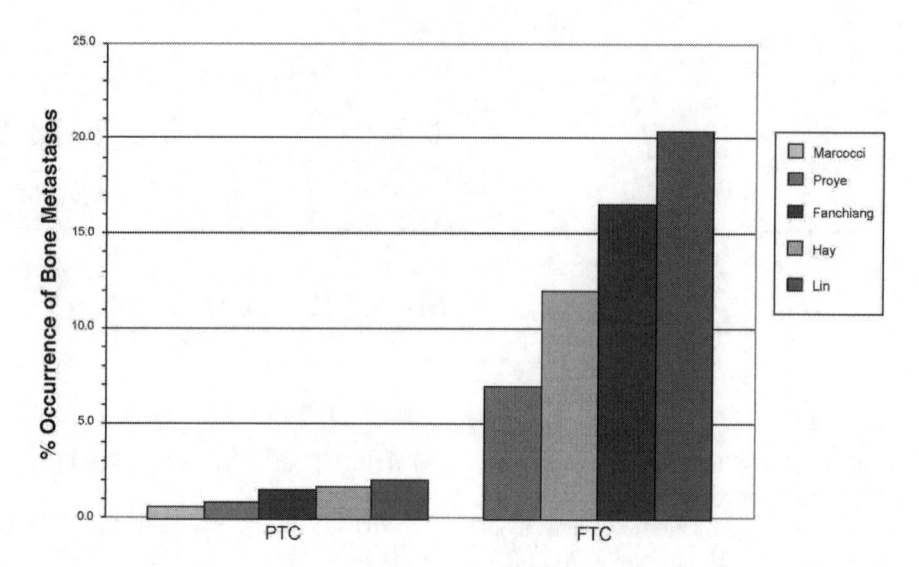

Fig. 1. Relative occurrence of papillary thyroid cancer (PTC) and follicular thyroid cancer (FTC) bone metastases across selected studies *(3–7)*. (Color illustration appears in insert following p. 198.)

there is a frequent inability to retrospectively validate suspected cases that requires exclusion of numerous cases from final statistical analysis. Cohorts within these studies are often assembled over multiple decades during which the methods of evaluation, histopathological categorization, and treatment have evolved *(10)*. Moreover, many excellent studies do not specifically consider bone metastases independent of other distant metastases, which further complicates the understanding of true incidence *(10)*. Few have examined the incidence and behavior of bone metastases from poorly, undifferentiated, and medullary thyroid cancers. Instead, most studies report only the complications of differentiated thyroid carcinomas, specifically papillary and follicular types.

Although the 10-yr survival of patients with differentiated thyroid carcinoma without distant metastases is as high as 95% *(11)*, the occurrence of bone metastases is an ominous sign and portends significantly reduced survival *(12,13)*. Like incidence data, metastatic survival data (survival after the metastases development) also varies across studies. Determining a true survival rate is problematic. Total survival, i.e., survival including the time following cancer diagnosis, but before diagnosis of bone metastases, is frequently not reported. Instead, metastatic survival (i.e., survival reported from the time of diagnosis of metastases) is more common. Detection strategies and therapeutic modalities have changed and evolved over the often lengthy retrospective periods of study. As a result, there is a wide variability in reported survival rates. One recent review cited a mean metastatic survival of 48 mo *(9)*. Our review across selected series reporting bone metastases from differentiated thyroid cancer indicates an average 5- and 10-yr survival of 55% and 22%, respectively (Fig. 2).

PROGNOSTIC FACTORS

Identification of factors that predict survival and the natural history of bone metastases has been a common goal of numerous retrospective studies. Prognostic variables are frequently strongly interrelated and difficult to analyze independently *(16)*. Univariate analysis remains the primary means for data evaluation throughout the majority of published studies. Although univariate analysis allows the identification of interesting data trends, it cannot adequately account for the interrelationship among variables. Conclusions drawn through this method of analysis must therefore be considered with an appropriate perspective. To date, only four studies have accumulated a cohort sufficient to enable successful multivariate analysis of endpoints regarding bone metastases of thyroid cancer *(10,15,17,18)*. As previously noted, even these studies are limited by methodologic constraints and subject to bias. Several others use multivariate analysis but do not specifically separate data about bone metastases from data regarding all distant metastases, limiting their usefulness in this evaluation *(16,19,20)*. Thus, the extant data concerning bone metastases from thyroid cancer are imperfect. Prospective data are unlikely to ever be available. Consequently, no general consensus exists regarding how to translate these numerous and sometimes contradictory findings into treatment guidelines. That notwithstanding, several important prognostic features of differentiated thyroid cancer have been identified and warrant further discussion.

Age

Age has been identified as an important factor in bone metastasis survival. Several authors have noted a significant

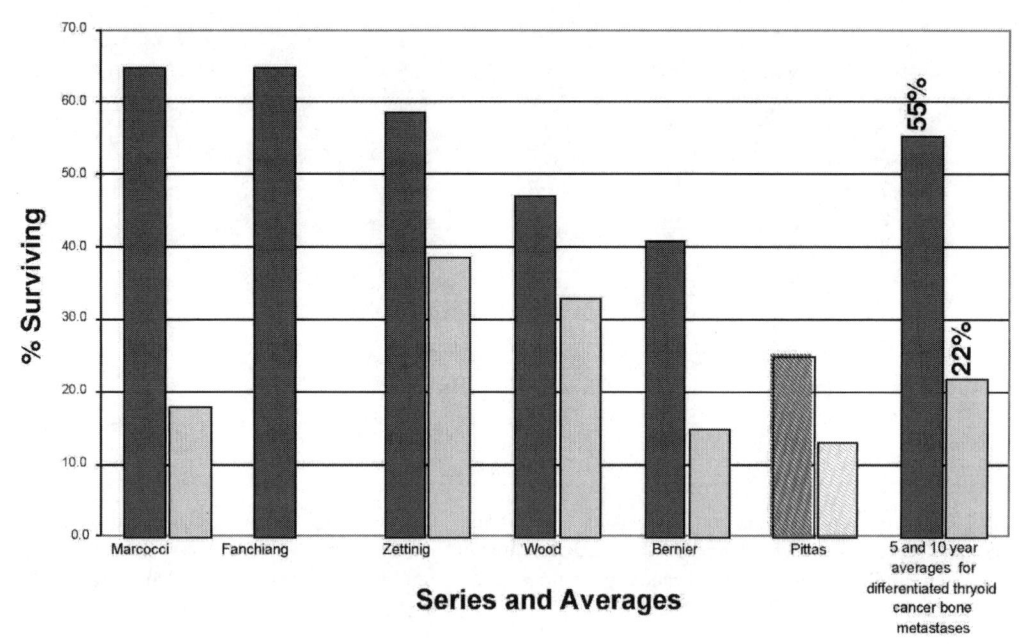

Fig. 2. The 5- and 10-yr metastatic survival data from the time of bone metastasis diagnosis. Solid bars represent data of metastatic survival in only differentiated thyroid cancer. The hashed bars represent a single study of metastatic survival in patients with differentiated, poorly differentiated, and undifferentiated thyroid cancer bone metastases. The average metastatic survival rate considers only those series limited to differentiated thyroid cancer *(3,5,8,10,14,15)*. (Color illustration appears in insert following p. 198.)

worsening of survival when bone metastases occur after the age range of 40–45 *(15,17,19–24)*. Schlumberger found that long-term prognosis is particularly favorable in the young, especially children. His data indicate this fact despite typically more advanced disease at presentation *(25)*. Schlumberger has also observed that increasing age inversely affects iodine avidity. He notes that 90% of tumors in those less than 40 yr old but only 56% of tumors in those older than 40 remained iodine-avid *(16)*. Petrich noted that age greater than 45 increased the required cumulative dose of radioiodine to treat patients with three or less bone metastases from 300 mCi to over 1000 mCi *(26)*. In addition, Casara reported a clear relationship between advancing age, loss of iodine avidity, and incidence of bone metastases *(18)*. The latter study showed an age-dependent increase in the prevalence of bone metastases of 1%, 45%, and 50% in patients younger than 40, 45–60, and above 60 years of age, respectively. Decreased iodine uptake in 6%, 29%, and 45% of patients, respectively, was also noted across the same age strata. However, age at diagnosis was not a significant independent variable in a multivariate analysis conducted by Pittas in patients with bone metastases *(10)*. However, only 13% of the cohort in that study was less than 45 yr old. A more recent study by Bernier examined data from 109 patients, all of whom had bone metastases from differentiated thyroid cancer and found that survival decreased from a median of 15.2 to 3.3 yr when bone metastases were diagnosed after age 45 *(15)*. This relationship appears quite compelling, but these data were highly significant only in univariate analysis, and the observation did not maintain its significance after multivariate analysis. What is not clear from these studies is the degree to which age alone can be separated as an independent variable from other simultaneous and confounding factors. How best to understand age as a predictor of survival remains somewhat unclear.

Natural History of Thyroid Cancer Bone Metastases

Certain characteristics of bone metastases from thyroid cancer may affect pathobiologic behavior and, in turn, tumor natural history and patient survival. Bone metastases may present synchronously (at the onset of diagnosis) or metachronously (after diagnosis). Synchronous bone metastases occur in 37–90% of patients *(3,4,8,10,15,26–28)* who develop bone metastases (Fig. 3) and are frequently symptomatic at presentation (Fig. 4). However, in most studies, treatment outcomes are rarely stratified based on whether metastases present early or late in the course of the disease *(26)*. Schlumberger and Casara report cohorts in whom bone metastases did not become manifest, and were therefore not treated for 5–7 yr from the time of initial thyroid cancer diagnosis *(18,30)*. The majority of the tumors in these series did not demonstrate significant radioiodine avidity and were associated with poor outcomes. In contrast Petrich et al. examined 107 patients with "early" bone metastases diagnosed within 4 mo of initial onset of primary thyroid cancer. Radioiodine uptake by bone metastases in this cohort was 94.4%.

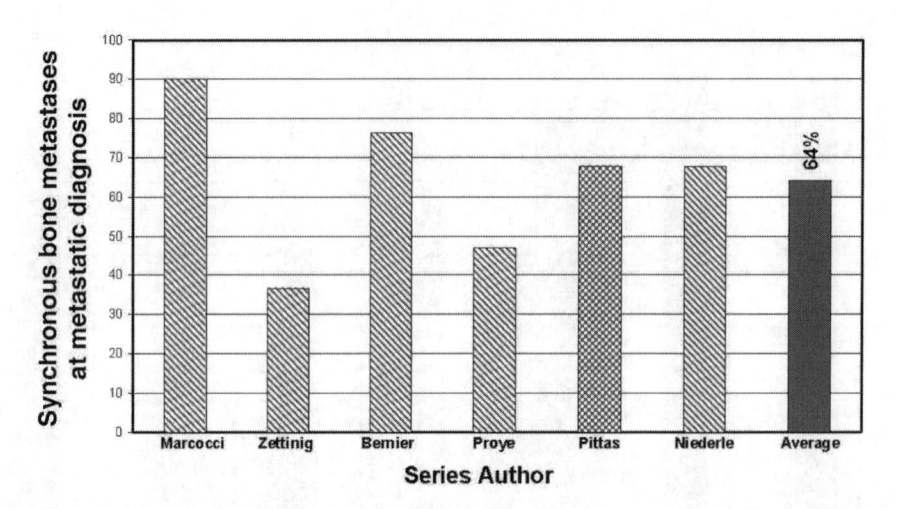

Fig. 3. Percent incidence of synchronous bone metastases of thyroid cancer among patients with thyroid cancer bone metastases. Diagonally hashed bars represent data from studies of only differentiated thyroid cancer. A single study in patients with differentiated, poorly differentiated, and undifferentiated thyroid cancer bone metastases is represented by a checkered bar. Average of all studies shown is represented by a solid bar *(3, 4,8,10,15,28)*. (Color illustration appears in insert following p. 198.)

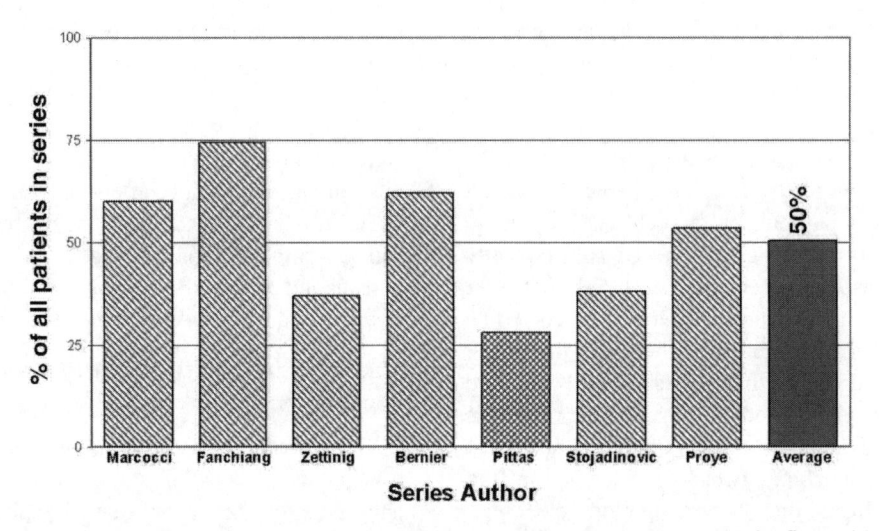

Fig. 4. Percentage of patients in selected series presenting with symptomatic bone metastases as the first evidence of thyroid cancer. Diagonally hashed bars represent data of only differentiated thyroid cancer. A single study in patients with differentiated, poorly differentiated, and undifferentiated thyroid cancer bone metastases is represented by a checkered bar. The average rate of all studies shown is represented by a solid bar *(3–5,8,10,15,29)*. (Color illustration appears in insert following p. 198.)

Remission rates following aggressive radioiodine therapy in this series were over 50%, even when extraskeletal metastases were present. These results far exceed the usual range of 10–35% for radioiodine-induced remission of thyroid cancer bone metastases *(26,31)*. Petrich et al. concluded that iodine-avid "early" metastases from differentiated thyroid cancer may be treated with radioiodine with a greater expectation of remission than that suggested by data where "early" and "late" metastases of thyroid cancer are not specifically stratified *(26)*. However, these data are limited by a relatively scant definition of "remission" and are again, in this case, the product of univariate analysis.

TREATMENT OF BONE METASTASES

Radioactive Iodine Therapy

Another major issue surrounded by ongoing contention is whether radioiodine is effective for the treatment of bone metastases from differentiated thyroid cancer. As noted, the multivariate data analysis of Schlumberger et al. and others have shown that radioiodine improves survival in combined data from patients with lung and bone metastases of differentiated thyroid cancer *(16)*. However, this evidence does not consider treatment outcomes in the patient subset with only bone metastases. Schlumberger and Hay expressed skepticism regarding the magnitude of benefit following radioiodine treatment in patients with bone metastases from thyroid cancer *(32)*. However, Schlumberger et al. have noted that bone metastases at the skull base are typically more responsive to therapy than bone metastases elsewhere *(16)*. Both Proye et al. and Schlumberger et al. have observed that thyroid cancer bone metastases demonstrate a more favorable response to treatment with radioiodine when metastases are only visible by isotope scan, not on plain radiographs *(4,20,33)*. In a series of 28 patients with differentiated thyroid cancer bone metastases, Proye has noted that 17% of metastases only visible by isotope scan completely resolved after radioiodine therapy. However, no metastases visible by radiograph had a complete response to radioiodine *(4)*. An analysis of two large cohorts from the Mayo Clinic *(17,19)* of patients with bone and other distant metastases of differentiated thyroid cancer showed no benefit from radioiodine *(4)*. Data from the Memorial Sloan-Kettering Cancer Center, specifically in patients with bone metastases from differentiated thyroid cancer, also showed no improvement from radioiodine treatment *(10)*. With multivariate analysis, the latter study did show a better prognosis in patients with bone metastases associated with preserved iodine uptake. A more recent multivariate analysis by Bernier demonstrated that a cumulative radioiodine dose of more than 200 mCi was linked with improved survival *(15)*.

There may not be adequate information in the literature to definitively settle the question of whether radioiodine therapy for all bone metastases confers a survival benefit. However, what is not often emphasized in studies that attempt to assess a "cure," is the extent of "control" gained through the appropriate use of radioiodine over disease progression, symptoms, and advanced complications of metastases *(34)*. Sarlis has noted anecdotal reports of long progression-free intervals following repeated radioiodine doses with lifetime cumulative doses reaching as high as 4500 mCi *(34)*.

The literature suggests strongly that younger patients with early iodine-avid bone metastases who do not have extraskeletal metastases have the best chance of response to radioiodine therapy. As patients diverge from this archetype, this response may become less robust, but there is no literature that absolutely allows quantification or prediction of this divergence.

Adjunctive Treatments

Recent studies have shown the benefits of adjunctive therapies, such as external-beam radiotherapy, arterial embolization, and surgical metastectomy, for the management of thyroid cancer bone metastases. Surgical resection with curative intent (i.e., complete surgical removal of all metastatic tissue) has been advocated for solitary distant bone metastasis, palliation of symptomatic lesions, and treatment lesions that are not iodine-avid *(4,28,29)*. Data from the Japanese Bone Tumor Registry suggests that surgery for thyroid cancer bone metastases may be indicated more often than for other types of cancer that metastasize to bone *(35)*. Bernier has published multivariate data demonstrating survival benefit from curative resection in patients less than 45 yr old when diagnosed with bone metastasis *(15)*. In another recent study, Zettinig found that even more aggressive surgical treatment of bone metastases from differentiated thyroid cancer was effective. In that series, 21 patients underwent resection of up to five bone metastases with the intention of eradicating disease. Univariate analysis of this cohort identified complete surgical removal of all bone metastases and the absence of extraskeletal metastases with improved survival *(8)*. A major limitation of all these studies is the relative paucity of resectable bone lesions, which have been estimated to be fewer than 10% *(29)*. In these studies, bone metastasis surgery was performed, in addition to other adjunctive therapies, including radioiodine treatment. This approach suggests a role in selected patients without further extraskeletal metastases for surgical management to achieve a cure.

Several other adjunctive treatments have emerged and are cited in recent literature. Selective arterial embolization—traditionally used for the treatment of vascular anomalies—has been useful therapy for bone metastases of thyroid cancer. Data have suggested that it is efficacious in two settings: as aggressive treatment for bone lesions not amenable to surgical cure and in combination with surgery to reduce vascular supply to bone lesions preoperatively. Additionally, data indicate embolization is effective for rapid palliation of pain and neurological symptoms in patients with vertebral metastases *(36)*.

Eustatia-Rutten et al. have shown that embolization provided rapid symptomatic relief from complicated bone metastases of thyroid cancer in 60% of their cases. Although this study did not show an improvement in overall survival after embolization, it demonstrated a clear increase in the duration of symptomatic relief *(37)*. Studies by van Tol et al. have shown that arterial embolization in combination with radioiodine treatment resulted in a significantly larger decrease in serum thyroglobulin than treatment with radioiodine alone. In that study, thyroglobulin decreased by 88.7% in the embolization group compared to only an 18.6% decrease in the group treated with radioiodine (Fig. 5; *38*). The research cited above have all shown embolization as largely safe and effective with minimal complications. However, one case suggests the development of acute respiratory distress syndrome (ARDS) from presumed pulmonary thyroglobulin aggregates after embolization of a large sacral metastasis *(39)*.

Reports examining the use of vertebroplasty, kyphoplasty, radiofrequency ablation, and percutaneous ethanol injection for the treatment of bone metastases have included small numbers of patients with bone metastases from thyroid cancer *(1,40,41;* see Chapter 54*)*. These methods are most

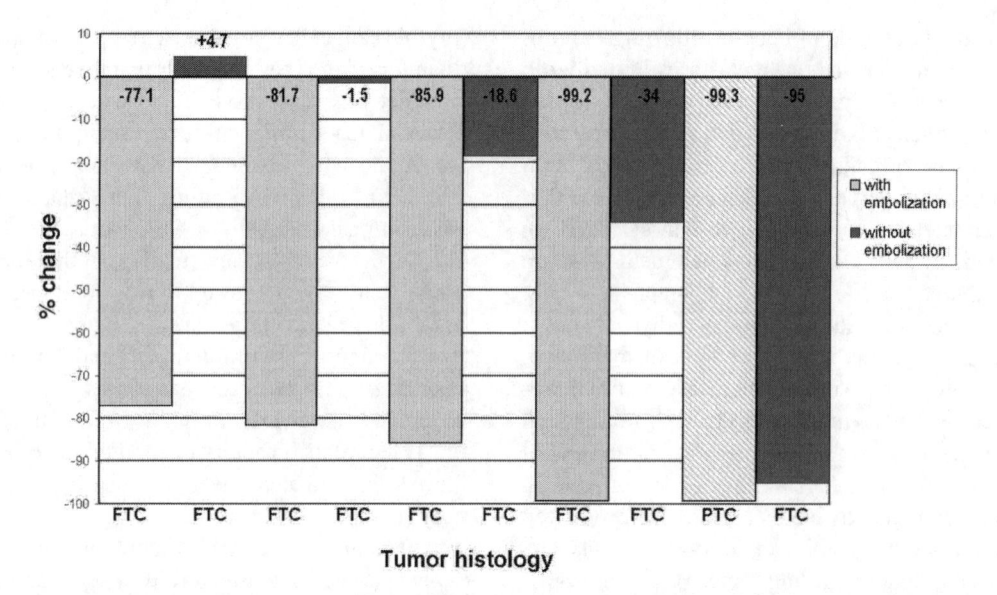

Fig. 5. Reduction of thyroglobulin levels with and without embolization of differentiated thyroid cancer metastases. Diagnonal striped bar, papillary thyroid carcinoma. Solid bars, follicular thyroid carcinoma *(38)*. (Color illustration appears in insert following p. 198.)

commonly used as part of a combined supportive approach with lesions that are refractory or not amenable to more definitive intervention. Relevant data suggest that they are effective in palliating bone pain, which has been reported as otherwise uncontrolled in up to 70% of patients with bone metastases *(1)*. These series are primarily composed of patients with bone metastases from nonthyroid cancers. Despite the relative underrepresentation of thyroid cancer patients in the studies, they appear to be generalizable to thyroid cancer metastases.

External-beam radiotherapy has been used as an adjunctive treatment in complicated thyroid cancer. A recent review has again supported its use, specifically with thyroid cancer bone metastases not amenable to surgery or radiiodine therapy *(33)*.

BISPHOSPHONATE THERAPY

One successful intervention, borrowed from the general oncology armamentarium, has been bisphosphonate therapy for the treatment of bone metastases of thyroid cancer. Developed three decades ago, early bisphosphonates inhibited osteoclast function through their incorporation into cytotoxic analogs of adenosine triphosphate *(65)*. Bisphosphonate potency was subsequently found to be determined by the chemical structure of its side chains. The discovery of the importance of structure has allowed the more recent development of the most potent bisphosphonates known. These newer agents contain a basic nitrogen group in their side chain and are therefore referred to as "aminobisphosphonates." Aminobisphosphonates possess additional mechanisms of action compared to older bisphosphonates. They appear to inhibit farnesyl diphosphonate synthase and disrupt the mevalonate pathway in osteoclasts. The mevalonate pathway is responsible for posttranslational prenylation of guanosine triphosphate-binding proteins, such as Ras and Rho, which are essential for osteoclast function and survival *(65,66)*. Loss of protein prenylation inhibits formation of a ruffled border and tight-sealing zone, preventing normal osteoclast-mediated bone resorption. Aminobisphosphonates also prevent osteoclast function through several other mechanisms. Inhibition of the mevalonate pathway induces a wide array of disruptions in integrin expression, metalloproteinase activity, and causes induction of osteoclast apoptosis through bcl-2-mediated activation of caspase 3-like proteases *(67)*. Recent studies in multiple myeloma also suggest that pamidronate—one of the potent aminobisphosphonates—allows recognition and direct cytolysis of both tumor and osteoclasts by $\gamma\delta T$ cells *(68)*.

The use of pamidronate to specifically treat thyroid cancer bone metastases has been shown as beneficial in at least one small study *(69)*. This included 10 patients with symptomatic osseous metastases of thyroid cancer who had exhausted conventional means of therapy and were treated with monthly intravenous 90-mg doses of pamidronate for 1 year. Of the 10 patients, 2 showed partial radiographic regression of their bone lesions. Five additional patients showed stabilization of bone metastasis during treatment. All patients given pamidronate had significant reductions in bone pain. An average pain reduction of over 30% occurred after 3 mo of therapy. Treatment was well-tolerated with minimal side effects *(69)*.

Zolendronic acid, a newer and even more potent aminobisphosphonate, is now also available. Zolendronic acid has the advantage of more rapid administration in a 15-min infusion (vs 2 h for pamidronate) and has been shown to be superior to pamidronate in reducing skeletal complications in patients with breast cancer *(70)*. It has demonstrated more potent antiresorptive and antitumor effects in numerous preclinical studies *(9)*. In addition, zolendronic acid has been safe and efficacious in patients with impaired creatinine clearance as low as 43 mL per minute without dose adjustment *(71,72)*.

The importance of bisphosphonates for the management of skeletal cancer-related complications cannot be overstated. But although generally well-tolerated, recent reports have raised concern regarding possible involvement of both zolendronic acid and pamidronate with osteonecrosis of the jaw *(73–75)*. However, these are uncontrolled and anecdotal reports that cannot establish a causal association. This complication has been almost exclusively reported in cancer patients taking numerous medications who typically had some preceding oral trauma or chronic morbidity. Novartis, the manufacturer of both medications, has recently funded a retrospective chart review at one of the country's largest regional cancer centers to determine outcomes following the use of these agents *(73)*. Although any adverse findings from such a study would create the need for further caution, bisphosphonates will almost certainly remain critically important agents in the treatment of skeletal complications of cancer.

MECHANISMS OF BONE METASTASIS

The development of metastases requires interactions between both the invading malignant cell and the new host tissue. Stephen Paget recognized this while studying breast cancer and described the "seed and soil hypothesis" in the late 19th century. "When a plant goes to seed, its seeds are carried in all direction; but they can only grow if they fall on congenial soil" *(42)*. This simple observation remains illustrative and applicable to thyroid cancer metastases.

The process of metastasis has been frequently characterized to include multiple distinct steps *(9,43)*. Before metastasis can develop, a primary tumor must first lose cell–cell and cell–matrix cohesion, develop motility, chemotaxis, and ultimately, local invasiveness. Tumor dissemination requires entry and successful passage through the vascular or lymphatic compartments, as well as successful extravasation and implantation into a distant end organ. Once in its new location, a metastatic cell only becomes a mature secondary malignancy if it has the ability to prosper in its new environment *(44)*. Each step in this process requires numerous and unique changes in the expression of genes, enzymes, adhesion, and signaling molecules; without these changes, metastasis cannot occur *(45)*. Much has been published describing the mechanisms that underlie metastasis in such cancers as breast, prostate, and multiple myeloma. These mechanisms, and how they relate to thyroid cancer, remain in the early stages of study. Understanding of how thyroid cancer develops and metastasizes remains incomplete.

Recent findings have begun to shed some light on this process. Follicular carcinoma typically shows underexpression of caveolin-1 and -2. These genes affect tumor suppression in conjunction with PTEN. Paradoxically, caveolin-1 and -2 are overexpressed in papillary and anaplastic thyroid carcinomas and portend a worse prognosis *(46,47)*. Focal adhesion kinase (FAK) is involved in adhesion, motility, and anchorage-dependent growth. FAK may impact tissue invasion and metastasis in thyroid cancer. FAK is overexpressed in the most aggressive differentiated thyroid cancers but has limited expression in noninvasive neoplastic thyroid tissue *(48)*. Metastin—a product of the *KIS-1* gene— appears to act as a metastasis suppressor in an in vivo model of differentiated thyroid cancer metastasis *(49)*. Recombinant metastin has been shown to inhibit tumor cell growth and migration in this model. Thus, downregulation of metastin expression may be required before distant metastases can develop. Chen et al. has shown differential expression of several genes in the metastases of follicular thyroid cancer previously implicated in carcinogenesis of other types of malignancy. They showed that fibronectins, cell surface proteins that control cell adhesion and migration, are expressed to a lesser degree in follicular thyroid cancer *(50)*. Bone sialoprotein, which is overexpressed in thyroid carcinomas *(51)*, has been demonstrated to increase invasiveness of thyroid cancer cells in the invitro assays through interaction with integrin $\alpha v \beta 3$ *(52)*. Expression of integrin $\alpha v \beta 3$ in tumor cells increases bone adhesion and accelerates development of osteolytic lesions *(53)*.

Many mechanisms involved in the complex process of metastasis continue to be described in many nonthyroid cancers. How many, if any, of these important mechanistic cellular changes occur with ubiquity across disparate tumor types, including thyroid cancer, is still unclear. However, what seems apparent is that better understanding of how these cellular processes contribute to the generation of tumorigenesis and metastasis will allow the development of specific targeted treatments in not only these malignancies but in thyroid cancer as well.

OSTEOTROPISM AND THE DEVELOPMENT OF METASTASES

The skeleton is a common site of distant metastasis for several malignancies, including thyroid cancer. As with other cancers that metastasize to bone, the spine is an especially typical site for the metastases of thyroid cancer. Data from 10 series representing patients with 930 bone metastases of differentiated thyroid cancer identify the axial skeleton as the most common site of bone metastases (Fig. 6). As predicted by Paget, this frequent osteotropism results from the behavior of the metastatic cell and is also dependent on

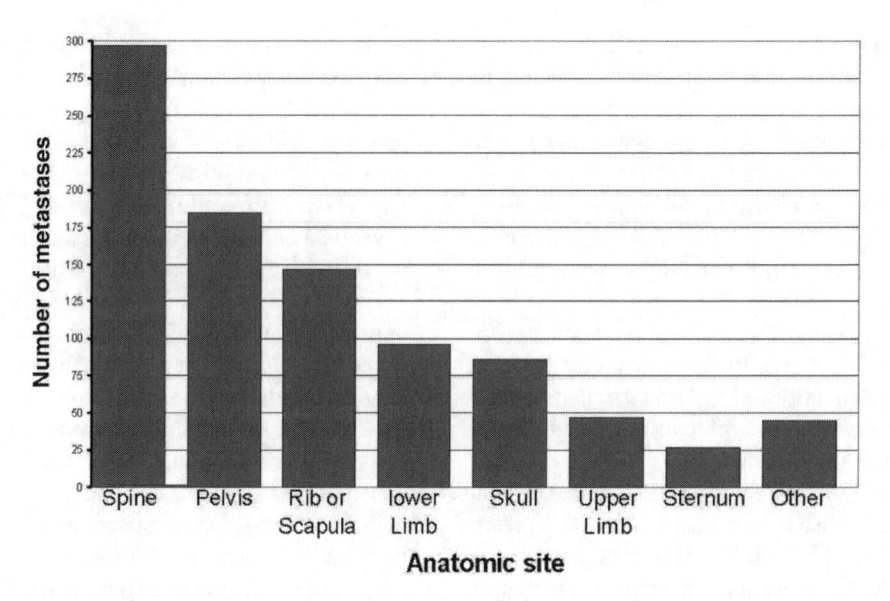

Fig. 6. Distribution of 930 bone metastases from thyroid cancer by anatomic site across 10 selected studies (3,5–8,10,13,15,28,54). (Color illustration appears in insert following p. 198.)

properties inherent to the osseous microenvironment. The combination of both produces the profound tropism of cancers to bone.

The skeleton is richly supplied with blood but is a more frequent site of metastasis than other highly vascular organs that receive an even larger percentage of total cardiac output *(55)*. Bone contains numerous sinusoids that are lined with an epithelium lacking a basement membrane. A mechanically favorable environment is thus created that is hospitable to osseous metastasis *(56)*. Cancer cells express surface adhesion molecules, which facilitate binding to bone matrix and stroma. Adhesion causes tumor cells to increase production of angiogenic and bone-resorbing factors *(56)*. The bone matrix and bone marrow possess immense stores of immobilized growth factors, cytokines, and mitogenic peptides. These are readily released following invasion by metastatic cells and facilitate proliferation of nascent metastases *(57)*. Production and release of stored transforming growth factors β, insulin-like growth factors I and II, fibroblast growth factors, platelet-derived growth factors, and bone morphogenetic proteins are readily subverted by an invading tumor. This results in disruption of normal bone homeostasis and enhanced survival of the metastatic cell. Mobilization of these factors may occur via direct interaction of tumor cells with the bone or indirectly through cytokine-stimulated bone resorption by osteoclasts or bone formation by osteoblasts.

Osseous metastases develop as lytic, blastic, or mixed lesions. This is largely dependent on the direction in which a tumor is able to tip the equilibrium that controls bone resorption and formation. Bone metastases from thyroid cancer are almost exclusively osteolytic *(13,58)*, however, there are rare reports of osteoblastic bone lesions in metastases associated with medullary thyroid cancer *(59)*. In well-studied models of bone metastases, activation of the receptor activator of nuclear factor (NF)-κB (RANK) by its cognate ligand (RANK-L) causes recruitment and terminal differentiation of osteoclast precursors into mature osteoclasts. The direct action of the osteoclast mediates osteolytic bone disease. RANK-L is expressed on the surface of stromal cells and osteoblasts and is released as a soluble ligand by activated Tcells. The binding of RANK-L to RANK induces cell signaling through the NF-κB and Jun N-terminal kinase pathways, leading to osteoclast differentiation *(43,57)*. This process is opposed by a soluble "decoy receptor" osteoprotegerin (OPG), which is produced by osteoblast precursors, bone stromal cells, and some tumors. OPG binds to and immobilizes RANK-L, preventing its binding with RANK. The signal for terminal differentiation of osteoclast progenitor cells and osteoclast-mediated bone resorption is thereby modulated by OPG.

The RANK/RANK-L/OPG mechanism appears common to all osteolytic tumors. Control of this interaction appears to depend on autocrine-, paracrine-, and juxtacrine-acting factors that vary based on tumor type *(59)*. Many of these factors have been identified in the bone metastases of myeloma, breast, and prostate cancers but remain virtually unstudied in thyroid cancer. In mouse models of metastasis, osseous implantation of PC-3 prostate cancer cells—known to elaborate RANK-L, interleukin (IL)-1 and tumor necrosis factor α produced purely osteolytic bone lesions. Implantation of LAPC-9 prostate cancer cells that elaborate OPG and no detectable RANK-L or IL-1, resulted in purely osteoblastic bone lesions *(60,61)*. In other mouse models, the treatment of osteolytic metastases with OPG dramatically reduced skeletal tumor burden and caused significant decreases in tumor-associated osteoclasts *(62)*.

Osteolytic lesions depend not only on exuberant osteoclast activity, mediated by the RANK/OPG system, but on the dysregulation of normal osteoblast function as well. In multiple myeloma, which is almost exclusively osteolytic, suppression of osteoblast function has been shown to occur through a tumor-mediated effect on the Wnt signaling pathway. This pathway is a critical element involved in the growth and differentiation of osteoblasts. The Wnt pathway is directly inhibited in multiple myeloma by tumoral secretion of DKK1—a product of the dickopf-1 gene (60). Cytokine and signaling pathways that control osteoblastic metastases have only recently been described. Endothelin-1 and the platelet-derived growth factor are now thought to be important mediators of osteoblastic metastases in breast cancer (57,63,64). How the dysregulation of these pathways may contribute to the rare occurrence of osteoblastic thyroid cancer bone metastases remains unclear.

It is likely that osteolytic bone metastases in thyroid cancer are mediated by osteoclasts controlled by the RANK/RANKL/OPG system, as is the case with other well-studied cancers. However, direct study of this mechanism in thyroid cancer metastases is still lacking. Our understanding of how thyroid cancer metastasizes to bone, and the exact mechanisms that underlie its successful osseous proliferation, remain largely inferential, based on our understanding of other malignancies. Similarly, treatments for bone metastases of thyroid cancer, other than radioiodine, have been largely drawn from successful therapy developed for other cancer types. Only further direct study of the genetic and cellular processes of thyroid cancer and its metastases will allow the identification of novel targets for therapy and provide insight for new and unique treatment options.

CLINICAL RECOMMENDATIONS

Considerable data exist regarding the natural history and treatment of bone metastases from thyroid cancer. However, the relative rarity of thyroid cancer, inherent limitations of existing literature, and lack of controlled studies makes it difficult to derive an evidence-based approach. Nevertheless, treatment decisions must be made. Therefore, the approach used at our institution for the treatment of patients who develop bone metastases from differentiated thyroid cancer is now summarized.

Typically, total thyroidectomy and ^{131}I scanning and therapy precede any treatment of distant metastases. However, this may not occur if the advanced stage of disease allows only palliative care. Whenever the presence of bone metastases are suspected or confirmed, we fully stage each patient to help determine the extent of disease, regardless of whether metastases are synchronous or metachronous. Our practice is to obtain a withdrawal or recombinant human thyrotropin-stimulated serum thyroglobulin level, magnetic resonance image (MRI) or sonogram of the neck, and noncontrast-enhanced computed tomography (CT) scan of the head, chest, and abdomen.

Skeletal radiographic survey and radionuclide bone scanning may be useful in circumstances where bone metastases are suspected. 18-Fluoro-deoxyglucose-positron emission tomography (FDG-PET) scanning is also an effective means of visualizing otherwise occult extrathyroidal lesions. We find FDG-PET particularly valuable when "fused" with MRI or CT images, allowing more precise lesional localization. The evolution of ultrasensitive thyroglobulin assays has reduced our routine dependence on radioiodine whole-body scanning. However, whole-body scans are helpful when metastases arise metachronously, the disease is persistent or has proven poorly responsive to previous radioiodine treatment, or when a specific determination of iodine avidity is desired. In these instances, a negative whole-body scan may strongly support a decision to defer further radioiodine therapy. In such cases, we would explore alternative means of treatment, such as surgical extirpation, external radiation, or other techniques (e.g., radiofrequency ablation).

Radioiodine still remains the primary treatment in the majority of circumstances. We believe that age less than 45, limited early metastases confined only to the skeleton, and iodine-avid lesions not visible on plain radiograph all suggest potentially favorable responses to radioiodine therapy. In this setting, we make every attempt to provide radioiodine therapy, utilizing dosimetry to calculate the greatest tolerable activity permissible. We incorporate a low-iodine diet in the pretherapy plan to maximize radioiodine avidity by the tumor. If bone lesions are few in number, we consider aggressive surgical metastectomy with curative intent before radioiodine therapy. Data to support this decision are limited, but we believe that in addition to providing a potential surgical cure, metastectomy represents an effective method to debulk tumor mass and may contribute to the successful treatment of remaining micrometastases with radioiodine. Presurgical embolization to reduce vascular supply has proven effective (in our experience) to reduce operative blood loss. Embolization, radiofrequency ablation, and external-beam therapy have all proven beneficial when surgery is not possible or the response to radioiodine is incomplete or absent. These interventions have also been effective as palliative therapy for selected symptomatic lesions in the setting of refractory diseases.

Intravenous bisphosphonate therapy with zolendronic acid is used for patients with known bone metastases. Yet, little data exist to guide such therapy in thyroid cancer. Our practice is to treat with monthly 4-mg infusions for 1 yr and reassess fully before continuing bisphosphonate therapy. How long intravenous zolendronic acid should be continued is unknown. Patients with thyroid cancer that is complicated by osseous metastases may have longer survival rates than patients with bone metastases from other primary tumors, such as breast cancer. Therefore, guidelines for the use of intravenous zolendronic acid in other tumors may not be applicable. This issue remains poorly studied. Our present practice is to continue zolendronic acid therapy, if required after the intial year, at a reduced frequency of 4 mg intravenously every 3–4 mo. Serum electrolytes, creatinine, and blood urea nitrogen are assessed immediately prior to each dose. Some have advocated following bone turnover markers during aggressive bisphosphonate therapy, but it is not clear how these values should guide treatment. We do not believe there is sufficient human data at this time to support the prophylactic use of bisphosphonates in the absence of proven bone metastases from thyroid cancer. We do, however, fully evaluate all patients with histologically or biologically aggressive thyroid cancer for osteoporosis and vitamin D deficiency, as well as begin oral bisphosphonates, calcium, and oral vitamin D supplementation as indicated.

The decision regarding which patients should undergo complete evaluation for osseous metastases is frequently difficult. We aggressively examine those patients whose primary tumor is large or demonstrates vascular extensive local invasion or multiple positive lymph node metastases. Patients with potentially more aggressive tumor variants (e.g., tall-cell or columnar-cell carcinomas) also are reviewed carefully. Patients with known pulmonary metastases seem particularly prone to developing osseous metastases. Patients with known brain, liver, renal, or other parenchymal metastases also require extensive evaluation.

In general, we recommend that the initial osseous metastasis be confirmed by an aspiration or biopsy to prove it is, in fact, derived from a thyroid primary. Tissue diagnosis of subsequent lesions may be unnecessary, depending on clinical context. This is particularly true when subsequent lesions demonstrate radioiodine avidity. Although unlikely, metastases from nonthyroid primary malignancies may occur in the presence of thyroid cancer. For this reason, the clinician should consider appropriate cancer screening, as indicated by the clinical setting, and scrupulously explore the derivation of new metastases if this suspicion is high.

Cases of dramatic response to radioiodine in combination with adjunctive therapy have been described; however, the appearance of bone metastases of differentiated thyroid cancer usually suggests the inexorable progression of disease. Cure is possible, but it is usually unlikely. Our focus, in those cases, turns to containment of existing disease, symptomatic palliation, and aggressive management of lesions that impair quality of life or are at a high risk of fracture. The data reviewed here is extensive, but it does not allow definitive recommendations based purely on evidence. Nonetheless, it does provide a framework for decision-making relating to typically complex clinical situations that require case-by-case consideration. It is doubtful that large multicenter prospective trials will ever be conducted to directly address the many remaining questions about the optimal treatment of bone metastases from differentiated thyroid cancer. Thus, we agree completely with J. Jeffrey Ruegemer, who in his 1988 review of data from the Mayo Clinic quoted A. L. Vickery: "In the meantime, decisions must be made on the basis of imperfect data" *(19,76)*.

REFERENCES

1. Halpin RJ, Bendok BR, Liu JC. Minimally invasive treatments for spinal metastases: vertebroplasty, kyphoplasty, and radiofrequency ablation. J Support Oncol 2004; 2:339–351; discussion 352–355.
2. Hundahl SA, Fleming ID, Fremgen AM, Menck HR. A National Cancer Data Base report on 53,856 cases of thyroid carcinoma treated in the U.S., 1985-1995. Cancer 1998; 83:2638–2648.
3. Marcocci C, Pacini F, Elisei R, et al. Clinical and biologic behavior of bone metastases from differentiated thyroid carcinoma. Surgery 1989; 106:960–966.
4. Proye CA, Dromer DH, Carnaille BM, et al. Is it still worthwhile to treat bone metastases from differentiated thyroid carcinoma with radioactive iodine? World J Surg 1992; 16:640–645; discussion 645–646.
5. Fanchiang JK, Lin JD, Huang MJ, Shih HN. Papillary and follicular thyroid carcinomas with bone metastases: a series of 39 cases during a period of 18 years. Changgeng Yi Xue Za Zhi 1998; 21: 377–382.
6. Hay ID, Rock MG, Sim FH, et al., editors. Metastatic Bone Cancer: Thyroid Cancer. New York, NY: Raven Press, 1988.
7. Lin JD, Huang MJ, Juang JH, et al. Factors related to the survival of papillary and follicular thyroid carcinoma patients with distant metastases. Thyroid 1999; 9:1227–1235.
8. Zettinig G, Fueger BJ, Passler C, et al. Long-term follow-up of patients with bone metastases from differentiated thyroid carcinoma—surgery or conventional therapy? Clin Endocrinol (Oxf) 2002; 56:377–382.
9. Lipton A. Pathophysiology of bone metastases: how this knowledge may lead to therapeutic intervention. J Support Oncol 2004; 2: 205–213; discussion 213–214, 216–217, 219–220.
10. Pittas AG, Adler M, Fazzari M, et al. Bone metastases from thyroid carcinoma: clinical characteristics and prognostic variables in one hundred forty-six patients. Thyroid 2000; 10:261–268.
11. Schlumberger MJ. Papillary and follicular thyroid carcinoma. N Engl J Med 1998; 338:297–306.
12. Mazzaferri E. Radioiodine and Other Treatment and Outcomes, 8th ed. Philadelphia, PA: Williams & Wilkins, 2000.
13. Castillo LA, Yeh SD, Leeper RD, Benua RS. Bone scans in bone metastases from functioning thyroid carcinoma. Clin Nucl Med 1980; 5: 200–209.
14. Wood WJ, Jr., Singletary SE, Hickey RC. Current results of treatment for distant metastatic well-differentiated thyroid carcinoma. Arch Surg 1989; 124:1374–1377.
15. Bernier MO, Leenhardt L, Hoang C, et al. Survival and therapeutic modalities in patients with bone metastases of differentiated thyroid carcinomas. J Clin Endocrinol Metab 2001; 86:1568–1573.
16. Schlumberger M, Challeton C, De Vathaire F, et al. Radioactive iodine treatment and external radiotherapy for lung and bone metastases from thyroid carcinoma. J Nucl Med 1996; 37:598–605.
17. Dinneen SF, Valimaki MJ, Bergstralh EJ, et al. Distant metastases in papillary thyroid carcinoma: 100 cases observed at one institution during 5 decades. J Clin Endocrinol Metab 1995; 80:2041–2045.
18. Casara D, Rubello D, Saladini G, et al. Distant metastases in differentiated thyroid cancer: long-term results of radioiodine treatment and statistical analysis of prognostic factors in 214 patients. Tumori 1991; 77: 432–436.
19. Ruegemer JJ, Hay ID, Bergstralh EJ, et al. Distant metastases in differentiated thyroid carcinoma: a multivariate analysis of prognostic variables. J Clin Endocrinol Metab 1988; 67:501–508.

20. Schlumberger M, Tubiana M, De Vathaire F, et al. Long-term results of treatment of 283 patients with lung and bone metastases from differentiated thyroid carcinoma. J Clin Endocrinol Metab 1986; 63:960–967.
21. Tubiana M, Schlumberger M, Rougier P, et al. Long-term results and prognostic factors in patients with differentiated thyroid carcinoma. Cancer 1985; 55:794–804.
22. Samaan NA, Schultz PN, Hickey RC, et al. The results of various modalities of treatment of well differentiated thyroid carcinomas: a retrospective review of 1599 patients. J Clin Endocrinol Metab 1992; 75:714–720.
23. Maheshwari YK, Hill CS, Jr., Haynie TP, III, et al. 131I therapy in differentiated thyroid carcinoma: M. D. Anderson Hospital experience. Cancer 1981; 47:664–671.
24. Mazzaferri EL, Jhiang SM. Long-term impact of initial surgical and medical therapy on papillary and follicular thyroid cancer. Am J Med 1994; 97:418–428.
25. Schlumberger M, De Vathaire F, Travagli JP, et al. Differentiated thyroid carcinoma in childhood: long term follow-up of 72 patients. J Clin Endocrinol Metab 1987; 65:1088–1094.
26. Petrich T, Widjaja A, Musholt TJ, et al. Outcome after radioiodine therapy in 107 patients with differentiated thyroid carcinoma and initial bone metastases: side-effects and influence of age. Eur J Nucl Med 2001; 28:203–208.
27. Tickoo SK, Pittas AG, Adler M, et al. Bone metastases from thyroid carcinoma: a histopathologic study with clinical correlates. Arch Pathol Lab Med 2000; 124:1440–1447.
28. Niederle B, Roka R, Schemper M, et al. Surgical treatment of distant metastases in differentiated thyroid cancer: indication and results. Surgery 1986; 100:1088–1097.
29. Stojadinovic A, Shoup M, Ghossein RA, et al. The role of operations for distantly metastatic well-differentiated thyroid carcinoma. Surgery 2002; 131:636–643.
30. Schlumberger M, Challeton C, De Vathaire F, Parmentier C. Treatment of distant metastases of differentiated thyroid carcinoma. J Endocrinol Invest 1995; 18:170–172.
31. Sherman SI. The management of metastatic differentiated thyroid carcinoma. Rev Endocr Metab Disord 2000; 1:165–171.
32. Wartofsky L, Sherman SI, Gopal J, et al. The use of radioactive iodine in patients with papillary and follicular thyroid cancer. J Clin Endocrinol Metab 1998; 83:4195–4203.
33. Brierley JD, Tsang RW. External-beam radiation therapy in the treatment of differentiated thyroid cancer. Semin Surg Oncol 1999; 16:42–49.
34. Sarlis NJ, Gourgiotis L. Unresolved issues, dilemmas and points of interest in thyroid cancer: A current perspective. Hormones 2004; 3:149–170.
35. Manabe J. Treatment modalities for metastatic bone tumors and associated issues: focusing on surgical indications and techniques for metastatic lesions in limb bones. J Orthop Sci 2000; 5:524–531.
36. Smit JW, Vielvoye GJ, Goslings BM. Embolization for vertebral metastases of follicular thyroid carcinoma. J Clin Endocrinol Metab 2000; 85:989–994.
37. Eustatia-Rutten CF, Romijn JA, Guijt MJ, et al. Outcome of palliative embolization of bone metastases in differentiated thyroid carcinoma. J Clin Endocrinol Metab 2003; 88:3184–3189.
38. Van Tol KM, Hew JM, Jager PL, et al. Embolization in combination with radioiodine therapy for bone metastases from differentiated thyroid carcinoma. Clin Endocrinol (Oxf) 2000; 52:653–659.
39. Elshafie O, Hussein S, Jeans WD, Woodhouse NJ. Massive rise in thyroglobulin with adult respiratory distress syndrome after embolisation of thyroid cancer metastasis. Br J Radiol 2000; 73:547–549.
40. Nakada K, Kasai K, Watanabe Y, et al. Treatment of radioiodine-negative bone metastasis from papillary thyroid carcinoma with percutaneous ethanol injection therapy. Ann Nucl Med 1996; 10:441–444.
41. Goetz MP, Callstrom MR, Charboneau JW, et al. Percutaneous image-guided radiofrequency ablation of painful metastases involving bone: a multicenter study. J Clin Oncol 2004; 22:300–306.
42. Paget S. The distribution of secondary growths in cancer of the breast. Lancet 1889; 1:571–572.
43. Guise TA, Mundy GR. Cancer and bone. Endocr Rev 1998; 19:18–54.
44. Fidler IJ. The pathogenesis of cancer metastasis: the "seed and soil" hypothesis revisited. Nat Rev Cancer 2003; 3:453–458.
45. Ramaswamy S, Ross KN, Lander ES, Golub TR. A molecular signature of metastasis in primary solid tumors. Nat Genet 2003; 33:49–54.
46. Aldred MA, Ginn-Pease ME, Morrison CD, et al. Caveolin-1 and caveolin-2, together with three bone morphogenetic protein-related genes, may encode novel tumor suppressors down-regulated in sporadic follicular thyroid carcinogenesis. Cancer Res 2003; 63:2864–2871.
47. Aldred MA, Huang Y, Liyanarachchi S, et al. Papillary and follicular thyroid carcinomas show distinctly different microarray expression profiles and can be distinguished by a minimum of five genes. J Clin Oncol 2004; 22:3531–3539.
48. Owens LV, Xu L, Dent GA, et al. Focal adhesion kinase as a marker of invasive potential in differentiated human thyroid cancer. Ann Surg Oncol 1996; 3:100–105.
49. Stathatos N, Bourdeau I, Saji M, et al. Metastin receptor (GPR 54) activation inhibits growth and migration of thyroid cancer cells an increases expression of endogenous AKT and calcineurin inhibitors. In 86th Annual Meeting of the Endocrine Society, New Orleans, LA: 2004.
50. Chen KT, Lin JD, Chao TC, et al. Identifying differentially expressed genes associated with metastasis of follicular thyroid cancer by cDNA expression array. Thyroid 2001; 11:41–46.
51. Bellahcene A, Albert V, Pollina L, et al. Ectopic expression of bone sialoprotein in human thyroid cancer. Thyroid 1998; 8:637–641.
52. Karadag A, Ogbureke K, Fedarko N, Fisher LW. Bone sialoprotein, matrix metalloproteinase 2, and alpha(v)beta3 integrinin osteotropic cancer cell invasion. J Nat Cancer Ins 2004; 96:956–965.
53. Pecheur I, Peyruchaud O, Serre CM, et al. Integrin alpha(v)beta3 expression confers on tumor cells a greater propensity to metastasize to bone. Faseb J 2002; 16:1266–1268.
54. Bru A, Combes PF, Naja A. Localizations and radiological aspects of osseous metastases from thyroid cancers. J Radiol Electrol Med Nucl 1963; 44:872–876.
55. Choong PF. The molecular basis of skeletal metastases. Clin Orthop 2003(415 Suppl):S19–S31.
56. Orr FW, Lee J, Duivenvoorden WC, Singh G. Pathophysiologic interactions in skeletal metastasis. Cancer 2000; 88(12 suppl):2912–2918.
57. Roodman GD. Mechanisms of bone metastasis. N Engl J Med 2004; 350:1655–1664.
58. McCormack KR. Bone metastases from thyroid carcinoma. Cancer 1966; 19:181–184.
59. Ernst S. Osteolytic bone metastases in medullary thyroid carcinoma. Strahlenther Onkol 1991; 167:549–552.
60. Tian E, Zhan F, Walker R, et al. The role of the Wnt-signaling antagonist DKK1 in the development of osteolytic lesions in multiple myeloma. N Engl J Med 2003; 349:2483–2494.
61. Lee Y, Schwarz E, Davies M, et al. Differences in the cytokine profiles associated with prostate cancer cell induced osteoblastic and osteolytic lesions in bone. J Orthop Res 2003; 21:62–72.
62. Morony S, Capparelli C, Sarosi I, et al. Osteoprotegerin inhibits osteolysis and decreases skeletal tumor burden in syngeneic and nude mouse models of experimental bone metastasis. Cancer Res 2001; 61:4432–4436.
63. Mohammad KS, Guise TA. Mechanisms of osteoblastic metastases: role of endothelin-1. Clin Orthop 2003(415 Suppl):S67–S74.
64. Guise TA, Yin JJ, Mohammad KS. Role of endothelin-1 in osteoblastic bone metastases. Cancer 2003; 97:779–784.

65. Green JR. Bisphosphonates in cancer therapy. Curr Opin Oncol 2002; 14:609–615.
66. Dunford JE, Thompson K, Coxon FP, et al. Structure-activity relationships for inhibition of farnesyl diphosphate synthase in vitro and inhibition of bone resorption in vivo by nitrogen-containing bisphosphonates. J Pharmacol Exp Ther 2001; 296:235–242.
67. Green JR, Clezardin P. Mechanisms of bisphosphonate effects on osteoclasts, tumor cell growth, and metastasis. Am J Clin Oncol 2002; 25(6 suppl 1):S3–S9.
68. Das H, Wang L, Kamath A, Bukowski JF. Vgamma2 Vdelta2 T-cell receptor-mediated recognition of aminobisphosphonates. Blood 2001; 98:1616–1618.
69. Vitale G, Fonderico F, Martignetti A, et al. Pamidronate improves the quality of life and induces clinical remission of bone metastases in patients with thyroid cancer. Br J Cancer 2001; 84:1586–1590.
70. Rosen LS, Gordon DH, Dugan W, Jr., et al. Zoledronic acid is superior to pamidronate for the treatment of bone metastases in breast carcinoma patients with at least one osteolytic lesion. Cancer 2004; 100:36–43.
71. Skerjanec A, Berenson J, Hsu C, et al. The pharmacokinetics and pharmacodynamics of zoledronic acid in cancer patients with varying degrees of renal function. J Clin Pharmacol 2003; 43:154–162.
72. Berenson J, Major P, Miller W, et al. Effect of renal function on the pharmacokinetics (PK), pharmacodynamics (PD), and sefety of zoledronic acid in cancer patietns with bone metastases. In Proceedings of the American Association for Cancer Research, 2002:167a.
73. Schwartz HC. Osteonecrosis and bisphosphonates: correlation versus causation. J Oral Maxillofac Surg 2004; 62:763–764.
74. Marx RE. Pamidronate (Aredia) and zoledronate (Zometa) induced avascular necrosis of the jaws: a growing epidemic. J Oral Maxillofac Surg 2003; 61:1115–1117.
75. Tarassoff P, Csermak K. Avascular necrosis of the jaws: risk factors in metastatic cancer patients. J Oral Maxillofac Surg 2003; 61: 1238–1239.
76. Vickery AL, Jr., Wang CA, Walker AM. Treatment of intrathyroidal papillary carcinoma of the thyroid. Cancer 1987; 60:2587–2595.

54
Adjunctive Local Approaches to Metastatic Thyroid Cancer

Leonard Wartofsky

INTRODUCTION

The overwhelming majority of differentiated thyroid cancers are curable, and this optimistic outlook applies particularly to stage I, II, and most stage III tumors. Stage IV tumors are typically and clearly in a different category, as the prognosis is significantly worse once distant metastases are present. In the author's view, a worse prognosis is not a justification for therapeutic nihilism but instead demands more aggressive therapy, with the hopeful expectation of improving outcome and prognosis. Not infrequently, some stage I and II patients have local disease that is resistant to ablation by conventional surgery and radioiodine.

This chapter attempts to summarize some approaches used to eradicate or at least control local foci of both distant and regional metastatic disease. In many cases, these local approaches are viewed as preferable alternatives to surgery or radioactive iodine administration. Repeat surgery may be declined by the patient or may be burdened with higher risk after multiple prior dissections or following external radiation therapy. In addition, external radiation may not be an option because of proven radioresistance of the particular cancer. Radioiodine treatment may be an unappealing option when a patient may have already approached or exceeded their maximally safe cumulative dose of radioiodine or when ^{131}I treatment is not feasible because the metastases are not iodine-avid. (External radiation therapy is discussed in detail in Chapters 51, 63, 72, and 81.) Chemotherapeutic approaches are another option (see Chapters 52, 73, 82, and 87), with potential molecularly targeted therapies (see Chapter 86). However, the local approaches described below may be used with chemotherapy or when chemotherapy is either ineffective or too toxic.

ETHANOL ABLATION

The percutaneous injection of 95% ethanol into hyperfunctioning thyroid nodules began in Europe and has achieved only modest use in the United States (1,2; see Chapter 17). Benign cysts and even "cold nodules" have been managed by ethanol injection after initially proven by fine-needle aspiration to be benign. The procedure may have to be repeated several times to be effective, and the instillations of alcohol may be very painful to the patient. Much of this pain is believed to be from leakage of ethanol to surrounding soft tissues. In addition to local pain, some fever and hematoma formation are common; albeit rare in experienced hands, damage to the recurrent laryngeal nerve with vocal cord paralysis is possible.

Gangi et al. (3) may have been the first to employ ethanol injection into bone metastases under computed tomography (CT) guidance to achieve pain relief. From the Mayo Clinic, Lewis et al. (4) were the first group to publish a report of percutaneous ethanol injection of thyroid cancer metastases in cervical lymph nodes. A total of 14 patients with 29 metastatic nodes were described. 20 patients who had 23 nodes injected were reported from the same group several months later by Hay at the meetings of the American Thyroid Association (5), and it is unclear if any of these represent the same patients. In the initial analysis, the patients were not considered candidates for either surgery or further radioiodine therapy. A 25-gauge needle was used and placed under sonographic guidance by a radiologist, with the needle penetrated deeply into the node. After the first injection of 0.05–0.1 mL of ethanol, the needle was repositioned, followed by an additional 3–10 injections of small amounts of ethanol. A total of 0.1–0.8 mL was used with each patient undergoing up to four treatment visits. Responses to ethanol were assessed by follow-up ultrasonographic measurement at an average of 18 mo posttreatment. Lymph node volumes were decreased from a mean basal value of 492 to 76 mm^3 1 yr later and lowered further to 20 mm^3 after 2 yr. As mentioned above, patients experienced some local pain, and a few had transient pain radiating to the jaw or chest, but they observed no major complications and achieved excellent control of metastatic lymph node disease in 12 of 14 patients. No serum thyroglobulin (Tg) data before and after the ethanol ablations were provided by the authors.

In the presentation by Hay (5) of 20 patients, decreases in node size were described in all 23 nodes injected, with 6 disappearing completely. At subsequent reevaluation of

From: *Thyroid Cancer: A Comprehensive Guide to Clinical Management*, 2/e
Edited by: L. Wartofsky and D. Van Nostrand © Humana Press Inc., Totowa, NJ

16 patients, 7 had nodes that required a second injection of ethanol. However, successful control was achieved in 15 of these 16 patients, with only 1 requiring additional surgical intervention. An average 0.7-mL dose of ethanol was injected in two occasions with no significant complications. Our own experience at the Washington Hospital Center has been similar to that of the Mayo group in a small and limited personal series of patients with local lymph node metastases. Ethanol injection has also been used for distant bone metastases by Nakada et al. (6).

EMBOLIZATION OF METASTASES

The earliest applications of embolization therapy were for vascular malformations and hemangiomas. Materials used for embolization have included polyvinyl alcohol beads (Ivalon) and gelfoam. Embolization has been employed for such benign tumors as parathyroid adenomas and uterine fibroids. The earliest malignant tumors treated were craniofacial and head and neck tumors, with bone metastases from renal carcinoma treated shortly thereafter. Embolization is the most safe and effective when a single feeding artery to a tumor can be identified that does not also supply a more critical distal tissue. Thus, bone metastases have been particularly suitable for embolization therapy, and this approach is discussed at greater length in Chapter 53. Once bone metastases occur with thyroid cancer, prognosis is sufficiently worse (7) to warrant aggressive and innovative therapeutic methods. After an analysis of prognostic factors associated with survival, Bernier et al. also recommended that this type of therapy, particularly in young patients, should be as aggressive as possible (8).

Perhaps the earliest description of embolization for thyroid cancer metastatic to bone was by Camille et al. in 1980 (9) in a report of four patients with metastases to the spine and pelvis. Smit et al. (10) studied four patients with follicular carcinoma metastases to the spine with cord compression. They postulated that they would achieve maximal tumor destruction by first administering radioiodine, then embolizing the lesions about 3–6 d later. Selective catheterization of the vessel(s) "feeding" the tumor was performed after magnetic resonance or CT imaging to identify the best vessel and determine that there was no downstream vital structure (e.g., spinal cord). Pain was the predominant symptom in their patients, and embolization was associated with significant reduction in pain. Recurrent pain or persistence of tumor based on rising Tg or visible growth on imaging were an indication for repeat embolization, with or without additional radioiodine. Pain relief is observed faster than seen after radioiodine or external radiation therapy, and a reduction (but not elimination) may be seen in serum Tg. One possible complication of embolization is a "postembolization syndrome" believed owing to acute tumor necrosis and associated with pain and fever.

Smit et al. speculated that a potential negative aspect of embolization might be the creation of tumor tissue hypoxia, which might then drive angiogenesis and neovascularization. They suggested a possible role for adjunctive antiangiogenesis chemotherapy. Some benefit in this regard might also derive from bisphosphonate therapy, with recent reports of thyroid cancer metastases treated with both pamidronate (11,12) and zoledronic acid (13,14) to reduce pain and tumor growth (see Chapter 53).

The same group (Smit et al.) reported on an updated larger patient series with follow-up periods of 2 mo to 8.6 yr (15). There were 16 patients treated with a total of 41 separate embolizations for pain, spinal cord compression, or both. They noted reduced or stable tumor size on CT in 18 of 22 treatments and considered the procedure successful overall in 24 of the 41 treatments. They did not confirm greater efficacy of treatment when combined with radioactive iodine therapy, but there was an apparently longer duration of benefit. Intervals of success were 6.5 mo for embolization alone and 15 mo for embolization coupled with either radioiodine or external radiation. Otherwise, there was no clear additional benefit in patients who had adjunctive surgery or external radiation. The patients tolerated the procedures well, and there was only one case of the postembolization syndrome.

Van Tol et al. (16) examined five patients with symptomatically painful bone metastases to determine whether there was any benefit from adjunctive radioactive iodine therapy. The patients had 5.55-GBq ablation and embolization 4–6 wk later with polyvinyl alcohol particles, then administered a second dose of 5.55 GBq of radioiodine 3 mo later. The response relating to tumor metastasis size and serum Tg was assessed with the latter parameter vs that in a control group of six patients relatively matched for disease who were treated without embolization. The combination therapy led to a median tumor volume reduction of 52.5% and a significantly improved average Tg decrement of 88.7%, in contrast to an 18.6% reduction in the control group. Although there was pain relief and some neurologic symptoms with embolization, other than the more dramatic drop in serum Tg, the degree of improvement was probably not different from that seen with radioiodine alone. One patient developed postembolization syndrome. Early measurement of serum Tg after embolization may be misleading, as a striking rise in levels may occur shortly after therapy (17), which can be seen after radioiodine as well.

In several patients, additional radioiodine or surgery was required for recurrence, but all of the combination-treatment patients were alive at the end of the study. During the longer follow-up period of the six control patients, all eventually died after a median period of 52 mo. As mentioned above, the prognosis for patients with bone metastases is not good. For both the treating clinician and the patient with extensive bone metastases, perhaps the most important issue to consider is that these therapies are only palliative and not curative.

In the series by Eustatia-Rutten et al. *(15)*, 9 of 16 patients died during the follow up period and the other five had progression of their disease.

OTHER PALLIATIVE APPROACHES TO SPINAL METASTASES

Vertebroplasty and Kyphoplasty

Back pain is the typical symptom that leads to the discovery of spinal metastases of thyroid cancer. A solitary metastatic lesion in the spine may be managed surgically by shelling out the tumor in the involved vertebral body and replacing it with bone cement, with or without reinforcement by a titanium cage or plates, as needed.

Most of the pain associated with spinal metastases is caused by compression fractures of the vertebral bodies. Both acute and chronic pain may result from these fractures, along with deformities, limitations in mobility, and a higher mortality rate. In addition to the adjunctive measures of external radiation therapy and bisphosphonates mentioned above, a benefit may be achieved by aggressive surgical approaches to the spine, especially in younger patients. An excellent overview of these procedures has appeared by Halpin et al. *(18)*, and these techniques are also discussed by Hodak and Burman in Chapter 53.

In brief, vertebroplasty is an attempt to stabilize and strengthen bone weakened by metastatic cancer and relieve pain from compression fractures. The procedure is done by a minimally invasive percutaneous approach, injecting polymethylmethacrylate into the vertebral body. The vertebral bodies need to be incompletely compressed to technically inject the material; local infection, low-platelet count, or coagulation problems are contraindications to the procedure *(19)*.

The literature indicates excellent results in selected patients, and 90% of subjects had pain reduction and improved mobility within 24 h of the procedure. The methacrylate cement fills the vertebral body, and the pain relief may be the result of destruction of nerve endings, stabilization, or actual tumor necrosis from ischemia. This procedure is burdened with many potential minor and major complications *(18,19)* and should be reserved to centers with experienced staff and success with the technique.

Kyphoplasty involves the same principle as vertebroplasty—stabilizing the vertebrae by percutaneously injecting methacrylate—but the procedure differs in two ways. The vertebral body is first expanded by the insertion via cannula of a balloon that is inflated to expand the body, then deflated prior to the cement injection *(20,21)*. Second, the cement is a more viscous or dense form than that used for vertebroplasty. Kyphoplasty is generally more effective than vertebroplasty in restoring greater height of the vertebral body and relieving pain and is the preferred procedure in many cases. Like vertebroplasty, kyphoplasty can predictably reduce pain and deformity and also improve mobility. Some of the same contraindications exist. In the series by Ledlie and Fenfro *(21)*, there were only six patients with metastatic cancer, but they had an excellent result. Four indicated the disappearance of pain, and one had reduction of pain. The same caveats regarding performance by experienced operators apply to reduce the potential complication rate.

Radiofrequency Ablation

Radiofrequency ablation (RFA) is performed either under general anesthesia or with local anesthesia and conscious sedation. Originally, the tumor metastases that were managed by RFA included liver and bone *(18,22–24)*, but it was rapidly adapted and applied to a wide variety of solid tumors, including lung metastases *(25,26)*. It is particularly effective in bone and may be combined with vertebroplasty *(27,28)*. The procedure is based essentially on inducing coagulation necrosis of tumor by the generation of heat from an electrode inserted percutaneously. Basically, it is similar to an electrocautery in that no heat actually flows through the device. Rather, high-frequency alternating current travels through the needle probe device, which serves as an antenna that elicits heat by friction, then the heat denatures the protein of the tumor. Coagulation necrosis occurs when tissues reach 50–52°C over 4–5 min. At this time, the devices are approved by the Food and Drug Administration for the treatment of bone and soft-tissue metastases. The equipment used at our medical center is provided by Rita Medical Systems and includes their Generator Model 1500 that provides 460-kHz frequency, with a maximum power of 150 W and the Starburst XL probe. Other workers have employed a Boston Scientific RF 3000 Radiofrequency Generator with a LaVeen Needle Electrode system.

RFA is done as an outpatient procedure, with assistance by an anesthetist for conscious sedation and CT guidance for placement of the probe. Fentanyl and Versed may be titrated to achieve adequate sedation. The lesions to be treated may have been identified by CT or 18-fluorodeoxyglucose positron emission tomography, biopsy be confirmed, and in the case of differentiated thyroid cancer, would likely be associated with high and rising serum Tg levels. The lesions should be sufficiently distant from key adjacent structures, such as the spinal cord, major blood vessels, or nerves. Halpin et al. *(18)* pointed out that a layer of cortical or cancellous bone between tumor in a vertebral body and the spinal cord or nerve roots can serve as a protective insulator. Specific details about how the procedure is typically done for thyroid cancer are described by Dupuy et al. *(29)* and for bone metastases, by Callstrom et al. *(30)*. As also done for liver metastases, the procedure involves introduction of the electrode through a nick in the skin using guidance by ultrasound, CT, or both. The Starburst XL described above is a 14-gauge 6.4-F needle with an active electrode trocar tip and nine electrodes that spread out into a spherical formation in the tissue being treated. This generates a necrotic core of 5-cm diameter; however, size is adjustable based on the length of the exposed electrode. The insulated needle tip is placed into the lesion, and the electrode is advanced through the soft portion of the lesion until the electrode tips butt against the interface between soft tissue and bone, precluding further advancement. The position of the needle tip is confirmed by ultrasound or CT with continuous real-time monitoring to ensure a proper electrode position. The temperature goal is 100°C, which is variably maintained for at least 3–5 min with a range of 5–15 min.

One treatment may be sufficient for small lesions, whereas larger lesions require the patient to return for multiple therapies. After the ablative procedure, the spread electrodes are withdrawn back into the needle, and the needle is removed. With bone lesions, postprocedure pain may be a problem for several hours and can be controlled by a local injection of Marcaine and intravenous fentanyl, with or without Versed. Some patients tolerate the procedure amazingly well.

Laser Thermal Ablation

For over a decade, laser thermal ablation has been used for the treatment of various metastases and primary hepatomas (31,32) and more recently was shown to be effective for thyroid malignancies (33,34). The technique involves ultrasound-guided insertion of 21-gauge spinal needles into the lesion(s) within the sheath, of which a 300-μm diameter quartz optical fiber is threaded. The energy for the ablation is provided by a Nd:YAG laser with an output of 3–5 W. Patients described the sensation as painful but tolerable. With larger lesions, the needles are slightly withdrawn and repositioned for several additional treatments.

Details of the procedure can be reviewed in the most recent report by Pacella et al. (35), who described the results of percutaneous laser thermal ablation of 25 patients, 16 of whom had benign "hot" nodules, 8 had "cold" nodules, and only one had thyroid cancer, an anaplastic carcinoma. The patients were deemed poor candidates for surgery. Nodule size was reduced by an average of 3.3 mL in the hot nodules and 7.7 mL in the cold nodules. The sole anaplastic carcinoma experienced necrosis of 32 mL of tissue. The therapy was considered relatively ineffective for the hot nodules (which would still require ^{131}I therapy), and there are clearly insufficient data on thyroid cancer to warrant its use. Rather, controlled clinical trials should be performed to determine whether this therapeutic modality will have any future role in the management of metastatic thyroid cancer.

Any of the above local ablative techniques may be applied to the management of any type of thyroid cancer. The greatest benefit or indication for these local procedures lies in the patient who has demonstrable tumor burden and who cannot tolerate or refuses surgical approaches. It should be noted that most of these procedures will be palliative but not curative.

REFERENCES

1. Bennedbaek FN, Hegedus L. Treatment of rrecurrent thyroid cysts with ethanol: a randomized double-blind controlled trial. J Clin Endocrinol Metab 2003; 88:5773–5777.
2. Guglielmi R, Pacella CM, Bianchini A, et al. Percutaneous ethanol injection treatment in benign thyroid lesions: Role and efficacy. Thyroid 2004; 14:125–131.
3. Gangi A, Kastler B, Klinkert A, Dietemann JL. Injection of alcohol into bone metastases under CT guidance. J Comput Assist Tomogr 1994; 18:932–935.
4. Lewis BD, Hay ID, Charboneau JW, et al. Percutaneous ethanol injuection for treatment of cervical lymph node metastases in patients with papillary thyroid carcinoma. Am J Roentgenol 2002; 178: 699–704.
5. Hay I, Charboneau W, Lewis B, et al. Successful ultrasound-guided percutaneous ethanol ablation of neck nodal metastases in 20 patients with postoperative TNM Stage I papillary thyroid carcinoma resistant to conventional therapy. Los Angeles, CA: 74th Meeting, American Thyroid Association, 2002; Abstract 176.
6. Nakada K, Kasai K, Watanabe Y, et al. Treatment of radioiodine-negative bone metastasis from papillary thyroid carcinoma with percutaneous ethanol injection therapy. Ann Nucl Med 1996; 10: 441–444.
7. Schlumberger M, Challeton C, De Vathaire F, et al. Radioactive iodine treatment and external radiotherapy for lung and bone metastases from thyroid carcinoma. J Nucl Med 1996; 37:598–605.
8. Bernier M-O, Leenhardt L, Hoang C, et al. Survival and therapeutic modalities in patients with bone metastases of differentiated thyroid carcinoma. J Clin Endocrinol Metab 2001; 86:1568–1573.
9. Camille RR, Leger FA, Merland JJ, et al. Recent advances in the treatment of bone metastases from cancer of the thyroid. Chirurgie 1980; 106:32–36.
10. Smit JW, Vielvoye GJ, Goslings BM. Embolization for vertebral metastases of follicular thyroid carcinoma. J Clin Endocrinol Metab 2000; 85:989–994.
11. Vitale G, Fonderico F, Martignetti A, et al. Pamidronate improves the quality of life and induces clinical remission of bone metastases in patients with thyroid cancer. Br J Cancer 2001; 84:1586–1590.
12. Rosen HN, Moses AC, Garber J, et al. Randomized trial of pamidronate in patients with thyroid cancer: Bone density is not reduced by suppressive doses of thyroxine, but is increased by cyclic intravenous pamidronate. J Clin Endocrinol Metab 1998; 83: 2324–2330.
13. Rosen LS, Gordon D, Tchekmedyian S, et al. Zoledronic acid versus placebo in the treatment of skeletal metastases in patients with lung cancer and other solid tumors: A phase III, double-blind, randomized trial—The Zoledronic acid lung cancer and other solid tumors study group. J Clin Oncol 2003; 21:3150–3157.
14. Rosen LS, Gordon D, Tchekmedyian NS, et al. Long-term efficacy and safety of zoledronic acid in the treatment of skeletal metastases in patients with non-small cell lung carcinoma and other solid tumors. Cancer 2004; 100:2613–2621.
15. Eustatia-Rutten CF, Romijn JA, Guijt MJ, et al. Outcome of palliative embolization of bone metastases in differentiated thyroid carcinoma. J Clin Endocrinol Metab 2003; 88:3184–3189.
16. Van Tol KM, Hew JM, Jager PL, et al. Embolization in combination with radioiodine therapy for bone metastases from differentiated thyroid carcinoma. Clin Endocrinol 2000; 52:653–659.
17. Elshafie O, Hussein S, Jeans WD, Woodhouse NJ. Massive rise in thyroglobulin with adult respiratory distress syndrome after embolisation of thyroid cancer metastasis. Br J Radiol 2000; 73:547–549.
18. Halpin RJ, Bendok BR, Liu JC. Minimally invasive treatments for spinal metastases: vertebroplasty, kyphoplasty, and radiofrequency ablation. J Support Oncol 2004; 2:339–355.

19. Peh WC, Gilula LA. Percutaneous vertebroplasty: Indications, contraindications, and technique. Br J Radiol 2003; 76:69–75.
20. Ahmad Z, Abbasi F, Mitsunaga M, Portner B. Pain reduction and functional improvement after kyphoplasty: a retrospective study of 50 patients. Arch Phy Med Rhab 2003; 84:A21.
21. Ledlie JT, Fenfro M. Balloon kyphoplasty: one-year outcomes in vertebral body height restoration, chronic pain, and activity levels. J Neurosurg 2003; 98:36–42.
22. McGahan JP, Dodd GD. Radiofrequency ablation o the liver: current status. AJR Am J Roentgenol 2001; 176:3–16.
23. Dupuy DE. Minimally invasive therapies in the treatment of bone malignancies. Crit Rev 1998; 75:161–171.
24. Goetz MP, Callstrom MR, Charboneau JW, et al. Percutaneous image-guided radiofrequency ablation of painful metastases involving bone: a multicenter study. J Clin Oncol 2004; 22:300–306.
25. Schaefer O, Lohrmann C, Ghanem N, Langer M. CT-guided radiofrequency heat ablation of malignant lung tumors. Med Sci Monit 2003; 9:127–131.
26. Dupuy DE, Zagoria RJ, Akerley W, et al. Percutaneous radiofrequency ablation of malignancies in the lung. Am J Roentgenol 2000; 174:57–59.
27. Schaefer O, Lohrmann C, Markmiller M, et al. Technical innovation: combined treatment of a spinal metastasis with radiofrequency heat ablation and vertebroplasty. Am J Roentgenol 2003; 180: 1075–1077.
28. Halpin RJ, Bendok BB, Sato KT, et al. Combination treatment of vertebral metastases using image-guided percutaneous radiofrequency ablation and vertebroplasty: a case report. Surg Neurol 2005; 63: 469–474.
29. Dupuy DE, Monchik JM, Decrea C, Pisharodi L. Radiofrequency ablation of regional recurrence from well-differentiated thyroid malignancy. Surgery 2001; 130:971–977.
30. Callstrom MR, Charboneau JW, Goetz MP, et al. Painful metastases involving bone: Feasibility of percutaneous CT- and US-guided radiofrequency ablation. Radiology 2002; 224:87–97.
31. Pacella CM, Bizzarri G, Ferrari FS, et al. Interstitial photocoagulation with laser in the treament of liver metastases. Radiol Med 1996; 92: 438–447.
32. Pacella CM, Bizzarri G, Magnolfi F, et al. Laser thermal ablation in the treatment of small hepatocellular carcinoma: Results in 74 patients. Radiology 2001; 221:712–720.
33. Guglielmi R, Pacella CM, Dottorini MF, et al. Severe thyrotoxicosis due to hyperfunctioning liver metastases from follicular carcinoma treatment with 131-I and interstitial laser ablation. Thyroid 1999; 9: 173–177.
34. Pacella CM, Bizzarri G, Guglielmi R., et al. Thyroid tissue: US-guided percutaneous interstital laswer ablation—a feasibility study. Radiology 2000; 217:673–677.
35. Pacella CM, Bizzarri G, Spiezia S, et al. Thyroid tissue: US-guided percutaneous laser thermal ablation. Radiology 2004; 232:272–280.

Part V
Well-Differentiated Thyroid Cancer
Follicular Carcinoma

55
Follicular Thyroid Carcinoma
Clinical Aspects

Leonard Wartofsky

INTRODUCTION

Several excellent general reviews regarding follicular thyroid carcinoma (FTC) are recommended *(1–4)*. Similarly to papillary thyroid carcinoma (PTC), follicular carcinoma is also a relatively well-differentiated thyroid cancer. Together, both types of tumor represent the most common malignancy of the endocrine system *(5)*. Controversies exist over how aggressively to approach the early management of PTC (i.e., subtotal vs total thyroidectomy) or whether to administer radioiodine ablation, but this debate is significantly less of an issue with well-differentiated FTC. This is so because there is general recognition that FTC behaves in a more aggressive manner, with the propensity to invade both the thyroid capsule and blood vessels and show up as metastases in sites distant from the neck. Hence, in order to identify and treat such metastases with radioiodine, there is greater justification for ensuring that there are no remaining normal thyroid follicular cells in the neck that would be competing for the tracer isotope. Thus, total thyroidectomy and radioiodine ablation may be justified by data that indicate a somewhat worse prognosis for FTC than PTC, but either tumor may be fully curable if caught at an early stage. Establishing a specific and clear distinction between the behavior of these two types of thyroid cancer from the published literature is somewhat difficult because most describe their experience with patients who have differentiated thyroid cancer (DTC), thereby grouping FTC with PTC. However, there are differences between the presentation and behavior of these two cancer types, and these differences are emphasized in this chapter.

As described in Chapter 57 (Pathology of FTC), the diagnostic distinction between FTC and PTC is based on their appearance under the microscope. Classic PTC demonstrates overlapping or palisading nuclei, many that show nuclear clefts and intranuclear cytoplasmic inclusions or vacuoles, whereas FTC does not exhibit the latter nuclear features. Although most PTCs are not encapsulated, FTC typically is. The pathologist's description of tumor invasion into or through the capsule is a key aspect of the histopathologic diagnosis. FTC is generally described as one or the other of two general types—well-encapsulated and minimally invasive or more poorly differentiated, less well-encapsulated, and more widely invasive. A third potentially more invasive form of FTC, as classified by the World Health Organization *(6)*, is the Hürthle cell (Askanazy cell or oncocytic) variant, which is described further below and in Chapter 58.

Distinction between the former well-encapsulated, minimally invasive FTC and benign follicular adenomata may be difficult, and not surprisingly, this type of FTC tends to have an excellent prognosis. Williams et al. *(7)* have proposed to label these questionably invasive tumors as "well-differentiated follicular tumor of indeterminate malignant potential." Such a designation is clearly less helpful to the clinician, rendering the decision more difficult regarding the need for radioiodine ablation and a meaningful discussion of prognosis with the patient. Clearly, there are patients with the so-called minimally invasive tumors who subsequently present with distant metastases. Baloch and LiVolsi *(8)* have elegantly summarized the controversy in pathologic diagnosis and provided useful recommendations on the distinction between these various forms of follicular neoplasm. An Armed Forces Institute of Pathology review of 95 cases of minimally invasive FTC concluded that the prognosis was so good that aggressive surgical management was not necessary for a positive outcome *(9)*. A significant problem in interpreting the literature extant on disease-free survival and outcomes with various therapeutic FTC approaches is the great variability in histologic description and classification. Clearly there is a correlation between invasiveness and prognosis. D'Avanso et al. *(10)* reviewed 132 patients who were stratified into three groups: minimally invasive (only capsular invasion), moderately invasive (blood vessel invasion with or without capsular invasion), or widely invasive. The 5-yr survival rates were 98%, 80%, and 38%, respectively.

From: *Thyroid Cancer: A Comprehensive Guide to Clinical Management, 2/e*
Edited by: L. Wartofsky and D. Van Nostrand © Humana Press Inc., Totowa, NJ

CLINICAL PRESENTATION

FTC typically presents as a single, painless thyroid nodule in an older (age >55 yr) patient. Although it is more common in women by twofold or more, men tend to have a worse prognosis. Lymphadenopathy from involved cervical nodes is uncommon, but distant metastases will be present in the lung or bone in 10–20% of patients at the time of initial presentation (11–15). FTC tends to occur in endemic (iodide-deficient) goiters and in preexisting adenomatous goiters. Iodide deficiency or the secondary thyrotropin (TSH) stimulation associated with it appear to be etiologically related to the development of these tumors (16). In one recent series from Norway, decreased risk was linked with the use of iodized salt, and increased risk was shown in areas of endemic goiter (17). In areas of iodide sufficiency in the western hemisphere, papillary carcinoma seems to be more common. The frequency of thyroid cancer in the United States appears to have increased each year over the past two decades; it is estimated that there will be 25,690 new cases in 2005 (5). Of this total number, it is predicted that a smaller proportion will be from FTC, with a higher proportion of PTC. A decline in the reported frequency of pure FTC may also be partly related to more rigid pathological diagnostic criteria. In many hospitals, follicular tumors are more often misdiagnosed (i.e., false-positive) because of confusion with other lesions, such as benign follicular adenomas, adenomatoid goiter, or the follicular variants of either papillary or medullary carcinoma (18).

In addition to iodide deficiency and endemic goiter, there are several other possible predisposing factors for FTC, including advancing age, female gender, and radiation exposure to the head and neck. The greater frequency in women and the somewhat increased presentation of thyroid cancer during pregnancy implies an association with higher endogenous estrogen levels. The high levels of human chorionic gonadotropin (hCG) that occur in early pregnancy could be another etiological or permissive factor, as hCG binds to the TSH receptor and can constitute a stimulus to both hormone production and thyroid hypertrophy. Nevertheless, pregnancy does not appear to have an adverse impact on ultimate outcome (19). Moreover, men with FTC have a worse prognosis for long-term survival than women (20).

The not-uncommon occurrence of FTC in an adenomatous goiter suggests a pathogenetic evolution of these cancers from lesions that were originally benign. Both follicular adenomas and carcinomas appear to have monoclonal origin. Evolution of an adenoma into a malignant lesion could occur via mutational or translocational activation of oncogenes, particularly the *ras* oncogene that has been specifically identified in follicular tumors (21,22). Evolution of adenoma into carcinoma could occur through the genetic loss of tumor suppressor genes that, taken together with *ras* oncogene activation, would lead to clonal expansion and the growth of a malignant subclone of cells. Certain cytogenetic alterations have been linked to more aggressive tumor behavior (23). Much current investigation is also focusing on mutations of the TSH receptor in various thyroid disorders, and there may be mutations of the TSH receptor or the a subunit of the stimulatory G protein, which could also lead to tumorigenesis (22,24). A patient with an activating mutation of the TSH receptor in a tumor metastatic to lungs and lymph nodes sufficient to cause thyrotoxicosis has been described (25).

THYROID FUNCTION TESTS AND EVALUATION

At presentation, all routine blood thyroid function tests are within normal limits, including the serum TSH (except in the presence of severe iodine deficiency and endemic goiter). Serum thyroglobulin (Tg) may be elevated, but a diagnosis should not be inferred from serum Tg levels. Utility of Tg monitoring is discussed elsewhere (Chapters 23 and 30) and may be adversely affected by interfering antithyroglobulin antibodies, which usually falsely lower serum Tg levels. This may be more problematic with immunoluminometric assays than with highly specific radioimmunoassays for Tg (26). Unfortunately, as much as 25–35% of thyroid cancer patients may have underlying Hashimoto's disease with positive antithyroglobulin autoantibodies. While it has been hoped that management of such patients might be facilitated by measurement of Tg mRNA in serum (27), this method has not yet lived up to its expectations (see Chapter 31 by Ringel). Other, but unproven, techniques may allow distinction between circulating Tg derived from benign vs malignant thyroid tissue (28). Another potentially useful assay demanding further study relates to the measurement of carcinoembryonic antigen (CEA) mRNA in blood. CEA has proven a useful tumor marker for medullary thyroid cancer and other nonthyroid tumors. However, Sato et al. also described measurement of the CEA mRNA as allowing designation between benign follicular adenomas and FTC (29).

Continuous periodic monitoring of serum Tg as the marker for residual or recurrent disease is critically essential to the basic management of patients with thyroid cancer. Patients with known metastatic or residual thyroid cancer should be followed by an endocrinologist or thyroid specialist, in addition to their primary care physician. The physician should ensure that serum Tg is measured only in a high-quality laboratory. Ideally, this measurement should be in the same laboratory at each follow-up interval, and the laboratory should provide companion Tg levels upon remeasurement of stored serum from the prior venapuncture. In the postoperative state, a clearly measurable or rising serum Tg when the patient is TSH-suppressed on levothyroxine implies residual disease and may be a definite clue to future recurrence. Yet, serum Tg levels are usually most useful when measured while the patient is hypothyroid, e.g., during preparation for follow-up scanning. The current availability of recombinant human (rh) TSH has facilitated monitoring Tg before and after rhTSH stimulation (*30–33*; see Chapter 11). The management dilemma presented by patients with negative radioiodine scan surveys but elevated serum Tg is discussed in Chapter 39.

Nuclear medicine studies have limited use in the evaluation of patients with thyroid nodules that may harbor a FTC. The radioiodine uptake is normal, and an isotopic scan discloses a "cold" nodule that corresponds to the palpable lesion. In a multinodular gland, there may be other "hot" or autonomously hyperfunctional nodules, but malignancy in the latter is very rare.

Thyroid ultrasound imaging is useful to confirm the presence of the nodule or nodules detected on physical examination to determine the nodule(s) size and if there is multinodularity. Ultrasonography cannot reliably distinguish between benign and malignant lesions, but a purely cystic (anechoic) lesion only rarely harbors a malignancy, and a clear area around a solid (echogenic) lesion may represent an intact capsule ("halo" sign), suggesting benignancy.

Although the diagnostic *sine qua non* for evaluating thyroid nodules is usually the cytological examination derived from fine-needle aspiration (FNA), this technique also does not reliably distinguish between benign and malignant follicular neoplasms (see below and Chapters 17 and 57). There is a very close similarity in the appearance of follicular cells in benign adenomata and those of follicular carcinoma, making it impossible in most cases to distinguish between the two with a cytological examination after FNA. Some cytopathologists may detect a greater degree of nuclear "atypia" and an increased rate of mitoses in malignant lesions, but the distinction may be so difficult that it may even be treacherous.

Instead, the diagnosis is based on histological, not cytologic, criteria, including evidence for either capsular or vascular invasion. Relating to the Hürthle cell variant of FTC, Renshaw *(34)* has proposed that the application of specific cytologic criteria could designate benign Hürthle cell adenomas from carcinoma. However, this is disputed by Skoog and Tani in an accompanying editorial *(35)*. The authors urge caution in accepting these criteria as sufficiently accurate and express hope that molecular markers will soon serve this function.

Numerous investigators are currently exploring different potential tumor markers and genetic analysis to distinguish benign from malignant lesions *(36,37)*. In one report *(38)*, estimates of telomerase activity appeared to show some promise. The many advances in the application of molecular markers to the diagnosis of malignancy in thyroid nodules are discussed at length in Chapter 19; only a few brief comments are addressed here.

In one early study examining the presence of PAX8-PPARγ1 in thyroid sections from adenomata and carcinomas, a greater number of the malignant lesions were found to have this fused gene *(39)*. However, although this finding tended to be confirmed by Marques et al. *(40)* in FNA aspirates of follicular neoplasms, it was not sufficiently specific to reliably separate malignant from benign lesions. Greater promise of potential utility and reliability as both a sensitive and specific presurgical marker for follicular thyroid cancer is suggested by a number of reports that have looked at the presence of polypeptide, Galectin-3 *(41,42)*. Prior studies had shown Galectin-3 expression in other thyroid cancers. The specificity for distinguishing follicular adenoma from minimally invasive follicular carcinoma appears certain to promote growing application of this approach to both presurgical FNA aspirates and surgical pathologic tissues of controversial diagnosis.

Cytological differentiation of follicular adenoma from carcinoma has been difficult, but frozen-section analysis is even worse in most *(43)*, but not all *(44)*, hands. An experienced pathologist should be able to diagnose the more aggressive and invasive type of follicular carcinoma, which often presents with distant metastases to bone or lung. Although local lymph node invasion can be discovered during thyroidectomy in possibly 5–10% of follicular cancers, it is much less common than in the papillary variety, which may present with involved cervical nodes in 35–45% of patients. In addition to the typically higher frequency of metastases to bone (spine, skull, and pelvis) and the lungs, other less common sites for distant metastases include the brain and rarely, the liver.

As outlined above, and apart from Hürthle cell cancers, there are two major types of true follicular carcinoma: a minimally invasive, encapsulated type and a more aggressive, invasive form, which often presents with distant metastases. Histologically, the encapsulated type may closely resemble a benign follicular adenoma. (See Chapter 57 for a full description of the pathological features.) On rare occasions, even a small, well-encapsulated follicular carcinoma may present with distant metastases in bone or lung, presumably from poorly understood differences in host factors.

Pathologically, follicular cancer cells do not demonstrate any typical or pathognomonic features of papillary cancer, such as crowded, overlapping cells with nuclear clefts or grooves and large intranuclear clear inclusions ("Orphan Annie eyes"). Invaginations of cytoplasm into the nuclei-forming vacuoles, which are also common in papillary cancer, are seen only rarely in follicular carcinoma. These tumors are usually composed of follicular elements but not the papillated structures often found with PTC. In contrast to PTC, both lymph node invasion and thyroidal multicentricity are uncommon.

Possible confusion with papillary cancer could occur in tumors with the greatest degree of potential overlapping characteristics, i.e., the follicular variant of papillary carcinoma (FVPTC; *45,46*). However, these tumors exhibit biological behavior much more similar to papillary than to follicular carcinoma, including a pattern of metastasis to regional nodes, rather than hematogenous spread to distant sites, as well as a better prognosis. Intraoperative frozen-section or FNA cytology has been indicated to help distinguish FVPTC from a real follicular lesion and thus better guide the surgical procedure (47).

Zidan et al. (48) have proposed that the distinction between FVPTC and PTC is moot because with comparable treatment, the two have similar prognosis and survival. In their series, more advanced age was the most impressive negative prognostic factor, and the presence or degree of either distant metastases or local lymph node metastases did not significantly differ. In a subsequent communication (49), LiVolsi strongly disagreed with the interpretation of Zidan et al. Additionally, a close relationship to FTC is suggested by observations that some chromosomal aberrations in FVPTC seem to resemble FTC to a greater level than PTC (50). However, other authors (51) have confirmed the conclusions of Zidan et al., with comparable outcome measures seen with FVPTC as with PTC but not with FTC (52). Another study also indicated that FVPTC had an even more benign course than PTC (53).

The initial evaluation of a patient proven to have FTC should include a chest radiograph. Notably, however, even if interpreted as negative, the lungs may still demonstrate radionuclide uptake, suggesting metastases on the postoperative ^{131}I scan. If pulmonary metastases are evident, a chest computed tomography scan provides excellent anatomical imaging as a baseline study for future comparisons after therapy. Pulmonary metastases may be particularly difficult to fully eliminate, as demonstrated in children and young adults (54–57). The mainstay of follow-up, however, is periodic serial monitoring of serum Tg levels and isotopic (^{131}I) scans. The frequency of both depends on tumor staging and the specific clinical circumstances (e.g., low vs high risk) of each patient, as discussed in Chapters 9, 23, and 60. Cancer recurrences after initial thyroidectomy and radioiodine ablation and therapy are most likely to occur within the first 18–60 mo. Patients with known tumor based on rising serum Tg levels but negative radioiodine scans may be studied with other imaging techniques, such as ^{201}Tl, sestamibi, or 18-fluorodeoxyglucose (see Chapter 35). Hürthle cell variants often do not concentrate radioiodine.

Tumor staging is important to establish prognosis, but preference and application of staging methods remain somewhat controversial (58–60; see Chapter 9). The TNM (tumor, nodes, and metastasis) system remains the most widely applied of all staging systems for thyroid carcinoma in use (61,62). This system allows determination of the category of relative risk (low vs high) and provides prognostic indicators for recurrence and death from the tumor. Prognostic indicators have been incorporated into systems that consist of a scale of risk. The AGES system, devised and advocated by the Mayo Clinic (63), incorporates the risks contributed by patient age, tumor grade, extracapsular invasion, and tumor size. Such systems provide useful parameters in the discussion of prognosis with patients in reasonably precise terms, considering the wide variability and uncertainty underlying prognosis of any malignancy. In the review of differing staging systems by DeGroot and colleagues (64), the TNM system was thought to provide the best risk stratification, at least for PTC. The practical importance and clinical relevance of risk stratification to treatment and management was carefully analyzed by Shaha in a retrospective review of more than 1000 patients with DTC (65).

SUMMARY

Although most primary thyroidal cancers arise from *follicular* epithelium, the most common type of thyroid malignancy is the well-differentiated papillary carcinoma, which accounts for about 70–80% of thyroid tumors, with true follicular carcinomas accounting for only 10–15% of all thyroid cancers. Follicular cancer is more common in older patients and spreads via blood vessel invasion, often presenting with metastases in lungs or bone. Rarely, the mass of functioning metastatic cancer may be so great as to cause thyrotoxicosis. FTC may be contrasted with PTC, which occurs more frequently in younger patients, is slowly growing and less aggressive, and has a more favorable prognosis. Certain characteristics are associated with a worse prognosis with follicular tumors, including a more invasive or metastatic tendency, male gender, and larger size, especially with lesions larger than 4 cm in diameter. Although age over 50 is generally considered to be an independent adverse risk factor, this was not found to be the case by Besic et al. (65a) who warned that younger patients with large tumors or distant metastases are also at risk of poor outcomes. Unlike papillary carcinoma, follicular carcinoma is much less likely to occur because of prior radiation exposure to the head and neck.

The management of FTC differs from that of PTC in one important way: the requirement for the early operative management of FTC to consist of a total, rather than subtotal, thyroidectomy (66). This difference relates to the propensity of FTC to be angioinvasive and present with distant metastases and the need to destroy all residual thyroid tissue in the neck to visualize these distant metastases with radioiodine scanning. However, one review of 82 patients with FTC found that the extent of surgery did not affect the rate of disease-free survival, which was more directly related to radioiodine therapy (67).

Thyroidectomy is then followed by radioiodine ablation of any remnant tissue. This procedure is a prerequisite to the potential need to more effectively treat distant metastases in lung or bone with radioiodine by removing all residual thyroid tissue that might compete for radioiodine (68,69). Traditionally, ablation is effected postoperatively while patients are hypothyroid from levothyroxine withdrawal. However, sufficient data are now available on the efficacy of employing rhTSH for ablation (as summarized in Chapter 27) to imply that this will be the leading method of the future.

Depending on the surgical techniques, a considerable portion of the contralateral thyroid lobe may remain after a subtotal thyroidectomy or so-called near-total thyroidectomy. Because of the need to destroy all remaining thyroid tissue to achieve satisfactory surveillance scanning, most experts would consider a completion thyroidectomy. Alternatively, other investigators have advocated radioiodine ablation of larger remnants of the thyroid, rather than introducing the risks that are inherent with a completion thyroidectomy (70). Patients with FTC are more likely to have advanced disease (stage III or IV) at presentation, placing them at a higher risk than patients with PTC (58). One reported 10-yr overall survival rate for follicular cancer was 85% (71), whereas papillary cancers tend to have a more favorable prognosis with a 93% 10-yr survival (99), especially if less than 1.5 cm in size and, if so, may not require aggressive management with radioiodine. Subsequent surveillance to determine a cancer cure or recurrence involves follow-up evaluations with ^{131}I scanning and measurement of serum Tg as a tumor marker for recurrence. Traditionally, periodic evaluations consisted of allowing TSH to rise following discontinuation of L-thyroxine therapy. The availability of recombinant human TSH (rhTSH) (30–33) has radically altered routine follow-up evaluations for residual or recurrent disease. Several authoritative review articles have appeared in recent years (1–3,72,73), as well as guidelines for management from both the United States (74) and the United Kingdom (75).

REFERENCES

1. Kinder BK. Well differentiated thyroid cancer. Curr Opin Oncol 2003; 15:71–77.
2. Haigh PI. Follicular thyroid carcinoma. Curr Treat Options Oncol 2002; 3:349–354.
3. Mazzaferri EL, Kloos RT. Current approaches to primary therapy for papillary and follicular thyroid cancer. J Clin Endocrinol Metab 2001; 86:1447–1463.
4. Schlumberger MJ. Papillary and follicular thyroid carcinoma. N Engl J Med 1998; 338:297–306.
5. Jemal A, Murray T, Ward E, et al. Cancer statistics, 2005. CA Cancer J Clin 2005; 55:10–30.
6. Hedinger CE Williams ED, Sobin LH. Histological typing of thyroid tumors. In Hedinger CE, editor. International Histological Classification of Tumors, vol. 11. Berlin, Germany: Springer-Verlag, 1988.
7. Williams ED, Abrosimov A, Bogdanova TI, et al. Two proposals regarding the terminology of thyroid tumors. Int J Surg Pathol 2000; 8:181–183.
8. Baloch AZ, LiVolsi VA. Follicular-patterned lesions of the thyroid: The bane of the pathologist. Am J Clin Pathol 2002; 117:143–150.
9. Thompson LDR, Wierneke JA, Paal E, et al. A clinicopathologic study of minimally invasive follicular carcinoma of the thyroid gland with a review of the English literature. Cancer 2001; 91:505–524.
10. D'Avanzo A, Treseler P, Ituarte PHG, et al. Follicular thyroid carcinoma: histology and prognosis. Cancer 2004; 100:1123–1129.
11. Jensen MH, Davis RK, Derrick L. Thyroid cancer: a computer-assisted review of 5287 cases. Otolaryngol Head Neck Surg 1990; 102:51–65.
12. Ruegemer JJ, Hay ID, Bergstralh EJ, et al. Distant metastases in differentiated thyroid carcinoma: a multivariate analysis of prognostic variables. J Clin Endocrinol Metab 1988; 67:501–508.
13. Schlumberger M, Tubiana M, de Vathaire F, et al. Long-term results of treatment of 283 patients with lung and bone metastases from differentiated thyroid carcinoma. J Clin Endocrinol Metab 1986; 63:960–966.
14. Young RL, Mazzaferri EL, Rahe AJ, Dorfman SG. Pure follicular carcinoma: impact of therapy in 214 patients. J Nucl Med 1980; 21:733–737.
15. Simpson WJ, McKinney SE, Carruthers JS, et al. Papillary and follicular thyroid cancer: prognostic factors in 1578 patients. Am J Med 1987; 83:479–488.
16. Franceschi S. Iodine intake and thyroid carcinoma—a potential risk factor. Exper Clin Endocrinol Diab 1998; 106(Suppl 3):S38–S44.
17. Galanti MR, Hansson L, Bergstrom R, et al. Diet and the risk of papillary and follicular thyroid carcinoma: a population-based case-control study in Sweden and Norway. Cancer Causes Control 1997; 8:205–214.
18. LiVolsi VA, Asa SL. The demise of follicular carcinoma of the thyroid gland. Thyroid 1994; 4:233–236.
19. Moosa M, Mazzaferri EL. Outcome of differentiated thyroid cancer diagnosed in pregnant women. J Clin Endocrinol Metab 1997; 82:2862–2866.
20. Eichhorn W, Tabler H, Lippold R, et al. Prognostic factors determining long-term survival in well-differentiated thyroid cancer: An analysis of four hundred eighty-four patients undergoing therapy and aftercare at the same institution. Thyroid 2003; 13:949–958.
21. Farid NR, Shi Y, Zou M. Molecular basis of thyroid cancer. Endocr Rev 1994; 15:202–232.
22. Challeton C, Bounacer A, DuVillard JA, et al. Pattern of ras and gsp oncogene mutations in radiation-associated human thyroid tumors. Oncogene 1995; 11:601–603.
23. Roque L, Clode A, Beige G, et al. Follicular thyroid carcinoma: chromosome analysis of 19 cases. Genes Chromosomes Cancer 1998; 21:250–255.
24. Russo D, Aruri F, Schlumberger M, et al. Activating mutations of the TSH receptor in differentiated thyroid carcinoma. Oncogene 1995; 11:1907–1911.
25. Russo D, Tumino S, Arturi F, et al. Detection of an activating mutation of the thyrotropin receptor in a case of an autonomously hyperfunctioning thyroid insular carcinoma. J Clin Endocrinol Metab 1997; 82:735–738.
26. Spencer CA, Takeuchi M, Kazaroxyan M, et al. Serum thyroglobulin autoantibodies: prevalence, influence on serum thyroglobulin measurement, and prognostic significance in patients with differentiated thyroid carcinoma. J Clin Endocrinol Metab 1998; 83:1121–1127.
27. Ringel MD, Ladenson PW, Levine MA. Molecular diagnosis of residual and recurrent thyroid cancer by amplification of thyroglobulin messenger ribonucleic acid in peripheral blood. J Clin Endocrinol Metab 1998; 83:4435–4442. Editorial comment by Haber RS. The diagnosis of recurrent thyroid cancer—a new approach. J Clin Endocrinol Metab 1998; 83:4189–4190.
28. Maruyama M, Kato R, Kobayashi S, Kasuga Y. A method to differentiate between thyroglobulin derived from normal thyroid tissue and from thyroid carcinoma based on anlysis of reactivity to lectins. Arch Path Lab Med 1998; 122:715–720.
29. Sato T, Harao M, Nakano S, et al. Circulating tumor cells detected by reverse transcription-polymerase chain reaction for carcinoembryonic antigen mRNA: Distinguishing follicular thyroid carcinoma from adenoma. Surgery 2005; 137:552–558.
30. Wartofsky L. Using baseline and recombinant human TSH-stimulated thyroglobulin measurements to manage thyroid cancer without diagnostic 131-I scanning. J Clin Endocrinol Metab 2002; 87: 1486–1489.
31. Robbins RJ, Robbins AK. Recombinant human thyrotropin and thyroid cancer management. J Clin Endocrinol Metab 2003; 88: 1933–1938.

32. Wartofsky L and the rhTSH-Stimulated Thyroglobulin Study Group. Management of low risk well differentiated thyroid cancer based only upon thyroglobulin measurement after recombinant human thyrotropin. Thyroid 2002; 12:583–592.
33. Mazzaferri EL, Robbins RJ, Spencer CA, et al. A consensus report on the role of serum thyroglobulin as a monitoring method for low risk patients with papillary thyroid carcinoma. J Clin Endocrinol Metab 2003; 88:1433–1441.
34. Renshaw A, Gould EW. Why there is the tendency to "over-diagnose" the follicular variant of papillary thyroid carcinoma. Am J Clin Pathol 2002; 117:19–21.
35. Skoog L, Tani E. Hurthle cell carcinoma: time for a drastic change? Cancer 2002; 96:259–260.
36. Arturi F, Russo D, Giuffrida D, et al. Early diagnosis by genetic analysis of differentiated thyroid cancer metastases in small lymph nodes. J Clin Endocrinol Metab 1997; 82:1638–1641.
37. Winzer R, Schmutzler C, Jakobs TC, et al. Reverse transcriptase-polymerase chain reaction analysis of thyrocyte-relevant genes in fine-needle aspiration biopsies of the human thyroid. Thyroid 1998; 8: 981–987.
38. Umbricht CB, Saji M, Westra WH, et al. Telomerase activity: a marker to distinguish follicular thyroid adenoma from carcinoma. Cancer Res 1997; 57:2144–2147.
39. Kroll TG, Sarraf P, Pecciarini L, et al. PAX8-PPARγ1 fusion in oncogene human thyroid carcinoma. Science 2000; 289:1357–1360.
40. Marques AR, Espadinha C, Catarino AL, et al. Expression of PAX8-PPARγ1 rearrangements in both follicular thyroid carcinomas and adenomas. J Clin Endocrinol Metab 2002; 87:3947–3952.
41. Bartolazzi A, Gasbarri A, Papotti M, et al. Application of an immunodiagnostic method for improving diagnosis of nodular thyroid lesions. Lancet 2001; 357:1644–1650.
42. Saggiorato E, Cappia S, De Giuli P, et al. Galectin-3 as a presurgical immuno cytodiagnostic marker of minimally invasive follicular thyroid carcinoma. J Clin Endocrinol Metab 2001; 86:5152–5158.
43. Collins SL. Thyroid cancer: controversies and etiopathogenesis of thyroid cancer. In Falk S, editor. Thyroid Disease: Endocrinology, Surgery, Nuclear Medicine, and Radiotherapy, 2nd ed. New York: Raven Press, 1997:495–564.
44. Paphavasit A, Thompson GB, Hay ID, et al. Follicular and Hürthle cell thyroid neoplasms: is frozen section evaluation worthwhile? Arch Surg 1997; 132:674–678.
45. Tielens ET, Sherman SI, Hruban RH, Ladenson PW. Follicular variant of papillary thyroid carcinoma: a clinical pathologic study. Cancer 1994; 73:424–431.
46. Baloch ZW, Gupta PK, Yu GH, et al. Follicular variant of papillary carcinoma. Cytologic and histologic correlation. Am J Clin Path 1999; 111:216–222.
47. Kesmodel SB, Terhune KP, Canter RJ, et al. The diagnostic dilemma of follicular variant of papillary thyroid carcinoma. Surgery 2003; 134: 1005–1012.
48. Zidan J, Karen D, Stein M, et al. Pure versus follicular variant of papillary thyroid carcinoma; clinical features, prognostic factors, treatment, and survival. Cancer 2003; 97:1181–1185.
49. LiVolsi VA and reply by Zidan J. (Letters) Pure versus follicular variant of papillary thyroid carcinoma. Cancer 2003; 98:1997–1998.
50. Wreesman VB, Ghossein RA, Hezel M, et al. Follicular variant of papillary thyroid carcinoma: genome-wide appraisal of a controversial entity. Genes Chromosomes Cancer 2004; 40:355–364.
51. Burningham AR, Krishnan J, Davidson BJ, Ringel MD, Burman KD. Papillary and follicular variant of papillary carcinoma of the thyroid: Initial presentation and response to therapy. Otolaryngol Head Neck Surg 2005; 132:840–844.
52. Passler C, Prager G, Scheuba C, et al. Follicular variant of papillary thyroid carcinoma: a long-term follow-up. Arch Surg 2003; 138: 1362–1366.
53. Jain M, Khan A, Patwardhan N, et al. Follicular variant of papillary thyroid carcinoma: a comparative study of histopathologic features and cytology results in 141 patients. Endocr Pract 2001; 7:79–184.
54. Vassilopoulou-Sellin R, Klein MJ, Smith TH, et al. Pulmonary metastases in children and young adults with differentiated thyroid cancer. Cancer 1993; 71:1348–1352.
55. Samuel AM, Rajashekharrao B, Shah DH. Pulmonary metastases in children and adolescents with well-differentiated thyroid cancer. J Nucl Med 1998; 39:1531–1536.
56. Feinmesser R, Lubin E, Segal K, Noyek A. Carcinoma of the thyroid in children—a review. J Fed Endocrinol Metab 1997; 10:561–568.
57. Hung W, Sarlis NJ. Current controversies in the management of pediatric patients with well-differentiated nonmedullary thyroid cancer: A review. Thyroid 2002; 12:683–702.
58. Sherman SI, Brierley JD, Sperling M, et al. Prospective multicenter study of thyroid carcinoma treatment: Initial analysis of staging and outcome. Cancer 1998; 83:1012–1021.
59. Cady B. Staging in thyroid carcinoma. Cancer 1998; 83:844–847.
60. Sherman SI. Editorial: Staging in thyroid carcinoma—a reply. Cancer 1998; 83:848–850.
61. Brierley JD, Panzarella T, Tsang RW, et al. A comparison of different staging systems predictability of patient outcome: thyroid carcinoma as an example. Cancer 1997; 79:2414–2423.
62. Loh K-C, Greenspan FS, Gee L, et al. Pathological tumor-node-metastasis (pTNM) staging for papillary and follicular thyroid carcinomas: a retrospective analysis of 700 patients. J Clin Endocrinol Metab 1997; 82:3553–3562.
63. Hay ID, Bergstralh EJ, Goellner JR, et al. Predicting outcome in papillary thyroid carcinoma: Development of a reliable prognostic scoring system in a cohort of 1779 patients treated surgically at one institution during 1940 through 1989. Surgery 1993; 114:1050–1058.
64. DeGroot LJ, Kaplan EL, Straus FH, Shukla MS. Does the method of management of papillary thyroid carcinoma make a difference in outcome? World J Surg 1994; 18:123–130.
65. Shaha AR. Implications of prognostic factors and risk groups in the management of differentiated thyroid cancer. Laryngoscope 2004; 114: 393–402.
66. Schwartz AE, Clark OH, Ituarte P, LoGerfo P. Thyroid surgery—the choice. J Clin Endocrinol Metab 1998; 83:1097–1105.
67. Taylor T, Specker B, Robbins J, et al. Outcome after treatment of high-risk papillary and non-Hürthle cell follicular thyroid carcinoma. Ann Intern Med 1998; 129:622–627.
68. Lin JD, Kao PF, Chao TC. The effects of radioactive iodine in thyroid remnant ablation and treatment of well differentiated thyroid carcinoma. Br J Radiol 1998; 71:307–313.
69. Pelikan DM, Lion HL, Hermans J, Goslings BM. The role of radioactive iodine in the treatment of advanced differentiated thyroid carcinoma. Clin Endocrinol 1997; 47:713–720.
70. Lin JD, Chao TC, Huang MJ, et al. Use of radioactive iodine for thyroid remnant ablation in well-differentiated thyroid carcinoma to replace thyroid reoperation. Am J Clin Oncol 1998; 21:77–81.
71. Hundahl SA, Fleming ID, Fremgen AM, Menck HR. A national cancer data base report on 53, 856 cases of thyroid carcinoma treated in the U.S., 1985-1995. Cancer 1998; 83:2638–2648.
72. Grebe SKG, Hay ID. Follicular thyroid cancer. Endocrinol Metab Clin North Am 1995; 24:761–801.
73. Goldman ND, Coniglio JU, Falk SA. Thyroid cancers I: Papillary, follicular, and Hürthle cell. Otolaryngol Clin North Am 1996; 29: 593–609.
74. National Comprehensive Cancer Network (NCCN) Thyroid Carcinoma: Clinical Practice Guidelines 2005. J Natl Comprehensive Cancer Network 2005; 3:404–457.
75. British Thyroid Association. Guidelines for the management of differentiated thyroid cancer in adults. Available at: www.british-thyroid-association.org/guidelines.htm, 2002.

56
Surgical Management of Follicular Cancer

Orlo H. Clark

Follicular thyroid cancers are derived from follicular epithelium within the thyroid gland, accounting for about 10% of all thyroid cancers, but this percentage seems to be decreasing (1). Follicular thyroid cancers differ from the more common follicular adenomas because the follicular cells in the cancers invade the vessels, capsule, or both. Most follicular thyroid cancers have a microfollicular histological pattern, and some are associated with RAS and PAX8/PPARγ mutations. These tumors are usually unifocal and encapsulated. In contrast to papillary thyroid cancers that often metastasize to regional lymph nodes, follicular thyroid cancers infrequently involve the lymph nodes (<10% of patients) but more frequently hematogenously metastasize to lung and bones (2). Follicular thyroid tumors that contain papillary elements are considered to be papillary thyroid cancer, as are follicular variants of papillary thyroid cancer (FVPTC) (3). In fact, when a young patient is reported to have follicular thyroid cancer with numerous regional lymph node metastases, upon review, this tumor is usually reclassified as a FVPTC. Crile and Hazard (4) stated that follicular thyroid cancers in children behave like papillary thyroid cancer and commonly have lymph node metastases. In retrospect, it is likely that some of these tumors were actually FVPTC.

Patients with follicular thyroid cancer are generally considered to have a worse prognosis than patients with papillary thyroid cancer (5). However, most of the difference in prognosis is related to the patients' older age and more advanced tumor stage at presentation (6). Tumor size and the presence of distant metastases were more important prognostic indicators than age in one recent series of patients (6a). The survival rates of patients with follicular and papillary thyroid cancer when compared at similar age and disease stage are alike (7–9). Patients who have follicular cancer that is small, with minimal capsular invasion, have an excellent prognosis (9). Yet, older patients with follicular cancer larger than 4 cm, with angioinvasion, distant metastasis, or extensive capsular invasion have a poor prognosis (2,3,5,7,10–12).

Hürthle cell cancer is included within the category of follicular thyroid cancer by the World Health Organization classification (see Chapter 58). Like other follicular thyroid carcinomas, Hürthle cell tumors are considered malignant when angioinvasion, capsular invasion, or distant metastases occurs. Both Hürthle cell and follicular thyroid cancers originate from follicular thyroid epithelium and usually increase cyclic adenosine monophosphate and thyroglobulin production in response to thyrotropin (TSH; 13). Hürthle cell cancers, however, are more likely to be multifocal, to involve regional lymph nodes, to occur after radiation exposure, to recur locally, and more likely to be lethal (14). DeGroot and colleagues (15) reported a mortality rate of 24% in patients with Hürthle cell carcinoma vs 12.5% in patients with follicular carcinoma. Others have also found a higher mortality in patients with Hürthle cell cancer than in patients with other well-differentiated thyroid cancers (16). Only about 9% of Hürthle cell carcinomas take up radioiodine, whereas about 75% of follicular cancers take up radioiodine (17,18). Interestingly, all deaths and recurrences in patients with follicular carcinoma, as reported by DeGroot and colleagues (15) and our group (14), occurred within 15 yr, whereas recurrences and deaths from papillary thyroid cancer are expected to continue during a 40 yr follow-up period.

Similarly to papillary thyroid cancer, the optimal surgical management of follicular and Hürthle cell thyroid cancers is controversial (18a). However, more experts agree that total or near-total thyroidectomy should be conducted because of the risk of distant metastases and apparently more aggressive behavior of these tumors. The problem of managing most patients with follicular or Hürthle cell cancers is that diagnosis is usually not made preoperatively by fine-needle aspiration (FNA) cytology or frozen-section examination but only after permanent histological sections are available. Therefore, the surgeon must have a plan of action for patients with follicular neoplasms. Regarding patients with follicular neoplasm by FNA, the author usually recommends a sensitive TSH test and radioiodine scan if the lesion is smaller than 3 cm. When the scan demonstrates a "hot" nodule, the patient can be observed, as these tumors rarely ever represent thyroid cancer (approx 1%). When the nodule is "cold" on scintiscan, thyroid lobectomy and isthmusectomy is advised. As mentioned, about 20% of such nodules are cancerous, and this estimate increases with older patients or when the tumor is larger than 4 cm in maximal diameter *(11,19)*. In about half of the 20% with cancer, the diagnosis can be made intraoperatively because of regional nodal involvement (usually in patients with FVPTC) or because of local invasion. The diagnosis in such patients should be confirmed by frozen section of the enlarged node or of tissue at the site of apparent invasion. For most patients with follicular or Hürthle cell neoplasms, frozen-section examination wastes unnecessary time and money, as the pathologist usually cannot distinguish between benign and malignant lesions until the permanent sections are obtained.

Before surgery, the potential situation can be discussed with patients, and they can be told that pathologists cannot determine whether a tumor is benign or malignant during the operative procedure. This author prefers to perform a thyroid lobectomy. In the 10% of patients who have cancer on permanent section, a complete total thyroidectomy is suggested. Some surgeons advise a near-total thyroidectomy for all patients with follicular or Hürthle cell neoplasms; however, this recommendation subjects all patients to bilateral procedures and the need for lifelong thyroid hormone replacement therapy. Additionally, near-total or subtotal thyroidectomy is probably not as effective as a total thyroidectomy for follicular thyroid cancer, because the remnant normal thyroid tissue usually has to be ablated before possible distant metastases can be detected with radioiodine scanning.

Many patients with follicular thyroid cancer have minimal capsular invasion *(9)*. These patients have such an excellent prognosis that thyroid lobectomy often provides definitive treatment. However, some pathologists use different definitions of "minimal capsular invasion" *(12)*. Thyroid cancer can be considered minimally invasive when it is seen to invade through only the capsule. When there is angioinvasion with or without capsular invasion, these tumors are thought to be moderately invasive. When there is extensive invasion, this author designates these as "widely invasive" *(10)*. Kahn and Perzin *(12)* reported the presence of metastatic disease in 14% of patients with capsular invasion vs about 50% for patients with angioinvasion and was found in 75% with the presence of both angioinvasion and invasion into extrathyroidal tissue.

In contrast to patients with typical follicular thyroid cancer, in patients with Hürthle cell neoplasms, regional nodal metastases can be searched for in the central neck and tracheoesophageal groove. As previously mentioned, patients with Hürthle cell neoplasms are more likely to have nodal metastases (~30%), and these metastases often cannot be ablated with radioiodine *(15–18)*. When a Hürthle cell neoplasm is known to be Hürthle cell cancer, the patient can be treated similarly to a patient with a medullary thyroid cancer. Therefore, a total thyroidectomy and thorough ipsilateral central neck dissection should be performed to avoid tumor recurrence in this area, as others have advocated for medullary cancer *(19)*.

Postoperatively, we manage patients with follicular thyroid cancer similarly to those with papillary thyroid cancer. In brief, a serum thyroglobulin is obtained to ensure the level is less than 3 ng/mL. In the author's experience, the serum thyroglobulin is repeated when the patient is rendered hypothyroid in preparation for radioiodine scanning or therapeutic treatment with ^{131}I. For low-risk patients, treatment is suggested with an outpatient dose of ^{131}I (>30 mCi). We recommend treatment with 100–200 mCi of ^{131}I for high-risk patients (>45 yr), patients whose tumors are angioinvasive or have extensive capsular invasion, a combination of both, are larger than 4 cm, or have distant metastases. Dose recommendations vary, as discussed in Chapters 44–48. Clinically, solitary distant metastases should be removed surgically, and radioiodine should be used to destroy and ablate any residual microscopic disease.

REFERENCES

1. LiVolsi VA, Asa SL. The demise of follicular carcinoma of the thyroid gland. Thyroid 1994; 4:233–236.
2. D'Avanzo A, Ituarte P, Treseler P, et al. Prognostic scoring systems in patients with follicular thyroid cancer: a comparison of different staging systems in predicting the patient outcome. Thyroid 2004; 14: 453–458.
3. Evans HL. Follicular neoplasms of the thyroid: a study of 44 cases followed for a minimum of 10 years, with emphasis on differential diagnosis. Cancer 1984; 54:535–540.
4. Crile G Jr, Hazard JB. Relationship of the age of the patients to the natural history and prognosis of carcinoma of the thyroid. Ann Surg 1953; 138:33–38.
5. Grebe SK, Hay ID. Follicular thyroid cancer. Endocrinol Metab Clin North Am 1995; 24:761–801.
6. Donohue JH, Goldfien SD, Miller TR, et al. Do the prognoses of papillary and follicular thyroid carcinomas differ? Am J Surg 1984; 148:168–173.
6a. Besic N., Zgajnar J, Hoevar M, Frkovic-Grazio S. Is patient's age a prognostic factor for follicular thyroid carcinoma in the TNM classification system? Thyroid 2005; 15:439–448.
7. Brennan MD, Bergstralh EJ, van Heerden JA, McConahey WM. Follicular thyroid cancer treated at the Mayo Clinic, 1946 through 1970: initial manifestations, pathologic findings, therapy, and outcome. Mayo Clin Proc 1991; 66:11–22.
8. Mazzaferri EL. Treating differentiated thyroid carcinoma: where do we draw the line? Mayo Clin Proc 1991; 66:105–111.
9. van Heerden JA, Hay ID, Goellner JR, et al. Follicular thyroid carcinoma with capsular invasion alone: a nonthreatening malignancy. Surgery 1992; 112:1130–1136; discussion 1136–1138.
10. D'Avanzo A, Treseler P, Ituarte PH, et al. Follicular thyroid carcinoma: histology and prognosis. Cancer 2004; 100:1123–1129.

11. Emerick GT, Duh QY, Siperstein AE, et al. Diagnosis, treatment, and outcome of follicular thyroid carcinoma. Cancer 1993; 72: 3287–3295.
12. Kahn NF, Perzin KH. Follicular carcinoma of the thyroid. Pathol Ann 1996; 18:221–253.
13. Clark OH, Gerend PL. Thyrotropin receptor-adenylate cyclase system in Hürthle cell neoplasms. J Clin Endocrinol Metabol 1985; 61: 773–778.
14. Grossman RF, Clark OH. Hürthle cell carcinoma. Cancer Control J Moffitt Cancer Center 1997; 4:13–17.
15. DeGroot LJ, Kaplan EL, Shukla MS, et al. Morbidity and mortality in follicular thyroid cancer. J Clin Endocrinol Metab 1995; 80: 2946–2953.
16. Azadian A, Rosen IB, Walfish PG, Asa SL. Management considerations in Hürthle cell carcinoma. Surgery 1995; 118:711–714; discussion 714–715.
17. Cooper DS, Schneyer CR. Follicular and Hürthle cell carcinoma of the thyroid. Endocrinol Metab Clin North Am 1990; 19:577–591.
18. Kushchayeva Y, Duh Q-Y, Kebebew E, Clark OH: Hurthle cell carcinoma: Predictive factors of outcome. World J Surg 2004; 28:1266–1270.
18a. Chao T-C, Lin J-D, Chen M-F. Surgical treatment of Hurthle cell tumors of the thyroid. World J Surg 2005; 29:164–168.
19. Yen TWF, Shapiro SE, Gagel RF, et al. Medullary thyroid carcinoma: Results of a standardized surgical approach in a contemporary series of 80 consecutive patients. Surgery 2003; 134:890–901.

57
Pathology of Follicular Cancer

Yolanda C. Oertel

Follicular carcinomas are rare in today's industrialized nations *(1,2)*. This cancer type does not have the nuclear features of papillary carcinoma, usually has no papillae, lacks amyloid and calcitonin, and does not contain the numerous spindle cells, giant cells, and mitotic figures of undifferentiated (anaplastic) carcinoma. Most published classifications are based on the degree of cancer invasiveness, but histological patterns of the neoplasm may also provide clues to its likely behavior *(3)*. At present, evaluating the neoplasm's relationship to the surrounding tissues has proved to be the most useful guide to categorizing these tumors *(4–7)*.

Inspection of the tissues usually reveals a single, spherical, solid, fleshy neoplasm, with pink-to-tan cut surfaces (if fresh) or pale tan-to-pale gray surfaces (if fixed in formaldehyde; *8*). Tumors composed of oxyphilic cells (Askanazy/Hürthle cells) are brown. If the tumor contains a considerable amount of colloid, the cut surface may appear translucent and gelatinous. Small hemorrhages may be present, along with focal scarring (especially in the center). A few cancers present as multiple neoplastic nodules, with "daughter nodules" around the nodule with the thickest capsule. Cystic change and focal necrosis sometimes occur. The tumors are usually encapsulated, but if a tumor is quite invasive, only remnants of the capsule can be detected. Capsules vary in thickness (are often thick), and when a small tumor has a thick capsule, the pathologist should suspect carcinoma, not adenoma *(9,10)*.

A moderate proportion of follicular carcinomas occurs in association with multiple adenomatoid nodules (or adenomas). It can be difficult to decide which tumor is malignant upon gross examination; thus, systematic sectioning of such a specimen is essential.

Follicular carcinomas can be considered minimally or widely invasive *(1,7,11)*. Assessment is performed after surgical resection of the tumor (or occasionally at autopsy) and requires multiple sections of the periphery of the neoplasm to exclude an adenoma. A total of 10 tissue blocks from the periphery of the tumor is desirable *(4)*, or more if the tumor is particularly cellular or contains many mitotic figures.

For small tumors, the entire neoplasm should be embedded in such a way as to enable multiple views of its periphery to be obtained *(12)*.

Minimally invasive carcinoma (or encapsulated carcinoma) has tiny scattered foci of vascular and capsular invasion at its periphery (see Figs. 1 and 2). Rarely, capsular extension in one or two places without evident vascular invasion is found *(3,4)*. When only capsular penetration appears to be present, the patient probably does not have distant spread *(13)*, but the pathologist should search vigorously for vascular invasion *(4,5)*. Therefore, if a tumor is not evaluated systematically, it may be mistaken for an adenoma *(12)*. Differentiating capsular invasion from invasion of small vessels in the capsule may be difficult to impossible. Therefore, discussion of such phenomena must be evaluated with caution *(2,5,13)*. Widely invasive carcinoma is uncommon, with extensive protrusion into surrounding tissues and/or extension into multiple vessels (often large vascular spaces; Fig. 3). Moderately invasive carcinoma can occupy the region between these extremes and is difficult to define exactly; thus, such neoplasms are categorized with the widely invasive tumors.

Cells of follicular carcinoma are often small and monotonous in histological sections, with uniform round nuclei, stippled chromatin, and central nucleoli. The nucleoli vary considerably in size from one carcinoma to another. Mitotic figures range greatly in number in each tumor; atypical mitoses are rare. Scattered large or bizarre nuclei may occur, but they appear in atypical adenomas, as well as in the carcinomas, and their prognostic significance is uncertain *(14,15)*. Cytoplasm is lightly eosinophilic or amphophilic but rarely clear. Papillae are usually absent, but if present, they are few, small, and simple *(1)*. Psammoma bodies are also often nonexistent; when present, they lie in the colloid of the neoplastic follicles *(1)*.

Assessing differentiation by examining routine histological sections can be beneficial, especially when combined with immunohistochemical staining using antithyroglobulin *(15,16)*. Patterns within a neoplasm may be uniform or

From: *Thyroid Cancer: A Comprehensive Guide to Clinical Management, 2/e*
Edited by: L. Wartofsky and D. Van Nostrand © Humana Press Inc., Totowa, NJ

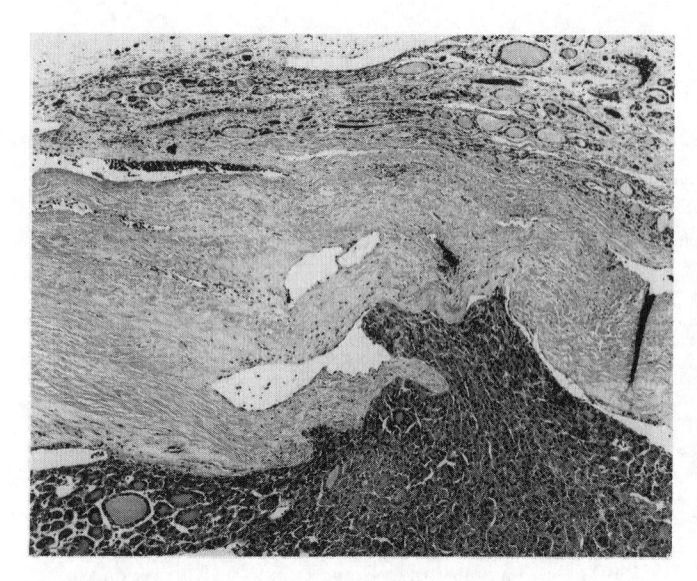

Fig. 1. Minimally invasive follicular carcinoma. The cancer extends into a vessel in the thick capsule (hematoxylin and eosin [H&E] stain).

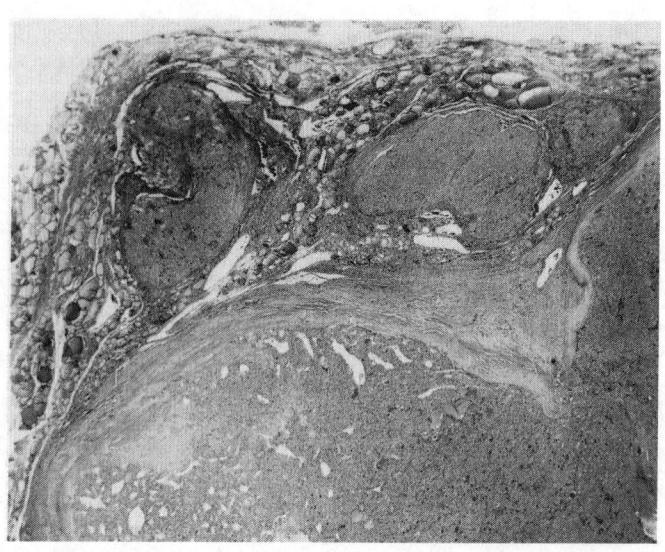

Fig. 3. Widely invasive follicular carcinoma. Vessels are distended by the carcinoma (superior part of the field; H&E stain).

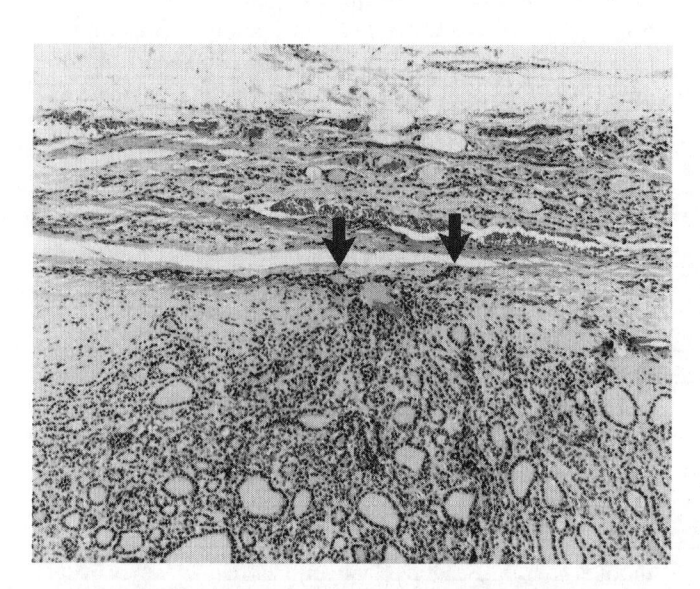

Fig. 2. Minimally invasive follicular carcinoma. There is subtle infiltration of the tumor capsule (arrows; H&E stain).

notably heterogeneous. Consequently, biopsies have limited value in determining the degree of differentiation.

Well-differentiated follicular carcinomas are composed entirely (or almost entirely) of either empty or colloid-filled follicles (16). These may vary from minute microfollicles (easily visualized with the PAS technique, showing the tiny droplets of colloid) to follicles even larger than those of normal thyroid tissue (1). Most cancers with a follicular pattern are predominantly microfollicular (2). Large amounts of immunoreactive thyroglobulin are present in the cells and follicles of many of these tumors. Some investigators report that a predominantly follicular pattern has a more favorable prognosis (3,4). Moderately differentiated follicular carcinomas are those in which follicular elements of any size are mixed with solid islands of cells and/or cords of cells (trabeculae; 16). Both the solid regions and trabeculae may contain some microfollicles. Considerable thyroglobulin is present in some areas, but it is sparse or absent in others. Some neoplastic cells may be elongated, even spindled, especially in regions where the cells form trabeculae. Such parts are different from undifferentiated carcinomas with better organization, a lack of numerous mitotic figures, and a lack of necrosis.

Poorly differentiated follicular carcinoma is a solid and/or trabecular neoplasm that contains some microfollicles, lacks the cellular characteristics of papillary carcinoma, is devoid of the usual features of anaplastic thyroid carcinoma, and may have focal thyroglobulin production (16). Obviously, this type of cancer overlaps (or is the same as) the poorly differentiated carcinoma (insular carcinoma, "Wuchernde struma").

Metastases to cervical lymph nodes are rare (4,8,17) and often accompanied by direct extrathyroidal extension of the cancer. The presence of such nodal involvement should provoke a review of the histological features of the resected tissues. If nodes contain follicular carcinoma, the prognosis is likely worse (18,19).

Assessing nuclear ploidy has not provided a reliable means of differentiating follicular adenomas from follicu-

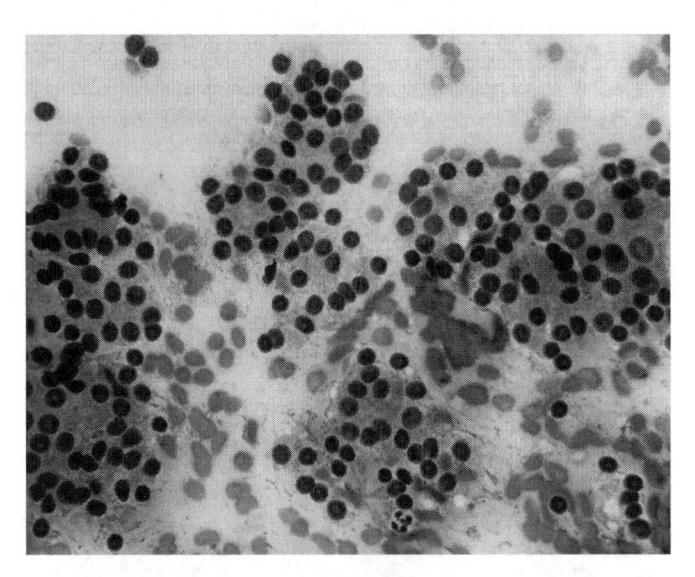

Fig. 4. Follicular neoplasm. Hypercellular smear with neoplastic cells arranged predominantly in rosettes. Resected specimen revealed a follicular adenoma (Diff-Quik stain).

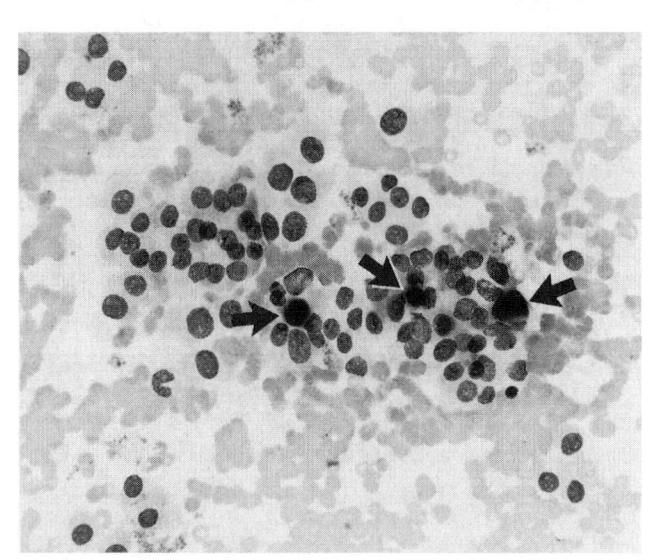

Fig. 5. Follicular neoplasm. Aspirate contains rosettes and three follicles with inspissated colloid (arrows). Resected specimen revealed a follicular adenoma (Diff-Quik stain).

lar carcinomas (18,20,21), and the prognostic value is uncertain (20,22). Argyrophilic staining of nucleolar-organizing regions might be useful to recognize the malignant follicular neoplasms (23,24), but thus far, it is only one of various special techniques not yet proven sufficiently to consider its use on a routine basis.

Aspirates from these lesions are diagnosed as follicular neoplasms, which include both follicular adenomas and carcinomas (25–27). Our reports state that "to differentiate between an adenoma and a carcinoma, multiple sections through the capsule of the surgically excised specimen are required." Upon aspiration, these neoplasms bleed easily; therefore, many specimens are diluted by blood and may be interpreted as unsatisfactory. If the physician performing the aspiration is experienced and exceptionally careful, a specimen with tumor cellularity may be obtained.

In the hypocellular smears, the presence of a few microfollicles with inspissated colloid should raise the possibility of a follicular neoplasm. Some follicular cells arranged in rosettes and tubules may also be seen.

The hypercellular smears contain many follicular cells set in rosettes and tubules (Fig. 4), microfollicles (often with inspissated dark blue colloid; Fig. 5), and tissue fragments.

The neoplastic follicular cells are enlarged and have delicate, pale pink or bluish cytoplasm (a scant-to-moderate amount), with poorly demarcated borders. The nuclei are enlarged, the chromatin varies in density, and it usually has a mottled appearance. The nuclear borders are slightly irregular, and nucleoli may be visible. In some tumors (both benign and malignant), the variation in nuclear size may be marked.

Colloid is usually absent, except for the droplets of inspissated colloid observed in some neoplastic microfollicles.

Follicular carcinoma with oxyphilic cells (Askanazy/Hürthle cells) are composed mostly or completely of these distinctive cells. Recognizing the malignant potential of a tumor depends on evidence of aggressive behavior at its periphery (1,28). Trabecular patterns are common. Bizarre, large, and/or hyperchromatic nuclei may be striking histological features, but these are more common in the benign proliferations of oxyphilic cells. The proliferative cell nuclear antigen is reported to be present at higher levels in indeterminate and malignant oxyphilic cell neoplasms, compared to oxyphilic cell adenomas (29). Metastases to cervical lymph nodes are more common than with the usual follicular carcinoma, especially after the patient has undergone surgery to treat the cancer. Some studies suggest that oxyphilic follicular carcinomas are more aggressive than typical nonoxyphilic follicular carcinomas. The presence of nondiploid cells in an oxyphilic carcinoma indicates a poorer prognosis than that with diploid nuclei (30).

The cytological smears show tumor cellularity and often a monotonous cell population. In most cases, the cells are large (but can be small) and have generous amounts of grayish-pink to grayish-blue cytoplasm, large round nuclei, and prominent nucleoli. Binucleation is common. They are arranged in large tissue fragments, small clusters, or as single entities (25). Frequently, the cellular borders are well demarcated (Fig. 6). The neoplastic follicles are common but appear empty (Fig. 7). Some follicles with inspissated blue colloid may be seen.

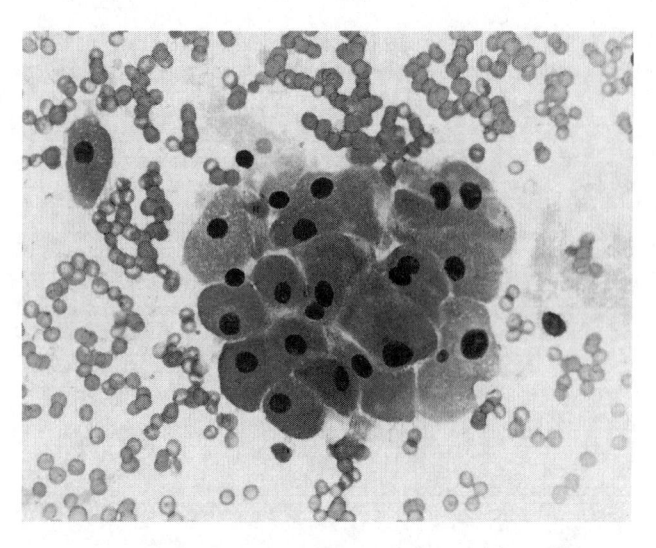

Fig. 6. Follicular neoplasm with oxyphilic cells. Smear shows neoplastic cells with abundant dense cytoplasm and well-demarcated borders (Diff-Quik stain).

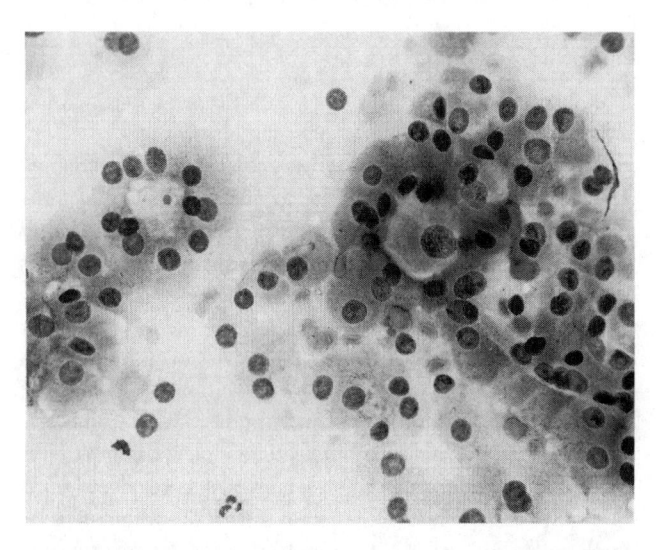

Fig. 7. Follicular neoplasm with oxyphilic cells. Smear shows large neoplastic cells with abundant cytoplasm and conspicuous nucleoli. Three empty follicles are visible in the superior half of the field (Diff-Quik stain).

REFERENCES

1. Franssila KO, Ackerman LV, Brown CL, Hedinger CE. Follicular carcinoma. Semin Diagn Pathol 1985; 2:101–122.
2. LiVolsi VA. Surgical pathology of the thyroid. Major Probl Pathol 1990; 22:173–212.
3. D'Avanzo A, Treseler P, Ituarte PHG, et al. Follicular thyroid carcinoma: Histology and prognosis. Cancer 2004; 100:1123–1129.
4. Thompson LDR, Wieneke JA, Paal E, et al. A clinicopathologic study of minimally invasive follicular carcinoma of the thyroid gland with a review of the English literature. Cancer 2001; 91:505–524.
5. Shaha AR. Invited commentary: Minimally invasive follicular thyroid carcinoma. Surgery 2001; 130:119–120.
6. Saadi H, Kleidermacher P, Esselstyn C Jr. Conservative management of patients with intrathyroidal well-differentiated follicular thyroid carcinoma. Surgery 2001; 130:30–35.
7. Franc B, De La Salmonière P, Lange F, et al. Interobserver and intraobserver reproducibility in the histopathology of follicular thyroid carcinoma. Hum Pathol 2003; 34:1092–1100.
8. Rosai J, Carcangiu ML, DeLellis RA. Tumors of the thyroid gland. In Rosai J, Sobin LH, editors. Atlas of Tumor Pathology, 3rd Ser, Fasc 5. Washington, DC: A. F. I. P., 1992.
9. Evans HL. Follicular neoplasms of the thyroid: a study of 44 cases followed for a minimum of 10 years, with emphasis on differential diagnosis. Cancer 1984; 54:535–540.
10. Yamashita T, Fujimoto Y, Kodama T, et al. When is total thyroidectomy indicated as a treatment of "follicular carcinoma"? World J Surg 1988; 12:559–564.
11. Grebe SKG, Hay ID. Follicular thyroid cancer. Endocrinol Metab Clin North Am 1995; 24:761–801.
12. Yamashina M. Follicular neoplasms of the thyroid. Total circumferential evaluation of the fibrous capsule. Am J Surg Pathol 1992; 16:392–400.
13. van Heerden JA, Hay ID, Goellner JR, et al. Follicular thyroid carcinoma with capsular invasion alone: a nonthreatening malignancy. Surgery 1992; 112:1130–1138.
14. Hazard JB, Kenyon R. Atypical adenoma of the thyroid. Arch Pathol Lab Med 1954; 58:554–563.
15. Jorda M, Gonzalez-Campora R, Mora J, et al. Prognostic factors in follicular carcinoma of the thyroid. Arch Pathol Lab Med 1993; 117:631–635.
16. Harach HR, Franssila KO. Thyroglobulin immunostaining in follicular thyroid carcinoma: relationship to the degree of differentiation and cell type. Histopathology 1988; 13:43–54.
17. Schroder S, Pfannschmidt N, Dralle H, et al. The encapsulated follicular carcinoma of the thyroid: a clinicopathologic study of 35 cases. Virchows Arch A Pathol Anat Histopathol 1984; 402:259–273.
18. Schroder S. Pathological and Clinical Features of Malignant Thyroid Tumors: Classification, Immunohistology, Prognostic Criteria. New York: Gustav Fischer, 1988.
19. Segal K, Arad A, Lubin E, et al. Follicular carcinoma of the thyroid. Head Neck 1994; 16:533–538.
20. Grant CS, Hay ID, Ryan JJ, et al. Diagnostic and prognostic utility of flow cytometric DNA measurements in follicular thyroid tumors. World J Surg 1990; 14:283–290.
21. Oyama T, Vickery Jr AL, Preffer FI, Colvin RB. A comparative study of flow cytometry and histopathologic findings in thyroid follicular carcinomas and adenomas. Hum Pathol 1994; 25:271–275.
22. Hruban RH, Huvos AG, Traganos F, et al. Follicular neoplasms of the thyroid in men older than 50 years of age: a DNA flow cytometric study. Am J Clin Pathol 1990; 94:527–532.
23. Ruschoff J, Prasser C, Cortez T, et al. Diagnostic value of AgNOR staining in follicular cell neoplasms of the thyroid: comparison of evaluation methods and nucleolar features. Am J Surg Pathol 1993; 17:1281–1288.
24. Shem-Tov Y, Straus M, Talmi YP, et al. Nucleolar organizer regions in follicular tumors of the thyroid. Head Neck 1994; 16:420–423.
25. Tuleke MA, Wang HH. ThinPrep® for cytologic evaluation of follicular thyroid lesions: Correlation with histologic findings. Diagn Cytopathol 2004; 30:7–13.
26. Greaves TS, Olvera M, Florentine BD, et al. Follicular lesions of thyroid: a 5-year fine-needle aspiration experience. Cancer 2000; 90: 335–341.
27. Baloch ZW, Fleisher S, LiVolsi VA, Gupta PK. Diagnosis of "follicular neoplasm": a gray zone in thyroid fine-needle aspiration cytology. Diagn Cytopathol 2002; 26:41–44.
28. Carcangiu ML, Bianchi S, Savino D, et al. Follicular Hürthle cell tumors of the thyroid gland. Cancer 1991; 68:1944–1953.
29. Tateyama H, Yang Y-P, Eimoto T, et al. Proliferative cell nuclear antigen expression in follicular tumours of the thyroid with special reference to oxyphilic cell lesions. Virchows Arch A Pathol Anat Histopathol 1994; 424:533–537.
30. Ryan JJ, Hay ID, Grant CS, et al. Flow cytometric DNA measurements in benign and malignant Hürthle cell tumors of the thyroid. World J Surg 1988; 12:482–487.

58
Hürthle Cell Carcinoma

Kenneth D. Burman and Leonard Wartofsky

INTRODUCTION

The Hürthle cell variant of follicular carcinoma is composed of large acidophilic, Askanazy, or oncocytic cells that are considered altered follicular cells *(1,2)*. For instance, Hürthle cells bind thyrotropin (TSH) and have TSH receptors, like other types of follicular thyroid cells *(3,4)*. Similar to other follicular neoplasms, Hürthle cell carcinoma is more common in women than men, but the patients tend to be older than those with typical follicular thyroid carcinoma (FTC; see Chapter 55). Hürthle cells contain many mitochondria (which are the basis for the abundant, eosinophilic, and granular cytoplasm), frequently eccentric nuclei, and visible nucleoli. The Hürthle cell carcinoma variant of follicular carcinoma discussed here is to be distinguished from the variant of papillary thyroid cancer, "Hürthle cell papillary thyroid carcinoma," which also contains an abundance of oxyphilic cells *(4a)*. The central genetic or environmental factors that allow a thyrocyte to differentiate into a Hürthle cell are unknown, and Hürthle cells may occur in a variety of thyroid disorders. Solitary thyroid nodules may have a predominance of Hürthle cells, to the exclusion of more typical thyrocytes, and these lesions are often highly cellular with minimal colloid. When such a lesion is aspirated for cytologic examination, the interpretation would likely be "suggestive of a Hürthle cell neoplasm," because as with follicular tumors, a definite diagnosis of benign or malignant would be difficult or impossible to make. Hürthle cell neoplasms may be benign or malignant, and the distinction is based on the demonstration of vascular or capsular invasion, metastatic capacity, and growth rate, similarly to other follicular neoplasms *(5)*.

When patients with Hürthle cell carcinoma are stratified regarding low vs high risk, there does not appear to be a significantly worse prognosis than that for follicular carcinoma *(6;* see Chapters 55 and 64). In contrast to other follicular carcinomas, they have a higher rate of bilaterality or multicentricity. One recent report suggested that the distinction could be inferred from the size of the lesion; those tumors larger than 4 cm are considered invariably malignant *(7)*.

With the use of fine-needle aspiration (FNA) cytology some solitary thyroid nodules may also have a more varied appearance, where Hürthle cells intermingle with thyrocytes, macrophages, and lymphocytes and have moderate amounts of colloid. In such circumstances, the cytology may be more difficult to interpret, and when insufficient Hürthle cells are present the tumor is characterized as a Hürthle cell neoplasm. Furthermore, Hürthle cells may be found in the thyroid glands of patients with Hashimoto's thyroiditis and other benign thyroid disorders but usually in this circumstance, the Hürthle cells are scattered and are not the predominant cell type *(4)*.

The typical Hürthle cell neoplasm is composed mostly of these distinctive cells and is generally considered to be a variant of follicular carcinoma. Recognizing the malignant potential of a tumor depends on the evidence of aggressive behavior at its periphery *(8–15)*. Bizarre, large, and/or hyperchromatic nuclei may be a striking histological feature, and these are more common than in benign proliferations of oxyphilic cells.

Metastases to cervical lymph nodes are more frequent than with the usual follicular carcinoma, especially after the patient has undergone surgery. Notwithstanding the comments above, there are some studies that suggest oxyphilic follicular carcinomas are more aggressive than typical nonoxyphilic follicular carcinomas. Particularly, the presence of nondiploid cells in an oxyphilic carcinoma indicates a poorer prognosis than that with diploid nuclei *(16)*. Papillary carcinomas may also contain significant populations of these cells *(4a)*. Whether they are more aggressive than a nonoxyphilic cancer with otherwise similar characteristics remains uncertain.

However, what does appear clear is that without specific attention to risk stratification, Hürthle cell malignancies will tend to have a worse prognosis than other follicular tumors in many *(17,18)*, but not all, studies *(19)*. This may be partly because of their greater tendency to be locally invasive and propensity to concentrate radioiodine less avidly, thereby rendering them more difficult to manage with isotopic scanning and therapy *(20,21)*. Yet, this is not universal, and some

From: *Thyroid Cancer: A Comprehensive Guide to Clinical Management, 2/e*
Edited by: L. Wartofsky and D. Van Nostrand © Humana Press Inc., Totowa, NJ

Hürthle cell cancers will trap iodine (22). In a review of 89 cases of Hürthle cell carcinoma seen at the MD Anderson Cancer Center, Lopez-Penabad et al. (23) expressed a rather pessimistic assessment of the efficacy of currently available therapies for this variant of FTC. There was a 40% cause-specific mortality over their long follow-up interval, with no improvement in mortality rates found over the prior 50 yr. Larger tumor size and more advanced age were negative prognostic indicators. Additionally, in the setting of metastatic disease, there was no further survival advantage seen with more extensive surgery, external radiation therapy, chemotherapy, or even radioactive iodine therapy.

CLINICAL PRESENTATION

Hürthle cell carcinomas may represent about 3–5% of all types of thyroid carcinomas. Most Hürthle cell carcinomas appear to be a more aggressive kind of follicular carcinoma, with more frequent recurrences, higher morbidity, and higher mortality, but this is controversial (8,9). The tumors are frequently multifocal and bilateral.

Thompson and associates (9–11) suggested that it is difficult to differentiate benign from malignant Hürthle cell tumors. The implication of their studies is that even experienced pathologists may not be able to make a reliable distinction. Carcangiu and coworkers (12) and Grant and associates (13) support the concept that strict histological criteria and adequate sampling may be able to differentiate Hürthle cell carcinoma from adenoma in nearly all cases. Grant et al. (13) reviewed the world literature and observed that only 6 of 642 patients with apparent benign Hürthle cell adenomas were found to have a recurrence, thereby indicating that the tumor was a carcinoma, with an incidence of less than 1%. Gosain and Clark (14) found no patients with Hürthle cell adenoma in whom recurrences were observed. Similarly, Bondeson and coworkers (16) studied 42 patients diagnosed with Hürthle cell adenoma over a 2–20-yr period and found no recurrences.

The above reports help to support the contention that Hürthle cell adenomas can be accurately diagnosed and distinguished from carcinoma on histological examination by experienced pathologists. As with other follicular carcinomas, the major histological criteria that separate a Hürthle cell adenoma from a carcinoma are vascular and/or capsular invasion. However, subtleties do remain. For example, does the capsular invasion have to be completely through the capsule, or is invasion into, but not through, the capsule enough to make the diagnosis? It is also important to ensure that sufficient histologic sections were taken and examined. Notwithstanding these concerns, it is likely that experienced pathologists can reliably make this differential diagnosis.

The absence of radioiodine uptake by residual or metastatic follicular cancer renders management much more difficult, but not impossible. Typically, these tumors are less avid for radioactive iodine and therefore respond less often than the usual follicular carcinoma. Several groups are currently evaluating the thyroidal sodium iodide symporter (Na^+/I^- symporter [NIS]) function and expression in Hürthle cell carcinomas relative to FTC (3,4,8). These studies are exploring methods for the management of follicular cancers that have lost their ability to either trap iodide (and be treatable with radioiodine) or to synthesize and release thyroglobulin. The ability of both normal and malignant thyroid cells to concentrate iodide is dependent on expression of the NIS gene (24,25). The loss of this gene during tumor dedifferentiation can account for the tumor's failure to concentrate iodide. Gene therapy or redifferentiation therapy with retinoic acid, depsipeptide, and other agents had been thought to hold promise for the restoration of both radioiodine uptake for potential treatment and thyroglobulin production for monitoring recurrence (26–31). However, a recent analysis of results with retinoic acid was less than optimistic (32).

It is reasonable to assume that one major reason why these tumors do not respond as well to therapy is because they do not concentrate radioiodine as well as usual follicular carcinomas. It may be appropriate to approach Hürthle cell carcinomas as if they were medullary carcinomas, i.e., with more aggressive diagnostic procedures and treatment (14,33).

In most clinical circumstances, patients diagnosed with a Hürthle cell neoplasm by FNA should undergo surgery somewhat promptly. We recommend a near-total to total thyroidectomy by an experienced thyroid surgeon. It is important to discuss with the patient the alternative approaches of a near-total thyroidectomy compared to a lobectomy with isthmusectomy (33a). If only a lobectomy and isthmusectomy are performed, and if the lesion is found to be cancerous, then a subsequent completion thyroidectomy must be performed. This completion thyroidectomy frequently causes mental and psychosocial distress to the patient, especially if the requirement for this procedure is not expected by the patient. However, only about 20% of Hürthle cell neoplasms diagnosed by FNA are found to be malignant. If a total thyroidectomy is conducted initially, then in 80% of cases, this procedure would be unnecessarily aggressive and exposes the patient to a higher risk of temporary and permanent hypocalcemia, along with recurrent laryngeal nerve paralysis.

The decision regarding which operation is needed for a patient with a solitary thyroid nodule and an FNA consistent with Hürthle cell neoplasm is difficult. A frozen-section interpretation is often problematic and therefore not helpful (34). It is important to candidly discuss the advantages and disadvantages of each approach with the patient and family and arrive at a mutual decision. The initial operation should include an ipsilateral central node dissection. Obviously, the surgeon must be allowed to exercise judgment at the time of surgery about the precise operative procedures. Soh and Clark (3,33) suggest that a routine modified radical neck dissection be performed when the tumor is found in the central compartment or cervical nodes.

Because these tumors are somewhat less differentiated than most papillary thyroid cancers and FTCs, there is a reasonable chance that they can be detected by 18-fluorodeoxyglucose positron emission tomography (FDG-PET) when they do not concentrate radioiodine. Lowe et al. (35) found PET scanning to be useful to identify both local and metastatic disease, thereby facilitating disease management. Growth of Hürthle cell tumors has been described to reflect the net of proliferative vs apoptotic indices, and it may become feasible to exploit these characteristics to distinguish benign from malignant lesions (36).

McDonald and coworkers (37) reviewed 40 cases of Hürthle cell carcinoma, noting that this number represented 4% of all thyroid cancers in their experience. Their median follow-up interval after thyroidectomy was 8.5 yr. Vascular or capsular invasion was observed in 32 patients, extrathyroidal invasion in 11, and regional lymph node involvement in 2. One patient had distant metastases at presentation, and only nine patients received ^{131}I. Of 34 subjects analyzed, 5 died of thyroid cancer, 9 died of nonthyroidal causes, 4 were alive with existing disease, and 16 were alive without evidence of disease. At about an average of 4 yr, nine patients had recurrences and five had distant disease. Recurrent disease was associated with mortality in half of these patients. Risk factors assessed at initial presentation were useful to help predict recurrence. Low-risk tumors did not recur (e.g., tumors less than 5-cm diameter, lack of distant metastases, men younger than 41 yr, and women younger than 51 yr). Tumor size and the presence of distant metastases were more important prognostic indicators than age in one recent series of patients (37a).

Bhattacharyya (38) performed a retrospective review of the Surveillance, Epidemiology, and End Results database for cases between 1973 and 1998, finding that 3% of cases represented Hürthle cell carcinoma, and 555 of the patients (377 women, 178 men) were analyzed. Outcomes in 411 were compared to outcomes in 411 matched patients with follicular carcinoma; 5- and 10-yr mortality rates were 15% and 29% vs 11% and 45%, respectively. The survival time was also not different, with an average of 109 mo for Hürthle cell carcinoma and 113 mo for follicular cancer. For the patients with Hürthle cell carcinoma patients, increased mortality was associated with larger tumor size and male gender, but not the presence of local invasion. In a small patient series, Lopez-Penabad et al. (23) observed the worst prognosis in older patients with larger tumors and local extension. Similar findings were reported by Kushchayeva et al. in a series of 33 patients (38a).

Because some Hürthle cell carcinomas were found to have *ret/PTC* gene rearrangements similar to papillary thyroid cancers (39), as well as a propensity to spread to local lymph nodes like papillary cancers, it may be that there can be subspecies of what we have presumed to be classic Hürthle cell carcinoma that represent variants of either follicular or papillary thyroid cancer (4a). Such differences might account for our difficulty in comparing individual reports in the literature with mortality and morbidity rates, of which some but not all support the view that Hürthle cell carcinoma is linked with a poorer prognosis than the usual FTC or papillary thyroid cancer.

Following appropriate surgery for Hürthle cell carcinoma, radioiodine scanning and therapy is recommended. Scan preparation would be routine and is usually performed about 6 wk after surgery. A diagnostic radioiodine scan is important before therapy to help determine the avidity of the remaining thyroid cells for radioiodine and to define the nature and extent of remaining thyroid tissue or disease. Assuming that there is visible uptake, the diagnostic scan is then followed by radioiodine therapy, usually with 100–150 mCi ^{131}I. A posttreatment scan is performed approx 7–10 d after treatment. (These protocols are detailed in Chapter 45.)

As described above, many Hürthle cell cancers will not trap radioiodine, and sometimes only as little as 10% of Hürthle cell cancers will trap and respond to radioiodine. This number seems low in our experience and, of course, somewhat depends on the dose of ^{131}I used for scanning, the length of time that the patient did not receive thyroid hormone, the extent of TSH elevation, and possibly the assiduous adherence to a low-iodine diet. Based on published reports, it may be difficult to adequately assess these factors. Perhaps in some cases, lack of apparent iodine avidity by the tumor may not be an accurate representation of the tumor's true properties.

For surveillance over the subsequent 5 yr after initial surgery and ablation, we recommend following the patient with physical examinations, thyroid function tests, and thyroglobulin monitoring about every 3–6 mo for the first several years, and possibly every 4–6 mo for the next several years if there has been no evidence of disease recurrence. Our approach of utilizing radioiodine scans is consistent with that of Besic et al. (22). In the initial year or two of surveillance, levothyroxine therapy is used in a dosage designed to achieve suppressed TSH in most patients (0.1 µU/mL or lower), depending on the clinical context. Thyroglobulin levels are analyzed at the same time as thyroid function tests, and the thyroglobulin level during L-thyroxine suppression must be less than 2 ng/mL (according to the assay). Thyrogen testing may be employed as outlined by a consensus group of thyroid cancer investigators (40). The latter follow-up would generally include a repeat whole-body ^{131}I scan in 1 yr, then 3–5 yr later. Given the aggressive nature of this tumor, we may also obtain occasional radiographs of the chest. An imaging study of the neck, such as an magnetic resonance image or sonogram, is routinely performed, especially if the tumor is not iodine-avid, if the thyroglobulin level is increasing, or if palpable cervical abnormalities become manifest. In women, particularly those who are postmenopausal, suppressive doses of levothyroxine therapy should be accompanied by measures to prevent osteoporosis (daily oral ingestion of 1–1.5 g of calcium, 400 U of vitamin D, exercise against gravity, and the possible addition of a bisphosphonate; *41*).

Other scanning agents may have reasonably good utility for the detection of Hürthle cell carcinoma. In a study comparing radioiodine and thallium scanning to that with ^{99m}Tc-MIBI, Yen et al. *(42)* reported a 100% specificity and an 82% sensitivity for ^{99m}Tc-MIBI in patients with Hürthle cell carcinoma. The utility of FDG-PET scanning has already been mentioned *(35)* and was also reported earlier *(43)* to have an 80% specificity and a 92% sensitivity for this tumor. The issue of which scanning agent to employ arises when serum thyroglobulin levels indicate residual or recurrent disease. Despite the proven value of PET scanning, because of its cost and lack of widespread availability, we believe that radioiodine scanning should be attempted first, followed by ^{99m}Tc-MIBI, before utilizing FDG-PET.

Hürthle cell cancer is discussed further in Chapters 55–57. These and other follicular cancers that do not concentrate radioiodine may be treated with chemotherapy (see Chapter 52), external radiation therapy *(44–47*; see Chapter 63), or redifferentiation therapy with retinoic acid or other agents could be attempted *(26–30)*. However, although external radiation therapy may cause apparent tumor regression and provide palliation and reduced recurrence rate, even in Hürthle cell carcinoma *(48)*, the effect may be transitory with little improvement in survival rate *(49)*.

REFERENCES

1. Umbricht CB, Saji M, Westra WH, et al. Telomerase activity: a marker to distinguish follicular thyroid adenoma from carcinoma. Cancer Res 1997; 57:2144–2147.
2. Watson RG, Brennan MD, Goellner JR, et al. Invasive Hürthle cell carcinoma of the thyroid: natural history and management. Mayo Clin Proc 1984; 59:851–855.
3. Soh EY, Clark OH. Surgical considerations and approach to thyroid cancer. Endocrinol Metab Clin North Am 1996; 25:115–139.
4. Cooper DS, Schneyer CR. Follicular and Hürthle cell carcinoma of the thyroid. Endocrinol Metab Clin North Am 1990; 19:577–591.
4a. Beckner ME, Heffess CS, Oertel JE. Oxyphillic papillary thyroid carcinomas. Am J Clin Pathol 1995; 103:280–287.
5. Bronner MP, LiVolsi VA. Oxyphilic (Askenasy/Hürthle cell) tumors of the thyroid: microscopic features predict biologic behavior. Surg Pathol 1988; 1:137–150.
6. Sanders LE, Silverman M. Follicular and Hürthle cell carcinoma: predicting outcome and directing therapy. Surgery 1998; 124:967–974.
7. Chen H, Nicol TL, Zeiger MA, et al. Hürthle cell neoplasms of the thyroid: are there factors predictive of malignancy? Ann Surg 1998; 227:542–546.
8. Azadian A, Rosen IB, Walfish PG, Asa SL. Management considerations in Hürthle cell carcinoma. Surgery 1995; 118:711–714; discussion 714–715.
9. Gundry SR, Burney RE, Thompson NW, Lloyd R. Total thyroidectomy for Hürthle cell neoplasm of the thyroid. Arch Surg 1983; 118:529–532.
10. Thompson NW, Dunn EL, Batsakis JG, Nishiyama RH. Hürthle cell lesions of the thyroid gland. Surg Gynecol Obstet 1974; 139:555–560.
11. McLeod MK, Thompson NW. Hürthle cell neoplasms of the thyroid. Otolaryngol Clin North Am 1990; 23:441–452.
12. Carcangiu ML, Bianchi S, Savino D, et al. Follicular Hürthle cell tumors of the thyroid gland. Cancer 1991; 68:1944–1953.
13. Grant CS, Barr D, Goellner JR, Hay ID. Benign Hürthle cell tumors of the thyroid: a diagnosis to be trusted? World J Surg 1988; 12:488–495.
14. Gosain AK, Clark OH. Hürthle cell neoplasms. Malignant potential. Arch Surg 1984; 119:515–519.
15. Carcangiu M. Hürthle cell carcinoma: clinic-pathologic and biological aspects. Tumori 2003; 89:529–532.
16. Bondeson L, Bondeson AG, Ljungberg O, Tibblin S. Oxyphil tumors of the thyroid: follow-up of 42 surgical cases. Ann Surg 1981; 194:677–680.
17. Samaan NA, Schultz PN, Haynie TP, Ordonez NG. Pulmonary metastasis of differentiated thyroid carcinoma: treatment results in 101 patients. J Clin Endocrinol Metab 1985; 60:376–380.
18. Samaan NA, Schultz PN, Hickey RC, et al. The results of various modalities of treatment of well differentiated thyroid carcinoma: a retrospective review of 1599 patients. J Clin Endocrinol Metab 1992; 75:714–720.
19. Har-El G, Hadar T, Segal K, et al. Hürthle cell carcinoma of the thyroid gland: a tumor of moderate malignancy. Cancer 1986; 57:1613–1617.
20. Thoresen SO, Akslen LA, Glattre E, et al. Survival and prognostic factors in differentiated thyroid carcinoma: a multivariate analysis of 1055 cases. Br J Surg 1989; 59:231–235.
21. Sugino K, Ito K, Mimura K, et al. Hürthle cell tumor of the thyroid: Analysis of 188 cases. World J Surg 2001; 25:1160–1163.
22. Besic N, Vidergar-Kralj B, Frkovic-Grazio S, et al. The role of radioactive iodine in the treatment of Hürthle cell carcinoma of the thyroid. Thyroid 2003; 13:577–584.
23. Lopez-Penabad L, Chiu AC, Hoff AO, et al. Prognostic factors in patients with Hürthle cell neoplasms of the thyroid. Cancer 2003; 97:1186–1194.
24. Arturi F, Russo D, Schlumberger M, et al. Iodide symporter gene expression in human thyroid tumors. J Clin Endocrinol Metab 1998; 83:2493–2496.
25. Dadachova E, Carrasco N. The Na/I symporter (NIS): imaging and therapeutic applications. Sem Nucl Med 2004; 34:23–31.
26. Grunwald F, Pakos R, Bender H, et al. Redifferentiation therapy with retinoic acid in follicular thyroid cancer. J Nucl Med 1998; 39:1555–1558.
27. Grunwald F, Menzel C, Bender H, et al. Redifferentiation therapy-induced radioiodine uptake in thyroid cancer. J Nucl Med 1998; 39:1903–1906.
28. Schmutzler C, Wnzer R, Meissner-Weigl J, Kohrle J. Retinoic acid increases sodium/iodide symporter mRNA levels in human thyroid cancer cell lines and suppresses expression of functional symporter in nontransformed FRTL-5 rat thyroid cells. Biochem Biophys Res Comm 1997; 240:832–838.
29. Park J-W, Clark OH. Redifferentiation therapy for thyroid cancer. Surg Clin N Am 2004; 84:921–943.
30. Braga-Basaria M, Ringel MD. Beyond radioiodine: a review of potential new therapeutic approaches for thyroid cancer. J Clin Endocrinol Metab 2003; 88:1947–1960.
31. Spitzweg C, Morris JC. Gene therapy for thyroid cancer: current status and future prospects. Thyroid 2004; 14:424–434.
32. Gruning T, Tiepolt C, Zophel K, et al. Retinoic acid for redifferentiation of thyroid cancer—does it hold its promise? Eur J Endocrinol 2003; 148:395–402.
33. Clark OH, Hoelting T. Management of patients with differentiated thyroid cancer who have positive serum thyroglobulin levels and negative radioiodine scans. Thyroid 1994; 4:501–505.

33a. Chao T-C, Lin J-D, Chen M-F. Surgical treatment of Hürthle cell tumors of the thyroid. World J Surg 2005; 29:164–168.
34. Chen H, Nicol TL, Udelsman R. Follicular lesions of the thyroid. Does frozen section evaluation alter operative management? Ann Surg 1995; 222:101–106.
35. Lowe VJ, Mullan BP, Hay ID, et al. 18-F-FDG PET of patients with Hürthle cell carcinoma. J Nucl Med 2003; 44:1402–1406.
36. Lazzi S, Spina d, Als C, et al. Oncocytic (Hürthle cell) tumors of the thyroid: Distinct growth patterns compared with clinicopathological features. Thyroid 1999; 9:97–103.
37. McDonald MP, Sanders LE, Silverman ML, et al. Hürthle cell carcinoma of the thyroid gland: prognostic factors and results of surgical treatment. Surgery 1996; 120:1000–1004; discussion 1004–1005.
37a. Besic N, Zgajnar J, Hoevar M, Frkovic-Grazio S. Is patient's age a prognostic factor for follicular thyroid carcinoma in the TNM classification system? Thyroid 2005; 15:439–448.
38. Bhattacharyya N. Survival and prognosis in Hürthle cell carcinoma of the thyroid gland. Arch Otolaryngol Head Neck Surg 2003; 129:207–210.
38a. Kushchayeva Y, Duh Q-Y, Kebebew E, Clark OH. Prognostic indications for Hürthle cell cancer. World J Surg 2004; 28:1266–1270.
39. Belchetz G, Cheung CC, Freeman J, et al. Hürthle cell tumors: using molecular techniques to define a novel classification system. Arch Otolaryngol Head Neck Surg 2002; 128:237–240.
40. Mazzaferri EL, Robbins RJ, Spencer CA, et al. A consensus report on the role of serum thyroglobulin as a monitoring method for low risk patients with papillary thyroid carcinoma. J Clin Endocrinol Metab 2003; 88:1433–1441.
41. Burman K. How serious are the risks of thyroid hormone over-replacement? Thyroid Today 1995; 18:1–6.
42. Yen TC, Lin HD, Lee CH, et al. The role of technetium-99m sestamibi whole-body scans in diagnosing metastatic Hürthle cell carcinoma of the thyroid gland after total thyroidectomy: A comparison with iodine-131 and thallium-201 whole-body scans. Eur J Nucl Med 1994; 21:981–983.
43. Plotkin M, Hautzel H, Krause BJ, et al. Implication of 2-18 Fluor-2-deoxyglucose positron emission tomography in the follow-up of Hürthle cell thyroid cancer. Thyroid 2002; 12:155–161.
44. Simpson WJ, Panzarella T, Carruthers JS, et al. Papillary and follicular thyroid cancer: impact of treatment in 1578 patients. Int J Radiat Oncol Biol Physiol 1988; 14:1063–1075.
45. Brierley JD, Tsang RW. External-beam radiation therapy in the treatment of differentiated thyroid cancer. Semin Surg Oncol 1999; 16:42–49.
46. Ford D, Giridharan S, McConkey C, et al. External beam radiotherapy in the management of differentiated thyroid cancer. Clin Oncol 2003; 15:337–341.
47. Schuck A, Biermann M, Pixberg MK, et al. Acute toxicity of adjuvant radiotherapy in locally advanced differentiated thyroid carcinoma. First results of the multicenter study of differentiated thyroid carcinoma (MSDS). Strahlenther Onkol 2003; 179:832–839.
48. Foote RL, Brown PD, Garces YI, et al. Is there a role for radiation therapy in the management of Hürthle cell carcinoma? Intern J Radiat Oncol Biol Phys 2003; 56:1067–1072.
49. Lin JD, Tsang NM, Huang MJ, Weng HF. Results of external beam radiotherapy in patients with well differentiated thyroid carcinoma. Jpn J Clin Oncol 1997; 27:244–247.

59
Radionuclide Imaging, Ablation, and Treatment in Follicular Thyroid Carcinoma

Douglas Van Nostrand

INTRODUCTION

Radioisotopic scanning with radioiodine and other agents, radioisotope "stunning," advantages of ^{123}I vs ^{131}I, and radioiodine therapy (including dosimetry) are addressed in separate chapters (26, 27, 32, 33, 36, 44–48) in this volume. This brief chapter relates primarily to special aspects of follicular thyroid cancer (FTC) relative to papillary thyroid carcinoma (PTC). Although papillary and follicular well-differentiated thyroid cancers are histologically different, their biological behavior is similar. As a result, most published reports do not differentiate between the two, describing outcomes for "differentiated thyroid carcinoma," and this is also true for the literature involving radionuclide imaging, ablation, and treatment. Accordingly, the other chapters discussing these issues for papillary carcinoma are applicable to patients with follicular carcinoma. However, several differences are related to these two types of thyroid malignancy that are noteworthy.

First, FTC is significantly less likely to metastasize to local cervical lymph nodes than PTC. For example, whereas PTC may metastasize to cervical lymph nodes in as many as 35–45% of patients, metastases to cervical lymph nodes is found in patients with FTC in only 5–17% of patients (1–5). Consequently, radioiodine uptake in lymph node metastases is much less likely to be visualized on imaging studies in patients with follicular carcinoma than is typical in papillary carcinoma. This difference is probably related to the degree of differentiation or undifferentiation of follicular cells. Histologically, FTC typically demonstrates a microfollicular pattern but follicular tumors with less radioiodine uptake tend to show more solid growth with macrofollicles and high levels of cellular atypia. FTC is also more likely to be unifocal, whereas papillary cancers are often multicentric, particularly with several satellite microcarcinomata.

Second, FTC is angioinvasive and may therefore metastasize hematogenously to the lung, bone, liver, brain, and kidney (2). Thus, distant metastases in these various sites is visualized more frequently on radionuclide imaging in patients with follicular cancer, but not papillary carcinoma.

Another distinction with papillary carcinoma relates to the variant of follicular carcinoma, known as Hürthle cell carcinoma (see Chapter 58), which is considered somewhat less differentiated, often losing the ability to transport iodide via the sodium iodide symporter (NIS). This property is reflected by a lower frequency of radioiodine uptake (3–7). Papillary and non-Hürthle cell follicular carcinoma may have radioiodine uptake in 60% and 64% of patients, respectively; Hürthle cell carcinoma may take up radioiodine in 36% of patients (3). This may make both imaging and treatment with radioiodine more problematic in these patients. However, because of variability in patient populations, patient age, sample size, and possibly diagnostic criteria for Hürthle cell carcinoma, the frequency of radioiodine uptake in Hürthle cell carcinoma is still debatable. For example, Besic et al. (4) reported uptake in 69% (11 of 16) patients with Hürthle cell carcinoma and concluded that radioiodine therapy may be effective in a significant number of these patients.

The biological behavior of FTC certainly appears to differ from PTC regarding prognostic factors associated with tumor recurrence (5) and survival (6). In one large follow-up series of 1578 patients, thyroid cancer was the cause of death in just over half of the PTC deaths and in two thirds of FTC deaths (7). The follicular variant of papillary carcinoma is discussed in Chapters 23, 25 and is generally considered to behave more like PTC (8) although multicentricity, lymph node metastases and local soft tissue invasion may be seen less often than in PTC (9).

Nevertheless, and despite the above clear differences between PTC and FTC, for all practical purposes, they are similarly regarded in terms of radionuclide imaging, ablation, and treatment at most medical centers. In addition to those cited in this text, excellent general reviews on FTC are available (10,11), and the reader is referred to the most recently published guidelines for management of thyroid cancer in the United States and the United Kingdom, which include guidelines for radioisotopic scanning and treatment (12,13).

REFERENCES

1. Wartofsky L. Follicular thyroid carcinoma, clinical aspects. In Wartofsky L, editor. Thyroid Cancer: A Comprehensive Guide to Clinical Management. Totowa, NJ: Humana Press, 2000.
2. Mazzaferri EL. Radioiodine and other treatments and outcomes. In Braverman LE, Utiger RD, editors. Werner and Ingbar's The Thyroid: A Fundamental and Clinical Text. Philadelphia, PA: Lippincott-Raven Press, 1996.
3. Samaan NA, Schultz PN, Haynie TP, Ordonez NG. Pulmonary metastasis of differentiated thyroid carcinoma: treatment results in 101 patients. J Clin Endocrinol Metab 1985; 60:376–380.
4. Besic N, Vidergar-Kralj B, Frkovic-Grazio S, et al. The role of radioactive iodine in the treatment of Hurthle cell carcinoma of the thyroid. Thyroid 2003; 13:577–584.
5. Simpson WJ, McKinney SE, Carruthers JS, et al. Papillary and follicular thyroid cancer. Prognostic factors in 1,578 patients. Am J Med 1987; 83:479–488.
6. Eichhorn W, Tabler H, Lippold R, et al. Prognostic factors determining long-term survival in well-differentiated thyroid cancer. An analysis of 484 patients undergoing therapy and aftercare at the same institution. Thyroid 2003; 13:949–958.
7. Simpson WJ, Panzarella T, Carruthers JS, et al. Papillary and follicular thyroid cancer; impact of treatment in 1578 patients. Int J Radiat Oncol Biol Phys 1988; 14:1063–1075.
8. Zidan J, Karen D, Stein M, et al. Pure versus follicular variant of papillary thyroid carcinoma. Cancer 2003; 97:1181–1185.
9. Jain M, Khan A, Patwardhan N, et al. Follicular variant of papillary thyroid carcinoma: A comparative study of histopathologic features and cytology results in 141 patients. Endocr Pract 2001; 7:79–84.
10. Kinder BK. Well differentiated thyroid cancer. Current Opin Oncol 2003; 15:71–77.
11. Haigh PI. Follicular thyroid carcinoma. Curr Treat Options Oncol 2002; 3:349–354.
12. National Comprehensive Cancer Network (NCCN) Thyroid Carcinoma Guidelines 2005, J Natl Comprehensive Cancer Network 2005; 3:404–457.
13. British Thyroid Association. Guidelines for the management of differentiated thyroid cancer in adults. Available at: www.british-thyroid-association.org/guidelines.htm. Accessed 2002.

60
Follow-up Strategy in Follicular Thyroid Cancer

Henry B. Burch

INTRODUCTION

As with papillary thyroid cancer, the effort applied to the search for recurrent follicular thyroid cancer is determined by the prognostic risk of tumor recurrence and death from disease. The presence or absence of certain poor prognostic indicators is used to tailor the frequency and intensity of surveillance for tumor recurrence. As discussed below (see also Chapter 40), many of the same determinants of prognosis in papillary thyroid cancer are applicable to patients with follicular thyroid cancer. Based largely on tumor histology and findings at the time of surgery, patients with follicular thyroid cancer may be divided into two nonoverlapping subtypes: minimally invasive (the majority) and widely invasive tumors (the minority; *1*). Patients with widely invasive follicular cancer have a higher incidence of cancer-related death than patients with papillary thyroid cancer *(1,2)*. Conversely, patients with minimally invasive follicular thyroid cancer are at a relatively low risk for recurrence and cancer-related death *(3–6)*. This chapter reviews the rationale used to determine appropriate follow-up for patients with follicular thyroid cancer and provides a current overview of the tools available to assist in this objective.

SURVEILLANCE LEVEL

The higher rate of cancer-related death associated with widely invasive follicular thyroid cancer mandates a higher index of suspicion for recurrent disease than with papillary thyroid cancer. The propensity for early hematogenous spread also directs attention to distant sites, such as the lungs, bones, brain, and liver, in cases of suspected persistent or recurrent disease. Numerous unusual patterns of hematogenous metastasis have been described in patients with follicular thyroid cancer, including the skin, iris, pericardium, kidney, and paranasal sinuses *(7–11)*.

At this author's medical center, the approach to patients with widely invasive follicular thyroid cancer is near-total thyroidectomy, followed by radioiodine ablation with 150 mCi of ^{131}I. Patients with one or more poor prognostic factor (see Chapter 40) undergo whole-body scanning (WBS) every 6 mo for 18 mo, then annually for 5 yr. Thereafter, if there is no evidence of residual disease, WBS and serum thyroglobulin (Tg) levels are obtained at 3–5 yr intervals. The methods chosen to follow patients with smaller, minimally invasive tumors are dependent on the extent of initial therapy. Patients with minimally invasive disease are treated initially with total thyroidectomy and radioiodine ablation. Following treatment, they undergo WBS and serum Tg measurements annually for 2 yr, then at 3–5-yr intervals for two cycles, and are thereafter followed using serum Tg levels alone on thyroid hormone suppressive therapy. Notably, within the minimally invasive follicular thyroid cancer category, cases with tumor capsule invasion alone, without vascular invasion, have a particularly indolent course with normal disease-specific survival *(5)*, and the above surveillance approach may therefore be too aggressive. The availability of recombinant human TSH (rhTSH) (see Chapter 11) has radically altered routine follow-up evaluations for residual or recurrent disease *(12,13)*. When basal Tg levels are undetectable on levothyroxine suppressive therapy, 18–26% of patients may still have occult tumor which may be uncovered by measurement of Tg after rhTSH stimulation *(14)*. Indeed, rhTSH-stimulated Tg is sufficiently sensitive that abandonment of diagnostic scanning has been advocated by some *(15,16)* but not all *(17)* centers.

The National Comprehensive Cancer Network (NCCN) practice guidelines *(18)* recommend that patients with follicular thyroid cancer who have no gross residual disease receive a WBS and have their Tg level measured at 4–6 wk postoperatively, which determines subsequent management. Patients with a negative WBS in the thyroid bed and an undetectable Tg (with negative antithyroglobulin antibodies) are not given ^{131}I remnant ablation. Alternatively, patients with positive thyroid bed uptake are treated with remnant ablation, whereas a larger, treatment dose of radioiodine is used in patients with metastatic disease on WBS or a serum Tg level greater than 10 ng/mL *(18)*. For follow-up of follicular thyroid cancer patients, NCCN guidelines advise a physical exam every 3–6 mo for the first 2 yr, a WBS annually until a negative scan is obtained, and serum Tg measurement at 6 and 12 mo, and then annually if disease-free.

Adverse events appear to occur earlier in patients with follicular thyroid cancer compared to those with papillary thyroid cancer *(1,4,19,20)*. An extensive literature review for follicular thyroid cancer found that most recurrences and cancer-related deaths occur in the first 5 yr after diagnosis. In fact, 50–80% of adverse events took place in the first 2 yr after diagnosis *(1)*. A study involving 49 patients with follicular and Hürthle cell thyroid cancer found that all recurrences and deaths occurred within 13 yr of diagnosis, whereas papillary thyroid cancer patients at the same institution continued to experience adverse events throughout 40 yr of observation *(20)*.

SERUM TG AND ANTITHYROGLOBULIN ANTIBODY MEASUREMENT

Patients with follicular carcinomas generally have higher levels of serum Tg than those with papillary carcinoma *(21)*. Antithyroglobulin antibodies, present in up to 25% of patients with differentiated thyroid cancer *(22)*, tend to decrease following thyroidectomy and complete remnant ablation, disappearing at a median of 3 yr in one study *(23)*. Persistent or increasing antithyroglobulin antibodies may serve as a serum marker for persistent thyroid cancer *(24–26)*.

A recent study of 51 patients with differentiated thyroid cancer and undetectable serum Tg but positive antithyroglobulin antibodies found a higher incidence of recurrent disease (49% vs 3.4%) than in a group of patients with negative Tg and antithyroglobulin antibodies *(24)*. Another study involved 32 patients with positive antithyroglobulin antibodies before therapy. Each of 5 patients with persistent or progressive disease had persistently positive Tg antibody levels, compared to only 6 of the 27 patients deemed free of disease *(27)*. A third study examining 43 thyroid cancer patients with positive antithyroglobulin antibodies found that 5 of 19 (26%) patients with persistent antithyroglobulin antibodies had residual disease, compared to 0 of 23 patients whose antithyroglobulin antibodies decreased after therapy *(27)*. Apparently, the presence of functioning thyroid tissue—metastatic or otherwise—is necessary to perpetuate Tg antibody synthesis.

REFERENCES

1. Grebe SK, Hay ID. Follicular thyroid cancer. Endocrinol Metab Clin North Am 1995; 24:761–801.
2. Chow SM, Law SC, Au SK, et al. Differentiated thyroid carcinoma: comparison between papillary and follicular carcinoma in a single institute. Head Neck 2002; 24:670–677.
3. Davis NL, Bugis SP, McGregor GI, Germann E. An evaluation of prognostic scoring systems in patients with follicular thyroid cancer. Am J Surg 1995; 170:476–480.
4. Jorda M, Gonzalez-Campora R, Mora J, et al. Prognostic factors in follicular carcinoma of the thyroid. Arch Pathol Lab Med 1993; 117:631–635.
5. van Heerden JA, Hay ID, Goellner JR, et al. Follicular thyroid carcinoma with capsular invasion alone: a nonthreatening malignancy. Surgery 1992; 112:1130–1136.
6. Thompson LD, Wieneke JA, Paal E, et al. A clinicopathologic study of minimally invasive follicular carcinoma of the thyroid gland with a review of the English literature. Cancer 2001; 91:505–524.
7. Koller EA, Tourtelot JB, Pak HS, et al. Papillary and follicular thyroid carcinoma metastatic to the skin: a case report and review of the literature. Thyroid 1998; 8:1045–1050.
8. Ainsworth JR, Damato BE, Lee WR, Alexander WD. Follicular thyroid carcinoma metastatic to the iris: a solitary lesion treated with iridocyclectomy. Arch Ophthalmol 1992; 110:19–20.
9. Chiewvit S, Pusuwan P, Chiewvit P, et al. Metastatic follicular carcinoma of thyroid to pericardium. J Med Assoc Thai 1998; 81:799–802.
10. Lam KY, Ng WK. Follicular carcinoma of the thyroid appearing as a solitary renal mass. Nephron 1996; 73:323–324.
11. Altman KW, Mirza N, Philippe L. Metastatic follicular thyroid carcinoma to the paranasal sinuses: a case report and review. J Laryngol Otol 1997; 111:647–651.
12. Ladenson PW. Strategies for thyrotropin use to monitor patients with treated thyroid carcinoma. Thyroid 1999; 9:429–433.
13. Robbins RJ, Robbins AK. Recombinant human thyrotropin and thyroid cancer management. J Clin Endocrinol Metab 2003; 88:1933–1938.
14. Mazzaferri EL, Robbins RJ, Spencer CA, et al. A consensus report of the role of serum thyroglobulin as a monitoring method for low-risk patients with papillary thyroid carcinoma. J Clin Endocrinol Metab 2003; 88:1433–1441.
15. Wartofsky L. Editorial: Using baseline and recombinant human TSH-stimulated Tg measurements to manage thyroid cancer without diagnostic 131-I scanning. J Clin Endocrinol Metab 2002; 87:1486–1489.
16. Mazzaferri EL, Kloos RT. Is diagnostic iodine-131 scanning with recombinant human TSH useful in the follow-up of differentiated thyroid cancer after thyroid ablation? J Clin Endocrinol Metab 2002; 87:1490–1498.
17. Robbins RJ, Chon JT, Fleisher M, Larson SM, Tuttle RM. Is the serum thyroglobulin response to recombinant human thyrotropin sufficient, by itself, to monitor for residual thyroid carcinoma? J Clin Endocrinol Metab 2002; 87:3242–3247.
18. National Comprehensive Cancer Network (NCCN) Thyroid Carcinoma Guidelines 2005, J Natl Comprehensive Cancer Network 2005; 3:404–457.
19. Zidan J, Kassem S, Kuten A. Follicular carcinoma of the thyroid gland: prognostic factors, treatment, and survival. Am J Clin Oncol 2000; 23:1–5.
20. DeGroot LJ, Kaplan EL, Shukla MS, et al. Morbidity and mortality in follicular thyroid cancer. J Clin Endocrinol Metab 1995; 80:2946–2953.
21. Torrens JI, Burch HB. Serum thyroglobulin measurement. Utility in clinical practice. Endocrinol Metab Clin North Am 2001; 30:429–467.
22. Spencer CA, Takeuchi M, Kazarosyan M, et al. Serum thyroglobulin autoantibodies: prevalence, influence on serum thyroglobulin measurement, and prognostic significance in patients with differentiated thyroid carcinoma. J Clin Endocrinol Metab 1998; 83:1121–1127.
23. Chiovato L, Latrofa F, Braverman LE, et al. Disappearance of humoral thyroid autoimmunity after complete removal of thyroid antigens. Ann Intern Med 2003; 139:346–351.
24. Chung JK, Park YJ, Kim TY, et al. Clinical significance of elevated level of serum antithyroglobulin antibody in patients with differentiated thyroid cancer after thyroid ablation. Clin Endocrinol 2002; 57:215–221.
25. Kumar A, Shah DH, Shrihari U, et al. Significance of antithyroglobulin autoantibodies in differentiated thyroid carcinoma. Thyroid 1994; 4:199–202.
26. Rubello D, Girelli ME, Casara D, et al. Usefulness of the combined antithyroglobulin antibodies and thyroglobulin assay in the follow-up of patients with differentiated thyroid cancer. J Endocrinol Invest 1990; 13:737–742.
27. Rubello D, Casara D, Girelli ME, et al. Clinical meaning of circulating antithyroglobulin antibodies in differentiated thyroid cancer: a prospective study. J Nucl Med 1992; 33:1478–1480.

61
PET in Follicular Cancer, Including Hürthle Cell Cancer

I. Ross McDougall

INTRODUCTION

All the basic information regarding the role of positron emission tomography (PET) using 18-fluorodeoxyglucose (FDG) was reviewed in depth in the section on papillary cancer (see Chapter 34). The fundamental principles are identical. The main role is to find the source of thyroglobulin (Tg) production in a patient who is negative on a ^{131}I scan (i.e., whose cancer does not trap iodine) (see Chapter 39).

For the PET scan, 10–15 mCi (370–550 MBq) of FDG is injected intravenously in a patient who has fasted for 6 h. The patient should sit quietly in a dark, comfortable room without talking, eating, or chewing. Imaging is started 1 h later and includes the head, from the inferior margin of the brain, to the upper or mid-thigh. It is advisable for the patient not to exercise vigorously for 24 h before the investigation.

Most references cited in the earlier chapter included patients with both papillary and follicular cancers, and in most cases, it is not possible to separate the cancer types and analyze the results. Such was the case with Dietlin et al., who presented results in 58 patients: 38 had papillary cancer, 15 had follicular cancer, and 5 had variants of follicular cancer *(1)*. In another paper, there were 11 follicular and 3 Hürthle cell cancers of the total 51 patients *(2)*. Some reports simply state that patients had papillary or follicular cancer *(3)*. Other studies even include patients with anaplastic cancer, as well as differentiated cancer *(4)*.

The multicenter report by Grunwalt et al. allows the results of PET in different tumor types to be calculated *(5)*. There were 80 patients with follicular cancer, and 52 of these had a negative scan with radioiodine. PET had a sensitivity of 78%, a specificity of 100%, and a positive predictive value of 100%. In 28 patients with a well-differentiated cancer that was capable of trapping iodine, the PET scan was negative in 8 (29%).

Hürthle cell cancer is more aggressive than standard follicular cancer, but it is known as a variant of follicular cancer (see Chapter 58). The 5- and 20-yr survival rates for follicular cancer are 87% and 81% and fall to 81% and 65% for Hürthle cell cancer. The management of Hürthle cell cancer that has metastasized is difficult. The lesions seldom trap iodine and therefore represent a classic example of iodine-negative Tg-positive lesions. Treatment with high-dose ^{131}I is usually ineffective.

The results of PET are encouraging. Case reports indicated that FDG uptake was real *(6,7)*. In one series, 17 patients with Hürthle cell cancer were evaluated by PET *(8)*. There were 13 who had an elevated Tg level and PET was positive in all cases. Additional testing confirmed metastases in 10 of the 13. In two patients, there was no confirmation, and the last patient was considered to have a false-positive scan. There was suspicion of cancer but a low Tg in four patients. The PET scan was truly negative in three and falsely positive in the final patient. In the multicenter study presented above *(5)*, there were 20 patients with Hürthle cell cancer. The sensitivity of PET was 87%, and the specificity and positive predictive values were both 100% *(5)*. Lowe et al. used PET in 12 patients with Hürthle cell cancer, and a total of 14 scans were obtained *(9)*. PET identified sites of disease that were not detected by any other test in seven of the scans. In another seven, the extent of local and distant metastases was greater on PET scan. The results of the scan altered management in seven patients. As has been demonstrated for recurrences of papillary thyroid carcinoma of the thyroid *(10,11)*, dedicated combination PET with computed tomography may have application to the localization or confirmation of metastases of follicular thyroid cancer.

In summary, the role of PET in typical follicular cancer that does not trap iodine is the same as for papillary cancer. PET is an extremely valuable test for patients with metastatic Hürthle cell cancer.

REFERENCES

1. Dietlein M, Scheidhauer K, Voth E, et al. Fluorine-18 fluorodeoxyglucose positron emission tomography and iodine-131 whole-body scintigraphy in the follow-up of differentiated thyroid cancer. Eur J Nucl Med 1997; 24:1342–1348.

2. Giammarile F, Hafdi Z, Bournaud C, et al. Is [18F]-2-fluoro-2-deoxy-d-glucose (FDG) scintigraphy with non-dedicated positron emission tomography useful in the diagnostic management of suspected metastatic thyroid carcinoma in patients with no detectable radioiodine uptake? Eur J Endocrinol 2003; 149:293–300.
3. Conti PS, Durski JM, Bacqai F, et al. Imaging of locally recurrent and metastatic thyroid cancer with positron emission tomography. Thyroid 1999; 9:797–804.
4. Fridrich L, Messa C, Landoni C, et al. Whole-body scintigraphy with 99Tcm-MIBI, 18F-FDG and 131I in patients with metastatic thyroid carcinoma. Nucl Med Commun 1997; 18:3–9.
5. Grunwald F, Kalicke T, Feine U, et al. Fluorine-18 fluorodeoxyglucose positron emission tomography in thyroid cancer: results of a multicentre study. Eur J Nucl Med 1999; 26:1547–1552.
6. Blount CL, Dworkin HJ. F-18 FDG uptake by recurrent Hurthle cell carcinoma of the thyroid using high-energy planar scintigraphy. Clin Nucl Med 1996; 21:831–833.
7. Wiesner W, Engel H, von Schulthess GK, et al. FDG PET-negative liver metastases of a malignant melanoma and FDG PET-positive hurthle cell tumor of the thyroid. Eur Radiol 1999; 9:975–978.
8. Plotkin M, Hautzel H, Krause BJ, et al. Implication of 2-18fluor-2-deoxyglucose positron emission tomography in the follow-up of Hurthle cell thyroid cancer. Thyroid 2002; 12:155–161.
9. Lowe VJ, Mullan BP, Hay ID, et al. 18F-FDG PET of patients with Hurthle cell carcinoma. J Nucl Med 2003; 44:1402–1406.
10. Zimmer LA, McCook B, Meltzer C, et al. Combined positron emission tomography/computed tomography imaging of recurrent thyroid cancer. Otolaryngol Head Neck Surg 2003; 128:178–184.
11. Nahas Z, Goldenberg D, Fakhry C, et al. The role of positron emission tomography/computed tomography in the management of recurrent papillary thyroid carcinoma. Laryngoscope 2005; 155:237–243.

62
Follicular Thyroid Cancer
Special Aspects in Children and Adolescents*

Andrew J. Bauer

INTRODUCTION

Follicular thyroid cancer (FTC) in children is a disease that has received little specific scrutiny regarding surgical or medical management. More often, it has been grouped with papillary thyroid cancer (PTC) in articles addressing pediatric differentiated thyroid cancer and has been treated with the same regimens as for pediatric PTC.

A cumulative review of 22 studies covering a period from 1902 to 2002 reported on 1974 cases of differentiated, nonmedullary thyroid cancer in patients younger than 21 yr old. A 20% incidence (382 of 1974) of FTC was found in that age group *(1–11)*. The incidence over such a broad time period would likely be skewed by differences in the incidence of iodine deficiency, change in the histologic criteria for diagnosing FTC, and the increased exposure to ionizing radiation, both medically and environmentally.

However, evaluation of the five most recent reports, from 1972–2002, shows that the incidence has remained relatively stable at 19% (141 of 743) *(5–8,11)*. Although we can attempt to draw conclusions on the clinical nature of FTC in children, we caution that these observations are drawn from a small number of total cases and from medical centers in geographically diverse areas of the world. Furthermore, conclusions on the appropriate medical and surgical treatment are even more limited, as no single study to date has evaluated the long-term outcome of a large number of pediatric FTC in regard to treatment options.

In adults, FTC is generally considered more aggressive than PTC, usually presenting with a higher stage of disease. In the adult population, FTC is reported to have a 20-yr mortality as high as 92% when it presents with two or more negative prognostic factors. These include age more than 45 yr, tumor size greater than 4 cm, local invasion, or distant metastasis *(12,13)*. Lymph node metastasis is uncommon in adults, but pulmonary or bone metastasis occurs in up to 30% of adults, compared to 15% for PTC *(14)*.

In contrast, predicting the clinical behavior and prognosis in children and adolescents is more challenging. Most current pediatric thyroid cancer studies have not reported significant differences in clinical behavior between PTC and FTC and, as previously stated, both have been treated under the same regimens *(2–4,7,8)*. In the few studies that have performed uni- or multivariate regression analysis between pediatric PTC and FTC, no differences in disease-free survival have been found *(2,5,7)*. However, two studies have shown a lower time to recurrence *(15)* and a lower relapse rate (PTC vs FTC, 24.5% vs 9%; *9*). In the latter study, whereas the percentage of patients undergoing total thyroidectomy was similar between FTC and PTC (82% for both), FTC patients were more frequently treated with ^{131}I (82% vs 55%), which may have significantly affected recurrence rates.

In four studies comparing the clinical behavior of pediatric FTC to PTC, FTC was shown to be more common in the adolescent age group than in children younger than 10 yr old *(6,7)* and to have less frequent regional lymph node and distant metastasis compared to PTC *(6,7,10,11)*. This observation, however, is only based on 77 cases of FTC vs 326 cases of PTC *(6,9–11)*. An interesting observation in one study *(11)* is that FTC in adolescents may not show the increased female predominance that is present with PTC, raising the question whether the pathogenesis underlying the development of FTC may be less estrogen-sensitive. The authors also note a 50% incidence of iodine-deficient goiter in the population (Germany), but they do not comment on why the adolescent population appears to show a decreased incidence of FTC, a disease known to be more common in iodine-deficient states *(11)*.

The current evaluation and treatment of FTC in children is usually identical to pediatric PTC (see Chapter 41), but

---

*The opinions and assertions contained here are the private views of the author and are not to be construed as official or as reflecting the opinions of the Uniformed Services University of the Health Sciences, the Department of the Army, or the Department of Defense.

From: *Thyroid Cancer: A Comprehensive Guide to Clinical Management, 2/e*
Edited by: L. Wartofsky and D. Van Nostrand © Humana Press Inc., Totowa, NJ

some clinicians may opt for a less aggressive approach. Similar to pediatric PTC, the child often presents with an asymptomatic solitary nodule and undergoes radiologic evaluation (ultrasound), followed by fine-needle biopsy (FNB). It is important to realize that while the incidence of PTC is increased in children with a history of radiation exposure, FTC may also develop in these patients, but with a slightly lower incidence when compared to spontaneous tumors (10–17% vs 18–20%; *11*).

When the FNB is suspicious for a follicular neoplasm, the initial operation may be a total thyroidectomy followed by ^{131}I ablation. Some centers continue to perform a lobectomy and await a final pathology report for consideration of completion thyroidectomy. In this circumstance, it is unlikely that examination of tissue at frozen section will yield useful data, as the diagnosis of FTC relies on tissue analysis for extracapsular invasion. Thus, any discussion regarding further surgery should await the final pathology report.

The need for completion thyroidectomy in the case of a small lesion reported as FTC is also controversial. Because the long-term prognosis is excellent in lesions smaller than 4 cm, and no studies show that the extent of surgery or the use of ^{131}I in these cases improves prognosis, some experts would simply follow such patients after a lobectomy, without adjunctive therapy. Most, however, would at least treat the condition with thyroxine at a dose sufficient to keep the serum thyrotropin at the lower extreme of the normal range. In the end analysis, the risk of a second surgery must be weighed against the benefit of less aggressive surgery (lobectomy). This consideration is necessary, as 10–15% of FTC may be multifocal *(10)*, and suppressive thyroid hormone therapy is needed whether a lobectomy or total thyroidectomy has been performed. Should subsequent radioiodine therapy be indicated, some workers are beginning to employ recombinant human TSH to facilitate radioiodine therapy in lieu of withdrawal of thyroxine therapy *(16)*.

There are many unanswered questions in regard to the best approach to medical and surgical management of pediatric FTC and this disease should be thought of with cautious respect. Understanding the limitations of our knowledge of the clinical behavior of FTC must be balanced with the risks of aggressive surgery, which may differ among medical centers. However, although there may be a lower incidence of local and distant metastasis for pediatric FTC compared to PTC, the recurrence risk for these two forms of pediatric thyroid cancer may be the same: a 15% risk over 5 yr *(10)*.

In addition, knowledge of the long-term response to ^{131}I therapy in pediatric FTC is also quite limited. With increasing experience, we may learn that pediatric FTC may not be as responsive to long-term ^{131}I therapy as FTC in adults. With the absence of definitive data concerning, the long-term outcome of pediatric FTC in response to specific treatment regimens, it may be advisable to manage these patients conservatively.

REFERENCES

1. De Keyser L, Van Herle AJ. Differentiated thyroid cancer in children. Head Neck Surg 1985; 8:100–114.
2. Lee YM, Lo CY, Lam KY, et al. Well-differentiated thyroid carcinoma in Hong Kong Chinese patients under 21 years of age: A 35-year experience. J Am Coll Surg 2002; 194:711–716.
3. Landau D, Vini L, A'Hern R, Harmer C. Thyroid cancer in children: the Royal Marsden Hospital experience. Eur J Cancer 2000; 36:214–220.
4. Kowalski LP, Filho JG, Pinto CA, et al. Long-term survival rates in young patients with thyroid carcinoma. Arch Otolaryngol Head Neck Surg 2003; 129:746–749.
5. Jarzab B, Junak D, Wloch J, et al. Multivariate analysis of prognostic factors for differentiated thyroid carcinoma in children. Eur J Nucl Med 2000; 27:833–841.
6. Giuffrida D, Scollo C, Pellegriti G, et al. Differentiated thyroid cancer in children and adolescents. J Endocrinol Invest 2002; 25:18–24.
7. Kumar A, Bal CS. Differentiated thyroid cancer. Indian J Pediatr 2003; 70:707–713.
8. Haveman JW, Van Tol KM, Rouwe CW, et al. Surgical experience in children with differentiated thyroid carcinoma. Ann Surg Oncol 2003; 10:15–20.
9. Chow SM, Law S, Mendenhall WM, et al. Differentiated thyroid carcinoma in childhood and adolescence—clinical course and role of radioiodine. Pediatr Blood Cancer 2004; 42:176–183.
10. Welch-Dinauer C, Tuttle RM, Robie D, et al. Clinical features associated with metastasis and recurrence of differentiated thyroid cancer in children, adolescents, and young adults. Clin Endocrinol (Oxf) 1997; 49:619–628.
11. Farahati J, Bucsky P, Parlowsky T, et al. Characteristics of differentiated thyroid carcinoma in children and adolescents with respect to age, gender, and histology. Cancer 1997; 80:2156–2162.
12. DeGroot LJ, Kaplan EL, Shukula MS, et al. Morbidity and mortality in follicular thyroid cancer. J Clin Endocrinol Metab 1995; 80:2946–2953.
13. Brennan MD, Bergstralh EJ, van Heerden JA, McConahey WM. Follicular thyroid cancer treated at the Mayo Clinic, 1946 through 1970: Initial manifestations, pathologic findings, therapy, and outcome. Mayo Clin Proc 1991; 68:1944–1953.
14. D'Avanzo A, Treseler P, Ituarte PHG, et al. Follicular thyroid carcinoma: Histology and prognosis. Cancer 2004; 100:1123–1129.
15. La Quaglia MP, Corbally MT, Heller G, et al. Recurrence and morbidity in differentiated thyroid carcinoma in children. Surgery; 104:1149–1156.
16. Ralli M, Cohan P, Lee K. Successful use of recombinant human thyrotropin in the therapy of pediatric well-differentiated thyroid cancer. J Endocrinol Invest 2005; 28:270–273.

63
External Radiation Therapy of Follicular Carcinoma

James D. Brierley and Richard W. Tsang

INTRODUCTION

The role of external-beam radiotherapy (RT) in the management of follicular thyroid cancer can be subdivided regarding its purpose into adjuvant, radical, and palliative. The intent of adjuvant therapy is to improve the results of standard therapy, consisting of surgery and radioactive iodine; however, its exact role is controversial. Unlike radioactive iodine, external-beam RT is a local therapy. Therefore, its role is confined to cases where local therapy is required to maximize local regional control of the disease beyond what can be achieved with optimal surgery and radioactive iodine. Consequently, the role of RT is generally limited to patients deemed to have unresectable or residual disease after surgery or patients at high risk of locoregional recurrence. This risk includes older patients with extensive extrathyroidal extension of disease, residual disease following surgery, or extensive lymphatic spread.

RADICAL EXTERNAL-BEAM RT FOR GROSS DISEASE

Sheline et al. described their experience of RT in 58 patients treated between 1935 and 1964, examining its use for a variety of thyroid histologies and clinical situations (1). Despite limitations of the radiation equipment during this time period, the study indicated the effectiveness of RT in controlling gross residual disease. Nine patients had follicular tumors, four with gross disease, and one died from progressive tumor growth 3 yr later. However, three were free of disease 2–16 yr after radiation. Five other patients had infiltration of the trachea but no gross disease, two died of local disease, and three had no evidence of disease 5–18 yr after treatment. Although these data are relatively old, the results suggest that external-beam RT can control gross follicular thyroid cancer and may benefit patients with microscopic residual disease. Other studies have reported a complete clinical response rate for gross disease (2,3) that ranges from 40% to 60% after 5 yr (4,5). Yet these studies did not separate the treatment results of follicular and papillary tumors.

EXTERNAL-BEAM RT AS ADJUVANT THERAPY

As discussed in the section on papillary thyroid cancer, external-beam RT is a local therapy and would only be expected to be effective when there is a high risk of local recurrence. This is usually meant as residual disease after surgical resection in patients with extrathyroidal extension.

Mazzaferri and Jhiang studied 278 patients with follicular thyroid cancer among 1355 patients with differentiated thyroid cancer, 12% of whom had extrathyroidal extension, compared with 8% in patients with papillary thyroid cancer (6). The local recurrence rate was 38% in patients with extrathyroidal extension vs 25% in patients without extrathyroidal extension ($p = 0.001$). This difference was observed in papillary thyroid cancer, not follicular, but both histological types were associated with a higher risk of death from cancer in patients with extrathyroidal extension ($p = 0.001$).

Given the higher risk of extrathyroidal extension in follicular thyroid cancer compared to papillary, it might be considered easier to demonstrate a benefit from external-beam RT in patients with follicular thyroid cancer. However, as discussed below, the evidence for efficacy in follicular thyroid cancer is less strong than in papillary thyroid cancer. This variation might relate to insufficient data because of the smaller number of patients. In addition, the natural history of high-risk follicular thyroid cancer indicates there is a greater risk of distant metastases, resulting in tumor death. Therefore, it may be more difficult to show improved local control, and local issues may be less important to the patient if the predominant problem is the distant spread of disease-causing death.

In the *trans*-Canada study, Simpson et al. suggested that patients with microscopic residual follicular cancer following resection may improve with external-beam RT (7). The local control rates in patients treated by surgery and radioactive iodine were similar to those treated with the addition of external-beam radiation. This was the case despite the observation that patients given additional external-beam radiation tended to have more extensive disease. In the two studies that

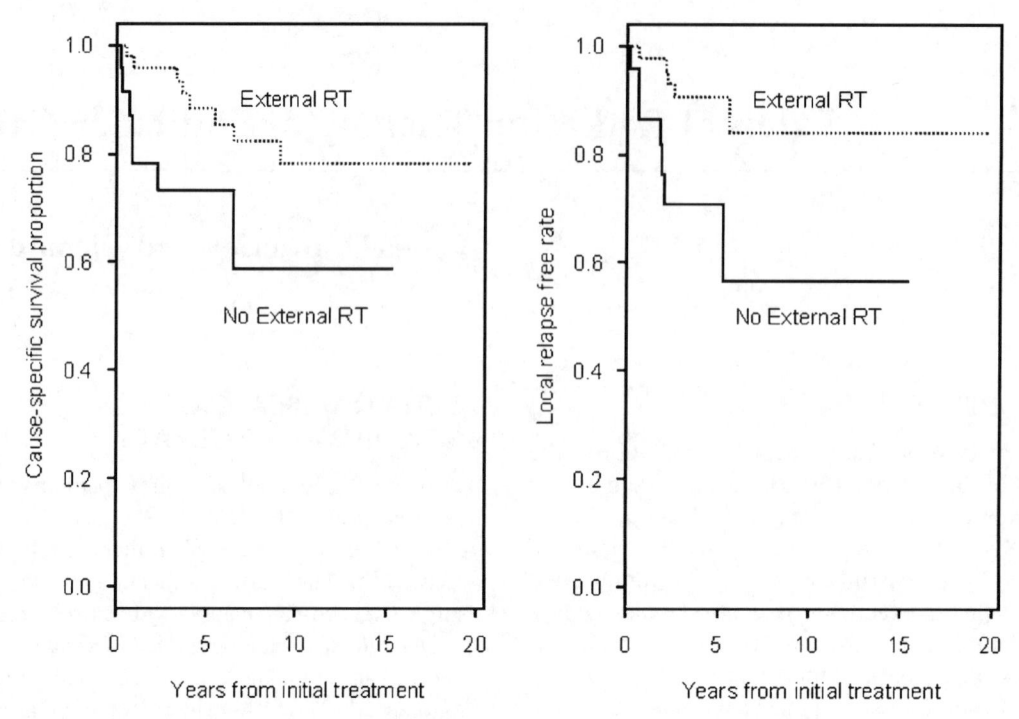

Fig. 1. Effect of the use of external-beam RT on cause-specific survival and LRFR in patients over age 60 who have differentiated thyroid cancer (papillary and follicular combined) with extrathyroidal extension and no evidence of gross residual disease *(10).*

Table 1
Results of Adjuvant External RT in High-Risk Follicular Thyroid Cancer From Retrospective Studies

Author (Reference)	10-yr Local Recurrence	
	Surgery With and Without ^{131}I	Surgery and RT, With and Without ^{131}I
Simpson *(7)*	53%	47%
Esik *(9)*	42%[a]	2%[a]
Ford *(25)*[b]	63%[a]	18%[a]
Phlips *(26)*	21%	3%
Brierley *(10)*[b]	34.3%	13.6%
Tubiana *(5)*[b]	21%	14%

[a]Compares low vs higher dose.
[b]Papillary and follicular histologies combined.

demonstrated a benefit of adjuvant external-beam radiation in papillary thyroid cancer, neither showed efficacy in follicular thyroid cancer *(4,8).*

Contrasting results were seen by Esik et al., who reported on a series of 56 patients with follicular cancer, of whom 43 patients had no gross residual disease *(9).* Patients treated with radiation had a significantly better local relapse-free rate (LRFR) when the dose was considered adequate, compared to those given an inadequate dose, but none of the patients received radioactive iodine *(9).*

Other reports that suggest a role for adjuvant external-beam radiation do not separate differentiated cancers into papillary or follicular *(5,10,11).* A recent analysis of patients with papillary or follicular carcinoma identified a high-risk subgroup who were older (≥60 yr) with extrathyroidal extension and no gross residual disease *(10).* Among the 70 patients with these features, 47 received RT and 23 did not. There was a higher cause-specific survival (81% and 64.6%, $p = 0.04$) and LRFR (86.4% and 65.7%, $p = 0.01$) in patients who received RT (Fig. 1, Table 1).

Despite the differing conclusions and lack of definitive data specific to follicular thyroid cancer, we believe that in patients at high risk of recurrence in the thyroid bed (older patients with gross extrathyroidal extension and gross or microscopic residual disease without metastatic disease), it is logical to assume that they may benefit from intensifying local regional therapy with the addition of external-beam radiation, combined with radioactive iodine. The thyroid bed alone is irradiated in patients at high risk of recurrence. The cervical lymph nodes are included in patients who have extensive nodal involvement with extranodal extension and soft-tissue invasion. RT to the cervical lymph nodes is also considered in patients with nodal disease that does not take up radioactive iodine, such as some Hürthle cell tumors, as discussed below.

HÜRTHLE CELL CARCINOMA

In a recent analysis of 18 patients with Hürthle cell carcinoma, who were treated at a single institution over a 50-yr period, external-beam radiation was suggested to impact a variety of situations. In nine patients in whom the RT served either as adjuvant or salvage following recurrence, there was a 50% local regional control rate at 5 yr. However, all 10 patients who died succumbed from metastatic disease. All patients who received palliative radiation experienced relief of pain or similar symptoms for a median of 12 mo. It was concluded that Hürthle cell carcinoma is a radiosensitive tumor, and patients with large invasive tumors may benefit from adjuvant external-beam radiation (12). This is particularly true when other adverse features are present, e.g., nodal metastases and vascular or extrathyroidal extension.

EXTERNAL-BEAM RT

The thyroid bed is a technically challenging volume to treat, as the thyroid bed curves around the vertebral body and includes the air column in the trachea. Sparing the spinal cord to a dose within tolerance while adequately treating the thyroid bed can be especially difficult. Various techniques have been described that produce adequate dose distribution (13). Advances in radiation methods that result in better dose distribution to the areas at risk and reduce the volume of normal tissues to a minimum are described in Chapter 84.

Well-planned external-beam RT has acceptable acute toxicity and rarely leads to serious complications. In patients assigned to the radiation arm of the German randomized control study (14; which closed because of poor accrual), it was noted that most patients experience mild-to-moderate side effects from adjuvant external-beam RT. At the first follow-up examination, most side effects had subsided and the early or acute toxicity was tolerable in these patients. Late toxicity was an infrequent problem; the most common issues were skin telangiectasia, increased skin pigmentation, soft-tissue fibrosis, and mild lymphedema, predominantly in the submental area. Esophageal and tracheal stenosis were extremely rare. Neither Tsang et al. (4) nor Farahati et al. (8) reported any Radiation Therapy Oncology Group grade IV late toxicity. If the external-beam radiation does not result in local control, and the patient relapses in the thyroid bed area, salvage surgery may still be possible with an experienced surgeon in postradiation surgery in the head and neck region.

PALLIATION

The effectiveness of ^{131}I for metastatic disease depends greatly on the site of metastasis. As a generalization, it is well known that lung metastases respond well to radioactive iodine. Although it has been noted that the outcome of patients with metastases from follicular histology is worse than for papillary thyroid histology, most studies on the management of metastases do not analyze the clinical outcome by histology.

In a series of patients with distant metastases, Casara et al. reported that those age 40 or older or those with bone metastases were much less likely to concentrate radioactive iodine and achieve a complete response (15). Only 3% of bone metastases were considered to have achieved a complete response following radioactive iodine. Similar poor control of bone metastases has been reported by others (16–18), and an aggressive surgical approach has been therefore recommended (18,19; see Chapter 53). Not all secondary bone tumors, however, are amenable to surgical resection. Thus, external-beam radiation, in addition to radioactive iodine, is appropriate and may result in long-term control (20). External-beam radiation also has an important role in palliating symptomatic bone pain or spinal cord compression.

Brain metastases from thyroid cancer are unusual. In a study of metastases in the brain from all histological tumor types (32 were differentiated), there was no benefit from external-beam radiation (21). In another series, external-beam RT resulted in complete response in three of four patients with measurable disease (22). External-beam RT should probably be offered if surgical resection is not possible; however, it is uncertain whether there is any clear benefit following complete excision of brain metastases. Single large, lung metastases-causing hemoptysis or obstruction may also respond to RT.

The role of RT in controlling gross residual disease after surgery and in unresectable disease has already been discussed. High-dose RT may not be considered appropriate for long-term control in patients with symptomatic recurrent disease, poor performance, or widespread incurable disease. Instead, a shorter course of RT may be effective in controlling such local symptoms as pain, skin ulceration, and obstruction.

REFERENCES

1. Sheline GE, Galante M, Lindsay S. Radiation therapy in the control of persistent thyroid cancer. Am J Roentgenol Radium Ther Nucl Med 1966; 97:923–930.
2. Glanzmann C, Lutolf UM. Long-term follow-up of 92 patients with locally advanced follicular or papillary thyroid cancer after combined treatment. Strahlenther Onkol 1992; 168:260–269.

3. O'Connell M, A'Hern RP, Harmer CL. Results of external beam radiotherapy in differentiated thyroid carcinoma: a retrospective study from the Royal Marsden Hospital. Eur J Cancer 1994; 30A:733–739.
4. Tsang RW, Brierley JD, Simpson WJ, Panzarella T, et al. The effects of surgery, radioiodine and external radiation therapy on the clinical outcome of patients with differentiated thyroid cancer. Cancer 1998; 82:375–388.
5. Tubiana M, Haddad E, Schlumberger M, et al. External radiotherapy in thyroid cancers. Cancer 1985; 55(9 Suppl):2062–2071.
6. Mazzaferri EL, Jhiang SM. Long-term impact of initial surgical and medical therapy on papillary and follicular thyroid cancer. Am J Med 1994; 97:418–428.
7. Simpson WJ, Panzarella T, Carruthers JS, et al. Papillary and follicular thyroid cancer: impact of treatment in 1578 patients. Int J Radiat Oncol Biol Phys 1988; 14:1063–1075.
8. Farahati J, Reiners C, Stuschke M, et al. Differentiated thyroid cancer. Impact of adjuvant external radiotherapy in patients with perithyroidal tumor infiltration (stage pT4). Cancer 1996; 77:172–180.
9. Esik O, Nemeth G, Eller J. Prophylactic external irradiation in differentiated thyroid cancer: a retrospective study over a 30-year observation period. Oncology 1994; 51:372–379.
10. Brierley JD, Tsang RW, Panzarella T. Analysis of prognostic factors and effect of treatment from a single institution on patients treated over forty years. Thyroid 2003; 13.
11. Sautter-Bihl ML, Raub J, Hetzel-Sesterheim M, Heinze HG. Differentiated thyroid cancer: prognostic factors and influence of treatment on the outcome in 441 patients. Strahlenther Onkol 2001; 177:125–131.
12. Foote RL, Brown PD, Garces YI, et al. Is there a role for radiation therapy in the management of Hurthle cell carcinoma? Int J Radiat Oncol Biol Phys 2003; 56:1067–1072.
13. Tsang RW, Brierley JD. The thyroid. In Cox JD, Kian Ang K, editors. Radiation Oncology. St Louis, MO: Mosby; 2003.
14. Schuck A, Biermann M, Pixberg MK, et al. Acute toxicity of adjuvant radiotherapy in locally advanced differentiated thyroid carcinoma. First results of the multicenter study differentiated thyroid carcinoma (MSDS). Strahlenther Onkol 2003; 179:832–839.
15. Casara D, Rubello D, Saladini G, et al. Distant metastases in diffentiated thyroid cancer: longterm results of radioiodine treatment. Tumori 1991; 77:432–436.
16. Brown AP, Greening WP, McCready VR, et al. Radioiodine treatment of metastatic thyroid carcinoma: the Royal Marsden Hospital experience. Br J Radiol 1984; 57:323–327.
17. Schlumberger M, Challeton C, De Vathaire F, et al. Radioactive iodine treatment and external radiotherapy for lung and bone metastases from thyroid carcinoma. J Nucl Med 1996; 37:598–605.
18. Proye CA, Dromer DH, Carnaille BM, et al. Is it still worthwhile to treat bone metastases from differentiated thyroid carcinoma with radioactive iodine? World J Surg 1992; 16:640–645; discussion 645–646.
19. Niederle B, Roka R, Schemper M, et al. Surgical treatment of distant metastases in differentiated thyroid cancer: indication and results. Surgery 1986; 100:1088–1097.
20. Brierley JD, Tsang RW. External-beam radiation therapy in the treatment of differentiated thyroid cancer. Seminars in Surgical Oncology 1999; 16:42–49.
21. Chiu AC, Delpassand ES, Sherman SI. Prognosis and treatment of brain metastases in thyroid carcinoma. J Clin Endocrinol Metab 1997; 82:3637–3642.
22. McWilliams RR, Giannini C, Hay ID, et al. Management of brain metastases from thyroid carcinoma: a study of 16 pathologically confirmed cases over 25 years. Cancer 2003; 98:356–362.
23. Ford D, Giridharan S, McConkey C, et al. External beam radiotherapy in the management of differentiated thyroid cancer. Clin Oncol (R Coll Radiol) 2003; 15:337–341.
24. Phlips P, Hanzen C, Andry G, et al. Postoperative irradiation for thyroid cancer. Eur J Surg Oncol 1993; 19:399–404.

64
Determinants of Prognosis in Patients With Follicular Thyroid Cancer

Henry B. Burch

INTRODUCTION

A large number of retrospective analyses have examined patient and tumor characteristics associated with a poor prognosis in patients with follicular thyroid cancer (1), and several recent reports have reinforced and extended these findings (2–6). Compared to patients with papillary thyroid cancer, follicular thyroid cancer patients are more likely to be older, male (although the male-to-female ratio remains <1), have unifocal disease, as well as distant metastases, and less likely to have direct tumor extension or cervical lymph nodes (7). Factors consistently found to negatively impact prognosis in follicular thyroid cancer include age older than 45, tumor size larger than 4 cm, local tumor extension beyond the thyroid, extensive capsular and vascular invasion, and the presence of distant metastases (Table 1). Tumor size and the presence of distant metastases were more important prognostic indicators than age in one recent series of patients (7a). In addition, certain variants of follicular thyroid cancer, including oxyphilic (Hürthle cell) carcinomas and insular carcinomas, are linked with a generally worse prognosis (8) (see Chapters 58 and 66).

EFFECT OF PROGNOSIS FACTORS ON SURVIVAL

The impact of clinical factors on survival is illustrated in a series of 100 patients with pure follicular thyroid cancer, who received treatment at the Mayo Clinic over a 35-yr period (9). The overall cancer-related mortality was 29% after 20 yr. However, patients with only one negative prognostic indicator had a 20-yr mortality of only 14%, whereas those patients with two or more predictors had a 92% risk of death from thyroid cancer at 20 yr. More recently, a study including 198 cases with follicular and oxyphilic (Hürthle cell) thyroid cancer found that patients ages younger than 40 yr, with tumors smaller than 5 cm and no local extension or distant metastases, had a 100% 15-yr survival. In contrast, older patients, those with larger tumors, or those with disease outside the thyroid had a 40% survival rate (3). A study of 215 patients with pure follicular thyroid cancer found that factors negatively influencing disease-specific survival included the presence of known postoperative residual macroscopic disease, extrathyroidal extension, distant metastases, or failure to treat with postoperative radioiodine therapy (6). A study from the University of San Francisco found that patients with tumor-specific deaths were 66 ± 9.3 yr old at the time of initial diagnosis, compared to 59 ± 10 yr for those with recurrence, and 42 ± 17 yr for those remaining disease-free (2). Similarly, these authors found that disease-free patients had initial tumor sizes of 3.0 ± 2.0 cm, compared to 4.8 ± 4.0 cm in those dying from their disease.

MINIMALLY INVASIVE FOLLICULAR THYROID CANCER

An important prognostic consideration in patients with follicular thyroid cancer is the degree of capsular and vascular invasion (see Chapter 57). Patients with minimally invasive follicular thyroid cancer have been often shown to have lower cause-specific mortality rates than those with widely invasive tumors (10–12). In fact, patients with minimal capsular invasion alone have a survival rate that approximates the rate of the general population (13). This finding has led some authorities to recommend avoidance of a "cancer" diagnosis in these patients owing to socioeconomic concerns, e.g., employability and insurability (14). A recent study compared clinical outcomes in 95 patients with minimally invasive follicular thyroid cancer to 35 patients initially thought to have minimally invasive disease but who were later reclassified because of evidence of invasion through the nodule capsule or into larger vessels (those with smooth muscle walls). These authors found an 82.1% disease-free survival at 18 yr in patients with minimally invasive disease vs 68.5% in those reclassified with more than minimally invasive disease (12).

Table 1
Poor Prognostic Factors for Differentiated Thyroid Cancer

Large tumors (>4.0 cm)
Male gender
Advanced tumor grade
Tumors with local extension
Distant metastases
Extensive vascular and capsular invasion

EFFECT OF THERAPY ON PROGNOSIS

As is the case with papillary thyroid cancer, retrospective assessment of the effect of therapy on prognosis is hampered by the fact that patients selected to receive more extensive treatment are likely to have more advanced disease. Therefore, a finding that shows no difference in survival between patients receiving or not receiving therapy (e.g., radioiodine ablation) might actually indicate a beneficial effect, as these patients would have been expected to have a shorter survival than those with less advanced disease.

Analyzing the effect of surgery on survival, one study found that among 214 patients operated on for follicular thyroid cancer, those treated with total thyroidectomy had survival rates similar to patients receiving less extensive procedures (15). Another study, after adjusting for other risk factors in a multivariate analysis, found no difference in survival between 19 patients undergoing lobectomy and 81 patients treated with a bilateral surgical procedure (9). Finally, a recent analysis of 215 patients with follicular thyroid cancer treated at a single institution found no difference in local-regional control or survival in patients undergoing subtotal thyroidectomy compared to those treated with total or near-total thyroidectomy (6).

Conversely, most studies have shown that patients with incomplete tumor removal have worse survival than those with no known residual macroscopic or microscopic disease after surgery (1). The use of radioiodine for remnant ablation after thyroidectomy has been found to have variable effects on survival, with a definite beneficial effect found in some studies (6,15,16), a marginal effect in one study (17), and no effect in yet another study (18). Despite this controversy, effective follow-up of patients with follicular thyroid cancer is greatly facilitated by the use of both near-total thyroidectomy and radioiodine ablation therapy (1,19). Detection of recurrent disease or metastases has been facilitated by the availability of recombinant human TSH (rhTSH) (see Chapter 11) employed for scanning or more simply, the measurement of serum thyroglobulin before and after rhTSH stimulation (20–22).

REFERENCES

1. Grebe SK, Hay ID. Follicular thyroid cancer. Endocrinol Metab Clin North Am 1995; 24:761–801.
2. Emerick GT, Duh QY, Siperstein AE, et al. Diagnosis, treatment, and outcome of follicular thyroid carcinoma. Cancer 1993; 72:3287–3295.
3. Rao RS, Parikh HK, Deshmane VH, et al. Prognostic factors in follicular carcinoma of the thyroid: a study of 198 cases. Head Neck 1996; 18: 118–124.
4. Lin JD, Huang MJ, Juang JH, et al. Factors related to the survival of papillary and follicular thyroid carcinoma patients with distant metastases. Thyroid 1999; 9:1227–1235.
5. Zidan J, Kassem S, Kuten A. Follicular carcinoma of the thyroid gland: prognostic factors, treatment, and survival. Am J Clin Oncol 2000; 23: 1–5.
6. Chow SM, Law SC, Mendenhall WM, et al. Follicular thyroid carcinoma: prognostic factors and the role of radioiodine. Cancer 2002; 95: 488–498.
7. Chow SM, Law SC, Au SK, et al. Differentiated thyroid carcinoma: comparison between papillary and follicular carcinoma in a single institute. Head Neck 2002; 24:670–677.
7a. Besic N, Zgajnar J, Hoevar M, Frkovic-Grazio S. Is patient's age a prognostic factor for follicular thyroid carcinoma in the TNM classification system? Thyroid 2005; 15:439–448.
8. LiVolsi VA. Follicular carcinoma of the thyroid. Pathology Case Rev 2003; 8:4–15.
9. Brennan MD, Bergstralh EJ, van Heerden JA, McConahey WM. Follicular thyroid cancer treated at the Mayo Clinic, 1946 through 1970: initial manifestations, pathologic findings, therapy, and outcome. Mayo Clin Proc 1991; 66:11–22.
10. Davis NL, Bugis SP, McGregor GI, Germann E. An evaluation of prognostic scoring systems in patients with follicular thyroid cancer. Am J Surg 1995; 170:476–480.
11. Jorda M, Gonzalez-Campora R, Mora J, et al. Prognostic factors in follicular carcinoma of the thyroid. Arch Pathol Lab Med 1993; 117: 631–635.
12. Thompson LD, Wieneke JA, Paal E, et al. A clinicopathologic study of minimally invasive follicular carcinoma of the thyroid gland with a review of the English literature. Cancer 2001; 91: 505–524.
13. van Heerden JA, Hay ID, Goellner JR, et al. Follicular thyroid carcinoma with capsular invasion alone: a nonthreatening malignancy. Surgery 1992; 112:1130–1136.
14. Feind C. Follicular thyroid cancer with capsular invasion alone: a nonthreatening malignancy. Surgery 1992; 112:1137–1138.
15. Young RL, Mazzaferri EL, Rahe AJ, Dorfman SG. Pure follicular thyroid carcinoma: impact of therapy in 214 patients. J Nucl Med 1980; 21: 733–737.
16. Samaan NA, Schultz PN, Hickey RC, et al. The results of various modalities of treatment of well differentiated thyroid carcinomas: a retrospective review of 1599 patients. J Clin Endocrinol Metab 1992; 75: 714–720.
17. DeGroot LJ, Kaplan EL, Shukla MS, et al. Morbidity and mortality in follicular thyroid cancer. J Clin Endocrinol Metab 1995; 80:2946–2953.
18. Jensen MH, Davis RK, Derrick L. Thyroid cancer: a computer-assisted review of 5287 cases. Otolaryngol Head Neck Surg 1990; 102: 51–65.
19. Mazzaferri EL, Kloos RT. Clinical review 128: Current approaches to primary therapy for papillary and follicular thyroid cancer. J Clin Endocrinol Metab 2001; 86:1447–1463.
20. Robbins RJ, Robbins AK. Recombinant human thyrotropin and thyroid cancer management. J Clin Endocrinol Metab 2003; 88: 1933–1938.
21. Mazzaferri EL, Robbins RJ, Spencer CA, et al. A consensus report of the role of serum thyroglobulin as a monitoring method for low-risk patients with papillary thyroid carcinoma. J Clin Endocrinol Metab 2003; 88:1433–1441.
22. Wartofsky L. Editorial: Using baseline and recombinant human TSH-stimulated Tg measurements to manage thyroid cancer without diagnostic 131-I scanning. J Clin Endocrinol Metab 2002; 87: 1486–1489.

Part VI
Variants of Thyroid Cancer

65
Miscellaneous and Unusual Types of Thyroid Tumors

Kenneth D. Burman, Matthew D. Ringel, and Barry M. Shmookler

INTRODUCTION

The majority of epithelial thyroid tumors maintain some degree of thyroid follicular cell function, as shown by thyroglobulin production and the ability to concentrate iodine. They also have typical histological appearances, such as those seen in papillary and follicular carcinomas. This chapter discusses a group of unusual primary thyroid neoplasms characterized by limited, or the absence of, differentiated thyroid cellular function and structure. In general, these tumors have more aggressive clinical courses than differentiated carcinomas. The term "poorly differentiated" is relatively nonspecific. To a pathologist, it might refer to the cellular architecture, whereas a clinician might believe a tumor is "poorly differentiated" when it traps radioiodine poorly. To both groups, however, the implication of more aggressive disease and poorer prognosis applies. This chapter also reviews tumors that metastasize to the thyroid gland. The thyroid tumors discussed in this chapter have been classified by the World Health Organization (WHO) under the category of "other" thyroid carcinomas, nonepithelial tumors, and in the case of several histological types to be discussed, variants of papillary and follicular carcinoma (1,2).

Most thyroid neoplasms originate from thyroid follicular epithelium, and poorly differentiated thyroid neoplasms represent 5–15% of all thyroid tumors (3,4), where the most common is probably anaplastic carcinoma (see Chapters 77–83). Based on the WHO recommendation, the previously described variants of spindle-cell and giant-cell carcinoma are now included under anaplastic carcinoma, whereas the small-cell carcinoma variant is not included because nearly all these tumors have been reclassified as non-Hodgkin's lymphomas (5–7). In addition, many tumors classified in the past as sarcomas have been reclassified as anaplastic carcinomas, but some sarcomas of the thyroid clearly exist. The important clinical and histological diagnostic features of these rare, often aggressive tumors are discussed, as well as the therapeutic options. Similar to the diagnosis and management of most cancers, the importance of approaching these patients in an organized multidisciplinary manner should be emphasized.

SQUAMOUS CELL CARCINOMA OF THE THYROID

Demographics

Primary squamous cell carcinoma of the thyroid is a rare disorder, containing cells of uncertain origin. The WHO classification defines squamous cell carcinoma as a tumor comprised entirely of cells that demonstrate intercellular bridges and/or form keratin (1). This definition of squamous cell carcinoma is quite important, as up to 43% of papillary carcinomas contain regions of squamous cell metaplasia, and many anaplastic carcinomas are partly comprised of squamoid regions (30,31; see Chapter 79). Adenosquamous cell carcinomas and adenoacanthomas, tumors containing regions of squamous cell carcinoma and adenocarcinoma (usually papillary), are also excluded by this WHO definition. Using these strict criteria, the incidence of squamous cell carcinoma of the thyroid is less than 1% of all thyroid malignancies (11,21). Squamous cell carcinoma appears to have a predilection to develop in thyroglossal duct remnants, accounting for an estimated 1% of thyroglossal duct tumors (see Chapter 43). The vast majority of thyroglossal duct neoplasms are papillary thyroid cancer, and approximately 6% have squamous cell origin (32). Care must be taken to exclude local extension or metastasis from a laryngeal or other head and neck carcinoma. Squamous cell carcinoma of the lung can also metastasize to the thyroid gland.

The demographics of this tumor are difficult to determine because of the rarity of pure squamous cell thyroid carcinomas. We have reviewed recent case reports of pure squamous cell carcinoma published in the English literature since 1970 (8,9,11,12,21,27,33–35). Cases reported as squamous cell carcinoma that did not clearly meet the WHO criteria were excluded. These excluded tumors were generally papillary, adenosquamous, or anaplastic carcinomas with a squamoid element. Table 1 summarizes the demographic information on pure squamous cell carcinoma. Similar to anaplastic carcinoma, the tumors usually present in the fifth, sixth, or seventh decades of life, but cases have been described in patients as young as 35 yr of age. The female:male ratio is 1.7:1.

From: *Thyroid Cancer: A Comprehensive Guide to Clinical Management, 2/e*
Edited by: L. Wartofsky and D. Van Nostrand © Humana Press Inc., Totowa, NJ

Table 1
Demographics of Patients With Squamous Cell Carcinoma of the Thyroid

First Author (Reference)	Number (n)	Age (years, mean)	Female (n)	Male (n)
Prakash (8)	1	38	1	0
Bahuleyan (9)	1	35	1	0
Harada (10,11)	2	71 (at death)	2	0
White (12)[a]	1	61	0	1
Kapoor (13)	1	45	1	0
Misonou (14)	1	61	1	0
Tsuchiya (15)	3	63	2	1
Kampsen (16)	2	65	2	0
Sarda (17)	7	46	5	2
Theander (18)	1	72	1	0
Chaudhary (19)	1	76	1	0
Budd (20)	2	59	1	1
Simpson (21)	8	60	3	5
Huang (22)	4	58	2	2
Bukachevsky (23)[b]	1	73	1	0
Korvonin (24)	4	62	3	1
Riddle (25)	1	66	0	1
Shimaoka (26)	3	60	1	2
Saito (27)	1	71	1	0
Zimmer (28)	1	64	1	0
Zhou (29)	4			
Total	50	59	30	16

[a]Thyroglossal duct tumor.
[b]Lingual thyroid cancer.

Clinical Characteristics

Several cases of squamous cell carcinoma have been associated with thyroiditis and squamous cell metaplasia, but the etiology of this rare variant remains obscure. One patient with adenosquamous thyroid carcinoma has been described after radiation therapy (34), but thus far, no cases have been described in several large cohorts of patients with Hodgkin's disease who were followed longitudinally, making a relationship with prior radiation therapy unlikely.

The origin of squamous cells within the thyroid remains controversial, and several hypotheses have been proposed. Squamous cell carcinoma has been found within thyroglossal duct remnants and lingual thyroid glands (12,33). These tumors were believed to derive from squamous epithelial cells in the walls of these cell rests. A few cases of pure squamous cell carcinoma appear to have developed from squamous metaplasia. However, as Klinck and Menk observed (36), this pattern of squamous metaplasia, leading to squamous cell carcinoma, has not been identified in other organs. Moreover, Harada and colleagues (11) did not identify any areas of squamous metaplasia in their series of squamous cell carcinomas. If squamous cell carcinoma commonly arose from squamous metaplasia, a higher occurrence of these cancers would be expected in clinical conditions associated with squamous metaplasia (e.g., thyroiditis, papillary thyroid carcinoma, and adenomatoid nodules), but this has not been reported.

Bond and colleagues (37) reported a variant thyroid epithelial cell population characterized by a squamoid appearance, the absence of thyroglobulin staining, and positive immunostaining for cytokeratin and vimentin. These cells had a higher proliferative capacity than the follicular cells in primary culture. The authors suggest that these cells may represent areas of squamous metaplasia within the thyroid gland; yet, they might also represent a small population of normal squamoid thyroid cells that grow well in the cell culture environment.

Zimmer et al. (28) described a 64-yr-old woman with an asymptomatic nodule who was determined to have squamous cell carcinoma of the thyroid gland as confirmed by cytokeratin staining and transmission electron microscopy. The patient developed local recurrence and expired 7 mo after resection from local invasion and airway obstruction. Zhou (29) reviewed the clinical records of four patients with squamous cell thyroid cancer. Two of the four patients had surgical excision plus radiotherapy but died of local tumor recurrence at 6 and 13 mo. One patient had surgery alone and died 4 mo later of respiratory distress. The fourth patient had radical surgery coupled with radiotherapy and chemotherapy and was disease-free at 26-mo follow-up.

Squamous cell thyroid carcinoma may also occur in association with a well-differentiated carcinoma (particularly papillary carcinoma), an adenoma, a multinodular goiter, or (occasionally) chronic autoimmune thyroiditis *(1,2,4)*. Because of the intimate relationship to neoplastic glandular elements, some squamous cancers have been called "adenosquamous carcinomas." Undifferentiated carcinoma may be evident, along with the predominant squamous carcinoma *(5)*. Squamous carcinoma with extensive spindle-cell change has been reported in association with tall-cell papillary carcinoma *(6)*. Mucin-producing carcinoma has been linked with squamous carcinoma *(2,38)*. The presence of mucosubstances in the thyroid presents a complex diagnostic problem, and uncertainty about such neoplasms continues *(39,40)*. Bland focal squamous metaplasia may occur in both follicular and papillary carcinomas, but this does not usually behave as squamous carcinoma.

Most patients with squamous cell carcinoma of the thyroid present with the rapid growth of a firm mass in a previously existing multinodular goiter. Symptoms generally begin over several weeks to months. The quick growth is often associated with pain, weight loss, night sweats, and local symptoms, e.g., dysphagia and dysphonia. Similar to some cases of anaplastic carcinoma, a syndrome of leukocytosis and non–parathyroid hormone–mediated hypercalcemia has been described *(25,27,41,42)*. At least one cell line derived from a patient with squamous cell thyroid carcinoma has been characterized to make an interleukin 1a–like factor and a colony-stimulating factor *(27)*. Although many patients develop distant metastases during the course of their illness, the majority of patients present with only local neck complaints.

The diagnosis of squamous cell carcinoma is usually made on fine-needle aspiration (FNA) cytology or at the time of surgery for progressive local symptoms. These lesions do not typically concentrate radioiodine and are "cold" on radionuclide scanning. Care must be taken to exclude the possibility of metastases from local head and neck tumors or lung carcinoma. Appropriate radiologic studies should be performed, such as neck and chest computed tomographic (CT) or magnetic resonance imaging (MRI) scans, bronchoscopy, endoscopy, and an otolaryngologic examination should be performed preoperatively to ensure that the tumor originated from the thyroid.

Treatment and Clinical Course

Squamous cell carcinoma of the thyroid has a clinical course that resembles anaplastic carcinoma. Complete surgical resection is the primary curative therapy, in combination with postoperative external-beam radiation therapy. Radioiodine scanning and treatment have limited value, as nearly all these tumors are not iodine-avid. A variety of chemotherapeutic regimens have been attempted to cure individual cases, including bleomycin, doxorubicin, and cisplatin, all with disappointing results. Thyroid hormone suppression is usually initiated, but the clinical utility of this treatment has not been documented well. These cancers, similar to anaplastic cancers, have likely sustained sufficient genetic alterations to lead to thyrotropin-independent growth. Palliative surgery and radiation therapy is appropriate in selected patients to avoid airway compromise and the inability to swallow.

Nearly all the patients reported with squamous cell carcinoma died within 16 mo of diagnosis. These deaths were caused by distant metastases or local complications of disease. The rare long-term survivors of these tumors are those who presented with earlier stage disease who had a near-complete or complete surgical resection. After surgery, these patients were generally treated with external-beam radiation.

Summary

Pure squamous cell carcinoma is a rare thyroid cancer with an extremely poor prognosis. Like anaplastic carcinoma, these tumors present as rapidly enlarging masses in older patients and are generally not responsive to radioiodine or conventional chemotherapy. Direct extension or metastases from other squamous cell carcinomas of the head, neck, and lungs must be ruled out before choosing a treatment plan. A cure seems possible only in those rare patients who present with surgically resectable disease. Generally, postoperative radiation therapy should be prescribed in these patients. Radioiodine and thyroid hormone suppression therapy have limited utility in this disease; however, thyroid hormone replacement is obviously required after thyroidectomy. Control of local disease is important to preserve the quality of life in patients with squamous cell carcinoma.

POORLY DIFFERENTIATED ("INSULAR") CARCINOMA

Demographics

Insular thyroid carcinoma was originally described by Langhans in 1907 *(43)* and termed "Wuchernde Struma" (see Chapters 23 and 25). Subsequently, in 1984, Carcangiu and colleagues *(44)* renamed this variant, poorly differentiated carcinoma (insular carcinoma) because of the solid clusters of polygonal cells characteristic of this tumor and resembling pancreatic islet cells. Insular carcinoma is included as a variant of follicular carcinoma by the WHO *(2)* and generally appears to be more aggressive than well-differentiated follicular carcinoma but less aggressive than anaplastic carcinoma. From a histologic standpoint, poorly differentiated carcinoma defines a group of follicular thyroid epithelium that retain sufficient differentiation to produce scattered small follicular structures and some thyroglobulin but that generally lack the typical morphological characteristics of papillary and follicular carcinoma *(45,46)*. Instead, the histological patterns are

Table 2
Clinical Presentation and Outcome of Insular Thyroid Cancer Compared With Differentiated Thyroid Carcinoma

Characteristic	Insular	Differentiated*	Outcome	Insular (%)	Differentiated (%)
Age (yr)	54	36	Died of disease	20	8
Size (cm)	4.7	2.5	Alive with disease	30	29
Intrathyroidal	34%	48%	No disease	44	63
Regional	36%	50%	Died with disease	6	0
Distant	30%	2%			

*Data on differentiated cancer reported by Mazzaferri and Jhiang (71).
Adapted from ref. 72 with permission of W. B. Saunders Co.

described as solid, insular (islands of cells separated by connective tissue and artifactual spaces), trabecular, and alveolar, with tiny scattered follicles containing colloid within the solid, insular, and trabecular regions. These patterns may mix with each other, and small foci of characteristic follicular and papillary carcinoma may also be found, even both within the same neoplasm. The Bcl-2 protein (a suppressor of apoptosis) has been described in a large proportion of these tumors, in contrast to undifferentiated carcinoma (47).

We have reviewed the literature concerning well-documented cases of insular carcinoma (44,45,48–70). The median age at presentation for the group is approx 54 yr, with a range of 12–78 yr. The incidence of this histological variant appears low. Mizukami and associates (56) identified only three cases of insular carcinoma of 800 thyroid tumors resected at their institution during 20 yr. Machens et al. (70) found that 14 of 127 differentiated thyroid cancers were the insular subtype. Higher rates have been described in other populations; however, many of these groups included tumors with other "poorly differentiated" appearances, such as solid, trabecular, and alveolar patterns. It remains unclear whether this group of tumors described as "poorly differentiated" is a spectrum of one tumor type identified during the dedifferentiating process or whether each histological type represents a specific entity.

Clinical Characteristics

The prognosis of insular carcinoma has been controversial because of the varied histological pattern and the evidence of well-differentiated papillary or follicular carcinoma that can be found within most of these neoplasms. Although the controversy is understandable, the presence of the "primordial cells" in these neoplasms must be taken into account and the fact that they display many characteristics differing from well-differentiated cancers (66–68).

We have compared the presenting characteristics and clinical outcomes of patients with insular carcinoma reported in the literature by Mazzaferri and Jhiang (71), who studied 1355 patients with well-differentiated thyroid cancer (Table 2). Many larger patient series are summarized in detail below. Patients with insular carcinoma tended to be older, had larger primary tumors, and were more likely to present with metastases, compared to patients with differentiated carcinoma. Often, there is a preceding history of goiter in adults with insular carcinoma. The male:female ratio is similar to well-differentiated carcinoma. In the three largest series, the female:male ratio was 2.1:1. The most common complaint was an enlarging mass, but metastases in the neck, mediastinum, and femur has been reported. The duration of enlargement appears variable, but most of these tumors are slow-growing nodules that often enlarge for months or years before clinical diagnosis. These lesions are not typically iodine- or technetium-avid relative to normal thyroid tissue, and FNA biopsy is usually suggestive of malignancy. Children with this entity tend to present with early nodal metastases, either in the neck or mediastinum (51,56,59). As with anaplastic and squamous cell carcinomas, insular carcinoma frequently develops in the setting of prior multinodular goiter, underscoring the importance of both long-term follow-up and the rapid recognition of changes in growth pattern.

Treatment and Clinical Course

The clinical course of insular thyroid carcinoma was initially described by Carcangiu in 1984 (44). In their series of 25 patients, 11 (44%) presented with intrathyroidal disease, 11 (44%) with neck metastases or invasion of local neck structures, and 4 (12%) with metastatic disease. With a mean follow-up of 3.5 yr (range of 1–8 yr), 11 (44%) died of disease and 7 (28%) were alive with disease. Of the four patients presenting with distant metastases, three died of disease during follow-up. The authors concluded that insular carcinoma was more aggressive than well-differentiated carcinoma but less aggressive than anaplastic carcinoma.

Falvo et al. (73) assessed 9 patients with insular thyroid cancer and compared their clinical characteristics to 27 patients of similar age and tumor size who had follicular and papillary cancer (follow-up range of 24–72 mo). All the patients underwent total thyroidectomy. Vascular invasion was observed in 44% of insular carcinomas ($p < 0.05$ vs papillary carcinomas). No significant differences were observed relating to multifocality, lymph node metastases, or TNM (tumor, nodes, metastasis) tumor stage. The death rate of patients with insular carcinoma (33.3%) was higher than that of patients with follicular ($p < 0.05$) and papillary carcinoma ($p < 0.01$). Distant metastases were observed in 66% of insular carcinomas ($p < 0.005$ vs follicular carcinoma and $p < 0.001$ vs papillary carcinoma). Two patients (22.2%) with insular carcinoma have remained disease-free ($p < 0.001$ vs those with follicular and papillary carcinomas). This study emphasized the poor prognostic features of insular thyroid cancer. Luna-Ortiz (74) have also concluded that insular thyroid cancer is generally aggressive, typically occurs later in life, and is frequently accompanied by a history of a chronic goiter.

Ashfaq and colleagues (58) examined 41 patients who had insular carcinoma with a mean follow-up of 4 yr (range, 1 mo to 12 yr). Clinical outcome information was available on 28 patients: 18% died of disease; 21% were alive with disease at the time of the study; 50% were alive with no evidence of disease; and 11% died of other causes but had known disease. Similar to the findings by Carcangiu and colleagues, only 41% of patients presented with intrathyroidal lesions. They reported no difference in clinical outcome between patients with a minor (10–40%) or predominant (50–90%) histological component of insular carcinoma. The majority of these patients were treated with thyroidectomy followed by radioiodine.

Papotti and coworkers (49) addressed the treatment of thyroid cancers containing a "primordial cell" component by considering two tumors groups: those comprised predominantly of insular carcinoma ($n = 31$) and those with predominant trabecular or solid patterns and a minor component of insular carcinoma ($n = 32$). The only presentation or outcome difference between the two groups was a higher recurrence rate among tumors with a predominant insular histology, with a mean follow-up of 4.6 yr. After surgery, 46 (72%) of the patients were free of disease, whereas 16 (28%) had evidence of metastases or invasion of local structures at presentation. Other than those with incidentally discovered malignancies at thyroidectomy, all patients received near-total thyroidectomy, followed by ^{131}I and subsequent L-thyroxine suppression therapy. Of the 46 patients initially rendered disease-free at surgery, 27 were free of disease at follow-up; 83% of the tumors were iodine-avid and produced measurable serum levels of thyroglobulin, which indicated differentiated follicular cell function. Of the total 63 patients in the study, 35 had persistent or recurrent disease. Of these 35 with recurrence, 30 had evidence of iodine uptake on diagnostic scan and were treated with ^{131}I. Iodine scanning and measurements of serum thyroglobulin showed 17% of those patients as cured, 27% were alive with disease, and 56% died of disease. Five patients with noniodine-avid recurrence or metastases were treated with chemotherapy and/or external-beam radiation therapy, three of whom were alive with disease 1–15 yr after presentation.

Chao et al. (69) have recently emphasized the aggressive clinical course of these patients. They studied eight patients with insular cancer and observed that local invasion into the strap muscles, pulmonary metastases, and local cervical nodes metastases were frequent. Four patients died of their disease. Machens et al. (70) retrospectively analyzed 127 patients with differentiated thyroid cancer and identified 14 with the insular subtype. Greater tumor size (>4 cm) and the presence of distant metastasis correlated with this subtype.

Similar data were reported by Sasaki and colleagues (60), who identified 44 cases of papillary or follicular carcinoma with an insular component. For the time period reviewed, this number represented 1.8% of thyroid carcinomas. Although the follow-up was variable, 17 patients died of their disease, 18 patients were free of disease, and 2 were alive with disease. Multivariate analysis revealed that the presence of insular carcinoma, as well as tumor size, the absence of a tumor capsule, vascular invasion, and necrosis within the tumor, were all independently associated with a worse prognosis. Many other groups have reported successful ^{131}I therapy in patients with metastatic disease. Metastatic insular carcinoma has been detected utilizing ^{99}Tc (48,55), and levels of serum thyroglobulin are also useful in monitoring patients for tumor recurrence. Table 2 compares the outcome of patients with insular carcinoma to the outcome of those with well-differentiated carcinoma, as reported by Mazzaferri and Jhiang (71). The follow-up related to insular carcinoma was shorter, and the treatment modalities were variable, compared to the cohort with well-differentiated tumors. Among patients presenting with metastatic insular thyroid carcinoma with relatively short follow-up periods (several years), 60% died of disease and 20% were alive with disease. The remaining 20% were believed to be cured from their metastatic carcinoma following treatment with ^{131}I.

Therapy with L-thyroxine is prudent in patients with insular thyroid carcinoma. Because many of these patients have tumors that display differentiated epithelial function, doses of L-thyroxine to fully suppress pituitary production of thyrotropin (TSH) is recommended. We believe that the target TSH level in these patients is a value less than 0.01 µU/mL, if tolerated and if the patient has no contraindications to such therapy related to age and cardiovascular status. This TSH level should be achieved relatively gradually with the levothyroxine dose sufficient to just suppress the TSH level to this range. The average daily dose of exogenous L-thyroxine required to suppress TSH in thyroid cancer patients is approx 2.1 µg/kg of body weight. Because the recurrence and mortality rates for this tumor are higher than for differentiated carcinoma, and as these carcinomas generally remain iodine-avid, aggressive surgical and ^{131}I therapy are appropriate. This should be followed by frequent monitoring for tumor recurrence with radioiodine scanning and measurements of serum thyroglobulin. We also believe that the adjunctive use of radiological procedures, e.g., neck sonogram, CT, and/or MRI, may be useful in diagnosing recurrent disease as early as possible. 18-Fluorodeoxyglucose positron emission tomography (FDG-PET) scans are often useful in detecting disease, especially in poorly differentiated thyroid cancers, such as the insular variety *(75)*.

Summary

Insular thyroid carcinoma is a histological variant with a clinical course more aggressive than well-differentiated carcinoma but less aggressive than anaplastic thyroid carcinoma. Therefore, insular carcinoma may represent an important intermediate stage in the dedifferentiation of thyroid carcinoma. Patients with insular carcinoma are more likely to present with metastases and to develop tumor recurrence than those with well-differentiated tumors, but the majority present with either intrathyroidal lesions or regional disease. These tumors generally maintain differentiated thyroid follicular cell function, allowing for ^{131}I therapy and scanning and measurement of serum thyroglobulin levels.

Most patients with local disease are successfully treated surgically and with ^{131}I therapy, followed by L-thyroxine suppression. Tumor recurrence rates appear to be higher among patients with local or regional disease than seen with more well-differentiated tumors. Patients with distant metastases treated with ^{131}I and thyroid hormone suppression appear to have a cure rate of approximately 20%, justifying aggressive treatment with surgery, ^{131}I, and thyroid hormone suppression.

TALL-CELL VARIANT OF PAPILLARY CARCINOMA

Demographics

The tall-cell variant of papillary carcinoma (TCV) was initially reported by Hazard in 1964 *(76)*, who defined a group of papillary tumors with certain characteristics in at least 30% of the tumor. These included papillary structures, epithelial cell height at least twice the cellular width, oxyphilic cytoplasm, and hyperchromic basilar nuclei. Hawk and Hazard *(77)* found that 9% of their papillary tumors met this definition. They also described these tumors as being grossly larger and more locally invasive than nontall-cell papillary carcinoma, affecting an older group of patients (mean age of 57 yr). Most studies report that TCV represents approximately 5–10% of thyroid carcinomas. The female predominance typically linked with other forms of thyroid cancer remains. The literature on TCV has been reviewed *(11,77–90)*.

Clinical Characteristics

At least 30% of the tumor must be composed of tall cells to be considered a TCV tumor (see Chapter 66). However,

Table 3
Clinical Presentation of TCV Compared With Differentiated Thyroid Cancer

Characteristic	TCV (n = 163)	Differentiated Thyroid Carcinoma* (n = 1355)
Age (yr)	51.8	36
Size (cm)	3.2	2.5
Intrathyroidal	33%	48%
Regional (neck)	19%	50%
Distant metastases	19%	2%
Female	74%	67%

*Data on differentiated cancer reported by Mazzaferri and Jhiang *(71)*.
Adapted from ref. 72 with permission of W. B. Saunders Co.

the inherent subjectivity involved in this diagnosis is of concern. For example, no studies have been published in which identical slides were sent in a blinded manner to multiple pathologists to determine the frequency of a TCV diagnosis. TCV must be differentiated from the less common columnar-cell variant, which is characterized by "tall" cells but with nuclear stratification, as opposed to basilar nuclei and scant, nonoxyphilic, but often vacuolated, cytoplasm. These two closely related variants of papillary carcinoma were recently described in the same patient, suggesting a similar pathogenesis *(91)*.

TCV has been found in combination with cell types other than the usual forms of papillary carcinoma. A recent report describes five TCV cases in tumors with regions of a variant of anaplastic carcinoma, described as spindle-cell squamous carcinoma *(92)*. These cases, in addition to the general occurrence of TCV within tumors containing usual papillary carcinoma and a high incidence of p53 mutations *(93)*, suggest that this lesion might represent a transition between papillary and anaplastic carcinoma, similar to the intermediate stage assigned to insular carcinoma. The similarities between TCV and the columnar-cell variant have been described above. These two variants have been classified separately but may represent similar "transition" tumors. The consistency and reliability in diagnosing TCV requires further study. The interobserver variability is unknown but may be quite important when attempting to compare published data on the frequency and clinical course of TCV.

Table 3 compares the presenting characteristics of 163 patients with TCV compiled from the literature to the patient cohort with typical differentiated papillary carcinoma, as reported by Mazzaferri and Jhiang *(71)*. Patients with TCV tend to be older, have larger lesions, and are more likely to have metastases outside of the neck than patients with well-differentiated tumors.

The aggressiveness of TCV has been debated in the literature since its initial description, particularly in younger patients (see below; *78,82*). The mechanism for this aggres-

Table 4
Clinical Outcomes of TCV Compared With Differentiated Thyroid Cancer

	All Patients (%)		Patients Over Age 50 (%)		Patients Under Age 50 (%)	
Outcomes	Tall Cell[a] (n = 148)	Differentiated[b] (n = 1355)	Tall Cell (n = 41)	Differentiated[b] (n = 222)	Tall Cell (n = 35)	Differentiated[b] (n = 1133)
Died of disease	19	8	21	19	6	2
Alive with disease	26	29	27	23	17	21
No disease	55	63	32	58	77	77

[a]Follow-up data included on 148 of 163 patients with TCV; presenting age included on 76 of 163.
[b]Data on differentiated cancer by Mazzaferri and Jhiang *(71)*.
Adapted from ref. *97* with permission of W. B. Saunders Co.

sive behavior is not known. However, *RET* rearrangements were recently identified in about 36% of TCV (14 of 39 cases). Interestingly, the prevalence of *RET/PTC1* and *RET/PTC3* abnormalities were almost equal in classic papillary and follicular thyroid cancer, whereas all the TCV-positive cases expressed the *RET/PTC3* rearrangement *(94)*.

Treatment and Clinical Course

Johnson and associates *(82)* attempted to define TCV prognosis by comparing 12 patients with TCV to a similar group of age- and gender-matched patients with typical papillary thyroid carcinomas. The groups were different in the extent of disease at presentation. All patients with usual papillary carcinoma had either intrathyroidal (58%) or regional lymphatic spread (42%). Of the patients with TCV, 25% had intrathyroidal disease, 33% had cervical lymphatic spread, and 42% had invasion into cervical soft tissue or distant metastases. Tumor size correlated with recurrence and tumor-related mortality. Clinical outcome was different between the TCV and usual papillary thyroid carcinoma only among patients older than 50 yr, but the authors concluded that TCV was more aggressive than typical papillary thyroid carcinoma.

Terry and colleagues *(78)* compared 19 patients with TCV to those with usual papillary carcinoma. The follow-up times were similar for both groups (62 and 93 mo, respectively). Patients with TCV had larger tumors than those with papillary carcinoma (4.2 vs 2.8 cm). Patients older than 50 yr with TCV had larger tumors than younger patients with TCV (5.6 vs 2.7 cm) and had a higher incidence of distant metastases and locally invasive disease. The authors performed a multivariate analysis on their data, comparing TCV to usual papillary carcinoma, and found that patients older than 50 with tumor size larger than 4 cm had an increased risk of tumor recurrence, but not mortality. Similar to Johnson and colleagues *(82)*, they could find no difference in the prognosis of patients younger than 50 with TCV vs usual papillary carcinoma.

Moreno Egea and colleagues *(95)* reported a series of five patients with TCV ages 58–73 yr. All these patients presented with large tumors and extrathyroidal disease.

When compared to 85 patients with typical papillary carcinoma, a statistically significant increase in tumor recurrence and mortality was reported. The patients in these series were treated with a variety of protocols; nearly all included thyroidectomy and ^{131}I therapy. Some patients received palliative external-beam radiation therapy to control local recurrence. When compared to the large cohort of Mazzaferri and Jhiang (Table 4), the clinical outcomes of patients under the age of 50 were indistinguishable from those with the usual forms of papillary carcinoma. Yet, older patients were more likely to have recurrence of their tumors. The patients with TCV were followed for a shorter time period, and treatment may have been more variable than in this reference group. Mortality and recurrence rates may rise as the follow-up period lengthens. The data suggest a poor prognosis for older patients with TCV that present with larger primary tumors. This tumor variant most commonly occurs in patients older than 50, but the distinction between younger and older patients may be important when determining the prognosis of younger patients with a small TCV tumor.

Sywak et al. *(96)* have also reviewed the literature and conclude (in a summary of 209 cases) that TCV is generally a more aggressive tumor, associated with distant metastases in 22% of cases and had a mean tumor-related mortality of 16%. They concluded that the histological diagnosis of TCV was a poor prognostic factor, regardless of patient age or tumor size. Further studies in this area are required, especially to examine this tumor in younger patients with smaller sized tumors, a group for whom the literature is less clear whether this tumor may frequently exhibit a more aggressive nature.

Surgical therapy followed by ^{131}I and L-thyroxine suppression is appropriate. These tumors typically produce thyroglobulin and are iodine-avid. Loss of these characteristics of differentiation should be taken as further dedifferentiation of the tumor.

TCV typically presents in older patients with a higher frequency of local adenopathy or invasion and distant metastases. It has been linked with well-differentiated papillary carcinoma and anaplastic carcinoma, suggesting that it may represent a "transition" histology between these two types.

These tumors generally maintain thyroglobulin production and iodine-avidity. Among older patients with thyroid cancer, TCV appears to have a higher recurrence rate and possibly a higher mortality than the usual form of papillary thyroid carcinoma. In the unusual younger patient who presents with a small locally confined TCV tumor, the prognosis appears similar to usual papillary carcinoma. Patients with TCV, probably regardless of size or invasive features, should be treated aggressively with thyroidectomy, ^{131}I, and long-term L-thyroxine suppression. Follow-up should include periodic ^{131}I scanning and determinations of serum thyroglobulin levels. Routine cervical sonogram, CT scans, and/or MRI can also help detect evidence of recurrence as soon as possible. When there are suggestive changes with these techniques, guided biopsies can be performed to confirm recurrent cancer and distinguish it from a benign reactive process.

COLUMNAR-CELL VARIANT OF PAPILLARY CARCINOMA

Demographics

The columnar-cell variant of papillary carcinoma is a rare tumor (46,91–93,98–103; see Chapter 66). Patients with columnar cell carcinoma had a mean age of 45 yr, with a range of 16–76 years and a female:male ratio of 1.4:1. As described above, the pathology is similar to that of TCV, as the height of the cells should be at least three times the width to qualify for diagnosis. The nuclei are stratified, not basilar, and the cytoplasm is clear, as opposed to pink (91,93,98,99, 102). These tumors form large distinct papillae, and the follicular cells are immunoreactive for thyroglobulin. The tumors are typically large, with a mean longest dimension of 5.4 cm. Cytopathology is most commonly consistent with papillary carcinoma.

Columnar-cell carcinoma has been described in an otherwise unremarkable well-differentiated papillary carcinoma (99), along with anaplastic carcinoma (93,102), or in combination with tall-cell carcinoma (91). Initial reports of the columnar-cell variant of papillary cancer suggested a highly aggressive neoplasm. However, Gaertner et al. (100) analyzed 16 cases of this rare tumor and concluded that extrathyroidal extension at the time of presentation, rather than cell type, was predictive of a more aggressive clinical course.

Clinical Characteristics

Neoplasms have been described where the columnar cell pattern was mixed with tall-cell papillary carcinoma (99, 104), as well as with solid regions of typical papillary carcinoma (99,100). Also, extensive insular and trabecular patterns have been seen adjacent to the columnar-cell pattern. Research suggests that the locally infiltrative tumors are usually fatal (91,93,98,99,102), but those that are encapsulated may be successfully resected (94,95).

Treatment and Clinical Course

In patients with large tumor masses, metastatic diseas was present in 29%, including six to the lungs, one to the adrenal glands, one to the brain, and two to bone. Patients were treated with thyroidectomy and radioactive iodine. Of the 24 patients described, 58% were free of disease at follow-up. Recurrences typically occurred within 2 yr of the initial surgery. In all, 38% (9 of 24) of the patients died of their columnar-cell carcinoma.

Treatment should be directed at early diagnosis by FNA cytology, followed by a complete surgical resection when possible. Treatment with ^{131}I is appropriate, along with subsequent L-thyroxine suppression. If the primary tumor is large, and a complete surgical resection is not possible, local palliative control with external-beam therapy has been utilized.

Swyak et al. (96) also reviewed the literature relating to columnar-cell thyroid cancer (41 cases). They confirmed a significant mortality rate of 32%. However, they also concluded that when the tumor was encapsulated at the original surgery, the prognosis was comparable to typical papillary thyroid cancer. However, patients with tumors that were not encapsulated had extrathyroidal spread in 67% and had distant metastases in 87%.

Summary

Columnar-cell carcinoma is a rare variant of papillar thyroid carcinoma that appears to have a course similar to TCV, consistent with dedifferentiation in comparison to well-differentiated papillary thyroid carcinoma. Early metastases and local tumor invasion are common; the key to curative therapy is early diagnosis followed by complete surgical resection.

DIFFUSE SCLEROSING VARIANT OF PAPILLARY CARCINOMA

Diffuse sclerosing variant of papillary thyroid cancer is rare and tends to occur in younger patients, with a mean age of approximately 31 yr (95,105–112). There were 13 patients (21%) younger than 20 yr old. Pathologically, diffuse sclerosing papillary carcinoma is characterized by pronounced fibrosis, numerous psammoma bodies, and extensive lymphocytic infiltrates (see Chapter 66). Mucin may be present; thus, these tumors may be misclassified as mucoepidermoid or anaplastic carcinomas. Although the prognostic significance of this variant is not clear, these tumors most commonly present as diffuse enlarging lobes or entire thyroid glands. Their clinical course is not yet well-characterized, but it appears that they behave similarly to well-differentiated papillary carcinomas (98) and should be treated with surgery, radioiodine, and thyroxine suppression.

Swyak et al. (96) suggested that diffuse sclerosing variant of papillary thyroid cancer ($n = 65$) had a tendency for intrathyroidal extension (40%) and a high propensity for nodal metastases (68%). However, tumor-related mortality was similar to that of well-differentiated thyroid cancer: 2% at 8 yr follow-up.

SOLID VARIANT OF PAPILLARY THYROID CARCINOMA

Until recently, this variant was poorly described in the literature; however, the apparent unique association between the solid variant of papillary carcinoma and the Chernobyl nuclear accident in 1986 has stimulated renewed interest in its pathogenesis and prognosis *(113–116)*. Although rare in adults, this histological pattern (see Chapter 66) is frequently identified in tumors in children but usually comprises a small amount of an otherwise well-differentiated tumor. The prognostic significance of these small regions is unclear but is not reported to impact survival.

The role of radiation exposure and the high prevalence of *ret/PTC3* gene rearrangements in solid variant tumors support the notion that this tumor type is a unique thyroid malignancy. Nikiforov and colleagues *(114,116)* compared the histologies of thyroid tumors removed from children who were exposed to the Chernobyl accident vs a control group of sporadic thyroid tumors removed from children from the United States. These investigators found that 37% of the "radiation-induced" tumors had solid variant as the predominant growth pattern, compared to 4% of the "sporadic" tumors. About 79% of the solid variant tumors had *ret/PTC3* gene rearrangements. These data support the hypothesis that rearrangements of this gene occurred in response to the radiation exposure and may be involved in the tumorigenesis. Increased p53 immunohistochemical staining has been reported in some solid regions of these tumors, raising the concern of more aggressive clinical behavior *(114,116)*.

Sywak et al. *(96)* also found that the solid variant of papillary thyroid cancer (in Chernobyl victims) had cervical lymph node metastases in 83% of patients. Long-term follow-up studies of these children are required. The impact of the solid variant histology in adults may differ from the impact in children as well, and it is unknown if patients with this disorder who had radiation-induced tumors from the Chernobyl accident have the same clinical course as those who develop it spontaneously.

MIXED MEDULLARY-FOLLICULAR CELL CARCINOMA

These variants of medullary thyroid carcinoma (MTC) display the microscopic features of both MTC and carcinomas of follicular cells *(1,2)*. The tumor regions are immunoreactive with calcitonin, whereas other regions have thyroglobulin production. Normal follicles may be "trapped" within any MTC and seemingly cause thyroglobulin immunoreactivity in MTC. This pattern differs from the mixed variants that have regions of follicular or papillary cancer adjacent to MTC regions *(117–124)*. Similar medullary-papillary cancers have been reported *(125–127)*. Occasionally, these mixed tumors can be suspected even on cytologic FNA samples *(128)*.

The pathogenesis of these tumors is uncertain. Care must be taken to exclude insular thyroid carcinoma, which may have a similar histological appearance to MTC but expresses only thyroglobulin. Paragangliomas may also present like MTC but are rare in the thyroid. The appearance of these mixed tumors suggests the presence of a progenitor thyroid cell that differentiates into follicular or C-cell lineages; yet, most researchers believe these cell types derive from separate lineages. Pappoti and associates *(117)* identified rare cells expressing both thyroglobulin and calcitonin in 2 of 11 cases. However, in some instances, the medullary-follicular cell carcinoma may represent a "collision tumor" of the thyroid.

Clinical recommendations are difficult to formulate for such rare tumors. As with most cases of MTC, aggressive surgical therapy is appropriate. Treatment with ^{131}I and L-thyroxine suppression, not performed for usual forms of MTC, are recommended for these rare lesions. Serum calcitonin and thyroglobulin measurements are helpful. The prevalence of mutations in the *ret* gene is not known, but familial occurrence of the medullary-follicular and medullary-papillary variants have been reported *(121,125)*. It would seem reasonable to examine the white blood cells of a patient with mixed medullary-follicular carcinoma for mutations in the *ret* oncogene and to ensure (to the extent possible) that this entity is not part of a familial syndrome. However, there are no specific studies addressing this issue.

MUCOEPIDERMOID CARCINOMA

Demographics

Mucoepidermoid carcinoma is a rare variant of thyroid carcinoma of uncertain cell lineage. A recent report of 6 new cases of mucoepidermoid carcinoma also identified 31 cases in the literature *(129)*. This type is more common in women than men (2.9:1), with the majority of patients presenting with a solitary "cold" nodule. There is no clear relationship with risk factors, such as a prior history of radiation therapy or a family history of thyroid cancer. The mean presenting age of patients with mucoepidermoid carcinoma is 42 yr (range, 10–71 yr) with four patients younger than 20 yr old. These neoplasms are usually a low grade of malignancy, and their histogenesis is uncertain. Sometimes the tumor is associated with papillary carcinoma (or even present as a metastatic focus in a papillary carcinoma; *129–137*). An adjacent undifferentiated (anaplastic) carcinoma has been reported *(134)*. The tumors are typically solid, firm, light-colored masses, not encapsulated, sometimes cystic, and can have mucus visible on the cut surfaces (see Chapter 66). Various sizes (1–8 cm) have been documented. A rare variant, sclerosing mucoepidermoid cancer with eosinophils, has also been described (136). This tumor usually occurs in patients with Hashimoto's thyroiditis, potentially representing metaplastic changes. Extensive eosinophil infiltration is noted in the stroma and tumor nests. The natural history of this variant needs to be further defined.

Clinical Presentation and Diagnosis

Most of the 31 patients presented with a painless neck mass or a slowly growing thyroid nodule (67,98,129,130,133, 135–137). When obtained, radioiodine scanning revealed a photopenic region corresponding to the nodule. FNA cytology has been diagnostic of carcinoma but is not specific for mucoepidermoid carcinoma (135). The diagnosis is usually made or confirmed histologically at the time of thyroidectomy. Both partial and near-total thyroidectomies have been performed, the former only for small, well-circumscribed tumors. At presentation, 17 of 31 (55%) had extrathyroidal disease, and all but one patient had disease confined to the neck. Patients with cervical node metastases or invasion of local structures were treated with surgery, followed by external-beam radiation therapy. There have been no reports of postoperative ^{131}I scanning after the usual preparation with thyroid hormone withdrawal.

Clinical Course and Treatment

Among patients with local adenopathy, complete remission rates are quite high, but the duration of follow-up is variable. These tumors appear to be more indolent than many other forms of dedifferentiating thyroid carcinoma. Similar to most other forms of thyroid cancer, cure depends on early diagnosis and surgical intervention. Patients with small primary tumors (<2 cm) confined to the thyroid appear to do well (129). Therapy for those patients with locally advanced disease (utilizing surgery and external-beam radiation) appears to induce remission in most patients. Several patients have either presented with or developed distant metastases. Treatment has not been reported; however, the lesions tend to be indolent, similar to well-differentiated thyroid carcinoma. The utility of thyroid hormone therapy and radioiodine scanning and treatment have not yet been evaluated in these tumors.

Summary

Mucoepidermoid thyroid carcinoma is a rare tumor that affects adults. It is commonly coincident with lymphocytic thyroiditis and shares some features with papillary thyroid carcinoma. It has been identified adjacent to well-differentiated papillary carcinoma and anaplastic carcinoma. The so-called "adenosquamous carcinoma" could represent an aggressive variant of mucoepidermoid carcinoma. These factors raise the possibility that this tumor represents a slowly growing variant of papillary carcinoma, but this is an unproven hypothesis. A cure seems possible with a complete surgical resection (when feasible) and external-beam radiation therapy for residual local disease. The role of ^{131}I therapy in mucoepidermoid carcinoma requires further evaluation.

SARCOMAS OF THE THYROID

True primary sarcomas of the thyroid gland are exceedingly rare. Some cases of sarcoma have been reclassified as anaplastic carcinoma and, in a few cells, display mixed immunohistochemical markers of epithelial and mesenchymal lineages (so-called "carcinosarcomas"). Careful ultrastructural and immunohistochemical analyses have convincingly described several cases of leiomyosarcoma (138–141), osteosarcoma (142,143), chondrosarcoma (141), fibrosarcomas (141), liposarcomas (144), and, most commonly, angiosarcomas (141,145–148). See Chapter 66. Angiosarcomas (malignant hemangioepitheliomas) have been found mostly in European Alpine regions known to be iodine-deficient.

In general, sarcomas often present in older patients with a long-standing history of a goiter. Three thyroid sarcomas have been described in those with a prior history of external-beam radiation therapy, including in a 23-yr-old patient, but no cases were reported among a large group of previously irradiated patients with Hodgkin's disease (144).

These tumors resemble sarcomas arising in other locations. Angiosarcomas typically have features of endothelial differentiation with immunoreactivity for factor VIII-related antigens, CD34 and CD31. Keratin immunoreactivity has been indicated in some cases. Because of this characteristic, some authors prefer to consider these neoplasms as angiomatoid carcinomas (145,149). There may be little importance in differentiating sarcomas from anaplastic carcinomas. Most patients presented with large primary tumors that invaded local structures and had lymphatic spread. The majority of these patients die from aggressive local or metastatic disease. Similar to anaplastic carcinoma, a cure seems possible only with complete surgical resection. Local control with radiation therapy seems advisable if the patient is clinically stable following surgical resection. The utility of chemotherapy for thyroid sarcomas has not been described.

Sarcomas may rarely metastasize to the thyroid gland. A primary originating organ, other than the thyroid, should be excluded in any patient presenting with thyroid sarcoma, as primary thyroid sarcomas are identical to sarcomas in other organs. Kaposi's sarcoma, a well-recognized secondary disease in patients with AIDS, has been found to infiltrate the thyroid. A case of thyroid infiltration by KS-causing hypothyroidism has been reported (148). An interesting association exists between systemic sarcomas and thyroid abnormalities. Of 610 patients with sarcoma, 28 (4.6%) had related significant thyroid disorder. The interval between diagnosis of the thyroid disorder and the sarcoma varied as long as

10–15 yr with thyroid disorders, including goiter, thyroiditis, and carcinoma *(150)*.

TERATOMAS OF THE THYROID

The diagnosis of teratoma, whether benign or malignant, requires demonstration of various cells with characteristics of the three germ-cell layers. Teratomas of the thyroid are rare, usually occur in childhood, and are most often benign. Most benign teratomas are found in infancy and are generally quite large, often greater than 10 cm. Buckley and colleagues *(151)* identified 139 cases of childhood thyroid teratoma, nearly all of which were benign, usually presenting as a mass causing local compressive symptoms. Thyroidal origin is inferred by identifying the blood supply as arising from the thyroidal vessels.

Among adults, teratomas are even more unusual than in children but are more commonly malignant. Bowker and Whittaker *(152)* recently reported a case of malignant teratoma in a 17-yr-old patient and reviewed nine other cases reported in the literature *(151–157)*. Adults with malignant thyroid teratoma had a mean age of 31.2 yr, with a range of 17–68 yr. There were no specific risk factors linked with malignant teratoma. The majority were quite large (up to 17 cm in diameter). Patients were treated with thyroidectomy, radiation, and chemotherapy. Cervical and/or distant metastases were found in all patients. No cases of long-term survival have been reported, and response to radiation therapy and chemotherapy appears to be transient. Only the patient described by Bowker and Whitaker was disease-free at 7-mo follow-up *(152)*. The remaining patients died within 22 mo of diagnosis. Children with rare malignant thyroid teratomas have a similarly poor prognosis.

RARE, MOSTLY BENIGN THYROID TUMORS

There are case reports of rare histological types of benign tumors involving the thyroid; we will mention a few nonepithelial varieties. Benign leiomyomas *(138,158,159)* and neurilemomas *(158–161)* have presented as slowly growing, palpable masses that were "cold" on radioiodine imaging. They were composed of spindle cells with abundant eosinophilic cytoplasm, but no atypia or evidence of increased mitotic activity. Immunoperoxidase staining confirmed the neural or smooth muscle nature of these tumors. The lack of extrathyroidal invasion and absence of recurrent disease after 1–6 yr of follow-up support a benign diagnosis. There has been one case of granulosa cell tumor of the thyroid in a girl treated for short stature with relatively high doses of ethinyl estradiol (0.1 mg daily) and medroxyprogesterone (10 mg) for several years *(162)*. This patient has also done well after surgical resection. Microscopically, this tumor resembled Hürthle cell adenoma because of the abundant eosinophilic cytoplasm.

HYALINIZING TRABECULAR NEOPLASMS, USUALLY ADENOMAS

These rare neoplasms are solid masses, often less than 3.0 cm in diameter, and are well circumscribed (usually encapsulated; *163–167*). Psammoma bodies may be scattered through the tumor. Most cells contain immunoreactive thyroglobulin and keratin. Calcitonin has never been demonstrated. Colloid is not present, but irregular masses of hyaline material are adjacent to the cell clusters. Nuclei often contain grooves and cytoplasmic inclusions that, in addition to the psammoma bodies, are reminiscent of papillary thyroid carcinoma. Thus, aspirates of these lesions have been confused with papillary neoplasms. Rarely, the tumors have been invasive, involving cervical lymph nodes, and have been termed the "cribiform variant of papillary carcinoma" *(168)*. An alteration resembling this hyalinizing tumor has been described in adenomatoid nodules in multinodular goiter *(167;* see Chapter 66).

Thymic and Related Neoplasms

Thymic, parathyroid, and salivary gland tissues may be found in the thyroid *(169–171)*. Therefore, it is not surprising that occasional neoplasms occur in the thyroid and inferior part of the neck that resemble the thymus *(172–175)*. Such tumors may be benign or malignant.

EMBRYOLOGIC THYROID REMNANTS

Thyroglossal Duct Cysts

The thyroglossal tract in adults may be a vestigial remnant or may be a more fully developed structure, composed of thyroid follicles, a duct (usually lined by ciliated pseudostratified columnar epithelium), connective tissue, and lymphoid tissue. The thyroid follicles in this tract may undergo any of the changes that occur in the gland proper, even papillary or follicular thyroid cancer *(176,177)*. When thyroid cancer occurs at the more proximal portion of this duct, it may actually involve the base of the tongue. Generally, the thyroglossal tract resides in the midline, and a thyroglossal tumor may move cephalad when the tongue is protruded because of the persistent connection between the mass and the tongue. When a tumor is present in the thyroglossal tract, it may be associated with a similar tumor within the thyroid gland itself. Thyroglossal tumors must be differentiated from thyroglossal cysts, branchial cleft cysts, and cystic hygromas (fluid-filled multiloculated lymphangiomas present at birth). Thyroid cancers that arise exclusively in the thyroglossal tract are rare and discussed at greater length in Chapter 43.

Clinical Presentation

The proper approach to thyroglossal duct tumors is largely unknown, but our approach is to perform FNA and base our therapeutic decision largely on the cytologic findings *(176–178)*. If the FNA is positive or suspicious for thyroid cancer, we generally recommend removal of the entire thyroglossal tract from the base of the tongue to the thyroid gland. If the FNA is diagnostic of thyroid cancer, the thyroid gland may be removed at the initial surgery. If the FNA is suspicious for thyroid cancer, we may recommend, in conjunction with discussions with the patient, removal of the thyroid gland at the initial operation. Some prefer a subsequent thyroidectomy when the diagnosis of thyroid cancer in the thyroglossal tract has been confirmed. Carcinoma that resides within the thyroglossal tract may emanate from the thyroid epithelium in this area or, alternatively, could arise within the thyroid gland and (rarely) metastasize to the thyroglossal tract. The diagnostic and therapeutic approach to thyroglossal duct tumors is controversial, as long-term controlled studies assessing various options have not been performed.

The natural history of thyroid carcinomas derived from the thyroglossal duct tract is poorly understood. Heshmati and coworkers *(179)* retrospectively reviewed thyroglossal carcinoma in 12 patients seen over a 44-yr period at the Mayo Clinic. Age at presentation ranged from 17 to 60 yr, with a mean of 40 yr. The patients were equally divided between men and women. The most common complaint was a midline neck mass. In all 12 cases, papillary thyroid cancer was found, and 3 patients also had involvement of the thyroid gland. Nine patients had a subtotal or near-total thyroidectomy. Despite that only three patients received postoperative radioactive iodine therapy, no patient had recurrence, distant metastases, or disease-specific mortality during a mean follow-up period of 13 yr.

The usual surgical approach included a Sistrunk procedure in combination with a thyroidectomy. Because these patients were reviewed over a long time period, especially before our improved understanding of thyroid cancer, we do not necessarily concur with their recommendations that radioactive iodine is not necessary and that these patients have an excellent prognosis. Tew and coworkers *(180)* found 90 thyroglossal duct cysts or nodules over a 30-yr period. Four patients had thyroid cancer in the thyroglossal duct cyst, an incidence similar to that of carcinoma arising in an intrathyroidal location. Mahnke and colleagues *(181)* estimate that approximately 150 cases of thyroid carcinoma from a thyroglossal tract have been reported. We tend to treat patients who have thyroglossal papillary thyroid cancer with a Sistrunk procedure, a total or near-total thyroidectomy, and most frequently, radioiodine therapy, based on the clinical findings. At present, there is no reason to expect these tumors will behave differently than an intrathyroidal papillary cancer. Size, capsular invasion, soft-tissue invasion, and vascular or nodal invasion should be considered in the decision how to treat a patient with thyroglossal papillary thyroid cancer.

In addition to papillary thyroid cancer, squamous cell carcinoma and lymphoma may arise within this tissue *(182,183)*.

Deshpande and Bobhate *(184)* believed that only nine cases of squamous cell carcinoma from a thyroglossal tract have been reported. This tumor is difficult to diagnose; we suggest that a Sistrunk procedure, along with a total or near-total thyroidectomy, be performed for these rare tumors.

METASTATIC CANCERS IN THE THYROID GLAND

Metastatic tumors in the thyroid gland occur in as many as 24% of subjects when examined at autopsy, but the clinical manifestations of these metastases certainly are uncommon. Generally, a metastatic tumor in the thyroid gland presents as a solitary nodule, which is usually hypofunctioning on radioisotope scans. Involvement of an existing adenomatoid nodule or adenoma is likely, thereby complicating the morphological features. The most common primary sites of such tumors are breast, kidney, lung, and skin (malignant melanoma; *185–187*). There is often widespread metastatic disease present, and the manifestations in the thyroid gland are clinically unimportant. Nevertheless, solitary thyroid metastasis to the thyroid gland may be the initial evidence of disease or the first presentation of recurrent disease. For example, we have seen a patient with acute myelogenous leukemia who had been treated earlier, and the first evidence of recurrent disease was in the thyroid gland.

Nakhjavani and colleagues *(186)* recently reported a total of 43 patients (23 women, 20 men) with tumors metastatic to the thyroid gland. Solitary thyroid nodules or a multinodular gland was the presentation in 40 patients, whereas the remaining three had tracheal compression, necessitating thyroid surgery. Renal cell carcinoma was found in 14 patients, lung cancer in 7, and breast cancer in 7. More rarely, parathyroid cancer, salivary gland tumors, ovarian or uterine cancer, skin cancer, and esophageal cancer were found. In some instances, the source of the tumor was identified concurrently with the thyroid gland metastases. However, renal cell carcinoma within the thyroid gland was found as long as 26 yr after the original tumor diagnosis; 15% of subjects had evidence of thyroidal involvement before the diagnosis of metastasis to other sites. Although the investigators suggest that a thyroidectomy was associated with enhanced survival, compared to a nonsurgical approach (to the thyroid gland), we believe that more information is required to adequately address this issue.

The diagnostic evaluation revolves around the FNA and examination of the cytological sample. In most cases, there is abundant cellularity, and the cells may be typical of the original site, especially when specific immunohistochemical stains are performed. Obviously, diagnostic evaluation for the original tumor site and for the presence of other metastatic sites is important before approaching management. Occasionally, it may be difficult to determine if the cytological specimen represents metastatic disease or if it is originating from the thyroid gland, such as an anaplastic thyroid carcinoma or the unusual clear-cell variant of follicular carcinoma.

The therapeutic approach depends on the clinical context and cytological examination. For example, if there is widespread metastasis from an obvious extrathyroidal site, and the thyroid nodule cytology examination suggests metastasis from the same site, it may not be appropriate to remove the thyroid gland. Alternatively, if the patient had renal cell carcinoma that was treated successfully several years earlier, and now the patient presents with a thyroid nodule, cytologically appearing to resemble renal cell carcinoma, it might be useful to perform a lobectomy for diagnostic reasons. In fact, if an evaluation confirms that this single thyroid nodule might be the only evidence of metastatic disease, some clinicians might approach the thyroid lesion for diagnostic and even therapeutic reasons. Our general opinion is that it is desirable to obtain as much information as possible from the thyroid cytological specimen, including specific staining, and that radiological evaluation for other sites of metastasis for staging will be useful. Once as much information as reasonably possible is obtained, a frank discussion of the prognosis should take place with the patient and their family. In general, the outlook of patients with metastasis to the thyroid gland is poor, but individual tumors or circumstances may require a different method of treatment *(188)*.

Tumors may also invade the thyroid gland by local extension. This mostly occurs with laryngeal, pharyngeal, and esophageal tumors, and such invasion may present as a neck mass in or around the thyroid gland. Cervical lymph node enlargement may also be noted. Radiological studies, e.g. CT (generally without contrast to avoid the iodine load), MRI, and direct visualization of the larynx or esophagus, may be useful. On thyroid isotope scanning, this invasion may present as a hypofunctioning area.

Occasionally, metastatic disease to the thyroid gland may cause destruction of the thyroid gland, with resultant leakage of iodothyronines into the circulation and hyperthyroidism *(189)*. This hyperthyroidism is thought to be a type of carcinoma-induced thyroiditis and may be associated with a low radioiodine uptake, but it has not been adequately studied using modern techniques.

Summary

This chapter has reviewed various types of unusual thyroid tumors and discussed their general pattern of clinical presentation and progression. Several general points should be made. There are no relevant controlled prospective studies assessing treatment modalities in any of these tumors; thus, we have to rely on clinical reports and experience. Furthermore, different institutions follow patients with any thyroid tumor, much less these relatively unusual disorders, in a variety of ways. After thyroidectomy, in addition to radioiodine scans and monitoring serum thyroglobulin levels, we think it is appropriate to clinically stage and monitor most patients with periodic radiologic studies, such as neck MRI or sonogram and chest CT (without contrast when ^{131}I scanning or treatment is being considered). In selected circumstances, tumor assessment at other distant locations, e.g., brain, liver, kidneys and bone, may also be needed. FDG-PET scans can help identify and/or follow sites of disease activity, especially if the PET activity can be fused digitally with a CT scan or MRI. In certain patients, it may also be beneficial to search for osseous metastases. TSH suppression by exogenous L-thyroxine therapy seems reasonable, based on the clinical context. When TSH is suppressed, preventative measures for osteoporosis should be undertaken, such as the ingestion of calcium and vitamin D and periodic bone mineral densities, as necessary. Some patients should receive treatment with a bisphosphonate with the proper prescribing precautions. It is also extremely important that these patients be addressed in a multidisciplinary manner, with necessary involvement of the patient in clinical decisions.

REFERENCES

1. Hedinger C, Williams E, Sobin L. Histological Typing of Thyroid Tumors. Berlin: Springer-Verlag, 1988.
2. Hedinger C, Williams ED, Sobin LH. The WHO histological classification of thyroid tumors: a commentary on the second edition. Cancer 1989; 63:908–911.
3. Mazzaferri E. Undifferentiated thyroid carcinomas and unusual thyroid malignancies. In Mazzaferri E, Samaan N, editors. Endocrine Tumors. Boston, MA: Blackwell Scientific Publications, 1993: 378–398.
4. Samaan NA, Ordonez NG. Uncommon types of thyroid cancer. Endocrinol Metab Clin North Am 1990; 19:637–648.
5. Holting T, Moller P, Tschahargane C, et al. Immunohistochemical reclassification of anaplastic carcinoma reveals small and giant cell lymphoma. World J Surg 1990; 14:291–294; discussion 295.
6. Schmid KW, Kroll M, Hofstadter F, Ladurner D. Small cell carcinoma of the thyroid. A reclassification of cases originally diagnosed as small cell carcinomas of the thyroid. Pathol Res Pract 1986; 181: 540–543.
7. Wolf BC, Sheahan K, DeCoste D, et al. Immunohistochemical analysis of small cell tumors of the thyroid gland: an Eastern Cooperative Oncology Group study. Hum Pathol 1992; 23:1252–1261.
8. Prakash A, Kukreti SC, Sharma MP. Primary squamous cell carcinoma of the thyroid gland. Int Surg 1968; 50:538–541.
9. Bahuleyan CK, Ramachandran P. Primary squamous cell carcinoma of thyroid. Indian J Cancer 1972; 9:89–91.
10. Harada T, Katagiri M, Tsukayama C, et al. Squamous cell carcinoma with cyst of the thyroid. J Surg Oncol 1989; 42:136–143.
11. Harada T, Shimaoka K, Katagiri M, et al. Rarity of squamous cell carcinoma of the thyroid: autopsy review. World J Surg 1994; 18: 542–546.
12. White IL, Talbert WM. Squamous cell carcinoma arising in thyroglossal duct remnant cyst epithelium. Otolaryngol Head Neck Surg 1982; 90:25–31.
13. Kapoor VK, Sharma D, Mukhopadhyay AK, Chattopadhyay TK. Primary squamous cell carcinoma of the thyroid gland—a case report. Jpn J Surg 1985; 15:60–62.
14. Misonou J, Aizawa M, Kanda M, et al. Pure squamous cell carcinoma of the thyroid gland—report of an autopsy case and review of the literature. Jpn J Surg 1988; 18:469–474.

15. Tsuchiya A, Suzuki S, Nomizu T, et al. Squamous cell carcinoma of the thyroid—a report of three cases. Jpn J Surg 1990; 20:341–345.
16. Kampsen EB, Jager N, Max MH. Squamous cell carcinoma of the thyroid: a report of two cases. J Surg Oncol 1977; 9:567–578.
17. Sarda AK, Bal S, Arunabh, et al. Squamous cell carcinoma of the thyroid. J Surg Oncol 1988; 39:175–178.
18. Theander C, Loden B, Berglund J, Seidal T. Primary squamous carcinoma of the thyroid—a case report. J Laryngol Otol 1993; 107:1155–1158.
19. Chaudhary RK, Barnes EL, Myers EN. Squamous cell carcinoma arising in Hashimoto's thyroiditis. Head Neck 1994; 16:582–585.
20. Budd DC, Fink DL, Rashti MY, Woo TH. Squamous cell carcinoma of the thyroid. J Med Soc N J 1982; 79:838–840.
21. Simpson WJ, Carruthers J. Squamous cell carcinoma of the thyroid gland. Am J Surg 1988; 156:44–46.
22. Huang TY, Assor D. Primary squamoous cell carcinoma of the thyroid gland: a report of four cases. Am J Clinic Pathol 1970; 55:93–98.
23. Bukachevsky RP, Casler JD, Oliver J, Conley J. Squamous cell carcinoma and lingual thyroid. Ear Nose Throat J 1991; 70:505–507.
24. Korovin GS, Kuriloff DB, Cho HT, Sobol SM. Squamous cell carcinoma of the thyroid: a diagnostic dilemma. Ann Otol Rhinol Laryngol 1989; 98:59–65.
25. Riddle PE, Dincsoy HP. Primary squamous cell carcinoma of the thyroid associated with leukocytosis and hypercalcemia. Arch Pathol Lab Med 1987; 111:373–374.
26. Shimaoka K, Tsukada Y. Squamous cell carcinomas and adenosquamous carcinomas originating from the thyroid gland. Cancer 1980; 46:1833–1842.
27. Saito K, Kuratomi Y, Yamamoto K, et al. Primary squamous cell carcinoma of the thyroid associated with marked leukocytosis and hypercalcemia. Cancer 1981; 48:2080–2083.
28. Zimmer PW, Wilson D, Bell N. Primary squamous cell carcinoma of the thyroid gland. Mil Med 2003; 168:124–125.
29. Zhou XH. Primary squamous cell carcinoma of the thyroid. Eur J Surg Oncol 2002; 28:42–45.
30. LiVolsi VA, Merino MJ. Squamous cells in the human thyroid gland. Am J Surg Pathol 1978; 2:133–140.
31. Katoh R, Sakamoto A, Kasai N, Yagawa K. Squamous differentiation in thyroid carcinoma with special reference to histogenesis of squamous cell carcinoma of the thyroid. Acta Pathol Jpn 1980; 39:306–312.
32. Motamed M, McGlashan JA. Thyroglossal duct carcinoma. Curr Opin Otolaryngol Head Neck Surg 2004; 12:106–109.
33. Renard TH, Choucair RJ, Stevenson WD, et al. Carcinoma of the thyroglossal duct. Surg Gynecol Obstet 1990; 171:305–308.
34. Bakri K, Shimaoka K, Rao U, Tsukada Y. Adenosquamous carcinoma of the thyroid after radiotherapy for Hodgkin's disease. A case report and review. Cancer 1983; 52:465–470.
35. Bakri KM, Shimaoka K, Gajera R, et al. Association of thyroid carcinoma with malignant lymphoma. Jpn J Clin Oncol 1983; 13:645–655.
36. Klinck GH, Menk KF. Squamous cells in the human thyroid. Mil Surg 1951; 109:406–414.
37. Bond JA, Wyllie FS, Ivan M, et al. A variant epithelial sub-population in normal thyroid with high proliferative capacity in vitro. Mol Cell Endocrinol 1993; 93:175–183.
38. Carcangiu ML, Steeper T, Zampi G, Rosai J. Anaplastic thyroid carcinoma. A study of 70 cases. Am J Clin Pathol 1985; 83:135–158.
39. Hadar T, Mor C, Shvero J, et al. Anaplastic carcinoma of the thyroid. Eur J Surg Oncol 1993; 19:511–516.
40. Tan RK, Finley RK, III, Driscoll D, et al. Anaplastic carcinoma of the thyroid: a 24-year experience. Head Neck 1995; 17:41–47; discussion 47–48.
41. Sato K, Fujii Y, Ono M, et al. Production of interleukin 1 alpha-like factor and colony-stimulating factor by a squamous cell carcinoma of the thyroid (T3M-5) derived from a patient with hypercalcemia and leukocytosis. Cancer Res 1987; 47:6474–6480.
42. Okabe T, Nomura H, Oshawa N. Establishment and characterization of a human colony-stimulating factor-producing cell line from a squamous cell carcinoma of the thyroid gland. J Natl Cancer Inst 1982; 69:1235–1243.
43. Langhans T. Uber die epithelialen formen der malignen struma. Virchow Arch Pathol Anat 1907; 385:125–141.
44. Carcangiu ML, Zampi G, Rosai J. Poorly differentiated ("insular") thyroid carcinoma. A reinterpretation of Langhans' "wuchernde Struma". Am J Surg Pathol 1984; 8:655–668.
45. Sakamoto A, Kasai N, Sugano H. Poorly differentiated carcinoma of the thyroid. A clinicopathologic entity for a high-risk group of papillary and follicular carcinomas. Cancer 1983; 52:1849–1855.
46. Hwang TS, Suh JS, Kim YI, et al. Poorly differentiated carcinoma of the thyroid retrospective clinical and morphologic evaluation. J Korean Med Sci 1990; 5:47–52.
47. Pilotti S, Collini P, Del Bo R, et al. A novel panel of antibodies that segregates immunocytochemically poorly differentiated carcinoma from undifferentiated carcinoma of the thyroid gland. Am J Surg Pathol 1994; 18:1054–1064.
48. Yen TC, King KL, Yang AH, et al. Comparative radionuclide imaging of metastatic insular carcinoma of the thyroid: value of technetium-99m-(V)DMSA. J Nucl Med 1996; 37:78–80.
49. Papotti M, Botto Micca F, Favero A, et al. Poorly differentiated thyroid carcinomas with primordial cell component. A group of aggressive lesions sharing insular, trabecular, and solid patterns. Am J Surg Pathol 1993; 17:291–301.
50. Killeen RM, Barnes L, Watson CG, et al. Poorly differentiated ('insular') thyroid carcinoma. Report of two cases and review of the literature. Arch Otolaryngol Head Neck Surg 1990; 116:1082–1086.
51. Justin EP, Seabold JE, Robinson RA, et al. Insular carcinoma: a distinct thyroid carcinoma with associated iodine-131 localization. J Nucl Med 1991; 32:1358–1363.
52. Ljungberg O, Bondeson L, Bondeson AG. Differentiated thyroid carcinoma, intermediate type: a new tumor entity with features of follicular and parafollicular cell carcinoma. Hum Pathol 1984; 15:218–228.
53. Pietribiasi F, Sapino A, Papotti M, Bussolati G. Cytologic features of poorly differentiated 'insular' carcinoma of the thyroid, as revealed by fine-needle aspiration biopsy. Am J Clin Pathol 1990; 94:687–692.
54. Flynn SD, Forman BH, Stewart AF, Kinder BK. Poorly differentiated ("insular") carcinoma of the thyroid gland: an aggressive subset of differentiated thyroid neoplasms. Surgery 1988; 104:963–970.
55. Zak IT, Seabold JE, Gurll NJ. Tc-99m MIBI scintigraphic detection of metastatic insular thyroid carcinoma. Clin Nucl Med 1995; 20:31–36.
56. Mizukami Y, Nonomura A, Michigishi T, et al. Poorly differentiated ('insular') carcinoma of the thyroid. Pathol Int 1995; 45:663–668.
57. Dominguez-Malagon H, Guerrero-Medrano J, Suster S. Ectopic poorly differentiated (insular) carcinoma of the thyroid. Report of a case presenting as an anterior mediastinal mass. Am J Clin Pathol 1995; 104:408–412.
58. Ashfaq R, Vuitch F, Delgado R, Albores-Saavedra J. Papillary and follicular thyroid carcinomas with an insular component. Cancer 1994; 73:416–423.
59. Kotiloglu E, Kale G, Senocak ME. Follicular thyroid carcinoma with a predominant insular component in a child: a case report. Tumori 1995; 81:296–298.
60. Sasaki A, Daa T, Kashima K, Yokoyama S, et al. Insular component as a risk factor of thyroid carcinoma. Pathol Int 1996; 46:939–946.
61. Pereira EM, Maeda SA, Alves F, Schmitt FC. Poorly differentiated carcinoma (insular carcinoma) of the thyroid diagnosed by fine needle aspiration (FNA). Cytopathology 1996; 7:61–65.
62. Begin LR, Allaire GS. Insular (poorly differentiated) carcinoma of the thyroid: an ultrastructural and immunocytochemical study of two cases. J Submicrosc Cytol Pathol 1996; 28:121–131.

63. Paik SS, Kim WS, Hong EK, et al. Poorly differentiated ("insular") carcinoma of the thyroid gland—two cases report. J Korean Med Sci 1997; 12:70–74.
64. Russo D, Tumino S, Arturi F, et al. Detection of an activating mutation of the thyrotropin receptor in a case of an autonomously hyperfunctioning thyroid insular carcinoma. J Clin Endocrinol Metab 1997; 82: 735–738.
65. Hassoun AA, Hay ID, Goellner JR, Zimmerman D. Insular thyroid carcinoma in adolescents: a potentially lethal endocrine malignancy. Cancer 1997; 79:1044–1048.
66. Papotti M, Torchio B, Grassi L, et al. Poorly differentiated oxyphilic (Hurthle cell) carcinomas of the thyroid. Am J Surg Pathol 1996; 20: 686–694.
67. Sobrinho-Simoes M, Sambade C, Fonseca E, Soares P. Poorly differentiated carcinomas of the thyroid gland: a review of the clinicopathologic features of a series of 28 cases of a heterogeneous, clinically aggressive group of thyroid tumors. Int J Surg Pathol 2002; 10: 123–131.
68. Sironi M, Collini P, Cantaboni A. Fine needle aspiration cytology of insular thyroid carcinoma. A report of four cases. Acta Cytol 1992; 36: 435–439.
69. Chao TC, Lin JD, Chen MF. Insular carcinoma: infrequent subtype of thyroid cancer with aggressive clinical course. World J Surg 2004; 28: 393–396.
70. Machens A, Hinze R, Lautenschlager C, Dralle H. Multivariate analysis of clinicopathologic parameters for the insular subtype of differentiated thyroid carcinoma. Arch Surg 2001; 136:941–944.
71. Mazzaferri EL, Jhiang SM. Long-term impact of initial surgical and medical therapy on papillary and follicular thyroid cancer. Am J Med 1994; 97:418–428.
72. Burman KD, Ringel MD, Wartofsky L. Unusual types of thyroid neoplasms. Endocrinol Metab Clin North Am 1996; 25:49–68.
73. Falvo L, Catania A, D'Andrea V, et al. Prognostic factors of insular versus papillary/follicular thyroid carcinoma. Am Surg 2004; 70: 461–466.
74. Luna-Ortiz K, Hurtado-Lopez LM, Dominguez-Malagon H, et al. Clinical course of insular thyroid carcinoma. Med Sci Monit 2004; 10: CR108–CR111.
75. Diehl M, Graichen S, Menzel C, et al. F-18 FDG PET in insular thyroid cancer. Clin Nucl Med 2003; 28:728–731.
76. Hazard JB. Classification and staging of thyroid cancer. J Surg Oncol 1981; 16:255–257.
77. Hawk WA, Hazard JB. The many appearances of papillary carcinoma of the thyroid. Cleve Clin Q 1976; 43:207–215.
78. Terry JH, St John SA, Karkowski FJ, et al. Tall cell papillary thyroid cancer: incidence and prognosis. Am J Surg 1994; 168:459–461.
79. Harach HR, Zusman SB. Cytopathology of the tall cell variant of thyroid papillary carcinoma. Acta Cytol 1992; 36:895–899.
80. Hicks MJ, Batsakis JG. Tall cell carcinoma of the thyroid gland. Ann Otol Rhinol Laryngol 1993; 102:402–403.
81. Robbins J, Merino MJ, Boice JD, Jr., et al. Thyroid cancer: a lethal endocrine neoplasm. Ann Intern Med 1991; 115:133–147.
82. Johnson TL, Lloyd RV, Thompson NW, et al. Prognostic implications of the tall cell variant of papillary thyroid carcinoma. Am J Surg Pathol 1988; 12:22–27.
83. Ain KB. Papillary thyroid carcinoma. Etiology, assessment, and therapy. Endocrinol Metab Clin North Am 1995; 24:711–760.
84. Ostrowski ML, Merino MJ. Tall cell variant of papillary thyroid carcinoma: a reassessment and immunohistochemical study with comparison to the usual type of papillary carcinoma of the thyroid. Am J Surg Pathol 1996; 20:964–974.
85. Ozaki O, Ito K, Mimura T, et al. Papillary carcinoma of the thyroid. Tall-cell variant with extensive lymphocyte infiltration. Am J Surg Pathol 1996; 20:695–698.
86. Segal K, Friedental R, Lubin E, et al. Papillary carcinoma of the thyroid. Otolaryngol Head Neck Surg 1995; 113:356–363.
87. Ruter A, Nishiyama R, Lennquist S. Tall-cell variant of papillary thyroid cancer: disregarded entity? World J Surg 1997; 21:15–20; discussion 21.
88. van den Brekel MW, Hekkenberg RJ, Asa SL, et al. Prognostic features in tall cell papillary carcinoma and insular thyroid carcinoma. Laryngoscope 1997; 107:254–259.
89. Gamboa-Dominguez A, Candanedo-Gonzalez F, Uribe-Uribe NO, Angeles-Angeles A. Tall cell variant of papillary thyroid carcinoma. A cytohistologic correlation. Acta Cytol 1997; 41:672–676.
90. Bocklage T, DiTomasso JP, Ramzy I, Ostrowski ML. Tall cell variant of papillary thyroid carcinoma: cytologic features and differential diagnostic considerations. Diagn Cytopathol 1997; 17:25–29.
91. Asklen L, Verhaug J. Thyroid carcinoma with mixed tall-cell and columnar-cell carcinoma: another variant of poorly differentiated carcinoma of the thyroid. Am J Clin Pathol 1990; 94:442–445.
92. Bronner MP, LiVolsi VA. Spindle cell squamous carcinoma of the thyroid: an unusual anaplastic tumor associated with tall cell papillary cancer. Mod Pathol 1991; 4:637–643.
93. Evans HL. Columnar-cell carcinoma of the thyroid. A report of two cases of an aggressive variant of thyroid carcinoma. Am J Clin Pathol 1986; 85:77–80.
94. Basolo F, Giannini R, Monaco C, et al. Potent mitogenicity of the RET/PTC3 oncogene correlates with its prevalence in tall-cell variant of papillary thyroid carcinoma. Am J Pathol 2002; 160:247–254.
95. Moreno Egea A, Rodriguez Gonzalez JM, Sola Perez J, et al. Prognostic value of the tall cell variety of papillary cancer of the thyroid. Eur J Surg Oncol 1993; 19:517–521.
96. Sywak M, Pasieka JL, Ogilvie T. A review of thyroid cancer with intermediate differentiation. J Surg Oncol 2004; 86:44–54.
97. Ringel MD, Burman KD, Shmookler BM. Unusual types of thyroid cancer. In Wartofsky L editor. Thyroid Cancer: A Comprehensive Guide to Clinical Management. Totowa, NJ: Humana Press editor, 1999: 421–451.
98. Sobrinho-Simoes M, Nesland JM, Johannessen JV. Columnar-cell carcinoma. Another variant of poorly differentiated carcinoma of the thyroid. Am J Clin Pathol 1988; 89:264–267.
99. Mizukami Y, Nonomura A, Michigishi T, et al. Columnar cell carcinoma of the thyroid gland: a case report and review of the literature. Hum Pathol 1994; 25:1098–1101.
100. Gaertner EM, Davidson M, Wenig BM. The columnar cell variant of thyroid papillary carcinoma. Case report and discussion of an unusually aggressive thyroid papillary carcinoma. Am J Surg Pathol 1995; 19: 940–947.
101. Ferreiro JA, Hay ID, Lloyd RV. Columnar cell carcinoma of the thyroid: report of three additional cases. Hum Pathol 1996; 27: 1156–1160.
102. Evans HL. Encapsulated columnar-cell neoplasms of the thyroid. A report of four cases suggesting a favorable prognosis. Am J Surg Pathol 1996; 20:1205–1211.
103. Hui PK, Chan JK, Cheung PS, Gwi E. Columnar cell carcinoma of the thyroid. Fine needle aspiration findings in a case. Acta Cytol 1990; 34:355–358.
104. Akslen LA, Varhaug JE. Thyroid carcinoma with mixed tall-cell and columnar-cell features. Am J Clin Pathol 1990; 94:442–445.
105. Caplan R, Wester K, Kisken W. Diffuse sclerosing variant of papillary thyroid carcinoma of the thyroid: fine needle aspiration findings in a case. Endocr Pract 1997; 3:287–292.
106. Chan JK, Tsui MS, Tse CH. Diffuse sclerosing variant of papillary carcinoma of the thyroid: a histological and immunohistochemical study of three cases. Histopathology 1987; 11:191–201.
107. Soares J, Limbert E, Sobrinho-Simoes M. Diffuse sclerosing variant of papillary thyroid carcinoma. A clinicopathologic study of 10 cases. Pathol Res Pract 1989; 185:200–206.
108. Wu PS, Leslie PJ, McLaren KM, Toft AD. Diffuse sclerosing papillary carcinoma of thyroid: a wolf in sheep's clothing. Clin Endocrinol (Oxf) 1989; 31:535–540.

109. Carcangiu ML, Bianchi S. Diffuse sclerosing variant of papillary thyroid carcinoma. Clinicopathologic study of 15 cases. Am J Surg Pathol 1989; 13:1041–1049.
110. Fujimoto Y, Obara T, Ito Y, et al. Diffuse sclerosing variant of papillary carcinoma of the thyroid. Clinical importance, surgical treatment, and follow-up study. Cancer 1990; 66:2306–2312.
111. Hayashi Y, Sasao T, Takeichi N, et al. Diffuse sclerosing variant of papillary carcinoma of the thyroid. A histopathological study of four cases. Acta Pathol Jpn 1990; 40:193–198.
112. Mizukami Y, Nonomura A, Michigishi T, et al. Diffuse sclerosing variant of papillary carcinoma of the thyroid. Report of three cases. Acta Pathol Jpn 1990; 40:676–682.
113. Furmanchuk AW, Averkin JI, Egloff B, et al. Pathomorphological findings in thyroid cancers of children from the Republic of Belarus: a study of 86 cases occurring between 1986 ('post-Chernobyl') and 1991. Histopathology 1992; 21:401–408.
114. Nikiforov YE, Erickson LA, Nikiforova MN, et al. Solid variant of papillary thyroid carcinoma: incidence, clinical-pathologic characteristics, molecular analysis, and biologic behavior. Am J Surg Pathol 2001; 25:1478–1484.
115. Klugbauer S, Lengfelder E, Demidchik EP, Rabes HM. High prevalence of RET rearrangement in thyroid tumors of children from Belarus after the Chernobyl reactor accident. Oncogene 1995; 11:2459–2467.
116. Nikiforov YE, Rowland JM, Bove KE, et al. Distinct pattern of ret oncogene rearrangements in morphological variants of radiation-induced and sporadic thyroid papillary carcinomas in children. Cancer Res 1997; 57:1690–1694.
117. Papotti M, Negro F, Carney JA, et al. Mixed medullary-follicular carcinoma of the thyroid. A morphological, immunohistochemical and in situ hybridization analysis of 11 cases. Virchows Arch 1997; 430:397–405.
118. Hales M, Rosenau W, Okerlund MD, Galante M. Carcinoma of the thyroid with a mixed medullary and follicular pattern: morphologic, immunohistochemical, and clinical laboratory studies. Cancer 1982; 50:1352–1359.
119. Kashima K, Yokoyama S, Inoue S, et al. Mixed medullary and follicular carcinoma of the thyroid: report of two cases with an immunohistochemical study. Acta Pathol Jpn 1993; 43:428–433.
120. Ljungberg O, Ericsson UB, Bondeson L, Thorell J. A compound follicular-parafollicular cell carcinoma of the thyroid: a new tumor entity? Cancer 1983; 52:1053–1061.
121. Mizukami Y, Michigishi T, Nonomura A, et al. Mixed medullary-follicular carcinoma of the thyroid occurring in familial form. Histopathology 1993; 22:284–287.
122. Tanaka T, Yoshimi N, Kanai N, et al. Simultaneous occurrence of medullary and follicular carcinoma in the same thyroid lobe. Hum Pathol 1989; 20:83–86.
123. Tanda F, Massarelli G, Minggloni V, et al. Mixed follicular-parafollicular carcinoma of the thyroid: a light, elctron microscopic and histoimmunologic study. Surg Path 1990; 3:65–74.
124. Papotti M, Volante M, Komminoth P, et al. Thyroid carcinomas with mixed follicular and C-cell differentiation patterns. Semin Diagn Pathol 2000; 17:109–119.
125. Lamberg BA, Reissel P, Stenman S, et al. Concurrent medullary and papillary thyroid carcinoma in the same thyroid lobe and in siblings. Acta Med Scand 1981; 209:421–424.
126. Lax SF, Beham A, Kronberger-Schonecker D, et al. Coexistence of papillary and medullary carcinoma of the thyroid gland-mixed or collision tumour? Clinicopathological analysis of three cases. Virchows Arch 1994; 424:441–447.
127. Pastolero GC, Coire CI, Asa SL. Concurrent medullary and papillary carcinomas of thyroid with lymph node metastases. A collision phenomenon. Am J Surg Pathol 1996; 20:245–250.
128. Duskova J, Janotova D, Svobodova E, et al. Fine needle aspiration biopsy of mixed medullary-follicular thyroid carcinoma. A report of two cases. Acta Cytol 2003; 47:71–77.
129. Wenig BM, Adair CF, Heffess CS. Primary mucoepidermoid carcinoma of the thyroid gland: a report of six cases and a review of the literature of a follicular epithelial-derived tumor. Hum Pathol 1995; 26: 1099–1108.
130. Rhatigan RM, Roque JL, Bucher RL. Mucoepidermoid carcinoma of the thyroid gland. Cancer 1977; 39:210–214.
131. Rocha AS, Soares P, Machado JC, et al. Mucoepidermoid carcinoma of the thyroid: a tumour histotype characterised by P-cadherin neoexpression and marked abnormalities of E-cadherin/catenins complex. Virchows Arch 2002; 440:498–504.
132. Cameselle-Teijeiro J, Febles-Perez C, Sobrinho-Simoes M. Cytologic features of fine needle aspirates of papillary and mucoepidermoid carcinoma of the thyroid with anaplastic transformation. A case report. Acta Cytol 1997; 41:1356–1360.
133. Cameselle-Teijeiro J, Chan JK. Cribriform-morular variant of papillary carcinoma: a distinctive variant representing the sporadic counterpart of familial adenomatous polyposis-associated thyroid carcinoma? Mod Pathol 1999; 12:400–411.
134. Cameselle-Teijeiro J, Febles-Perez C, Sobrinho-Simoes M. Papillary and mucoepidermoid carcinoma of the thyroid with anaplastic transformation: a case report with histologic and immunohistochemical findings that support a provocative histogenetic hypothesis. Pathol Res Pract 1995; 191:1214–1221.
135. Franssila KO, Harach HR, Wasenius VM. Mucoepidermoid carcinoma of the thyroid. Histopathology 1984; 8:847–860.
136. Chan JK, Albores-Saavedra J, Battifora H, et al. Sclerosing mucoepidermoid thyroid carcinoma with eosinophilia. A distinctive low-grade malignancy arising from the metaplastic follicles of Hashimoto's thyroiditis. Am J Surg Pathol 1991; 15:438–448.
137. Katoh R, Sugai T, Ono S, et al. Mucoepidermoid carcinoma of the thyroid gland. Cancer 1990; 65:2020–2027.
138. Thompson LD, Wenig BM, Adair CF, et al. Primary smooth muscle tumors of the thyroid gland. Cancer 1997; 79:579–587.
139. Kawahara E, Nakanishi I, Terahata S, Ikegaki S. Leiomyosarcoma of the thyroid gland. A case report with a comparative study of five cases of anaplastic carcinoma. Cancer 1988; 62:2558–2563.
140. Chetty R, Clark SP, Dowling JP. Leiomyosarcoma of the thyroid: immunohistochemical and ultrastructural study. Pathology 1993; 25:203–205.
141. Iida Y, Katoh R, Yoshioka M, et al. Primary leiomyosarcoma of the thyroid gland. Acta Pathol Jpn 1993; 43:71–75.
142. Lindahl F. Sarcoma of the thyroid gland: twenty-two cases in Denmark 1943–1968. Dan Med Bull 1976; 23:103–107.
143. Syrjanen KJ. An osteogenic sarcoma of the thyroid gland (report of a case and survey of the literature). Neoplasma 1979; 26:623–638.
144. Griem KL, Robb PK, Caldarelli DD, Templeton AC. Radiation-induced sarcoma of the thyroid. Arch Otolaryngol Head Neck Surg 1989; 115:991–993.
145. Mills SE, Gaffey MJ, Watts JC, et al. Angiomatoid carcinoma and 'angiosarcoma' of the thyroid gland. A spectrum of endothelial differentiation. Am J Clin Pathol 1994; 102:322–330.
146. Lamovec J, Zidar A, Zidanik B. Epithelioid angiosarcoma of the thyroid gland. Report of two cases. Arch Pathol Lab Med 1994; 118: 642–646.
147. Chan YF, Ma L, Boey JH, Yeung HY. Angiosarcoma of the thyroid. An immunohistochemical and ultrastructural study of a case in a Chinese patient. Cancer 1986; 57:2381–2388.
148. Mollison LC, Mijch A, McBride G, Dwyer B. Hypothyroidism due to destruction of the thyroid by Kaposi's sarcoma. Rev Infect Dis 1991; 13:826–827.
149. Mills SE, Stallings RG, Austin MB. Angiomatoid carcinoma of the thyroid gland. Anaplastic carcinoma with follicular and medullary features mimicking angiosarcoma. Am J Clin Pathol 1986; 86:674–678.
150. Merimsky O, Issakov J, Kollender Y, et al. Sarcoma and thyroid disorders: a common etiology? Oncol Rep 2002; 9:863–869.

151. Buckley NJ, Burch WM, Leight GS. Malignant teratoma in the thyroid gland of an adult: a case report and a review of the literature. Surgery 1986; 100:932–937.
152. Bowker CM, Whittaker RS. Malignant teratoma of the thyroid: case report and literature review of thyroid teratoma in adults. Histopathology 1992; 21:81–83.
153. Stone HH, Henderson WD, Guidio FA. Teratomas of the neck. Am J Dis Child 1967; 113:222–224.
154. Buckwalter JA, Layton JM. Malignant teratoma in the thyroid gland of an adult. Ann Surg 1954; 139:218–223.
155. Kimler SC, Muth WF. Primary malignant teratoma of the thyroid: case report and literature review of cervical teratomas in adults. Cancer 1978; 42:311–317.
156. Hajdu SI, Hajdu EO. Malignant teratoma of the neck. Arch Pathol 1967; 83:567–570.
157. O'Higgins N, Taylor S. Malignant teratoma in the adult thyroid gland. Br J Clin Pract 1975; 29:237–238.
158. Andrion A, Bellis D, Delsedime L, et al. Leiomyoma and neurilemoma: report of two unusual non-epithelial tumours of the thyroid gland. Virchows Arch A Pathol Anat Histopathol 1988; 413:367–372.
159. Hendrick JW. Leiomyoma of thyroid gland; report of case. Surgery 1957; 42:597–599.
160. Delaney WE, Fry KE. Neurilemoma of the thyroid gland. Ann Surg 1964; 160:1014–1017.
161. Goldstein J, Tovi F, Sidi J. Primary schwannoma of the thyroid gland. Int Surg 1982; 67:433–434.
162. Mahoney CP, Patterson SD, Ryan J. Granular cell tumor of the thyroid gland in a girl receiving high-dose estrogen therapy. Pediatr Pathol Lab Med 1995; 15:791–795.
163. Carney JA, Ryan J, Goellner JR. Hyalinizing trabecular adenoma of the thyroid gland. Am J Surg Pathol 1987; 11:583–591.
164. Sambade C, Franssila K, Carmeselle-Teijero, et al. Hyalinizing trabecular adenoma: a misnomer for a peculiar tumor of the thyroid gland. Endocr Pathol 1991; 2:83–91.
165. Goellner JR, Carney JA. Cytologic features of fine-needle aspirates of hyalinizing trabecular adenoma of the thyroid. Am J Clin Pathol 1989; 91:115–119.
166. Bondeson L, Bondeson AG. Clue helping to distinguish hyalinizing trabecular adenoma from carcinoma of the thyroid in fine-needle aspirates. Diagn Cytopathol 1994; 10:25–29.
167. Chan JK, Tse CC, Chiu HS. Hyalinizing trabecular adenoma-like lesion in multinodular goitre. Histopathology 1990; 16:611–614.
168. Chan JK, Loo KT. Cribriform variant of papillary thyroid carcinoma. Arch Pathol Lab Med 1990; 114:622–624.
169. Russell WO, Ibanez ML, Clark RL, White EC. Thyroid carcinoma. Classification, intraglandular dissemination, and clinicopathological study based upon whole organ sections of 80 glands. Cancer 1963; 16: 1425–1460.
170. LiVolsi V. Branchial and thymic remnants in the thyroid gland and cervical region: an explanation for unusual tumors and microscopic curiosities. Endocr Pathol 1993; 4:115–119.
171. Mizukami Y, Nonomura A, Michigishi T, et al. Ectopic thymic tissue in the thyroid gland. Endocr Pathol 1993; 4:162–164.
172. Harach HR, Saravia Day E, Franssila KO. Thyroid spindle-cell tumor with mucous cysts. An intrathyroid thymoma? Am J Surg Pathol 1985; 9:525–530.
173. Chan JK, Rosai J. Tumors of the neck showing thymic or related branchial pouch differentiation: a unifying concept. Hum Pathol 1991; 22:349–367.
174. Mizukami Y, Kurumaya H, Yamada T, et al. Thymic carcinoma involving the thyroid gland: report of two cases. Hum Pathol 1995; 26: 576–579.
175. Shek TW, Luk IS, Ng IO, Lo CY. Lymphoepithelioma-like carcinoma of the thyroid gland: lack of evidence of association with Epstein-Barr virus. Hum Pathol 1996; 27:851–853.
176. Pollock WF, Stevenson EO. Cysts and sinuses of the thyroglossal duct. Am J Surg 1966; 112:225–232.
177. Jaques DA, Chambers RG, Oertel JE. Thyroglossal tract carcinoma. A review of the literature and addition of eighteen cases. Am J Surg 1970; 120:439–446.
178. LiVolsi VA, Perzin KH, Savetsky L. Carcinoma arising in median ectopic thyroid (including thyroglossal duct tissue). Cancer 1974; 34: 1303–1315.
179. Heshmati HM, Fatourechi V, van Heerden JA, et al. Thyroglossal duct carcinoma: report of 12 cases. Mayo Clin Proc 1997; 72: 315–319.
180. Tew S, Reeve TS, Poole AG, Delbridge L. Papillary thyroid carcinoma arising in thyroglossal duct cysts: incidence and management. Aust N Z J Surg 1995; 65:717–718.
181. Mahnke CG, Janig U, Werner JA, Rudert H. Primary papillary carcinoma of the thyroglossal duct: case report and review of the literature. Auris Nasus Larynx 1994; 21:258–263.
182. Kwan WB, Liu FF, Banerjee D, et al. Concurrent papillary and squamous carcinoma in a thyroglossal duct cyst: a case report. Can J Surg 1996; 39:328–332.
183. Udoji WC. Thyroglossal duct cyst mass with Hashimoto's disease and non-Hodgkin's lymphoma. J Tenn Med Assoc 1996; 89:113–114.
184. Deshpande A, Bobhate SK. Squamous cell carcinoma in thyroglossal duct cyst. J Laryngol Otol 1995; 109:1001–1004.
185. Czech JM, Lichtor TR, Carney JA, van Heerden JA. Neoplasms metastatic to the thyroid gland. Surg Gynecol Obstet 1982; 155: 503–505.
186. Nakhjavani MK, Gharib H, Goellner JR, van Heerden JA. Metastasis to the thyroid gland. A report of 43 cases. Cancer 1997; 79:574–578.
187. Giuffrida D, Ferrau F, Pappalardo A, et al. Metastasis to the thyroid gland: a case report and review of the literature. J Endocrinol Invest 2003; 26:560–563.
188. Marallie E, Rigaud J, Mathonnet M, et al. Management and prognosis of metastases to the thyroid gland. J Am Coll Surg 2005; 200:203–207.
189. Miyakawa M, Sato K, Hasegawa M, et al. Severe thyrotoxicosis induced by thyroid metastasis of lung adenocarcinoma: a case report and review of the literature. Thyroid 2001; 11:883–888.

66
Pathology of Miscellaneous and Unusual Cancers of the Thyroid

James E. Oertel and Yolanda C. Oertel

METASTATIC (SECONDARY) NEOPLASMS

The most common metastatic neoplasms in the gland that may mimic primary tumors are those from the lung, breast, and kidney (1,2). These neoplasms have the usual range of histological patterns, depending on the primary sites. Involvement of an existing adenomatoid nodule or adenoma is likely, thereby complicating the morphological features. Immunohistochemical procedures are helpful in separating metastatic lesions from primary thyroid neoplasms when uncertainty exists with the interpretation. Data and materials must be evaluated carefully, however, because some nonspecific uptake of thyroglobulin may occur by the metastatic cells. Malignant melanoma involves the thyroid with moderate frequency, but the patient's clinical history allows this metastasis to be somewhat easy to diagnose.

Squamous Cell Carcinoma, Adenosquamous Carcinoma, and Mucin-Producing Carcinoma

These rare aggressive neoplasms usually occur in middle-aged or elderly patients, often in glands containing a well-differentiated carcinoma (especially papillary carcinoma), an adenoma, a multinodular goiter, or occasionally, chronic autoimmune thyroiditis (1,3,4). Because of the intimate relationship to neoplastic glandular elements, some squamous cancers have been called "adenosquamous carcinomas." Undifferentiated carcinoma may be evident, along with the predominant squamous carcinoma (5). Squamous carcinoma with extensive spindled cell change has been reported in association with tall-cell papillary carcinoma (6). An occasional squamous carcinoma of the thyroid has been linked with hypercalcemia and leukocytosis (7).

Mucin-producing carcinoma has been related to squamous carcinoma (1,8). The presence of mucosubstances in the thyroid is a complex problem, and uncertainty about such neoplasms continues (9,10).

Bland focal squamous metaplasia may occur in both follicular and papillary carcinomas, but usually this does not behave as squamous carcinoma.

Poorly Differentiated Carcinoma

Poorly differentiated carcinoma is proposed to include carcinomas of follicular thyroid epithelium that retain sufficient differentiation to produce small scattered follicular structures and thyroglobulin. However, this cancer type generally lacks the usual morphologic characteristics of papillary and follicular carcinoma (11–14). Instead, the histological patterns are described as solid, insular (islands of cells separated by connective tissue and artifactual spaces), trabecular, and alveolar (Fig. 1), with tiny scattered follicles containing colloid (Fig. 2) within the solid, insular, and trabecular regions. These patterns may mix with each other, and small foci of characteristic follicular and papillary carcinoma may also be found, even both within the same neoplasm. The Bcl-2 protein (a suppressor of apoptosis) has been described in a large proportion of these tumors, unlike undifferentiated carcinoma (15).

Much of the cancer may be composed of small, uniform cells with pale, scanty cytoplasm and small, spherical nuclei with uniformly dark, finely clumped chromatin (Fig. 2). Nuclear contours are smooth. These have been labeled "primordial cells" because of their resemblance to fetal thyroid cells (14). PAS-positive globules of thyroglobulin may lie next to the nuclei. Such cells may encompass a large proportion of the neoplasm. In addition, medium-sized to large cells with more varied nuclei may be present and may dominate some parts; their cytoplasm can be eosinophilic or clear. Although most of their nuclei are regular and round with smooth contours, some are spindled or large and pleomorphic. Such irregular cells are isolated, not present as regions of anaplastic carcinoma. Oxyphilic

From: *Thyroid Cancer: A Comprehensive Guide to Clinical Management, 2/e*
Edited by: L. Wartofsky and D. Van Nostrand © Humana Press Inc., Totowa, NJ

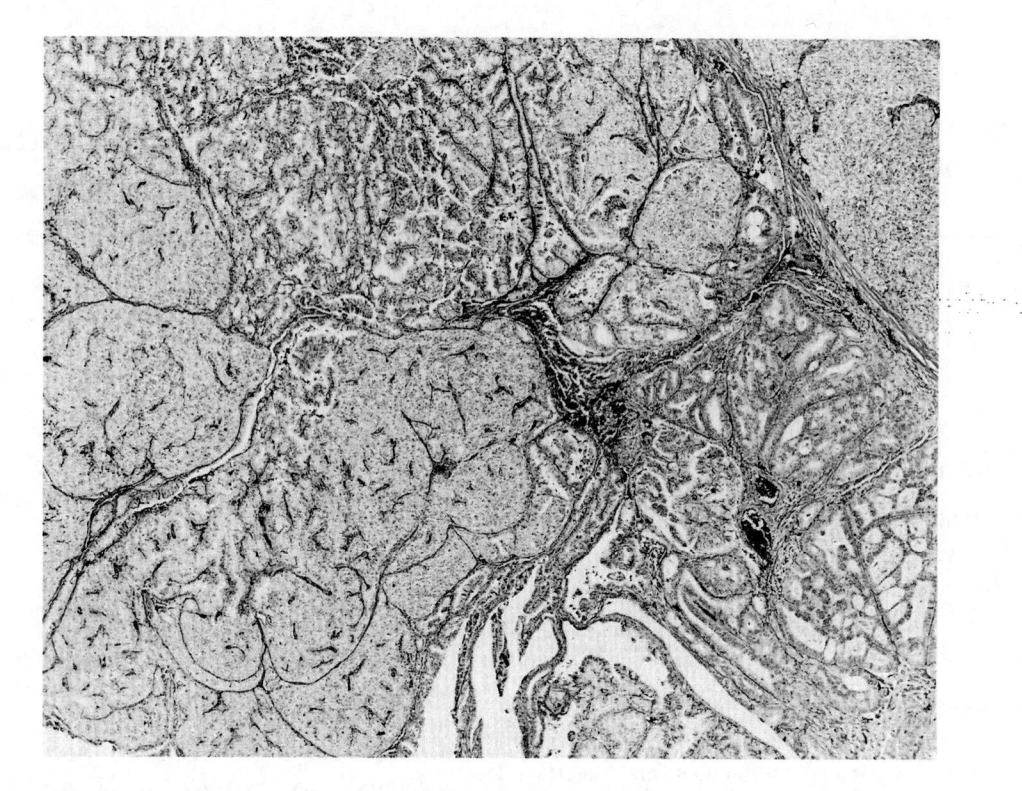

Fig. 1. Poorly differentiated carcinoma. Both insular and cribriform patterns are evident (hematoxylin and eosin [H&E] stain).

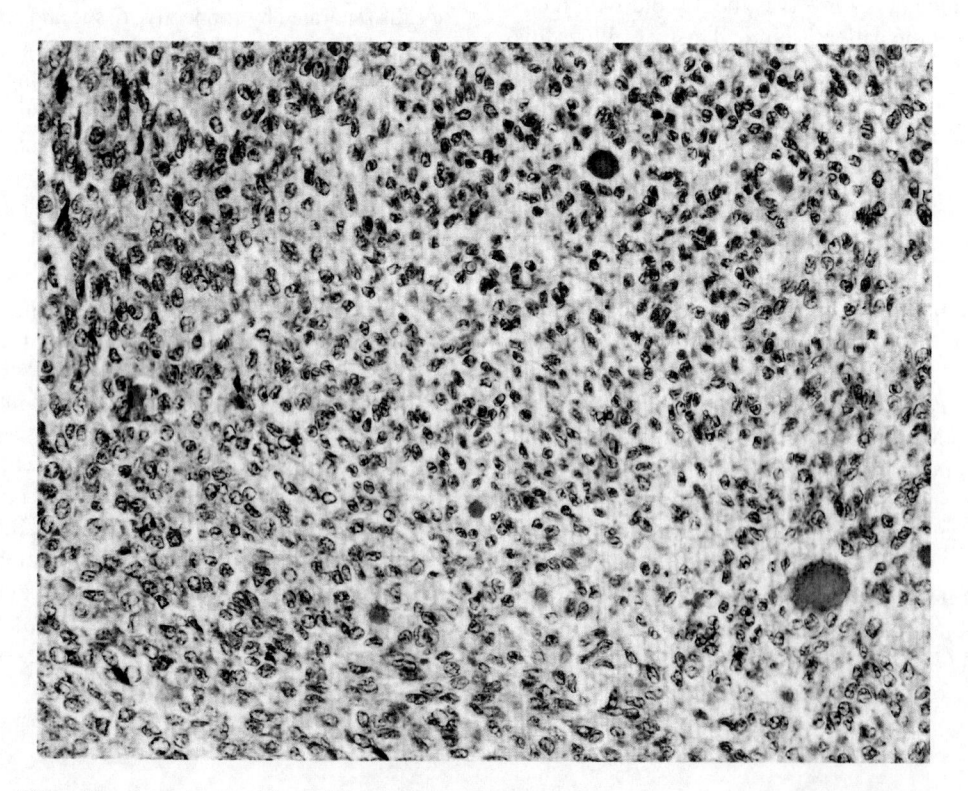

Fig. 2. Poorly differentiated carcinoma. The solid part has small- to medium-sized cells. Two small follicles are filled with dense colloid (H&E stain).

cell variants have been described *(16)*. In both small-cell and large-cell regions, necrosis may be present, either as large fields or as tiny foci (especially within the insular parts). Preservation of the neoplastic cells next to vessels in the regions of necrosis may cause a "peritheliomatous" pattern. Mitotic figures vary in number. Usually, nucleoli are tiny, but a few tumors have been described with conspicuous nucleoli. Most of the nuclei of these tumors are rounded and have rather evenly distributed heterochromatin (thereby resembling those of follicular carcinoma), but some portions of these tumors may contain nuclei that resemble those of papillary carcinoma.

Poorly differentiated carcinoma has been considered a controversial entity because of the varied histologic patterns present and the evidence of well-differentiated papillary or follicular carcinoma that can be found as small portions of most of these neoplasms. This is understandable but does not account for the presence of primordial cells in many of these neoplasms and the fact that they share many characteristics different from both well-differentiated and anaplastic cancers *(17)*.

We do not have much experience with the cytological appearance of these neoplasms. Reports *(18–20)* indicate that the smears are markedly cellular, with the cells in loose clusters, small sheets, or large sheets. Little colloid is evident, and necrosis and hemorrhage are common in the background. Microfollicles, rosettes, trabeculae, and papillae have been noted. Single cells may be present. The cells usually have scant, poorly defined cytoplasm and darkly stained, rounded nuclei. Nuclear grooves may be seen, and there are occasional intranuclear cytoplasmic inclusions. Nuclear overlapping can occur.

Angiosarcoma

This neoplasm has been regarded as rare, even in endemic goiter regions *(21,22)*; several tumors with histological features consistent with angiosarcoma have expressed immunoreactive keratins, as well as endothelial features (e.g., factor VIII-associated antigens and Weibel-Palade bodies). Authors have suggested that some of these neoplasms might be considered as angiomatoid carcinomas (a form of undifferentiated or anaplastic carcinoma; *23*), expressing epithelial markers and endothelial characteristics. Most patients are middle-aged or elderly, and most tumors are extremely aggressive, similar to typical anaplastic carcinomas.

Leiomyosarcoma

Leiomyosarcoma has been reported but is extremely rare. A characteristic histological pattern is not only required, but immunohistochemical and ultrastructural techniques are also needed to separate leiomyosarcoma from anaplastic carcinoma *(24)*.

Thyroglossal Duct Cancer

Nearly all the tumors arise in the thyroid tissue that accompanies the duct or cyst *(25,26)*. Most are papillary carcinomas *(26,27)*, a few are follicular carcinomas *(28)*, and an anaplastic carcinoma is rarely present *(29)*. Squamous carcinoma has been documented *(30)*, presumably arising from the respiratory epithelium of the thyroglossal duct or cyst.

Fine-needle aspiration is useful in diagnosing thyroglossal abnormalities *(31)*. If the aspirate consists of more than the usual hypocellular specimen from a cyst, then the standard criteria are applied for recognizing thyroid tumors.

Hyalinizing Trabecular Neoplasms

These rare neoplasms are solid masses, often less than 3 cm in diameter, and are well-circumscribed (usually encapsulated; *32,33*). The cut surfaces are light-colored, and vessels and small foci of fibrosis may be visible. Microscopically, the tumors consist of trabeculae and lobules of elongated, oval, or polygonal cells, usually medium-sized and with poorly defined borders. The groups of cells are surrounded by capillaries and variable amounts of eosinophilic, hyalinized material, which consists of clumps of type IV collagen and laminin. The numerous cytoplasmic microfilaments (presumably keratin) present in many of the epithelial cells also contribute to the eosinophilic zones.

The neoplastic cells have been described as eosinophilic, amphophilic, or clear with fine granules apparent in the cytoplasm. Nuclei appear rounded, oval, or elongated and often grooved. They may contain cytoplasmic inclusions and clear zones; in turn, these zones contain tiny rods composed of bundles of minute filaments (visible on electron microscopy; *34*). Variable numbers of small follicles occur in the trabeculae, some with colloid and some empty. Electron microscopy shows intercellular spaces surrounded by microvilli, presumably representing developing follicles. Psammoma bodies may be scattered throughout the tumor. Most cells contain immunoreactive thyroglobulin and keratin; calcitonin has never been demonstrated. Rarely, the tumors have been invasive and involved cervical lymph nodes. An alteration similar to this hyalinizing tumor has been described in the adenomatoid nodules of a nodular goiter *(34)*.

Aspirates of these lesions have been misinterpreted as follicular neoplasms, papillary carcinomas, and medullary carcinomas *(35)*. Moderate-to-marked cellularity is evident, with the cells forming clusters and follicles. Colloid is not present, but irregular masses of hyaline material are adjacent to the cell clusters. This material has been described

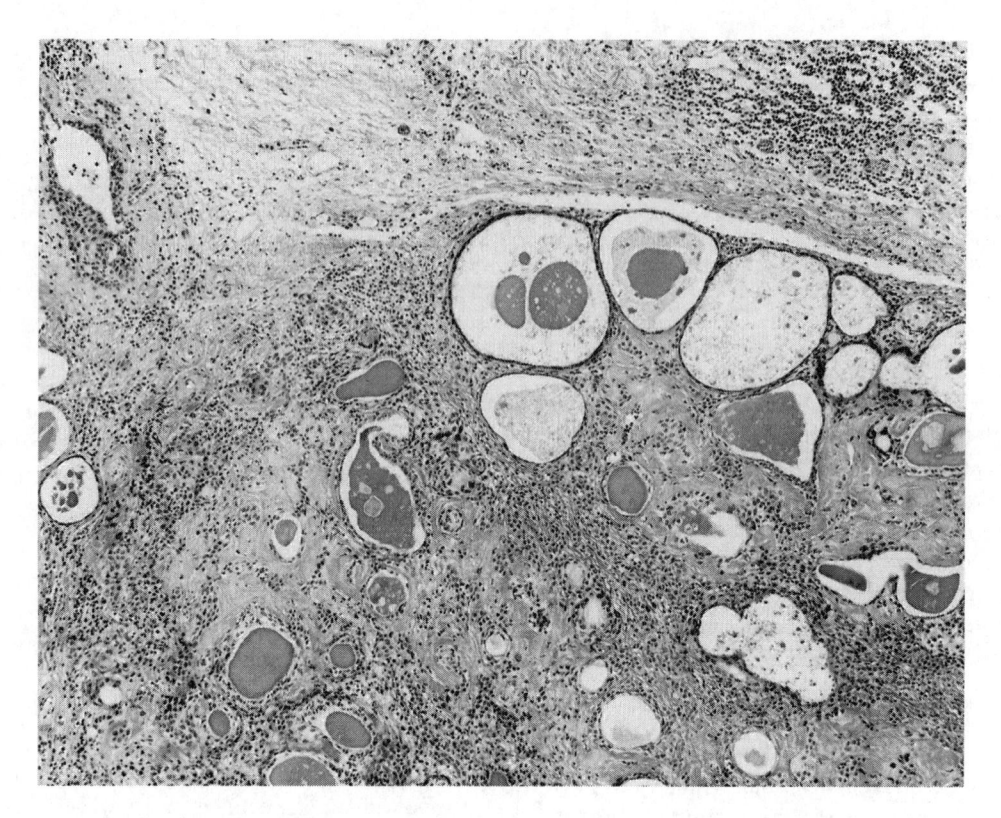

Fig. 3. Mucoepidermoid carcinoma. Dilated cystic spaces are visible (H&E stain).

with fringed or granular margins and a suggestion of a fibrillary structure. It is purple-red or magenta with May-Grunwald Giemsa stain *(36)* and pink to gray-blue with Papanicolaou stain *(35)*. Cells are rounded, polygonal, or elongated with cytoplasm of diverse density. Nuclei often contain grooves (in Papanicolaou-stained material) and cytoplasmic inclusions. Small psammoma bodies have been seen in some cases.

Neoplasms Associated with Familial Intestinal Adenomatous Polyposis

These rare neoplasms have trabecular, solid, papillary, and cribriform patterns that are formed by spindled, polygonal, and tall columnar cells and are different from the usual papillary and follicular carcinomas *(37–39)*. Small whorls of cells may be found, but these are not squamous foci. Cytoplasm is oxyphilic to amphophilic, sometimes clear. Nuclei are hyperchromatic, slightly irregular, and medium-sized; nucleoli vary in size and visibility. Cytoplasmic inclusions in the nuclei vary in number and size, and some nuclear grooves may be seen. Focal positivity for thyroglobulin can be found, but colloid is present in minimal amounts or absent.

These neoplasms are usually small and multiple, and the majority have occurred in girls and young women.

Mucoepidermoid Carcinoma

These neoplasms are rare, occur mostly in women, are usually of a low grade of malignancy, and can be associated with papillary carcinoma (or even present as a metaplastic focus in a papillary carcinoma; *40–43*). An associated undifferentiated (anaplastic) carcinoma has been reported *(44)*. Mucoepidermoid carcinomas are typically solid, firm, light-colored masses, not encapsulated, sometimes cystic, and can have mucus visible on the cut surfaces.

Microscopic examination reveals islands of epithelial cells anastomosing with each other. The cells also form pseudovascular and cribriform patterns, as well as irregular glandular spaces (Fig. 3). Mucous cells are scattered among the numerous cells with squamous characteristics. Many mucous cells line the glands and ducts. Squamous cells have diverse cytoplasm, ranging from pale to eosinophilic; some are keratinized. Keratin pearls may be present (Fig. 4), and some groups of cells have intercellular bridges by light microscopy. Mucous cells have pale, foamy, or granular cytoplasm, and intermediate forms between squamous and mucous cells may be recognized. Nuclei are round or ovoid, medium-sized, generally regular (occasionally atypical), and some contain grooves and cytoplasmic inclusions. Central nucleoli vary from incon-

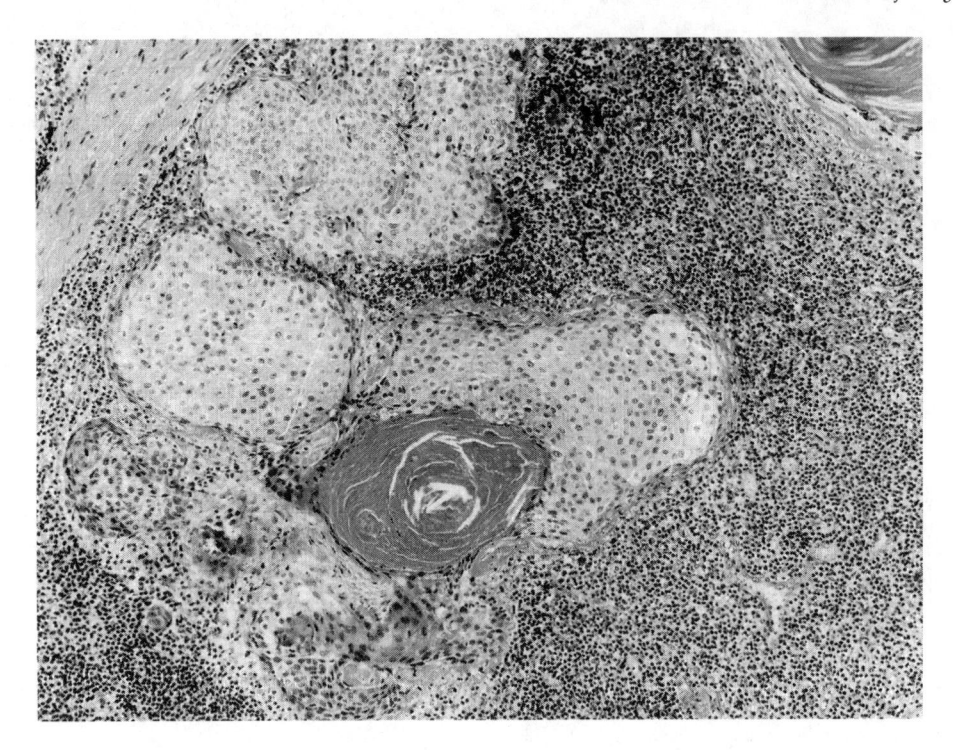

Fig. 4. Mucoepidermoid carcinoma. Nests of squamous cells and two keratin pearls lie in a heavy infiltrate of lymphocytes (H&E stain).

spicuous to large. Mitotic figures vary in number, depending on the case. Some cells have been reported to contain thyroglobulin *(41)*, but many do not *(42)*. Virtually all cells contain keratins. Ciliated cells may line the spaces, and within the spaces are colloid-like PAS-positive material, sulfated mucus-stained with Alcian blue and mucicarmine, along with cellular debris. Small PAS-positive hyaline bodies may be found in the nests and cords of cells. Psammoma bodies may occur *(41)*. Fibrous stroma (often dense) is present, and the tumor may be infiltrated by lymphocytes and both neutrophilic and eosinophilic granulocytes. Lymphocytic thyroiditis is usually present in the remainder of the thyroid gland. Metastases to lymph nodes in the neck have been reported.

Thymic and Related Neoplasms

Thymic, parathyroid, and salivary gland tissues may be found in the thyroid *(45–47)*; therefore, it is not surprising that occasional neoplasms occur in the thyroid and inferior part of the neck that resemble the thymus *(48–51)*. Such tumors may be benign or malignant.

Teratoma

Benign teratomas in newborns and infants may cause various obstruction phenomena, especially when cystic, and must be resected promptly. They do not recur or spread *(52)*.

Malignant teratomas have been seen in adults and are composed of primitive epithelial, mesenchymal, and neurectodermal elements *(53,54)*. They spread locally and may have metastases.

REFERENCES

1. Rosai J, Carcangiu ML, DeLellis RA. Tumors of the thyroid gland. In Rosai J, Sobin LH, editors. Atlas of Tumor Pathology, 3rd Ser, Fasc 5. Washington, DC: A. F. I. P., 1992.
2. Nakhjavani MK, Gharib H, Goellner JR, van Heerden JA. Metastasis to the thyroid gland: a report of 43 cases. Cancer 1997; 79: 574–578.
3. Huang T-Y, Assor D. Primary squamous cell carcinoma of the thyroid gland: a report of four cases. Am J Clin Pathol 1971; 55:93–98.
4. Harada T, Shimaoka K, Yakumaru K, Ito K. Squamous cell carcinoma of the thyroid gland: Transition from adenocarcinoma. J Surg Oncol 1982; 19:36–43.
5. Harada T, Ito K, Shimaoka K, et al. Fatal thyroid carcinoma. Anaplastic transformation of adenocarcinoma. Cancer 1977; 39: 2588–2596.
6. Bronner MP, LiVolsi VA. Spindle cell squamous carcinoma of the thyroid: an unusual anaplastic tumor associated with tall cell papillary cancer. Mod Pathol 1991; 4:637–643.
7. Riddle PE, Dincsoy HP. Primary squamous cell carcinoma of the thyroid associated with leukocytosis and hypercalcemia. Arch Pathol Lab Med 1987; 111:373–374.
8. LiVolsi VA. Surgical pathology of the thyroid. Major Probl Pathol 1990; 22:253–274.
9. Gherardi G. Signet ring cell 'mucinous' thyroid adenoma: a follicle cell tumour with abnormal accumulation of thyroglobulin

and a peculiar histochemical profile. Histopathology 1987; 11: 317–326.
10. Rigaud C, Bogomoletz WV. "Mucin secreting" and "mucinous" primary thyroid carcinomas: pitfalls in mucin histochemistry applied to thyroid tumours. J Clin Pathol 1987; 40:890–895.
11. Volante M, Landolfi S, Chiusa L, et al. Poorly differentiated carcinoma of the thyroid with trabecular, insular, and solid patterns. A clinicopathologic study of 183 patients. Cancer 2004; 100: 950–957.
12. Carcangiu ML, Zampi G, Rosai J. Poorly differentiated ("insular") thyroid carcinoma: a reinterpretation of Langhans' "wuchernde Struma." Am J Surg Pathol 1984; 655–668.
13. Hwang TS, Suh JS, Kim YI, et al. Poorly differentiated carcinoma of the thyroid: retrospective clinical and morphologic evaluation. J Korean Med Sci 1990; 5:47–52.
14. Papotti M, Botto Micca F, Pavero A, et al. Poorly differentiated thyroid carcinomas with primordial cell component: a group of aggressive lesions sharing insular, trabecular, and solid patterns. Am J Surg Pathol 1993; 17:291–301.
15. Pilotti S, Collini P, Del Bo R, et al. A novel panel of antibodies that segregates immunocytochemically poorly differentiated carcinoma from undifferentiated carcinoma of the thyroid gland. Am J Surg Pathol 1994; 18:1054–1064.
16. Papotti M, Torchio B, Grassi L, et al. Poorly differentiated oxyphilic (Hürthle cell) carcinomas of the thyroid. Am J Surg Pathol 1996; 20: 686–694.
17. Sobrinho-Simoes M. Poorly differentiated carcinomas of the thyroid. Endocr Pathol 1996; 7:99–102.
18. Pietribiasi F, Sapino A, Papotti M, Bussolati G. Cytologic features of poorly differentiated "insular" carcinoma of the thyroid, as revealed by fine-needle aspiration biopsy. Am J Clin Pathol 1990; 94: 687–692.
19. Sironi M, Collini P, Cantaboni A. Fine needle aspiration cytology of insular thyroid carcinoma: a report of four cases. Acta Cytol 1992; 36:435–439.
20. Pereira EM, Maeda SA, Alves F, Schmitt FC. Poorly differentiated carcinoma (insular carcinoma) of the thyroid diagnosed by fine needle aspiration (FNA). Cytopathology 1996; 7:61–65.
21. Rys̆ka A, Ludvíková M, Szépe P, Böör A. Epithelioid hemangiosarcoma of the thyroid gland. Report of six cases from a non-Alpine region. Histopathology 2004; 44:40–46.
22. Tötsch M, Dobler G, Feichtinger H, et al. Malignant hemangioendothelioma of the thyroid: its immunohistochemical discrimination from undifferentiated thyroid carcinoma. Am J Surg Pathol 1990; 14: 69–74.
23. Mills SE, Gaffey MJ, Watts JC, et al. Angiomatoid carcinoma and "angiosarcoma" of the thyroid gland: a spectrum of endothelial differentiation. Am J Clin Pathol 1994; 102:322–330.
24. Iida Y, Katoh R, Yoshioka M, et al. Primary leiomyosarcoma of the thyroid gland. Acta Pathol Jpn 1993; 43:71–75.
25. Ellis PDM, van Nostrand AWP. The applied anatomy of thyroglossal tract remnants. Laryngoscope 1977; 87:765–770.
26. LiVolsi VA, Perzin KH, Savetsky L. Carcinoma arising in median ectopic thyroid (including thyroglossal duct tissue). Cancer 1974; 34: 1303–1315.
27. Jaques DA, Chambers RG, Oertel JE. Thyroglossal tract carcinoma: a review of the literature and addition of eighteen cases. Am J Surg 1970; 120:439–446.
28. Case WG, Ausobsky J, Smiddy FG, High AS. Primary follicular adenocarcinoma arising in the thyroglossal tract. J R Coll Surg Edinb 1987; 32:250–251.
29. Woods RH, Saunders Jr JR, Pearlman S, et al. Anaplastic carcinoma arising in a thyroglossal duct tract. Otolaryngol Head Neck Surg 1993; 109:945–949.
30. Deshpande A, Bobhate SK. Squamous cell carcinoma in thyroglossal duct cyst. J Laryngol Otol 1995; 109:1001–1004.
31. Shaffer MM, Oertel YC, Oertel JE. Thyroglossal duct cysts: diagnostic criteria by fine-needle aspiration. Arch Pathol Lab Med 1996; 120: 1039–1043.
32. Carney JA, Ryan J, Goellner JR. Hyalinizing trabecular adenoma of the thyroid gland. Am J Surg Pathol 1987; 11:583–591.
33. Sambade C, Franssila K, Cameselle-Teijeiro J, et al. Hyalinizing trabecular adenoma: a misnomer for a peculiar tumor of the thyroid gland. Endocr Pathol 1991; 2:83–91.
34. Chan JKC, Tse CCH, Chiu HS. Hyalinizing trabecular adenoma-like lesion in multinodal goitre. Histopathology 1990; 16:611–614.
35. Goellner JR, Carney JA. Cytologic features of fine-needle aspirates of hyalinizing trabecular adenoma of the thyroid. Am J Clin Pathol 1989; 91:115–119.
36. Bondeson L, Bondeson A-G. Clue helping to distinguish hyalinizing trabecular adenoma from carcinoma of the thyroid in fine-needle aspirates. Diagn Cytopathol 1994; 10:25–29.
37. Chan JKC, Loo KT. Cribriform variant of papillary thyroid carcinoma. Arch Pathol Lab Med 1990; 114:622–624.
38. Harach HR, Williams GT, Williams ED. Familial adenomatous polyposis associated thyroid carcinoma: a distinct type of follicular neoplasm. Histopathology 1994; 25:549–561.
39. Mizukami Y, Nonomura A, Michigishi T, et al. Encapsulated follicular thyroid carcinoma exhibiting glandular and spindle cell components: a case report. Pathol Res Pract 1996; 192: 67–71.
40. Rhatigan RM, Roque JL, Bucher RL. Mucoepidermoid carcinoma of the thyroid gland. Cancer 1977; 39:210–214.
41. Sambade C, Franssila K, Basilio-de-Oliveira CA, Sobrinho-Simoes M. Mucoepidermoid carcinoma of the thyroid revisited. Surg Pathol 1990; 3:271–280.
42. Chan JKC, Albores-Saavedra J, Battifora H, et al. Sclerosing mucoepidermoid thyroid carcinoma with eosinophilia: a distinctive low-grade malignancy arising from the metaplastic follicles of Hashimoto's thyroiditis. Am J Surg Pathol 1991; 15:438–448.
43. Wenig BM, Adair CF, Heffess CS. Primary mucoepidermoid carcinoma of the thyroid gland: a report of six cases and a review of the literature of a follicular epithelial-derived tumor. Hum Pathol 1995; 26:1099–1108.
44. Cameselle-Teijeiro J, Febles-Pérez C, Sobrinho-Simoes M. Papillary and mucoepidermoid carcinoma of the thyroid with anaplastic transformation: a case report with histologic and immunohistochemical findings that support a provocative histogenetic hypothesis. Pathol Res Pract 1995; 191:1214–1221.
45. Russell WO, Ibanez ML, Clark RL, White EC. Thyroid carcinoma: classification, intraglandular dissemination, and clinicopathological study based upon whole organ sections of 80 glands. Cancer 1963; 16:1425–1460.
46. LiVolsi VA. Branchial and thymic remnants in the thyroid and cervical region: an explanation for unusual tumors and microscopic curiosities. Endocr Pathol 1993; 4:115–119.
47. Mizukami Y, Nonomura A, Michigishi T, et al. Ectopic thymic tissue in the thyroid gland. Endocr Pathol 1993; 4:162–164.
48. Harach HR, Saravia Day E, Franssila KO. Thyroid spindle-cell tumor with mucous cysts: an intrathyroid thymoma? Am J Surg Pathol 1985; 9:525–530.
49. Chan JKC, Rosai J. Tumors of the neck showing thymic or related branchial pouch differentiation: a unifying concept. Hum Pathol 1991; 22:349–367.
50. Mizukami Y, Kurumaya H, Yamada T, et al. Thymic carcinoma involving the thyroid gland: report of two cases. Hum Pathol 1995; 26: 576–579.

51. Shek TWH, Luk ISC, Ng IOL, Lo CY. Lymphoepithelioma-like carcinoma of the thyroid gland: lack of evidence of association with Epstein-Barr virus. Hum Pathol 1996; 27:851–853.
52. Bale GF. Teratoma of the neck in the region of the thyroid gland: a review of the literature and report of four cases. Am J Pathol 1950; 26:565–579.
53. Kimler SC, Muth WF. Primary malignant teratoma of the thyroid: case report and literature review of cervical teratomas in adults. Cancer 1978; 42:311–317.
54. Bowker CM, Whittaker RS. Malignant teratoma of the thyroid: case report and literature review of thyroid teratoma in adults. Histopathology 1992; 21:81–83.

Part VII
Undifferentiated Tumors
Medullary Thyroid Carcinoma

67
Clinical Aspects of Medullary Thyroid Carcinoma

Douglas W. Ball

INTRODUCTION

Medullary thyroid cancer (MTC), an uncommon neoplasm stemming from the calcitonin-producing thyroid parafollicular C cells, represents approximately 5% of thyroid cancer cases. Unique among all types of thyroid cancer is the close association of MTC with inherited tumor syndromes in about 20% of patients. Activating mutations in the *ret* proto-oncogene account for the hereditary basis of MTC and contribute significantly to sporadic tumor development as well. These findings have a major impact on the diagnosis and therapy of MTC.

GENETICS

MTC is traditionally classified as sporadic vs hereditary. The three autosomal dominant hereditary MTC syndromes, collectively referred to as multiple endocrine neoplasia type II (MEN2), are described in Table 1. MEN2A, which comprises MTC in 95% of affected individuals, pheochromocytoma in approx 50%, and hyperparathyroidism in 10–15%, is the most common MEN2 syndrome. MEN2B consists of MTC (often with early onset), pheochromocytoma, ganglioneuromas of the oral mucosa and gastrointestinal tract, a characteristic elongated facies, a marfanoid body habitus, and no increase in hyperparathyroidism. Familial medullary thyroid cancer (FMTC) is a term used to describe families with MTC, but no other associated manifestations (see ref. *1* for review). There is substantial overlap between *ret* mutations associated with MEN2A and FMTC. Two minor variants of MEN2A have been described: MEN2A associated with Hirschsprung's disease (hypoplasia of intestinal myenteric plexus) and MEN2A associated with the skin disorder, cutaneous lichen amyloidosis *(2,3)*.

The *ret* proto-oncogene encodes a receptor tyrosine kinase most closely related to the fibroblast growth factor receptor family. The physiologic role of *ret* is to activate growth-related signaling pathways in a limited range of neural crest–derived tissues that express the receptor. Downstream signaling pathways activated by *ret* include ras-mitogen-activated protein kinase and PI-3K/Akt *(4)*. Activating point mutations in *ret* lead to constitutive activity of the receptor, sometimes with altered substrate specificity. In the thyroid, these mutations lead to C-cell hyperplasia (CCH) and emergence of multiple foci of MTC.

The range of *ret* codon mutations seen in the various forms of hereditary and sporadic MTC is listed in Table 1 and has been reviewed recently *(4a)*. From the standpoint of genetic testing, it is fortunate that more than 97% of MEN2 families can be identified by analysis of six exons of the *ret* gene, including all the mutant codons described in Table 1 *(1)*. Exons 10 and 11 involve mutation sites at codons 609, 611, 618, 620, 630, and 634, which are associated with both MEN2A and FMTC. Each of these codons encodes a cysteine residue in the extracellular domain of *ret* that is associated with the three-dimensional ligand-binding pocket. Disruption of this pocket through mutation of any of these cysteine residues leads to ligand-independent dimerization and receptor activation. Exons 13–16 include intracellular domain mutation sites linked primarily with FMTC and, in the case of exon 16 (codon 918), MEN2B. The relatively limited variety of *ret* gene mutations within these six exons has facilitated genetic testing. Although a small percentage of MEN2 families have had no *ret* gene mutation detected, all affected families studied to date apparently exhibit genetic linkage to the *ret* gene locus *(1)*.

Specific germline *ret* mutations carry important implications regarding the penetrance of MTC and associated lesions. For example, the most common germline *ret* mutation site, codon 634 (exon 11), accounts for approx 60% of all MEN2 families *(5)*. Most of these families are classified as MEN2A, rather than FMTC. About 20% of individuals with a codon 634 mutation develop hyperparathyroidism, whereas this manifestation is otherwise uncommon with other *ret* mutations *(6)*. Patients with codon 634 mutations have significantly earlier progression from CCH to MTC and earlier lymph node involvement than patients with most other mutations related to MEN2A and FMTC. A large European consortium study reported by Machens and colleagues offers detailed clinical penetrance data, analyzed according to individual mutations *(5)*.

From: *Thyroid Cancer: A Comprehensive Guide to Clinical Management, 2/e*
Edited by: L. Wartofsky and D. Van Nostrand © Humana Press Inc., Totowa, NJ

Table 1
Classification of MTC

Type	Associated Lesion	Ret Gene Mutation (codon)	Clinical Behavior
Sporadic	None	Somatic (esp 918)	Intermediate
FMTC	None	Germline (609, 611, 618, 620, 634, 768, 790, 791, 804, 891)	Variable, less aggressive
MEN2A	Pheochromocytoma Hyperparathyroidism	Germline (609, 611, 618, 620, 630, 634, 790, 791, 804)	Intermediate
MEN2B	Pheochromocytoma Ganglioneuromatosis Marfanoid habitus	Germline (918, rarely 883)	More aggressive

In MEN2B, the great majority of patients exhibits a single mutation at codon 918 (methionine to threonine), resulting in an alteration of the substrate recognition pocket of the tyrosine kinase enzyme (7). Unlike MEN2A, MEN2B germline mutations frequently arise *de novo* in the presenting individual (e.g., are not detectable in either parent). The *de novo* mutation is noted at a much higher frequency in the allele inherited from the patient's father (8). An alternate mutation at codon 883 in exon 15 has been found in a small number of MEN2B families (9).

When MTC patients with a negative family history are investigated with germline *ret* testing, approx 3–6% are found to harbor such mutations (10). The *ret* mutations linked with cryptic heritable MTC tend to be disproportionately clustered in the intracellular domain (exons 13–15), linked with reduced MTC penetrance, compared to the more classic familial patterns associated with extracellular mutations in exons 10 and 11. Based on this relatively high frequency of detection in family history–negative patients and the important "multiplier effect" of identifying other family members at risk, germline *ret* testing is now recommended in all MTC patients, even in the absence of family history. Currently, a "complete" *ret* mutation test should include exons 10, 11, 13–15, and 16.

In sporadic MTC, acquired or somatic *ret* gene mutations (occurring in tumor DNA only) may also be critical to tumor pathogenesis. Approximately 50% of specimens contain *ret* mutations, most frequently the codon-918 mutation seen in MEN2B (11). However, the discovery that mutation-positive and -negative regions coexist in MTC tumors suggests that these mutations may not always be initiating or essential (12). To further assess this tumor heterogeneity phenomenon, Schilling and colleagues examined multiple lymph nodes from sporadic MTC patients for somatic codon-918 mutations. Of patients studied, 76% had concordant mutation results in all lymph nodes tested (43% all positive, 33% all negative; (13). Patients with somatic codon-918 mutations had a significantly increased rate of metastases to the lung, bone, or liver, along with reduced overall survival. Although the clinical utility of somatic *ret* mutation analysis is currently undefined, clinical trials are beginning to correlate somatic *ret* mutation status with response to therapy.

BIOCHEMISTRY

The characteristic secreted product of thyroid C cells and the most useful circulating marker for MTC is the polypeptide hormone, calcitonin. The mature 32-amino acid polypeptide is synthesized as a large 135-amino acid precursor, which is processed by prohormone convertases in the C cell. Calcitonin is encoded by a multiexon gene that produces two principal mRNA species. In addition to calcitonin itself, alternative splicing of the primary calcitonin transcript yields calcitonin gene-related peptide (CGRP). The resulting polypeptide hormones are unique and interact with distinct receptors. Calcitonin secretion predominates in normal thyroid C cells, whereas CGRP predominates in neural tissue (14). In MTC, abnormal RNA splicing permits an approximately equal ratio of calcitonin to CGRP, but CGRP measurement is not employed clinically. Although substantial elevations of calcitonin (>100 pg/mL) are usually diagnostic for MTC, modest elevations can be seen from extrathyroidal disorders, including pulmonary inflammatory diseases, small-cell lung cancer, gastrinoma, carcinoid tumors, and renal failure (15).

An important thyroidal cause of calcitonin hypersecretion is CCH. CCH may be genetic—as a precursor lesion in the three hereditary MTC disorders—or sporadic, either idiopathic or associated with such conditions as autoimmune thyroiditis, papillary thyroid cancer, or primary hyperparathyroidism (16). At low levels of calcitonin excess, CCH can be very difficult to distinguish from microscopic MTC. In otherwise healthy individuals, extrathyroidal sources of calcitonin are usually undetectable in serum, using a specific, highly sensitive assay. Thus, patients in remission following successful thyroidectomy characteristically have serum calcitonin values less than 1 pg/mL.

Current-generation calcitonin immunoradiometric assays (IRMA) with a detection limit of approx 1 pg/mL are significantly more sensitive and specific than older calcitonin radioimmunoassays. Use of the calcitonin IRMA has coincided with reduced use of provocative testing with the calcitonin secretogogues, calcium and pentagastrin in the United States, but several large European centers continue routine provocative testing. In normal adults given a pentagastrin infusion of 0.5 µg/kg, normal peak values are less than 30 pg/mL.

In addition to calcitonin, MTC cells express biochemical markers typifying secretory cells of the diffuse neuroendocrine system. Polypeptide hormones produced by MTC cells include somatostatin (17), adrenocorticotropic hormone (ACTH) (18), gastrin-releasing peptide (19), substance P (20), and vasoactive intestinal peptide (21). Other neuroendocrine markers include neuron-specific enolase, neural cell adhesion molecule, chromogranin A, prohormone convertases, synaptophysin, and the amine synthetic enzyme, L-dopa decarboxylase (22). Roughly 80% of MTCs express the thyroid and lung-related foregut thyroid transcription factor 1 (23). In addition, many MTC tumors express two surface markers that have been exploited for diagnostic and therapeutic purposes: carcinoembryonic antigen (CEA) and somatostatin receptor.

DIAGNOSIS

The clinical diagnosis of MTC can be challenging because of the potential for misdiagnosis as a more common form of thyroid cancer or metastatic tumor from another site. Early accurate diagnosis is critical to avoid the possibility of undiagnosed pheochromocytoma and to allow for an appropriate surgical approach. The important differences in surgical methods for MTC vs papillary and follicular cancer are detailed in Chapter 69.

Sporadic MTC

Clinical Presentation

Outside of the 20% of cases with known heritable disease, the diagnosis of MTC most commonly begins with the palpation of an asymptomatic thyroid nodule. Sporadic cases present frequently in the third to seventh decades of life, with a nearly equal prevalence in males and females. In most instances, the history and physical exam do not offer any distinctive information, compared to typical patients with thyroid nodules. A sufficiently detailed family history is warranted to detect the presence of thyroid cancer, pheochromocytoma, or hyperparathyroidism in first-degree relatives. Approximately 20% of patients present with locally advanced disease with dysphagia, painful lymph node metastases, or recurrent laryngeal nerve invasion. Rarely, individuals may present with a chief complaint related to a paraneoplastic manifestation of MTC, e.g., flushing, secretory diarrhea, or symptoms of hypercortisolism and the ectopic ACTH syndrome. If prominent, these paraneoplastic manifestations usually indicate a significant tumor burden.

An increasing number of patients with sporadic MTC are now being identified with primary tumors that are incidentally detected by imaging directed at another condition, such as carotid ultrasonography or staging of an unrelated tumor. Although the appearance of incidentally discovered MTC on ultrasound, computed tomography (CT), or 18-fluorodeoxyglucose positron emission tomograph (FDG-PET) is not sufficiently distinctive to provide a radiologic diagnosis, MTC lesions (like papillary thyroid cancer) may contain fine calcifications (24). Even clinically unapparent subcentimeter MTC lesions have a potential for metastasis and warrant appropriate surgical intervention.

A controversial approach to MTC diagnosis is the routine use of calcitonin testing in patients with nodular goiter. Two large European studies found significantly elevated calcitonin levels and MTC in a combined 0.6% of patients undergoing surgery for multinodular goiter. According to these authors, only one third of these MTC cases were diagnosed independently by fine-needle aspiration (FNA) biopsy (25,26). A follow-up Italian study found a 0.4% prevalence of significant hypercalcitoninemia and MTC in over 10,000 patients undergoing thyroidectomy for nodular thyroid disease (basal calcitonin range, 20–6200 pg/mL). In this subset of patients, 65% had a FNA result that was positive for MTC or other cancer (27). Currently, the American Thyroid Association does not recommend the calcitonin assay as part of the routine evaluation of nodular goiter, but some endocrinologists add this to standard assessment using FNA and thyrotropin, especially if any clinical features suggest MTC.

FNA

The standard diagnostic procedure of choice for sporadic MTC is thyroid FNA for cytological examination, either with direct palpation or ultrasound guidance. The sensitivity of thyroid cytopathology for MTC is theoretically equivalent to that in papillary cancer. In practice, the cytopathologist needs an adequate index of suspicion for atypical, cellular, and colloid-poor specimens to employ the diagnostic calcitonin immunostaining. In cases where there is clinical suspicion but insufficient cytologic material, a serum calcitonin level can help confirm or rule out the diagnosis. Occasionally, specimens are misdiagnosed as atypical follicular neoplasms or poorly differentiated/ anaplastic cancers. The practice of referring patients directly to thyroidectomy without preceding FNA cytology is especially discouraged. Where lymph node enlargement is first identified, rather than a thyroid nodule, FNA is favored over lymph node excisional biopsy to preserve the lymph node compartment for subsequent comprehensive neck dissection.

Calcitonin Testing

Virtually all patients with clinically evident MTC have elevated basal levels of calcitonin. For clinically occult, early MTC, basal calcitonin values may merge with the upper limit of the normal range, which is typically 8 pg/mL in men and 4 pg/mL in women. Although very rare, medullary microcarcinomas have been reported in patients with a normal basal calcitonin level (28). At what calcitonin level is the presence of MTC confirmed, and in what range is CCH or nonspecific elevation more likely? This question cannot be answered precisely owing to conflicting results in multiple studies (29). A reasonable generalization is that basal calcitonin IRMA values between 10 and 100 pg (prior to thyroidectomy) include both early MTC and CCH, with an overall prevalence of MTC in the 15–30% range (29). Above 100 pg/mL, MTC prevalence rises substantially; however, rare CCH cases can still be observed in this range.

Preoperative calcitonin levels generally correlate with tumor size. In a large French series, a calcitonin level above 1000 pg/mL corresponded to a median tumor diameter of 2.5 cm, calcitonin levels below 1000 pg/mL corresponded to an average size of 0.7 cm, and levels below 100 pg/mL, 0.3 cm. A calcitonin level greater than 1000 pg/mL was associated with a 10% risk of distant metastases vs 3% for levels less than 1000 (30). Similarly, the degree of preoperative calcitonin elevation is an important predictor of the chance of normalizing the serum calcitonin with surgery. The possibility of postoperative normalization falls from 97% (if the preoperative level is <50 pg/mL) to 42% (preoperative >50 pg/mL), and 8% (preoperative >4000 pg/mL; 30).

Other Preoperative Testing

In our institution, individuals with newly diagnosed MTC, even in the absence of a family history of MTC, are evaluated with *ret* proto-oncogene DNA testing, 24-h urine metanephrines, or plasma-fractionated metanephrines, serum calcium, and CEA, in addition to calcitonin.

Preoperative Imaging

The preoperative imaging work-up varies from patient to patient. At minimum, a high-quality thyroid and neck ultrasound is useful to detect multifocal thyroid involvement and metastasis to central compartment and jugular chain nodes. However, the absence of abnormal lymph nodes on palpation or ultrasound does not obviate the need for lymph nodal dissection. Lymph node prevalence in sporadic MTC can be estimated from the surgical and pathological data analyzed by Scollo et al. Both central compartment and ipsilateral jugular chain node involvement occurred in more that 50% of patients, whereas contralateral jugular chain nodes had a 25–30% prevalence (31). Chapter 69 provides a detailed description of operative management in MTC. In our institution, the choice of additional imaging modalities is guided by the degree of calcitonin elevation. Neck and chest CT with contrast and dual-phase (early and late) contrast scan of the abdomen are most commonly employed in preoperative staging. Magnetic resonance imaging has proven useful for identification of bone and bone marrow involvement (31a).

Hereditary MTC

Since the late 1990s, a consensus has emerged that *ret* proto-oncogene testing, rather than calcitonin-provocative testing, is the preferred method for diagnosis of hereditary MEN2. The sensitivity of *ret* testing is excellent, currently estimated at about 98% for known families (1). The test is widely available through commercial laboratories. Efficient family testing focuses on identifying the mutation in a known affected individual, then proceeding systematically through first-degree relatives. The primary goal of this testing is to identify presymptomatic young individuals at risk for MTC and allow for appropriate prophylactic thyroidectomy. Additional goals are identification of subjects with existing MTC requiring treatment, as well as subjects at risk for pheochromocytoma and hyperparathyroidism. Prophylactic thyroidectomy, at the stage of CCH or microscopic MTC, is associated with marked improvements in morbidity and mortality, compared with historical patterns of tumor detection later in life (1). Indeed, most individuals with FMTC and MEN2A have normal life expectancy after undergoing childhood prophylactic thyroidectomy.

The optimal timing of genetic testing (and prophylactic surgery) is somewhat controversial. These decisions are predicated on data for the earliest onset of MTC and nodal metastases for a particular *ret* mutation site. The most complete data currently available from Machens et al. indicate that for the most common mutation at codon 634, microscopic MTC can occur as early as age 15 mo, and lymph nodal metastases can begin as early as age 6, but ages 14–20 are more common (5). For other extracellular codons, including 609, 611, 618, and 620, no patients have been reported to develop MTC prior to age 6 (5). Smaller numbers of patients have been studied for the intracellular mutant codons 768, 790, 791, 804, and 891, associated predominantly with FMTC. With the exception of patients with codon-804 mutations that may variably develop cancer at an earlier age, few patients with these intracellular codon lesions have developed MTC prior to age 20. For individuals with a 918 mutation and the MEN2B phenotype, metastatic MTC has been reported in the first year of life.

Based on data for MTC onset and metastasis, an international consensus panel has recommended prophylactic thyroidectomy by age 5 for subjects harboring mutations in codon 611, 618, 620, or 634. For codons 609, 768, 790, 791, 804, and 891, no consensus was reached, with a range of 5–10 yr most commonly chosen (1). Because of frequent *de novo* mutations, patients with MEN2B are often initially suspected not on the basis of family history, but because of a characteristic elongated facies and oral ganglioneuromas involving the lips and tongue (see Fig. 1). DNA diagnosis then provides confirmation. Clearly, identification of MEN2B should be as early as possible, with surgical cure increasingly unlikely after the first 5 yr of life.

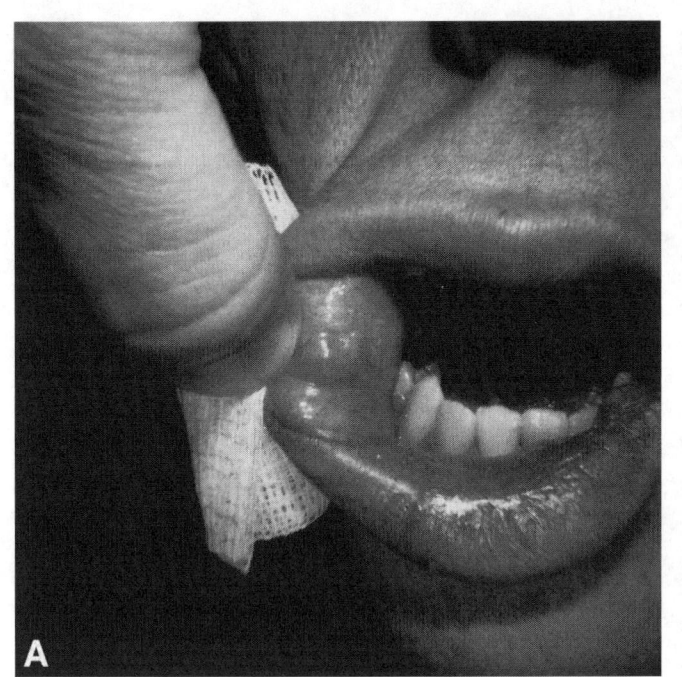

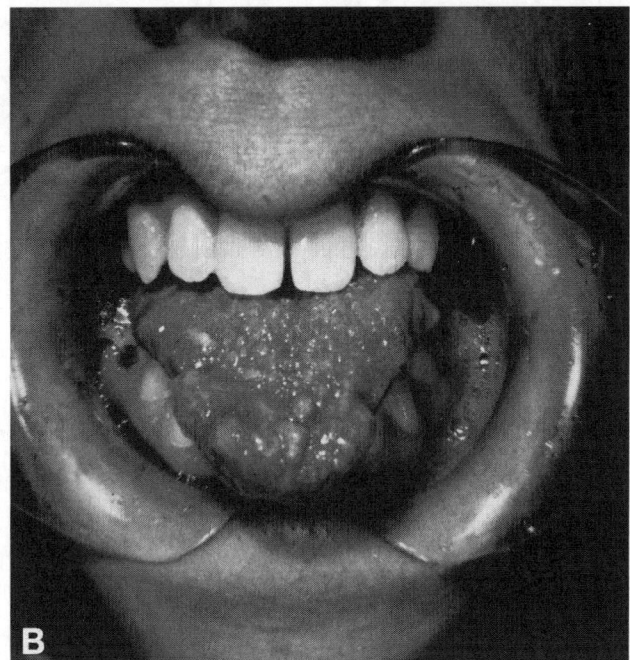

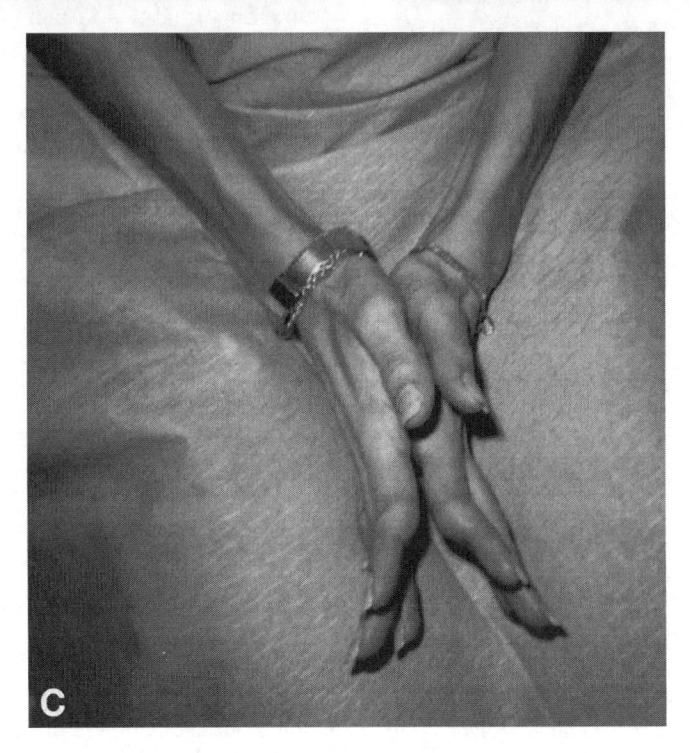

Fig. 1. Photograph of a patient with MEN2B showing the typical mucosal neuromas associated with a marfanoid habitus. (**A**) Lips; (**B**) tongue; (**C**) hyperextensibility of the hands.

Preoperative Studies

All patients diagnosed with hereditary MEN2 should have an assessment of catecholamine secretion prior to surgical procedures, as well as a determination of basal calcitonin, CEA, and serum calcium. For young patients undergoing prophylactic thyroidectomy, no imaging studies are usually employed. Patients in their teens and older, or patients with significant calcitonin elevations, are considered for imaging studies, as described above for sporadic disease. The choice of operation, particularly the extent of lymph nodal dissection and prophylactic parathyroid resection, depends on knowledge of the natural history of inherited MTC and the impact of different *ret* mutations. In general, this surgery should be performed in a specialized center by surgeons familiar with these issues, as discussed in Chapter 69.

TUMOR PROGRESSION AND COMPLICATIONS

Of typical patients with a palpable sporadic MTC who have undergone thyroidectomy and neck exploration, the majority have persistent increased calcitonin levels *(32)*. Those patients who prove to be node-negative with appropriate comprehensive lymph nodal exploration have a 95% chance of an undetectable basal calcitonin level *(31)*. In contrast, the presence of lymphadenopathy reduces the chance of calcitonin normalization to 32% *(31)*. Even patients considered to have complete resection at the time of surgery have a strong likelihood of persistent hypercalcitonemia. In the absence of overt adenopathy or extensive distant metastases, the clinical course is usually characterized by slow disease progression. Patients with minimal calcitonin elevations and no radiologically detectable metastasis after primary surgery have an 86% 10-yr survival rate and relatively little tumor-associated morbidity *(33)*. Similarly, a Memorial Sloan-Kettering series reported a 94% 5-yr survival in patients with nodal disease alone vs 41% in patients with stage IV disease *(34)*.

In addition to regional lymphadenopathy, the most common metastatic sites include lung and hilar or mediastinal lymph nodes, liver and abdominal lymph nodes, and bone. Lung and liver metastases occur in a diffuse, hematogenous pattern, usually with slow growth. Fortunately, modest metastatic burdens in the lung and to a lesser extent, liver, can be compatible with a long survival. Standard imaging modalities, e.g., contrast CT, magnetic resonance imaging (MRI), and PET, are quite insensitive for detecting early liver metastases *(35)*. The inclusion of an arterial phase-contrast protocol apparently improves sensitivity for liver metastasis detection. Laparoscopic liver visualization and biopsy or hepatic venous sampling are more invasive approaches to this diagnosis. Occasionally, liver metastases can become bulky and painful. Extensive liver metastases are also frequently associated with diarrhea. Although liver resection is not routinely advocated for MTC liver metastases because of the multifocality of the process, surgical debulking of symptomatic masses can provide useful palliation *(36)*.

The most frequent serious complications in advanced MTC relate to local tumor invasion into the thyroid bed, trachea, carotid sheath, and brachial plexus or progressive metastasis in the upper mediastinum, lung, or pericardium. Recurrent laryngeal nerve paresis, tracheal and esophageal invasion, superior vena cava syndrome, aspiration-related and postobstructive pneumonia, and hemoptysis all may be seen in patients with advanced disease and may contribute to disease mortality. Another significant cause of morbidity is lytic bone metastasis. MTC lesions are generally not considered radiation-sensitive, but external-beam radiation is a useful palliative measure for painful bone lesions or lytic metastases in weight-bearing sites.

The principal paraneoplastic humoral complications of MTC are flushing, diarrhea, and the ectopic ACTH syndrome. The etiology of flushing in MTC patients is still an issue of some debate. One likely mediator is CGRP—a potent vasodilator capable of inducing prolonged cutaneous erythema with intradermal administration *(37)*. Symptomatic flushing can sometimes be improved by subcutaneous octreotide injection *(38)*. Unfortunately, octreotide has little efficacy in MTC-associated diarrhea; some patients paradoxically worsen.

Like flushing, the pathophysiology of diarrhea in MTC requires further clarification. The small minority of MEN2A patients with Hirschsprung's disease, as well as MEN2B patients, have well-characterized abnormalities in enteric nerve development, with resulting obstruction and megacolon *(39)*. In contrast, there are no reproducible structural abnormalities in most MTC patients with diarrhea. Functional studies have not shown any consistent evidence for either malabsorbtion or a secretory abnormality in the small intestine. Instead, patients exhibit colonic hypermotility and a decreased ability to absorb water *(40)*. Intravenous CGRP can increase colonic output of water and electrolytes *(41)*; however, the relative importance of other mediators, including vasoactive intestinal peptide, histamine, and prostaglandins, remain unclear. Patients can be treated symptomatically with loperamide and diphenoxylate to lengthen colonic transit time. Calcitonin excess, *per se*, is not associated with any clinically significant changes in bone or mineral metabolism.

PROGNOSIS

MTC occupies an intermediate position among thyroid cancer histologic types regarding biologic behavior and long-term prognosis. Although there is intrinsic variability in patients' clinical course, prognostic factors apparent at the time of diagnosis and initial surgery have important utility in predicting long-term outcomes of MTC. An accurate understanding of prognostic factors and their influence in both sporadic and hereditary contexts is essential to select appropriate levels of therapeutic intervention.

Sporadic MTC

To date, the most comprehensive reviews of prognostic factors in MTC are based on nationwide cancer surveillance in Sweden, with follow-up for 30 yr *(42,43)*. These studies have revealed several important predictors of survival. Among all sporadic MTC patients, relative survival (the ratio between observed and expected survival) was 63% at 10 yr and 50%

at 20 yr. The most important prognostic factor was initial clinical stage (see Table 2). Stage III (nodal disease) and stage IV (distant metastases) were linked with relative hazards of 3.3 and 4.1, compared to patients with no nodal or distant disease. Similarly, a French study involving 79 patients with stage IV disease and a US study found a 5-yr survival of 35–40% *(34,38)*. Initial clinical stage remains highly predictive of future mortality, even up to 20 yr after diagnosis *(43)*. Other important negative prognostic indicators are tumor size (more than 3 cm), capsular invasion, weak or heterogeneous calcitonin staining, male gender, and older age. Alternatively, patients with a tumor less than 1 cm without known metastases do not differ in their survival rates vs the general population *(43,44)*. The impact of new molecular markers on MTC prognostic assessment is still unclear. Somatic mutations in *ret* at codon 918 appear to be associated with an adverse prognosis, but the impact in a large multivariate analysis is unknown. Although unproven, it is likely that different *ret* gene mutations will impact response to tyrosine kinase inhibitors and other experimental therapies.

Hereditary MTC

The significant improvement in outcome that was seen over the last three decades for patients with heritable MTC can be attributed to the success of presymptomatic screening programs, first with calcitonin secretogogues and more recently, genetic testing. Survival rates of MEN2A subjects identified in early childhood are projected to be indistinguishable from the general population *(43,44)*. Whether the MTC in MEN2A behaves intrinsically less aggressively than sporadic tumors when matched for clinical stage unsettled. Swedish MTC registry data suggest statistically similar outcomes for non-screened MEN2A and sporadic patients *(44)*. At either extreme of the hereditary MTC spectrum, FMTC associated with some intracellular codons appears significantly less aggressive than classic MEN2A in terms of disease latency and survival *(45)*. MEN2B is usually more aggressive *(1,5)*.

The age-specific likelihood that a MEN2A gene carrier would present with detectable calcitonin hypersecretion or with symptomatic MTC has been studied by Ponder and colleagues *(46)*. Approximately 65% of obligate gene carriers exhibit calcitonin hypersecretion at age 20 yr. By age 35, 95% of gene carriers have a positive provocative test. In contrast, the likelihood of a clinical presentation with MTC is only 25% at age 35 and only about 60% at age 70 *(46)*. However, these data cannot be extrapolated to less penetrant hereditary MTC associated with intracellular domain mutations.

CLINICAL SURVEILLANCE

Goals of clinical surveillance in MTC are to detect recurrences in patients in surgical remission, and importantly, to prevent morbidity from cancer progression in patients with persistent disease. It is reasonable to restage patients prior

Table 2
Clinical Staging of MTC

Stage I	CCH
Stage II	Tumors <1 cm and negative lymph nodes
Stage III	Tumors ≥1 cm or tumor of any size with positive nodes
Stage IV	Tumors of any size with metastases outside the neck or with extrathyroidal extension

Source: Clinical Tumor Staging, National Thyroid Cancer Treatment Cooperative Study. (Brierly JD, et al., Cancer 1997; 79:2414–2423.)

to performing neck reoperation to exclude stage IV, inoperable disease. An emerging aim of surveillance is to select patients who could potentially benefit from clinical trials of systemic therapies for MTC. The intensity of clinical surveillance depends on the risk of death and morbidity and possibility of beneficial intervention.

For patients with modest calcitonin elevations after primary surgery, follow-up testing utilizes a combination of biochemical tumor markers and radiologic studies to screen for disease progression. In one commonly used scheme, serum calcitonin, CEA, and thyroid function tests are obtained 6 wk after surgery, then at approx 6-mo intervals. The timing of the postoperative calcitonin nadir may be variable *(47)*, and calcitonin levels may vary considerably from measurement to measurement. This variability likely stems from uneven secretion by tumors, rather than assay variability. In contrast to calcitonin, CEA levels exhibit less inconsistency and, if elevated at baseline, are useful to detect disease progression. Both calcitonin and CEA, with repeated testing for outlying results, will identify most patients with progressive disease. A flat calcitonin level, coupled with rapid doubling in CEA, is particularly worrisome pattern over time. Overall, the most typical doubling time for calcitonin and CEA is approx 18 mo, reflecting the generally indolent course of this disease.

Of the available imaging modalities, high-quality neck ultrasound appears to have the greatest sensitivity for lymphadenopathy in the central compartment and jugular chains *(48)*. Because of variability in imaging protocols and interpretation, this type of ultrasound imaging is not available in all centers. Distinct advantages of ultrasound vs CT/MRI are precise lesional measurements, assessment of fatty hilum (characteristic of reactive nodes), and especially the ability to perform ultrasound-guided FNA of lymph nodes if needed. Neck CT and MRI are complementary to ultrasound by providing wider coverage in the neck and more detailed anatomic localization of lymph nodes once they are detected. Patients with small calcitonin elevations (<50 pg/mL) frequently do not have disease detectable by imaging. Patients with more significant elevations (>500 pg/mL) are often followed with periodic whole-body imaging, in addition to ultrasound, including either CT (neck, chest, and dual-phase abdomen) or FDG-PET.

Despite the wide range of imaging options now available, a vexing problem for clinicians and patients is occult residual MTC, i.e., elevated calcitonin and negative imaging studies. At low levels of calcitonin, this dilemma generally reflects low disease burden below threshold sensitivities of even sensitive techniques, such as neck ultrasound. Even with higher calcitonin levels and ostensibly greater disease burdens, patients may undergo frustrating and expensive rounds of unproductive imaging. The issue regarding which whole-body modality is best for imaging occult disease remains unsettled. There is general consensus that octreotide, dimercaptosuccinic acid, and ^{131}I meta-iodobenzylguanidine scintigraphy have lower overall sensitivity, whereas CT and FDG-PET have greater sensitivity overall (49). The choice between CT and FDG-PET is not clear-cut, and there are advantages at different metastatic sites for both modalities, as discussed in Chapter 71.

THERAPEUTIC SELECTION IN RESIDUAL MTC

Faced with a rising calcitonin level and/or metastatic lesions seen on imaging studies, patients and clinicians can choose between a course of "watchful waiting" or intervention with surgery, radiotherapy, or systemic therapy. (Specific surgical, radiation, and chemotherapeutic approaches to MTC are discussed in Chapters 69, 72, and 73). The decision to undertake these interventions presupposes an understanding of MTC natural history and the appropriate use of biochemical and imaging data, as well as an effective treatment option.

Patients with biochemical evidence of only persistent MTC and negative imaging studies are frequently managed expectantly. In patients with mild hypercalcitoninemia and negative imaging, an excellent overall prognosis supports this conservative approach (33,34). A more aggressive approach—neck reoperation with a potential curative intent—seems justified in some patients who have not had recommended primary surgery, as described in Chapter 69. However, the low-to-moderate success rates in normalizing the calcitonin level following repeat lymph nodal dissection suggests that this approach be used highly selectively (50–52).

Locoregional recurrence is frequently managed surgically. In the presence of stage IV disease, particularly with distant progression, the goals of neck surgery become focused on symptom palliation and, to a lesser extent, on the prevention of anticipated complications. The importance of locoregional control, even in patients with stage IV disease, has been emphasized (53). The limited role of adjuvant neck radiation following surgery is discussed in Chapter 72.

Patients with distant metastases should be considered as potential candidates for investigational systemic therapy, as no currently available regimen produces frequent durable responses. The decision to undertake such treatment is based on a variety of factors, including the rate of metastatic progression on interval scanning, study availability, comorbidities, and patient preference. Presently, numerous experimental therapies are being investigated for MTC. For example, interest is growing in the investigation of agents that target specific signaling pathways such as the activation of raf-1 which may inhibit cell growth in MTC (54). Other therapies are targeted at ret kinase inhibition, additional cellular kinases, tumor angiogenesis, and protein chaperone function. Conceivably, combinations of targeted treatment, or targeted and cytotoxic therapies, will prove most effective.

REFERENCES

1. Brandi ML, Gagel RF, Angeli A, et al. Guidelines for diagnosis and therapy of MEN type 1 and type 2. J Clin Endocrinol Metab 2001; 86: 5658–5671.
2. Frilling A, Becker H, Roehr H-D. Unusual features of multiple endocrine neoplasia. Henry Ford Hosp Med J 1992; 40:233–235.
3. Gagel RF, Levy ML, Donovan DT, et al. Multiple endocrine neoplasia type 2a associated with cutaneous lichen amyloidosis. Ann Intern Med 1989; 111:802–806.
4. De Vita G, Melillo RM, Carlomagno F, et al. Tyrosine 1062 of RET-MEN2A mediates activation of Akt (protein kinase B) and mitogen-activated protein kinase pathways leading to PC12 cell survival. Cancer Res 2000; 3727–3231.
4a. Kouvaraki MA, Shapiro SE, Perrier ND, et al. RET proto-oncogene: A review and update of genotype-phenotype correlations in hereditary medullary thyroid cancer and associated endocrine tumors. Thyroid 2005; 15:531–544.
5. Machens A, Niccoli-Sire P, Hoegel J, et al. Early malignant progression of hereditary medullary thyroid cancer. N Engl J Med. 2003; 349: 1517–1525.
6. Schuffenecker I, Virally-Monod M, Brohet R, et al. Risk and penetrance of primary hyperparathyroidism in multiple endocrine neoplasia type 2A families with mutations at codon 634 of the RET proto-oncogene. J Clin Endocrinol Metab 1998; 83: 487–491.
7. Santoro M, Carlomagno F, Romano A, et al. Activation of RET as a dominant transforming gene by germline mutations of MEN2A and MEN2B. Science 1995; 267:381–383.
8. Carlson KM, Bracamontes J, Jackson CE, et al. Parent-of-origin effects in multiple endocrine neoplasia type 2B. Am J Hum Genet 1994; 5:1076–1082.
9. Gimm O, Marsh DJ, Andrew SD, et al. Germline dinucleotide mutation in codon 883 of the RET proto-oncogene in multiple endocrine neoplasia type 2B without codon 918 mutation. J Clin Endocrinol Metab 1997; 82:3902–3904.
10. Wohllk N, Cote GJ, Bugalho MM, et al. Relevance of RET proto-oncogene mutations in sporadic medullary thyroid carcinoma. J Clin Endocrinol Metab 1996; 81:3740–3745.
11. Blaugrund JE, Johns MM Jr, Eby YJ, et al. RET proto-oncogene mutations in inherited and sporadic medullary thyroid cancer. Hum Mol Genet 1994; 3:1895–1897.
12. Eng C, Mulligan LM, Healey CS, et al. Heterogeneous mutation of the RET proto-oncogene in subpopulations of medullary thyroid carcinoma. Cancer Res 1996; 56:2167–2170.
13. Schilling T, Burck J, Sinn HP, et al. Prognostic value of codon 918 (ATG→ACG) RET proto-oncogene mutations in sporadic medullary thyroid carcinoma. Int J Cancer 2001; 95:62–66.
14. Amara SG, Jonas V, Rosenfeld MG, et al. Alternative RNA processing in calcitonin gene expression generates mRNAs encoding different polypeptide products. Nature 1982; 298:240–244.

15. Becker KL, Nash D, Silva OL, et al. Increased serum and urinary calcitonin in patients with pulmonary disease. Chest 1981; 79:211–216.
16. Perry A, Molberg K, Albores-Saavedra J. Physiologic versus neoplastic C-cell hyperplasia of the thyroid: separation of distinct histologic and biologic entities. Cancer 1996; 77:750–756.
17. Roos BA, Lindall A W, Ells J, et al. Increased plasma and tumor somatostatin-like immuno reactivity in medullary thyroid carcinoma and small cell lung cancer. J Clin Endocrinol Metab 1981; 52:187–194.
18. Melvin KE, Tashjian AH Jr, Cassidy CE, Givens JR. Cushing's syndrome caused by ACTH and calcitonin-secreting medullary carcinoma of the thyroid. Metabolism 1970; 19:831–838.
19. Kameya T, Bessho T, Tsumuraya M, et al. Production of gastrin-releasing peptide in medullary carcinoma of the thyroid. Virchows Arch [A] 1983; 401:99–107.
20. Skrabanek P, Cannon D, Dempsey J, et al. Substance P in medullary carcinoma of the thyroid. Experientia 1979; 35:1259–1260.
21. Said SI. Evidence for secretion of vasoactive intestinal peptide by tumours of pancreas, adrenal medulla, thyroid and lung. Clin Endocrinol (Oxf) 1976; 5(Suppl):201S–204S.
22. Baylin SB, Mendelsohn G. Medullary thyroid carcinoma: a model for the study of human tumor progression and cell heterogeneity. In Owens AH Jr, Coffey DS, Baylin SB, editors. Tumor Cell Heterogeneity, Origins and Implications. New York: Academic Press, 1982: 12.
23. Katoh R, Miyagi E, Nakamura N, et al. Expression of thyroid transcription factor-1 (TTF-1) in human C cells and medullary thyroid carcinomas. Hum Pathol 2000; 31:386–393.
24. McDonnell CH III, Fishman EK, Zerhouni EA. CT demonstration of calcified liver metastases in medullary thyroid carcinoma. J Comput Assist Tomogr 1986; 10:976–978.
25. Pacini F, Fontanelli M, Fugazzola L, et al. Routine measurement of serum calcitonin in nodular thyroid diseases allows the preoperative diagnosis of unsuspected sporadic medullary thyroid carcinoma. J Clin Endocrinol Metab 1994; 78:826–829.
26. Rieu M, Lame MC, Richard A, et al. Prevalence of sporadic medullary thyroid carcinoma: the importance of routine measurement of serum calcitonin in the diagnostic evaluation of thyroid nodules. Clin Endocrinol (Oxf) 1995; 42:453–460.
27. Elisei R, Bottici V, Luchetti F, et al. Impact of routine measurement of serum calcitonin on the diagnosis and outcome of medullary thyroid cancer: experience in 10,864 patients with nodular thyroid disorders. J Clin Endocrinol Metab 2004; 89:163–168.
28. Niccoli P, Wion-Barbot N, Caron P, et al. Interest of routine measurement of serum calcitonin: study in a large series of thyroidectomized patients. J Clin Endocrinol Metab 1997; 82:338–341.
29. Hodak SP, Burman KD. The calcitonin conundrum—is it time for routine measurement of serum calcitonin in patients with thyroid nodules? J Clin Endocrinol Metab 2004; 89:511–514.
30. Cohen R, Campos JM, Salaun C, et al. Preoperative calcitonin levels are predictive of tumor size and postoperative calcitonin normalization in medullary thyroid carcinoma. J Clin Endocrinol Metab 2000; 85:919–922.
31. Scollo C, Baudin E, Travagli JP, et al. Rationale for central and bilateral lymph node dissection in sporadic and hereditary medullary thyroid cancer. J Clin Endocrinol Metab 2003; 88:2070–2075.
31a. Mirallie E, Vuillez JP, Barber S, et al. High frequency of bone/bone marrow involvement in advanced medullary thyroid cancer. J. Clin Endocrinol Metab 2005; 90:779–788.
32. Wells SA Jr, Dilley WG, Farndon JA, et al. Early diagnosis and treatment of medullary thyroid carcinoma. Arch Intern Med 1995; 145:1248–1252.
33. van Heerden JA, Grant CS, Gharib H, et al. Long-term course of patients with persistent hypercalcitoninemia after apparent curative primary surgery for medullary thyroid carcinoma. Ann Surg 1990; 212: 395–400.
34. Ellenhorn JD, Shah JP, Brennan MF. Impact of therapeutic regional lymph node dissection for medullary carcinoma of the thyroid gland. Surgery 1993; 114:1078–1081.
35. Tung WS, Vesely TM, Moley JF. Laparoscopic detection of hepatic metastases in patients with residual or recurrent medullary thyroid cancer. Surgery 1995; 118:1024–1029.
36. Chen H, Roberts JR, Ball DW, et al. Effective long-term palliation of symptomatic, incurable metastatic medullary thyroid cancer by operative resection. Ann Surg 1998; 227:887–895.
37. Brain SD, Williams TJ, Tippins JR. Calcitonin gene-related peptide is a potent vasodilator. Nature 1985; 313:54–56.
38. Modigliani E, Cohen R, Joannidis S, et al. Results of long-term continuous subcutaneous octreotide administration in 14 patients with medullary thyroid carcinoma. Clin Endocrinol (Oxf) 1992; 36:183–186.
39. Cohen MS, Phay JE, Albinson C, et al. Gastrointestinal manifestations of multiple endocrine neoplasia type 2. Ann Surg 2002; 235: 648–654.
40. Rambaud JC, Jian R, Flourie B, et al. Pathophysiological study of diarrhoea in a patient with medullary thyroid carcinoma: evidence against a secretory mechanism and for the role of shortened colonic transit time. Gut 1988; 29:537–543.
41. Rolston RK, Ghatei MA, Mulderry PK, Bloom SR. Intravenous calcitonin gene-related peptide stimulates net water secretion in rat colon in vivo. Dig Dis Sci 1989; 34:612–616.
42. Bergholm U, Adami HO, Auer G, et al. Histopathologic characteristics and nuclear DNA content as prognostic factors in medullary thyroid carcinoma: a nationwide study in Sweden. The Swedish MTC Study Group. Cancer 1989; 64:135–142.
43. Bergholm U, Bergstrom R, Ekbom A. Long-term follow-up of patients with medullary carcinoma of the thyroid. Cancer 1997; 79: 132–138.
44. Modigliani E, Cohen R, Campos JM, et al. Prognostic factors for survival and for biochemical cure in medullary thyroid carcinoma: results in 899 patients. Clin Endocrinol (Oxf) 1998; 48:265–273.
45. Farndon JR, Leight GS, Dilley WG, et al. Familial medullary thyroid carcinoma without associated endocrinopathies: a distinct clinical entity. Br J Surg 1986; 73:278–281.
46. Ponder BA, Ponder MA, Coffey R, et al. Risk estimation and screening in families of patients with medullary thyroid carcinoma. Lancet 1989; 1:397–401.
47. Stepanas AV, Samaan NA, Hill CS Jr, Hickey RC. Medullary thyroid carcinoma: importance of serial serum calcitonin measurement. Cancer 1979; 43:825–837.
48. Kouvaraki MA, Shapiro SE, Fornage BD, et al. Role of preoperative ultrasonography in the surgical management of patients with thyroid cancer. Surgery 2003; 134:946–954.
49. Gotthardt M, Battmann A, Hoffken H, et al. 18F-FDG PET, somatostatin receptor scintigraphy, and CT in metastatic medullary thyroid carcinoma: a clinical study and an analysis of the literature. Nucl Med Commun 2004; 25:439–443.
50. Kebebew E, Kikuchi S, Duh QY, Clark OH. Long-term results of reoperation and localizing studies in patients with persistent or recurrent medullary thyroid cancer. Arch Surg 2000; 135:895–901.
51. Fleming JB, Lee JE, Bouvet M, et al. Surgical strategy for the treatment of medullary thyroid carcinoma. Ann Surg 1999; 230:697–707.
52. Moley JF, Dilley WG, DeBenedetti MK. Improved results of cervical reoperation for medullary thyroid carcinoma. Ann Surg 1997; 225: 734–740.
53. Yen TW, Shapiro SE, Gagel RF, et al. Medullary thyroid carcinoma: results of a standardized surgical approach in a contemporary series of 80 consecutive patients. Surgery 2003; 134:890–899.
54. Chen H, Kunnimalaiyaan M, Van Gompel JJ. Medullary thyroid cancer: The functions of raf-1 and human achaetescute homologue-1. Thyroid 2005; 15:511–521.

68
Pathology of Medullary Thyroid Cancer

James E. Oertel and Yolanda C. Oertel

In the 1950s, the physicians of the Cleveland Clinic defined medullary thyroid carcinoma as a clinicopathologic entity *(1,2)*. During the same decade, a few were recognized independently as unusual tumors that differed from the majority of thyroid neoplasms *(3)*. Subsequently, a thorough search of the literature revealed several other probable medullary carcinomas *(4)*; sporadic and hereditary forms were recognized. The latter is associated with other endocrine neoplasms, most frequently, pheochromocytoma (Fig. 1).

Histologically, medullary carcinoma consists of solid masses of rounded, polygonal, and/or spindled neoplastic cells of various sizes (Fig. 2), often mixed with amyloid, nearly always in the lateral lobes *(5)*, rarely in the isthmus *(4)*. Insular (micronodular and nesting) and trabecular (cordlike and ribbon-like) patterns are common. Arrangements described as rosettes, pseudorosettes, as well as glandular, tubular, and follicular structures are less obvious in many tumors *(4)*. Many medullary carcinomas contain microacini *(6)*, and some have desmoplastic stroma *(7)*. Other characteristics include pseudopapillary and papillary patterns, solid "small cell," "oat-cell," and "neuroblastoma-like" features, and more pleomorphic anaplastic patterns. "Plasmacytoid" cells, binucleated cells, and cells with large nuclei, even giant nuclei *(4)*, have been noted. Multinucleated neoplastic cells are present *(4)*. Similarities to Askanazy/Hürthle cells have been found along with squamous cell characteristics *(8,9)* and clear cells. Some tumors produce mucus, and rarely, a few form melanin granules. Amyloid deposits may be accompanied by giant cells of the foreign body type *(2,4)*; a minority lack amyloid *(4)*, and some are well-encapsulated. Within carcinomas, there may be focal necrosis, cystic change, desmoplastic stroma, irregular calcification, and psammoma bodies *(4)*. The pathologist should search for necrosis, because its presence may indicate a worse prognosis *(10)*.

Medullary carcinoma may occur in association with autoimmune thyroiditis. Other proliferative processes may also be present in the gland: adenomatoid nodules and adenomas *(2)* and other thyroid cancers. A few are small (Fig. 3) and thus can be discovered during autopsies, because of an operation for another thyroid disorder, during an evaluation for hypercalcemia, by finding elevated levels of calcitonin, or from the appearance of metastases. Such small tumors are unlikely to be encountered during aspiration.

Most medullary carcinomas are readily recognized on histologic examination because the usual features of papillary or follicular carcinomas are absent, and because amyloid is present. Any unusual thyroid carcinoma of uncertain classification should be evaluated for calcitonin because it may be medullary carcinoma (Fig. 4). A cytological diagnosis of medullary carcinoma is often a "diagnosis of exclusion." When examining wet smears under the microscope after performing the aspiration, the pathologist is surprised at the findings: the pattern is "unexpected," not fitting the usual nonneoplastic findings (adenomatoid nodule or chronic thyroiditis) or commonly seen neoplastic patterns (follicular neoplasms or papillary carcinoma).

Considering the rarity of these tumors, several years are usually needed to see more than a few. Our first 10 cases were all different, and only when we encountered additional cases did some patterns start reoccurring. In our experience, with over 30 diagnosed, these neoplasms may have the most varied cytological patterns of any thyroid neoplasm. However, they have a few aspects in common *(11–15)*: significant lack of cellular cohesiveness, pleomorphic multinucleated neoplastic cells scattered among the predominant cell population (Fig. 5), lack of prominent nucleoli, cells with plasmacytoid features, spindled cells (Fig. 6), and frequent binucleation (Fig. 7). Multinucleated histiocytes (usually associated with the presence of amyloid) are seen rarely. Calcitonin cytoplasmic granules (that stain pink if hematological stains are used) are found in approximately 30% of cases (Fig. 8).

Very few neoplasms have been reported where there is differentiation toward C cells (calcitonin production) and follicular cells (thyroglobulin production). The follicular elements have been described as similar to follicular *(16–18)* and papillary carcinoma *(18,19)*. Critical examination of such a neoplasm is needed to exclude collision tumors and nonspecific uptake of thyroglobulin by medullary carcinoma.

From: *Thyroid Cancer: A Comprehensive Guide to Clinical Management, 2/e*
Edited by: L. Wartofsky and D. Van Nostrand © Humana Press Inc., Totowa, NJ

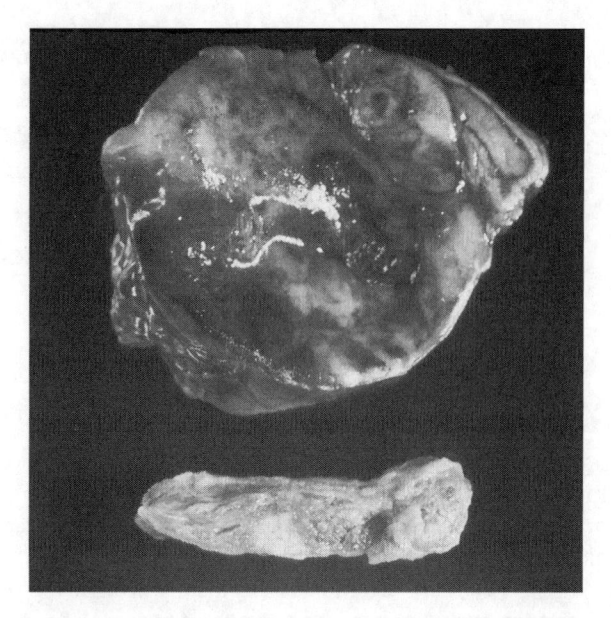

Fig. 1. A small medullary carcinoma lies in part of the thyroid lobe cut in cross-section. In the upper part, a pheochromocytoma replaces most of the adrenal gland. Hemorrhages are visible in the pheochromocytoma.

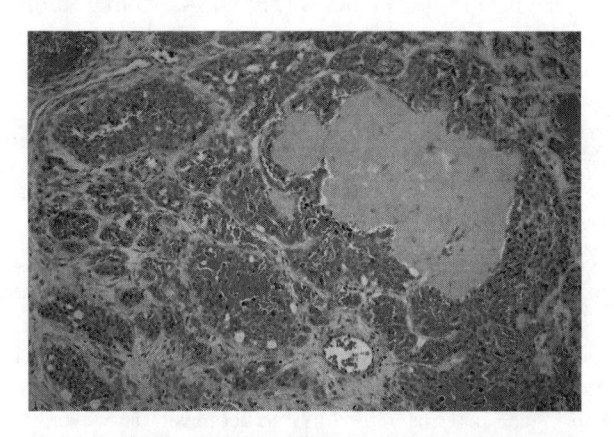

Fig. 2. Medullary carcinoma from a 47-yr-old woman. Note the deposit of amyloid (hematoxylin and eosin [H&E stain]).

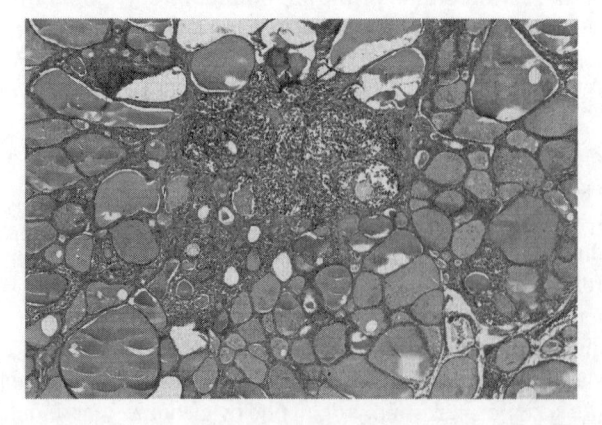

Fig. 3. A tiny medullary carcinoma was discovered incidentally in this thyroid of a 62-yr-old man (H&E stain).

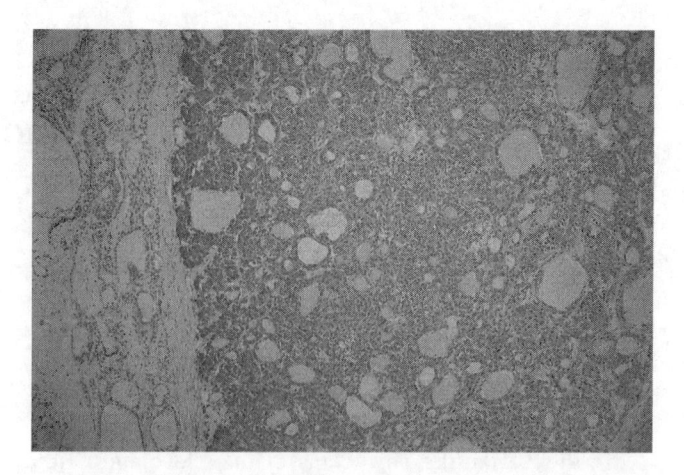

Fig. 4. Medullary carcinoma has trapped several normal thyroid follicles. The anticalcitonin procedure has stained the neoplastic cells.

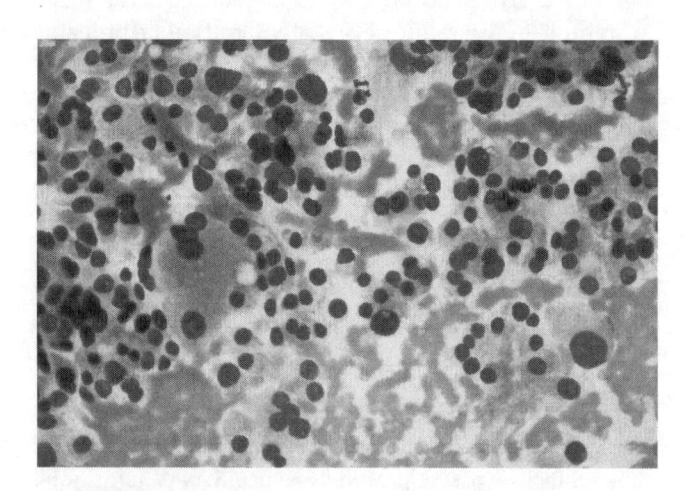

Fig. 5. Medullary carcinoma. Smear shows "tumor cellularity." Note loosely cohesive cells and the variation in nuclear size (Diff-Quik stain).

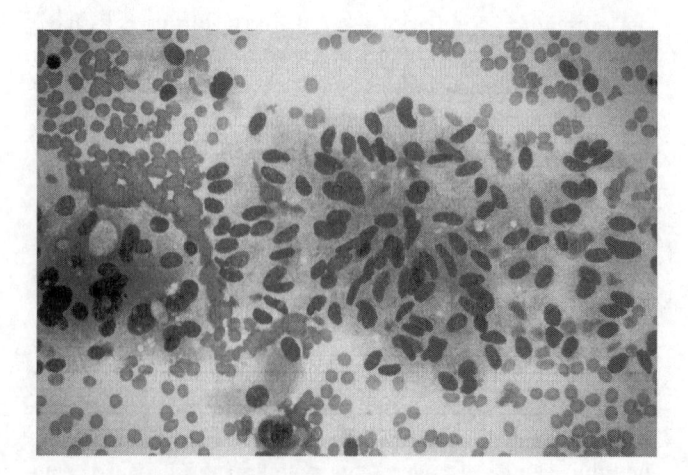

Fig. 6. Medullary carcinoma. Smear shows spindled cells with tenuous cytoplasm (Diff-Quik stain).

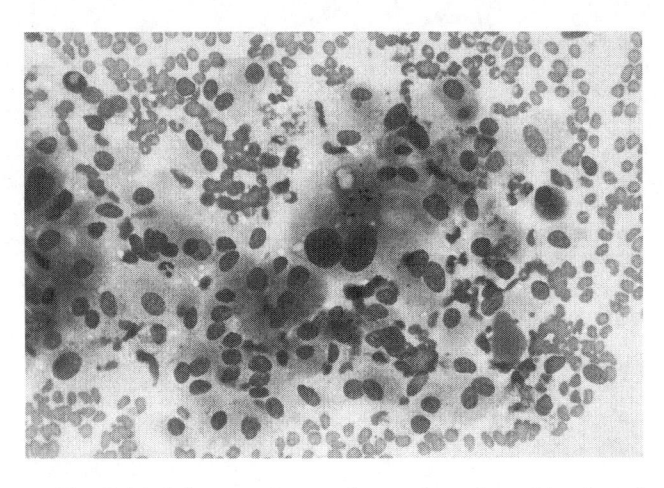

Fig. 7. Medullary carcinoma. Smear shows large binucleated cell with cytoplasmic vacuoles (Diff-Quik stain).

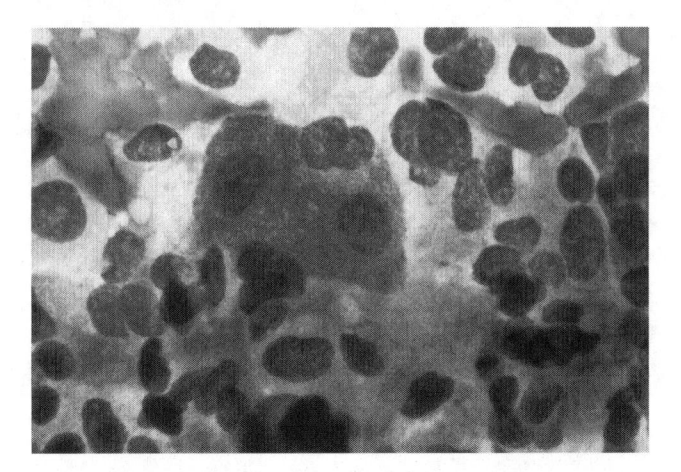

Fig. 8. Medullary carcinoma. Two of the neoplastic cells (with pink-staining cytoplasm) show calcitonin granules (Diff-Quik stain).

REFERENCES

1. Hazard JB, Crile Jr G, Dinsmore RS, et al. Neoplasms of the thyroid. Classification, morphology, and treatment. Arch Pathol Lab Med 1955; 59:502–513.
2. Hazard JB, Hawk WA, Crile G Jr. Medullary (solid) carcinoma of the thyroid: a clinicopathologic entity. J Clin Endocrinol Metab 1959; 19: 152–161.
3. Horn RC Jr. Carcinoma of the thyroid. Description of a distinctive morphological variant and report of seven cases. Cancer 1951; 4: 697–707.
4. Ljungberg O. On medullary carcinoma of the thyroid. APMIS Suppl 1972; (A)80:1–57.
5. Papotti M, Sambataro D, Pecchioni C, Bussolati G. The pathology of medullary carcinoma of the thyroid: review of the literature and personal experience on 62 cases. Endocr Pathol 1996; 7:1–20.
6. Sobrinho-Simoes M, Sambade C, Nesland JM, et al. Lectin histochemistry and ultrastructure of medullary carcinoma of the thyroid gland. Arch Pathol Lab Med 1990; 114:369–375.
7. Kaserer K, Scheuba C, Neuhold N, et al. Sporadic versus familial medullary thyroid microcarcinoma. A histopathologic study of 50 consecutive patients. Am J Surg Pathol 2001; 25:1245–1251.
8. Uribe M, Grimes M, Fenoglio-Preiser CM, Feind C. Medullary carcinoma of the thyroid gland: clinical, pathological, and immunohistochemical features with review of the literature. Am J Surg Pathol 1985; 9:577–594.
9. Dominguez-Malagon H, Delgado-Chavez R, Torres-Najera M, et al. Oxyphil and squamous variants of medullary thyroid carcinoma. Cancer 1989; 63:1183–1188.
10. Dottorini ME, Assi A, Sironi M, et al. Multivariate analysis of patients with medullary thyroid carcinoma: prognosis significance and impact on treatment of clinical and pathologic variables. Cancer 1996; 77: 1556–1565.
11. Papaparaskeva K, Nagel H, Droese M. Cytologic diagnosis of medullary carcinoma of the thyroid gland. Diagn Cytopathol 2000; 22:351–358.
12. Green I, Ali SZ, Allen EA, Zakowski MF. A spectrum of cytomorphologic variations in medullary thyroid carcinoma. Cancer (Cancer Cytopathol) 1997; 81:40–44.
13. Mendonca ME, Ramos S, Soares J. Medullary carcinoma of thyroid: a re-evaluation of the cytological criteria of diagnosis. Cytopathology 1991; 2:93–102.
14. Kumar PV, Hodjati H, Monabati A, Talei A. Medullary thyroid carcinoma. Rare cytologic findings. Acta Cytol 2000; 44:181–184.
15. Luboshitzky R, Dharan M. Mixed follicular-medullary thyroid carcinoma: A case report. Diagn Cytopathol 2004; 30:122–124.
16. Matias-Guiu X. Mixed medullary and follicular carcinoma of the thyroid. On the search for its histogenesis. Am J Pathol 1999; 155: 1413–1418.
17. Volante M, Papotti M, Roth J, et al. Mixed medullary-follicular thyroid carcinoma. Molecular evidence for a dual origin of tumor components. Am J Pathol 1999; 155:1499–1509.
18. Ljungberg O, Bondeson L, Bondeson A-G. Differentiated thyroid carcinoma, intermediate type: a new tumor entity with features of follicular and parafollicular cell carcinoma. Hum Pathol 1984; 15: 218–228.
19. Albores-Saavedra J, Gorraez de la Mora T, de la Torre-Rendon F, Gould E. Mixed medullary-papillary carcinoma of the thyroid: a previously unrecognized variant of thyroid carcinoma. Hum Pathol 1990; 21:1151–1155.

69
Medullary Carcinoma of the Thyroid
Surgical Management

Orlo H. Clark

ETIOLOGY AND DIAGNOSIS

Medullary thyroid cancer (MTC) accounts for about 6–10% of all thyroid malignancies. About 75% of patients with MTC have sporadic disease, and 25% have either familial MTC, multiple endocrine neoplasia (MEN) IIA, or IIB *(1)*. The different clinical types of MTC are associated with different but specific *ret* point mutations. About 50% of patients with sporadic MTC also have somatic *ret* mutations in their medullary cancer that appear to correlate with specific mutations *(2)*. For example, the 918 mutation associated with MENIIB when found as a somatic mutation in the tumor of MTC patients is linked with a worse prognosis *(2)*.

Most patients with MTC are first detected by fine-needle aspiration of a thyroid nodule. In patients with possible familial disease, MTC is detected by testing blood samples for a *ret* mutation or by basal and pentagastrin or calcium-stimulated calcitonin levels *(2–5)*. When suspected by cytological examination, the diagnosis of MTC should be confirmed by testing blood calcitonin and carcinoembryonic antigen (CEA) levels and/or with histochemical stains for calcitonin on the cytological specimen.

Because of possible MEN syndrome, all patients with suspected MTC by cytological examination should have their serum calcium levels tested to determine whether hyperparathyroidism is present and, more importantly, they must have a plasma and/or a 24-h urine test for catecholamine and metanephrine levels to rule out a pheochromocytoma. If present, surgical management of the pheochromocytoma takes precedence over medullary cancer. After appropriate α blockade, hydration, and often β blockade (for tachycardia), the pheochromocytoma should be removed. All patients with MTC should be retested for familial disease, as about 10% of patients with sporadic MTC have *de novo* germline mutations.

SURGICAL APPROACH

The preferred treatment for patients with MTC is total thyroidectomy and a meticulous central neck dissection, with or without removing the upper thymus *(6)*. The author requests an ultrasound examination of the thyroid and nodes preoperatively, and the central neck dissection is more vigorous on the side of any focal defects in the thyroid. Parathyroid glands should be marked but not removed unless the patient has primary hyperparathyroidism or the parathyroid gland or glands appear abnormal. However, any parathyroid gland that appears possibly devascularized should be autotransplanted into the neck muscle of patients with familial MTC, sporadic MTC, and MENIIB, and into the forearm of patients with MENIIA. The latter patients have an increased risk of developing hyperparathyroidism.

An ipsilateral modified neck dissection is recommended for: (1) patients with palpable cervical nodes, (2) patients with central neck nodes, and (3) patients with primary thyroid tumors greater than 1.5 cm in size. Studies by the Wells group *(7)* and at the Mayo Clinic *(8)* document that although about 70% of patients who had presented with nodal metastases are still alive at 10 yr, very few of these patients are calcitonin-negative. Patients with more than occult familial or bilateral disease need bilateral modified radical neck dissections. The parathyroid glands are at more risk in patients with MTC than in patients with papillary or follicular thyroid cancer because of the required meticulous central neck dissection. As previously mentioned, when a parathyroid gland cannot be saved on its vascular pedicle, it should be removed, washed in saline, biopsied to confirm it is parathyroid, and immediately autotransplanted to the sternocleidomastoid muscle on the side with less or no tumor. However, in patients with MENIIA, it should be autotransplanted to the forearm because subsequent hyperplasia and hyperfunction may develop.

Family members who are *ret* oncogene–positive or who have elevated basal calcitonin levels that increase in response to pentagastrin or calcium stimulation should have a total thyroidectomy and central neck dissection before age 6. Some authorities would recommend surgery even earlier.

From: *Thyroid Cancer: A Comprehensive Guide to Clinical Management, 2/e*
Edited by: L. Wartofsky and D. Van Nostrand © Humana Press Inc., Totowa, NJ

As mentioned above, an ultrasound is recommended to document whether there are any intrathyroidal nodules or adjacent lymph nodes preoperatively. The findings on ultrasound may modify the planned surgical approach in up to 40% of patients (9), and it clearly helps with planning the operation. The finding of lymph node metastases is likely to dictate both a central compartment and bilateral neck dissection (10), and a compartmentalized approach has been shown to minimize the risk of recurrence (11). Postoperatively, patients are followed with calcitonin and CEA levels. Magnetic resonance imaging or computed tomography are useful for documenting recurrent disease in the neck and/or mediastinum. Selective venous catheterization of the hepatic and cervical veins is useful for detecting distant metastases that are usually situated in the liver, lungs, or bone (12). Radiation therapy may be palliative in some patients (see Chapter 72).

REFERENCES

1. Jimenez C, Dang GT, Schultz PN, et al. A novel point mutation of the RET protooncogene involving the second intracellular tyrosine kinase domain in a family with medullary thyroid carcinoma. J Clin Endocrinol Metab 2004; 89:3521–3526.
2. Zedenius J, Larsson C, Bergholm U, et al. Mutations of codon 918 in the *ret* proto-oncogene correlate to poor prognosis in sporadic medullary thyroid carcinomas. J Clin Endocrinol Metab 1995; 80: 3088–3090.
3. Eng C. Seminars in medicine of the Beth Israel Hospital, Boston: the *ret* proto-oncogene in multiple endocrine neoplasia type 2 and Hirschsprung's disease. N Engl J Med 1996; 335:943–951.
4. Wells SA Jr, Chi DD, Toshima K, et al. Predictive DNA testing and prophylactic thyroidectomy in patients at risk for multiple endocrine neoplasia type 2A. Ann Surg 1994; 220:237–247; discussion 247–250.
5. Lips CJ, Landsvater RM, Hoppener JW, et al. Clinical screening as compared with DNA analysis in families with multiple endocrine neoplasia type 2A. N Engl J Med 1994; 331:828–835.
6. Kebebew E, Kikuchi S, Duh QY, Clark OH. Long-term results of reoperation and localizing studies in patients with persistent or recurrent medullary thyroid cancer. Arch Surg 2000; 135:895–901.
7. Kebebew E, Clark OH, Medullary thyroid cancer. In Clark OH, Duh Q-Y, Perrier ND, Jahan TM, editors. Endocrine Tumors. Hamilton, Ontario: BC Decker Inc., 2003: 23–36.
8. Gharib H, McConahey WM, Tiegs RD, et al. Medullary thyroid carcinoma: clinicopathologic features and long-term follow-up of 65 patients treated during 1946 through 1970. Mayo Clin Proc 1992; 67: 934–940.
9. Kouvaraki MA, Shapiro SE, Fornage BD, et al. Role of preoperative ultrasonography in the surgical management of patients with thyroid cancer. Surgery 2003; 134:946–955.
10. Scollo C, Baudin E, Travagli J-P, et al. Rationale for central and bilateral lymph node dissection in sporadic and hereditary medullary thyroid cancer. J Clin Endocrinol Metab 2003; 88:2070–2075.
11. Yen TWF, Shapiro SE, Gagel RF, et al. Medullary thyroid carcinoma: Results of a standardized surgical approach in a contemporary series of 80 consecutive patients. Surgery 2003; 134:890–901.
12. Gautvik KM, Talle K, Hager B, et al. Early liver metastases in patients with medullary carcinoma of the thyroid gland. Cancer 1989; 63: 175–180.

70
Radionuclide Imaging of Medullary Carcinoma
Utility of Radiolabeled Somatostatin Analogs and Other Radiotracers

Giuseppe Esposito

INTRODUCTION

Medullary thyroid cancer (MTC) has a favorable prognosis if locally confined at diagnosis. Its 10-yr survival rate decreases dramatically if distant metastases are present. Early recognition of residual/metastatic disease allows surgical excision of the tumor, which can be curative. If surgical excision cannot be done, chemotherapy and external-beam radiation have limited therapeutic success. The initial diagnostic evaluation should include neck ultrasound (US), computed tomography (CT), and/or magnetic resonance imaging (MRI). Nuclear medicine studies have an important role for the early localization of metastatic disease when it is suspected based on persistently elevated calcitonin or carcinoembryonic antigen (CEA) plasma levels following the initial surgery. For the evaluation of metastatic disease, nuclear medicine studies are used in conjunction with US, CT, and MRI, particularly if the extent and location of metastatic foci are still inconclusive.

Radiolabeled somatostatin analogs (RSAs) have become the most useful radiotracers for the detection of metastatic/recurrent MTC. Along with other neuroendocrine tumors (NETs), MTC can express different subtypes of somatostatin receptors (SSTRs), which are the targets of RSAs for diagnostic and therapeutic applications. Imaging with RSAs provides information on the receptor status of MTCs and other NETs to help decide which patients may benefit from treatment with either unlabeled somatostatin analogs (SAs) or RSAs.

Other radiotracers have proven to be useful in the diagnostic evaluation of MTC but do not offer the prognostic and therapeutic information like the RSAs. Among these, the most commonly used are pentavalent dimercaptosuccinic acid (DMSA) labeled with ^{99m}Tc and metaiodobenzylguanidine (MIBG) labeled with ^{131}I. This chapter focuses on the role of RSAs in the clinical evaluation of MTC and briefly reviews the role of other radiotracers in comparison with the RSAs. The use of 18-fluorodeoxyglucose positron emission tomography (FDG-PET) in the management of MTC is reviewed in detail in Chapter 71 and is only briefly presented in this chapter for comparison to the RSAs.

RADIOLABELED SOMATOSTATIN ANALOGS

^{111}In pentetreotide (Octreoscan®) is among the first and the most often used RSA. ^{111}In-labeling (2.83-d half-life) has replaced ^{123}I (13.3-h half-life). Compared to the ^{123}I formulation, Octreoscan® offers more flexibility in the imaging protocols, a more favorable body distribution, and a higher tumor–background ratio *(1)*.

Mechanism of Uptake

Pentetreotide is a synthetic analog of somatostatin—a 14-amino acid polypeptide normally produced by neurons and endocrine cells. There are five subtypes of SSTRs. Pentetreotide binds with higher affinity to the subtype II. After binding to the SSTRs, pentetreotide is internalized, then transferred into the nucleus. SSTRs are present on tumor cells that can be visualized with Octreoscan®: pituitary adenomas, meningiomas, pancreatic islet cells tumors, lung cancer (particularly small-cell lung cancer), carcinoids, and neuroendocrine cancers, including MTC and pheochromocytomas *(2,3)*. Lymphocytes are also rich in SSTRs, which explains the uptake of Octreoscan® in granulomas, lymphomas, autoimmune disorders (e.g., Graves' disease), and particularly in patients with Graves' ophthalmopathy *(1)*.

Dose and Normal Body Distribution

For diagnostic applications, Octreoscan® is administered intravenously at a dose of 222 MBq. It is important to discontinue any therapy with cold octreotide for 2 d before radiotracer administration because the latter will interfere with the uptake of Octreoscan®. Whole-body planar and single-photon emission computed tomography (SPECT) images are usually taken at 4 and 24 h after administration to allow clearance of background activity. The ^{111}In γ emissions at 171 and 245 keV are used for imaging.

From: *Thyroid Cancer: A Comprehensive Guide to Clinical Management, 2/e*
Edited by: L. Wartofsky and D. Van Nostrand © Humana Press Inc., Totowa, NJ

Octreoscan® is excreted mainly through the kidneys via glomerular filtration, but some degree of excretion occurs through the hepatobiliary route as well. During the first 4 h after administration, plasma radioactivity is mainly owing to unmetabolized Octreoscan®, which is mostly eliminated ultimately via the kidneys. Subsequent to the first 4 h from administration, metabolites appear in both plasma and urine. Spleen and kidneys represent the dose-limiting organs (4). Normal uptake is visualized in the pituitary gland, thyroid gland, spleen, liver, kidneys, and urinary bladder. The normal visualization of the kidneys on Octreoscan® images is primarily because of nonspecific tubular reabsorption of the radiotracer after glomerular filtration, but a small portion represents interaction with SSTRs in renal tissue. Activity in the gallbladder and bowel is sometimes visualized, particularly on images acquired after 24 h. This activity represents nonspecific uptake and excretion. In the normal thyroid, pituitary gland, and spleen, the uptake is the result of interaction with specific SSTRs (1). Diffuse breast uptake can be normally seen in young women. Uptake has been described in the nose and lung hila in patients with upper respiratory infections and appears to be from activated lymphocytes. After surgery or external radiation therapy, uptake of ^{111}In pentetretide has been described and may be secondary to the associated inflammatory/reactive changes (1).

Indications

Diagnosis

The reported sensitivity of Octreoscan® for MTC detection varies widely across studies (between 65% and 100%; 5–9). Sensitivity is lower for detection or localization of primary tumor in the thyroid gland and that of metastatic disease in the liver (10), probably because of the higher background activity present in the surrounding tissues of these organs. The ability to detect foci of metastatic disease strongly depends on the expression of somatostatin receptors on the tumor cells. Lower uptake levels of Octreoscan® are seen with less differentiated tumors that present with a lower calcitonin–CEA plasma ratio (11) and that likely express fewer SSTRs. Detection sensitivity is generally lower for MTC vs other NETs. Compared to other NETs, MTCs express lower densities of SSTRs and have greater variability in SSTR subtypes, with a lower expression rate of the subtypes II and V that bind octreotide with higher affinity (12,13). In addition, MTCs may also produce somatostatin, which would compete for receptor binding of Octreoscan® (13). Even with these potential limitations, Octreoscan® and other RSAs have a well-defined role as adjuncts to conventional imaging for the evaluation of metastatic MTC.

Octreoscan® may detect additional lesions when compared to conventional imaging. Krauz et al. (14) reported that pathological uptake was detected in 9 of 10 patients with persistent or recurrent MTC, and 5 of these foci were not seen by other diagnostic modalities (CT or MRI). In another series, tumor localization was demonstrated by octreotide scanning in 11 of 17 patients (5). In a prospective study of 18 patients with MTC (15), Octreoscan® outperformed MRI in some of the patients with minimal residual disease who were diagnosed by persistent elevation of calcitonin. The adjunctive role of Octreoscan® in cases not clarified by conventional imaging was evaluated by Baudin et al. (8) in patients in whom metastatic disease was suspected based of an increased calcitonin level. In 12 patients with metastatic disease identified by conventional imaging, Octreoscan® imaging did not add additional clinically relevant information, even though some smaller lesions were identified only by Octreoscan®. In 12 patients with negative or indeterminate results with conventional imaging, Octreoscan® was negative in 10 patients, but correctly identified disease in two patients.

Accuracy of Octreoscan® imaging was worse than that by conventional imaging, particularly for lesions less than 1 cm in size. In a series of 20 patients with elevated calcitonin levels after initial surgery (16), Octreoscan® detected 15 pathological uptake foci in 11 patients, and CT detected 17 foci in 11 patients. A false-positive scan occurred in one patient with sarcoidosis. The patients with true-positive Octreoscan® studies had significantly higher basal calcitonin and CEA levels than the patients with negative isotopic studies. The authors concluded that the sensitivity of Octreoscan® imaging for detection of metastatic disease is generally lower than conventional imaging but is more favorable in patients with high calcitonin serum levels. They also concluded that Octreoscan® should be used when conventional imaging is negative or ambiguous, or when treatment with somatostatin analogs is being considered.

In a retrospective study of 14 patients with recurrent metastatic MTC, Arslan et al. (17) compared Octreoscan® imaging with conventional imaging, including CT, MRI, and US. They found that Octreoscan® detected disease similar to other imaging in 78.5% of the patients but detected fewer lesions (44% vs 81%). As seen in other studies, Octreoscan® was able to detect a few lesions that were not revealed by conventional imaging. In fact, the highest sensitivities for lesion detection were reached with the combination of conventional and radionuclide imaging (85.7%).

The use of combined SPECT/CT acquisition can also increase the accuracy of Octreoscan® imaging. In a series of 72 patients, the combined acquisition affected diagnostic interpretation in 32% of patients and changed clinical management in 14% compared to routine acquisition protocols (14). Preoperative administration of Octreoscan® can increase the ability to detect disease and improve the yield of surgical therapy using handheld intraoperative probes to search for tumors that express SSTRs *(18,19)*.

Evaluation of Treatment With SAs

SAs have a role in the treatment of NETs, possibly controlling symptoms that derive from the hormonal production of NETs. The therapeutic potential of SAs is related to several mechanisms of antitumoral action. These are the inhibition of angiogenesis, antimitotic effect, regulation of the immune response, induction of apoptosis and inhibition of the release, and action of growth factors and growth hormones *(20)*. In MTC, results have been controversial pertaining to the ability to induce a therapeutic response *(21–24)*. The importance of nuclear medicine imaging with RSAs is in its potential to visualize tumors that express SSTRs. The degree of RSA uptake in the tumor foci is directly related to the number of SSTRs expressed in the tumor *(25,26)*. The possibility to stratify patients for treatment with SAs based on the results of nuclear medicine evaluation.

Treatment With RSAs

^{111}In Octreotide

The success of radioimmunotherapy in the treatment of B-cell lymphomas that are refractory to conventional chemotherapy or radiation therapy has drawn scientific and commercial interest in the use of radiolabeled peptides for therapeutic applications. ^{111}In Octreoscan® at high doses (20–74 GBq) has been among the first peptides used for therapeutic methods in oncology. It combines the pharmacologic action of the SA octreotide and radiotoxic effect of ^{111}In. The radiotoxic effect is because of the emission of Auger electrons. Auger electrons have a short range of action that is less than the diameter of a cell but are highly cytotoxic if emitted within the cell nucleus. After interaction with SSTRs, the ^{111}In–receptor–ligand complex is internalized and transported into the cell nucleus *(27)*. In cell cultures, internalization of Octreoscan® decreases cell survival vs cells that do not show internalization *(28)*.

Several phase I/II studies are being conducted to examine the value of radionuclide treatment with ^{111}In Octreoscan® in NETs that express SSTRs. Among various studies and different NETs, variable response rates have been observed (as high as ~60%) in patients refractory to other treatment modalities *(29–31)*. Most protocols fractionate a total cumulative dose of 20–74 GBq of ^{111}In Octreoscan®. The kidney is the dose-limiting organ, and the principal toxicity is derived from exposure of the hematopoietic system, but most patients experience only a temporary decline in blood counts, particularly platelets. Side effects related to the pharmacologic action of the SA usually include abdominal discomfort, nausea, flatulence, and diarrhea.

Other RSAs

Most NETs express SSTR 2 and interact with octreotide. The expression of SSTRs and the receptor subtypes may vary in the different NETs and within the same kind of NETs. The variability in receptor expression may be responsible for poor response to treatment with cold or radiolabeled octreotide. SAs that have broader spectrum of interaction among SSTRs subtypes have been synthesized and may prove useful to visualize and treat tumors with lower expression of SSTR type 2. Lanreotide is a SA with high affinity for different receptor subtypes *(2–5)*. It has been labeled with ^{111}In *(32)* and has shown discrepancies in tumor uptake when compared with ^{111}In-Octreoscan® in about one third of different tumor patients. Differences in affinity profiles with the five SSTR subtypes seem to explain these differences *(33)*.

SAs have also been labeled with other radionuclides, ^{90}Y, and more recently, ^{177}Lu, and are being tested as therapeutic agents *(34,35,35a)*. These radionuclides emit β radiation of longer range of action, which extends their effectiveness to nearby cells that do not internalize the receptor–radioligand complex ("crossfire"). This represents a theoretical advantage in larger tumors where the nonuniform vascularization leaves some tumor cells out of reach of the radioligand. A phase IIa clinical trial (Mauritius trial) in Europe administered doses of up to 232 mCi of ^{90}Y-lanreotide to 154 different tumor patients. In 63 of 154 patients (41%), disease remained stable, and regression was observed in 14% of the patients. Quantitative assessment of uptake from the different tumors showed that NETs accumulate ocreotide more than lanreotide, and that lanreotide accumulated better in radioiodine-negative thyroid cancer, hepatocellular cancer, lung cancers, and brain tumors *(33)*.

OTHER DIAGNOSTIC AGENTS

Pentavalent ^{99m}Tc DMSA appears to localize in MTC because of increased turnover of calcium and phosphate ions and has shown satisfactory tumor–background ratios to permit good scintigraphic images *(36)*. However, experience with DMSA has been limited by difficulties in the preparation and storage of the radioisotope *(37)*. Guerra and coworkers *(38)* found an overall 84% sensitivity of ^{99m}Tc (V) DMSA in 26 patients with MTC. Clarke and associates *(39)* found an even higher sensitivity of 95% ^{99m}Tc (V) DMSA for the detection of bone and soft-tissue metastases. The use of ^{99m}Tc (V) DMSA is limited by the fact that it is not commercially available in the United Stated but must be prepared in each laboratory by adding sodium bicarbonate to standard DMSA kits. The ratio of ^{99m}Tc (IV) DMSA to ^{99m}Tc (V) DMSA must be monitored using thin-layer chromatography. Small changes in bicarbonate/DMSA levels cause dramatic worsening of image quality and sensitivity. Overall, DMSA is less accurate than Octreoscan® to detect metastatic MTC (17), but the two methods combined may sometimes show additive value in the visualization of metastatic lesions.

MIBG is a radiolabeled norepinephrine analog taken up by cells through a specific energy-dependent transport mechanism in which the tracer competes with norepinephrine. Sensitivities for ^{131}I MIBG imaging are highest for detecting pheochromocytomas and less satisfactory for MTC (40). Several case reports confirm accurate localization of primary and recurrent MTC in sporadic and familial cases using ^{131}I MIBG (41,42). However, in a review of larger series (36), the diagnostic accuracy of MIBG was found to be limited by low overall sensitivity to find metastatic MTC. In a recent direct comparison, Octreoscan® imaging was more sensitive than MIBG in the detection of metastatic disease in different NETs, including MTC (43). In addition, imaging with ^{131}I MIBG is burdened with technical difficulties, resulting from the ^{131}I label. The thyroid gland must be blocked with cold iodine administration prior to the study. The high-energy γ rays (364 keV) of ^{131}I also make imaging technically difficult and patient dosimetry unfavorable.

Metastatic MTC may be visualized with anti-CEA monoclonal antibodies labeled with ^{99m}Tc, ^{131}I, or ^{111}In, particularly in tumors that have higher CEA–calcitonin plasma ratios (44). Phases I and II clinical trials have tested the efficacy of radioimmunotherapy with ^{131}I- or ^{90}Y-labeled anti-CEA monoclonal antibodies alone or in association with different chemotherapeutic regimens (45,46). Partial responses were achieved only at myeloablative doses. Other trials have then tested radioimmunotherapy in combination with autologous hematopoietic stem cell rescue (47), with only one durable partial remission and one minor response obtained in 12 patients. Better tumor–background ratios, better antitumor effect, and the possibility for outpatient treatment favor labeling with ^{90}Y compared to ^{131}I.

^{99m}Tc methylene diphosphonate (MDP) has been used for years for nonspecific, but extremely sensitive, detection of bone metastases of a variety of tumors, including MTC (39). Nonskeletal metastases of MTC may be seen using ^{99m}Tc MDP. This may be related to the propensity of MTC to calcify or the association with amyloid deposits (48).

The tumor-seeking properties of ^{201}Tl that localizes in hypercellular structures have been utilized in the evaluation of MTC (49). ^{99m}Tc sestamibi may also localize in MTC with very high calcitonin levels (50,51). In a direct comparison of ^{201}Tl, ^{99m}Tc sestamibi, and ^{99m}Tc-DMSA, overall sensitivity was better for sestamibi and DMSA (~80%) vs ^{201}Tl (73%; 52). In the same study, ^{99m}Tc sestamibi appeared less accurate in identifying lymphadenopathies, ^{201}Tl performed poorly in bone metastasis, and ^{99m}Tc sestamibi appeared better in nonlymphatic soft-tissue metastasis.

SAS IN DIFFERENTIATED THYROID CANCER

Octreoscan® imaging has proven useful to detect metastatic disease from thyroid cancer that has lost the ability to concentrate radioiodine and has become unresponsive to radioiodine treatment with ^{131}I. The utility of somatostatin analogs for this purpose will only be briefly mentioned here but is discussed in Chapter 35. In 48 patients with metastatic non-MTC as assessed by high thyroglobulin (TG) levels, Octreoscan® detected metastatic lesions in 74% of the patients when TG was less than 10 ng/mL and in 85% when TG was more than 10 ng/mL. Octreoscan® uptake was greater in Hürthle cell cancer ($n = 29$ patients), for which Octreoscan® had 95% sensitivity if TG was below 10 ng/mL (53). In a recent study, Stokkel et al. (54) were able to visualize metastatic thyroid cancer in 9 of 10 patients with elevated TG levels and ^{131}I-negative whole-body scans, in whom metastasis was detected by conventional imaging. In patients with ^{131}I-positive scans, Octreoscan® was positive in only two of five patients, suggesting that expression of SSTRs may be more frequent in less differentiated tumors that have lost the ability to trap iodine. In a series of 18 patients with iodine-negative thyroid cancer, Octreoscan® found metastatic disease in 14 of the patients who had metastatic disease already diagnosed by conventional imaging (55).

In eight of these patients, conventional and Octreoscan® imaging were concordant; in nine patients, conventional imaging showed more extensive disease than seen with Octreoscan®. In one patient, Octreoscan® was more accurate and showed more extensive disease than conventional imaging. Haslinghuis et al. (56) reported visualization of metastatic lesions in 75% of the patients with negative iodine uptake. FDG-PET is an important tool in the evaluation of metastatic thyroid cancer that does not concentrate iodine. FDG-PET is more accurate than imaging with RSAs in the diagnostic evaluation of patients with negative iodine scans and suspected or known metastatic disease (57). FDG-PET has shown a sensitivity of more than 65% for detection of metastatic disease in numerous studies (58). Virgolini et al. (59) reported detection of disease in 36 of 38 patients with iodine-negative metastatic thyroid cancer. Studies are needed to specifically evaluate the diagnostic and potential therapeutic role of the RSA studies in iodine-negative, FDG-PET-negative, metastatic thyroid cancer as suspected on the basis of elevated TG levels.

The ability to detect disease that has lost the ability to take up iodine may open new possibilities for treatment with high doses of Octreoscan® or with other SAs labeled with ^{111}In or ^{90}Y (55). However, considerable uncertainty exists as to whether treatment with RSAs of thyroid cancer that is refractory to radioiodine treatment will be effective. Gorges et al. (53) failed to obtain response in three patients treated with ^{90}Y-DOTATOC. Newer agents and the refinement of treatment protocols and of patient selection may improve the outcome with these novel therapeutic strategies.

SUMMARY AND FUTURE DIRECTIONS

For the diagnostic examination of MTC, nuclear medicine techniques are most useful in the evaluation of suspected metastatic disease as an adjunct to traditional radiologic evaluation, which includes neck US, CT, and MRI. A number of imaging agents are available in nuclear medicine, but RSAs offer the best combination of diagnostic accuracy, technical flexibility, and availability in comparison to other radiotracers. Overall, conventional imaging has a better diagnostic accuracy for the evaluation of metastatic disease and should always represent the first line in the diagnostic process. However, SAs may detect disease not identified by conventional imaging, particularly in cases of well-differentiated disease that maintains a high calcitonin–CEA plasma values.

The unique application of RSAs is in the ability to assess the expression of SSTRs on foci of metastatic disease that would then constitute targets for possible treatment with either cold or RSAs, thereby combining pharmacologic and radiotoxic actions on the tumor cells. The introduction of new SAs, which have either a wider spectrum of action among the different subtypes of SSTRs or greater specificity for single subtypes, may improve treatment and visualization of disease that expresses different subtypes. This is particularly true for MTC. Progress in the radiochemistry of SAs now offers the flexibility to label them with different radionuclides (^{111}In, ^{90}Y, and ^{177}Lu). It is conceivable that different SAs may be used for different tumors, according to the specific receptor subtype profiles. Technical advances in methods (PET, PET/CT, and SPECT/CT) have already made an impact in the management of different tumors. The role of FDG-PET in MTC and other NETs has been explored in Chapter 71. The synthesis of SAs labeled with positron emission emitters may bring exciting developments in the diagnostic and therapeutic management of patients with neuroendocrine and other tumors *(35)*.

REFERENCES

1. Krenning EP, Kwekkeboom DJ, Bakker WH, et al. Somatostatin receptor scintigraphy with [111In-DTPA-D-Phe1]- and [123I-Tyr3]-octreotide: the Rotterdam experience with more than 1000 patients. Eur J Nucl Med 1993; 20:716–731.
2. Reubi JC, Laissue J, Krenning E, Lamberts SW. Somatostatin receptors in human cancer: incidence, characteristics, functional correlates and clinical implications. J Steroid Biochem Mol Biol 1992; 43:27–35.
3. Reubi JC, Chayvialle JA, Franc B, et al. Somatostatin receptors and somatostatin content in medullary thyroid carcinomas. Lab Invest 1991; 64:567–573.
4. Krenning EP, Bakker WH, Kooij PP, et al. Somatostatin receptor scintigraphy with indium-111-DTPA-D-Phe-1-octreotide in man: metabolism, dosimetry and comparison with iodine-123-Tyr-3-octreotide. J Nucl Med 1992; 33:652–658.
5. Kwekkeboom DJ, Reubi JC, Lamberts SW, et al. In vivo somatostatin receptor imaging in medullary thyroid carcinoma. J Clin Endocrinol Metab 1993; 76:1413–1417.
6. Tisell LE, Ahlman H, Wangberg B, et al. Somatostatin receptor scintigraphy in medullary thyroid carcinoma. Br J Surg 1997; 84: 43–547.
7. Adams S, Baum RP, Hertel A, et al. Comparison of metabolic and receptor imaging in recurrent medullary thyroid carcinoma with histopathological findings. Eur J Nucl Med 1998; 25:1277–1283.
8. Baudin E, Lumbroso J, Schlumberger M, et al. Comparison of octreotide scintigraphy and conventional imaging in medullary thyroid carcinoma. J Nucl Med 1996; 37:912–916.
9. Kurtaran A, Scheuba C, Kaserer K, et al. Indium-111-DTPA-D-Phe-1-octreotide and technetium-99m-(V)-dimercaptosuccinic acid scanning in the preoperative staging of medullary thyroid carcinoma. J Nucl Med 1998; 39:1907–1909.
10. Frank-Rave K, Bihl H, Dorr, et al. Somatostatin receptor imaging in persistent medullary thyroid carcinoma. Clin Endocrinol 1995; 42:31–37.
11. Rougier P, Calmettes C, Laplanche A, et al. The values of calcitonin and carcinoembryonic antigen in the treatment and management of nonfamilial medullary thyroid carcinoma. Cancer 1983; 51:855–862.
12. Papotti M, Kumar U, Volante M, et al. Immunohistochemical detection of somatostatin receptor types 1–5 in medullary carcinoma of the thyroid. Clin Endocrinol (Oxf) 2001; 54:641–649.
13. Pacini F, Elisei R, Anelli S, et al. Somatostatin in medullary thyroid cancer. In vitro and in vivo studies. Cancer 1989; 63:1189–1195.
14. Krausz Y, Keidar Z, Kogan I, et al. SPECT/CT hybrid imaging with 111In-pentetreotide in assessment of neuroendocrine tumours. Clin Endocrinol (Oxf) 2003; 59:565–573.
15. Dorr U, Wurstlin S, Frank-Raue K, et al. Somatostatin receptor scintigraphy and magnetic resonance imaging in recurrent medullary thyroid carcinoma: a comparative study. Horm Metab Res Suppl 1993; 27:48–55.
16. Berna L, Chico A, Matias-Guiu X, et al. Use of somatostatin analogue scintigraphy in the localization of recurrent medullary thyroid carcinoma. Eur J Nucl Med 1998; 25:1482–1488.
17. Arslan N, Ilgan S, Yuksel D, et al. Comparison of In-111 octreotide and Tc-99m (V) DMSA scintigraphy in the detection of medullary thyroid tumor foci in patients with elevated levels of tumor markers after surgery. Clin Nucl Med 2001; 26:683–688.
18. Benevento A, Dominioni L, Carcano G, Dionigi R. Intraoperative localization of gut endocrine tumors with radiolabeled somatostatin analogs and a gamma-detecting probe. Semin Surg Oncol 1998; 15:239–244.
19. Benjegard SA, Forssell-Aronsson E, Wangberg B, et al. Intraoperative tumour detection using 111In-DTPA-D-Phe1-octreotide and a scintillation detector. Eur J Nucl Med 2001; 28:1456–1462.
20. Lamberts SW, Krenning EP, Reubi JC. The role of somatostatin and its analogs in the diagnosis and treatment of tumors. Endocr Rev 1991; 12:450–482.
21. Modigliani E, Cohen R, Joannidis S, et al. Results of long-term continuous subcutaneous octreotide administration in 14 patients with medullary thyroid carcinoma. Clin Endocrinol (Oxf) 1992; 36:183–186.
22. Mahler C, Verhelst J, de Longueville M, Harris A. Long-term treatment of metastatic medullary thyroid carcinoma with the somatostatin analogue octreotide. Clin Endocrinol (Oxf) 1990; 33:261–269.
23. Diez JJ, Iglesias P. Somatostatin analogs in the treatment of medullary thyroid carcinoma. J Endocrinol Invest 2002; 25:773–778.
24. Lupoli G, Cascone E, Arlotta F, et al. Treatment of advanced medullary thyroid carcinoma with a combination of recombinant interferon alpha-2b and octreotide. Cancer 1996; 78:1114–1118.
25. Janson ET, Westlin JE, Eriksson B, et al. [111In-DTPA-D-Phe1] octreotide scintigraphy in patients with carcinoid tumours: the predictive value for somatostatin analogue treatment. Eur J Endocrinol 1994; 131:577–581.

26. Lamberts SW, Hofland LJ, Nobels FR. Neuroendocrine tumor markers. Front Neuroendocrinol 2001; 22:309–339.
27. Hofland LJ, Lamberts SW. The pathophysiological consequences of somatostatin receptor internalization and resistance. Endocr Rev 2003; 24:28–47.
28. Janson ET, Westlin JE, Ohrvall U, et al. Nuclear localization of 111In after intravenous injection of [111In-DTPA-D-Phe1]-octreotide in patients with neuroendocrine tumors. J Nucl Med 2000; 41:1514–1518.
29. Valkema R, De Jong M, Bakker WH, et al. Phase I study of peptide receptor radionuclide therapy with [In-DTPA]octreotide: the Rotterdam experience. Semin Nucl Med 2002; 32:110–122.
30. De Jong M, Breeman WA, Bernard HF, et al. Therapy of neuroendocrine tumors with radiolabeled somatostatin-analogues. Q J Nucl Med 1999; 43:356–366.
31. McCarthy KE, Woltering EA, Anthony LB. In situ radiotherapy with 111In-pentetreotide. State of the art and perspectives. Q J Nucl Med 2000; 44:88–95.
32. Virgolini I, Szilvasi I, Kurtaran A, et al. Indium-111-DOTA-lanreotide: biodistribution, safety and radiation absorbed dose in tumor patients. J Nucl Med 1998; 39:1928–1936.
33. Virgolini I, Britton K, Buscombe J, et al. In- and Y-DOTA-lanreotide: results and implications of the MAURITIUS trial. Semin Nucl Med 2002; 32:148–155.
34. Virgolini I, Traub T, Novotny C, et al. Experience with indium-111 and yttrium-90-labeled somatostatin analogs. Curr Pharm Des 2002; 8:1781–1807.
35. Weiner RE, Thakur ML. Radiolabeled peptides in the diagnosis and therapy of oncological diseases. Appl Radiat Isot 2002; 57:749–763.
35a. Vainas I, Koussis CH, Pazaitou-Panayiotou K, et al. Somatostatin receptor expression in vivo and response to somatostatin analog therapy with or without other antineoplastic treatments in advanced medullary thyroid carcinoma. J Exp Clin Cancer Res 2005; 23:549–559.
36. Miyauchi A, Endo K, Ohta H, et al. 99mTc(V)-dimercaptosuccinic acid scintigraphy for medullary thyroid carcinoma. World J Surg 1986; 10:640–645.
37. Skowsky WR, Wilf LH. Iodine 131 metaiodobenzylguanidine scintigraphy of medullary carcinoma of the thyroid. South Med J 1991; 84:636–641.
38. Guerra UP, Pizzocaro C, Terzi A, et al. New tracers for the imaging of the medullary thyroid carcinoma. Nucl Med Commun 1989; 10:285–295.
39. Clarke SE, Lazarus CR, Wraight P, et al. Pentavalent [99mTc]DMSA, [131I]MIBG, and [99mTc]MDP—an evaluation of three imaging techniques in patients with medullary carcinoma of the thyroid. J Nucl Med 1988; 29:33–38.
40. Shapiro B, Copp JE, Sisson JC, et al. Iodine-131 metaiodobenzylguanidine for the locating of suspected pheochromocytoma: experience in 400 cases. J Nucl Med 1985; 26:576–585.
41. Sone T, Fukunaga M, Otsuka N, et al. Metastatic medullary thyroid cancer: localization with iodine-131 metaiodobenzylguanidine. J Nucl Med 1985; 26:604–608.
42. Ansari AN, Siegel ME, DeQuattro V, Gazarian LH. Imaging of medullary thyroid carcinoma and hyperfunctioning adrenal medulla using iodine-131 metaiodobenzylguanidine. J Nucl Med 1986; 27:1858–1860.
43. Kaltsas G, Korbonits M, Heintz E, et al. Comparison of somatostatin analog and meta-iodobenzylguanidine radionuclides in the diagnosis and localization of advanced neuroendocrine tumors. J Clin Endocrinol Metab 2001; 86:895–902.
44. Behr TM, Sharkey RM, Juweid ME, et al. Reduction of the renal uptake of radiolabeled monoclonal antibody fragments by cationic amino acids and their derivatives. Cancer Res 1995; 55:3825–3834.
45. Stein R, Chen S, Reed L, et al. Combining radioimmunotherapy and chemotherapy for treatment of medullary thyroid carcinoma: effectiveness of dacarbazine. Cancer 2002; 94:51–61.
46. Stein R, Govindan SV, Mattes MJ, et al. Targeting human cancer xenografts with monoclonal antibodies labeled using radioiodinated, diethylenetriaminepentaacetic acid-appended peptides. Clin Cancer Res 1999; 5(10 Suppl):3079S–3087S.
47. Juweid ME, Hajjar G, Stein R, et al. Initial experience with high-dose radioimmunotherapy of metastatic medullary thyroid cancer using 131I-MN-14 F(ab)2 anti-carcinoembryonic antigen MAb and AHSCR. J Nucl Med 2000; 41:93–103.
48. Johnson DG, Coleman RE, McCook TA, et al. Bone and liver images in medullary carcinoma of the thyroid gland: concise communication. J Nucl Med 1984; 25:419–422.
49. Koizumi M, Yamada Y, Nomura E, et al. Scintigraphic detection of recurrence of medullary thyroid cancer. Ann Nucl Med 1995; 9:101–104.
50. Learoyd DL, Roach PJ, Briggs GM, et al. Technetium-99m-sestamibi scanning in recurrent medullary thyroid carcinoma. J Nucl Med 1997; 38:227–230.
51. Lebouthillier G, Morais J, Picard M, et al. Tc-99m sestamibi and other agents in the detection of metastatic medullary carcinoma of the thyroid. Clin Nucl Med 1993; 18:657–661.
52. Adalet I, Kocak M, Oguz H, et al. Determination of medullary thyroid carcinoma metastases by 201Tl, 99Tcm(V)DMSA, 99Tcm-MIBI and 99Tcm-tetrofosmin. Nucl Med Commun 1999; 20:353–359.
53. Gorges R, Kahaly G, Muller-Brand J, et al. Radionuclide-labeled somatostatin analogues for diagnostic and therapeutic purposes in nonmedullary thyroid cancer. Thyroid 2001; 11:647–659.
54. Stokkel MP, Reigman HI, Verkooijen RB, Smit JW. Indium-111-Octreotide scintigraphy in differentiated thyroid carcinoma metastases that do not respond to treatment with high-dose I-131. J Cancer Res Clin Oncol 2003; 129:287–294.
55. Christian JA, Cook GJ, Harmer C. Indium-111-labelled octreotide scintigraphy in the diagnosis and management of non-iodine avid metastatic carcinoma of the thyroid. Br J Cancer 2003; 89:258–261.
56. Haslinghuis LM, Krenning EP, De Herder WW, et al. Somatostatin receptor scintigraphy in the follow-up of patients with differentiated thyroid cancer. J Endocrinol Invest 2001; 24:415–422.
57. Gabriel M, Froehlich F, Decristoforo C, et al. 99mTc-EDDA/HYNIC-TOC and (18)F-FDG in thyroid cancer patients with negative (131)I whole body scans. Eur J Nucl Med Mol Imaging 2004; 31:330–341.
58. Sarlis NJ, Gourgiotis L, Guthrie LC, et al. In-111 DTPA-octreotide scintigraphy for disease detection in metastatic thyroid cancer: comparison with F-18 FDG positron emission tomography and extensive conventional radiographic imaging. Clin Nucl Med 2003; 28:208–217.
59. Virgolini I, Patri P, Novotny C, et al. Comparative somatostatin receptor scintigraphy using In-111-DOTA-lanreotide and In-111-DOTA-Tyr3-octreotide versus F-18-FDG-PET for evaluation of somatostatin receptor-mediated radionuclide therapy. Ann Oncol 2001; 12 (Suppl 2):S41–S45.

71
PET in Medullary Thyroid Cancer

I. Ross McDougall

INTRODUCTION

The optimal treatment for medullary thyroid cancer is total thyroidectomy and central nodal lymphadenectomy at presentation when the primary cancer is small and has not metastasized significantly (1). In the three phenotypes of familial medullary cancer, i.e., familial medullary cancer, multiple endocrine neoplasia (MEN) IIA, and MENIIB, screening of families for patients with a mutation in the *RET* proto-oncogene and a genetic predisposition for the diseases allows surgery at an even earlier stage (2–4). Unfortunately, not all patients are treated at the optimal time. Some patients with sporadic medullary cancer have extensive local and distant metastases at the time of diagnosis. It is important to define the extent of disease when planning treatment. Other patients who have undergone appropriate surgery are found to have a measurable calcitonin level after the operation. This implies there is residual disease in the thyroid bed or lymph nodes or distant sites. It is helpful if the site or sites of calcitonin production can be identified when they are small and amenable to removal at a reoperation.

When a decision is reached to try and identify the sites of residual or recurrent cancer, there should be an organized approach that begins with a careful clinical examination. The surgical and pathological reports should be reviewed because they can provide clues to the most likely site of cancer. Radiological imaging includes ultrasound, computed tomography (CT), and magnetic resonance imaging (MRI). These are less useful postoperatively and are not effective when they do not include the anatomic region of the potential metastases. Possible methods for scintigraphic investigation include ^{201}Tl, ^{99m}Tc sestamibi, ^{99m}Tc tetrafosmin, or ^{99m}Tc pentavalent dimercaptosuccinate acid (DMSA; 5–7). Metaiodobenzylguanidine (MIBG) labeled with either ^{131}I or ^{123}I has been used to image pheochromocytoma, and these radiopharmaceuticals occasionally localize in medullary cancer (8). Antibodies against antigens from medullary cancer cells have been labeled with radiotracers and tested for imaging (see Chapter 70).

More recently, positron emission tomography (PET) after intravenous injection of F-18 fluorodeoxyglucose (FDG) has been investigated for this purpose. The number of patients with medullary cancer who have been studied using FDG-PET is considerably less than those with differentiated thyroid cancer. Nevertheless, Bockisch et al. indicate that PET is the most sensitive of these investigations, with a sensitivity and specificity of approx 80% (9). The results of several studies are summarized here, followed by information of a newer PET radiopharmaceutical, F-18 fluorodopa (18F-DOPA).

Seven patients with recurrent medullary thyroid cancer and rapidly increasing carcinoembryonic antigen (CEA) levels were evaluated using FDG and ^{99m}Tc-DMSA (10). DMSA identified only three lesions in two patients. PET found abnormalities in all patients, including 1 pulmonary, 3 skeletal, 20 mediastinal, 10 cervical, and 4 liver metastases. The authors confirmed tumor in 29 of these positive sites on PET, with 9 lymph node metastases removed by operation. In a report from different investigators, 20 patients were studied using FDG-PET (11). Some patients had abnormal ultrasound findings in the neck, and all had elevated calcitonin. FDG-PET identified the cancer in 13 of 17 patients, which were confirmed by other imaging tests or biopsy. Five patients had negative PET scans, and four were judged to be false-negatives. FDG-PET detected 12 of 14 cancer sites in the neck, 6 of 7 in the mediastinum, and both pulmonary and bone metastases. In two patients with elevated calcitonin levels, no site of cancer was found by any test. The sensitivity of FDG-PET was 76% (95% confidence interval, 53–94%).

A multi-institutional study examined 100 FDG-PET scans in 85 patients with elevated calcitonin or CEA levels, and several had abnormal ultrasound findings (12). Many authors of this report have published independent studies; therefore, some patients might be included in more than one article. There were 181 lesions that could be identified by one imaging test, and 55 sites were confirmed pathologically. FDG-PET detected 123 of the lesions (68%). In patients with proven sites of medullary cancer, the investigators identified 32 true-positive, 3 false-positive, 11 true-negatives, and 9 false-negative lesions. The sensitivity for proven cancers was 78%, and the specificity was 79%. In comparison to other diagnostic modalities, the sensitivities were 25% for ^{111}In octreotide, 33% for ^{99m}Tc-DMSA, 25% for ^{99m}Tc sestamibi, 50% for CT, and 82% for MRI.

In a separate investigation in 40 patients with elevated calcitonin values after thyroidectomy, FDG detected 270 foci, MRI identified 116 lesions, and CT found 141 *(13)*. Regarding lesions in the neck, PET, MRI, and CT found 98, 34, and 34, respectively. PET was also superior for detection of lesions in the mediastinum.

False-positive FDG-PET scans were discussed in detail in the section above on well-differentiated thyroid cancer (see Chapter 34), and causes include such inflammatory diseases as tuberculosis and histoplasmosis. Abnormal uptake of FDG-PET in neck muscles and brown fat that can be misinterpreted as nodal metastases are best recognized by PET or CT technology *(14,15)*. Cook et al. have summarized the problem areas *(16,17)*.

6-F-18 Fluorodopamine PET has been used as an alternative to FDG, and there are reports of its value in detecting recurrent medullary cancer and pheochromocytoma *(18)*. Hoergerle et al. used several imaging tests, including 18F-DOPA and FDG, ^{111}In octeotide, CT, and MRI, to evaluate sensitivity and specificity in detecting 27 known lesions *(19)*. There were 3 in the thyroid region, 16 in lymph nodes, and 8 were distant metastases. The tests were complementary, with the sensitivity of 18F-DOPA-PET being 63% vs 44% for FDG-PET and 52% for ^{111}In octeotide. Morphological procedures had the highest sensitivity at 81%, but their specificities were the lowest. The same authors reported a 100% sensitivity for 18F-DOPA-PET in 17 pheochromocytomas *(20)*, a sensitivity that was superior to that of MIBG. Other investigators have presented similar results *(21)*.

In summary, PET has a definite role in staging medullary cancer in patients who have a significant primary cancer and a high level of calcitonin. However, the main role of PET is to identify the site or sites of calcitonin production in patients who have had surgery and continue to have measurable calcitonin levels. FDG is the preferred radiopharmaceutical because it is widely available. Combined PET and CT have the advantage of demonstrating the exact anatomic position of abnormal accumulation of FDG. The results with 18F-DOPA are encouraging, and this might prove to be the agent of choice when it is approved and available for routine clinical use.

REFERENCES

1. Kebebew E, Ituarte PHG, Siperstein AE, et al. Medullary thyroid carcinoma. Clinical characteristics, treatment, prognostic factors, and a comparison of staging systems. Cancer 2000; 88:1139–1148.
2. Machens A, Niccoli-Sire P, Hoegel J, et al. Early malignant progression of hereditary medullary thyroid cancer. N Engl J Med 2003; 349: 1517–1525.
3. Eng C, Clayton D, Schuffenecker I, et al. The relationship between specific RET proto-oncogene mutations and disease phenotype in multiple endocrine neoplasia type 2. International RET mutation consortium analysis. JAMA 1996; 276:1575–1579.
4. Cote GJ, Gagel RF. Lessons learned from the management of a rare genetic cancer. N Engl J Med 2003; 349:1566–1568.
5. Forssell-Aronsson EB, Nilsson O, Bejegard SA, et al. 111In-DTPA-D-Phe1-octreotide binding and somatostatin receptor subtypes in thyroid tumors. J Nucl Med 2000; 41:636–642.
6. Adalet I, Demirkale P, Unal S, et al. Disappointing results with Tc-99m tetrofosmin for detecting medullary thyroid carcinoma metastases comparison with Tc-99m VDMSA and Tl-201. Clin Nucl Med 1999; 24: 678–683.
7. Adams BK, Fataar A, Byrne MJ, et al. Pentavalent technetium-99m (V)-DMSA uptake in a pheochromocytoma in a patient with Sipple's syndrome. J Nucl Med 1990; 31:106–108.
8. Baulieu JL, Guilloteau D, Delisle MJ, et al. Radioiodinated meta-iodobenzylguanidine uptake in medullary thyroid cancer. A French cooperative study. Cancer 1987; 60:2189–2194.
9. Bockisch A, Brandt-Mainz K, Gorges R, et al. Diagnosis in medullary thyroid cancer with [18F]FDG-PET and improvement using a combined PET/CT scanner. Acta Med Austriaca 2003; 30:22–25.
10. Adams S, Baum R, Rink T, et al. Limited value of fluorine-18 fluorodeoxyglucose positron emission tomography for the imaging of neuroendocrine tumours. Eur J Nucl Med 1998; 25:79–83.
11. Brandt-Mainz K, Muller SP, Gorges R, et al. The value of fluorine-18 fluorodeoxyglucose PET in patients with medullary thyroid cancer. Eur J Nucl Med 2000; 27:490–496.
12. Diehl M, Risse JH, Brandt-Mainz K, et al. Fluorine-18 fluorodeoxyglucose positron emission tomography in medullary thyroid cancer: results of a multicentre study. Eur J Nucl Med 2001; 28: 1671–1676.
13. Szakall S, Jr, Esik O, Bajzik G, et al. 18F-FDG PET detection of lymph node metastases in medullary thyroid carcinoma. J Nucl Med 2002; 43: 66–71.
14. Barrington S, Maisey MN. Skeletal muscle uptake of fluorine-18 FDG: effect of oral diazepam. J Nucl Med 1996; 37:1127–1129.
15. Cohade C, Mourtzikos KA, Wahl RL. "USA-Fat": prevalence is related to ambient outdoor temperature-evaluation with 18F-FDG PET/CT. J Nucl Med 2003; 44:1267–1270.
16. Cook G, Maisey MN, Fogelman I. Normal variants, artefacts and interpretative pitfalls in PET with 18-fluoro-2-deoxyglucose and carbon-11 methionine. Normal variants, artefacts and interpretative pitfalls in PET with 18-fluoro-2-deoxyglucose and carbon-11 methionine. Eur J Nucl Med 1999; 26:1363–1378.
17. Cook G, Wegner EA, Fogelman I. Pitfalls and artifacts in 18FDG PET and PET/CT oncologic imaging. Semin Nucl Med 2004; 34: 122–133.
18. Gourgiotis L, Sarlis NJ, Reynolds JC, et al. Localization of medullary thyroid carcinoma metastasis in a multiple endocrine neoplasia type 2A patient by 6-[18F]-fluorodopamine positron emission tomography. J Clin Endocrinol Metab 2003; 88:637–641.
19. Hoegerle S, Altehoefer C, Ghanem N, et al. 18F-DOPA positron emission tomography for tumour detection in patients with medullary thyroid carcinoma and elevated calcitonin levels. Eur J Nucl Med 2001; 28: 64–71.
20. Hoegerle S, Nitzsche E, Altehoefer C, et al. Pheochromocytomas: detection with 18F DOPA whole body PET—initial results. Radiology 2002; 222:507–512.
21. Ilias I, Yu J, Carrasquillo JA, et al. Superiority of 6-[18F]-fluorodopamine positron emission tomography versus [131I]-metaiodobenzylguanidine scintigraphy in the localization of metastatic pheochromocytoma. J Clin Endocrinol Metab 2003; 88: 4083–4087.

72
External Radiation Therapy of Medullary Cancer

James D. Brierley and Richard W. Tsang

GROSS RESIDUAL DISEASE

For patients with gross residual disease after surgery for medullary thyroid cancer (MTC), the local control rate after radiation therapy (RT) is unsatisfactorily low (20–25%; *1,2*). Therefore, every attempt should be made to diagnose MTC at an early stage, then to initiate a surgical management plan to achieve complete excision of the disease. When this is not possible, external RT may result in long-term local control, but in only a few patients. Innovative approaches with novel systemic agents *(3,4)* or radioimmunotherapy *(5,6)* are being investigated.

ADJUVANT THERAPY

External-beam RT has no role in postsurgical management of MTC patients with small intrathyroidal primary lesions, where spread to regional lymph nodes is absent. However, for patients with high-risk features, such as gross or microscopic residual disease, extrathyroidal invasion, or extensive regional lymph node involvement, postoperative adjuvant external RT to the thyroid bed and regional lymph nodes may be considered. With surgery alone, approximately half of these high-risk patients will have recurrences in the neck. Radiation doses of 4000 cGy in 2-Gy fractions to the cervical and superior mediastinal lymph nodes, followed by a boost to the thyroid bed to total a dose of 5000 cGy, has been associated with a 10-yr local regional control rate of 86% *(2)*. External-beam RT does not impact overall survival, but optimal local regional control is important because a relapse in neck tissues after prior extensive neck surgery may be difficult to treat, a potential deleterious impact on the patient's quality of life. However, it is important to note that patients at high risk of local regional relapse are also at high risk of distant metastases. Other investigators have confirmed similar results of improved local regional control in high-risk patients after radiation; these data are summarized in Table 1 *(1,7–9)*.

Following standard surgical therapy that generally involves total thyroidectomy and central and bilateral cervical lymph node dissection, a patient may continue to have high calcitonin levels with no clinically detectable metastasis. Imaging with radionuclides (e.g., metaiodobenzylguanidine) or somatostatin analogs (e.g., octreotide) may show abnormalities and help direct therapy *(10–12)* (see Chapter 70). If there is no evidence of disease below the clavicles, local regional neck radiation may be considered as an alternative to reoperation and meticulous neck dissection. Selective venous catheterization may occasionally locate the main source of calcitonin *(13,14)*. More recently, F-18 fluorodeoxyglucose positron emission tomography (FDG-PET) has shown promise in locating small tumor volumes and assisting the overall management of the patient *(15–19)* (see Chapter 71). These scans are generally more informative when the FDG-PET data is correlated directly with computed tomography findings *(17,19)*. The levels of calcitonin and carcinoembryonic antigen (CEA) in the blood correlate with tumor bulk, and patients with high calcitonin levels may be symptomatic with watery diarrhea. It is not unusual to see elevated but stable calcitonin and/or CEA levels for a long period of time (e.g., 5–10 yr) without obvious progression of disease *(20)*. Hence, the presence of asymptomatic subclinical metastatic disease is not an absolute contraindication to adjunctive local regional RT to the neck. However, cytotoxic treatment for an asymptomatic patient should be considered with some reluctance because the patient may have indolent disease *(9)*. Symptoms of diarrhea can be palliated with antidiarrheal drugs (e.g., diphenoxylate, loperamide) or somatostatin analogs *(21)*, with or without interferon *(3,22)*. A decline in the calcitonin level may not necessarily reflect tumor regression, as it can be secondary to dedifferentiation and could herald a more aggressive clinical course *(23)*. Therefore, RT for hypercalcitonemia should only occur in the adjuvant setting, when there is a high risk of recurrence in the neck from extensive extrathyroidal extension, extensive nodal disease, or both.

EXTERNAL-BEAM RT

The thyroid bed is a technically challenging volume to treat, as the thyroid bed curves around the vertebral body and includes the air column in the trachea. It can be difficult to adequately treat the thyroid bed and spare the spinal cord to

From: *Thyroid Cancer: A Comprehensive Guide to Clinical Management, 2/e*
Edited by: L. Wartofsky and D. Van Nostrand © Humana Press Inc., Totowa, NJ

Table 1
Results of Adjuvant External RT in High-Risk MTC From Retrospective Studies

	Surgery Alone 10-yr Local/Regional Recurrence Rate	Surgery and RT 10-yr Local/Regional Recurrence Rate
Brierley (2)	86%	52%
Fersht (9)	59%	29%
Mak (7)	76%	16%
Nguyen (8)	N/A	30%

N/A, not available.
Note: Non-randomized comparison.

a tolerable dose. A variety of techniques have been described that produce sufficient dose distribution (24). Advances in radiation techniques that result in better dosage to the areas at risk and reduce the volume of normal tissues to a minimum are described in Chapter 84. Well-planned external-beam RT has acceptable acute toxicity and rarely produces serious complications. In patients assigned to the radiation arm of a German randomized control study (that closed because of poor accrual), the majority of patients experienced mild-to-moderate side effects from adjuvant external-beam RT. At the first follow-up, most adverse effects had subsided, and the early or acute toxicity was tolerable in these patients. Late toxicity is infrequent; the most common manifestations are skin telangiectasia, increased skin pigmentation, soft-tissue fibrosis, and mild lymphedema, predominantly in the submental area. Esophageal and tracheal stenosis are extremely rare. Neither Tsang et al. (25) nor Farahati et al. (26) reported any grade IV (Radiation Therapy Oncology Group) late toxicity. If external-beam radiation does not lead to local control, and the patient relapses in the thyroid bed, salvage surgery may still be possible with an experienced surgeon in postradiation surgery to the head and neck region.

METASTATIC DISEASE

Metastasis is unfortunately common in sporadic MTC, and the most frequently involved organs are the liver, lung, and bone. Treatment is palliative and includes supportive measures, analgesic drugs, and possibly, hormonal therapy, chemotherapy, and local radiation. Hormonal therapy consists of somatostatin analogs (e.g., octreotide), reported to lessen symptoms and reduce calcitonin levels but generally does not induce tumor responses (3,21,27–29). A combination of octreotide and interferon α may result in a higher response rate (3,21,22). Compared with hormones, chemotherapy is associated with more toxicity and is documented to have a tumor response rate of only 15–30%. Active chemotherapeutic drugs include doxorubicin, either as single agent or with cisplatin (30), 5-fluorouracil combination therapy (31–34), and others (4,35,36) (see Chapter 73). Therefore, local radiation should be considered for metastasis. Unfortunately, neither the liver nor large volumes of the lung tolerate RT well. Thus, RT is usually reserved for painful osseous metastases. With bone lesions, a dose of 2000 cGy in five daily fractions or 3000 cGy in 10 fractions would typically result in pain relief. Single large lung metastases causing hemoptysis or obstruction may also respond to RT. Experimental therapy with targeted radiation by monoclonal antibodies (e.g., anti-CEA, or ^{111}In octreotide) conjugated to radionuclides are under investigation (5,6,37–40).

REFERENCES

1. Fife KM, Bower M, Harmer CL. Medullary thyroid cancer: the role of radiotherapy in local control. Eur J Surg Oncol 1996; 22:588–591.
2. Brierley JD, Tsang RW, Gospodarowicz MK, et al. Medullary thyroid cancer—analyses of survival and prognostic factors and the role of radiation therapy in local control. Thyroid 1996; 6:305–310.
3. Vitale G, Tagliaferri P, Caraglia M, et al. Slow release lanreotide in combination with interferon-alpha2b in the treatment of symptomatic advanced medullary thyroid carcinoma. J Clin Endocrinol Metab 2000; 85:983–988.
4. Kaczirek K, Schindl M, Weinhausel A, et al. Cytotoxic activity of camptothecin and paclitaxel in newly established continuous human medullary thyroid carcinoma cell lines. J Clin Endocrinol Metab 2004; 89:2397–2401.
5. Behr TM, Sharkey RM, Juweid ME, et al. Phase I/II clinical radio-immunotherapy with an iodine-131-labeled anti-carcinoembryonic antigen murine monoclonal antibody IgG. J Nucl Med 1997; 38: 858–870.
6. Juweid ME, Hajjar G, Stein R, et al. Initial experience with high-dose radioimmunotherapy of metastatic medullary thyroid cancer using 131I-MN-14 F(ab)2 anti-carcinoembryonic antigen MAb and AHSCR. J Nucl Med 2000; 41:93–103.
7. Mak A, Morrison W, Garden A, et al. The value of postoperative radiotherapy for regional medullary carcinoma of the thyroid. Int J Radiat Oncol Biol Phys 1994; 30:234.
8. Nguyen TD, Chassard JL, Lagarde P, et al. Results of postoperative radiation therapy in medullary carcinoma of the thyroid: a retrospective study by the French Federation of Cancer Institutes—the Radiotherapy Cooperative Group. Radiother Oncol 1992; 23:1–5.
9. Fersht N, Vini L, A'Hern R, Harmer C. The role of radiotherapy in the management of elevated calcitonin after surgery for medullary thyroid cancer. Thyroid 2001; 11:1161–1168.
10. Baudin E, Lumbroso J, Schlumberger M, et al. Comparison of octreotide scintigraphy and conventional imaging in medullary thyroid carcinoma. J Nucl Med 1996; 37:912–916.
11. Tisell LE, Ahlman H, Wangberg B, et al. Somatostatin receptor scintigraphy in medullary thyroid carcinoma. Br J Surg 1997; 84:543–547.
12. Parisella M, D'Alessandria C, van de Bossche B, et al. 99mTc-EDDA/HYNIC-TOC in the management of medullary thyroid carcinoma. Cancer Biother Radiopharm 2004; 19:211–217.
13. Abdelmoumene N, Schlumberger M, Gardet P, et al. Selective venous sampling catheterisation for localisation of persisting medullary thyroid carcinoma. Br J Cancer 1994; 69:1141–1144.
14. Ben Mrad MD, Gardet P, Roche A, et al. Value of venous catheterization and calcitonin studies in the treatment and management of clinically inapparent medullary thyroid carcinoma. Cancer 1989; 63: 133–138.

15. Schoder H, Yeung HW. Positron emission imaging of head and neck cancer, including thyroid carcinoma. Semin Nucl Med 2004; 34:180–197.
16. Crippa F, Alessi A, Gerali A, Bombardieri E. FDG-PET in thyroid cancer. Tumori 2003; 89:540–543.
17. Gotthardt M, Battmann A, Hoffken H, et al. 18F-FDG PET, somatostatin receptor scintigraphy, and CT in metastatic medullary thyroid carcinoma: a clinical study and an analysis of the literature. Nucl Med Commun 2004; 25:439–443.
18. Boer A, Szakall S, Jr., Klein I, et al. FDG PET imaging in hereditary thyroid cancer. Eur J Surg Oncol 2003; 29:922–928.
19. Bockisch A, Brandt-Mainz K, Gorges R, et al. Diagnosis in medullary thyroid cancer with [18F]FDG-PET and improvement using a combined PET/CT scanner. Acta Med Austriaca 2003; 30:22–25.
20. Girelli ME, Nacamulli D, Pelizzo MR, et al. Medullary thyroid carcinoma: clinical features and long-term follow-up of seventy-eight patients treated between 1969 and 1986. Thyroid 1998; 8:517–523.
21. di Bartolomeo M, Bajetta E, Buzzoni R, et al. Clinical efficacy of octreotide in the treatment of metastatic neuroendocrine tumors. A study by the Italian Trials in Medical Oncology Group. Cancer 1996; 77:402–408.
22. Lupoli G, Cascone E, Arlotta F, et al. Treatment of advanced medullary thyroid carcinoma with a combination of recombinant interferon alpha-2b and octreotide. Cancer 1996; 78:1114–1118.
23. Saad M, Orddonez N, Rashid R, et al. Medullary carcinoma: Prognostic factors and treatment. Int J Radiat Oncol Biol Phys 1984; 9:161–169.
24. Tsang RW, Brierley JD. The Thyroid. In Cox JD, Kian Ang K, editors. Radiation Oncology. St. Louis, MO: Mosby, 2003.
25. Tsang RW, Brierley JD, Simpson WJ, et al. The effects of surgery, radioiodine and external radiation therapy on the clinical outcome of patients with differentiated thyroid cancer. Cancer 1998; 82:375–388.
26. Farahati J, Reiners C, Stuschke M, et al. Differentiated thyroid cancer. Impact of adjuvant external radiotherapy in patients with perithyroidal tumor infiltration (stage pT4). Cancer 1996; 77:172–180.
27. Frank-Raue K, Ziegler R, Raue F. The use of octreotide in the treatment of medullary thyroid carcinoma. Horm Metab Res Suppl 1993; 27:44–47.
28. Mahler C, Verhelst J, de Longueville M, Harris A. Long-term treatment of metastatic medullary thyroid carcinoma with the somatostatin analogue octreotide. Clin Endocrinol (Oxf) 1990; 33:261–269.
29. Modigliani E, Cohen R, Joannidis S, et al. Results of long-term continuous subcutaneous octreotide administration in 14 patients with medullary thyroid carcinoma. Clin Endocrinol (Oxf) 1992; 36:183–186.
30. Shimaoka K, Schoenfeld DA, DeWys WD, et al. A randomized trial of doxorubicin versus doxorubicin plus cisplatin in patients with advanced thyroid carcinoma. Cancer 1985; 56:2155–2160.
31. Schlumberger M, Abdelmoumene N, Delisle MJ, Couette JE. Treatment of advanced medullary thyroid cancer with an alternating combination of 5 FU-streptozocin and 5 FU-dacarbazine. The Groupe d'Etude des Tumeurs a Calcitonine (GETC). Br J Cancer 1995; 71:363–365.
32. Orlandi F, Caraci P, Berruti A, et al. Chemotherapy with dacarbazine and 5-fluorouracil in advanced medullary thyroid cancer. Ann Oncol 1994; 5:763–765.
33. Bajetta E, Rimassa L, Carnaghi C, et al. 5-Fluorouracil, dacarbazine, and epirubicin in the treatment of patients with neuroendocrine tumors. Cancer 1998; 83:372–378.
34. Di Bartolomeo M, Bajetta E, Bochicchio AM, et al. A phase II trial of dacarbazine, fluorouracil and epirubicin in patients with neuroendocrine tumours. A study by the Italian Trials in Medical Oncology (I.T.M.O.) Group. Ann Oncol 1995; 6:77–79.
35. Wu LT, Averbuch SD, Ball DW, et al. Treatment of advanced medullary thyroid carcinoma with a combination of cyclophosphamide, vincristine, and dacarbazine. Cancer 1994; 73:432–436.
36. Ekman ET, Lundell G, Tennvall J, Wallin G. Chemotherapy and multimodality treatment in thyroid carcinoma. Otolaryngol Clin North Am 1990; 23:523–527.
37. Juweid M, Sharkey RM, Behr T, et al. Radioimmunotherapy of medullary thyroid cancer with iodine-131-labeled anti-CEA antibodies. J Nucl Med 1996; 37:905–911.
38. Stein R, Juweid M, Zhang CH, Goldenberg DM. Assessment of combined radioimmunotherapy and chemotherapy for treatment of medullary thyroid cancer. Clin Cancer Res 1999; 5:3199S–3206S.
39. Monsieurs M, Brans B, Bacher K, et al. Patient dosimetry for 131I-MIBG therapy for neuroendocrine tumours based on 123I-MIBG scans. Eur J Nucl Med Mol Imaging 2002; 29:1581–1587.
40. Buscombe JR, Caplin ME, Hilson AJ. Long-term efficacy of high-activity 111In-pentetreotide therapy in patients with disseminated neuroendocrine tumors. J Nucl Med 2003; 44:1–46.

73
Medullary Carcinoma of the Thyroid
Chemotherapy

Lawrence S. Lessin

Like other neuroendocrine tumors, medullary thyroid carcinoma (MTC) runs a protracted course. Early detection and surgery provides the only curative approach. Extension of the tumor beyond the thyroid capsule is the most significant prognostic indicator, and when present, the disease cannot be cured by surgery alone. For local and distant metastases of MTC that cannot be treated by surgery or external-beam radiation therapy, chemotherapy is used. Doxorubicin used either alone or in combination is the most widely applied chemotherapeutic agent. Responses are assessed by the degree of or decrease in tumor mass, reduction in symptoms, or decline in levels of calcitonin and carcinoembryonic antigen (CEA) tumor markers.

Controversy exists regarding the chemosensitivity of medullary carcinoma. Gottlieb and Hill (1) treated a variety of thyroid cancers with doxorubicin (including MTC) and found three partial responses of five patients treated. Disease-related diarrhea improved not only in tumor responders but also in one patient who did not achieve a response (see Table 1). Benker and Reinwein (2) and De Besi and colleagues (3) treated MTC with doxorubicin alone and found a higher response rate than in differentiated and anaplastic carcinomas. In contrast, Scheruble and colleagues (4) treated 10 patients with advanced MTC with combination chemotherapy using doxorubicin, bleomycin, and vindesine; the observed response rate was poor, with only one partial response. Although six patients in the latter series had stable disease, calcitonin and CEA tumor markers continued to rise. Similarly, Athanassiades and associates (5) treated six patients with doxorubicin and cisplatinum and found no response. Droz and coworkers (6) reported their experience over a 10-yr period using five different protocols, with both single-agent and combination chemotherapy. Of 41 treatments, only two partial responses were noted, and both occurred in patients receiving doxorubicin at a dose rate of 60 mg/m^2 every 4 wk. Response duration was brief, lasting only 3 mo in both cases. Porter and Ostrowski (7) treated a patient who had MTC with low-dose doxorubicin at 15 mg/m^2 per week and achieved a complete response; the patient remained in remission for 18 mo.

Although there are no definitive phase III trial data, combination chemotherapy appears to have no advantage over single-agent doxorubicin in the treatment of advanced MTC. Massart and colleagues (8) showed overexpression of the *MDR-1* gene in a human MTC cell line, which could explain its multidrug resistance. They also showed that in vitro resistance to doxorubicin can be partially reversed by the blockage of the MDR-1 pump with cyclosporin A or verapamil.

Etoposide has been used as single-agent chemotherapy by Hoskin and Harmer (9) and by Kelsen et al. (10), based on its activity in other neuroendocrine tumors. However, only minor responses were seen. A complete response was reported by Sigurdur and Petursson (11) using darcarbazine and 5-fluorouracil; pulmonary and subcutaneous metastases remained in remission for 10 mo, along with suppression of CEA and calcitonin tumor markers. Burgess and colleagues (12), reporting for the M.D. Anderson group, treated nine patients with metastatic MTC with a four-drug combination, including doxorubicin, carboplatin, imidazole carboxamide, and vincristine. Five patients responded for a median of 5 mo at the time of the report, with sustained decreases in calcitonin and/or CEA.

In a European multicenter study by the *Groupe d'Etude des Tumeurs a Calcitonine*, Nocera and colleagues treated 20 patients with advanced metastatic MTC using alternating doublets of doxorubicin and streptozotocin and 5-fluorouracil and dacarbazine (13). They observed three partial responses and 10 long-term stabilizations, with acceptable toxicity. The principal toxicity was myelosuppression, and the authors considered this regimen to be effective and tolerable. New protocols are assessing the role of high-dose chemotherapy with hematopoietic stem cell rescue (autologous transplant) in metastatic MTC. Although anecdotal responses have been reported, this approach is investigational and the potential benefit has yet to be determined.

From: *Thyroid Cancer: A Comprehensive Guide to Clinical Management, 2/e*
Edited by: L. Wartofsky and D. Van Nostrand © Humana Press Inc., Totowa, NJ

Table 1
Chemotherapeutic Trials in Treatment of Medullary Thyroid Cancer

Author (Ref.)	Agent Used	Patient Response
Gottlieb and Hill (1)	Doxorubicin 60–75 mg/m^2 q3 wk	3 of 5
Shimaoka (15)	Doxorubicin 60 mg/m^2 q3 wk; doxorubicin	1 of 4
	60 mg/m^2 plus cisplatin 40 mg/m^2/q3 wk	2 of 6
Benker and Reinwein (2)	Doxorubicin at various dose schedule	8 of 20
Hoskin and Harmer (9)	Doxorubicin, bleomycin, and vincristine	5 of 13
Droz et al. (16)	Doxorubicin 60 mg/m^2 q4 wk	2 of 18
Scheruble et al. (4)	Doxorubicin 50 mg/m^2, cisplatin 60 mg/m^2, and vindesine 3 mg/m^2	1 of 10
Athanassiades et al. (5)	Doxorubicin 50 mg/m^2 and cisplatin 70 mg/m^2 q3 wk	0 of 6
Frame et al. (17)	Doxorubicin 20 mg/m^2 and streptozotocin 1000 mg/m^2	1 of 5
De Besi et al. (3)	Doxorubicin 60 mg/m^2, bleomycin 30 U × 3 d, and cisplatin 60 mg/m^2	3 of 9
Burgess et al. (12)	Doxorubicin 45–70 mg/m^2, carboplatin 600–750 mg/m^2, DTIC 600–800 mg/m^2, vincristine, 2 mg, all q21 d	4 of 9
Nocera et al. (13)	Doxorubicin—streptozotocin, alternating with 5-fluorouracil and decarbazine	3 of 20

Because MTC is a neuroendocrine tumor, the somatostatin analog, octreotide, has been employed since 1977, when Muller and colleagues (14) reported reduction in tumor markers in a patient treated with octreotide. Mahler and colleagues (15) reported symptomatic improvement of diarrhea with octreotide and reduction in tumor markers but only minimal or no decrease in tumor mass. Tachyphylaxis, which occurs with continued use of octreotide, can be temporarily overcome by increasing the dose. As medullary carcinoma is often indolent, quality-of-life assessment is important in treatment evaluation. Octreotide relieves symptoms of diarrhea leading to avoidance of electrolyte depletion, weight gain, and enhanced quality of life with minimal side effects. Interferon-α has been combined with octreotide to control symptoms but without significant measurable response in tumor mass.

Lanreotide, another somatostatin analog, has been used singly and in combination with interferon-α 2b in patients with advanced, MTC. Vitale et al. studied the combination of slow-release lanreotide and interferon-α 2b in seven patients with metastatic symptomatic MTC (16). Although no objective complete or partial responses were seen, disease stabilization and minor tumor regression were observed in five of seven patients. Flushing and diarrhea decreased in the majority of patients, and reduction of fatigue and improvement of performance status was seen in six of seven patients. Plasma calcitonin levels decreased significantly in six of seven patients.

Moley and colleagues have found that most MTCs have activating mutations in the RET proto-oncogene that encodes for a transmembrane tyrosine kinase (22). An orally administered tyrosine kinase inhibitor, Imatinib (Gleevec®) approved by the FDA for treatment of chronic myelocytic leukemia and gastrointestinal stromal tumor, produces inhibition of MTC cell growth, as shown in their in vitro studies. Two other investigational tyrosine kinase inhibitors have shown similar effects (21). Based on these findings, Moley et al. are currently conducting a clinical trial in patients with measurable metastatic MTC, utilizing relatively high-dose (800 mg) oral Imatinib (22). Skinner et al. studied the IC50 of Imatinib and its effects on MTC cell line proliferation and viability. The concentrations required to significantly inhibit RET tyrosine kinase and induce MTC cell necrosis were in the range of 25–100 µM, levels, which could not be clinically achievable in vivo (23).

In summary, chemotherapy may be active against MTC. Monotherapy with doxorubicin is equivalent to, and less toxic than, combination chemotherapy, and response rates are as high as 40%. Octreotide can be effectively used to control diarrhea as a side effect of this cancer. Tyrosine kinase inhibitors that are active in vitro against MTC and its RET proto-oncogene product are currently being evaluated in clinical trials.

REFERENCES

1. Gottlieb JA, Hill CS. Chemotherapy of thyroid cancer with Adriamycin: experience with 30 patients. N Engl J Med 1974; 290:193–197.
2. Benker G, Reinwein D. Ergebnisse der Chemotherapie des Schilddrusenkarzinoms. Dtsch Med Wochenschr 1983; 11:403–406.
3. DeBesi P, Busnardo B, Toso S, et al. Combined chemotherapy with bleomycin, Adriamycin and platinum in advanced thyroid cancer. J Endocrinol Invest 1991; 14:475–480.
4. Scherubl H, Rane F, Ziebler R. Combination chemotherapy of advanced medullary and differentiated thyroid cancer. J Cancer Res Clin Oncol 1990; 116:21–23.

5. Athanassiades P, Piperingos G, Pandos P, et al. Serial serum calcitonin concentrations to evaluate response to therapy of patients with medullarty thyroid carcinoma. Chemioterapia 1988; 7:195–197.
6. Droz JP, Schlumberger M, Rougier P, et al. Chemotherapy in metastatic non-anaplastic thyroid cancer: experience at the Institut Gustave-Roussy. Tumori 1990; 76:480–483.
7. Porter AT, Ostrowski MJ. Medullary carcinoma of the thyroid treated by low-dose Adriamycin. Br J Clin Pract 1990; 44:517–518.
8. Massart C, Gibassier J, Raoul M, et al. Cyclosporin A, verapamil and S9788 reverse doxorubicin resistance in a human medullary thyroid carcinoma cell line. Anti-cancer Drugs 1995; 6:135–146.
9. Hoskin PJ, Harmer C. Chemotherapy for thyroid cancer. Radiother Oncol 1987; 10:187–194.
10. Kelsen D, Fiore J, Heelan R, et al. Phase II trial of etoposide in APUD tumors. Cancer Treatm Rep 1987; 71:305–307.
11. Sigurdur R, Petursson. Metastatic medullary thyroid carcinoma complete response to combination chemotherapy with dacarbazine and 5-fluorouracil. Cancer 1988; 62:1899–1903.
12. Burgess MA, Sellin RV, Gagel RF. Chemotherapy for medullary carcinoma of the thyroid with doxorubicin, imadazole carboximide, vincristine and cyclophosphamide. Proc Annu Meet Am Soc Clin Oncol 1995; 14:417.
13. Nocera M, Baudin E, Pellegriti G, et al. Treatment of advanced medullary thyroid cancer with an alternating combination of doxorubicin-streptozocin and 5 FU-dacarbazine. Groupe d'Etude des Tumeurs a Calcitonine (GETC). Br J Cancer 2000; 83:715–718.
14. Muller OA, Landgraf R, Zeigler R, Scariba PC. Effects of somatostatin on calcitonin and ectopic ACTH release in a patient with medullary thyroid carcinoma. Acta Endocrinol 1977; 84(Suppl):49–50.
15. Mahler C, Verhelst J, DeLongueville M, Harris A. Long-term treatment of metastatic medullary thyroid carcinoma with the somatostatin analogue octreotide. Clin Endocrinol 1990; 33:261–269.
16. Vitale G, Tagliaferri P, Caraglia M, et al. Slow release lanreotide in combination with interferon-alpha2b in the treatment of symptomatic advanced medullary thyroid carcinoma. J Clin Endocrinol Metab 2000; 85:983–988.
17. Shimaoka K, Schoenfeld D, De Wys W, et al. A randomized trial of doxorubicin vs doxorubicin plus cisplatin in patients with advanced thyroid carcinoma. Cancer 1985; 56:2155–2160.
18. Droz JP, Rougier P, Goddefroy V, et al. Chemotherapy for medullary cancer of thyroid: phase II trials with adriamycin and cisplatinum administered as monochemotherapy. Bull Cancer 1984; 71:195–199.
19. Frame J, Kelsen D, Kemeny N, et al. A phase II trial of streptozotocin and Adriamycin in advanced APUD tumors. Am J Clin Oncol 1988; 11:490–495.
20. Stein R, Chen S, Reed L, et al. Combining radioimmunotherapy and chemotherapy for treatment of medullary thyroid carcinoma; effectiveness of dacarbazine. Cancer 2002; 94:51–61.
21. Cohen MS, Hussain HB, Moley JF. Inhibition of medullary thyroid carcinoma cell proliferation and RET phosphorylation by tyrosine kinase inhibitors. Surgery 2002; 132:960–966.
22. Moley JF. Medullary thyroid carcinoma. Curr Treat Options Oncol 2003; 4:339–347.
23. Skinner MA, Safford SD, Freemerman AJ. RET tyrosine kinase and medullary thyroid cells are unaffected clinical doses of ST1571. Anticancer Res 2003; 23:3601–3606.

Part VIII
Undifferentiated Tumors
Thyroid Lymphoma

74
Thyroid Lymphoma

Steven I. Sherman

EPIDEMIOLOGY

Primary thyroidal non-Hodgkin's lymphoma, albeit rare, is an important component of the differential diagnosis for thyroid nodules or malignancy, mainly because of the different prognosis and treatment approach *(1,2)*. Only about 2% of extranodal lymphomas arise as primary malignancies within the thyroid gland and represent no more than 5% of all thyroid malignancies *(3)*. In a Danish epidemiological survey, the annual incidence rate was estimated as 2.1 per million people, with a 4:1 female predominance *(4)*. Most other retrospective series have confirmed this markedly higher frequency of disease in women *(5–9)*. The mean and median ages at diagnosis are between 65 and 75 yr, suggesting that women present at a significantly older age than men *(4–9)*; like anaplastic carcinoma, presentation before age 40 is extremely rare.

Preexisting Hashimoto's thyroiditis is the only notable risk factor for primary thyroidal lymphoma, as patients with Hashimoto's have at least a 60-fold relative risk for developing non-Hodgkin's lymphoma of the thyroid *(4,10,11)*. Background chronic thyroiditis is often seen in surgical specimens *(12)*. Worldwide, the frequency of thyroid lymphoma appears higher in areas with a greater prevalence of thyroiditis. Along with an increasing frequency of thyroiditis, lymphoma may also occur more commonly after iodine supplementation *(13)*. The development of lymphoma in the setting of Hashimoto's thyroiditis has not been adequately explained. One potential mechanism may be the result of chronic antigenic stimulation in thyroiditis, enhancing the probability of neoplastic transformation *(14)*. There appears to be no clear association between exposure to ionizing radiation and lymphoma *(15)*, but individual cases have been described. Karyotypic chromosomal abnormalities are rarely reported.

HISTOLOGY, GRADE, AND CLASSIFICATION

Primary thyroidal lymphoma almost always has a B-cell lineage *(4,8,9)*. In contrast, occasional T-cell lymphomas have been reported, particularly in areas that are endemic for human T-cell lymphotropic virus-I-associated adult T-cell leukemia/lymphoma *(16,17)*. Diffuse, large-cell histologies (formerly described as histiocytic lymphomas) generally predominate, accounting for about 70–80% of tumors *(5,7,8,18)*. Less typical histologies include follicular or nodular patterns, mixed lesions, lymphomas with plasmacytoid features, signet cell lymphomas, and lymphocytic lymphomas *(19)*. Differing classification schemes have been proposed, adding considerable confusion to the literature on thyroid lymphomas. Using the National Cancer Institute Working Formulation, about 70% of thyroid lymphomas are intermediate-grade, with the remaining cases evenly divided among low-grade, high-grade, and undefined histologies *(6–8,20)*. In contrast, using the Kiel classification, approx 65% are low-grade, 30% high-grade, and 5% undefined *(21)*. The predictive value of tumor grading is unclear. One study suggested that Working Formulation high-grade tumors have a far worse prognosis than low- or intermediate-grade tumors *(21)*, whereas other studies have failed to demonstrate a significant difference based on either the Working Formulation *(5,7)* or Kiel classification *(6)*.

It has been suggested that the B-cell thyroid lymphomas should be grouped with mucosa-associated lymphoid tissue (MALT) lymphomas, considering the histologic and prognostic similarities *(22)*. Classically, MALT lymphomas contain small- to medium-sized centrocyte-like cells, often with plasmacytoid features, and they are associated with reactive germinal centers and lymphoepithelial lesions *(8)*. Likely, high-grade lesions arise from the transformation of low-grade MALT lymphomas, given the high frequency of tumors and both histologies sharing identical immunoglobulin light-chain restriction *(4,22)*. Molecular abnormalities associated with MALT lymphomas (including thyroid) have been a loss of *bcl-2* expression and an increase in *p53* inactivation with higher grade disease *(24,25)*. Epstein-Barr virus gene expression has been found in thyroid lymphomas, but the pathogenic significance is unknown *(26)*. Several studies have indicated that as many as 70–80% of thyroid lymphomas have histologic appearance consistent with MALT neoplasms (4,27). However, a multicenter immunohistochemical analysis from the Eastern Cooperative Oncology Group indicated a far smaller frequency of less than 10% (8). Consistent with the concept of thyroid lymphoma as a MALT lesion is the 10–60% prevalence of concomitant or metasynchronous gastrointestinal tract lymphomas, considerably higher than typically found in nodal non-Hodgkin's lymphomas (28,29). Yet, this finding has been disputed in other studies.

CLINICAL PRESENTATION

Similar to anaplastic carcinoma, symptoms of thyroid lymphoma are usually rapidly expanding bilateral goiter, occurring in 90–100% of patients (4,5,7,9,27,30). Symptoms and signs owing to compression of surrounding structures are also common, e.g., dysphagia, dyspnea, stridor, hoarseness, neck pain, and venous dilatation from superior vena cava obstruction. Although these symptoms are usually present for only a few months, long-standing goiter is found in 10–20% of patients, generally in association with hypothyroidism. Occasionally, lymphoma can present as a solitary nodule or with unilateral involvement, rather than as a diffuse, firm, or hard goiter. On examination, the thyroid is commonly fixed to underlying structures and does not move well with deglutition. Substernal extension is typical. When a distinct intrathyroidal mass is identified, the diameter is typically larger than 5 cm, but the exact borders of the goiter often cannot be recognized. Regional adenopathy in cervical or supraclavicular chains can be palpated in about half of patients. In the setting of stridor and hoarseness, laryngoscopy can often identify vocal cord paresis (31). Aside from the local manifestations, up to 10% of patients may report "B" symptoms, including fever, sweats, and weight loss. Symptoms from hypothyroidism may be present in up to 10% of patients because of coexisting thyroiditis, not destructive infiltration by lymphoma (20). In rare cases, thyrotoxic findings occur in association with the rapid destruction of follicles and release of preformed hormone into circulation (32) or from preexisting Graves' disease (33).

LABORATORY STUDIES

No laboratory abnormalities are specific to, or diagnostic of, thyroid lymphoma (4). When present, primary hypothyroidism is associated with an elevated serum thyrotropin (TSH), with minimal increases found in up to 50% of patients. A serum concentration of lactate dehydrogenase greater than 500 U/L is seen in about 25%, increased levels of serum uric acid in about 15%, and higher serum concentrations of immunoglobulin (Ig) A, IgM, or IgG in approximately 30% of patients (4). Elevated liters of antithyroid antibodies (antithyroglobulin and antimicrosomal) have been seen in up to 95% of patients (4,20).

IMAGING STUDIES

Radiographic and scintigraphic imaging studies are useful in defining the extent of disease, planning therapy, and monitoring response to treatment but are unable to distinguish lymphoma from other thyroid malignancies or thyroiditis (34,35). However, the computed tomography (CT) findings in lymphoma may be distinguished from those in anaplastic carcinoma by the presence of calcifications and necrosis in the latter tumor (35). Common CT findings have been described (36) and include the so-called "donut sign" because of the tendency of lymphoma to completely encircle the trachea. CT and magnetic resonance imaging are superior to ultrasound given their greater ability to detect malignant invasion of the trachea, substernal extension of disease, and involvement of mediastinal and abdominal nodal groups. However, ultrasound may show other clues that suggest the presence of lymphoma. In one series, the thyroid ultrasound showed a characteristic asymmetrical pseudocystic pattern in 93% of patients with thyroid lymphomas (15). Radioiodine scanning has no role in thyroid lymphoma, given the lack of iodine-concentrating ability in lymphocytes. By contrast, ^{67}Ga imaging detects abnormal uptake in about 90% of patients with thyroid lymphoma (37–39), and the degree of ^{67}Ga uptake can correlate with responses to therapy (39). However, it is quite nonspecific, with frequent uptake noted in Hashimoto's thyroiditis. A similar problem exists with F-18 deoxyglucose positron emission tomography (PET) scanning, as both Hashimoto's disease and lymphoma can cause diffuse uptake throughout the gland (40,41; see Chapter 76). In contrast, MALT lymphomas of the thyroid generally produce false-negative PET imaging. Other radionuclides that may detect thyroid lymphoma include ^{201}Tl and ^{99m}Tc-MIBI, but sensitivity and specificity are unknown (42).

DIAGNOSIS

Lymphoma should be part of the working differential diagnosis of a solitary thyroid nodule, a dominant nodule in a multinodular goiter, or in any patient with Hashimoto's thyroiditis whose chronic goiter enlarges or produces new symptoms. The diagnosis of lymphoma can often be established by cytologic examination of material obtained by fine-needle aspiration, particularly in the common large-cell histologic types (43–45). Given the frequent coexistence of chronic autoimmune thyroiditis, small-cell lymphomas are more difficult to diagnose cytologically, and immunohistochemical staining to demonstrate lymphocyte monoclonality may be necessary. Occasionally, large-bore needle biopsy or surgical excision may be needed to obtain sufficient material for immunohistochemical staining. Alternatively, the presence of lymphoma cannot be completely ruled out by an aspirate that shows thyroiditis; clinical judgement, open surgical biopsy, and follow-up are often necessary.

STAGING

The Ann Arbor stage classification is most widely used for primary thyroid lymphoma (20,46). Approximately half of patients present with disease that is limited to the thyroid gland, designated as stage IE. Another 45% have disease limited to the thyroid and locoregional nodes, classified as stage IIE and occasionally subdivided based on disease in mediastinal nodes. Only about 5% of patients present with additional disease located in nodal groups on both sides of the diaphragm (stage IIIE) or with diffuse organ involvement (stage IV). Extranodal sites reported are bone marrow, gastrointestinal tract, lungs, liver, pancreas, and kidney (4,19,31,47). Given these potential sites of disease involvement, the initial staging work-up for a patient diagnosed with primary thyroid lymphoma should probably include a complete blood count, serum chemistries (including TSH, lactate dehydrogenase, and uric acid), chest radiograph, and CT of the neck, chest, and abdomen. There is no consensus regarding the routine use of bone marrow examination, gallium scintigraphy, or lymphangiography, and these studies should probably be used selectively.

SURGICAL MANAGEMENT

As with anaplastic carcinoma, airway management is often a primary focus of the initial therapy of thyroid lymphoma. Severe airway compromise that requires tracheostomy can be anticipated in up to 25% of patients. Given the rapidly growing nature of the disease, it is often necessary to perform an emergent procedure, with an attendant increased risk of complication. Therefore, early consideration should be given to elective tracheostomy in patients at risk for airway obstruction. Surgery is also occasionally required for establishment of the diagnosis. Beyond airway management and diagnosis, controversy exists about the appropriate extent of further surgery for thyroid lymphoma. Several recent studies have failed to demonstrate a significant survival advantage from more extensive surgery, such as total thyroidectomy in stages IE and IIE, particularly when concurrent prognostic factors (e.g., initial tumor bulk or extrathyroidal invasion) are considered (5,9,18). However, for stage IE patients who have disease confined within the gland, without invasion across the thyroid gland capsule, thyroidectomy followed by adjuvant radiotherapy may be appropriate (6,48). The difficulty in making this distinction is that thyroidectomy is often required to determine whether the disease extends outside of the gland capsule (48). Radical procedures that increase the risk to surrounding structures, like recurrent laryngeal nerves, para-thyroid glands, or the upper aerodigestive tract, should be avoided. For patients with stage IE MALT lymphoma, surgery has been associated with prolonged relapse-free survival (13).

RADIATION THERAPY

External-beam radiotherapy has been the traditional primary therapy for stages IE and IIE of disease, administered alone or in combination with other modalities, in 70% of all patients (19). Radiotherapy may be as effective as surgery for stage IE MALT lymphoma (49). Disagreement prevails regarding the appropriate amount and duration of therapy, as well as the optimal extent of the radiation fields. Decreased relapse-free survival has been reported for patients treated with less than 30 Gy, compared with those who received more than 30 Gy (9). However, decreased doses have been often prescribed for patients presenting with the most advanced disease or who are too sick to tolerate full radiation dosing, making the analysis biased against lower doses. External radiotherapy delivering 40 Gy over a 4- to 5-wk period may be associated with a 55–70% 5-yr survival, with 90% survival for stage IE disease (30,50,51). Some authors advocate irradiating the thyroid bed and bilateral neck, emphasizing that most treatment failures tend to occur in distant sites (5,9,30). Others routinely recommend including the superior mediastinum in the radiation field (18).

CHEMOTHERAPY

More advanced lymphoma (stage IIIE or IV) or disease presenting in older patients is often treated with chemotherapy. For patients who develop distant recurrence after primary therapy for stage IE or IIE, chemotherapy is also indicated. Treatment regimens used in recent reports include CHOP (cyclophospharnide, doxorubicin, vincristine, and prednisone), ProMACE-CytaBOM (prednisone, methotrexate, doxorubicin, cyclophospharnide, etoposide, cytosine arabinoside, vincristine, and bleomycin), BACOP (bleomycin, doxorubicin, cyclophospharnide, vincristine, and prednisone), C-MOPP (cyclophospharnide, vincristine, prednisone, and procarbazine), and CVP (cyclophospharnide, vincristine, and prednisone). Because the amount of patients treated with any given regimen is small, it has not been possible to identify a superior drug combination.

PROGNOSIS

Using both chemotherapy and radiotherapy, the results of multiple studies that incorporated combined multimodality therapy (CMT) for stages IE and IIE disease have been recently summarized (52–54). Distant recurrence occurred significantly less frequently following CMT than either radiotherapy or chemotherapy alone. The benefit appeared limited to patients with disease extending into the mediastinum. Given the limitations of detecting distant micrometastases by current imaging modalities, the addition of a brief course of chemotherapy to local radiation may improve long-term outcome (7,18). The disease-specific 5-yr survival of all patients with primary thyroid lymphoma is 45–65%

(4,6,9,18,19,54). For patients with stage IE or IIE disease, the corresponding 5-year estimates are 55–80% and 20–50%, respectively *(4–7,9,18,54)*. In contrast, 5-yr disease-specific survival for patients with either stage IIIE or IV disease is only 15–35% *(4,6)*. Following initial therapy, about 85% of stage IE or IIE patients achieve complete remission *(6,18)*. However, at least half relapse within 5 yr, which is more likely to occur outside of the initial radiation fields and in distant sites. Relapse-free survival may be increased to 80% after initial combined modality therapy *(18)*. Once relapse occurs, occasional complete response and long-term survival can be obtained with chemotherapy and/or radiotherapy, but the median survival is about 7 mo following relapse *(9)*.

REFERENCES

1. Wirtzfeld DA, Winston JS, Hicks WL Jr., Loree TR. Clinical presentation and treatment of non-Hodgkin's lymphoma of the thyroid gland. Ann Surg Oncol 2001; 8:338–341.
2. Ansell SM, Grant CS, Habermann TM. Primary thyroid lymphoma. Semin Oncol 1999; 26:316–323.
3. Freeman C, Berg JW, Cutler SJ. Occurrence and prognosis of extranodal lymphomas. Cancer 1972; 39:252–260.
4. Pedersen RK, Pedersen NT. Primary non-Hodgkin's lymphoma of the thyroid gland: a population based study. Histopathology 1996; 28: 5–32.
5. Junor EJ, Paul J, Reed NS. Primary non-Hodgkin's lymphoma of the thyroid. Eur J Surg Oncol 1992; 18:313–321.
6. Pyke CM, Grant CS, Habermann TM, et al. Non-Hodgkin's lymphoma of the thyroid: is more than biopsy necessary? World J Surg 1992; 16:604–609.
7. Skarsgard ED, Connors JM, Robins RE. A current analysis of primary lymphoma of the thyroid. Arch Surg 1991; 126:1199–1203.
8. Wolf BC, Sheahan K, DeCoste D, et al. Immunohisto-chemical analysis of small cell tumors of the thyroid gland: an Eastern Cooperative Oncology Group study. Hum Pathol 1992; 23:1252–1261.
9. Logue JP, Hale RJ, Stewart AL, et al. Primary malignant lymphoma of the thyroid: a clinicopathological analysis. Int J Radiol Oncol Biol Phys 1992; 22:929–933.
10. Hyjek E, Isaacson PG. Primary B cell lymphoma and its relationship to Hashimoto's thyroiditis. Hum Pathol 1988; 19:1315–1326.
11. Holm LE, Blomgren H, Lowhagen T. Cancer risks in patients with chronic lymphocytic thyroiditis. N Engl J Med 1985; 312:601–604.
12. Harach HR, Williams ED. Thyroid cancer and thyroiditis in the goitrous region of Salta, Argentina, before and after iodine prophylaxis. Clin Endocrinol (Oxf) 1995; 43:701–706.
13. Thieblemont C, Mayer A, Dumontet C, et al. Primary thyroid lymphoma is a heterogeneous disease. J Clin Endocrinol Metab 2002; 87: 105–111.
14. Burke JS, Butler JJ, Fuller ML. Malignant lymphomas of the thyroid: a clinical pathologic study of 35 patients including ultrastructural observations. Cancer 1977; 39:1587–1602.
15. Matsuzuka F, Miyauchi A, Katayama S, et al. Clinical aspects of primary thyroid lymphoma: Diagnosis and treatment based on our experience of 119 cases. Thyroid 1993; 3:93–99.
16. Mizukami Y, Michigishi T, Nonomura A, et al. Primary lymphoma of the thyroid: a clinical, histological, and immunohistochemical study of 20 cases. Histopathology 1990; 17:201–209.
17. Ohsawa M, Noguchi S, Aozasa K. Immunologic type of thyroid lymphoma in an adult T-cell leukemia endemic area in Japan. Leuk Lymphoma 1995; 17:341–344.
18. Tsang RW, Gospodarowicz MK, Sutcliffe SB, et al. Non-Hodgkin's lymphoma of the thyroid gland: prognostic factors and treatment outcome. The Princess Margaret Hospital Lymphoma Group. Int J Radiat Oncol Biol Phys 1993; 27:599–604.
19. Derringer GA, Thompson LD, Frommelt RA, et al. Malignant lymphoma of the thyroid gland: A clinicopathologic study of 108 cases. Am J Surg Path 2000; 24:623–639
20. Mazzaferri EL, Oertel YC. Primary malignant thyroid lymphoma and related lymphoproliferative disorders. In Mazzaferri EL, Samaan NA, editors. Endocrine Tumors. Boston, MA: Blackwell Scientific Publications, 1993:348–377.
21. Aozasa K, Inoue A, Tajima K, et al. Analysis of 79 patients with emphasis on histologic prognostic factors. Cancer 1986; 58:100–104.
22. Isaacson P, Wright DH. Extranodal malignant lymphoma arising from mucosa-associated lymphoid tissue. Cancer 1984; 53:2515–2524.
23. Chan JKC, Ng CS, Isaacson PG. Relationship between high-grade lymphoma and low-grade B-cell mucosa-associated lymphoid tissue lymphoma (MALToma) of the stomach. Am J Pathol 1990; 136: 1153–1164.
24. Ashton-Key M, Biddolph SC, Stein H, et al. Heterogeneity of bcl-2 expression in MALT lymphoma. Histopathology 1995; 26:75–78.
25. Du M, Peng H, Singh N, et al. The accumulation of p53 abnormalities is associated with progression of mucosa-associated lymphoid tissue lymphoma. Blood 1995; 86:4587–4593.
26. Lam KY, Lo CY, Kwong DL, et al. Malignant lymphoma of the thyroid. A 30-year clinicopathologic experience and an evaluation of the presence of Epstein-Barr virus. Am J Clin Pathol 1999; 112:263–270.
27. Laing RW, Hoskin P, Hudson BV, et al. The significance of MALT histology in thyroid lymphoma: a review of patients from the BNLI and Royal Marsden Hospital. Clin Oncol (R Coll Radiol) 1994; 6: 300–304.
28. Anscombe AM, Wright DH. Primary malignant lymphoma of the thyroid—a tumour of mucosa-associated lymphoid tissue: review of seventy-six cases. Histopathology 1985; 9:81–97.
29. Herrmann R, Panahon AM, Barcos MP, et al. Gastro-intestinal involvement in non-Hodgkin's lymphoma. Cancer 1980; 46:215–222.
30. Sippel RS, Gauger PG, Angelos P, et al. Palliative thyroidectomy for malignant lymphoma of the thyroid. Ann Surg Oncol 2002; 9: 907–911.
31. Tupchong L, Hughes F, Harmer CL. Primary lymphoma of the thyroid: clinical features, prognostic factors, and results of treatment. Int J Radiat Oncol Biol Phys 1986; 12:1813–1821.
32. Jennings AS, Saben M. Thyroid lymphoma in a patient with hyperthyroidism. Am J Med 1984; 76:551–552.
33. Zeki K, Eto S, Fujihira T, et al. Primary malignant lymphoma of the thyroid in a patient with longstanding Graves' disease. Endocrinol Jpn 1985; 32:435–440.
34. Podoloff DA. Is there a place for routine surveillance using sonography, CT, or MR imaging for early detection (notably lymphoma) of patients affected by Hashimoto's thyroiditis? AJR Am J Roentgenol 1996; 167:1337–1338.
35. Ishikawa H, Tamaki Y, Takahashi M, et al. Comparison of primary thyroid lymphoma with anaplastic thyroid carcinoma on computed tomographic imaging. Radiation Med 2002; 20:9–15.
36. Kim HC, Han MH, Kim KH, et al. Primary thyroid lymphoma: CT findings. Eur J Radiol 2003; 46:233–239.
37. Higashi T, Ito K, Nishikawa Y, et al. Gallium-67 imaging in the evaluation of thyroid malignancy. Clin Nucl Med 1988; 13:792–798.
38. Higashi T, Ito K, Mimura T, et al. Clinical evaluation of 67-Ga scanning in the diagnosis of anaplastic carcinoma and malignant lymphoma of the thyroid. Radiology 1981; 141:491–497.
39. Nishiyama Y, Yamamoto Y, Yokoe K, et al. Diagnosis of thyroid lymphoma and follow-up evaluation using Ga-67 scintigraphy. Ann Nucl Med 2003; 17:351–357.

40. Mikosch P, Wurtz FG, Gallowitsch HJ, et al. F-18 FDG-PET in a patient with Hashimoto's thyroiditis and MALT lymphoma recurrence of the thyroid. Wien Med Wochenschr 2003; 153: 89–92.
41. Schmid DT, Kneifel S, Stoeckli SJ, et al. Increased 18F-FDG uptake mimicking thyroid cancer in a patient with Hashimoto's thyroiditis. Eur Radiol 2003; 13:2119–2121.
42. Scott AM, Kostakoglu L, O'Brien JP, et al. Comparison of technetium-99m-MIBI and thallium-201-chloride uptake in primary thyroid lymphoma. J Nucl Med 1992; 33:1396–1398.
43. Cha C, Chen H, Westra WH, Udelsman R. Primary thyroid lymphoma: can the diagnosis be made solely by fine-needle aspiration. Ann Surg Oncol 2002; 9:298–302.
44. Van den Bruel A, Drijkoningen M, Oyen R, et al. Diagnostic fine-needle aspiration cytology and immunocytochemistry analysis of a primary thyroid lymphoma presenting as an anatomic emergency. Thyroid 2002; 12:169–173.
45. Sangalli G, Serio G, Zampatti C, et al. Fine needle aspiration cytology of primary lymphoma of the thyroid: a report of 17 cases. Cytopathology 2001; 12:257–263.
46. Carbone PP, Kaplan HS, Musshoff K, et al. Report of the committee on Hodgkin's disease staging classification. Cancer Res 1971; 31: 1860–1861.
47. Evans TR, Mansi JL, Bevan DH, et al. Primary non-Hodgkin's lymphoma of the thyroid with bone marrow infiltration at presentation. Clin Oncol (R Coll Radiol) 1995; 7:54–55.
48. Friedberg MH, Coburn MC, Monchik JM. Role of surgery in stage IE non-Hodgkin's lymphoma of the thyroid. Surgery 1994; 116: 1061–1066.
49. Tsang RW, Gospodarowicz MK, Pintilie M, et al. Localized mucosa-associated lymphoid tissue lymphoma treated with radiation therapy has excellent clinical outcome. J Clin Oncol 2003; 21:4157–4164.
50. Vigliotti A, Kong JS, Fuller LM, Velasquez WS. Thyroid lymphomas stages IE and IIE: comparative results for radiotherapy only, combination chemotherapy only, and multimodality treatment. Int J Radiat Oncol Biol Phys 1986; 12:1807–1812.
51. Compagno J, Oertel JE. Malignant lymphoma and other lymphoproliferative disorders of the thyroid gland. Am J Clin Pathol 1980; 74:1–11.
52. Doria R, Jekel JF, Cooper DL. Thyroid lymphoma. The case for combined modality therapy. Cancer 1994; 73:200–206.
53. Belal AA, Allam A, Kandil A, et al. Primary thyroid lymphoma: a retrospective analysis of prognostic factors and treatment outcome for localized intermediate and high grade lymphoma. Am J Clin Oncol 2001; 24:299–305.
54. DiBiase SJ, Grigsby PW, Guo C, et al. Outcome analysis for stage IE and IIE thyroid lymphoma. Am J Clin Oncol 2004; 27:178–184.

75
Pathology of Lymphoma of the Thyroid

Yolanda C. Oertel and James E. Oertel

The thyroid may be involved secondarily by lymphoma from other sites in the body or by leukemic infiltrates (1). Most primary thyroidal lymphomas are B-cell types, but both Hodgkin's lymphoma (2,3) and T-cell lymphoma (4) may occur. Gross examination reveals homogeneous, pale, and firm tissue that has replaced the thyroid irregularly. If advanced autoimmune thyroiditis is also present, the lymphoma probably cannot be distinguished from the inflammatory infiltrate without histologic examination. Microscopically, the regions of autoimmune thyroiditis reveal either the usual benign lymphoplasmacytic infiltrates or the common alterations of the follicular epithelial cells (e.g., oxyphilic cell metaplasia).

The lymphoma usually consists of a monotonous infiltrate of abnormal lymphoid cells which replace the thyroid parenchyma, fill and distend some thyroid follicles (Figs. 1 and 2), permeate the walls of some of the larger vessels, and may extend into the juxtathyroidal tissues. Antikeratin antibodies can demonstrate displaced and distorted follicular epithelium, visible against the lymphomatous infiltrate. Cervical lymph nodes may be involved.

Smears from the aspirates may show predominantly chronic lymphocytic thyroiditis, and it is necessary to perform multiple aspirates until the lymphomatous regions are sampled. The latter show a monotonous lymphoid population (5), readily observed mitotic figures, and a conspicuous absence of follicular epithelial cells.

The lymphoma may be diffuse or follicular (nodular). Separating the lymphoma from an adjacent infiltrate of autoimmune thyroiditis requires careful appraisal of the abnormal cells in the routine histologic sections and the use of immunohistochemical and/or molecular genetic techniques. These demonstrate the abnormal phenotypes of the lymphoma and the varied nonneoplastic cells of any existing autoimmune thyroiditis.

Some thyroid lymphomas present as aggressive neoplasms, often in the elderly, typically with a short history of thyroid enlargement (6), and with extension to cervical tissues outside of the gland. The histological features in a moderate proportion of these cases have been interpreted as showing high-grade malignancy, but this did not influence the outcome in treated patients.

A considerable number of thyroid lymphomas are of intermediate- or low-grade malignancy and may have a history consistent with long-standing autoimmune thyroiditis. A few have been discovered in glands resected because of Hashimoto's thyroiditis. Cases of this type, along with careful evaluation of many other examples of lymphoma, have led to the concept that a thyroid involved from autoimmune disease is comparable to mucosa-associated lymphoid tissue (MALT), such as the Peyer's patches of the intestine (7). Thus, it has been suggested that the majority of thyroidal lymphomas are MALT lymphomas (7,8), composed of centrocyte-like cells (similar to the cells just outside the lymphoid follicles—the parafollicular lymphoid cells). These lymphomas may tend to be localized for extended periods of time, possibly explaining why some thyroid lymphomas have been cured by surgery alone. Thyroid lymphomas may spread to other sites of MALT. The centrocyte-like cells are varied in their morphology, which may be the source of the different cellular types described in various reports of thyroid lymphomas. They may undergo plasmacytic differentiation, which is a frequent finding in thyroid lymphomas (2,8). Such cells are usually monotypic with immunoglobulin light-chain restriction. The lymphoma cells may extend into the reactive lymphoid follicles of the autoimmune thyroiditis, thereby explaining the follicular (nodular) pattern of some lymphomas (9). Also, persisting lymphoid follicles have been reported in the rare plasmacytomas of the thyroid (10), possibly supporting the theory that plasmacytomas of the thyroid are mature MALT lymphomas. When a high-grade lymphoma is present, there is often evidence that it has arisen from a low-grade MALT lymphoma (11).

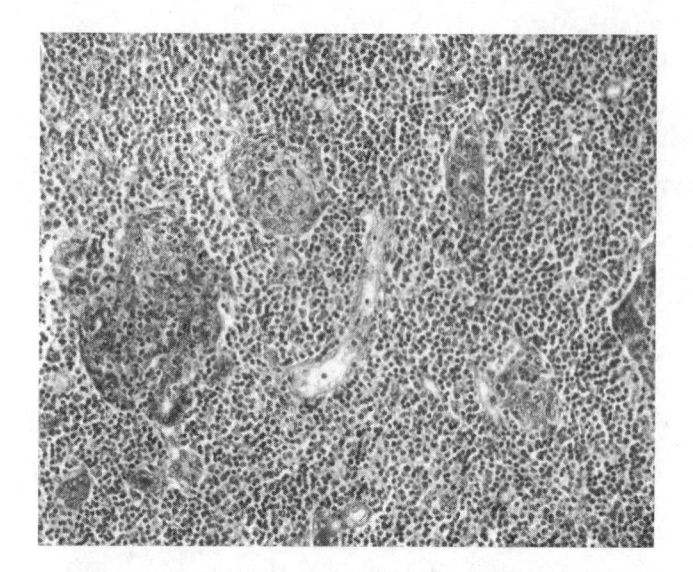

Fig. 1. Malignant lymphoma. A number of thyroid follicles are formed by metaplastic epithelial cells, presumably because of previous Hashimoto's thyroiditis. Both the interstitial tissue and the altered follicles are extensively infiltrated by the lymphoma (hematoxylin and eosin [H&E] stain).

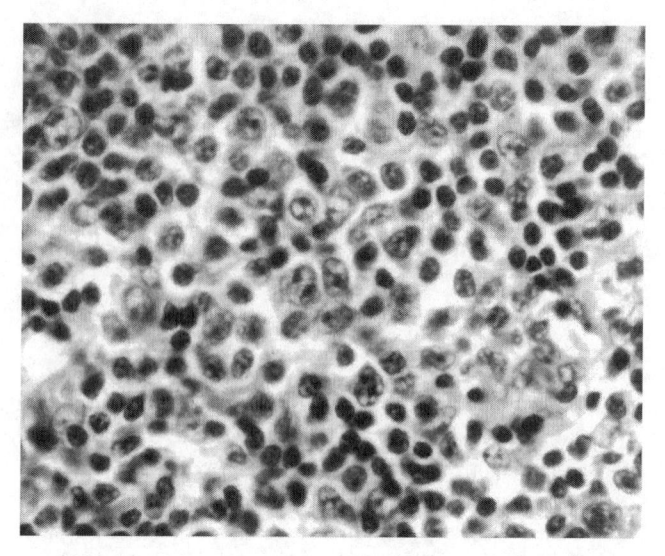

Fig. 2. Malignant lymphoma. Many abnormal lymphoid cells are visible. The smallest cells are likely normal lymphocytes that accompany the malignant infiltrate (H&E stain).

REFERENCES

1. Naylor B. Secondary lymphoblastomatous involvement of the thyroid gland. Arch Pathol Lab Med 1959; 67:432–438.
2. Compagno J, Oertel JE. Malignant lymphoma and other lymphoproliferative disorders of the thyroid gland: a clinicopathologic study of 245 cases. Am J Clin Pathol 1980; 74:1–11.
3. Feigen GA, Buss DH, Paschal B, et al. Hodgkin's disease manifested as a thyroid nodule. Hum Pathol 1982; 13:774–776.
4. Mizukami Y, Michigishi T, Nonomura A, et al. Primary lymphoma of the thyroid: a clinical, histological and immunohistochemical study of 20 cases. Histopathology 1990; 17:201–209.
5. Lerma E, Arguelles R, Rigla M, et al. Comparative findings of lymphocytic thyroiditis and thyroid lymphoma. Acta Cytol 2003; 47:575–580.
6. Van den Bruel A, Drijkoningen M, Oyen R, et al. Diagnostic fine needle aspiration cytology and immunocytochemistry analysis of a primary thyroid lymphoma presenting as an anatomic emergency. Thyroid 2002; 12:169–173.
7. Isaacson PG. Lymphomas of mucosa-associated lymphoid tissue (MALT). Histopathology 1990; 16:617–619.
8. Anscombe AM, Wright DH. Primary malignant lymphoma of the thyroid—a tumor of mucosa-associated lymphoid tissue: review of seventy-six cases. Histopathology 1985; 9:81–97.
9. Isaacson PG, Androulakis-Papachristou A, Diss TC, et al. Follicular colonization in thyroid lymphoma. Am J Pathol 1992; 141:43–52.
10. Aozasa K, Inoue A, Yoshimura H, et al. Plasmacytoma of the thyroid gland. Cancer 1986; 58:105–110.
11. Pedersen RK, Pedersen NT. Primary non-Hodgkin's lymphoma of the thyroid gland: a population based study. Histopathology 1996; 28:25–32.

76
FDG-PET Scanning in Lymphoma and Lymphoma of the Thyroid

I. Ross McDougall

INTRODUCTION

Medicare and most insurance companies have approved reimbursement for F-18 fluorodeoxyglucose positron emission tomography (FDG-PET) for imaging patients who have lymphoma. The instruments and methods are described in Chapter 34. In brief, the patients fast for 6 h and are intravenously administered 10–15 mCi (370–550 MBq) of FDG. After resting in a quiet and warm environment, the patient is imaged from the base of the skull to the mid-thighs. The use of combined PET/computed tomography (CT) improves the diagnostic accuracy, reduces the number of false-positive results, and also increases the throughput of patients (1).

At Stanford University Medical Center, the management of lymphoma is the primary indication for FDG-PET scans, and the images are all combined PET/CT. The test is important to establish the stage of disease, to determine the response to therapy, to decide whether to stop chemotherapy, continue, or change to a different regimen, and to detect recurrence. Comprehensive reviews of this issue are available (2,3).

A brief discussion of the general utility of FDG-PET scanning in lymphomas will help to place the potential efficacy of PET for thyroid lymphomas into context. FDG-PET has been shown to be better than CT or ^{67}Ga for staging both Hodgkin's disease and non-Hodgkin's lymphoma. In an investigation on cost-effectiveness, $30,000 was saved in 18 patients when PET was the first test and the additional work-up was based on PET results (3). PET can alter management by increasing the stage of disease in some patients and decreasing it in others. Several reports indicate a sensitivity range from 85% to 90% and a specificity greater than 90% (5–8). At the end of treatment, FDG-PET is predictive of the patient's outcome. A high probability of recurrence is found with persistent uptake of FDG in a lesion. This association contrasts with such anatomic imaging as CT, which can show a residual mass that may represent cancer or scar tissue.

PET was conducted 1–3 mo after completion of chemotherapy in 93 patients with non-Hodgkin's lymphoma (9). In those with negative scans, there was an 85% progression-free survival, compared to 4% of those who had a positive scan. Initial data are available showing that PET can be used mid-therapy to determine the response to treatment and to consider a change in management. Relapse occurred in all 33 patients with a positive PET in mid-treatment vs 7 of 37 in whom the test was negative (10). PET was used after one cycle of chemotherapy in 30 patients (11). Of 15 patients with a positive scan, 13 relapsed in comparison to 2 of 15 when the scan was negative (12). In the latter study, the PET results demonstrated great potential utility in predicting outcome of chemotherapy for lymphoma. FDG-PET has also been shown to have a better sensitivity for the early detection of recurrent disease than CT (13,14).

The superiority of FDG-PET over ^{67}Ga is demonstrated in several studies. In a comparison of 51 patients, PET increased the stage of disease in 13 patients (15). In a similar study of 50 patients, PET identified more lesions in 19 patients (8). Figure 1 is a typical PET scan in lymphoma.

Thyroid lymphoma is uncommon. The typical patient is an older woman, generally with clinical or immunological evidence of preexisting chronic lymphocytic thyroiditis (16–19). The gland enlarges rapidly. There can be evidence of pressure on the trachea and esophagus, and the patient may be hoarse (20–22). The differential diagnosis is a rapidly growing primary cancer of the thyroid, anaplastic cancer, Reidel's thyroiditis, and when there is pain, subacute thyroiditis. Diagnosis is made by fine-needle aspiration. Some patients have the disease confined to the thyroid (stage IE), and they have an excellent prognosis. The role of scintigraphic imaging tests is not to make a specific diagnosis but to determine the stage and response to treatment.

The use of ^{67}Ga in diagnosing lymphoma of the thyroid has been examined in eight patients with a prior diagnosis of Hashimoto's thyroiditis (23). Seven of the eight patients had "strong or very strong" uptake in the thyroid. Unfortunately,

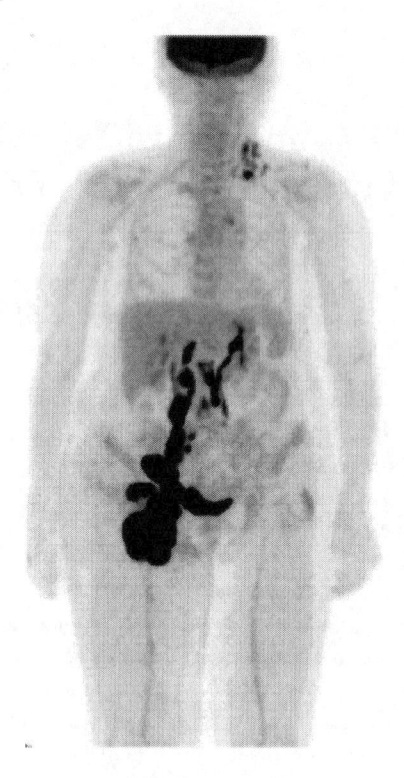

Fig. 1. This patient is an 85-yr-old woman who had a lump in her right groin for 2 mo. The diagnosis was B-cell non-Hodgkin's lymphoma. The FDG-PET scan demonstrates intense uptake in lymph nodes in the right inguinal, external and internal iliac, and para-aortic beds, as well as the left supraclavicular nodes. The images were obtained 1 h after injection of 15 mCi (550 MBq) FDG.

there can also be uptake of ^{67}Ga in benign chronic lymphocytic thyroiditis (24). Therefore, the specificity of the test is poor. FDG-PET is positive in the primary lesion, but it is also positive in uncomplicated autoimmune thyroiditis and could be misinterpreted to be cancerous (25–27). Thus, the main role of an FDG-PET scan is to identify disease sites outside of the thyroid (Fig. 1).

A meta-analysis of outcome demonstrated that patients treated with local external radiation had worse outcomes than those treated with combination of radiation and chemotherapy (28). The implication was that some patients had disease outside the radiotherapy port. The study predated the use of PET, and PET is sensitive for detecting lymphoma. There are no data specifically related to the thyroid, but the latter analysis predicts that it would be valuable and helpful to tailor treatment for individual patients.

One report involved the use of PET for the follow-up of thyroid lymphoma, but it is concerning (29). The patient had Hashimoto's thyroiditis and developed a thyroid mass 4 yr later. She had an operative biopsy, but not thyroidectomy. The pathology was diffuse large B-cell lymphoma. She was treated with cyclophosphamide, doxorubicin, vincristine, and prednisone. The PET scan was obtained 4 mo after therapy, showing intense uptake in the left lower lobe of the thyroid. This was excised and displayed only necrosis. Evidence indicates that uptake of FDG can be seen up to 6 wk after radiation therapy or surgery, whereas this false-positive result was after a longer delay. Hence, some caution should be taken in the interpretation of PET in lymphoma of the thyroid. The test should provide useful information of the response of lesions outside of the thyroid.

In summary, a wealth of information on the use of FDG-PET in lymphoma is present in the literature, but little published data exists on the specific use of PET scanning in thyroid lymphomas. Because PET is positive in chronic lymphocytic thyroiditis, it should not be used to establish a diagnosis of intrathyroidal lymphoma. Its main role lies in disease staging and in the follow-up after radiochemotherapy.

REFERENCES

1. Nahas Z, Goldenberg D, Fakhry C, et al. The role of positron emission tomography/computed tomography in the management of recurrent papillary thyroid carcinoma. Laryngoscope 2005; 115:237–243.
2. Schiepers C, Filmont JE, Czernin J. PET for staging of Hodgkin's disease and non-Hodgkin's lymphoma. Eur J Nucl Med Mol Imaging 2003; 30(Suppl 1):S82–S88.
3. Israel O, Keidar Z, Bar-Shalom R. Positron emission tomography in the evaluation of lymphoma. Semin Nucl Med 2004; 34:166–179.
4. Hoh CK, Glaspy J, Rosen P, et al. Whole-body FDG-PET imaging for staging of Hodgkin's disease and lymphoma. J Nucl Med 1997; 38: 343–348.
5. Stumpe KD, Urbinelli M, Steinert HC, et al. Whole-body positron emission tomography using fluorodeoxyglucose for staging of lymphoma: effectiveness and comparison with computed tomography. Eur J Nucl Med 1998; 25:721–728.
6. Buchmann I, Reinhardt M, Elsner K, et al. 2-(fluorine-18)fluoro-2-deoxy-D-glucose positron emission tomography in the detection and staging of malignant lymphoma. A bicenter trial. Cancer 2001; 91: 889–899.
7. Najjar F, Hustinx R, Jerusalem G, et al. Positron emission tomography (PET) for staging low-grade non-Hodgkin's lymphomas (NHL). Cancer Biother Radiopharm 2001; 16:297–304.
8. Wirth A, Seymour JF, Hicks RJ, et al. Fluorine-18 fluorodeoxyglucose positron emission tomography, gallium-67 scintigraphy, and conventional staging for Hodgkin's disease and non-Hodgkin's lymphoma. Am J Med 2002; 112:262–268.
9. Spaepen K, Stroobants S, Dupont P, et al. Prognostic value of positron emission tomography (PET) with fluorine-18 fluorodeoxyglucose ([18F]FDG) after first-line chemotherapy in non-Hodgkin's lymphoma: is [18F]FDG-PET a valid alternative to conventional diagnostic methods? J Clin Oncol 2001;19:414–419.
10. Spaepen K, Stroobants S, Dupont P, et al. Early restaging positron emission tomography with (18)F-fluorodeoxyglucose predicts outcome in patients with aggressive non-Hodgkin's lymphoma. Ann Oncol 2002; 13:1356–1363.
11. Kostakoglu L, Leonard JP, Kuji I, et al. Comparison of fluorine-18 fluorodeoxyglucose positron emission tomography and Ga-67 scintigraphy in evaluation of lymphoma. Cancer 2002; 94:879–888.
12. Kostakoglu L, Coleman M, Leonard JP, et al. PET predicts prognosis after 1 cycle of chemotherapy in aggressive lymphoma and Hodgkin's disease. J Nucl Med 2002; 43:1018–1027.

13. Dittmann H, Sokler M, Kollmannsberger C, et al. Comparison of 18FDG-PET with CT scans in the evaluation of patients with residual and recurrent Hodgkin's lymphoma. Oncol Rep 2001; 8: 1393–1399.
14. Bangerter M, Kotzerke J, Griesshammer M, et al. Positron emission tomography with 18-fluorodeoxyglucose in the staging and follow-up of lymphoma in the chest. Acta Oncol 1999; 38:799–804.
15. Kostakoglu L, Goldsmith SJ. Positron emission tomography in lymphoma: comparison with computed tomography and Gallium-67 single photon emission computed tomography. Clin Lymphoma 2000; 1:67–74; discussion 75–76.
16. Anscombe AM, Wright DH. Primary malignant lymphoma of the thyroid—a tumour of mucosa-associated lymphoid tissue: review of seventy-six cases. Histopathology 1985; 9:81–97.
17. Burke J, Butler JJ, Fuller LM. Malignant lymphomas of the thyroid. A clinical pathologic study of 35 patients including ultrastructure observations. Cancer 1977; 39:1587–1602.
18. Compagno J, Oertel JE. Malignant lymphoma and other lymphoproliferative disorders of the thyroid gland. A clinicopathologic study of 245 cases. Am J Clin Pathol 1980; 74:1–11.
19. Matsuzuka F, Miyauchi A, Katayama S, et al. Clinical aspects of primary thyroid lymphoma: diagnosis and treatment based on our experience of 119 cases. Thyroid 1993; 3:93–99.
20. Belal AA, Allam A, Kandil A, et al. Primary thyroid lymphoma: a retrospective analysis of prognostic factors and treatment outcome for localized intermediate and high grade lymphoma. Am J Clin Oncol 2001; 24:299–305.
21. Logue JP, Hale RJ, Stewart AL, et al. Primary malignant lymphoma of the thyroid: a clinicopathological analysis. Int J Radiat Oncol Biol Phys 1992; 22:929–933.
22. Souhami L, Simpson WJ, Carruthers JS. Malignant lymphoma of the thyroid gland. Int J Radiat Oncol Biol Phys 1980; 6:1143–1147.
23. Higashi T, Itoh K, Ozaki O, et al. Ga-67 scintigram in evaluation of malignant lymphoma of the thyroid originating from chronic thyroiditis. Rinsho Hoshasen 1989; 34:977–981.
24. Nishiyama Y, Yamamoto Y, Yokoe K, et al. Diagnosis of thyroid lymphoma and follow-up evaluation using Ga-67 scintigraphy. Ann Nucl Med 2003; 17:351–357.
25. Yasuda S, Ide M, Takagi S, Shohtsu A. Cancer screening with whole-body FDG PET. Kaku Igaku 1996; 33:1065–1071.
26. Schmid DT, Kneifel S, Stoeckli SJ, et al. Increased 18F-FDG uptake mimicking thyroid cancer in a patient with Hashimoto's thyroiditis. Eur Radiol 2003; 13:2119–2121.
27. Yasuda S, Shohtsu A, Ide M, et al. Chronic thyroiditis: Diffuse uptake of FDG at PET. Radiology 1998; 207:775–778.
28. Doria R, Jekel JF, Cooper DL. Thyroid lymphoma. The case for combined modality therapy. Cancer 1994; 73:200–206.
29. Marchesi M, Biffoni M, Biancari F. False-positive finding on 18F-FDG PET after chemotherapy for primary diffuse large B-cell lymphoma of the thyroid: a case report. Jpn J Clin Oncol 2004; 34:280–281.

Part IX
Undifferentiated Tumors
Anaplastic Thyroid Cancer

77
Anaplastic Carcinoma
Clinical Aspects

Steven I. Sherman

Anaplastic carcinoma describes an undifferentiated malignancy derived from more well-differentiated thyroid follicular epithelium. In contrast to the generally indolent nature of differentiated thyroid carcinoma, anaplastic carcinoma represents one of the most aggressive human neoplasms, with a disease-specific mortality of at least 90%. Early recognition of the disease is essential to allow prompt initiation of therapy and to achieve a significant tumor response.

Traditional descriptions of undifferentiated thyroid carcinomas divided anaplastic lesions into two categories based on histologic features. The spindle-cell, giant-cell, and squamoid tumors belonged to the typically more aggressive subtype, occurring in older patients and rapidly leading to death. These various histologic types continue to be classified as anaplastic carcinomas. The small-cell histology, however, was thought to be associated with relatively improved survival (1). Later studies with electron microscopy and immunocytochemical markers for lymphoid and neuroendocrine cell lineage demonstrated that most of these small-cell tumors were, in fact, lymphomas or medullary carcinomas. For example, of the three long-term survivors with small-cell carcinoma reported from the Mayo Clinic in 1985 (1), two were later reported to have lymphoma and one had medullary carcinoma (2). Therefore, current nosology for undifferentiated thyroid carcinomas does not include small-cell variants (3). Histopathologic subtypes continue to be described, but the biologic and clinical relevance of these subdivisions is unclear.

The age-adjusted annual incidence of anaplastic carcinoma is about two cases per million people in the United States (4), accounting for only 2–5% of all thyroid malignancies. A similarly low incidence and frequency among thyroid malignancies has been described from a national cancer registry in Norway (5). Higher incidence may exist in iodine-deficient areas of the world (6), with reduction subsequently found after iodine supplementation. The mechanism underlying this association with iodine deficiency is not clear. Given the diagnostic confusion in older series that combined anaplastic and medullary carcinomas with lymphoma as one disease entity, earlier estimates of a 20–30% frequency range among all thyroid malignancies were inaccurate.

Patients with anaplastic carcinoma often present at an age that is two decades older than those with differentiated carcinomas. Among 9 recent series on 473 patients with anaplastic carcinoma, the overall weighted mean age at diagnosis was 66 yr. In the five studies that provided sufficient age data, only 7.5% of the patients were diagnosed before the age of 50 yr. Women comprised 60% of all anaplastic carcinoma patients in these series—a frequency generally lower than that indicated for differentiated carcinomas. However, in one recent study on 15,700 patients with thyroid carcinoma in the United States, 68% of the 251 anaplastic carcinomas occurred in women (7). In this same study, 87% of the patients with anaplastic disease were non-Hispanic whites, a significantly higher frequency than the 79% for papillary and follicular carcinomas ($p < 0.005$; 7). No other large study has systematically reported on the ethnic distribution of anaplastic carcinoma.

In 20–30% of cases of anaplastic carcinoma, a coexisting differentiated carcinoma can be readily identified (1,4,8–10), and a higher frequency of coexisting disease was found following more extensive pathologic examination (11). The great majority of these coexistent differentiated tumors are of papillary histology, but follicular tumors have also been seen (see Chapter 79). Most impressively, nearly 10% of patients with oxyphilic (Hürthle cell) carcinomas may develop anaplastic foci (12). In most of these cases, the undifferentiated malignancy represents the dominant tumor within the thyroid and is generally the histology found in metastases (8). Cases have also been described of patients with a primary differentiated carcinoma within the thyroid, with subsequent development of anaplastic foci in distant metastases (13). In 20% of patients, a clinical history of

From: *Thyroid Cancer: A Comprehensive Guide to Clinical Management, 2/e*
Edited by: L. Wartofsky and D. Van Nostrand © Humana Press Inc., Totowa, NJ

antecedent thyroid neoplasia can be obtained. Molecular abnormalities that commonly occur with differentiated carcinomas can be identified in a coexistent anaplastic carcinoma, supporting the concept of disease progression (14). It has been suggested that anaplastic carcinoma develops from more differentiated tumors because of one or more dedifferentiating steps, particularly the loss of the tumor suppressor protein, p53 (4,15–18).

Radiation's effect to the thyroid gland in possibly inducing anaplastic transformation has been debated. Both ^{131}I and external-beam radiotherapy have been implicated as associated with a greater risk of developing anaplastic carcinoma (19–21). However, multiple studies examining the long-term follow-up of patients treated with ^{131}I for differentiated carcinoma have failed to identify a higher frequency of subsequent development of anaplastic carcinoma. Evidence for a catalytic event or environmental exposure that leads to dedifferentiation remains elusive. Therefore, the exact mechanism of anaplastic transformation of differentiated carcinoma is uncertain.

The clinical manifestations of anaplastic carcinoma reflect the locally invasive and mass effects from growth of primary tumor in the thyroid, as well as at metastatic sites. Nearly all patients present with symptoms of an enlarging primary tumor in the neck. Metastases to cervical and mediastinal lymph nodes are common at presentation, with less than 5% of patients who have disease limited to the thyroid gland (11). Direct extrathyroidal invasion into surrounding structures can be documented in up to 90% of patients (10,22). Potential sites of direct invasion can include perithyroidal fat and muscles, larynx, trachea, esophagus, great vessels of the neck and mediastinum, sternum, and vertebral column. Distant metastases are found at initial disease presentation in 15–50% of patients (1,8,9). As with differentiated carcinoma, the most common location for distant metastases from anaplastic carcinoma is pulmonary, identified in as many as 90% of patients with distant disease (8,9). Both intrapulmonary mass lesions and pleural involvement can be seen. Metastases to the bone (5–15%) and brain (5%) are less commonly found and even more rarely are the skin, liver, kidneys, stomach, pancreas, heart, tonsil, small bowel, mesentery, and adrenal glands (8–10,23–28). In rare cases, patients have presented without clinical evidence of a thyroid tumor *per se* but are identified subsequently because of evaluation (either pre- or postmortem) for a metastatic undifferentiated carcinoma of unknown primary (11).

The primary clinical manifestation of anaplastic carcinoma is generally a rapidly enlarging neck mass, reported in about 75% of patients. Often, the dramatic speed of tumor growth can be documented by marking the cutaneous outline of the tumor on a daily basis. In up to half of patients, a goiter has been recognized. A history of previous thyroid surgery, either for differentiated carcinoma or an apparently benign tumor, can often be elicited. Owing to the enlarging goiter, patients often complain of symptoms from compression or invasion of the upper aerodigestive tract. Dyspnea is reported by about 36% of patients, followed by dysphagia (30%), hoarseness (28%), cough (26%), and neck pain (17%). One case of dyspnea has been described secondary to an intralaryngeal metastasis that functions like a ball valve, obstructing airflow during inspiration (29). Less frequently, patients note hemoptysis, chest pain, bone pain, headache, confusion, or abdominal pain from metastases (23,28,30). Constitutional symptoms can include weight loss, fatigue, and fever of unknown origin (30–33). Rarely, rapid growth of the primary tumor can cause a nonspecific thyroiditis, with symptoms of thyrotoxicosis from follicular disruption and release of preformed thyroid hormone (23,34,35).

On physical examination, the goiter is typically quite hard, often nodular, and generally enlarged bilaterally. Softer, fluctuant masses have been associated with focal tumor necrosis (11). However, anaplastic carcinoma can also present as a solitary nodule or a diffuse nonnodular goiter. Often, the neck mass is found to be fixed to surrounding or underlying structures and does not move with deglutition. By the time of presentation, the primary tumor is typically greater than 5 cm in diameter, but exact measurements are often difficult to obtain, given the indistinct tumor borders because of regional invasion. Metastatic adenopathy may be detected on physical exam in either the neck, supraclavicular fossae, or axillae, but half of patients will not have palpable adenopathy. Other findings of local disease involvement are stridor from tracheal compression or invasion, tracheal deviation, vocal cord paralysis from laryngeal invasion or involvement of recurrent laryngeal nerves, and venous dilatation and superior vena cava syndrome from retrosternal tumor growth. Cutaneous findings can include ulceration, atrophy, or erythema of the skin overlying the primary tumor, as well as metastatic nodules on the chest and abdominal walls (11,36). Focal neurologic abnormalities may indicate brain metastases (28).

The diagnosis of anaplastic carcinoma is usually established by tissue examination and is often available from cytopathologic and electron microscopic review of fine-needle aspiration specimens (see Chapter 79). Laboratory testing rarely has diagnostic value in patients with anaplastic carcinoma. Serum thyroid hormone and thyrotropin levels are generally normal, except in the rare cases of thyrotoxicosis owing to necrosis (23,34,35). Increased serum levels of thyroglobulin can be seen; however, coexisting differentiated tumor cells are the likely source, rather than the anaplastic component of the tumor, perhaps from necrosis of those cells. In contrast, serum concentrations of the neuroendocrine markers, calcitonin, carcinoembryonic antigen, and neuron-specific enolase are usually normal *(37)*. Nonspecific markers of systemic illness, such as an elevated erythrocyte sedimentation rate, increased serum C-reactive protein, anemia, and hypoalbuminemia, can be mildly abnormal. Hypercalcemia in the absence of obvious osseous metastases can be secondary to the secretion of parathyroid hormone-related peptide *(38,39)*. Marked leukocytosis has been reported in several patients in whom elevated serum levels of granulocyte macrophage colony-stimulating factor or granulocyte colony-stimulating factor were found *(26,33,38,40,41)*.

Diagnostic imaging is useful to define the extent of disease, plan therapy, and monitor the response to treatment. Computed tomography (CT) of the neck and mediastinum can accurately identify tumor invasion of great vessels and upper aerodigestive tract structures and is superior to palpation for the detection of pathologic adenopathy *(42; see Chapter 38)*. Typical findings include masses that are isodense or slightly hyperdense relative to skeletal muscle, dense calcifications, and frequent necrosis. Similarly, neck ultrasonography can correctly establish pathologic involvement of locoregional nodes (see Chapter 37); both ultrasound and CT can help to guide fine-needle aspiration to solid nonnecrotic tumor for diagnosis *(43,44)*. Although ultrasound cannot distinguish benign from malignant intrathyroidal tumors—as both tend to produce hypoechoic lesions—extrathyroidal invasion can support the diagnosis of carcinoma *(45)*.

Routine chest radiographs can readily diagnose most instances of pulmonary metastases, considering the typical macronodular appearance of these lesions *(1)*. In patients with bony metastases, skeletal radiographs demonstrate lytic lesions. Scintigraphic imaging with radioiodine or pertechnetate usually reveals hypofunctioning or "cold" foci that correspond to palpable tumor *(1)*. In the setting of thyrotoxicosis from necrotic thyroiditis, depressed radioiodine uptake has been reported *(34)*. ^{67}Ga imaging has demonstrated positive uptake in 16 of 19 cases of anaplastic carcinoma, with one false-negative and two equivocal images *(46)*. Marked positivity was also noted in lymphoma, chronic thyroiditis, and metastases to the thyroid from other malignancies but was absent from all 19 differentiated carcinomas. However, ^{67}Ga uptake in metastatic foci may not be sufficiently sensitive to supplant radiographs and CT *(46)*. A reciprocal relationship has been noted between radioiodine uptake and uptake of F-18 fluorodeoxyglucose (FDG), the agent employed for positron emission tomography (PET), owing to the loss of the iodide symporter as tumors dedifferentiate, whereas glucose uptake remains avid. Indeed, anaplastic carcinoma cells in culture avidly import glucose from the circulation and would therefore be expected to be imaged effectively by FDG-PET scanning *(48)*. This is the case for most patients, as described in Chapter 80.

Prognostic factors and outcomes were reported in an updated review of 516 patients (171 men; 345 women) with anaplastic thyroid cancer from the Surveillance, Epidemiology, and End Results (SEERS) database of the National Cancer Institute *(48)*. At presentation, 43% of patients already had evidence of distant metastases, and cause-specific mortality for all patients was 68% at 6 months and 81% at one year. Poor prognostic factors included age > 60 yr, extrathyroidal tumor, and male sex, while improved survival benefit was shown by surgical resection, external beam radiotherapy or combination surgical resection with radiotherapy. These data tend to support an early aggressive therapeutic approach in younger patients.

REFERENCES

1. Nel CJ, van Heerden JA, Goellner JR, et al. Anaplastic carcinoma of the thyroid: a clinicopathologic study of 82 cases. Mayo Clin Proc 1985; 60:51–58.
2. Rosai J, Saxén EA, Woolner L. Session III: Undifferentiated and poorly differentiated carcinoma. Semin Diag Pathol 1985; 2:123–136.
3. Rosai J, Carcangiu ML, DeLellis RA. Tumors of the thyroid gland Rosai J, editor. Atlas of Tumor Pathology, Washington, DC: Armed Forces Institute of Pathology; 1992.
4. Wiseman SM, Loree TR, Rigual NR, et al. Anaplastic transformation of thyroid cancer: review of clinical, pathologic, and molecular evidence provides new insights into disease biology and future therapy. Head Neck 2003; 25:662–670.
5. Akslen LA, Haldorsen T, Thoresen SO, Glattre E. Incidence of thyroid cancer in Norway 1970–1985. APMIS 1990; 98:549–558.
6. Harach HR, Escalante DA, Onativia A, et al. Thyroid carcinoma and thyroiditis in an endemic goitre region before and after iodine prophylaxis. Acta Endocrinol (Copenh) 1985; 108:55–60.
7. Gilliland FD, Hunt WC, Morris DM, Key CR. Prognostic factors for thyroid carcinoma: A population-based study of 15,698 cases from the Surveillance, Epidemiology and End Results (SEER) program 1973–1991. Cancer 1997; 79:564–573.
8. Carcangiu ML, Steeper T, Zampi G, Rosai J. Anaplastic thyroid carcinoma: A study of 70 cases. Am J Clin Pathol 1985; 83:135–158.
9. Venkatesh YSS, Ordonez NG, Schultz PN, et al. Anaplastic carcinoma of the thyroid: a clinicopathologic study of 121 cases. Cancer 1990; 66:321–330.
10. Tan RK, Finley RK, Driscoll D, et al. Anaplastic carcinoma of the thyroid: a 24-year experience. Head Neck 1995; 17:41–47.
11. Aldinger KA, Samaan NA, Ibanez ML, Hill CSJ. Anaplastic carcinoma of the thyroid: a review of 84 cases of spindle and giant cell carcinoma of the thyroid. Cancer 1978; 41:2267–2275.
12. Chiu AC, Oliveira AA, Schultz PN, et al. Prognostic clinicopathologic features in Hürthle cell neoplasia. Thyroid 1996; 6:S29.
13. Moore JH Jr., Bacharach B, Choi HY. Anaplastic transformation of metastatic follicular carcinoma of the thyroid. J Surg Oncol 1985; 29:216–221.
14. Begum S, Rosenbaum E, Henrique R, et al. BRAF mutations in anaplastic thyroid carcinoma: implications for tumor origin, diagnosis and treatment. Mod Pathol 2004; 17:1359–1363.
15. Nakamura T, Yana I, Kobayashi T, et al. p53 gene mutations associated with anaplastic transformation of human thyroid carcinomas. Jpn J Cancer Res 1992; 83:1293–1298.

16. Ito T, Seyama T, Mizuno T, et al. Unique association of p53 mutations with undifferentiated but not with differentiated carcinomas of the thyroid gland. Cancer Res 1992; 52:1369–1371.
17. Ito T, Seyama T, Mizuno T, et al. Genetic alterations in thyroid tumor progression: association with p53 gene mutations. Jpn J Cancer Res 1993; 84:526–531.
18. Moretti F, Farsetti A, Soddu S, et al. p53 re-expression inhibits proliferation and restores differentiation of human thyroid anaplastic carcinoma cells. Oncogene 1997; 14:729–740.
19. Nêmec J, Nierdle B, Cenkova V, et al. Early manifestation of anaplastic thyroid carcinoma after radioiodine treatment for toxic nodular goiter. Neoplasma 1971; 18:325–333.
20. Gétaz EP, Shimaoka K. Anaplastic carcinoma of the thyroid in a population irradiated for Hodgkin disease, 1910–1960. J Surg Oncol 1979; 12:181–189.
21. Komorowski RA, Hanson GA, Garancis JC. Anaplastic thyroid carcinoma following low-dose irradiation. Am J Clin Pathol 1978; 70:303–307.
22. Tennvall J, Lundell G, Hallquist A, et al. Combined doxorubicin, hyperfractionated radiotherapy, and surgery in anaplastic thyroid carcinoma. Report on two protocols. Cancer 1994; 74:1348–1354.
23. Nishiyama RH, Dunn EL, Thompson NW. Anaplastic spindle-cell and giant-cell tumors of the thyroid gland. Cancer 1972; 30:113–127.
24. Hadar T, Mor C, Har-El G, Sidi J. Anaplastic thyroid carcinoma metastatic to the tonsil. J Laryngol Otol 1987; 101:953–956.
25. Phillips DL, Benner KG, Keeffe EB, Traweek ST. Isolated metastasis to small bowel from anaplastic thyroid carcinoma. With a review of extra-abdominal malignancies that spread to the bowel. J Clin Gastroenterol 1987; 9:563–567.
26. Murabe H, Akamizu T, Kubota A, Kusaka S. Anaplastic thyroid carcinoma with prominent cardiac metastasis, accompanied by a marked leukocytosis with a neutrophilia and high GM-CSF level in serum. Intern Med 1992; 31:1107–1111.
27. Hadar T, Mor C, Shvero J, et al. Anaplastic carcinoma of the thyroid. Eur J Surg Oncol 1993; 19:511–516.
28. Chiu AC, Delpassand ES, Sherman SI. Prognosis and treatment of brain metastases in thyroid carcinoma. J Clin Endocrinol Metab 1997; 82:3637–3642.
29. Lee WC, Walsh RM. Anaplastic thyroid carcinoma presenting as a pharyngeal mass with ball-valve type obstruction of the larynx. J Laryngol Otol 1996; 110:1078–1080.
30. Lip GY, Jaap AJ, McCruden DC. A presentation of anaplastic carcinoma of the thyroid with symptomatic intra-abdominal metastases. Br J Clin Pract 1992; 46:143–144.
31. Glikson M, Feigin RD, Libson E, Rubinow A. Anaplastic thyroid carcinoma in a retrosternal goiter presenting as fever of unknown origin. Am J Med 1990; 88:81–82.
32. Hanslik T, Gepner P, Franc B, et al. Anaplastic cancer of the thyroid gland disclosed by prolonged fever or hyperleukocytosis. Two cases (letter). Ann Med Interne (Paris) 1996; 147:122–124.
33. Chang TC, Liaw KY, Kuo SH, et al. Anaplastic thyroid carcinoma: review of 24 cases, with emphasis on cytodiagnosis and leukocytosis. Taiwan I Hsueh Hui Tsa Chih 1989; 88:551–556.
34. Murakami T, Noguchi S, Murakami N, et al. Destructive thyrotoxicosis in a patient with anaplastic thyroid cancer. Endocrinol Jpn 1989; 36:905–907.
35. Oppenheim A, Miller M, Anderson GH, Jr., et al. Anaplastic thyroid cancer presenting with hyperthyroidism. Am J Med 1983; 75:702–704.
36. Barr R, Dann F. Anaplastic thyroid carcinoma metastatic to skin. J Cutan Pathol 1974; 1:201–206.
37. Schlumberger M, Caillou B. Miscellaneous tumors of the thyroid. In Braverman LE, Utiger RD, editors. Werner and Ingbar's The Thyroid. 7th ed. Philadelphia, PA: Lippincott-Raven; 1996:961–965.
38. Yazawa S, Toshimori H, Nakatsuru K, et al. Thyroid anaplastic carcinoma producing granulocyte-colony-stimulating factor and parathyroid hormone-related protein. Intern Med 1995; 34:584–588.
39. Takashima S, Morimoto S, Ikezoe J, et al. Occult anaplastic thyroid carcinoma associated with marked hypercalcemia. J Clin Ultrasound 1990; 18:438–441.
40. Iwasa K, Noguchi M, Mori K, et al. Anaplastic thyroid carcinoma producing the granulocyte colony stimulating factor (G-CSF): report of a case. Surg Today 1995; 25:158–160.
41. Oka Y, Kobayashi T, Fujita S, et al. Establishment of a human anaplastic thyroid cancer cell line secreting granulocyte colony-stimulating factor in response to cytokines. In Vitro Cell Dev Biol Anim 1993; 29A:537–542.
42. Takashima S, Morimoto S, Ikezoe J, et al. CT evaluation of anaplastic thyroid carcinoma. AJR Am J Roentgenol 1990; 154:1079–1085.
43. Gatenby RA, Mulhern CB, Jr., Richter WP, Moldofsky PJ. CT-guided biopsy for the detection and staging of tumors of the head and neck. Am J Neuroradiol 1984; 5:287–289.
44. Sutton RT, Reading CC, Charboneau JW, et al. US-guided biopsy of neck masses in postoperative management of patients with thyroid cancer. Radiology 1988; 168:769–772.
45. Leisner B. Ultrasound evaluation of thyroid diseases. Horm Res 1987; 26:33–41.
46. Higashi T, Ito K, Nishikawa Y, et al. Gallium-67 imaging in the evaluation of thyroid malignancy. Clin Nucl Med 1988; 13:792–799.
47. Schonberger J, Ruschoff J, Grimm D, et al. Glucose transporter 1 gene expression is related to thyroid neoplasms with an unfavorable prognosis: an immunohistochemical study. Thyroid 2002; 12:747–754.
48. Kebebew E, Greenspan FS, Clark OH, Woeber KA, McMillan A. Anaplastic thyroid carcinoma: Treatment outcome and prognostic factors. Cancer 2005; 103:1330–1335.

78
Surgical Management of Anaplastic Thyroid Carcinoma

Orlo H. Clark

The treatment of patients with anaplastic thyroid cancer, like the treatment of patients with papillary thyroid cancer, is controversial. The reason for the controversy is that anaplastic carcinoma is one of the most aggressive and potentially deadly malignancies. Most patients with anaplastic thyroid cancer have a poor prognosis regardless of treatment and usually die of suffocation from local tumor invasion; the median survival time is about 6 mo (1,2), and the overall mortality rate is about 97% (1–3). At initial examination, patients usually have a large (5–10 cm) fixed mass, and about 30% will already have distant, usually pulmonary, metastases (1,4). Most patients with anaplastic thyroid cancer will also have coexistent well-differentiated thyroid cancer (4–7). Apparently, 1% of differentiated thyroid cancers transform into anaplastic cancers (8). Some of these tumors demonstrate progression from well-differentiated papillary cancers through the insular variant, then into anaplastic cancer (9). Serial transplantation of differentiated thyroid tumors also leads to anaplastic transformation (10,11). Anaplastic thyroid cancers are more likely to have p53 and platelet-derived growth factor mutations than differentiated thyroid cancers (12–14).

Anaplastic thyroid cancers occur most often in older patients, especially in areas of endemic goiter (15). Iodine deficiency appears to be an important factor, and the incidence of anaplastic cancer is decreasing in the United States despite the aging population. Radiation has also been implicated as a causative agent; however, in more than 70% of patients with anaplastic cancer, there is no history of radiation having been administered (16,17). Once anaplastic thyroid cancer is recognized, curative treatment is unlikely; thus, prevention of endemic goiter and diagnosis by fine-needle aspiration biopsy and removal of suspicious differentiated thyroid nodules is recommended. Even when anaplastic thyroid cancers are found incidentally when removing a differentiated thyroid cancer, the outcome is guarded. However, patients who have tumors that can be completely resected and are younger have a slightly better prognosis (18–20). An updated analysis (21) of the SEER database (2) indicated that age less than 60 yr, tumor confined to the thyroid, female sex, surgical resection, external beam radiotherapy or combination surgical resection with radiotherapy were favorable prognostic factors.

Most patients with anaplastic thyroid cancer are not difficult to diagnose. They are usually older patients, and 80% report a long history of goiter or a thyroid nodule (1,2). A typical history is that the thyroid goiter or nodule suddenly begins to grow rapidly and patients develop pain, dysphagia, and/or hoarseness. Some patients may experience symptoms of hyperthyroidism with pseudothyrotoxicosis and can be misdiagnosed with subacute thyroiditis. Fine-needle aspiration cytology is usually definitive, but tumor cells may be scant in large tumors because of hemorrhagic necrosis.

Based on the large size of these tumors at presentation, computed tomography or magnetic resonance imaging is recommended to document the extent of the disease. It can also determine if there is intratracheal growth or invasion. Although most of these tumors do not have thyrotropin receptors, take up radioiodine, or make thyroglobulin, some of these tumors will, as they have originated from more differentiated tumors. Therefore, documenting thyroid function and serum thyroglobulin levels is also recommended.

Once the diagnosis has been made by cytological examination or open biopsy, treatment with multimodality therapy seems necessary because the results of other treatments are dismal. A cooperative prospective study has been done in Sweden (19), where 33 patients were treated for a rapidly enlarging thyroid mass with adriamycin to both enhance the external radiation therapy and also to potentially limit the growth or speed of disseminated cancer. After 4 wk of combined radiation and chemotherapy with this approach, as much thyroid and tumor should be removed as safely as possible. Complications should be avoided, as most patients receive palliative, not curative therapy. From a technical point of view when conducting thyroidectomy in these patients, in contrast to other patients with thyroid cancer, the least involved lobe should be removed first, because this orients the surgeon to the trachea. Once this portion of the thyroid gland has been taken away, removing the side that is more involved with tumor often becomes easier.

From: *Thyroid Cancer: A Comprehensive Guide to Clinical Management, 2/e*
Edited by: L. Wartofsky and D. Van Nostrand © Humana Press Inc., Totowa, NJ

In the Swedish study of patients with anaplastic thyroid cancer, 29 of the 33 patients had the diagnosis established by fine-needle aspiration and cytologic examination *(19)*. No patients failed to complete the protocol because of toxicity. Definitive resection or debulking was done in 23 of the 33 (70%) of patients. After thyroidectomy, radiation and chemotherapy were readministered for 2 more wk. Recent experimental data suggests that the mechanism of action of doxorubicin (Adriamycin® may be via *Fas*-mediated apoptosis *(20)*. In the Swedish study to date, complete local control was obtained in 16 of 33 (48%) of the patients, and four patients had no evidence of disease at 2 yr. Only 8 of 33 (24%) patients died of local failure. Researchers reported that debulking surgery appeared to be a prerequisite for local control, as found in other studies *(22)*. These results are more encouraging than the dismal outcome seen at the Mayo Clinic of 134 cases over a 50-yr experience *(23)*.

REFERENCES

1. Haigh PI, Ituarte PH, Wu HS, et al. Completely resected anaplastic thyroid carcinoma combined with adjuvant chemotherapy and irradiation is associated with prolonged survival. Cancer 2001; 91: 2335–2342.
2. Gilliland FD, Hunt WC, Morris DM, Key CR. Prognostic factors for thyroid carcinoma: A population-based study of 15,698 cases from the Surveillance, Epidemiology and End Results (SEER) program 1973–1991. Cancer 1997; 79:564–573.
3. Junor EJ, Paul J, Reed NS. Anaplastic thyroid carcinoma: 91 patients treated by surgery and radiotherapy. Eur J Surg Oncol 1992; 18: 83–88.
4. Nicolosi A, Addis E, Massidda B, et al. Anaplastic carcinoma of the thyroid: our experience. Minerva Chir 1992; 47:1161–1167.
5. Nel CJ, van Heerden JA, Goellner JR, et al. Anaplastic carcinoma of the thyroid: a clinicopathologic study of 82 cases. Mayo Clinic Proc 1985; 60:51–58.
6. Carcangiu ML, Steeper T, Zampi G, Rosai J. Anaplastic thyroid carcinoma: a study of 70 cases. Am J Clin Pathol 1985; 83:135–158.
7. Miura D, Wada N, Chin K, et al. Anaplastic thyroid cancer: cytogenetic patterns by comparative genomic hybridization. Thyroid 2003; 13:283–290.
8. Cohn KH, Backdahl M, Forsslund G, et al. Biologic considerations and operative strategy in papillary thyroid carcinoma: arguments against the routine performance of total thyroidectomy. Surgery 1984; 96:957–971.
9. Vanderlaan BFAM, Freeman JL, Tsang RW, Asa SL. The association of well-differentiated thyroid carcinoma with insular or anaplastic thyroid carcinoma: evidence for dedifferentiation in tumor progression. Endocr Pathol 1993; 4:215–221.
10. Ito T, Seyama T, Mizuno T, et al. Unique association of p53 mutations with undifferentiated but not with differentiated carcinomas of the thyroid gland. Cancer Res 1992; 52:1369–1371.
11. Parid NR, Shi Y, Zou M. Molecular basis of thyroid cancer. Endocr Rev 1994; 15:202–232.
12. Fagin JA, Matsuo K, Karmakar A, et al. High prevalence of mutations of the p53 gene in poorly differentiated human thyroid carcinomas. J Clin Invest 1993; 91:179–184.
13. Heldin NE, Gustavsson B, Claesson-Welsh L, et al. Aberrant expression of receptors for platelet-derived growth factor in an anaplastic thyroid carcinoma cell line. Proc Nat Acad Sci USA 1988; 85:9302–9306.
14. Fagin JA. Tumor suppressor genes in human thyroid neoplasms: p53 mutations are associated undifferentiated thyroid cancers. J Endocrinol Invest 1995; 18:140–142.
15. Williams ED. Thyroid cancer: pathologic and natural history. Recent Res Cancer Res 1980; 73:47–55.
16. Baker HW. Anaplastic thyroid cancer twelve years after radioiodine therapy. Cancer 1969; 23:885–890.
17. Samaan NA, Schultz PN, Haynie TP, Ordonez NG. Pulmonary metastasis of differentiated thyroid carcinoma: treatment results in 101 patients. J Clin Endocrinol Metab 1985; 60:376–380.
18. Levendag PC, De Porre PM, van Putten WL. Anaplastic carcinoma of the thyroid gland treated by radiation therapy. Int J Radial Oncol Biol Phys 1993; 26:125–128.
19. Tennvall J, Lundell G, Hallquist A, et al. Combined doxorubicin, hyperfractionated radiotherapy, and surgery in anaplastic thyroid carcinoma: report on two protocols—the Swedish Anaplastic Thyroid Cancer Group. Cancer 1994; 74:1348–1354.
20. Massart C, Barbet R, Genettet N, Gibassier J. Doxorubicin induces Fas-mediated apoptosis in human thyroid carcinoma cells. Thyroid 2004; 14:263–270.
21. Kebebew E, Greenspan FS, Clark OH, Woeber KA, McMillan A. Anaplastic thyroid carcinoma: Treatment outcome and prognostic factors. Cancer 2005; 103:1330–1335.
22. Schlumberger M, Parmentier C, Delisle MJ, et al. Combination therapy for anaplastic giant cell thyroid carcinoma. Cancer 1991; 67: 564–566.
23. McIver B, Hay ID, Giuffrida DF, et al. Anaplastic thyroid carcinoma: A 50-year experience at a single institution. Surgery 2001; 130: 1028–1034.

79
Pathology of Anaplastic Carcinoma

James E. Oertel and Yolanda C. Oertel

Anaplastic carcinoma (undifferentiated carcinoma) is now rare, extremely malignant, and is usually fatal *(1–4)*. The thyroid gland has often been enlarged for years, containing multiple nodules or a low-grade, well-differentiated carcinoma that has grown slowly.

These cancers usually infiltrate the thyroid parenchyma and the juxtathyroidal tissues. Metastases to the regional lymph nodes and lungs are common. The neoplastic tissue is pale, firm or hard, and opaque. Foci of hemorrhage and necrosis are frequent and these parts are soft. Extensive dense fibrosis may be evident on gross examination. Foci of calcification are rare, and occasionally, there are regions of metaplastic cartilage and/or bone.

Varied histological patterns are present: (1) rounded to irregular medium- to giant-sized cells with eosinophilic cytoplasm and large or giant nuclei (often bizarre); (2) fusiform (spindle) cells in a fascicular or storiform pattern (Fig. 1); and (3) medium- to large-sized cells with squamoid characteristics (Fig. 2). Some of these cells may have clear cytoplasm. The neoplastic giant cells may have a single nucleus or may be multinucleated. These various cellular types can be mixed together, and transitional forms can be seen *(5)*. The implication of an alveolar or trabecular pattern may be evident. Bizarre nuclei, often vesicular, are common; large nucleoli may be present. There are numerous mitotic figures, and some are atypical. "Osteoclast-type" giant cells of histiocytic origin exist in a few tumors *(6;* Fig. 1).

Neoplastic cells may replace some portions of vessel walls, and small clusters of neoplastic cells may extend into individual thyroid follicles. Polymorphonuclear leukocytes can infiltrate the tumor and can be large in number near the necrotic regions.

A paucicellular variant has been reported *(7)*, and coagulative necrosis and fibrosis are extensive. The sparse neoplastic cells have atypical nuclei. Such tumors resemble Riedel's fibrous thyroiditis, especially when chronic inflammatory cells are scattered throughout the neoplasm. Regardless of the cell types present, some undifferentiated carcinomas are associated with large amounts of hyalinized fibrous tissue, sometimes as dense nodules *(8)*.

Immunoreactive thyroglobulin is typically absent; when present, it is evident only in some larger "epithelioid" cells. Immunoreactive keratin may be demonstrated and is the most common marker that suggests epithelial characteristics *(5,9)*. Immunoreactive vimentin is often detected and may be expressed in the same cells as keratin. Interpretation of such findings can be difficult because both normal thyroid epithelium and remnants of well-differentiated carcinoma (or a benign nodule) may be trapped within the aggressive neoplasm. In addition, the neoplastic cells may absorb these substances nonspecifically from neighboring thyroid tissue.

Evidence of a previous nodular goiter or a follicular or papillary carcinoma may be often found if multiple sections of the neoplasm are taken *(3,10)*. The tumors with substantial spindle-cell or giant- and spindle-cell components may be mistaken for soft-tissue neoplasms, but they are usually not recognizable as one of the well-characterized sarcomas.

Most so-called "small-cell carcinomas" diagnosed in the past were malignant lymphomas. Small-cell carcinoma almost certainly exists, but it is rare. Extensive study of such a lesion may show foci of well-differentiated, poorly differentiated (insular), or medullary carcinoma. Therefore, critical analysis suggests that only a few small-cell cancers exist and belong with the undifferentiated carcinomas *(11–14)*.

In middle-aged or elderly patients, a portion of an otherwise well-differentiated carcinoma may be anaplastic carcinoma, which has grave prognostic implications. If such a focus is only a few millimeters in diameter, it may have little effect on the patient's long-term survival, but in some patients, this is unfortunately not true *(15)*. The same concept applies for a tiny anaplastic carcinoma discovered in a thyroid that was removed for multinodular goiter.

Cytological smears may show marked cellularity or necrosis and hemorrhage (Fig. 3), depending on the part of the mass sampled *(16,17)*. Leukocytes can be numerous. Spindled and giant cells are present *(18)*; the latter may be multinucleated histiocytes (Fig. 4) or (more often) bizarre neoplastic cells with one or several nuclei. Abnormal mitotic figures may be seen. The smears may show cells from a follicular neoplasm or papillary carcinoma if one coexists

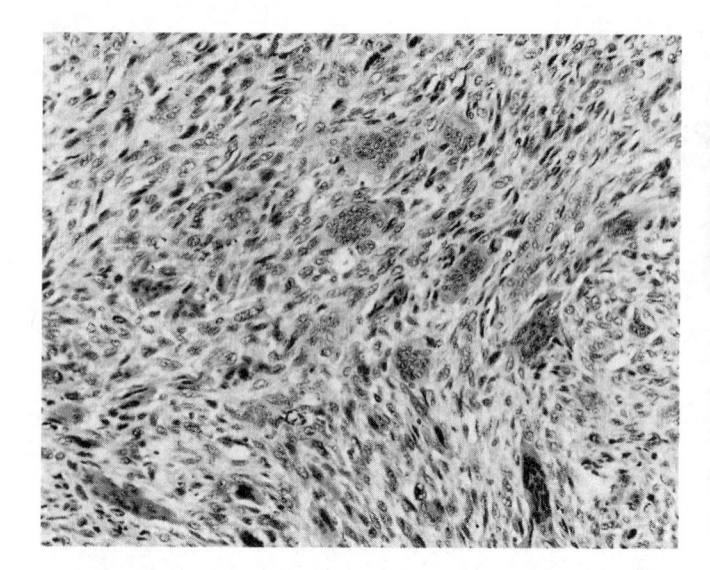

Fig. 1. Undifferentiated carcinoma. Spindled cells and osteoclast-type giant cells are present (hematoxylin and eosin [H&E] stain).

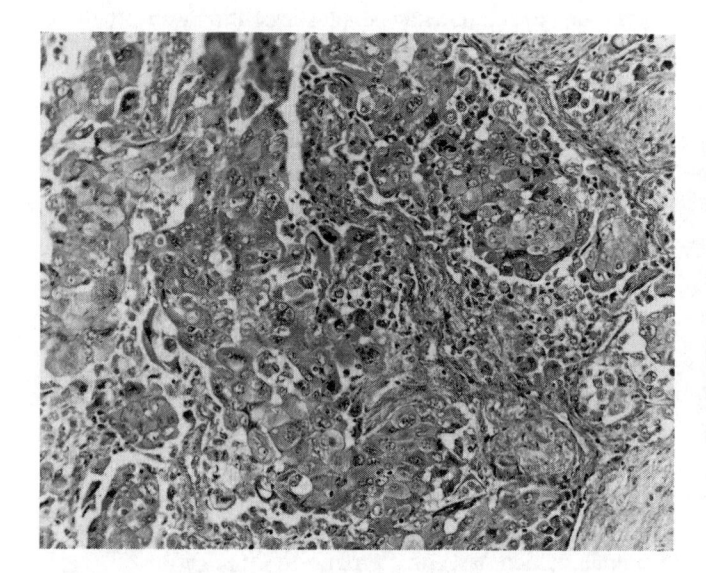

Fig. 2. Undifferentiated carcinoma. Part of the neoplasm has a "squamoid" appearance (H&E stain).

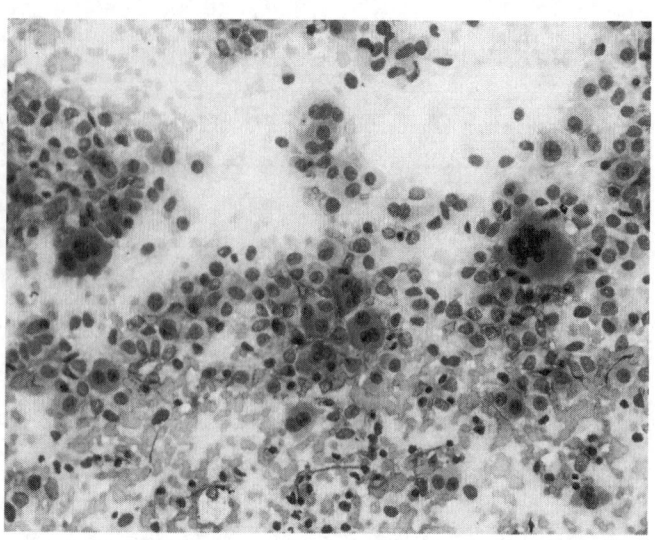

Fig. 3. Undifferentiated carcinoma. Hypercellular aspirate with marked variation in the size of the neoplastic cells. Multinucleated cells are evident (Diff-Quik stain).

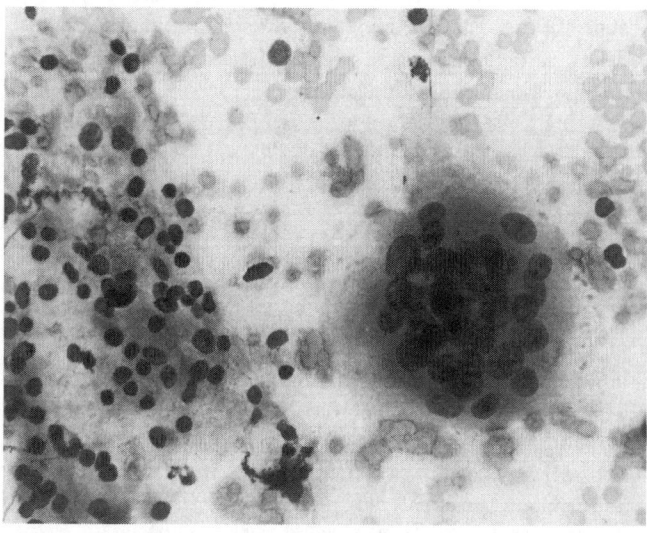

Fig. 4. Undifferentiated carcinoma. Hypercellular aspirate with an osteoclast-type cell on the right (Diff-Quik stain).

with the anaplastic carcinoma *(19)*. Therefore, this possibility illustrates the requirement that several aspirations should be performed when a fast-growing mass is present. Also, these neoplasms may be hemorrhagic or fibrotic; thus, the epithelial cells may be sparse or diluted by blood.

REFERENCES

1. McIver B, Hay ID, Giuffrida DF, et al. Anaplastic thyroid carcinoma: A 50-year experience at a single institution. Surgery 2001; 130: 1028–1034.
2. LiVolsi VA. Surgical pathology of the thyroid. Major Probl Pathol 1990; 22:253–274.
3. Rosai J, Carcangiu ML, DeLellis RA. Tumors of the thyroid gland. In Rosai J, Sobin LH, editors. Atlas of Tumor Pathology. Washington, DC: AFIP, 1992.
4. Tan RK, Finley RK III, Driscoll D, et al. Anaplastic carcinoma of the thyroid: a 24-year experience. Head Neck 1995; 17:41–48.
5. Wiseman SM, Loree TR, Rigual NR, et al. Anaplastic transformation of thyroid cancer: Review of clinical, pathologic, and molecular evidence provides new insights into disease biology and future therapy. Head Neck 2003; 25:662–670.
6. Gaffey MJ, Lack EE, Christ ML, Weiss L. Anaplastic thyroid carcinoma with osteoclast-like giant cells: a clinicopathologic,

immunohistochemical, and ultrastructural study. Am J Surg Pathol 1991; 15:160–168.
7. Wan S-K, Chan JKC, Tang S-K. Paucicellular variant of anaplastic thyroid carcinoma: a mimic of Riedel's thyroiditis. Am J Clin Pathol 1996; 105:388–393.
8. Chetty R, Mills AE, LiVolsi VA. Anaplastic carcinoma of the thyroid with sclerohyaline nodules. Endocr Pathol 1993; 4:110–114.
9. Ordonez NG, El-Naggar AK, Hickey RC, Samaan NA. Anaplastic thyroid carcinoma: immunocytochemical study of 32 cases. Am J Clin Pathol 1991; 96:15–24.
10. van der Laan BFAM, Freeman JL, Tsang RW, Asa SL. The association of well-differentiated thyroid carcinoma with insular or anaplastic thyroid carcinoma: evidence for dedifferentiation in tumor progression. Endocr Pathol 1993; 4:215–221.
11. Cameron RG, Seemayer TA, Wang N-S, et al. Small cell malignant tumors of the thyroid: a light and electron microscopic study. Hum Pathol 1975; 6:731–740.
12. Luna MA, Mackay B, Hill CS, et al. The quarterly case: malignant small cell tumor of the thyroid. Ultrastruct Pathol 1980; 1:265–270.
13. Mambo NC, Irwin SM. Anaplastic small cell neoplasms of the thyroid: an immunoperoxidase study. Hum Pathol 1984; 15:55–60.
14. Wolf BC, Sheahan K, DeCoste D, et al. Immunohistochemical analysis of small cell tumors of the thyroid gland: an eastern cooperative oncology group study. Hum Pathol 1992; 23:1252–1261.
15. Aldinger KA, Samaan NA, Ibanez M, Hill CS Jr. Anaplastic carcinoma of the thyroid: a review of 84 cases of spindle and giant cell carcinoma of the thyroid. Cancer 1978; 41:2267–2275.
16. Schneider V, Frable WJ. Spindle and giant cell carcinoma of the thyroid: cytologic diagnosis by fine needle aspiration. Acta Cytol 1980; 24:184–189.
17. Brooke PK, Hameed M, Zakowski MF. Fine-needle aspiration of anaplastic thyroid carcinoma with varied cytologic and histologic patterns: a case report. Diagn Cytopathol 1994; 11:60–63.
18. Us-Krasovec M, Golouh R, Auersperg M, et al. Anaplastic thyroid carcinoma in fine needle aspirates. Acta Cytol 1996; 40:953–958.
19. Vinette DSJ, MacDonald LL, Yazdi HM. Papillary carcinoma of the thyroid with anaplastic transformation: diagnostic pitfalls in fine-needle aspiration biopsy. Diagn Cytopathol 1991; 7:75–78.

80
PET Scanning in Anaplastic Cancer of the Thyroid

I. Ross McDougall

The role of positron emission tomography (PET) in differentiated and medullary cancers has been presented (see also Chapters 34 and 71). The latter chapters contain descriptions of methodology that are not presented again at length here. Briefly, the patient should fast and have a normal fasting serum glucose value. A range of 10–15 mCi (370–555 MBq) of F-18 Fluorinedeoxyglucose (FDG) is injected intravenously, and scanning commenced after a delay of 60 min, but some authorities prefer a delay of 90–120 min. It is important that the patient is resting in a quiet environment, not speaking or chewing during the hour between injection and scanning. The scan should usually be obtained from the base of the skull to the upper thighs. Attenuation correction is appropriate, or use of instrumentation for combined PET/computed tomography (CT) that includes attenuation correction is advisable.

From the original descriptions of the value of PET in well-differentiated thyroid cancer, it became apparent that there was a reciprocal relationship between PET scan uptake vs that seen on a whole-body radioiodine scan, which depended on the degree of cancer differentiation (1). Thus, well-differentiated cancers can trap radioiodine, but not FDG, and poorly differentiated cancers show avid uptake of FDG, but they do not tend to trap iodine (1,2). Iodine is concentrated by the sodium iodide symporter (NIS) (3). Glucose is taken into cells by glucose transporters, including GLUT 1–5 and GLUT 7. As cancers become more dedifferentiated, the quantity of NIS at the laterobasal membrane of follicular cells decreases, and its appropriate cellular positioning can be lost (4,5).

As cancers become more anaplastic, expression of glucose transporters increases. In one study, the quantity of GLUT 1 was studied in 45 thyroid cancers (6), 5 of which were anaplastic, and the remaining were graded for their degree of aggressiveness. All anaplastic cancers demonstrated more membranous and cytoplasmic GLUT 1, and the quantity of GLUT 1 in differentiated cancer cells was linearly related to the grade of malignancy. These data indicate that FDG-PET scan should be a powerful and accurate imaging modality in patients with anaplastic cancer. There are not many reports

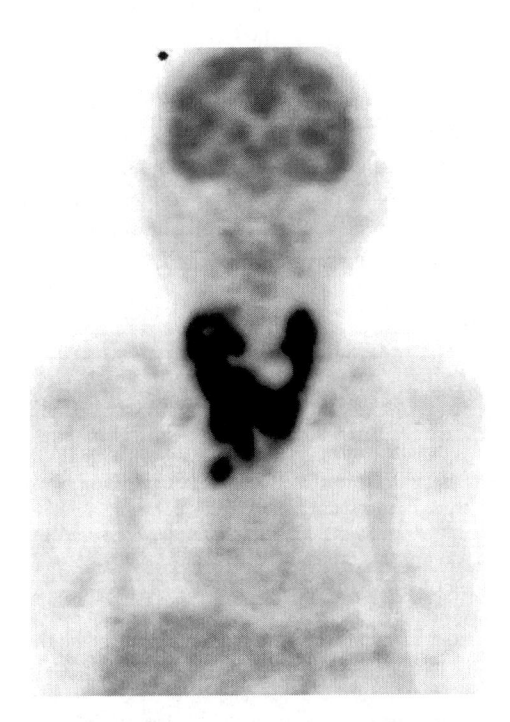

Fig. 1. The illustration shows a FDG scan in an elderly woman with a rapidly growing thyroid mass. The patient had difficulty breathing and swallowing. Fine-needle aspiration demonstrated anaplastic thyroid cancer. Intense uptake of FDG with irregular edges is noted.

on this topic because anaplastic cancer is relatively rare, accounting for 1–3% of thyroid cancers, and PET scan is a fairly new investigative tool (7,8). However, the cancers show intense trapping and concentration of FDG, and standard uptake values are among the highest seen (Fig. 1).

Anaplastic cancer is an extremely fast-growing cancer that is locally invasive and usually causes a rapid death by local compressive effects. It is estimated that about 80% of patients have regional nodal metastases, and 50% have distant metastases at presentation. PET can be used to stage the disease (9,10). This can help make a decision whether to operate first or to treat with systemic chemotherapy. When distant lesions are found, it may not be appropriate to conduct extensive surgery on the primary lesion except for palliative purposes. Several case reports attest to the value of FDG-PET *(11–13)*. Evidence shows that the prognosis in well-differentiated thyroid cancer can be related to the uptake of FDG, lesions showing a high uptake, which indicates that they will not trap iodine and consequently have a more bleak outcome *(14,15)*. Further research is needed to determine the correlation between the uptake of FDG and outcome or prognosis for anaplastic cancers.

PET has also been valuable in the evaluation of thyroid cancers that fall on the interface between differentiated and anaplastic tumors, such as the insular variant of papillary thyroid cancer *(16,17)*.

In summary, FDG-PET scanning has a role in defining the local, regional, and distant sites of metastases in patients with poorly differentiated (insular) cancer and anaplastic cancer. Combined ^{18}FDG PET with computed tomography *(18)* may prove to be even more efficacious.

REFERENCES

1. Joensuu H, Ahonen A. Imaging of metastases of thyroid carcinoma with fluorine-18 fluorodeoxyglucose. J Nucl Med 1987; 28:910–914.
2. Feine U. Fluor-18-deoxyglucose positron emission tomography in differentiated thyroid cancer. Eur J Endocrinol 1998; 138:492–496.
3. Dai G, Levy O, Carrasco N. Cloning and characterization of the thyroid iodide transporter. Nature 1996; 379:458–460.
4. Min JJ, Chung JK, Lee J, et al. Relationship between expression of the sodium/iodide symporter and 131I uptake in recurrent lesions of differentiated thyroid carcinoma. Eur J Nucl Med 2001; 28:639–645.
5. Lazar V, Bidart JM, Caillou B, et al. Expression of the Na+/I– symporter gene in human thyroid tumors: a comparison study with other thyroid-specific genes. J Clin Endocrinol Metab 1999; 84:3228–3234.
6. Schonberger J, Ruschoff J, Grimm D, et al. Glucose transporter 1 gene expression is related to thyroid neoplasms with an unfavorable prognosis: an immunohistochemical study. Thyroid 2002; 12:747–754.
7. Hundahl SA, Fleming ID, Fremgen AM, Menck HR. A National Cancer Data Base report on 53,856 cases of thyroid carcinoma treated in the U.S., 1985-1995. Cancer 1998; 83:2638–2648.
8. Kitagawa W, Shimizu K, Akasu H, Tanaka S. Endocrine surgery. The ninth report: the latest data on and clinical characteristics of the epidemiology of thyroid carcinoma. J Nippon Med Sch 2003; 70:57–61.
9. Lind P, Kresnik E, Kumnig G, et al. 18F-FDG-PET in the follow-up of thyroid cancer. Acta Med Austriaca 2003; 30:17–21.
10. Kumnig G. Value of F-18 fluorodeoxyglucose positron emission tomography in thyroid carcinoma. Wien Med Wochenschr 2002; 152:280–285.
11. Jadvar H, Fischman AJ. Evaluation of rare tumors with [F-18]fluorodeoxyglucose positron emission tomography. Clin Positron Imaging 1999; 2:153–158.
12. Kresnik E, Gallowitsch HJ, Mikosch P, et al. Fluorine-18-fluorodeoxyglucose positron emission tomography in the preoperative assessment of thyroid nodules in an endemic goiter area. Surgery 2003; 133:294–299.
13. McDougall IR, Davidson J, Segall GM. Positron emission tomography of the thyroid, with an emphasis on thyroid cancer. Nucl Med Commun 2001; 22:485–492.
14. Wang W, Larson SM, Fazzari M, et al. Prognostic value of [18F]fluorodeoxyglucose positron emission tomographic scanning in patients with thyroid cancer. J Clin Endocrinol Metab 2000; 85:1107–1113.
15. Wang W, Larson SM, Tuttle RM, et al. Resistance of [18f]-fluorodeoxyglucose-avid metastatic thyroid cancer lesions to treatment with high-dose radioactive iodine. Thyroid 2001; 11:1169–1175.
16. Diehl M, Graichen S, Menzel C, et al. F-18 FDG PET in insular thyroid cancer. Clin Nucl Med 2003; 28:728–731.
17. Zettinig G, Leitha T, Niederle B, et al. FDG positron emission tomographic, radioiodine, and MIBI imaging in a patient with poorly differentiated insular thyroid carcinoma. Clin Nucl Med 2001; 26:599–601.
18. Nahas Z, Goldenberg D, Fakhry C, et al. The role of positron emission tomography/computed tomography in the management of recurrent papillary thyroid carcinoma. Laryngoscope 2005; 115:237–243.

81
External Radiation Therapy of Anaplastic Thyroid Cancer

James D. Brierley and Richard W. Tsang

CERVICAL RADIATION THERAPY

As discussed in Chapters 22 and 24, complete surgical resection provides the best chance of cure; however, for anaplastic thyroid cancer, this is only possible in few patients. As anaplastic thyroid cancer does not concentrate ^{131}I radiotherapy, external-beam radiation therapy (RT) is the mainstay for local control and palliation of symptoms to maintain quality of life.

In a series of 91 patients, with an overall survival of 11% at 3 yr, 95% had external-beam radiation (1). Complete response to RT occurred in 40%, but 10% progressed locally during their radiation. Although there was a tendency of improved survival with an increase in the radiation dose, this was not statistically significant. There were 70 patients of whom information was available: 36% relapsed locally, 29% at distant sites, and 36% both locally and at distant sites. This study demonstrated that radiation alone can result in a complete response, but long-term local control remains a problem. Even if this is achieved, distant metastases almost invariably result in death.

In a phase II study of hyperfractionated radiotherapy without chemotherapy in 17 patients (60.8 Gy in 32 fractions daily over 20–24 d), complete response was reported in 3 (17.6%) patients, and there was a partial response in 7 (41.2%; 2). Despite this response rate, the median survival was only 10 wk, and the toxicity was unacceptable. The majority of patients developed grade 3 or 4 toxicity, and death occurred in five patients before the toxicity resolved. The ineffectiveness of radiation alone has led to the development of both novel fractionation schedules and concurrent chemotherapy regimens. Because anaplastic thyroid cancer grows rapidly, hyperfractionated and accelerated radiation regimens have been used, sometimes in combination with chemotherapy and surgical resection. The rationale for altered fractionation is that in rapidly growing tumors, giving the radiation as quickly as possible counteracts any tumor repopulation by the rapidly multiplying cancer cells. The results of published studies on altered fractionation with and without chemotherapy are summarized in Table 1.

The most successful regimen in obtaining local control is that described in a series of publications from Sweden. Combined hyperfractionated radiation and concurrent chemotherapy (often with doxorubicin) are given preoperatively, followed by surgical resection. In the first two of three consecutive series, further radiation and chemotherapy were given after surgical resection. In the third series, a higher dose of preoperative treatment was administered, and there was no post-resection therapy. In a total of 55 patients treated between 1985 and 1999, surgery was possible in 40 patients. Although this aggressive approach resulted in an impressive local recurrence-free rate of 60%, the median survival was still only 3.5 mo, with a 9% survival at 2 yr (3).

In a study of 33 patients with an overall median survival of 3.8 mo, Haigh et al. identified a small and highly selected subgroup of 8 patients with anaplastic thyroid cancer (4) who had an estimated 5-yr survival of 50%. These patients underwent surgical resection with no residual disease or only microscopic residual disease and subsequently received combined chemotherapy and RT. In another recent report of 32 patients, 82% had tumors less than 4 cm, and 31% were able to undergo a total thyroidectomy (5). A total of 23 patients were treated between 1981 and 1999, most of whom had twice-daily radiation and concurrent chemotherapy, with a 2-yr survival rate of 52%.

In contrast to these two small studies, a large series of 134 patients treated at the Mayo Clinic (6) with multimodality therapy did not have improved survival when compared to standard care. Yet, there was a small nonsignificant improvement in median survival in patients who received radiation in comparison to those who did not (3 vs 5 mo; $p = 0.08$). However, in a small number of patients (13 of 134) who were able to receive debulking surgery, radiation, and chemotherapy, the 1-yr survival was 23% vs 9% overall ($p = 0.019$). These studies suggest that hyperfractionated radiation and chemotherapy may result in a better outcome but only in a select series of patients who have small tumors amenable to surgical resection with at least minimal residual disease. In an analysis of 516 patients with anaplastic thyroid cancer from the Surveillance, Epidemiology, and End Results (SEER) database of the National Cancer Institute (11), the best outcomes were seen in younger patients (less than 60 yr) who had surgical resection, external beam radiotherapy or combination surgical resection with radiotherapy.

From: *Thyroid Cancer: A Comprehensive Guide to Clinical Management, 2/e*
Edited by: L. Wartofsky and D. Van Nostrand © Humana Press Inc., Totowa, NJ

Table 1
Local Control and Survival Following Fractionated Radiation and Concurrent Chemotherapy in Anaplastic Thyroid Cancer

Author (Ref.)	Patients	Local Control	Median Survival (mo)	2-yr Survival	Fractionation	Concurrent Chemotherapy
Haigh (4)	33	N/S	3.8	20%	Not stated	Yes
Heron (5)	32	N/S	N/S	48%[a]	Daily	In 15
Juror (1)	91	28%	5	11%[b]	Daily	In 18
Kim (8)	19	68%	6	20%	Hyperfractionated	Yes
McIver (6)	29	N/S	5	9%[a]	Daily[c]	In 13
Mitchell (2)	17	76%	2.5	N/S	Accelerated	No
Schlumberger (9)	20	N/S	N/S	15%[d]	Hypofractionated	Yes
Tennvall (3)	55	60%	2–4.5	9%	Hyperfractionated	Yes
Wong (10)	32	22%	6	18%	Accelerated/hyperfractionated	Yes

[a]At 1 yr.
[b]At 3 yr.
[c]For the group as a whole (134 patient) median survival was 3 mo.
[d]At 20 mo.
N/S, Not specified.

Generally, patients with good performance status and no evidence of distant metastatic disease may benefit from an aggressive approach, using high-dose altered fractionated RT with or without concurrent chemotherapy. Currently, at Princess Margaret Hospital, where patients rarely have potentially resectable disease, patients with good performance status are considered for accelerated hyperfractionated radiation without chemotherapy, 60 Gy in 40 fractions over 4 wk, with 2 fractions of 1.5 Gy/d. The rationale is that anaplastic thyroid cancer has a low response rate to chemotherapy, and combining hyperfractionated radiation with chemotherapy results in moderately severe toxicity. Therefore, by not giving concurrent chemotherapy, a higher dose of radiation can be given more safely without the risk of interruption and intensive support measures. For patients with poor performance status, palliative radiation at a lower dose (e.g., 2000 cGy in 5 daily fractions) is given.

EXTERNAL-BEAM RT

The thyroid bed is a technically challenging volume to treat, as the thyroid bed curves around the vertebral body and includes the air column in the trachea. It can be difficult to adequately treat the thyroid bed and spare the spinal cord to a dose within tolerance. A variety of techniques have been described that produce adequate dose distribution (7). Advances in radiation techniques that result in better dose distribution to the areas at risk and reduce the volume of normal tissues to a minimum are described in Chapter 84. Well-planned external-beam RT has acceptable acute toxicity and rarely produces serious complications.

METASTASES

Unlike papillary and follicular carcinoma, the prognosis for patients who have developed distant metastases from anaplastic thyroid cancer is extremely poor. The surgical resection of bone metastases, even if the lesion is apparently solitary, is not warranted unless there is a significant risk of a pathological fracture. Therefore, external-beam radiation has an important role in palliation of bone metastases. Similarly, in patients with brain metastases, whole-brain radiation should be considered, except in the elderly, who do not tolerate whole-brain radiation well.

REFERENCES

1. Junor E, Paul J, Reed N. Anaplastic thyroid carcinoma: 91 patients treated by surgery and radiotherapy. Eur J Surg 1992; 18:83–88.
2. Mitchell G, Huddart R, Harmer C. Phase II evaluation of high dose accelerated radiotherapy for anaplastic thyroid carcinoma. Radiother Oncol 1999; 50:33–38.
3. Tennvall J, Lundell G, Wahlberg P, et al. Anaplastic thyroid carcinoma: three protocols combining doxorubicin, hyperfractionated radiotherapy and surgery. Br J Cancer 2002; 86:1848–1853.
4. Haigh PI, Ituarte PH, Wu HS, et al. Completely resected anaplastic thyroid carcinoma combined with adjuvant chemotherapy and irradiation is associated with prolonged survival. Cancer 2001; 91:2335–2342.
5. Heron DE, Karimpour S, Grigsby PW. Anaplastic thyroid carcinoma: comparison of conventional radiotherapy and hyperfractionation chemoradiotherapy in two groups. Am J Clin Oncol 2002; 25:442–446.
6. McIver B, Hay ID, Giuffrida DF, et al. Anaplastic thyroid carcinoma: a 50-year experience at a single institution. Surgery 2001; 130:1028–1034.
7. Tsang RW, Brierley JD. The thyroid. In Cox JD, Kian Ang K, editors. Radiation Oncology. St. Louis, MO: Mosby; 2003.
8. Kim JH, Leeper RD. Treatment of locally advanced thyroid carcinoma with combination doxorubicin and radiation therapy. Cancer 1987; 60:2372–2375.
9. Schlumberger M, Parmentier C, Delisle MJ, et al. Combination therapy for anaplastic giant cell thyroid carcinoma. Cancer 1991; 67:564–566.
10. Wong CS, Van Dyk J, Simpson WJ. Myelopathy following hyperfractionated accelerated radiotherapy for anaplastic thyroid carcinoma. Radiother Oncol 1991; 20:3–9.
11. Kebebew E, Greenspan FS, Clark OH, Woeber KA, McMillan A. Anaplastic thyroid carcinoma: Treatment outcome and prognostic factors. Cancer 2005; 103:1330–1335.

82
Chemotherapy for Anaplastic Thyroid Cancer

Lawrence S. Lessin

Anaplastic carcinoma of the thyroid is one of the most aggressive human cancers, with a median survival of 4–6 mo after diagnosis. It is relatively resistant to chemotherapy alone. Shimaoka and associates (1) reported the response of anaplastic thyroid cancer to chemotherapy in a randomized trial conducted by the Eastern Cooperative Oncology Group. Of the 39 patients with anaplastic thyroid cancer enrolled in the study, 21 were treated with doxorubicin alone, and 18 were treated with a combination of doxorubicin and cisplatin. Only one patient showed partial response to doxorubicin alone, compared to three complete responses and three partial responses in the combination arm. However, patients treated with combination chemotherapy did not have a statistically longer duration of response, nor of time to relapse. Investigators concluded that combination chemotherapy is superior to single-agent treatment in anaplastic carcinoma, with a higher response rate but no survival advantage.

Tamura and colleagues (2) conducted a study of the Japanese Society of Thyroid Surgery in which 17 patients with anaplastic thyroid carcinoma were treated with a regimen of infusional cisplatin and bolus doxorubicin on day 1, bolus etoposide on days 1–3, and peplomycin (a bleomycin analog) on days 1–5, with granulocyte colony-stimulating factor (G-CSF) support. Of 10 patients with measurable lesions, 2 had brief partial responses lasting 2–3 mo. Despite G-CSF support, all patients experienced major neutropenia.

In 2000, the Collaborative Anaplastic Thyroid Cancer Health Intervention Trials Group, reported a phase II study of paclitaxel, given as a 96-h infusion, in 20 patients with anaplastic thyroid cancer (3). Doses of paclitaxel were increased from 120 mg/m^2 (7 patients) to 140 mg/m^2 (13 patients) over 96 h by continuous infusion. Nine additional patients were treated off protocol with 225 mg/m^2 as one-hour weekly infusions. The total response rate was 53%, with one complete response and nine partial responses. Two of the seven patients who relapsed after prior partial responses to the 96-hour infusion had subsequent partial responses to the 1-h higher dose weekly infusions. One patient who did not respond to this infusion had a partial response on the weekly higher dose regimen. Toxicities did not exceed grade 2 in the 96-h infusions, but grade 3 neurotoxicity was common in the weekly 225 mg/m^2 1-h infusion group.

Because single-modality treatment with radiotherapy, surgery, or chemotherapy has not improved survival, investigators have assessed the potential synergy of chemotherapy and radiation, often combined with surgical debulking. Studies of chemoradiotherapy for anaplastic thyroid carcinoma, usually given concomitantly, are summarized in Table 1.

COMBINED CHEMOTHERAPY AND RADIATION THERAPY

Combined chemoradiotherapy for the treatment of anaplastic thyroid cancer has been reported since the 1970s. Tennvall and Tallroth and their collaborators (4–7) documented a series of investigations relating to combined modality therapy for anaplastic thyroid cancer. In the early 1970s, combined chemotherapy and radiation with single-agent methotrexate was tested, achieving seven responses in eight patients, but none survived their disease. Severe side effects (mucositis and cytopenias) were encountered; thus, the chemotherapy regimen was changed to a combination of bleomycin, cyclophosphamide, and 5-fluorouracil (BCF; 5). With this regimen, seven of nine patients had a response, and one underwent surgical debulking after completion of chemoradiotherapy and survived for 14 yr without recurrence. Remissions observed in other patients were transient. Considering this experience, surgery was incorporated early in the treatment protocol using the same combination chemotherapy and hyperfractionated (twice-daily) radiotherapy (7). There were 20 patients treated, and 75% achieved a response, of which 3 remained in complete remission for more than 6 yr. Again, combination chemotherapy with BCF and hyperfractionated radiation therapy produced severe local and systemic toxicity.

In 1983, Kim and Leeper (8) used a combined modality regimen with low-dose doxorubicin (10 mg/m^2/wk) as a bolus injection before hyperfractionated radiation therapy. Their initial report stated that eight of nine patients achieved complete remission at primary tumor sites, and six of eight

From: *Thyroid Cancer: A Comprehensive Guide to Clinical Management*, 2/e
Edited by: L. Wartofsky and D. Van Nostrand © Humana Press Inc., Totowa, NJ

Table 1
Studies of Combination Chemoradiotherapy for Anaplastic Thyroid Cancer

Author (Reference)	Regimen	Response Rate: Patients
Kim and Leeper (8)	Doxorubicin 10 mg/m^2/wk; RT 160 cGy BID × 3 d/wk (total: 5760 cGy)	9 of 11
Kim and Leeper (9)	Same	16 of 19
Tennvall et al. (4)	Pre- and postoperative RT 100 cGy BID; doxorubicin 20 mg/wk IV to total dose 750 mg/m^2	14 of 20
Tennvall et al. (5)	Bleomycin, cytoxan, 5-fluorouracil with concomitant RT 200 cGy qd, (total 3000–4000 cGy)	7 of 9
Tennvall et al. (7)	*Protocol A:* Pre- and postoperative chemoradiotherapy using doxorubicin 20 mg/m^2/wk and RT 100 cGy qd (total 4600 cGy) with debulking surgery (total treatment duration of 10 wk)	8 of 16
	Protocol B: Pre- and postoperative chemoradiotherapy using doxorubicin 20 mg/wk and hyperfractionated RT 130 cGy BID (total 4600 cGy with debulking surgery (total treatment duration of 8 wk)	11 of 17
Schlumberger et al. (17)	*Protocol 1:* (<65 yr) doxorubicin 60 mg/m^2 and cisplatin 90 mg/m^2 q4 wk plus RT 175 cGy qd (total 1225 cGy)	10 of 12
	Protocol 2: (>61 yr) mitozantrone 14 mg/m^2 q4 wk plus RT 175 cGy qd (total 1225 cGy)	4 of 8
Tennvall et al. (10)	*Protocol C:* Preoperative chemotherapy with doxorubicin 20 mg/m^2 per week and hyperfractionated RT 60 cGy qd (total 4600 cGy) with debulking surgery	17 of 22

patients remained free of local disease in the neck until the time of death from distant metastases. In this study, only one of nine patients had complete surgical resection, and the rest had only biopsy or partial resection. Owing to the low dose of doxorubicin used and the hyperfractionation of radiation therapy, both acute and late-phase normal tissue toxicity were low. After 1983, Kim and Leeper (9) began a prospective study of therapy for anaplastic thyroid cancer and published their data in 1987 after treatment of 19 patients. Complete response was achieved in 84%, and the local control rate was 68% at 2 yr. Median survival was about 1 yr, which was significantly longer than the 4-mo median survival observed in historical controls. These authors also noted that if tumor volume exceeded more than 200 cm^3 when beginning radiation, there was no significant response to combined modality treatment.

After Kim and Leeper published their findings in 1983, the Tennvall-Tallroth group studied 16 patients who were treated with low-dose doxorubicin and radiation before and after surgery, instead of the BCF regimen, and confirmed the improved efficacy and reduced toxicity (4,5).

In 2002, Tennvall et al. summarized their experience of combined neoadjuvant doxorubicin with daily and hyperfractionated radiation therapy and debulking surgery in 55 consecutive patients with anaplastic thyroid cancer from 1984 to 1999 (10). Three protocols were used sequentially (as shown in Table 1). All utilized weekly doxorubicin combined with radiation therapy, initially once a day at 1.0 or 1.3 cGy (protocol A), then later at 1.6 cGy hyperfractionated (protocol B), divided in preoperative and postoperative treatments to a total dose of 4600 cGy. In protocol C, all radiation therapy was given presurgery. Surgery was performed in 40 of 55 patients. No patient failed to complete the protocol because of toxicity. Death was attributed to local failure in 13 of 55 (24%) patients, 5 patients survived for more than 2 yr, and 60% had no signs of local recurrence (5 of 16 in protocol A, 11 of 17 in protocol B, and 17 of 22 in protocol C). In the 40 patients who had debulking surgery, 33 showed no evidence of local recurrence, including 17 of 17 treated with protocol C.

In a retrospective nonrandomized study examining the sequence effect of therapies, Besic et al. (11) determined that initiating therapy with chemotherapeutic agents and radiation initially with surgery performed subsequently, tended to be associated with more optimal outcome. Regardless, prognosis remains grim for this tumor and multimodal approaches to therapy for patients with the poorest prognostic indices offer the best hope of at least temporary remission (12,13).

Heron et al. (14) published the results of a comparative trial of therapy for 32 patients with anaplastic carcinoma over a 47 year period at the University of Pittsburgh. Treatment consisted of either conventional radiation therapy or hyperfractionation chemoradiotherapy. Less than half of the patients had surgery, and radiotherapy techniques varied with the chemotherapeutic agents including doxorubicin, vincristine, paclitaxel, and cisplatin. In those patients who did not receive chemotherapy, overall 2-year survival was 44% compared to 52% for those receiving chemotherapy, and 10 patients survived more than two years. They concluded that "among patients with anaplastic thyroid cancer, surgery, hyperfractionated radiotherapy in conjunction with chemotherapy is associated with better overall survival, but not progression-free survival, compared to conventional radiotherapy."

DRUG RESISTANCE

Anaplastic thyroid cancer is relatively resistant to chemotherapy. The mechanism of drug resistance was studied by Yamashita and coworkers *(15)* who assessed expression of the *MDR-1* tumor resistance gene and its *p-glycoprotein* gene product in relation to chemotherapy response. Anaplastic thyroid carcinoma showed low expression of MDR-1, and no relationship was found between response to chemotherapy and *MDR-1* expression or p-glycoprotein. Asakawa and colleagues *(16)* utilized an in vitro chemosensitivity assay on anaplastic thyroid cancers from 14 patients. These assays demonstrated chemoresistance to doxorubicin, cisplatin, etoposide, cyclophosphamide, and carboplatin in the majority of tumors. Only one patient had in vitro sensitivity to doxorubicin, but no clinical response was seen. None of the in vitro–resistant patients had a clinical response to chemotherapy. The investigators suggest that in vitro chemosensitivity testing may prevent administration of ineffective chemotherapy; however, this remains to be established.

Newer approaches to therapy are on the horizon and are discussed below in Chapter 85. Based on cell culture and animal studies on anaplastic thyroid cancer, these may include such agents as gemcitabine *(18,19)*, tyrosine kinase inhibitors *(20,21)*, combretastatin *(22)*, VEGF (vascular endothelial growth factor) inhibitors *(23)*, thalidomide, and histone deacetylase inhibitors *(24,25)*. General overviews of anaplastic cancer are available in the recent literature *(26,27)* as well as in Chapter 77, with discussion of surgical management in Chapter 78 and external radiation therapy in Chapter 80.

In summary, anaplastic thyroid cancer, although relatively chemoresistant, has shown a response to combined modality therapy, including surgery and chemoradiation. Even in patients with distant metastases, local control with combined treatment may prevent distressing upper airway obstruction and improve the quality of life.

REFERENCES

1. Shimaoka K, Schoenfeld D, De Wys W, et al. A randomized trial of doxorubicin vs. doxorubicin plus cisplatin in patients with advanced thyroid carcinoma. Cancer 1985; 56:2155–2160.
2. Tamura K, Shimaoka K, Mimura T, et al. Intensive chemotherapy for anaplastic thyroid carcinoma: combination of cisplatin, doxorubicin, etoposide and peplomycin with granulocyte-colony stimulating factor. Jpn J Clin Oncol 1995; 25:203–207. [*Also*, Proc Annu Meet Am Soc Clin Oncol 1996; 15A:906.]
3. Ain KB, Egorin MJ, DeSimone PA. Treatment of anaplastic thyroid carcinoma with paclitaxel; phase 2 trial using ninety-six-hour infusion. Collaborative Anaplastic Thyroid Cancer Health Intervention Trials (CATCHIT) Group. Thyroid 2000; 10:587–594.
4. Tennvall J, Lundell G, Hallquist A, et al. and the Swedish Anaplastic Thyroid Cancer Group. Combined doxorubicin, hyperfractionated radiotherapy and surgery in anaplastic thyroid carcinoma: report on two protocols. Cancer 1994; 74:1348–1354.
5. Tennvall J, Anderson T, Aspengren K, et al. Undifferentiated giant and spindle cell carcinoma of the thyroid: report on two combined treatment modalities. Acta Radiol Oncol 1979; 18:408–416.
6. Tennvall J, Tallroth F, Hassan E, et al. Anaplastic thyroid carcinoma—doxorubicin, hyperfractionated radiotherapy and surgery. Acta Oncol 1990; 29:1025–1028.
7. Tennvall J, Lundell G, Hallquist A, et al. and the Swedish Anaplastic Thyroid Cancer Group. Combined doxorubicin, hyperfractionated radiotherapy and surgery in anaplastic thyroid carcinoma: report on two protocols. Cancer 1994; 74:1348–1354.
8. Kim JH, Leeper RD. Treatment of anaplastic giant and spindle cell carcinoma of the thyroid gland with combination adriamycin and radiation therapy: a new approach. Cancer 1983; 52:954–957.
9. Kim JH, Leeper RD. Treatment of locally advanced thyroid carcinoma with combination doxorubicin and radiation therapy. Cancer 1987; 60:2372–2375.
10. Tennvall J, Lundell G, Wahlberg P, et al. Anaplastic thyroid carcinoma: three protocols combining doxorubicin, hyperfractionated radiotherapy and surgery. Br J Cancer 2002; 86:1848–1853.
11. Besic N, Auersperg M, Us-Krasovec M, et al. Effect of primary treatment on survival in anaplastic thyroid carcinoma. Eur J Surg Oncol 2001; 27:260–267.
12. Sugitani I, Kasai N, Fujimoto Y, Yanagisawa A. Prognostic factors and therapeutic strategy for anaplastic carcinoma of the thyroid. World J Surg 2001; 25:617–622.
13. Busnardo B, Daniele O, Pelizzo MR, et al. A multimodality therapeutic approach in anaplastic thyroid cancer: study on 39 patients. J Endocrinol Invest 2000; 23:755–761.
14. Heron DC, Karimpour S, Grigsby PW. Anaplastic thyroid Carcinoma; comparison of conventional radiotherapy and hyperfractionation chemoradiotherapy in two groups. Am. J Clin Oncol 2002; 25:442–446.
15. Yamashita T, Watanabe M, Onodera M, et al. Multidrug resistance gene and p-glycoprotein expression in anaplastic carcinoma of the thyroid. Cancer Detect Prevent 1994; 18:407–413.
16. Asakawa H, Kobayashi T, Komoike Y, et al. Chemosensitivity of anaplastic thyroid carcinoma and poorly differentiated thyroid carcinoma. Anticancer Res 1997; 17:2757–2762.
17. Schlumberger M, Parmentier C, Delisle MJ, et al. Combination therapy for anaplastic giant cell thyroid carcinoma. Cancer 1991; 67: 564–566.
18. Ringel MD, Greenberg M, Chen X, et al. Cytotoxic activity of 2′,2′-difluorodeoxycytidine (gemcitabine) in poorly differentiated thyroid carcinoma cells. Thyroid 2000; 10:865–869.
19. Celano M, Calvagno MG, Bulotta S, et al. Cytotoxic effects of gemcitabine-loaded liposomes in human anaplastic thyroid carcinoma cells. BMC Cancer 2004; 4:63.
20. Schoenberger J, Grimm D, Kossmehl P, et al. Effects of PTK787/ZK222584, a tyrosine kinase inhibitor, on the growth of a poorly differentiated thyroid carcinoma: an animal study. Endocrinology 2004; 145:1031–1038.
21. Podtcheko A, Ohtsuru A, Tsuda S, et al. The selective tyrosine kinase inhibitor, ST1571, inhibits growth of anaplastic thyroid cancer cells. J Clin Endocrinol Metab 2003; 88:1889–1896.

22. Dziba JM, Marcinek R, Venkataraman G, et al. Combretastatin A4 phosphate has primary antineoplastic activity against human anaplastic thyroid carcinoma cell lines and xenograft tumors. Thyroid 2002; 12:1063–1070.
23. Bauer AJ, Terrell R, Doniparthi NK, et al. Vascular endothelial growth factor monoclonal antibody inhibits growth of anaplastic thyroid cancer xenografts in nude mice. Thyroid 2002; 12: 953–961.
24. Imanishi R, Ohtsuru A, Iwamatsu M, et al. A histone deacetylase inhibitor enhances killing of undifferentiated thyroid carcinoma cells by p53 gene therapy. J Clin Endocrinol Metab 2002; 87: 4821–4824.
25. Greenberg VL, Williams JM, Cogswell JP, et al. Histone deacetylase inhibitors promote apoptosis and differential cell cycle arrest in anaplastic thyroid cancer cells. Thyroid 2001; 11:315–325.
26. McIver B, Hay ID, Giuffrida DF, et al. Anaplastic thyroid carcinoma: a 50-year experience at a single institution. Surgery 2001; 130: 1028–1034.
27. Pasieka JL. Anaplastic thyroid cancer. Curr Opin Oncol 2003; 15: 78–83.

83
Anaplastic Carcinoma
Prognosis

Steven I. Sherman

All studies that have examined the outcome of patients with anaplastic carcinoma have demonstrated the bleak prognosis associated with this disease. Product-limit estimates of median survival from diagnosis range from 3 to 7 mo, and the 1- and 5-yr survival probabilities are 20–35% and 5–10%, respectively (1–6). The cause of death is related to upper airway obstruction and suffocation in 50–60% (often despite the presence of a tracheostomy), along with a combination of complications of local and distant disease in the remaining patients (2,7). Examination of survival curves from these studies reveals two distinct components: a sharp initial decline for the first 18–24 mo, followed by a slower rate of death over the ensuing years (Fig. 1). Perhaps 5% of patients with anaplastic carcinoma may survive many years after initial diagnosis and treatment without evidence of recurrent disease (2,6).

Several important prognostic clinical parameters have been identified in retrospective studies. Among clinical features that can be evaluated at disease presentation, various univariate analyses have suggested that greater extent of disease and larger primary tumor size increases the risk of death from anaplastic carcinoma. In the most recent series from the University of Texas M.D. Anderson Cancer Center, patients with disease initially confined to the neck had a mean survival of 8 mo, compared with 3 mo if the disease extended beyond the neck ($p < 0.001$; 8). These results are consistent with other reports that patients with disease either confined to the thyroid or in locoregional metastases survived longer than those with distant metastases (1,10,11). Patients whose primary tumor was less than 6 cm in maximum diameter have had a 25% 2-yr survival, compared with 3–15% for those with tumors larger than 6 cm (1,2). Other prognostic variables that may also predict worse prognosis include older age at diagnosis, male gender, and dyspnea as a presenting symptom.

In another study, patients who survived longer than 2 yr after diagnosis of anaplastic carcinoma had an average age at diagnosis of only 54 yr, significantly younger than the 64 yr for the group who died before 24 mo ($p < 0.01$; 8), but no major age-related effect was noted in other studies (1,2,12,13). A threefold longer survival was noted for women compared with men in one report (2), but no effect regarding gender was found in others, including two recent large epidemiologic surveys (1,8,10–13). In an updated report from the Surveillance, Epidemiology, and End Results (SEER) database of 516 patients with anaplastic thyroid cancer (13a), the best outcomes were seen in younger women patients (less than 60 yr) who had surgical resection, external beam radiotherapy or combination surgical resection with radiotherapy. Only one study addressed the predictive value of presenting symptoms, with a relative mortality rate of 2 for dyspnea but no impact of dysphagia or hoarseness (13). Patients who previously had been treated for differentiated carcinoma and subsequently developed anaplastic disease had outcomes similar to those without a previously treated differentiated cancer (8,12).

Several approaches to prognostic classification have been applied to anaplastic carcinoma. All anaplastic carcinomas are classified as stage IV disease—the highest stage—in both the TNM (tumor, node, metastasis)-based staging approach, adopted by the Union Internationale Centre Cancer and the American Joint Commission on Cancer, and the staging scheme, as used by the National Thyroid Cancer Treatment Cooperative Study Registry (6,14). The prognostic scoring system, introduced by the European Organization for Research on Treatment of Cancer, gives 45 points for a diagnosis of anaplastic carcinoma (15). Additional points are given for advanced age and extrathyroidal invasion; virtually all these patients are staged as either 4 or 5 (6). In an earlier M.D. Anderson series, patients with anaplastic disease were divided into four groupings (16):

Stage I: Disease confined to the thyroid.
Stage II: Disease in locoregional nodes.
Stage III: Disease extending to soft tissues in the neck.
Stage IV: Distant metastases.

Using this classification, advancing stage was significantly associated with shorter survival (8). In the absence of

From: *Thyroid Cancer: A Comprehensive Guide to Clinical Management, 2/e*
Edited by: L. Wartofsky and D. Van Nostrand © Humana Press Inc., Totowa, NJ

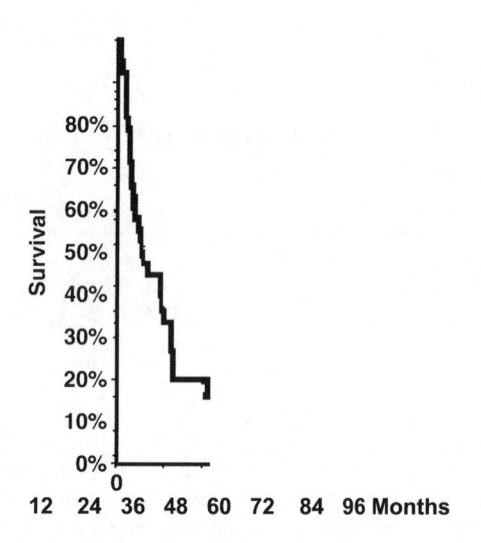

Fig. 1. Product-limit survival for 46 patients with anaplastic thyroid carcinoma. (Adapted from ref. 6.)

a comparison of the predictive value of these differing staging approaches, it is impossible to recommend one approach over another (6). The impact of treatment on survival is unclear. With the exception of patients whose tumors are small and confined entirely within the thyroid, attempts at total thyroidectomy and complete tumor resection are not associated with prolonged survival (1,8,13). External-beam radiotherapy, administered in conventional doses, also does not appear to affect survival. Although a complete response may be obtained in up to 40% of patients irradiated, most relapse locally with or without distant disease (13). Treatment with single-agent chemotherapy does not appear to improve survival or local control of neck disease, but about 20% may have some degree of response in distant metastases (17).

The introduction of hyperfractionated radiotherapy, combined with radiosensitizing doses of doxorubicin, may increase the local response rate to approx 80%, with a subsequent median survival of 1 yr, but distant metastases remain the leading cause of death (18). Similar improvement in local disease control has been reported with the combination of hyperfractionated radiotherapy and radiosensitizing doxorubicin, followed by debulking surgery in responsive patients (3). Hyperfractionated radiotherapy with doxorubicin and cisplatin, administered both before and after the radiation, has recently been associated with a 3-yr survival of nearly 30%. However, the best outcomes were limited to patients who had apparently complete surgical resection (19). Yet, the addition of larger doses of mitoxantrone or bleomycin/cyclophosphamide/5-fluorouracil is not linked with improved control of distant disease or improved survival (7).

A recent phase II study of paclitaxel demonstrated stabilization of disease in about half of patients treated with 96-h continuous infusions, but 1-yr survival was not affected by therapy (20). In a phase I study of the angiogenesis inhibitor combretastatin A-4 phosphate, prolonged complete remission was described in one patient with anaplastic thyroid carcinoma. This response led to two phase II studies that are currently ongoing with this novel drug (21). Using anaplastic carcinoma cell lines in culture and in xenograft models, other agents with reported activity have included liposomal gemcitabine (22), imatinib mesylate (23), histone deacetylase inhibitors (24), geldanamycin (25), farnesyl transferase inhibitors (26), and gefitinib (27), but evidence of clinical efficacy is lacking.

In summary, improved survival has only been demonstrated for patients with disease localized to the thyroid who receive aggressive local intervention. Better therapies for distant metastases are needed that can be combined with multimodality treatment of local neck disease.

REFERENCES

1. McIver B, Hay ID, Giuffrida DF, Dvorak CE. Anaplastic thyroid carcinoma: a 50-year experience at a single institution. Surgery 2001; 130:1028–1034.
2. Tan RK, Finley RK, Driscoll D, et al. Anaplastic carcinoma of the thyroid: a 24-year experience. Head Neck 1995; 17:41–47.
3. Tennvall J, Lundell G, Wahlberg P, et al. Anaplastic thyroid carcinoma: three protocols combining doxorubicin, hyperfractionated radiotherapy and surgery. Br J Cancer 2002; 86:1848–1853.
4. Hadar T, Mor C, Shvero J, et al. Anaplastic carcinoma of the thyroid. Eur J Surg Oncol 1993; 19:511–516.
5. Spires JR, Schwartz MR, Miller RH. Anaplastic thyroid carcinoma: association with differentiated thyroid cancer. Arch Otolaryngol Head Neck Surg 1988; 114:40–44.
6. Sherman SI, Brierley J, Sperling M, Maxon III HR. Initial analysis of staging and outcomes from a prospective multicenter study of treatment of thyroid carcinoma. Thyroid 1996; 6:S39.
7. Tallroth E, Wallin G, Lundell G, et al. Multimodality treatment in anaplastic giant cell thyroid carcinoma. Cancer 1987; 60:1428–1431.
8. Venkatesh YSS, Ordonez NG, Schultz PN, et al. Anaplastic carcinoma of the thyroid: a clinicopathologic study of 121 cases. Cancer 1990; 66:321–330.
9. Nishiyama RH, Dunn EL, Thompson NW. Anaplastic spindle-cell and giant-cell tumors of the thyroid gland. Cancer 1972; 30:113–127.
10. Gilliland FD, Hunt WC, Morris DM, Key CR. Prognostic factors for thyroid carcinoma: A population-based study of 15, 698 cases from the Surveillance, Epidemiology and End Results (SEER) program 1973–1991. Cancer 1997; 79:564–573.
11. Akslen LA, Haldorsen T, Thoresen S, Glattre E. Survival and causes of death in thyroid cancer: a population-based study of 2479 cases from Norway. Cancer Res 1991; 51:1234–1241.
12. Carcangiu ML, Steeper T, Zampi G, Rosai J. Anaplastic thyroid carcinoma: A study of 70 cases. Am J Clin Pathol 1985; 83:135–158.
13. Junor EJ, Paul J, Reed NS. Anaplastic thyroid carcinoma: 91 patients treated by surgery and radiotherapy. Eur J Surg Oncol 1992; 18:83–88.
13a. Kebebew E, Greenspan FS, Clark OH, Woeber KA, McMillan A. Anaplastic thyroid carcinoma: Treatment outcome and prognostic factors. Cancer 2005; 103:1330–1335.
14. Greene FL, Page DL, Fleming ID, et al., editors. Manual for Staging of Cancer, American Joint Commission on Cancer, 6th ed. New York: Springer-Verlag, 2002.

15. Byar DP, Green SB, Dor P, et al. A prognostic index for thyroid carcinoma. A study of the E. O. R. T. C. thyroid cancer cooperative group. Eur J Cancer 1979; 15:1033–1041.
16. Aldinger KA, Samaan NA, Ibanez ML, Hill CSJ. Anaplastic carcinoma of the thyroid: a review of 84 cases of spindle and giant cell carcinoma of the thyroid. Cancer 1978; 41:2267–2275.
17. Ahuja S, Ernst H. Chemotherapy of thyroid carcinoma. J Endocrinol Invest 1987; 10:303–310.
18. Kim JH, Leeper RD. Treatment of locally advanced thyroid carcinoma with combination doxorubicin and radiation therapy. Cancer 1987; 60: 2372–2375.
19. De Crevoisier R, Baudin E, Bachelot A, et al. Combined treatment of anaplastic thyroid carcinoma with surgery, chemotherapy, and hyperfractionated accelerated external radiotherapy. Int J Radiat Oncol Biol Phys 2004; 60:1137–1143.
20. Ain KB, Egorin MJ, DeSimone PA. Treatment of anaplastic thyroid carcinoma with paclitaxel: phase 2 trial using ninety-six-hour infusion. Collaborative Anaplastic Thyroid Cancer Health Intervention Trials (CATCHIT) Group. Thyroid 2000; 10:587–594.
21. Dowlati A, Robertson K, Cooney M, et al. A phase I pharmacokinetic and translational study of the novel vascular targeting agent combretastatin a-4 phosphate on a single-dose intravenous schedule in patients with advanced cancer. Cancer Res 2002; 62:3408–3416.
22. Celano M, Calvagno MG, Bulotta S, et al. Cytotoxic effects of gemcitabine-loaded liposomes in human anaplastic thyroid carcinoma cells. BMC Cancer 2004; 4:63.
23. Podtcheko A, Ohtsuru A, Tsuda S, et al. The selective tyrosine kinase inhibitor, STI571, inhibits growth of anaplastic thyroid cancer cells. J Clin Endocrinol Metab 2003; 88:1889–1896.
24. Furuya F, Shimura H, Suzuki H, et al. Histone deacetylase inhibitors restore radioiodide uptake and retention in poorly differentiated and anaplastic thyroid cancer cells by expression of the sodium/iodide symporter thyroperoxidase and thyroglobulin. Endocrinology 2004; 145: 2865–2875.
25. Park JW, Yeh MW, Wong MG, et al. The heat shock protein 90-binding geldanamycin inhibits cancer cell proliferation, down-regulates oncoproteins, and inhibits epidermal growth factor-induced invasion in thyroid cancer cell lines. J Clin Endocrinol Metab 2003; 88:3346–3353.
26. Yang HL, Pan JX, Sun L, Yeung SC. p21 Waf-1 (Cip-1) enhances apoptosis induced by manumycin and paclitaxel in anaplastic thyroid cancer cells. J Clin Endocrinol Metab 2003; 88:763–772.
27. Schiff BA, McMurphy A, Jasser SA, et al. Epidermal growth factor receptor (EGF-R) is over expressed in anaplastic thyroid cancer, and the EGF-R inhibitor Iressa (ZD 1839) inhibits the growth of anaplastic thyroid cancer. Clin Cancer Res 2004; 10:8594–8602.

Part X
New Frontiers and Future Directions

84
Advances in Radiation Therapy

James D. Brierley and Richard W. Tsang

INTRODUCTION

Before discussing recent advances in radiation therapy, it is important to consider the basic principles. The design for a proper course of radiation therapy must consider the extent of extrathyroidal disease and the location of lymph node disease, as well as the radiation tolerance of normal tissues and organs. The accepted terminology to describe the radiation dose and target volume in the planning of radiotherapy is summarized in Table 1. The principle is to deliver the prescribed dose to the entire clinical target volume (CTV) with a reasonable dose uniformity (±5%). Custom-designed fields should be used to conform to the target volume while keeping the volume of irradiated normal tissues to a minimum. In general, the aim should be to deliver 5000–6000 rad (50–60 Gy) to the CTV and 6000–7000 rad (60–70 Gy) to the gross tumor volume (GTV) in 1800–2000 rad (1.8–2.0 Gy) fractions over 5–7 wk *(1–6)*. External radiation therapy is delivered with linear accelerators generating X-ray beams in the megavoltage range of 4–25 MV (photons).

RADIATION TREATMENT PLANNING

Major advances have occurred in planning radiation treatment; effective treatment requires an understanding of the planning process. This process must have simulation in the desired treatment position with an appropriate immobilization mask to ensure day-to-day reproducibility. Simulation is performed with a computer tomography (CT) simulator, which simulates the actual geometric characteristics of the linear accelerator while imaging the area of interest. At simulation, reference marks are placed on the patient's mask to reproduce and align the beam profiles accurately. CT simulation allows planning treatment in three dimensions (3D) that are performed on the computer (i.e., "virtual simulation"). The process involves designating various target volumes (Table 1), critical structures and normal organs of interest, beam profiles and other modifying devices, such as wedges and shielding, and then displaying these outlines in different 3D perspectives (axial, coronal, and sagittal)

(see Fig. 1). Dose distributions of the treatment plan can be displayed in isodose lines and dose-volume histograms for both the target volume and normal organ(s) of interest. The most common method of planning external radiation therapy is based on the CT simulator. Important future advances are already in progress, directly integrating other imaging modalities such as magnetic resonance imaging and positron emission tomography using functional imaging agents (e.g., F-18 fluorodeoxyglucose).

TREATMENT VOLUMES

The CTV of the typical thyroid bed is an inverse "U"-shaped volume on an axial image, and the spinal cord is the critical dose-limiting normal organ *(1,3)*. Lymph nodes directly adjacent to the thyroid bed (including zone 6, central compartment; zone 3, mid-jugular; and zone 4, supraclavicular) are generally included into the CTV. At the Princess Margaret Hospital, the current technique involves CT planning with a conformal set of multiple photon beams *(9,10;* see Fig. 2). The maximum dose to the spinal cord typically varies between 50% and 70% of the prescribed dose; the objective is to keep the spinal cord total dose to less than 45–46 Gy *(1,3,7)*. When there is no significant posterior extension of disease, an alternative technique is to treat with lateral beams angled caudally to avoid the shoulders. Additional established methods and techniques are well-described by other investigators *(1,3,7)*. When it is necessary to treat the high cervical lymph nodes (e.g., zone 2 or upper jugular) and/or the superior mediastinal lymph nodes, it is customary to have a multiphase plan, such as treating a large CTV to a certain dose (e.g., 45–46 Gy; see Fig. 3), then a second "cone-down" phase (boost) to a smaller volume, designated as a gross tumor volume or a separate high-risk CTV *(1,3)*.

ADVANCES IN RADIATION THERAPY PLANNING AND DELIVERY

Another specialized treatment technique termed "intensity modulated radiation therapy" (IMRT) attempts to

Table 1
Definition of Radiation Therapy Terms

Term	Definition*	Comment
Absorbed dose	The energy deposited by ionizing radiation per unit mass of material (J/kg), expressed in the SI unit, the gray (Gy)	1 Gy = 100 cGy 1 Gy = 100 rad
Gross tumor volume (GTV)	The gross demonstrable extent and location of the malignant growth	Includes the extrathyroidal disease and any involved regional nodes Determined by clinical examination and imaging tests
Clinical target volume (CTV)	A tissue volume that contains a demonstrable GTV and/or subclinical malignant disease that must be eliminated. This volume must be treated adequately to achieve the aim of radical therapy	Includes the thyroid bed and any extrathyroidal tissues and lymph nodes with suspected involvement or at high risk of subclinical involvement
Planning target volume (PTV)	PTV is a geometric concept used for treatment planning, and it is defined to select appropriate beam sizes and arrangements to ensure that the prescribed dose is actually delivered to the CTV	Includes internal margin (e.g., to account for organ motion) and set-up margin (e.g., uncertainties in patient positioning and beam alignment)

*As defined in Report 62 of the International Commission on Radiation Units and Measurements.

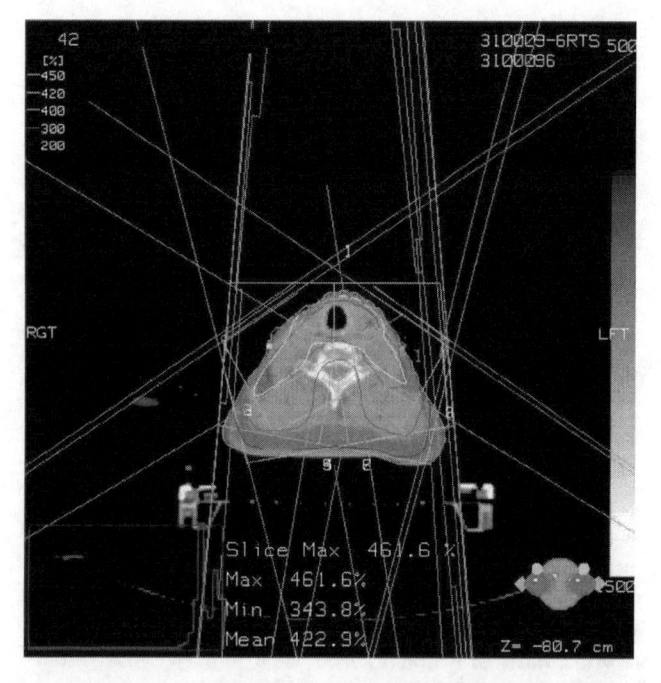

Fig. 1. These axial CT-planning images of a five-field conformal technique were used at Princess Margaret Hospital to treat the thyroid bed and adjacent regional lymph nodes. Note the inverse U-shaped high-dose volume. (Color illustration appears in insert following p. 198.)

achieve better conformation of the high-dose region to the target by additionally varying the fluence intensity within each beam (1,7). By setting the target dose(s) to the various tumor target volume(s), and the dose limits to the designated normal organs at risk, the computer perform iterations to establish the optimal beam arrangement and individual beam intensity profile. IMRT is capable of further reducing the spinal cord dose, compared with 3D conformal radiotherapy (1,7). IMRT is becoming increasing available (1,7) and is the standard of care in many radiation oncology centers including the Princess Margaret Hospital.

TOXICITY OF EXTERNAL RADIATION THERAPY

Well-planned external radiation therapy has moderate yet acceptable acute toxicity and rarely produces serious complications (3,6). It does not preclude future surgical intervention if required. During the course of radiation, moderate skin erythema will develop, and dry desquamation or occasionally patchy moist desquamation of the skin occurs. Mucositis of the esophagus, trachea and larynx, leading to dysphagia of solid foods, dryness, pain and irritation, and dysphonia, usually occur toward the end of the course and requires symptomatic management with soft diet and analgesics. Depending on the superior extent of the fields, change of taste and xerostomia may occur. Late toxicity is dose-dependent and generally infrequent, and the most common is mild lymphedema that is usually seen just below the chin, skin telangiectasias, skin pigmentation, and soft-tissue fibrosis, particularly in patients treated after cervical lymph node dissections. Esophageal and tracheal stenosis is extremely rare with conventional fractionation. Tsang et al. (6) found no Radiation Therapy Oncology Group grade IV toxicity in patients given 4000–5000 rads (40–50 Gy) in 200–250-rad (2–2.5 Gy) fractions to the neck and superior mediastinum. Farahati et al. (8) observed no irreversible late toxicity in 99 patients given 5000–6000 rads (50–60 Gy) in 180–200-rads (1.8–2.0 Gy) fractions to a large volume. Asymptomatic pulmonary fibrosis at the

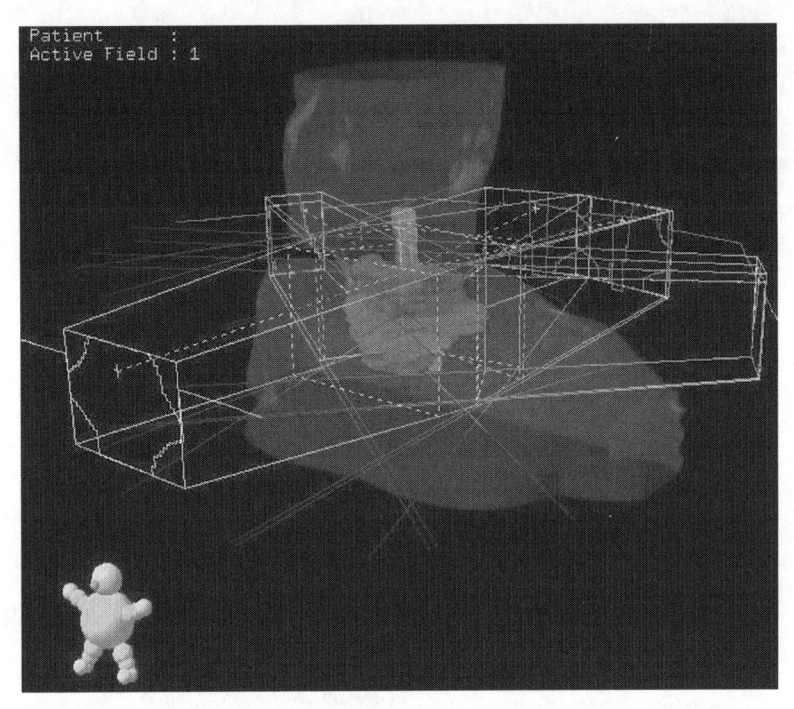

Fig. 2. This 3D view of the conformal five-field beam arrangement was designed to achieve dose uniformity for the thyroid bed CTV and spare the spinal cord. The plan consists of an anterior beam and four posterior oblique beams with segmentation, all shaped with multileaf collimators to conform to the shape of the CTV. (Color illustration appears in insert following p. 198.)

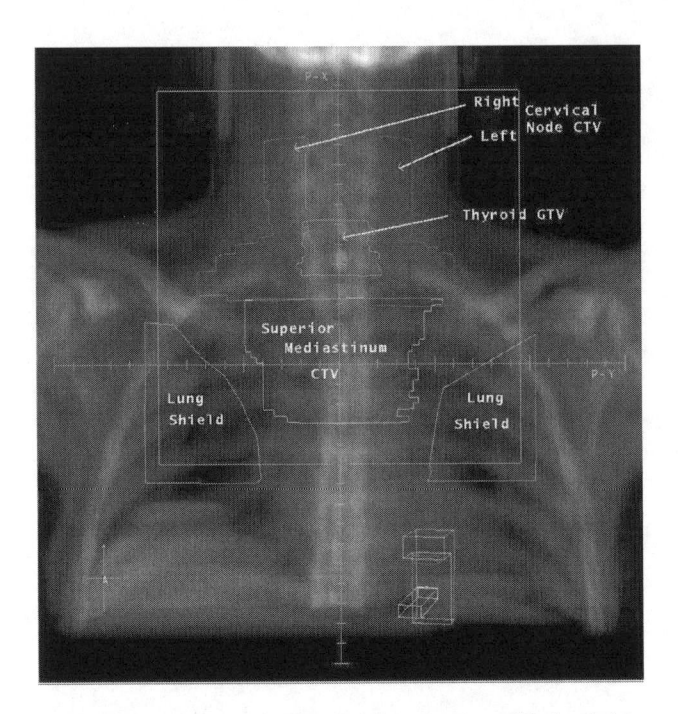

Fig. 3. Digitally reconstructed radiograph from CT simulation of an anterior beam targeting the thyroid bed and cervical and superior mediastinal lymph nodes. This volume can be safely treated to 4500–4600 rad (45–46 Gy), and any gross disease or high-risk area can be boosted with a conformal technique (avoiding the spinal cord) to a higher dose. (Color illustration appears in insert following p. 198.)

lung apices is expected, seen commonly on CT scan in subsequent follow-up and should not be mistaken for lung metastasis.

REFERENCES

1. Nutting CM, Convery DJ, Cosgrove VP, et al. Improvements in target coverage and reduced spinal cord irradiation using intensity-modulated radiotherapy (IMRT) in patients with carcinoma of the thyroid gland. Radiother Oncol 2001; 60:173–180.
2. O'Connell M, A'Hern RP, Harmer CL. Results of external beam radiotherapy in differentiated thyroid carcinoma: a retrospective study from the Royal Marsden Hospital. Eur J Cancer 1994; 30A:733–739.
3. Harmer C, Bidmead M, Shepherd S, et al. Radiotherapy planning techniques for thyroid cancer. Br J Radiol 1998; 71:1069–1075.
4. Brierley JD, Tsang RW. External-beam radiation therapy in the treatment of differentiated thyroid cancer. Semin Surg Oncol 1999; 16: 42–49.
5. Brierley JD, Tsang RW. External radiation therapy in the treatment of thyroid cancer. In Burman KD editor. Thyroid Cancer II, Endocrinology Metabolism Clinical North America. Philadelphia, PA: W. B. Saunders Co. 1996:141–157.
6. Tsang RW, Brierley JD, Simpson WJ, et al. The effects of surgery, radioiodine and external radiation therapy on the clinical outcome of patients with differentiated thyroid cancer. Cancer 1998; 82:375–388.
7. Posner MD, Quivey JM, Akazawa PF, et al. Dose optimization for the treatment of anaplastic thyroid carcinoma: a comparison of treatment planning techniques. Int J Radiat Oncol Biol Phys 2000; 48: 475–483.
8. Farahati J, Reiners C, Stuschke M, et al. Differentiated thyroid cancer. Impact of adjuvant external radiotherapy in patients with perithyroidal tumor infiltration (stage pT4). Cancer 1996; 77:172–180.

85
New Approaches in Nuclear Medicine for Thyroid Cancer

Douglas Van Nostrand

INTRODUCTION

In 1899, Charles Duell, Director of the United States Patent office, stated: "Everything that can be invented has been invented." In terms of a complete listing of specific potential advances in nuclear medicine, I am certain to miss the target as much as Mr. Duell did, but I will not miss the target regarding the general potential for advancements in nuclear medicine for the diagnosis and treatment of thyroid cancer. In Chapter 12, Henry Wagner quoted the president and CEO of General Electric Medical, Joseph M. Hogan, who stated, "In the years to come, we envision a health care system that uses molecular medicine to diagnose and treat patients before symptoms appear and treatments that are tailored to an individual based on his or her genetic makeup." Indeed, molecular approaches to medicine are being applied now and will be an important part of the future, and nuclear medicine using radiotracers will play a major role in molecular medicine.

This chapter briefly reviews only a few of the many exciting areas of research and development underway in nuclear medicine relating to equipment, imaging, and therapy. The role of nuclear medicine in the diagnosis, evaluation, and treatment of patients who have thyroid cancer has never been more exciting.

EQUIPMENT

The major advancements in equipment in the near future will be in positron emission tomography (PET) scanners and single-photon emission computer tomography (SPECT) cameras.

The equipment employed for PET will continue to improve rapidly, and some advancements will likely include integration of different imaging modalities, expanding capabilities, increasing software speed, development of specialized scanners, design of better detectors, implementation of respiratory gating, and development of time-of-flight scanners. The benefits of both PET and CT scanners into a single unit have already been proven; this is not just a convenience to the patient but is also a major advancement that improves the sensitivity and specificity of the PET and CT findings. Although combining a PET and magnetic resonance imaging (MRI) is more difficult, such a scanner has already been achieved for small-scale animal research with a single slice system [1]. The utility of PET will increase to include the ability to perform a biopsy or fine-needle aspiration of a nodule or a suspected metastasis that is localized only by a PET scanner. This will be very important to help in the management of "PET-positive CT-negative" or "PET-positive MRI-negative" abnormalities. PET-CT capabilities will also continue to expand in the planning of external radiation therapy for cancers (including thyroid cancer). PET-CT scanners will improve the delineation of tumor treatment target volumes by combining anatomic localization and volumes with heretofore unavailable *functional* volumes. PET software will have better and faster processing algorithms. As a result, acquisition times and processing times will be reduced.

Scanners will also be developed with specialized functions. Micro-PET scanners with exquisite resolution are already available for imaging small animals (e.g., rodents) for research. Naviscan has already developed a PET scanner, which is approximately the size of a mammography unit and images the breast and other areas of the body, such as joints in humans. The Food and Drug Administration has already approved this unit, and other specialized PET scanners will be developed. Conceivably, a specialized PET scanner could be designed to maximize the imaging of a nodule within the thyroid with a positron-emitting radionuclide labeled to a peptide, an antibody, or a reporter probe unique to thyroid cancer cells, resulting in "hot-spot" imaging.

Detectors will also improve. Although it is beyond the scope of this chapter, new designs of detectors are already underway. For the past 15 yr, the block-type detector for the organization of the crystals has dominated [2]. With new variants of the block design such as quadrant sharing and high-resolution research tomography [3], improved positional information may be obtained without loss in energy resolution. This can also enable the simultaneous acquisition of emission and transmission data, which then may decrease the whole-body acquisition times to 5 or 10 min, with minimal

From: *Thyroid Cancer: A Comprehensive Guide to Clinical Management, 2/e*
Edited by: L. Wartofsky and D. Van Nostrand © Humana Press Inc., Totowa, NJ

or no compromise in image quality *(4)*. This will not only lower imaging time for the patient but can also help to reduce the cost of a PET exam.

Respiratory motion has been a major problem for PET-CT imaging of the chest, creating artifacts on the fusion of PET and CT images of the lung. This may be important in the evaluation of thyroid cancer metastases in these areas. New respiratory gating techniques may reduce respiratory artifacts.

Finally, perhaps "time-of-flight" PET scanners may become a reality. These imaging systems, which Ter-Pogossian et al. *(5)* first considered in 1980, would harness the difference in the arrival times of the two 180° annihilation photons from the positron emitter. This difference in time would allow the localization of the annihilation site along the path of the two photons.

Equipment development will not be limited just to PET scanners but will also involve SPECT cameras. SPECT-CT scanners have already been introduced and will develop in many of the same areas as PET-CT. This will then allow the further expansion of single-photon emission radiotracers.

IMAGING

Regarding nuclear medicine imaging for patients who have thyroid cancer, the potential is unlimited. The future includes the development of numerous molecular imaging probes and additional positron emitters.

Molecular Imaging

With the dawn of molecular imaging, an ever-increasing array of molecular probes will be developed to image such processes as tumor metabolism, cellular proliferation, specific cell surface receptors, inflammation, angiogenesis, tumor hypoxia, and apoptosis. Receptor-targeted radiopeptide imaging, bispecific antibodies, and PET reporter-gene reporter-probe imaging represent three promising areas.

Receptor-Targeted Radiopeptide Imaging

Receptor-targeted radiopeptides have already been used and hold great promise not only for imaging but also for therapy *(6)*. Peptides are molecules that are derived from amino acids and have typically 2–50 amino acids linked together. Peptides have many important functions, such as modulating and regulating cellular function and intracellular communication. Table 1 lists many receptors expressed on human tumors. Some advantages of radiolabeled peptides include: (1) rapid diffusion and localization, (2) quick clearance from the body, (3) rapid internalization, (4) potentially long residence time, (5) possibly easy chemical synthesis, (6) lack of immunogenicity, and (7) metabolic stability.

To date, the best example of the future use of receptor-targeted radiopeptides for imaging and treatment of cancers, specifically thyroid cancer, involves the somatostatin receptors. The prototype of the somatostatin receptor-targeted

Table 1
Expression of Various Peptide Receptors in Various Tumors

Peptides	Tumors
Somatostatin	Neuroendocrine tumors, thyroid cancer
VIP/PACAP	Adenocarcinomas
CCK/gastrin	Medullary thyroid cancer
LHRH	Breast and prostate cancer
α-MSH	Melanoma
Bombesin/GRP	Medullary thyroid cancer
Neurotensin	Ewing sarcoma, medullary thyroid cancer
Opioid	Breast cancer
Substance P	Medullary thyroid cancer
GLIP-1	Insulinoma
Oxytocin	Endometrium, breast cancer
Neuropeptide Y	Breast cancer

radiopeptide is ^{111}In-DTPA octreotide (^{111}In-pentetreotide), Octreoscan®, which has been used in medullary thyroid carcinoma and even well-differentiated thyroid carcinoma (see Chapters 35 and 70). Radiolabeled octreotide has also been used by harnessing the therapeutic benefits of the auger electrons from ^{111}In and the β-emission from ^{90}Yttrium. The therapeutic benefits of auger electrons are discussed further below. Another radiolabeled somatostatin analog, ^{177}Lu-1,4,7,10-tetra-azacyclododecane-N,N',N'',N'''-tetra-acetic acid^0 (DOTA), Tyr^3-octreotate (^{177}Lu-DOTATATE), has been used to treat five patients with nonradioiodine-avid well-differentiated thyroid cancer with some success *(7)*. We are only beginning to address the potential application of receptor-targeted radiopeptides for imaging and treatment.

Bispecific Antibodies

The use of antibodies for diagnosis and therapy had been significantly improved because of monoclonal antibody technology. However, the percent of injected dose of the monoclonal antibody that targets a gram of tumor is low and ranges from 0.001% to 0.01% of injected activity per gram of tumor *(8)*. Multiple strategies have been evaluated to improve target organ activity and to decrease background activity. One such strategy is bispecific antibodies, which has been reported by Reardon et al. *(9)* and modified by Khaw et al. *(10)*. The goal with bispecific antibodies is that two antibodies are linked with one of the antibodies specific for the target and the other for radiolabeled chelates. This can significantly increase the sensitivity for detection and localization of specific antigens.

Reporter Gene Imaging

Reporter gene imaging is one of the most exciting areas for future research and development for thyroid cancer *(11)*. In brief, the concept is the placement of a gene (the reporter gene) into the nucleus of a cell, and the DNA of that gene is transcribed into its corresponding mRNA, which then makes its specific protein (the reporter protein). A radiolabeled chemical (the reporter probe), specifically designed to metabolize or bind to the reporter protein, is administered and metabolized or bound to the reporter protein. Then a PET scanner or SPECT camera images the radiolabeled emissions.

Specifically, genetic material may be placed into cells directly (in vivo) or indirectly (in vitro) by gene therapy vectors, which are the delivery systems. The gene therapy vectors may be generally classified as nonviral or viral vectors. Nonviral vectors may include a broad spectrum of methods, including DNA–protein complexes, liposomes, and naked DNA. Viral vectors use the gene-delivery mechanisms of various viruses and are efficient delivery systems. Once delivered, the DNA reporter gene is then transcribed with the production of the corresponding mRNA, which makes one of three broad categories of reporter proteins: enzymes, receptors, or transporters. A radiolabeled reporter probe is then administered and depending on the type of reporter protein, is (1) enzymatically metabolized within the cell; (2) attached to a receptor (e.g., on the cell wall); or (3) transported across the cell wall into the cytoplasm of the cell.

The prototype for the "enzyme" reporter gene is the herpes simplex type 1 virus thymidine kinase (HSV1-tk) and has been used as a therapeutic gene. After gene expression within the cell and after the administration of an acycloguanosine (e.g., ganciclovir), the ganciclovir enters the cell. It is monophosphorylated by the HSV1-tk enzyme to ganciclovir triphosphate, which kills the cell. Derivatives of acycloguanosine can also be radiolabeled with positron emitters that allow PET imaging of the reporter protein of the HSV1-tk.

The prototype for the "receptor" reporter gene is SSTr2, an analog of somatostatin (i.e., octreotide). As already noted above, imaging with somatostatin analogs has potential application for various types of thyroid cancers, and the SSTr2 as part of a PET reporter-gene reporter-probe system has already been labeled with the positron emitters of ^{64}Cu and ^{68}Ga *(12,13)*, as well as ^{99m}Tc for SPECT imaging *(14)*.

The prototype for a gene to transport a protein is the sodium iodide symporter (NIS). This is one of the most interesting genes for thyroid cancer, with possible application to thyroid cancer cells that do not organify iodine. For example, NIS incorporation into medullary carcinoma could allow a method for visualization and treatment of this tumor. Indeed, Chen et al. *(15)* have reported preliminary data indicating that the transduction of the NIS gene is sufficient to induce iodide transport in medullary thyroid carcinoma cells both in vitro and in vivo. A more in-depth discussion of the role of NIS in nuclear medicine is available *(16)*.

The potential clinical utility of PET reporter genes and PET reporter probes will be in imaging and therapy. Relevant areas include: (1) avoidance of invasive procedures for gene therapy monitoring, (2) pretherapy diagnosis, (3) treatment evaluation of other gene therapy at the biochemical level, (4) patient follow-up, and (5) prognostic indicators *(11)*.

Although promising and exciting, molecular imaging, such as for tumor metabolism, cellular proliferation, specific cell surface receptors, inflammation, angiogenesis, tumor hypoxia, apoptosis, receptor-targeted radiopeptides, bispecific antibodies, and gene expression is complicated, and there are many hurdles still to overcome. The combination of radioisotopes with chemicals is complex; the molecular targeting is difficult; increasing specificity and reducing nonspecific binding is problematic; and a radioconjugate can even irradiate itself and decompose. The important difference is that unlike the initial years of the development of radiotracers, when nuclear medicine was the only imaging modality that imaged physiologic processes, these newer imaging modalities can image molecular processes. These include targeted MRI imaging, targeted echocardiographic nanotechnology, optical coherence imaging, and optical imaging. While each new approach has its limitations, the future for radiotracers in nuclear medicine is extremely exciting and only in its infancy.

PET Radiotracers

^{18}F is the most widely used positron emitter and has the most extensive database on targetry, target chemistry, and radiochemistry available *(17)*. ^{18}F will continue to be evaluated and used with many new carriers, of which several have already been discussed. However, PET radiotracers are not limited to ^{18}F. Pagani et al. *(18)* have reviewed alternative positron emitters and the effects of their physical properties on image quality and potential clinical applications.

Glaser et al. *(19)* have recently reviewed the potential role of the positron-emitting halogens of ^{75}Br, ^{76}Br, and ^{124}I. Bromines have two advantages over other halogenation reactions. First, the chemistry of bromine is easier for synthesis than fluorine. Second, bromine radiotracers are anticipated to be much more stable in vivo owing to the higher binding energy of bromine-carbon. However, there are always trade-offs. The targetry and target chemistry of bromine is more difficult, requiring relatively higher beam energy for production, which is available in only a few centers. For imaging thyroid cancer, ^{124}I holds the most exciting promise. Although the first scan with ^{124}I in an animal was performed in 1959 *(20)*, and the first treatment in a thyroid cancer patient was performed with ^{124}I in 1960 *(21)*, the use and availability of ^{124}I has been limited. Yet, at the time of this book's publication, ^{124}I is now routinely produced commercially by one company: Eastern Isotopes, Inc. This should significantly increase the availability of ^{124}I, the breadth and extent of ^{124}I research, and the clinical utility of ^{124}I. Relative to ^{123}I and ^{131}I, the imaging of the positron emitter ^{124}I with a PET scanner will have several advantages. These include superior sensitivity, the ability to estimate "functional volume" of thyroid tissue *(19)*, and the ability to perform

Table 2
Additional Examples of Future Nuclear Medicine Research and Development for Thyroid Cancer

Further evaluation of the utility of ^{123}I for surveillance scans for metastatic well-differentiated thyroid cancer.
Further clarification of the role of alternative imaging modalities, such as F-18 flurodeoxyglucose and other radioisotopes.
Further evaluation and implementation of mechanisms to improve radioiodine uptake and retention time in metastasis.
Better identification of patients for radioiodine treatment.
Evaluation of the best radioisotope for the treatment of thyroid cancer.
Evaluation of the clinical effectiveness of "blind treatments" (thyroglobulin-positive radioiodine-negative) and if so, better identification of those patients who will benefit.
Evaluation of the efficacy of fractionated prescribed activity.
Evaluation of methods to reduce side effects secondary to radioiodine treatments.
Development of better methods to assess bone marrow reserve after previous radioiodine treatments.
Evaluation of the relationship of total bone marrow accumulative radiation-absorbed dose relative to time.
Further comparisons of outcome and side effects of radioiodine treatments with prescribed activities determined by various approaches (e.g., empiric fixed, Benua-Leeper, MIRD, Thomas-Maxon, and combinations of each)

lesional and whole-body dosimetry (22). ^{124}I will also have the advantages of excellent tomographic images and the ability to fuse with CT and MRI.

In addition to the use of ^{124}I as a radioiodine element for imaging itself, ^{124}I has also been labeled to other carriers, including antibodies, reporter genes, peptides, and amino acids. Examples include 5-{^{124}I}iodo-2′-deoxyurindine (^{124}I-IUdR) which is a thymidine analog, and 1-{2-fluoro-2-deoxy-B-D-arabinofuranoysl}-5-[^{124}I] iodouracil (^{124}I-FIAU), used for reporter gene imaging with HSV1-tk expression as discussed above. Additional examples include ^{124}I-metaiodobenzylguanidine (^{124}I MIBG) for possibly imaging medullary thyroid carcinoma, and ^{124}I annexin-V for imaging apoptosis during oncolytic therapy. ^{124}I will likely be labeled to other carriers as yet unreported, and it holds great promise for the imaging of thyroid cancer.

In addition to the development of areas noted above, many other areas involving nuclear medicine imaging of thyroid cancer, albeit perhaps less glamorous, will be evaluated with future resolution of many questions and problems. Some of these are listed in Table 2.

THERAPY

The most exciting aspect of nuclear medicine is radiotherapy and specifically "FedEX'ing" radiation to the cell for more localized radiation therapy. A limitation of external-beam radiotherapy is that it is "external" and thus must also pass through and irradiate normal tissue. Significant advancements, such as intensity modulated radiation therapy, γ knife, and cyber-knife have reduced the radiation exposure to the normal tissue; however, the ideal is to deliver the radiation by a carrier directly to the cell. In other words, the ideal is to "FedEX" the package by a vehicle to a specific address, with minimal travel time and minimal errors in delivery. The "package" is the radiation. The "vehicles" are carriers, such as peptides, antibodies, and receptor probes, and the "addresses" are receptors, antigens, or reporter genes. Improvements in specifically delivering or "FedEX'ing" radiation to the cell will come at many different points in the transportation and delivery process. Some developments in the "vehicles" and "addresses" have already been discussed above, and what is in the "packages" is discussed below.

"The Radiation Package" to "FedEX" to the Cell

The radioisotopes predominantly used for therapy have been ^{131}I and ^{90}Y, but the options are far more extensive. Humm (23) classified many potential radioisotopes for therapy by the distance of the principal radiation emitted, and Ackery tabulated them (see Table 3; 24). Humm restricted the list to radioisotopes with half-lives that are most valuable for therapy, i.e., 6 h to 4 wk.

It is important to have an armamentarium of different therapeutic radioisotopes because one will want to package different radioisotopes, depending on the therapeutic objectives and the address to which the package is being sent. Sisson et al. (25) noted that as a tumor becomes smaller and smaller, the β and γ energy from ^{131}I deposited within the actual tumor decreases. For a sphere of 0.5 mm in diameter, less than 40% of the energy of ^{131}I is deposited within that sphere (25). Accordingly, one may wish to use a different radionuclide or even a combination of radioisotopes, based on the tumor size. For smaller tumors, one may wish the principal radiation emitted to travel and deposit most of its energy over a short distance. For large bulky tumors, one may wish to use a radioisotope that deposits its energy over a longer distance, which would also harness the crossfire effect. This effect is the deposit in one cancer cell of the energy of a β or γ ray originating from another cancer cell.

One type of radioisotope that deposits significant amounts of energy over short distances is the α-emitter (25a). Typically, α-emitters travel a short distance of 50–90 μm (1 μm is 1/1000 of 1 mm) and may deposit as much as 800 keV or approx 0.25 Gy in a distance of 10-μm. A nucleus may

Table 3
Potential Radioisotopes for Therapeutic Application

α	β (mean range of <200 μm)	β (mean range of >200 μm to <1 mm)	β (mean range of >1 mm)	Electron capture-internal conversion
^{211}At	^{33}P	^{47}Sc	^{32}P	^{67}Ga
^{212}Bi(^{212}Pb)	^{121}Sn	^{67}Cu	^{89}Sr	^{71}Ge
^{223}Ra	^{177}Lu	^{77}As	^{90}Y	^{77}Br
	^{191}Os	^{105}Rh	^{114m}In	^{103}Pd
^{225}Ac	^{199}Au	^{109}Pb	^{188}Ret	^{119}Sb
		^{111}Ag		^{123}I
		^{131}I		^{125}I
		^{143}Pr		^{131}Cs
		^{153}Sm		^{193m}Pt
		^{161}Te		^{197}Hg
		^{186}Re		

Ac, actinium; Ag, silver; At, astatine; Au, gold; Bi, bismuth; Br, bromine; Cs, cesium; Cu, copper; Ga, gallium; Ge, germanium; Hg, mercury; I, iodine; In, indium; Lu, lutetium; Os, osmium; P, phosphorus; Pd, palladium; Pr, praseodymium; Pt, platinum; Ra, radium; Re, rhenium; Rh, rhodium; Sb, antimony; Sm, samarium; Sn, tin; Sr, strontium; Te, tellurium.

measure in the order of 10 μm. For certain cells, this may require only approx 3–6 α "hits" per nucleus to reduce the fraction of surviving cells by an average of 37%. In addition, this is enough energy to give multiple double-strand breaks in DNA, which may result in irreparable radiation damage (23). To appreciate the potential benefit of α-emitters, it would require 400 β-particles to deposit the same energy in a nucleus as one β-particle. As Kassis et al. (26) have stated, it make take up to 20,000 β-particles to traverse a cell nucleus to sterilize that cell whereas it may take only 1–4 α-emitters to traverse a cell nucleus to kill that cell. One of the α-emitters that has excellent potential is ^{211}At, and has been used in a human (27).

At the other end of the spectrum of radionuclides are those that decay by electron capture, such as ^{123}I. Although ^{123}I is not typically associated with therapeutic potential, ^{123}I can have a significant therapeutic effect if it is packaged into a carrier and "FedEX'ed" to the nucleus of a cell to be treated. When a radioisotope such as ^{123}I decays by electron capture, a low-energy characteristic X-ray is emitted as the electrons are rearranged in their orbits to replace the electron that was just absorbed into the nucleus. For heavy elements, the energy of this X-ray could be sufficient to be used for medical imaging. However, for ^{123}I, the energies of the characteristic X-rays are too small (maximum of about 30 keV) for conventional devices, such as the γ camera. Yet, in many of the decays, and especially for those originating from beyond the L electron orbit, the expected characteristic X-ray never makes it out of the atom. Instead, its energy interacts with another electron from that same atom and "ejects" that electron out of the atom entirely. This ejected electron is called an "Auger Electron." In fact, there is a cascade of Auger electrons of progressively lower energy that are emitted following each decay. Although most Auger electrons have very low energy (typically about 15 eV to several keV, they also travel only a short range over which they deposit their energy; typically less than 1 nm or about the diameter of the DNA helix. Consequently, the cytotoxic effect of ^{123}I can be significantly enhanced if it can be concentrated in proximity to the DNA relative to other cellular locations. The killing effects of an Auger electrons from ^{123}I have been confirmed with the conjugation of ^{123}I with deoxyuridine (28), and significant damage can be potentially achieved if the "package" is delivered close to the cellular DNA.

Thus, with more radioisotopes available and with better selection of the isotope based on the objectives and the "address" of the thyroid cancer, a greater therapeutic potential with less untoward effects is possible. Of course, "FedEX'ing" radiation to the cell is complicated, and there are many major foreseen and unforeseen problems to be solved. The process of combining elements with chemicals is complex; molecular targeting is difficult; nonspecific binding is problematic, and the radiochemical or conjugate can even irradiate itself and decompose. But with a firm faith in the ingenuity of man, this author believes that these hurdles will be overcome. If not, then different and even better approaches will be identified and successfully implemented.

Redifferentiation

Well-differentiated thyroid cancer may dedifferentiate and lose its ability to take up radioiodine, and future efforts will be made to redifferentiate these cells to take up radioiodine. Initial success of redifferentiation has already been achieved and are reviewed in Chapter 86. In brief, Grunwald et al. *(29)* administered retinoic acid to 12 patients, of which 4 had improved radioiodine uptake, and 2 patients had radioiodine uptake reestablished to allow radioiodine therapy. Schmutzler has extensively reviewed the use of retinoids *(30)*. In addition to retinoic acid, many other approaches have been evaluated. Furuya et al. *(31)* demonstrated accumulation of ^{125}I in poorly differentiated papillary and anaplastic thyroid cancer cells after reexpression of thyroid-specific genes by mRNA-induced histone deacetylase inhibitors. Chen et al. *(32)* was able to create iodide uptake in medullary thyroid carcinoma cells after transfer of the NIS gene. Misaki et al. *(33)* showed that tumoricidal cytokines may enhance radioiodine uptake, but this occurred in cultured thyroid cancer cells.

Enhancers

In addition to the mechanisms to restore radioiodine uptake, the future is bright regarding potential mechanisms to enhance radioiodine retention. For example, Koong et al. *(34)* have demonstrated the utility of lithium in enhancing the efficacy of increasing the retention of radioiodine. Zarnegar et al. *(35)* demonstrated that an increase in NIS and a decrease in pendrin activity may be associated with increased radioactive iodine effectiveness and could make radioiodine therapy more beneficial in patients with thyroid cancer.

Radiosensitizers

Radiosensitizers act to accentuate the effects of radiation, and several hold great potential. Kvols has selectively reviewed radiosensitizers (e.g., chemotherapeutic agents) that could increase the impact of radiotherapy *(36)*.

Miscellaneous

As noted in the imaging section, many other less dramatic but equally important clinical questions and problems involving therapy in nuclear medicine will be evaluated in the future and hopefully solved (see Table 2).

SUMMARY

The future of nuclear medicine in the diagnosis, management, and treatment of thyroid cancer is bright and exciting; this promise is also true for nuclear medicine innovations that will be applied to other realms of medicine. Indeed, the overall future of medicine warrants the cliché: It will be beyond our wildest imagination. Who thought: We would communicate in a way similar to Dick Tracy's two-way wrist radio? We could visit the Titanic in a Jules Verne-like vessel? We could go to the moon as H.G. Wells described? or We could sweep over the outside of our patients with an imaging scanner like Dr. McCoy on the Starship Enterprise and give Captain Kirk the diagnosis in a matter of minutes or even seconds? It is only a matter of time before patients in a remote location will be able to test or image themselves for a specific molecular or bodily function by an implanted device or by sweeping a scanner over the outside of their body, with the data transmitted halfway around the world to a computer. In fact, it is already being done. Charles Duell could not have been more wrong.

REFERENCES

1. Shao Y, Cherry SR, Farahani K. Simultaneous PET and MR imaging. Phys Med Biol 1997; 42:1965–1970.
2. Guy MJ, Castellano-Smith IA, Flower MA, et al. DETECT—dual energy transmission estimation CT—for improved attenuation correction in SPECT and PET. IEEE Trans Nucl Sc 1998; 45:1261–1267.
3. Wong WH, Uribe J, Hicks K, Hu G. An analog decoding GBO block detector using circular photomultipliers. IEEE Trans Nucl Sc 1997; 42:1095–1101.
4. Nahmias C, Nutt R, Hichwa RD, et al. PET tomograph designed for five minute routine whole-body studies. J Nucl Med 2002; 43:S36.
5. Ter-Pogossian MM, Mullani NA, Ficke DC, et al. Photon time of flight assisted positron emission tomography. J Comp Assist Tomogr 1981; 5:227–239.
6. Mäcke HR, Muller-Brand J. Receptor-targeted radiopeptide therapy. In Ell PJ, Gambhir SS, editors. Nuclear Medicine in Clinical Diagnosis and Treatment, 3rd ed., vol. 1. New York: Churchill Livingstone, 2004:459–472.
7. Teunissen JJM, Kwekkeboom DJ, Kooij PPM, et al. Peptide receptor radionuclide therapy for non-radioiodine-avid differentiated thyroid carcinoma. J Nucl Med 2005; 46:107S–114S.
8. Chang CH, Sharkey RM, Rossi EA, et al. Molecular advances in pretargeting radioimmuotherapy with bispecific antibodies. Mol Cancer Ther 2002; 1:530–563.
9. Reardon DT, Meares CF, Goodwin DA, et al. Antibodies against metal chelated. Nature 1985; 316:265–268.
10. Khaw BA, Kilbanov A, O'Donnell SM, et al. Gamma imaging with negatively charge-modified monoclonal antibody; Modification with synthetic polymers. J Nucl Med 1991; 32:1742–1751.
11. Peñuelas I, Boán JF, Martí-Climent MJ, et al. Positron emission tomography and gene therapy: basic concepts and experimental approaches for in vivo gene expression imaging. Mol Imag Biol 2004; 6:225–238.
12. Anderson CJ, Dehdashti F, Cutler, PD, et al. 64 Cu-TETA-octreotide as a PET imaging agent for patients with neuroendocrine tumors. J Nucl Med 2001; 42:213–221.
13. Henze M, Schuhmacher J, Hipp P, et al. PET imaging of somatostatin receptors using 68Ga-DOTA-D-Phel-Tyr3-octreotide: first results in patients with meningiomas. J Nucl Med 2001; 42:1053–1056.
14. Zinn KR, Chaudhuri TR. The type 2 human somatostatin receptor as a platform for reporter gene imaging. Eur J Nucl Med 2002; 29: 388–399.
15. Chen LB, Zhu RS, Lu HK, et al. Iodide uptake in medullary thyroid carcinoma cells after transfer of human sodium/iodide symporter gene. J Nucl Med 2004; 5S:337P.
16. Chung JK, Sodium iodide symporter: its role in nuclear medicine. J Nucl Med 2002; 43:1188–1200.
17. Stöcklin G Pike VW. Radiopharmaceuticals for positron emission tomography. In Cox P, editor. Methodological Aspects. Developments in Nuclear Medicine. Dordrecht: Kluwer Academic Publishers, 1993: p. 24.
18. Pagani M, Stone-Elander S, Larsson SA. Alternative positron emission tomography with non-conventional positron emitters: effects of

their physical properties on image quality and potential clinical applications. Eur J Nucl Med 1997; 24:1031–1327.
19. Glaser M, Luthra M, Brady F. Applications of positron-emitting halogens in PET oncology (review). Int J Oncol 2003; 22:253–267.
20. Newery GR. Cyclotron-produced isotopes in clinical and experimental medicine. Br J Radiol 1959; 32:633–641.
21. Phillips AF, Haybittle JL, Newbery GR. Use of iodine-124 for the treatment of carcinoma of the thyroid. Acta Unio Inern Contra Cancrum 1960; 16:1434–1438.
22. Sgouros G, Kolbert KS, Sheikh A, et al. Patient-specific dosimetry for I-131 thyroid cancer therapy using I-124 PET and 3-dimensional-internal dosimetry (3D-ID) software. J Nucl Med 2004; 45:1366–1372.
23. Humm JL. Dosimetric aspects of radiolabeled antibodies for tumor therapy. J Nucl Med 1986; 27:1490–1497.
24. Ackery D. Principles of radionuclide therapy. In Ell PJ, Gambhir SS, editors. Nuclear Medicine in Clinical Diagnosis and Treatment, 3rd ed., vol. 1. New York: Churchill Livingstone, 2004: pp. 359–362.
25. Sisson JC, Jamadar DDA, Kazerooni EA, et al. Treatment of micronodular lung metastases of papillary thyroid cancer: Are the tumors too small for effective irradiation from radioiodine? Thyroid 1998; 8:215–221.
25a. Couturier O, Supiot S, Degraef-Mougin M, et al. Cancer radioimmunotherapy with alpha-emitting nuclides. Europ J Nucl Med Mol Imaging 2005; 32:601–614.
26. Kassis AI, Adelstein SJ. Radiobiologic principles of radionuclide therapy. J Nucl Med 2005; 46:4S–12S.
27. Brown I. Astatine-211: its possible applications in cancer therapy. Appl Radiat Isot 1986; 37:789–798.
28. Makrigiorgos GM, Kassis AI, Baranowska-Kortylewicz J, et al. Radiotoxicity of 5-{^{123}I}iodo-2′-deoxyuridine in V79 cells: a comparison with 5-{^{125}I}iodo-2′-deoxyuridine. Radiat Res 1989; 118:532–544.
29. Grunwald F, Pakos E, Bender H, et al. Redifferentiation therapy with retinoic acid in follicular thyroid cancer. J Nucl Med 1998; 39:1555–1558.
30. Schmutzler C. Regulation of the sodium/iodide symporter by retinoids: a review. Exp Clin Endocrinol Diabetes 2001; 109:41–44.
31. Furuya F, Shimura H, Suzuki H, et al. Histone deacetylase inhibitors restore radioiodide uptake and retention in poorly differentiated and anaplastic thyroid cancer cells by expression of the sodium/iodide symporter thyroperoxidase and thyroglobulin. Endocrinology 2004; 145:2865–2875.
32. Chen LB, Zhu RS, Lu HK, et al. Iodide uptake in medullary thyroid carcinoma cells after transfer of human sodium/iodide symporter gene. J Nucl Med 2004; 5S:337P.
33. Misaki T, Miyamoto S, Alam MS, et al. Tumoricidal cytokines enhance radioiodine uptake in cultured thyroid cancer cells. J Nucl Med 1996; 37:646–648.
34. Koong SS, Reynolds JC, Movius EG, et al. Lithium as a potential adjuvant to 131-I therapy of metastatic, well differentiated thyroid carcinoma. J Clin Endocrinol Metab 1999; 84:912–916.
35. Zarnegar R, Brunaud L, Kanauchi H, et al. Increasing the effectiveness of radioactive iodine therapy in the treatment of thyroid cancer using Trichostatin A, a histone deacetylase inhibitor. Surgery 2002; 132:984–990.
36. Kvols LK. Radiation sensitizers: a selective review of molecules targeting DNA and non-DNA targets. J Nucl Med 2005; 46:187S–190S.

86
Alternative Options and Future Directions for Thyroid Cancer Therapy

Matthew D. Ringel

INTRODUCTION

The unique features of thyroid cells have enabled clinicians to specifically target therapy for patients with differentiated thyroid cancers. The retained expression and function of the thyrotropin (TSH) receptor and sodium-iodide symporter (NIS) in most thyroid cells have allowed the successful use of TSH-suppressive doses of levothyroxine (L-T4) and radioiodine. These targeted treatments, in combination with surgery, have led to long-term survival rates for patients with early stage thyroid cancers that approach 98% at 20 yr (1–4). However, this excellent prognosis is not shared by individuals with aggressive metastatic thyroid cancers, nor by those with malignancies that dedifferentiate and lose expression and function of the TSH receptor and NIS. Indeed, patients with these more aggressive thyroid cancers typically have a poor response to traditional therapies, resulting in a much higher incidence of cancer-related death. Alternative therapies using nontargeted cytotoxic chemotherapeutic agents have been largely disappointing.

Therefore, a major effort is underway to develop therapies for these more aggressive thyroid cancers that are designed to selectively halt or reverse the malignancy in a manner analogous to ^{131}I and TSH suppression therapy for typical thyroid cancers. Proper targeting therapy for these tumors requires clarification of the pathways most critical for tumor progression and tumor cell survival, as well as the mechanisms responsible for the loss of TSH receptor and NIS expression (Table 1) (5). Analysis of these agents in thyroid cancer patients requires early assessment of patients who are not responding to traditional therapies and access to clinical trials and clinical trial expertise. This chapter reviews the potential targets for alternative therapies. Specific clinical trials will not be reviewed in detail, as these are frequently changing over time.

CLINICAL TRIALS FOR CANCER

Thyroid cancer patients are most frequently treated by endocrinologists and nuclear medicine physicians, rather than medical and/or radiation oncologists. For patients with more aggressive thyroid cancers, it is important that the management team includes physicians who are comfortable with, and have access to, cancer clinical trials. Clinical trials are divided into phase I, II, and III studies. Phase I studies are the first human studies of an agent or combination of agents. These studies are designed to assess toxicity of the new therapeutic option. These trials are of greatest risk to the patients but may be very appealing if the therapy has been tested against thyroid cancer cells and animal models with encouraging results, and if the agent has particular logic for use as thyroid cancer therapy. Phase II studies are focused more on particular diseases for which there were clinical responses in phase I studies or strong logic based on mechanism of action. Phase III trials are generally large and often multi-institutional studies designed to determine if an agent or combination of agents is appropriate for FDA approval to use as treatment for a specific disease.

Several resources are available to identify clinical trials through the National Cancer Institute of the National Institutes of Health and from the Association of Clinical Oncologists. Physicians who care for patients with aggressive thyroid cancers should become familiar with these resources or enlist the help of an appropriate consultant involved in clinical trials to facilitate enrollment of patients if this becomes necessary.

INDIVIDUALIZED CANCER THERAPY

In the age of molecular targeting of therapies, an important concept when considering new therapy options is the notion of individualizing treatments based on the characteristics of a certain cancer. It may be possible to determine the best therapies for a patient's specific cancer through the development of microarrays to establish the gene expression profile of a cancer, proteomics to identify the protein expression profile, and now functional proteomics to detect patterns of pathway activation (5a). This goal, although not yet clinically available, is being utilized in clinical trials, where patients whose tumors display particular genotypes are considered for therapy with specific targeted agents.

From: *Thyroid Cancer: A Comprehensive Guide to Clinical Management, 2/e*
Edited by: L. Wartofsky and D. Van Nostrand © Humana Press Inc., Totowa, NJ

Table 1
Targets for Thyroid Cancer Therapies

Enhancing iodine uptake
Angiogenesis inhibitors
Tyrosine kinase receptor blockers
Signaling molecule inhibitors
Apoptosis sensitizers
Enhanced chemotherapy effects
Immunotherapy
Multimodality therapy

APPROACHES TO NOVEL THERAPIES

Increasing Iodine Uptake in Iodine Nonresponsive Thyroid Cancer

Initial work to devise therapies for iodine nonresponsive thyroid cancer was focused on enhancement of radioiodine retention or uptake into thyroid cancer cells. Over the past decade, advances in the understanding of the molecular biology of reduced iodine uptake that is characteristic of some thyroid cancers have greatly improved the ability to devise therapeutic strategies. The cloning of the *NIS* gene and its promoter, along with the development of reliable antibodies to allow protein detection, have shown that abnormalities in the *NIS* gene and protein expression and protein localization are common in thyroid cancer *(6–8)*. Recent data strongly suggest that the reduced *NIS* expression found in many thyroid cancers is most frequently from hypermethylation of the *NIS* promoter *(9,10)*. This epigenetic event results in gene silencing and reduced levels of *NIS* expression. Taking advantage of this knowledge, several investigators have treated thyroid cancer cell lines with demethylating agents or histone deacetylase (HDAC) inhibitors, e.g., 5-acacytidine and depsipeptide, respectively. Reduced methylation of the *NIS* promoter, reexpression of the *NIS* gene, increased iodine uptake, and enhanced efficacy of radioactive iodine therapy in vitro were demonstrated *(9,10)*. 5-Azacytidine is being used as a parent compound to develop new agents because of the rapid induction of resistance to this drug in vivo. Depsipeptide, an HDAC inhibitor, is one of several agents with similar activity currently in a clinical trial, albeit not in a combination with ^{131}I therapy.

Retinoid receptor agonists have been reported to enhance iodine uptake in vitro and in patients with thyroid cancers that do not respond to radioiodine. The initial studies appeared quite promising, both in vitro and in human studies *(11,12)*. However, it has become clear in subsequent larger studies that the benefit of more generalized retinoic acid receptor agonists appears to be limited for most patients, but a subset may still respond *(13)*. Over time, it has been recognized that thyroid cancers express a number of different retinoid receptors. The development of specific receptor-subtype agonists has led to several studies evaluating their effect in vitro. Initial results have been promising, both as enhancers of iodine uptake and as primary therapy for thyroid cancer *(14)*.

NIS gene therapy presents another alternative approach to increase *NIS* expression in cancers and enhance iodine uptake and therapeutic effect of radioactive iodine. The ability to target gene expression in cells is determined by the specificity of the promoter that drives the gene expression in the gene vector utilized. In the case of thyroid cells, several specific promoters exist, particularly the thyroglobulin gene promoter. Numerous in vitro and transgenic animals have been created using vectors that link the thyroglobulin promoter to a gene of interest, enabling thyroid-specific expression of that gene. Gene therapy has therefore been utilized for years in the laboratory to enhance expression of proteins in thyroid cells, including *NIS*. By placing this thyroglobulin promoter-*NIS* fusion gene into a gene therapy vector (such as a virus), it is possible to enhance expression of *NIS* in thyroid cells in vivo. In animal models, several groups have successfully induced *NIS* expression in thyroid cancer cells with low endogenous *NIS* levels by direct injection of the virus into tumors *(15,16,16a)*. This direct injection approach may be clinically problematic, as most patients with metastatic thyroid cancer have multiple small lesions in the neck and/or the lungs that are not amenable to direct injection. Thus, systemic therapy (inhaled or intravenous) is the goal. Unfortunately, the development of a systemic approach to gene therapy has been hampered by the potent immune response triggered by the viral vector and an extensive hepatic first-pass effect. Research using nonviral gene transporters is ongoing and holds promise as a less antigenic delivery method for future therapy. If this problem can be solved, gene therapy may become a useful method for increasing *NIS* expression in thyroid cancers, subsequently enhancing iodine uptake for treatment and monitoring.

Therapy Targeted Against Angiogenesis

The excessive growth and metabolic activity of cancer cells creates a need for access to nutrients and oxygen. Cancer cells invade and grow in regions that are not typically rich in blood vessels. Thus, to maintain growth and to invade, they need to create new blood vessels (neovascularization) to survive and grow. This process, known as angiogenesis, is therefore central to the ability of cancers to progress. Disruption of this process has been a strategy for new cancer therapies.

Thyroid cancer, in particular, is often a highly vascular tumor. This is specifically true for follicular thyroid cancers and poorly differentiated papillary and anaplastic thyroid cancers, where vascular invasion and local invasion are prevalent. Central to this process are the vascular endothelial growth factor (VEGF) and platelet-derived growth factor receptors, creating targets for agents directed against angiogenesis. Indeed, thyroid cancers are characterized by increased expression of angiogenic proteins and expression levels in tumors and serum correlate with more aggressive clinical behavior. These factors have increased the interest in this approach for thyroid cancer therapy.

Combretastatin A4 phosphate is a vascular-targeted compound that appears to have activity against human poorly differentiated thyroid cancer in clinical trials. Combretastatins are tubulin-binding proteins isolated from the African Willow. This family of compounds is vascular-targeted but also has direct cellular cytotoxic effects. In a recent phase I clinical trial, three of six thyroid cancer patients, including one with anaplastic thyroid cancer, had partial or complete responses to combretastatin A4 *(17,18)*. At follow-up, a phase II trial of combretastatin A4 for anaplastic or progressive thyroid cancer was initiated, and the results are currently pending. The primary toxicity of this compound is cardiac, causing both vascular events and arrhythmias. Thus, patients need to be cleared by a cardiac evaluation prior to starting this agent.

VEGF, as mentioned before, is an important stimulator of new blood vessel formation. Expression of VEGF and its receptors are stimulated by hypoxia through activation of a family of hypoxia-inducible transcription factors. VEGF-neutralizing antibodies, such as bevacizumab (Avastin, Genenetech) and receptor blockers, such as Semaxanib (Sugen) have demonstrated activity against thyroid cancer xenografts in vivo *(19,20,20a)*. Different from combretastatins, these agents appear to have minimal in vitro cytotoxic effect. Treatment with these agents reduced expression of vascular proteins and new blood vessels in treated tumors. Thalidomide is another vascular-targeted agent used in clinical trials for a variety of cancers, but it is not well-studied for thyroid cancers.

Overall, the concept of vascular targeting for thyroid cancer is evolving. Similar to other novel therapies, predictors of response (e.g., the degree of neovascularization) may be important in selecting appropriate patients for these agents. In addition, combination therapy may be the method that will maximize the efficacy of these treatments.

Therapy Targeted Against Cell-Signaling Pathways

Thyroid cancers are characterized by gene mutations that alter cell-signaling pathways. In general, these mutations either enhance activity of signaling proteins (oncogenes) or result in loss of expression of negative regulators of cell signaling (tumor suppressors). In either case, the end result is the unregulated activation of signaling pathways that lead to tumor formation, enhanced cell proliferation, resistance to cell death, angiogenesis, and metastatic potential. Over the past few decades, the genetic alterations responsible for most thyroid cancers have been identified. Overexpression or oncogenic rearrangements have been characterized in tyrosine kinase receptors (e.g., *RET*, *cMET*, and IGF-1; *21–23*), activating mutations of downstream serine-threonine kinases, including *RAS (24,25)* and *BRAF (26–32)*, and loss of tumor suppressor expression *(33–35)*. Several of these genetic abnormalities are specific for thyroid cancer (e.g., RET/PTC rearrangements), whereas other are common to other malignancies (e.g., *RAS*, *BRAF*, and *PTEN* mutants). Some appear to be induced by environmental factors, such as exposure to ionizing radiation, but others are induced through uncertain mechanisms. In rare cases, germline genetic alterations have been found to confer risk to thyroid cancer in families (including the loss of *PTEN* expression in Cowden's syndrome) and activating mutations of *RET* medullary thyroid cancer and multiple endocrine neoplasia syndromes. Oncogene expression is maintained in primary and metastatic thyroid cancers, suggesting that these pathways may be critical to the aggressive phenotype of some thyroid cancers. Importantly, with this expanding knowledge, there is now a unique opportunity to develop and test therapies targeted against these signaling molecules for the treatment of established thyroid cancer and the chemoprevention for individuals at risk for thyroid cancer development.

The presence of specific oncogenes is not unique to thyroid cancer. Indeed, kinase inhibitors have been developed for other cancers and have been used as beneficial therapeutic alternatives. The most successful have been inhibition of BCR/ABL and C-KIT in chronic myelogenous leukemia and gastrointestinal stromal tumors using STI-571—a specific inhibitor of these two kinases *(36–38)*. This success has resulted in the development of innumerable new kinase inhibitors, each with their own specific pattern of activity. Of particular interest for thyroid cancer are agents that inhibit tyrosine kinase receptors involved in thyroid cancer pathogenesis and progression. Indeed, several agents designed to block epidermal growth factor (EGF) receptor activity have demonstrated a high affinity to the *RET* tyrosine kinase, as well as the ability to inhibition *RET* function, suggesting the potential for clinical trials for medullary and papillary thyroid cancers that have activation of the *RET*-signaling cascade through mutations and gene rearrangements, respectively *(39, 40,40a)*.

In addition to *RET* inhibition, other tyrosine kinase receptors are overactivated in thyroid cancers, specifically the EGF receptor and the family of VEGF receptors. Several inhibitors of these pathways have been developed, including molecules that block the activity of the receptor directly and antibodies that bind VEGF itself to reduce cell signaling. Several of these agents have been studied in thyroid cancer in vitro and in vivo, and beneficial effects have been reported *(19,20)*.

Tyrosine kinase receptors activate numerous downstream signaling pathways. Among these, principal pathways are the *RAS*/MAP kinase and the PI3 kinase/Akt. Along with the activation from tyrosine kinase receptors, genetic abnormalities in the genes encoding RAS and its downstream target, *BRAF*, have been described in follicular and papillary thyroid cancers, respectively. Akt activation occurs because of loss of PTEN activity in Cowden's syndrome; activation of this pathway is reported to have a unique role in cell invasion. For these reasons, direct disruption of these signaling molecules has been utilized as an alternative targeting strategy for cancer therapy. One potential problem with this approach is the absence of clear specificity for the cancer cells. These signaling molecules are activated by a large number of receptors and external stimuli. Thus, they represent important regulators of many signaling pathways and are important for nearly all cells. Therefore, distinct from inhibition of receptors only expressed in cancer cells, the specificity of these agents depends on the level of pathway activity in cancer cells vs noncancer cells. Despite this reservation, inhibitors of *BRAF*, *RAS*, and Akt have all been developed utilizing several different strategies. Indeed, clinical trials involve agents that block the mechanism of activation (e.g., farnesyl transferase inhibitors; *41,42*), compounds that inhibit carrier proteins for these molecules that stabilize their structures (heat-shock protein-binding agents; *43,44*), and direct blockers of their expression *(44a)*. Phase I and II studies have demonstrated a high level of activity against various cancers with this approach. The side-effect profile has been acceptable, and they are therefore moving ahead with further clinical trials.

Because inhibition of these signaling pathways enhances the sensitivity of cells to apoptosis (programmed cell death), the most effective use of these drugs will likely be in combination with other approaches, such as radioiodine, radiation therapy, and cytotoxic chemotherapy. Although these agents are presented as individual compounds, many are currently in clinical trials in combination with chemotherapy agents.

Therapies Designed to Induce Cell Death

Cell growth is characterized by a skew in the balance of cell cycle proteins toward proliferation and away from apoptosis. The mechanisms that lead to this alteration are manifold and include the production of proteins that block external stimuli for apoptosis, expression of intracellular proteins that are antiapoptotic, and persistent expression of proteins to maintain chromosome length. In thyroid cancer, each of these mechanisms has been clearly described and is thought to have an important role in tumor progression and resistance to therapy. The pathways activated in thyroid cancer are potent apoptosis inhibitors, as well as growth activators. Thus, many families of agents described earlier also induce cell death by inducing apoptosis (programmed cell death), inhibiting antiapoptotic pathways, or causing cell necrosis. In addition to these agents, several other novel compounds have been created to more directly target cell survival pathways.

Tumor necrosis factor (TNF) and the FAS ligand are two common initiators of programmed cell death. Thyroid cancer cells are remarkably resistant to these two apoptosis inducers through both intracellular mechanisms and release of inhibitory proteins. Downstream of the TNF receptors is a related effector molecule—the TNF-related apoptosis-inducing ligand (TRAIL) receptor. Direct activation of this receptor is possible using recombinant human TRAIL, and its use has induced apoptosis in a number of apoptosis-resistant cell lines, including thyroid cancer cells *(45–47)*. Another approach to inhibit antiapoptotic-signaling molecules is to directly block endogenous inhibitors, such as BCL-2. BCL-2 is upregulated by Akt and RAS and is therefore felt to be involved in the inhibition of apoptosis common to most cancer cells and the more specific antiapoptotic effect of thyroid cancer oncogenes. BCL-2 levels can be reduced using an antisense RNA compound (e.g., olbermersen sodium, Genasense, Genta), which then sensitizes cancer cells to apoptotic stimuli. This approach has been recently reported in clinical trials but not yet for thyroid cancer *(48)*. Another way to sensitize thyroid cancer cells to apoptosis is to block proteins that stabilize intracellular signaling molecules or receptors simultaneously in cancer cells, but not in benign cells. Heat-shock protein 90 (Hsp90) is a chaperone protein that stabilizes intracellular proteins. This agent is active in thyroid cancer cells in vitro *(44)*. Its activity is predicted by the intracellular levels of Hsp90 and by the ability of a Hsp90 to interact with other proteins in a cancer cell–specific manner *(43)*, making this agent a potential cancer-targeted apoptosis-sensitizer.

Gene therapy can be utilized to carry vectors that induce cytotoxicity directly or after incubation of cancer cells with an activator of the newly expressed protein ("suicide gene therapy") *(48a)*. Similar to the reexpression of NIS, this model utilizes a vector that couples a "suicide gene" to the thyroglobulin gene promoter to induce thyroid-specific expression of this gene. The most commonly reported method is to induce thyroid cell expression of thymidine kinase by infecting thyroid cancer cells. These cells are infected with a virus carrying a transgene that couples the thyroglobulin promoter to the gene encoding thymidine kinase—a protein that is not normally expressed in mammalian cells. Expression of thymidine kinase uniquely sensitizes the cancer cells to the antiviral drug ganciclovir *(49)*. This approach has been used as primary therapy, as treatment to sensitize cancer cells to radiation therapy, and to sensitize cells to immunomodulators, such as TNF and tumor vaccines *(50,52,52a)*.

Other Potential Therapies for Thyroid Cancer

As noted above, thyroid cancer cells are typically remarkably resistant to cytotoxic chemotherapies. There are many potential mechanisms for this resistance, including oncogene expression and resistance to apoptosis. Another possibility is that the thyroid cancer cells express proteins specific for drug resistance. Indeed, thyroid cancer, and many other malignant cells, express a family of multiple drug-resistant genes that lead to chemotherapy resistance. Some of these proteins specifically cause resistance to compounds, with documented activity against anaplastic thyroid cancer (e.g., taxanes and doxorubicin; *53–57*). Cancer cells will likely develop new methods to resist the antitumor effect of the newer targeted agents as well. Thus, the use of antisense RNA and other approaches targeted against drug resistant mechanisms represents an important direction for cancer therapy. Clearly, these agents would be used to enhance the activity of chemotherapies against resistant thyroid cancer cells.

Immunotherapy has been an important area of research relating to thyroid cancer for decades *(58,59)*. The development of vaccines directed against specific antigens expressed by tumor cells to target cytotoxic immune responses has been the focus of therapy for many different types of cancer. For thyroid cancer, an important clue could be the development of thyroiditis reported in patients treated with inteferons or interleukins. These reports have led to elevated interest in this area of therapeutic research. One potential advantage of this option is to tailor therapy for a patient based on the specific antigens expressed by their specific tumor. As new therapies develop, this individualized therapy is an important concept.

Multimodality Therapies

Because cancer cells display abnormalities on multiple levels to allow for tumor progression and the development of drug resistance, the most effective therapeutic options are likely to require multiple agents and/or modalities. These may include several targeted agents, immunotherapy, radiation therapy, and/or radioiodine. The importance of animal models to help discern the most beneficial regimens cannot be overstated, as each combination will require clinical study to determine safety and efficacy. It is also important to recognize that cancer cells are not static cells. They display genomic instability and are also prone to epigenetic modifications that allow them to alter their expression profiles over time. This ability to modify targets may be combated by combination therapies in some cases. Thus, ultimately, combination therapy with agents targeted against several different pathways may be needed to treat patients with these aggressive tumors.

REFERENCES

1. Sherman SI, Brierley JD, Sperling M, et al. Prospective multicenter study of thyroid carcinoma treatment: initial analysis of staging and outcome. National Thyroid Cancer Treatment Cooperative Study Registry Group. Cancer 1998; 83:1012–1021.
2. Hundahl SA, Fleming ID, Fremgen AM, Menck HR. A National Cancer Data Base report on 53,856 cases of thyroid carcinoma treated in the U.S., 1985–1995. Cancer 1998; 83:2638–2648.
3. Hundahl SA, Cady B, Cunningham MP, et al. Initial results from a prospective cohort study of 5583 cases of thyroid carcinoma treated in the United States during 1996. U.S. and German Thyroid Cancer Study Group. An American College of Surgeons Commission on Cancer Patient Care Evaluation study. Cancer 2000; 89:202–217.
4. Mazzaferri EL, Jhiang SM. Long-term impact of initial surgical and medical therapy on papillary and follicular thyroid cancer. Am J Med 1994; 97:418–428.
5. Braga-Basaria M, Ringel MD. Clinical review 158: Beyond radioiodine: a review of potential new therapeutic approaches for thyroid cancer. J Clin Endocrinol Metab 2003; 88:1947–1960.
5a. Uhlen M, Bjorling E, Agaton C, et al. A human protein atlas for normal and cancer tissues based on antibody proteomics. Mol Cell Proteomics 2005; Aug 27; [Epub].
6. Dohan O, Baloch Z, Banrevi Z, et al. Rapid communication: predominant intracellular overexpression of the Na(+)/I(−) symporter (NIS) in a large sampling of thyroid cancer cases. J Clin Endocrinol Metab 2001; 86:2697–2700.
7. Jhiang SM. Regulation of sodium/iodide symporter. Rev Endocr Metab Disord 2000; 1:205–215.
8. Ringel MD, Anderson J, Souza SL, et al. Expression of the sodium iodide symporter and thyroglobulin genes are reduced in papillary thyroid cancer. Mod Pathol 2001; 14:289–296.
9. Venkataraman GM, Yatin M, Marcinek R, Ain KB. Restoration of iodide uptake in dedifferentiated thyroid carcinoma: relationship to human Na+/I-symporter gene methylation status. J Clin Endocrinol Metab 1999; 84:2449–2457.
10. Furuya F, Shimura H, Suzuki H, et al. Histone deacetylase inhibitors restore radioiodide uptake and retention in poorly differentiated and anaplastic thyroid cancer cells by expression of the sodium/iodide symporter thyroperoxidase and thyroglobulin. Endocrinology 2004; 145:2865–2875.
11. Grunwald F, Pakos E, Bender H, et al. Redifferentiation therapy with retinoic acid in follicular thyroid cancer. J Nucl Med 1998; 39: 1555–1558.
12. Schmutzler C, Winzer R, Meissner-Weigl J, Kohrle J. Retinoic acid increases sodium/iodide symporter mRNA levels in human thyroid cancer cell lines and suppresses expression of functional symporter in nontransformed FRTL-5 rat thyroid cells. Biochem Biophys Res Commun 1997; 240:832–838.
13. Gruning T, Tiepolt C, Zophel K, et al. Retinoic acid for redifferentiation of thyroid cancer—does it hold its promise? Eur J Endocrinol 2003; 148:395–402.
14. Haugen BR, Larson LL, Pugazhenthi U, et al. Retinoic acid and retinoid X receptors are differentially expressed in thyroid cancer and thyroid carcinoma cell lines and predict response to treatment with retinoids. J Clin Endocrinol Metab 2004; 89:272–280.
14a. Elisei R, Vivaldi A, Agate L, et al. All-trans-retinoic acid treatment inhibits the growth of retinoic acid receptor β messenger ribonucleic acid expressing thyroid cancer cell lines but does not reinduce the expression of thyroid-specific genes. J Clin Endocrinol Metab 2005; 90:2403–2411.
15. DeGroot LJ, Zhang R. Clinical review 131: Gene therapy for thyroid cancer: where do we stand? J Clin Endocrinol Metab 2001; 86:2923–2928.
16. Schmutzler C, Koehrle J. Innovative strategies for the treatment of thyroid cancer. Eur J Endocrinol 2000; 143:15–24.
16a. Cengic N, Baker CH, Schutz M, et al. A novel therapeutic strategy for medullary thyroid cancer based on radioiodine therapy following tissue-specific sodium iodide symporter gene expression. J Clin Endocrinol Metab 2005; 90:4457–4464.
17. Dowlati A, Robertson K, Cooney M, et al. A phase I pharmacokinetic and translational study of the novel vascular targeting agent combretastatin a-4 phosphate on a single-dose intravenous schedule in patients with advanced cancer. Cancer Res 2002; 62: 3408–3416.
18. Cooney MM, Radivoyevitch T, Dowlati A, et al. Cardiovascular safety profile of combretastatin a4 phosphate in a single-dose phase I study in patients with advanced cancer. Clin Cancer Res 2004; 10: 96–100.
19. Soh EY, Eigelberger MS, Kim KJ, et al. Neutralizing vascular endothelial growth factor activity inhibits thyroid cancer growth in vivo. Surgery 2000; 128:1059–1065; discussion 1065–1066.
20. Bauer AJ, Terrell R, Doniparthi NK, et al. Vascular endothelial growth factor monoclonal antibody inhibits growth of anaplastic thyroid cancer xenografts in nude mice. Thyroid 2002; 12:953–961.
20a. Straight AM, Oakley K, Moores R, et al. Aplidin reduces growth of anaplastic thyroid cancer xenografts and the expression of several angiogenic genes. Cancer Chemother Pharmacol 2005; Jul 5:1–8.
21. Farid NR. Molecular pathogenesis of thyroid cancer: the significance of oncogenes, tumor suppressor genes, and genomic instability. Exp Clin Endocrinol Diabetes 1996; 104(Suppl 4):1–12.

22. Segev DL, Umbricht C, Zeiger MA. Molecular pathogenesis of thyroid cancer. Surg Oncol 2003; 12:69–90.
23. Fagin JA. Perspective: lessons learned from molecular genetic studies of thyroid cancer—insights into pathogenesis and tumor-specific therapeutic targets. Endocrinology 2002; 143:2025–2028.
24. Namba H, Rubin SA, Fagin JA. Point mutations of ras oncogenes are an early event in thyroid tumorigenesis. Mol Endocrinol 1990; 4: 1474–1479.
25. Lemoine NR, Mayall ES, Wyllie FS, et al. High frequency of ras oncogene activation in all stages of human thyroid tumorigenesis. Oncogene 1989; 4:159–164.
26. Cohen Y, Xing M, Mambo E, et al. BRAF mutation in papillary thyroid carcinoma. J Natl Cancer Inst 2003; 95:625–627.
27. Fukushima T, Suzuki S, Mashiko M, et al. BRAF mutations in papillary carcinomas of the thyroid. Oncogene 2003; 22:6455–6457.
28. Kimura ET, Nikiforova MN, Zhu Z, et al. High prevalence of BRAF mutations in thyroid cancer: genetic evidence for constitutive activation of the RET/PTC-RAS-BRAF signaling pathway in papillary thyroid carcinoma. Cancer Res 2003; 63:1454–1457.
29. Nikiforova MN, Kimura ET, Gandhi M, et al. BRAF mutations in thyroid tumors are restricted to papillary carcinomas and anaplastic or poorly differentiated carcinomas arising from papillary carcinomas. J Clin Endocrinol Metab 2003; 88:5399–5404.
30. Trovisco V, Vieira de Castro I, Soares P, et al. BRAF mutations are associated with some histological types of papillary thyroid carcinoma. J Pathol 2004; 202:247–251.
31. Xing M, Vasko V, Tallini G, et al. BRAF T1796A transversion mutation in various thyroid neoplasms. J Clin Endocrinol Metab 2004; 89:1365–1368.
32. Xu X, Quiros RM, Gattuso P, et al. High prevalence of BRAF gene mutation in papillary thyroid carcinomas and thyroid tumor cell lines. Cancer Res 2003; 63:4561–4567.
33. Fagin JA. Tumor suppressor genes in human thyroid neoplasms: p53 mutations are associated undifferentiated thyroid cancers. J Endocrinol Invest 1995; 18:140–142.
34. Liaw D, Marsh DJ, Li J, et al. Germline mutations of the PTEN gene in Cowden disease, an inherited breast and thyroid cancer syndrome. Nat Genet 1997; 16:64–67.
35. Fagin JA, Matsuo K, Karmakar A, et al. High prevalence of mutations of the p53 gene in poorly differentiated human thyroid carcinomas. J Clin Invest 1993; 91:179–184.
36. Druker BJ. STI571 (Gleevec) as a paradigm for cancer therapy. Trends Mol Med 2002; 8:S14–S18.
37. Mauro MJ, O'Dwyer M, Heinrich MC, Druker BJ. STI571: a paradigm of new agents for cancer therapeutics. J Clin Oncol 2002; 20:325–334.
38. Sawyers CL. Cancer treatment in the STI571 era: what will change? J Clin Oncol 2001; 19:13S–16S.
39. Carlomagno F, Vitagliano D, Guida T, et al. ZD6474, an orally available inhibitor of KDR tyrosine kinase activity, efficiently blocks oncogenic RET kinases. Cancer Res 2002; 62:7284–7290.
40. Vitagliano D, Carlomagno F, Motti ML, et al. Regulation of p27Kip1 protein levels contributes to mitogenic effects of the RET/PTC kinase in thyroid carcinoma cells. Cancer Res 2004; 64:3823–3829.
40a. Cuccuru G, Lanzi C, Cassinelli G, et al. Cellular effects and antitumor activity of RET inhibitor RPI-1 on MEN2A-associated medullary thyroid carcinoma. J Natl Cancer Inst 2004; 96:980–991.
41. O'Regan RM, Khuri FR. Farnesyl transferase inhibitors: the next targeted therapies for breast cancer? Endocr Relat Cancer 2004; 11: 191–205.
42. Mazieres J, Pradines A, Favre G. Perspectives on farnesyl transferase inhibitors in cancer therapy. Cancer Lett 2004; 206:159–167.
43. Workman P. Altered states: selectively drugging the Hsp90 cancer chaperone. Trends Mol Med 2004; 10:47–51.
44. Ringel MD, Ladenson PW. Controversies in the follow-up and management of well-differentiated thyroid cancer. Endocr Relat Cancer 2004; 11:97–116.
44a. Mandal M, Kim S, Younes MN, et al. The Akt inhibitor KP372-1 suppresses Akt activity and cell proliferation and induces apoptosis in thyroid cancer cells. Br J Cancer 2005; 92:1899–1905.
45. Ahmad M, Shi Y. TRAIL-induced apoptosis of thyroid cancer cells: potential for therapeutic intervention. Oncogene 2000; 19: 3363–3371.
46. Mitsiades CS, Poulaki V, Mitsiades N. The role of apoptosis-inducing receptors of the tumor necrosis factor family in thyroid cancer. J Endocrinol 2003; 178:205–216.
47. Park JW, Wong MG, Lobo M, et al. Modulation of tumor necrosis factor-related apoptosis-inducing ligand-induced apoptosis by chemotherapy in thyroid cancer cell lines. Thyroid 2003; 13: 1103–1110.
48. Manion MK, Hockenbery DM. Targeting BCL-2-related proteins in cancer therapy. Cancer Biol Ther 2003; 2:S105–S114.
48a. Spitzweg C and Morris JC. Gene therapy for thyroid cancer: current status and future prospects. Thyroid 2004; 14:424–434.
49. Shimura H, Suzuki H, Miyazaki A, et al. Transcriptional activation of the thyroglobulin promoter directing suicide gene expression by thyroid transcription factor-1 in thyroid cancer cells. Cancer Res 2001; 61:3640–3646.
50. Tanaka K, Towata S, Nakao K, et al. Thyroid cancer immuno-therapy with retroviral and adenoviral vectors expressing granulocyte macrophage colony stimulating factor and interleukin-12 in a rat model. Clin Endocrinol (Oxf) 2003; 59:734–742.
51. Barzon L, Bonaguro R, Castagliuolo I, et al. Gene therapy of thyroid cancer via retrovirally-driven combined expression of human interleukin-2 and herpes simplex virus thymidine kinase. Eur J Endocrinol 2003; 148:73–80.
52. Barzon L, Bonaguro R, Castagliuolo I, et al. Transcriptionally targeted retroviral vector for combined suicide and immunomodulating gene therapy of thyroid cancer. J Clin Endocrinol Metab 2002; 87: 5304–5311.
52a. Barzon L, Pacenti M, Taccaliti A, et al. A pilot study of combined suicide/cytokine gene therapy in two patients with end-stage anaplastic thyroid carcinoma. J Clin Endocrinol Metab 2005; 90:2831–2834.
53. Asakawa H, Kobayashi T, Komoike Y, et al. Establishment of anaplastic thyroid carcinoma cell lines useful for analysis of chemosensitivity and carcinogenesis. J Clin Endocrinol Metab 1996; 81: 3547–3552.
54. Dapas B, Perissin L, Pucillo C, et al. Increase in therapeutic index of doxorubicin and vinblastine by aptameric oligonucleotide in human T lymphoblastic drug-sensitive and multidrug-resistant cells. Antisense Nucleic Acid Drug Dev 2002; 12:247–255.
55. Massart C, Gibassier J, Raoul M, et al. Effect of S9788 on the efficiency of doxorubicin in vivo and in vitro in medullary thyroid carcinoma xenograft. Anticancer Drugs 1996; 7:321–330.
56. Sekiguchi M, Shiroko Y, Arai T, et al. Biological characteristics and chemosensitivity profile of four human anaplastic thyroid carcinoma cell lines. Biomed Pharmacother 2001; 55:466–474.
57. Sugawara I, Masunaga A, Itoyama S, et al. Expression of multidrug resistance-associated protein (MRP) in thyroid cancers. Cancer Lett 1995; 95:135–138.
58. Casterline PF, Jaques DA, Blom H, Wartofsky L. Anaplastic giant and spindle-cell carcinoma of the thyroid: a different therapeutic approach. Cancer 1980; 45:1689–1692.
59. Schott M, Seissler J. Dendritic cell vaccination: new hope for the treatment of metastasized endocrine malignancies. Trends Endocrinol Metab 2003; 14:156–162.

87
Potential Approaches to Chemotherapy of Thyroid Cancer in the Future

Lawrence S. Lessin

INTRODUCTION

Cytotoxic chemotherapy is generally employed in patients with advanced metastatic thyroid cancers that are refractory to treatment with radioiodine. Although clinical remissions and even complete responses have been seen with various chemotherapeutic agents, this therapy does not produces any significant prolongation of survival in these patients (see Chapters 52, 73, and 82). Likely, effective drug therapy of thyroid cancer depends on development of specific targeted agents that are active against aberrant genes, gene products, growth processes, and signaling pathways in thyroid cancer (1).

CHEMOTHERAPY RESISTANCE

Resistance to chemotherapy in advanced thyroid cancer has been attributed to several mechanisms. Overexpression of the multidrug resistance (*MDR-1*) gene in poorly differentiated, anaplastic, and medullary thyroid cancers (MTC) leads to active transport of most anticancer drugs out of thyroid cancer cells via a transmembrane pump (2). Although inhibition of this pump by cyclosporine A or verapamil can overcome MDR-1-induced resistance in vitro, clinical studies with these agents in other cancers have not shown clinical benefit.

A second resistance mechanism involves mutations of normally occurring genes, which control apoptosis and its signaling pathways for programmed cell death. In Chapter 86, and in a recent review, Ringel summarizes the multiple antiapoptotic factors and pathways involved in cancer cell proliferation and survival (3). Synthesis of Bcl-2, an endogenous inhibitor of apoptosis, can be blocked by an antisense RNA specific to Bcl-2. This antisense drug (Genasense), active in lymphoproliferative disorders and prostate cancer, has not yet been studied in thyroid cancers. When nonspecific cytotoxic agents are combined with Bcl-2 antisense RNA, antiapoptotic pathways may be overcome, and tumor response initiated.

Santini et al. strove to overcome relative chemotherapy resistance to their epirubicin–cisplatin regimen for poorly differentiated thyroid cancer by increasing plasma thyrotropin (TSH) levels with either recombinant TSH or reduction of L-thyroxine dosage (4). Overall response rate in this refractory disease was 37%, and 50% of the 14 patients studied exhibited a decrease in serum thyroglobulin levels. Improved response in these patients was attributed to a synergistic effect of elevated TSH and chemotherapy on tumor cells.

Stassi, Todaro, and colleagues studied thyroid cancer chemotherapy resistance associated with autocrine production of interleukin (IL)-2 and IL-10 by thyroid cancer cells (5). They found that malignant cells from papillary, follicular, and anaplastic thyroid cancers all had high expression of Bcl-2 or Bcl-XL, which can prevent drug-induced cytotoxicity. All the tumors produced IL-4 and IL-10, which upregulate Bcl-2 and Bcl-XL. Monoclonal antibodies to IL-4 and IL-10 led to decreased expression of Bcl-2 and Bcl-XL and produced death of thyroid cancer cells with sensitization of the remaining tumor cell population to cytotoxic drug-induced apoptosis. The authors suggest that IL-4 and IL-10 represent therapeutic targets for the treatment of thyroid cancers, as well as another potential approach to decrease cytotoxic drug resistance.

Targeted Therapies for Thyroid Cancers

In a recent review, Burman summarized the major cellular pathways and potential molecules or actions that may serve as specific targets for anticancer therapy. Table 1, adapted from Burman (1) after Braga-Basaria and Ringel (2), lists some of these pathways and targets.

Tyrosine Kinase Inhibitors (TKIs)

Moley et al. are currently investigating the potential role of oral imatinib mesylate (STI571, Gleevec) in the therapy of patients with advanced, metastatic, carcinoembryonic antigen, CEA and calcitonin-positive medullary thyroid cancer (MTC) (6; see Tables 2 and 3). Imatinib, a TKI developed to specifically inhibit the BCR/Abl and C-kit of chronic myelogenous leukemia (CML), has produced dramatic

Table 1
Molecular Mechanisms as Potential Targets for Anticancer Agents

Pathways	Target, Agent, or Action
Ras	Antisense mRNA; tyrosine kinase (TK) inhibition
Farnesyl transferase inhibition	Specific inhibition
Raf	Antisense mRNA; specific Raf kinase inhibition
Tyrosine kinases	Specific inhibition through VEGF, EGFR, and RET-TK
Antibodies	Directed against protein and/or receptor; VEGF, EGF, Her2/neu
Angiogenesis	Direct inhibition of angiogenesis; tubulin-binding proteins
Apoptosis	Recombinant soluble TRAIL; TRM-1 binding to TRAIL-R1 receptor; Bcl-2 inhibition
Cyclooxygenase-2 inhibitor	Inhibition of enhanced apoptosis and decreased angiogenesis
Histone deacetylase	Inhibition

Adapted from Burman (1) after Braga-Basaria and Ringel (3).
Abbreviations: VEGF, vascular endothelial growth factor; EGFR, epidermal growth factor receptor; EGF, epidermal growth factor; TRAIL, tumor necrosis factor-related apoptosis-inducing ligand.

Table 2
New Antineoplastic Agents for Advanced Thyroid Cancer

Agent	Class	Thyroid Cancer Type (Ref.)
Imatinib mesylate	Tyrosine kinase inhibitor	MTC (6,7)
Combretastatin A4 phosphate	Tubulin-binding agent	ATC (13,14)
Gemcitabine-loaded liposomes	Antimetabolite	ATC (17,18)
Irinotecan	Topoisomerase I inhibitor	MTC (19)
Depsipeptide	Histamine deacetylase inhibitor	PTC, FTC, HCTC (16)
Manumycin	Farnesyl transferase inhibitor	ATC (9,10)

MTC, medullary thyroid cancer; ATC, anaplastic thyroid cancer; PTC, papillary thyroid cancer; FTC, follicular thyroid cancer; HCTC, Hürthle cell thyroid cancer.

clinical responses in CML, gastrointestinal stromal tumors (GIST) and dermatofibrosarcoma proliferans. In vitro, imatinib inhibits the RET-tyrosine kinase of MTC and prevents human MTC xenograft growth in nude mice. In vitro studies with MTC cell lines have shown growth inhibition by imatinib and other TKIs, but LD-50 concentrations are difficult to achieve in patients without unacceptable toxicity (7).

Several new TKIs are now in clinical trials involving patients with CML and GIST who have relapsed after initial responses to imatinib. These agents may also have activity against RET-TK and other tyrosine kinases involved in thyroid cancer growth. The orally active TKI, PTK 787/ZK 22584, inhibits vascular endothelial growth factor-induced tyrosine kinase and thereby interferes with neoangiogenesis and tumor growth of ML-1 follicular carcinoma xenografts in nude mice (8). As these TKIs lead to tumor growth suppression via promotion of apoptosis or inhibition of angiogenesis without complete tumor resolution, their principal role will likely be as synergistic agents with either cytoxic drugs or other specifically targeted agents.

Manumycin

This farnesyl transferase inhibitor, when combined with Paclitaxel, has been shown to inhibit both anaplastic thyroid cancer growth and angiogenesis (9). It has also been found that manumycin can enhance the cytotoxic effect of paclitaxel against six anaplastic thyroid cancer cell lines. In vitro studies revealed activation of caspace-3-induced apoptosis by the manumycin–pactitaxel combination (10). Clinical trials of this agent are planned.

Combretastatin A4 Phosphate

This tubulin-binding protein is a vascular-targeted compound with cytoxic effects against thyroid cancer cell lines and xenografts (11,12). Responses have been seen in thyroid

Table 3
Current Clinical Trials in Thyroid Cancer

Protocol	Lead Institution	Tumor Types Eligible
Phase II study of cisplatin, doxorubicin and tamoxifen in patients with incurable thyroid cancer (and other tumors)	Ottawa Regional Cancer Center, Ottawa, Canada	Refractory DTC, ATC, MTC
Phase II study of thalidomide in patients with radioiodine-unresponsive papillary, follicular, or medullary carcinoma	University of Kentucky Medical Center, Lexington, KY	Advanced PTC, FTC, MTC
Phase II study of vaccine therapy with tumor-specific mutated Ras peptides in combination with interleukin-2 and/or GM-CSF in adult metastatic solid tumors	National Cancer Institute, Bethesda, MD	Advanced MTC, ATC, poorly differentiated TC
Phase I study of recombinant Fowlpox-CEA-Trican vaccine with or without GM-CSF, or R-Fowlpox-GM-CSF in patients with advanced/metastatic CEA expressing solid tumors	Fox Chase Cancer Center, Philadelphia, PA	Advanced MTC
Phase I study of depsipeptide (NSC630176, FR901228) to treat thyroid and other advanced cancers	National Cancer Institute, Bethesda, MD	Advanced nonmedullary thyroid cancer
Phase II study of FR901228 (Depsipeptide) in patients with progressive recurrent and/or metastatic nonmedullary thyroid cancer, refractory to radioiodine	Memorial Sloan-Kettering Cancer Center, New York, NY	Advanced, nonmedullary thyroid cancer
Phase II study of induction chemotherapy with doxorubicin and cisplatin, followed by combretastatin A4 phosphate and radiotherapy in patients with newly diagnosed, regionally advanced ATC	Ireland Cancer Center, Case-Western Reserve University, Cleveland, OH	Regionally advanced ATC
Phase II study of imatinib (Gleevec) in metastatic, imeasurable MTC	Siteman Cancer Center Washington University, St. Louis, MO	Advanced metastatic MTC
Phase II study of irinotecan in patients with metastatic or inoperable locoregional MTC	Kimmel Cancer Center of Johns Hopkins Hospital, Baltimore, MD	Metastatic or inoperable MTC

DTC, differentiated thyroid cancer; ATC, anaplastic thyroid cancer; MTC, medullary thyroid cancer; PTC, papillary thyroid cancer; FTC, follicular thyroid cancer; GM-CSF, granulocyte macrophage-colony stimulating factor.

cancer patients in a phase I trial of this agent (13,14). A phase II study of this compound, in combination with doxorubicin, cisplatin, and radiation therapy in newly diagnosed patients with regionally advanced anaplastic thyroid cancer, is underway (see Table 3).

Depsipeptide

Depsipeptide (NSC 630176, FR901228) is an histamine deactylase inhibitor with potent cytotoxic activity against human tumor cell lines and xenografts (15). This drug is a P-glycoprotein substrate. In a current phase I trial at the National Cancer Institute, the drug was active against cutaneous T-cell lymphoma when given as a 4-h infusion on days 1 and 5 of a 21-d cycle, with a maximum tolerated dose of 17.8 mg/m^2. Dose-limiting toxicities were fatigue, nausea and/or vomiting, and thrombocytopenia (16). The in vitro activity of this agent against anaplastic thyroid cancer cell lines and tumor xenografts has led to a phase II study at Memorial Sloan-Kettering Cancer Center. This trial (Table 3) is open to patients with progressive, recurrent, and/or metastatic nonmedullary thyroid cancer, refractory to radioiodine.

NEW CLINICAL TRIALS

Rapid expansion of knowledge regarding genetic mutations, aberrant gene products and expression, altered signaling pathways, and tumor growth mechanisms (e.g., neoangiogenesis) have presented numerous new drug targets for treatment of advanced thyroid cancers. A multitude of new agents currently in preclinical testing will yield several agents each year that are suitable for phase I clinical trials. Agents with preclinical evidence of efficacy and acceptable toxicity in phase I studies will move on to phase II efficacy clinical trials. Table 2 lists new drugs that are potentially applicable to treatment of advanced thyroid cancers. Some, such as the TKI imatinib mesylate, are specific to a single histologic type, MTC. Others are to be tested against a spectrum of differentiated and anaplastic thyroid cancers. Table 3 lists "current" phase I and II clinical trials in thyroid cancer, obtained from the National Cancer Institute. For a continuing updated list of thyroid cancer clinical trials, the reader is directed to *www.cancer.gov* and *www.clinicaltrials.gov*. For recent abstracts of preclinical and clinical studies in progress, the research meeting proceedings of American Association for Cancer Research can be searched at www.aacr.org and for the American Society of Clinical Oncology, www.asco.org.

REFERENCES

1. Burman KD. A new paradigm in the treatment of carcinoma: specific molecular targeting. Endocrinology 2004; 145:1027–1030.
2. Massart C, Gibassier J, Raoul M, et al. Cyclosporin A, verapamil and S9788 reverse doxorubicin resistance in a human medullary thyroid carcinoma cell line. Anticancer Drugs 1995; 6:135–146.
3. Braga-Basaria M, Ringel MD. Clinical review 158: Beyond radioiodine: a review of potential new therapeutic approaches for thyroid cancer. J Clin Endocrinol Metab 2003; 88:1947–1960.
4. Santini F, Bottici V, Elisei R, et al. Cytotoxic effects of carboplatinum and epirubicin in the setting of an elevated serum thyrotropin for advanced poorly differentiated thyroid cancer. J Clin Endocrinol Metab 2002; 87:4160–4165.
5. Stassi G, Todaro M, Zerilli M, et al. Thyroid cancer resistance to chemotherapeutic drugs via autocrine production of interleukin-4 and Interleukin-10[1]. Cancer Res 2003; 63:6784–6790.
6. Moley JF. Medullary thyroid carcinoma. Curr Treat Options Oncol 2003; 4:339–347.
7. Skinner MA, Safford SD, Freemerman AJ. RET tyrosine kinase and medullary thyroid cells are unaffected clinical doses of ST1571. Anticancer Res 2003; 23: 3601–3606.
8. Schoenberger J, Grimm D, Kossmehl P, et al. Effects of PTK787/ZK222584, a tyrosine kinase inhibitor, on the growth of poorly differentiated thyroid carcinoma: an animal study. Endocrinology 2004; 145:1031–1038.
9. Xu G, Pan J, Martin C, Yeung SC. Angiogenesis inhibition in the in vivo antineoplastic effect of manumycin and paclitaxel against anaplastic thyroid carcinoma. J Clin Endocrinol Metab 2001; 86: 1769–1777.
10. Yeung SC, Xu G, Pan J, et al. Manumycin enhances the cytotoxic effect of paclitaxel on anaplastic thyroid carcinoma cells. Cancer Res 2000; 60:650–656.
11. Dziba JM, Marcinek R, Venkataraman G, et al. Combretastatin A4 phosphate has primary antineoplastic activity against human anaplastic thyroid carcinoma cell lines and xenograft tumors. Thyroid 2002; 12:1063–1070.
12. Nelkin BD, Ball DW. Combretastatin A-4 and doxorubicin combination treatment is effective in a preclinical model of human medullary thyroid carcinoma. Oncol Rep 2001; 8:157–160.
13. Dowlati A, Robertson K, Cooney M, et al. A phase I pharmacokinetic and translational study of the novel vascular targeting agent combretastatin A-4 phosphate on a single-dose intravenous schedule in patients with advanced cancer. Cancer Res 2002; 62:3408–3416.
14. Cooney MM, Radivoyevitch T, Dowlati A, et al. Cardiovascular safety profile of combretastatin A4 phosphate in a single-dose phase I study in patients with advanced cancer. Clin Cancer Res 2004; 10:96–100.
15. Ueda H, Nakajima H, Hori Y, et al. FR901228, a novel antitumor bicyclic depsipeptide produced by Chromobacterium violaceum No. 968. I. Taxonomy, fermentation, isolation, physico-chemical and biological properties, and antitumor activity. J Antibiot (Tokyo) 1994; 47:301–310.
16. Marshall JL, Rizvi N, Kauh J, et al. A phase I trial of depsipeptide (FR901228) in patients with advanced cancer. J Exp Ther Oncol 2002; 2:325–332.
17. Celano M, Calvagno MG, Bulotta S, et al. Cytotoxic effects of gemcitabine-loaded liposomes in human anaplastic thyroid carcinoma cells. BMC Cancer 2004; 4:63.
18. Ringel MD, Greenberg J, Chen X, et al. Cytotoxic activity of 2'2'-difluorodeoxycytidine (gemcitabine) in poorly differentiated thyroid carcinoma cells. Thyroid 2000; 10:865–869.
19. Kaczirek K, Schindl M, Weinhausel A, et al. Cytotoxic activity of camptothecin and paclitaxel in newly established continuous human medually thyroid carcinoma cell lines. J Clin Endocrinol Metab 2004; 89:2397–2401.

Part XI
Resources for Patients with Thyroid Cancer

88
Low Iodine Diets

Kenneth D. Burman

INTRODUCTION

In patients with thyroid cancer, radioactive iodine scans and treatment must be performed in conjunction with thyrotropin (TSH) stimulation *(1–5)*. Classically, serum TSH elevations and stimulation of thyroid cells by TSH have been achieved by withdrawing the patient from thyroid hormone supplementation, thereby allowing the patient to become hypothyroid. Alternatively, TSH elevations can be accomplished by the administration of recombinant human TSH *(4)*. Regardless of the method, to maximize efficacy, it is important that the accompanying radioactive iodine scan (or treatment) be performed when the patient's total-body iodine stores are relatively depleted *(6–8)*.

Administered radioactive iodine competes with the unlabeled serum iodine concentrations for available sites in thyroid follicular cells by affecting iodide uptake and transport by the sodium-iodide symporter (NIS). Consequently, as the competition provided by unlabeled iodine in the serum decreases, the transport of radioiodine and avidity of the thyroid tissue for the radioactive iodine increases *(9–16)*. Also, a general principle is that unlabeled ^{127}I (naturally occurring) and labeled radioactive iodine (^{123}I or ^{131}I) are handled identically by the body and thyroid tissue. In the starkest example, administration of a radiocontrast agent that contains a large amount of unlabeled iodine can provide such an excess of iodine that the ability of thyroid tissue to trap radioactive iodine is compromised to less than 1%. The mechanism of this decreased radioactive iodine uptake is thought mainly to be related to downregulation of NIS but is also related to the competition of both labeled and unlabeled iodine for the thyroid NIS *(9–16)*.

In contrast, decreased iodine stores in the body and lowered serum iodine are thought to enhance the action of NIS. This principle lies at the center of the rationale for low iodine diets. This belief, yet unproven, is that a low iodine diet can benefit ultimate outcome and prognosis in relation to increasing thyroidal radioiodine uptake and improving the long-term effect of radiation on residual thyroid tissue. This rule guides most centers managing patients with thyroid cancer to recommend that patients undergoing diagnostic radioiodine scans or treatment adhere to a low iodine diet for at least 2 wk prior to study.

IODINE METABOLISM

Iodine* is a chemical element found in a wide variety of foods and chemical agents (e.g., radiocontrast dye). The nonradioactive form of iodine has a molecular weight of 127 (i.e., ^{127}I), and the most common radioisotopes in clinical use are ^{123}I and ^{131}I, with the former used only for diagnostic purposes and the latter for both diagnosis and treatment.

In normal subjects, dietary iodine is absorbed through the small intestine and transported in the plasma to the thyroid, where it is concentrated, oxidized, and then incorporated into thyroglobulin as thyroxine (T4), tri-iodothyronine (T3), and inactive lesser iodinated analogs. When the stored thyroid hormones are needed, partly under the influence of TSH stimulation, thyroglobulin is subjected to proteolysis, and the stored thyroid hormones are then released. Following secretion into the blood, the predominant thyroid hormones, T4 and T3, are deiodinated by specific enzymes located mainly in the liver and kidney; thus, free iodine is released. Serum iodine is then passively filtered through the kidney, where it is excreted. Under normal conditions, the thyroid gland traps about 10–30% of the iodine that is available, and the normal thyroid gland contains approx 5–10 mg of iodine, most of which is stored, as noted in colloid (i.e., in thyroglobulin) as T4 and T3.

As described, the thyroid gland avidly traps iodine because of the presence of NIS, and a small amount of iodine is similarly trapped by the salivary glands. The kidneys passively filter and excrete the iodine in the blood; the breasts trap and secrete a small amount of iodine, especially during lactation

---

*Throughout this chapter iodine and iodide are used interchangeably although in vivo there are differences in their activities.

(9–16). Renal excretion varies with filtered load and reflects 97% of dietary intake, with less than about 3% excreted in the stool. Renal iodide is passively reabsorbed and depends on the glomerular filtration rate. Patients with significant renal disease excrete less iodine in their urine.

The protein responsible for iodide transport, NIS, is located at the basolateral plasma membrane of thyrocytes. TSH and iodine deficiency upregulate NIS, and iodine excess suppresses it (9–11,14–18).

In subjects with an intact thyroid gland, excess iodine can cause hyperthyroidism (primarily in the setting of underlying autonomous function, as in Graves' disease or toxic nodular disease), and deficient iodine exposure can cause goiters and hypothyroidism. The range of iodine intake that may be related to thyroid dysfunction is highly variable and partially depends on genetic factors.

The National Health and Nutrition Examination Surveys (NHANES III) demonstrated that the median national urinary iodine excretion in the United States in samples collected between 1988 and 1994 was 145 µg/L. Iodine intake had been higher in the previous decades. The median urine excretion in men was 160 µg/L and in women, 130 µg/L. Less than 50 µg/L of iodine was excreted by 8.1% of men and 15.1% of women. For women of childbearing age (14–44 yr), urinary iodine concentration in the 2.5–97.5 percentiles was 18–650 µg/L. For pregnant women, the range was 42–550 µg/L (19–22). The iodine content in the US diet varies based on various nonmedical reasons. Iodine content in various foods changes periodically based on commercial reasons, and the consumer is largely unable to track these changes.

THYROID CANCER

When patients with thyroid cancer are prepared for ^{131}I therapy, they have already had most or all of their thyroid gland removed surgically, and their 24-h radioactive iodine uptake typically ranges from approx 0.1% to 10% (2,5,23). As noted above, there is a virtual equilibrium between the amounts of nonradioactive iodine ingested daily in food, drink, and other exogenous sources and that ultimately excreted in the urine per day. Therefore, measuring urine iodine content can accurately reflect what the dietary consumption has been for the previous time period, probably about 7–14 d. Either the 24-h urine iodine can be measured, or a random urine sample can be assessed with the urine concentration estimated by conversion to microgram per liter. This latter measurement is adequate (and much easier) for thyroid cancer patients because only an estimate is needed, and most patients excrete about 1 L of urine daily. Typically, the urine iodine excretion is expressed per gram of urine creatinine. In customary circumstances, every thyroid cancer patient prepared for a radioactive scan and/or treatment should have a urine iodine measurement to ensure the subsequent radioactive iodine therapy will be administered under optimal conditions. Adherence to a low iodine diet for about 2 wk can decrease the urine iodine concentration to less than 200 µg/L and possibly even less than 50 µg/L.

Iodine exists ubiquitously in the environment in food, water, chemicals, and medications. Significant iodine deficiency that lasts for several months may cause goiter and/or hypothyroidism, especially in individuals with underlying autoimmune thyroid disease (24–27). If newborns are born to mothers with significant iodine deficiency, the neonates may display goiters and profound hypothyroidism, including mental retardation (28–32). The minimum daily requirement for iodine has been set at 150 µg/d for those living in the United States; however, pregnant and lactating women should probably increase their intake further to at least 220 and 290 µg/d, respectively. However, in select circumstances, such as preparation for ^{131}I scan and/or therapy in a thyroid cancer patient, judicious use of a low iodine diet for a short period of time is not considered detrimental. Of course, the issue of iodine deficiency is not relevant to the thyroid cancer patient who no longer has a thyroid gland and is taking exogenous thyroid hormone.

IODINE SOURCES

Amiodarone is an antiarrhythmic agent widely used in both Europe and the United States (33). The drug contains 37.2% iodine and is typically prescribed in doses of 300–1200 mg/d, providing 100–400 mg of iodine and an estimated 900 µg of free iodide. In the setting of iodine-induced thyroid disease or to reduce iodine intake to facilitate scanning and therapy, the drug usually cannot be discontinued because of medical reasons. Amiodarone therapy will completely abrogate the ability to treat a patient with radioactive iodine. In fact, even if it can be stopped, it takes months or years for the urine iodine to decrease sufficiently to allow radioactive iodine therapy. Radioactivity should not be administered to pregnant or lactating women.

Additionally, the various intravenous contrast dyes contain significant amounts of iodine and should be avoided for at least 6–8 wk prior to starting a low iodine diet (34–37). Radiocontrast dyes contain approximately 180,000–320,000 µg of iodine. The majority of this iodine is organic iodine, but significant quantities of free iodide are present or are released via hepatic deiodination and generation of free iodide.

It is unknown how long it takes to dissipate this iodine following radiocontrast dye administration or ingestion. In individuals with normal renal function, it probably requires about 4–8 wk, but this issue has not been adequately studied. The most practical manner to ensure the body's iodine stores are decreased is to assess urine iodine content. The usual contrast agent employed for magnetic resonance imaging (e.g., gadolinium) does not contain iodine.

Table 1
Common Sources of Iodine in North America

Dietary iodine	Daily intake (µg)
Dairy products	52
Grains	78
Meat	31
Mixed dishes	26
Vegetables	20
Desserts	20
Eggs	10
Iodized salt	380

Table 2
General Food Types to Avoid or Use When Adhering to a Low Iodine Diet

Food Items	Avoid	Permitted
Drinks	Soda, hot chocolate, and vegetable juices	Coffee, tea, and other juices
Breads	Commercial pastries, breads, and dough	Homemade pastries prepared properly
Meat	Canned and processed meats and dinners	Fresh unsalted meat
Fruits	Canned or preserved fruits	Fresh fruits
Vegetables	Canned or frozen vegetables	Fresh vegetables
Cereals	Dry or hot cereals	Puffed wheat and rice
Dairy products	Eggs and cream	Milk, yogurt, and nondairy creamer
Spices	Pickles, soy sauce, mustard, and ketchup	Nonpreserved herbs and spices

Taken from ref. 5.

A wide variety of other substances contain significant iodine, such as medication pills or tablets coated with red dye. It is important to examine the contents of food and medications to determine if that particular agent contains considerable amounts of iodine. Common iodide-containing drugs are listed in Tables 1–3. Antitussives contain 15–325 mg of iodine per teaspoon and may provide about 90–3900 mg per day. Patients should also be asked whether they are taking any so-called "alternative" medications that may contain iodine and multivitamins, which are often supplemented with iodine.

Iodochlorhydroxyquin may be contained in topical antifungal and bacteriostatic creams or solutions. Povidone-iodine solution (Betadine) is commonly used as a topical antiseptic. High blood iodide levels have been reported following topical and intravaginal application of Povidone. Antiamebic drugs with the active compound iodoquinol contain organic iodine. In typical dosages, they provide 19.5 mg of iodine daily, usually for a 20-d course.

LOW IODINE DIET

The types of food to avoid include iodized salt and processed, packaged, or preserved canned foods (6–8) (Table 2). Salt, *per se*, does not have to be avoided. Only iodized salt, and noniodized salt is readily available in most food stores. It is critically important that the patient read all food labels to avoid those that contain iodized salt. Even water may contain iodine, as it is known to be bacteriocidal and added to water in the US public park system; distilled water is therefore most desirable. Potassium iodate is commonly used in flour as a dough conditioner or preservative and pastry food or mixes should also be avoided. Unsalted butter or margarine is also preferable. Even fresh fish may contain large amounts of iodine, and kelp (seaweed) should definitely be avoided. Dairy products, particularly milk, may contain significant quantities of iodine, possibly because of the use of iodophors used in the procurement process or iodine antisepsis of dairy farm equipment.

Table 3
Iodine Content of Radiocontrast Dyes and Medications

Substance	Iodine Content	Usual Dose	Total Dose of Iodine (mg)
Radiologic contrast dyes			
Cholecystographic dyes			
Iopanoate, ipodate, tyropanoate, iodoxamate	55–70%	3–9 g	1650–6300
Diatrizoate, iodamide, iothalamate	45–60%	1–70 g	450–4200
Lymphangiographic dye			
Lipiodol (iodized poppyseed oil)	45–60%	1–70 g	450–4200
Myelographic dye			
Metrizamide	48%	5–15 mL	1100–3000
Iodide containing drugs			
Oral agents			
Amiodarone	75 mg/200-mg tablet	300–1200 mg/d (initial)	75–300/d
Benziodarone	49 mg/100-mg tablet	100–200 mg/d	49–98/d
Iodine-containing cough medications	15–325 mg/teaspoon	1–2 teaspoon/q4h	90–3900/d
Potassium iodide			
Calcium iodide			
Iodinate glycerol			
Iodochlorhydroxyquin (antiamebic)	104 mg/tablet	600–650 mg tid × 20 d	312/d
Iodine-containing vitamins (prenatal vitamins)	0.15 mg/tablet	1/d	0.15/d
Quadrinal (KI)	320 mg/tablet 160 mg/5 mL	1 tablet qid or 10 mL q4h	1280–1920/d
Kelp tablets	0.15 mg/tablet	1 or more/d	≥0.15/d
Antithyroidal preparations			
Lugol solution	8.4 mg/drop*	15 drops qid	378/d*
SSKI	38 mg/drop*	5 drops qid	760/d*
Topical iodine preparations			
Iodohydroxyquinolone	12 mg/g	4 g/d	4800/d
Povidone-iodine (Betadine)	10 mg/mL	Variable	
Ophthalmic solution			
Echothiophate iodide	5–40 µg/drop*	2 drops qid	0.40–0.320/d*
Idoxuridine solution	18 µg/drop*	2 drops qid	0.144/d*

*Varies according to drop size. Taken from ref. 38.

There are multiple appropriate methods to employ a low iodine diet prior to radioiodine scan and/or treatment. We generally initiate the low iodine diet approximately 2 wk prior to the diagnostic scan and continue until 1–2 d after the radioiodine treatment.

With the advent of the ability to perform diagnostic scans or therapies with recombinant human TSH stimulation, rather than after T4 withdrawal, the issue of iodine contained within the L-T4 molecule arose. Thus, the patients will be continuing to take exogenous L-T4 with its significant iodine content during a thyrogen-stimulated radioiodine scan or treatment. The iodine generated from the T4 therapy constitutes an added burden (Table 3). Consequently, it is strongly urged that these patients maintain a low iodine diet prior to their isotopic studies. L-T4 contains approx 66% iodine, and if a patient takes 150 µg L-T4 daily, then this medication will contribute about 100 µg of iodine intake, in addition to that from dietary intake. Therefore, patients taking L-T4 therapy while maintaining a low iodine diet will necessarily have a higher iodine intake than if they showed similar dietary adherence in preparation for a withdrawal scan. Another option is to switch the patients from T4 to T3 (which contains one less iodine molecule) during the interval for the scan and/or therapy. In either case, the amount of iodine provided by the thyroid hormone, together with that in a strict low iodine diet (39), will still be relatively low, and the radioactive iodine scan and treatment should be effective. We typically continue the patient on levothyroxine therapy during recombinant human TSH stimulation without switching to triiodothyronine.

In summary, adherence to a low iodine diet seems prudent for a thyroid cancer patient being prepared for radioiodine scan and treatment. Further studies are needed that assess the efficacy of these recommendations, with a focus on the optimal goal of 24-h iodine intake, as expressed by urine measurements.

REFERENCES

1. Haugen BR, Pacini F, Reiners C, et al. A comparison of recombinant human thyrotropin and thyroid hormone withdrawal for the detection of thyroid remnant or cancer. J Clin Endocrinol Metab 1999; 84: 3877–3885.
2. Mazzaferri EL, Jhiang SM. Long-term impact of initial surgical and medical therapy on papillary and follicular thyroid cancer. Am J Med 1994; 97:418–428.
3. Bal C, Padhy AK, Jana S, et al. Prospective randomized clinical trial to evaluate the optimal dose of 131 I for remnant ablation in patients with differentiated thyroid carcinoma. Cancer 1996; 77:2574–2780.
4. Ladenson PW, Braverman LE, Mazzaferri EL, et al. Comparison of administration of recombinant human thyrotropin with withdrawal of thyroid hormone for radioactive iodine scanning in patients with thyroid carcinoma. N Engl J Med 1997; 337:888–896.
5. Burman KD. Low iodine diet. In Van Nostrand D, Bloom G, Wartsofsky L, editors. Thyroid Cancer: A Guide for Patients. Baltimore, MD: Keystone Press, Inc., 2004:83–88.
6. Ain KB, Dewitt PA, Gardner TG, Berryman SW. Low-iodine tube-feeding diet for iodine-131 scanning and therapy. Clin Nucl Med 1994; 19:504–507.
7. Maxon HR, Thomas SR, Boehringer A, et al. Low iodine diet in I-131 ablation of thyroid remnants. Clin Nucl Med 1983; 8:123–126.
8. Goslings BM. Proceedings: Effect of a low iodine diet on 131-I therapy in follicular thyroid carcinomata. J Endocrinol 1975; 64:30P.
9. Baker CH, Morris JC. The sodium-iodide symporter. Curr Drug Targets Immune Endocr Metabol Disord 2004; 4:167–174.
10. Haberkorn U, Beuter P, Kubler W, et al. Iodide kinetics and dosimetry in vivo after transfer of the human sodium iodide symporter gene in rat thyroid carcinoma cells. J Nucl Med 2004; 45:827–833.
11. Ward LS, Santarosa PL, Granja F, et al. Low expression of sodium iodide symporter identifies aggressive thyroid tumors. Cancer Lett 2003; 200:85–91.
12. Rudnicka L, Sinczak A, Szybinski P, et al. Expression of the Na(+)/I(−) symporter in invasive ductal breast cancer. Folia Histochem Cytobiol 2003; 41:37–40.
13. Upadhyay G, Singh R, Agarwal G, et al. Functional expression of sodium iodide symporter (NIS) in human breast cancer tissue. Breast Cancer Res Treat 2003; 77:157–165.
14. Dohan O, De la Vieja A, Paroder V, et al. The sodium/iodide Symporter (NIS): characterization, regulation, and medical significance. Endocr Rev 2003; 24:48–77.
15. Wagner S, Aust G, Schott M, et al. Regulation of sodium-iodide-symporter gene expression in human thyrocytes measured by real-time polymerase chain reaction. Exp Clin Endocrinol Diabetes 2002; 110: 398–402.
16. Smyth PP, Dwyer RM. The sodium iodide symporter and thyroid disease. Clin Endocrinol (Oxf) 2002; 56:427–429.
17. Lacroix L, Pourcher T, Magnon C, et al. Expression of the apical iodide transporter in human thyroid tissues: a comparison study with other iodide transporters. J Clin Endocrinol Metab 2004; 89:1423–1428.
18. Smit JW, Schroder-van der Elst JP, Karperien M, et al. Iodide kinetics and experimental (131)I therapy in a xenotransplanted human sodium-iodide symporter-transfected human follicular thyroid carcinoma cell line. J Clin Endocrinol Metab 2002; 87:1247–1253.
19. Hollowell JG, Staehling NW, Flanders WD, et al. Serum TSH, T(4), and thyroid antibodies in the United States population (1988 to 1994): National Health and Nutrition Examination Survey (NHANES III). J Clin Endocrinol Metab 2002; 87:489–499.
20. Hollowell JG, Staehling NW, Hannon WH, et al. Iodine nutrition in the United States. Trends and public health implications: iodine excretion data from National Health and Nutrition Examination Surveys I and III (1971–1974 and 1988–1994). J Clin Endocrinol Metab 1998; 83:3401–3408.
21. Oddie TH, Fisher DA, McConahey WM, Thompson CS. Iodine intake in the United States: a reassessment. J Clin Endocrinol Metab 1970; 30: 659–665.
22. Soldin OP, Soldin SJ, Pezzullo JC. Urinary iodine percentile ranges in the United States. Clin Chim Acta 2003; 328:185–190.
23. Mazzaferri EL, Jhiang SM. Differentiated thyroid cancer long-term impact of initial therapy. Trans Am Clin Climatol Assoc 1994; 106: 151–168; discussion 168–170.
24. Heinisch M, Kumnig G, Asbock D, et al. Goiter prevalence and urinary iodide excretion in a formerly iodine-deficient region after introduction of statutory Iodization of common salt. Thyroid 2002; 12: 809–814.
25. Azizi F, Navai L, Fattahi F. Goiter prevalence, urinary iodine excretion, thyroid function and anti-thyroid function and anti-thyroid antibodies after 12 years of salt iodization in Shahriar, Iran. Int J Vitam Nutr Res 2002; 72:291–295.
26. Wu T, Liu GJ, Li P, Clar C. Iodised salt for preventing iodine deficiency disorders. Cochrane Database Syst Rev 2002:CD003204.
27. Zimmermann MB, Hess S, Zeder C, Hurrell RF. Urinary iodine concentrations in swiss schoolchildren from the Zurich area and the Engadine valley. Schweiz Med Wochenschr 1998; 128:770–774.
28. Delange F, Wolff P, Gnat D, et al. Iodine deficiency during infancy and early childhood in Belgium: does it pose a risk to brain development? Eur J Pediatr 2001; 160:251–254.
29. Klett M, Ohlig M, Manz F, et al. Effect of iodine supply on neonatal thyroid volume and TSH. Acta Paediatr Suppl 1999; 88:18–20.
30. Liesenkotter KP, Gopel W, Bogner U, et al. Earliest prevention of endemic goiter by iodine supplementation during pregnancy. Eur J Endocrinol 1996; 134:443–448.
31. Glinoer D, De Nayer P, Delange F, et al. A randomized trial for the treatment of mild iodine deficiency during pregnancy: maternal and neonatal effects. J Clin Endocrinol Metab 1995; 80:258–269.
32. Delange F. The disorders induced by iodine deficiency. Thyroid 1994;4:107–128.
33. Bartalena L, Brogioni S, Grasso L, et al. Treatment of amiodarone-induced thyrotoxicosis, a difficult challenge: results of a prospective study. J Clin Endocrinol Metab 1996;81:2930–2933.
34. Henzen C, Buess M, Brander L. Iodine-induced hyperthyroidism (iodine-induced Basedow's disease): a current disease picture. Schweiz Med Wochenschr 1999; 129:658–664.
35. Kamel N, Uysal AR, Kologlu S, et al. Sodium ipodate in the treatment of toxic diffuse goiter. Short-term and long-term effects on thyrotoxicosis. Endocrinologie 1988; 26:99–105.
36. Laurberg P. Multisite inhibition by ipodate of iodothyronine secretion from perfused dog thyroid lobes. Endocrinology 1985; 117: 1639–1644.
37. Laurberg P. The effect of some iodine-containing radiocontrast agents on iodothyronine secretion from the perfused canine thyroid. Endocrinology 1982; 111:1904–1908.
38. Nuovo J, Wartofsky L. Iodine induced thyroid disease. In Principles and Practice of Endocrinology and Metabolism, 3rd ed. Becker KL, editor. Philadelphia, PA: Lippincott Williams and Wilkins; 2002.
39. Pearce EN, Pino S, He X, Bazrafshan HR, Lee SL, Braverman LE. Sources of dietary iodine: bread, cow's milk, and infant formula in the Boston area. J Clinic Endocrinol Metab 2004; 89:3421–3424.

89
Appendix A
Books and Manuals

Thyroid Cancer. Biersack HJ, Grunwald F. New York: Springer Verlag, 2005, 2nd Edition.

Thyroid Cancer: Diagnosis and Treatment. Clark OH, Noguchi S. Quality Medical Publishing, 2000.

Thyroid Cancer. Fagin JA. Springer, New York, 1998.

Werner and Ingbar's The Thyroid: A Fundamental and Clinical Text. Braverman LE, Utiger RD. Philadelphia: J. B. Lippincott, 2005, 9th Edition.

Thyroid Disease: The Facts. 3rd ed. Tunbridge WMG, Bayliss RIS. Oxford University Press, New York, NY, 1999.

Radiation Oncology. Cox J, Ang K. St. Louis, MO: C.B. Mosby, 2003.

Cancer: Principles and Practice of Oncology. DeVita Jr VT, Hellman S, Rosenberg SA. Philadelphia, PA: Lippincott Williams & Wilkins 2005, 7th Edition.

PUBLICATIONS FOR PATIENTS, FAMILY, AND FRIENDS

Thyroid Cancer: A Guide for Patients. Van Nostrand D, Bloom G, Wartofsky L, editors. Baltimore, MD: Keystone Press, 2004. Available through ThyCA (www.thyca.org) and all major book stores.

Collection of Low-Iodine Recipes. Guljord L, editor. ThyCa: Thyroid Cancer Survivors' Association, Inc., 4th edition, 2003. Communication information located in Appendix A.

Light of Life Foundation Cookbook. Communication information located in Appendix B.

What You Need to Know About Thyroid Cancer. Online pamphlet available at: www.cancer.gov/cancerinfo/wyntk/thyroid.

The Official Patient's Sourcebook on Thyroid Cancer. A reference manual for self-directed patient research. Parker JN, Parker PM. San Diego, CA: ICON Health Publishers, 2002.

The Thyroid, Cancer and You. Wolfe A. Xlibrus Corp, 2003 (www.xlibrus.com).

Thyroid for Dummies. Rubin A. New York, NY: Hungry Minds, Inc., 2001.

Your Thyroid: A Home Reference. Wood LC, Cooper DS, Ridgway EC. Ballantine Books, Boston, MA, 1996.

The Thyroid Cancer Book. Rosenthal S. St. Victoria, B.C.: Traffor Publishing, 2002.

The Thyroid Sourcebook for Woman. Rosenthal S. Lowell House, Lincolnwood, IL 1999.

The Thyroid Sourcebook: Everything You Need to Know. Rosenthal S, Volpe R. Lincolnwood, IL: Lowell House, 1998.

How Your Thyroid Works. Baskin JH. Adams Press, 1995. Out of print.

Could It Be My Thyroid? Rubenfeld S. Sheldon Rubenfeld Publisher, Houston, TX, 2003.

The Thyroid Guide. Ditkoff BA, Lo Gerfo PL. Harper Perennial, New York, NY, 2000.

The Thyroid Book: What Goes Wrong and How to Treat It. Surks MI. Consumer Reports Books, Yonkers, NY: 1993. Out of print.

The Thyroid Gland: A Book for Thyroid Patients. Hamburger J. Privately published, 1991.

21st Century Complete Medical Guide to Thyroid Cancer. Authoritative Federal Government Documents, Clinical References, and Practice Information for Patients and Physicians, CD rom, PM Medical Health News. This is a CD rom of official public domain US federal government files, much of which is already available free through the federal government at www.cancer.gov and other websites noted in Appendix B.

The Harvard Medical School Guide to Overcoming Thyroid Problems. Garber JR, McGraw-Hill, New York, 2005.

A large portion of this appendix was reproduced from *Thyroid Cancer: A Guide for Patients*, with permission from Keystone Press, Inc.

From: *Thyroid Cancer: A Comprehensive Guide to Clinical Management, 2/e*
Edited by: L. Wartofsky and D. Van Nostrand © Humana Press Inc., Totowa, NJ

90
Appendix B
Additional Sources of Information

THYROID AND/OR CANCER PROFESSIONAL ORGANIZATIONS

American Thyroid Association, Inc.: A professional medical society of physicians and scientists dedicated to the treatment and research of thyroid disease.
Address:
 6066 Leesburg Pike, Suite 550
 Falls Church, VA 22041
Communication data:
 Office: 703-998-8890
 For patients: 1-800-thyroid
 Fax: 703-998-8893
 E-mail: admin@thyroid.org
 Website: www.thyroid.org
Services:
 For general endocrinologist referrals and general thyroid information

American Association of Clinical Endocrinologists (AACE): This is a professional medical organization of more than 2500 clinical endocrinologists. The mission of the AACE is to (1) improve the care given to the endocrine patient; (2) increase the public's understanding of the function of a clinical endocrinologist; (3) increase the awareness of endocrine disease; and (4) to make available to patients the choice of care by a specialist trained in the treatment of endocrine disorders.
Address:
 1000 Riverside Ave., Suite 205
 Jacksonville, FL 32204
Communication data:
 Telephone: 904-353-7878
 Fax: 904-353-8185
 Website: www.aace.com
 To find an endocrinologist, go to www.aace.com/memsearch.php
 Clinical guidelines: www.aace.com/clin/guidelines/
 Radiation related terms and radiation risk: www.physics.isu.edu/radinf

Services:
 Find an endocrinologist
 Clinical guidelines
 Information on radiation related terms and radiation risk

The Endocrine Society
Address:
 8401 Connecticut Avenue, Suite 900
 Chevy Chase, MD 20815-5817
Communication data:
 Office: 301-941-0200
 Fax: 301-941-0259
 E-mail : endostaff@end-soc.org
 Website: www.endo-society.org
Service:
 The largest and most active professional organization of endocrinologists in the world. The Society is internationaly known as the leading source of state-of-the-art research and clinical advancements in endocrinology and metabolism. The Society is dedicated to promoting excellence in research, education and the care of patients with endocrine diseases such as thyroid cancer. The Society publishes four scientific journals and sponsors the largest and most comprehensive scientific meetings, workshops, and postgraduate courses on endocrine-related topics.

Thyroid Disease Manager: An up-to-date analysis of thyrotoxicosis, hypothyroidism, thyroid nodules, cancer, thyroiditis, and all aspects of human thyroid disease and thyroid physiology. It provides physicians, researchers, and trainees (as well as patients) around the world with an authoritative, current, complete, objective, free, and down-loadable source on the thyroid. This website contains a newly revised version of the textbook "The Thyroid and Its Diseases" and much supplementary information, all directed toward helping physicians care for their patients with thyroid problems. The website (www.thyroidmanager.org) is updated continually with important new information, and major revisions are done annually.
 Website: www.thyroidmanager.org

A large portion of this appendix was reproduced from *Thyroid Cancer: A Guide for Patients*, with permission from Keystone Press, Inc.

From: *Thyroid Cancer: A Comprehensive Guide to Clinical Management, 2/e*
Edited by: L. Wartofsky and D. Van Nostrand © Humana Press Inc., Totowa, NJ

Johns Hopkins Thyroid Tumor Center
  Communication data
    Website: www.thyroid-cancer.net
  Services:
    Find a thyroid cancer specialist near you
    Frequently asked questions
    Patient Tools

INFORMATION REGARDING CLINICAL TRIALS

National Institutes of Health (Developed by the National Library of Medicine): ClinicalTrials.gov provides regularly updated information about federally and privately supported clinical research in human volunteers. ClinicalTrials.gov gives you information about a trial's purpose, who may participate, locations, and phone numbers for more details.
  Website: www.clinicaltrials.gov

National Cancer Institute:
  Website: www.cancer.gov/search/clinical_trials/

PATIENT SUPPORT GROUPS AND INFORMATION SOURCES

The Hormone Foundation: The Hormone Foundation is an independent, nonprofit organization established by The Endocrine Society in 1997. Its mission is to serve as a resource for the public by promoting the prevention, treatment and cure of hormone-related conditions through public outreach and education. Through its public education campaigns, Web site, forums, media roundtables and publications, The Hormone Foundation is a leading source of hormone-related information for the public, physicians, allied health professionals and the media.
  Address:
    8401 Connecticut Avenue, Suite 900
    Chevy Chase, MD 20815-5817
  Communication data:
    Telephone: 1-800-HORMONE
    Website: www.hormone.org
  Services:
    Information on Clinical Trials
    Patient information factsheets and brochures
    Find an endocrinologist in your area; physician referral database

ThyCa: Thyroid Cancer Survivors' Association, Inc. (ThyCa): All volunteer, national, nonprofit organization of thyroid cancer survivors, family members, and health professionals advised by nationally recognized leaders in the field of thyroid cancer, dedicated to education, communication, and support for thyroid cancer survivors, families, and friends.
  Address:
    Box 1545
    New York, NY 10159-1545
  Communication data:
    Telephone: 1-877-588-7904 (toll free)
    Fax: 1-630-604-6078
    E-mail: thyca@thyca.org
    Website: www.thyca.org
  Services (more information available through the website or the above communication data):
    Local support groups coast to coast
    E-mail discussion groups
    Person-to-person support with toll-free survivors' telephone line
    Website with over 300 pages plus extensive links list
    Low iodine diet cookbook and other free publications
    Newsletter, which is free online
    National and regional conferences and workshops
    Thyroid cancer awareness materials
    Thyroid Cancer Awareness Week and Month
    Thyroid Cancer Research Funds

States with local ThyCa support groups are: Alabama, Arizona, California, Colorado, Connecticut, Delaware, District of Columbia, Florida, Georgia, Hawaii, Idaho, Illinois, Iowa, Kansas, Kentucky, Maryland, Massachusetts, Michigan, Minnesota, Missouri, Nebraska, New Hampshire, New Jersey, New York, North Carolina, Ohio, Pennsylvania, Rhode Island, Texas, Vermont, Virginia, Washington, and Wisconsin.

Canadian Thyroid Cancer Support Group (Thry'vors) Inc.: Formed by a group of Canadian thyroid cancer patients who came together in a common search for information and support in dealing with treatment, recovery, and long-term monitoring of thyroid cancer. Thry'vors offers information and support to those affected by thyroid cancer through our website at www.thryvors.org and through an Internet-based listserv. The listserv, available through yahoo.groups (full address below), allows thyroid cancer patients, regardless of whether they are newly diagnosed, on the road to recovery, or long-term survivors, as well as their caregivers, friends, or family, to give and receive emotional support. Here they can post messages, listen, ask questions, and/or exchange experiences and information with those who have "been there." Access to our listserv is through: groups.yahoo.com/group/Thryvors.
  Address:
    P.O. Box 23007
    550 Eglinton Ave. W.
    Toronto, ON M5N 3A8
  Communication data:
    Telephone: 416-487-8267 (during office hours only)
    E-mail: thryvors@sympatico.ca
    Website: www.thryvors.org
    groups.yahoo.com/group/Thryvors

Light of Life Foundation: This foundation improves the quality of life and promotes research and education about thyroid cancer.

Address:
P.O. Box 163
Manalapan, NJ 07726
Communication data:
Telephone: 1-877-565-6325
Fax: 732-536-4824
Website: www.checkyourneck.com
E-mail: info@checkyourneck.com

Thyroid Foundation of America: Provides health education and support to thyroid patients.
Address:
1 Longfellow Place, #1518
Boston, MA 02114
Communication data:
Telephone: 800-832-8321
Fax: 617-534-1515
E-mail: info@allthyroid.org
Website: www.allthyroid.org

Thyroid Foundation of Canada (TFC) La Fondation canadiennne de la Thyroide: The Thyroid Foundation of Canada is the oldest North American patient education association. The TFC promotes awareness and education about thyroid disease including thyroid cancer.
Address:
797 Princess Street, Suite 304
Kingston, Ontario, Canada, K7L-1G1
Communication data:
Office: 613-544-8364
1-800-267-8822
Fax: 613-544-9731
Website: www.thryoid.ca

American Foundation of Thyroid Patients
Address:
P.O. Box 4914
Odessa, TX 79760
Communication data:
Telephone: 432-694-9966
E-mail: thyroid@flash.net
Website: www.thyroidfoundation.org

Thyroid Federation International: A worldwide network of affiliated thyroid patient organizations.
Address:
797 Princess Street, Suite 304
Kingston, Ontario, Canada K7L-1G1
Communication data:
Telephone: +1-613-544-8364
Fax: +1-613-544-9731
E-mail: tfi@on.aibn.com
Website: www.thyroid-fed.org

American Cancer Society
Communication data:
Telephone: 1-800-ACS-2345
Website: www.cancer.org: Enter type of cancer or other. On next page click on thyroid carcinoma.
Information on cancer, employment, insurance, law, Americans with Disabilities Act, diet, vitamins/supplements, and complementary treatment approaches.

National Cancer Institute at the National Institutes of Health
Address:
31 Center Drive, MSC 2580
Bethesda, MD 20892-2580
Communication data:
Telephone: 800-4-Cancer (800-422-6237) or 301-496-4000, ext. 5803
Website: www.cancer.gov/cancerinfo
Click on "Types of Cancer." Under alphabetical list of cancers, click on "T." Then click on thyroid cancer.
Radiation Therapy Website: www.nci.nih.gov/cancerinfo/radiation-therapy-and-you.
Fax: 301-480-2321
E-mail: cancergovstaff@mail.nih.gov
Services:
Information on types of cancers, treatment, clinical trials, and research.

National Coalition for Cancer Survivorship: The oldest survivor-led advocacy organization working exclusively on behalf of people with all types of cancer and their families, is dedicated to assuring quality cancer care for all Americans.
Address:
1010 Wayne Avenue, Suite 770
Silver Spring, MD 20910
Communication data:
Office: 301-650-9127
Fax: 301-565-9670
E-mail: info@canceradvocacy.org
Website: www.canceradvocacy.org

COMMERCIAL ORGANIZATIONS

Genzyme Corporation (manufacturers of Thyrogen®)
Address:
500 Kendall Square
Cambridge, MA 02142
Communication data:
Telephone: 800-745-4447
Website: www.thyrogen.com
Information about Thyrogen:
Genzyme's Patient Information Kit provides understanding about Thyrogen.

Abbott Laboratories (manufacturers of Synthroid®)
Address:
Abbott Laboratories
Abbot Park, IL
Communication data:
Telephone for customer service: 800-255-5162.
Websites: www.abbott.com (general website for Abbot Laboratories), www.synthroid.com. The latter website has excellent information on Synthroid. This website has excellent addition information.

MISCELLANEOUS WEBSITES

American Cancer Society (ACS)	www.cancer.org
American Medical Association	www.ama-assn.org
Cancer.Gov	www.cancer.gov
Cancer Information Service (NIH)	http://cis.nci.nih.gov
Cancer Medicine Textbook (Holland and Frei)	www.hollandandfrei.com
Cancernetwork.com	www.cancernetwork.com
Centers for Disease Control and Prevention (CDC)	www.cdc.gov
Centers for Medicare and Medicaid Services (CMS)	cms.hhs.gov
Clinical Trials.gov	www.clinicaltrials.gov
Combined Health Information Database (CHID)	www.chid.nih.gov
Doctor's Guide	www.docguide.com
eMedguides.com	www.emedguides.com
eMedicine.com	www.emedicine.com
First Gov	www.firstgov.gov
Food and Drug Administration (FDA)	www.fda.gov
Health Finder	www.healthfinder.gov
Health.Gov	www.health.gov
HealthLinks	http://healthlinks.washington.edu
Health Resources and Services Administration (HRSA)	www.hrsa.gov
HealthWeb	healthweb.org
Medscape	www.medscape.com
Intelihealth	www.intelihealth.com
Martindale's Health Science Guide	www.martindalecenter.com
MedicineNet.com	www.medicinenet.com
Medline Plus	www.medlineplus.gov
MedNews	www.newswise.com/menu-med.htm
MedWeb	www.medweb.emory.edu/MedWeb
Merck Manual Home Edition Interactive Version	www.merck.com/immhe/index.html
Merck Manual of Diagnosis and Therapy	www.merck.com/pubs/mmanual
Merck Manual of Geriatrics	www.merck.com/pubs/mm_geriaterics/contents.html
National Center for Complementary and Alternative Medicine	nccam.nih.gov
National Health Information Center	www.health.gov/nhic
National Institutes of Health (NIH)	www.nih.gov
National Institute of Mental Health	www.nimh.nih.gov
National Library of Medicine	www.nlm.nih.gov
NCC Health	www.cnn.com/HEALTH
NIH Disease/Health Topic Index	www.nih.gov/health
Office of the Surgeon General	surgeongeneral.gov
OncoLink	www.oncolink.upenn.edu
PubMed	www.ncbi.nlm.nih.gov/entrez/query.fcgi
Reuters Health	www.reutershealth.com
Virtual Hospital	www.vh.org
WebMD	my.webmd.com
Women's Complete Healthbook—American Medical Women's Association	www.amwa-doc.org/publications/wchb/index.htm
Yahoo Health News	dailynews.yahoo.com/headlines/health

Appendix C

Forms and Instructions for Patients Treated with Radioactivity

John E. Glenn

The following four examples may be copied or adapted for your use when hospitalizing patients for radioactive iodine ablation or therapy.

EXAMPLE 1

Written Instructions for the Patient at Home

The main protection for family and friends is for you to avoid close contact for about 3 d after coming home.

There is one critical person who is at potential great risk of harm. Nursing an infant or small child after receiving radioactive iodine will transfer the radioactive iodine from the mother to the child in the milk. Radioactive iodine ingested by the child will expose the thyroid of the child to potentially harmful levels of radiation. Lifelong medication may be required to prevent serious effects, both mentally and physically, if the child's thyroid receives a high dose of radiation.

Although there is no evidence that the amount of radiation received by those people coming close to you will do detectable harm, it is reasonable to take certain precautions for at least 3 d following release.

Once you get home:

1. Keep a safe distance from other people.
   a. Sleep alone for three nights.
   b. Avoid kissing and sexual intercourse for 7 d.
   c. Minimize time in public places, including public transportation, theaters, and sporting events for 3 d. You can eat meals with your family during this time.
   d. Stay at least 3 ft away from people if you will be involved with them for more than 1 h in the first 3 d.
2. You may care for children during this time, but time spent holding a child on a lap or lying next to you should be minimized.
3. Breastfeeding must be avoided, because it could seriously harm the infant.
4. Wash hands frequently for several days. Sweat contains some minuscule amount of radioactive iodine.
5. Wash bed linens and clothes separately for 3 d. After 3 d, resume normal care.
6. Use a separate bathroom for 3 d, if possible. Urine contains excreted radioactive iodine. Flush twice when using the toilet. If separate facilities are not available, good hygiene habits are adequate to minimize exposure.

These guidelines will limit exposure to others far below acceptable levels. Radioactive iodine will disappear completely through your own body excretions and as part of the physical nature of radioactive decay. If you wish to be very cautious, maintain these restrictions for 7 d.

EXAMPLE 2

Information Concerning Your Hospitalization

1. There will be restrictions on visitors during your hospitalization. Minors (under age 18) and pregnant women will not be permitted to visit. All visits will be restricted to a few minutes, and persons must remain a marked distance away. You are encouraged to tell friends and family not to visit.
2. Any personal belongings that you bring will be checked for radioactive iodine before you leave. Belongings that cannot be cleaned to acceptable release levels, such as radios, magazines, books, and so on, may have to be held for you until the radioactive iodine has decayed. Therefore, you should not bring any belongings with you that you cannot afford to be without for possibly a few weeks.
3. Nurses will be able to provide medical care but will use gloves and shoe covers when entering your room.
4. Housekeeping will be limited in your room. Housekeeping personnel are not permitted to enter the room, and all items must be measured using radiation detection instruments before leaving the room.
5. You may use the toilet without concern about the radioactive iodine. Sit while using the toilet. All other normal sanitary practices should be followed. The toilet should be flushed three times with the lid down.

A large portion of this appendix was reproduced from *Thyroid Cancer: A Guide for Patients*, with permission from Keystone Press, Inc.

From: *Thyroid Cancer: A Comprehensive Guide to Clinical Management, 2/e*
Edited by: L. Wartofsky and D. Van Nostrand © Humana Press Inc., Totowa, NJ

EXAMPLE 3

Questionnaire Concerning Hospitalization for Patients Administered Radioactive Iodine

By answering the following questions and agreeing to follow the guidelines, you may be able to be released earlier because of your limited contact with other people.

1. Are you a woman nursing a small child or infant?

    Yes ____ No ____

    Note: Nursing an infant or small child after receiving radioactive iodine will transfer the radioactive iodine from the mother to the child through the milk. Radioactive iodine ingested by the child will expose the thyroid of the child to potentially harmful levels of radiation. Lifelong medication may be required to prevent serious effects both mentally and physically if the child's thyroid receives a high dose of radiation. **If you are nursing a child, inform Nuclear Medicine personnel, and your administration will be at a later date after you have permanently ceased nursing this child.**

2. Can you take care of yourself except for brief visits and not be in the same room with another person for more than 3 h total during each of the first 2 d?

    Yes ____ No ____

    If no, briefly explain circumstances: _____
    _____
    _____

3. Will you be able to maintain distance from other people, including:
    Sleeping alone for at least one night (recommend 3 nights)?
    Avoiding kissing and sexual intercourse for at least 3 d?
    Staying at least 3 ft away from people if you will be involved with them for more than 1 h a day in the first 3 d?

    Yes ____ No ____

    If no, briefly explain circumstances: _____
    _____
    _____

4. Will you avoid travel by airplane or mass transit for the first day?

    Yes ____ No ____

    If no, briefly explain circumstances: _____
    _____
    _____

5. Will you avoid prolonged travel in an automobile with others for the at least first 2 d?

    Yes ____ No ____

    If no, briefly explain circumstances: _____
    _____
    _____

6. Will you have sole use of a bathroom for at least 2 d?

    Yes ____ No ____

    If no, briefly explain circumstances: _____
    _____
    _____

I have read these guidelines, understand the instructions, and agree to avoid contacts in accordance with my answers to items 2 through 6. (*Note:* If you cannot manage at home and avoid close contact, it may be necessary for you to remain in the hospital up to an additional 24 h.)

Signature: _____   Date: _____

(Patient or other person in accordance with hospital informed consent policy.)

Appendix C

EXAMPLE 4

Worksheet to Determine Acceptable Dose Rates for Release of Patients Administered Radioactive Iodine

Regulatory Limit

10 CFR 35.75 permits release of patients if the total effective dose equivalent to any other individual from exposure to the released individual is not likely to exceed 0.5 rad.

Acceptable Methods

Acceptable methods are described in Regulatory Guide 8.39 *"Release Of Patients Administered Radioactive Materials."*

Calculations

Calculations will be based on Equation B-1 from Regulatory Guide 8.39.

$$D(t) = \frac{34.6 \, \Gamma Q_0 \, T_p \, E \, (1 - e^{-0.693 t/T_p})}{r^2}$$

where

$D(t)$ = Accumulated dose to time t, in rad.
34.6 = Conversion factor of 24 h/d times the total integration of decay (1.44).
Γ = Exposure rate constant for a point source, rad/mCi × h at 1 cm.
Q_0 = Initial activity at the start of the time interval.
T_p = Physical half-life in days.
E = Occupancy factor that accounts for different occupancy times and distances when an individual is around a patient.
r = Distance in centimeters. This value is typically 100 cm.
t = exposure time in days.

The dose rate in rad/h for the effective remaining activity Q_m at time t_m (when a measurement is made) is by the definition of Γ:

$$\frac{dD(t)}{dt} = \frac{\Gamma Q_m}{r^2} \quad \text{or} \quad Q_m = \frac{dD(t)}{dt} \times \frac{r^2}{\Gamma}$$

and since the dose to infinity after the dose rate measurement at time t_m is:

$$D_\infty = \frac{34.6 \, \Gamma \, Q_m \, T_p \, E \, (1 - 0)}{r^2}$$

Then $D_\infty = (dD/dt) * 34.6 * T_p * E$

For the purposes of this worksheet:

D_{max} = 500 mrad
T_p = 8.08 d
And the acceptable dose rate is therefore:

$dD/dt = 500/(34.6*8.08*E) = 1.79/E$ mrad/h

E = 0.25 or 0.125 depending on the patient circumstances.

Evaluation (Sign for the appropriate dose rate for this administration)

1. If the patient has not submitted information about possible contacts with other people, we can assume without further justification the occupancy factor is 0.25. [Reference: Regulatory Guide 8.39 "Release Of Patients Administered Radioactive Materials" and 10 CFR 35.75]

    E = 0.25. The measured dose rate at 1 m must be equal to or less than 1.79/0.25 = 7.1 millirad/h

    Signature of person making evaluation _____

EXAMPLE FOUR (continued)

2. If the patient has submitted information about possible contacts with other people and has answered yes to all questions 2–6 of the questionnaire, we can assume the occupancy factor is 0.125. [Reference: Section B.1.2, "Occupancy Factors To Consider for Patient-Specific Calculations," Regulatory Guide 8.39 *"Release Of Patients Administered Radioactive Materials."*]

   E = 0.125. The measured dose rate at 1 meter must be equal to or less than 1.79/0.125 = 14.3 mrad/h.

   Signature of person making evaluation _____

3. If the patient has submitted information about possible contacts with other people but has answered no to any of the questions 2–6 of the questionnaire, the Radiation Safety Officer will make the determination of acceptable dose rate. [Reference: Section B.1.2, Regulatory Guide 8.39 *"Release Of Patients Administered Radioactive Materials."*]

   The measured dose rate at 1 m must be equal to or less than ___ mrad/h
   Basis:
   _____
   _____
   _____

   Signature of person making evaluation _____

Index

A

Adenoma, thyroid, 563
Adhesion molecules, 24, 25
AEC, *see* Atomic Energy Commission
AGES system, thyroid cancer staging, 91
Akt
 therapeutic targeting, 668
 thyroid cancer role, 58
AMES system, thyroid cancer staging, 88
Amifostine, salivary gland protection in radioiodine therapy, 464
Amiodarone, iodine content, 678
Anaplastic thyroid cancer
 chemotherapy,
  combination with radiotherapy, 643, 644
  drug resistance, 644, 645
 classification, 629
 clinical presentation, 629, 630
 coexisting differentiated tumors, 629, 630
 computed tomography, 631
 diagnosis, 630, 631
 epidemiology, 629
 external beam radiation therapy, 641, 642
 histopathology, 629, 635, 636
 in children, 629, 630
 metastasis, 630
 p53 mutation, 49
 positron emission tomography, 631, 639, 640
 prognosis, 629, 635, 647, 648
 staging, 92, 647
 surgical management, 633, 634
Anger, H., nuclear medicine contributions, 123, 125
Angiogenesis
 growth factors, 19, 36, 50
 therapeutic targeting, 666, 667, 672, 673
Angiosarcoma, thyroid, 574
Apoptosis, 55–59
 cancer defects, 56
 morphological features, 55
 pathways, 19, 56
 suppressors, 56
 thyroid cancer,
  pathogenesis, 58, 59
  therapeutic targeting, 59, 60, 668
Atomic Energy Commission (AEC), historical perspective, 120, 121
Aurora B, 218

B

Bcl-2
 cell cycle regulation, 58
 expression in thyroid cancer, 86
Benua protocol, dosimetry
 advantages and limitations, 442
 data collection, 435, 436
 modifications, 436–439
Bernard, Claude, physiology contributions, 118
Bispecific antibodies, molecular imaging, 658
Bisphosphonates, bone metastasis management, 502, 503
Bladder cancer, radioiodine therapy risks, 479, 480
Bleomycin, thyroid cancer management, 492
Bone metastasis, 497–506
 age as prognostic factor, 498, 499
 arterial embolization, 501
 bisphosphonate therapy, 502, 503
 external beam radiation therapy, 501, 502
 frequency, 497, 498
 mechanisms, 503–505
 natural history, 499
 palliative therapy for spinal metastasis
  kyphoplasty, 511
  laser thermal ablation, 512
  radiofrequency ablation, 511, 512
  vertebroplasty, 511
 radioiodine scanning, 166
 radioiodine therapy
  bone marrow suppression,
   literature review, 473–476
   prevention, 476, 477
  outcomes, 415, 418–421, 500, 501
 recommendations for management, 505, 506
 resection, 501
 survival, 498
BRAF
 mutations in thyroid cancer, 16, 23, 44, 49
 pediatric thyroid cancer mutations, 34, 35

Index

therapeutic targeting, 668
thyroid nodule malignancy marker, 217
Brain metastasis, radioiodine scanning, 167
Breast cancer, radioiodine therapy risks, 480

C

Cadherin, *see* E-Cadherin
Calcitonin
   medullary thyroid cancer marker, 582, 583
   surveillance, 587
   testing, 583, 584
Capecitabine, thyroid cancer management, 493
Carboplatin, thyroid cancer management, 493
Carcinoembryonic antigen (CEA),
   surveillance, 587
   thyroid nodule malignancy marker, 203
   tumor marker applications, 518
Carney complex, 34, 98
Caspases and apoptosis, 56, 57
Cassen, Benedict, nuclear medicine contributions, 123
CD30, thyroid nodule malignancy marker, 218
CD44
   expression in thyroid cancer, 24, 25
   thyroid nodule malignancy marker, 215
CD97, thyroid nodule malignancy marker, 216
CEA, *see* Carcinoembryonic antigen
Cell cycle
   gene expression and repair, 41, 42
   mitosis versus meiosis, 41
   phases, 41
   regulation, 18, 19, 35, 41, 50
Cell signaling, *see* Signal transduction
Cell surface adhesion molecules, 24, 25
Ceruloplasmin, thyroid nodule malignancy marker, 218
Chemotherapy
   agents
      bleomycin, 492, 609
      capecitabine, 493
      carboplatin, 493
      cisplatin, 492
      combretastatin, 672
      depsipeptide, 673
      doxorubicin, 491, 609, 610
      epirubicin, 491
      etoposide, 492
      gemcitabine, 493
      irinotecan, 492, 493
      lovastatin, 58
      manumycin, 58, 672
      methotrexate, 493
      mitoxantrone, 491, 492
      octreotide, 610
      paclitaxel, 58
      topotecan, 492, 493
   anaplastic thyroid cancer
      apoptosis induction, 58–59
      combination with radiotherapy, 643, 644
      drug resistance, 644, 645
   external-beam radiation therapy combination, 494, 495
   future prospects, 671–674
   medullary thyroid cancer, 609, 610
   resistance mechanisms, 671
   salvage therapy in thyroid cancer, 491
   single modality treatment outcomes, 494
   thyroid lymphoma, 617
Chernobyl accident, *see* Radiation-induced thyroid cancer
Children, *see* Pediatric thyroid cancer
Cisplatin, thyroid cancer management, 492
CK19, thyroid nodule malignancy marker, 218
Classical pattern, papillary thyroid cancer, 263, 264
Classification, thyroid tumors, 85–86
Clear-cell papillary carcinoma, pathology, 268
Clinical trials
   classification, 665
   novel trials in thyroid cancer, 673, 674
   thyroid cancer resources, 685
Colorectal cancer, radioiodine therapy risks, 479
Columnar-cell carcinoma, papillary thyroid cancer
   clinical characteristics, 560
   demographics, 560
   pathology, 269
   prognosis, 560
   treatment, 560
Combretastatin A4 phosphate, angiogenesis inhibition, 667, 672, 673
Computed tomography (CT)
   ablation therapy guidance, 364, 365
   advantages and limitations in thyroid cancer, 360, 361
   anaplastic thyroid cancer, 631
   comparison with other imaging techniques, 238, 239, 241, 361, 362
   follow-up of thyroid cancer, 362
   indications, 230, 241
   medullary thyroid cancer surveillance, 587, 588
   neck anatomy, 359, 360

positron emission tomography combination, 319, 604, 657
post-therapy imaging, 363
preoperative staging of thyroid cancer, 363
principles, 360
prospects in thyroid cancer, 657, 658
recurrent thyroid cancer interpretation, 363, 364
thyroid cancer findings, 362, 363
thyroid lymphoma, 616
Conjunctivitis, radioiodine side effect, 460, 461
Contrast agents, iodine content, 678
Cowden syndrome, 25, 34, 98
COX-2, *see* Cyclooxygenase-2
CT, *see* Computed tomography
Curie, Marie and Pierre, 118–119
Cyclin D
    cell cycle control, 18, 19, 50
    overexpression in thyroid cancer, 24
Cyclooxygenase-2 (COX-2), thyroid nodule malignancy marker, 215
Cystic carcinoma, papillary thyroid cancer, 267

D

Dentures, radioiodine uptake, 170
Depsipeptide, thyroid cancer trials, 673
Diffuse capillary carcinoma, papillary thyroid cancer, 267, 268, 560, 561
DNA methylation, thyroid cancer role, 19
DNA microarray, thyroid nodule analysis, 218, 219
Dosimetry
    Benua protocol
        advantages and limitations, 442
        data collection, 435, 436
        modifications, 436–439
    children, 314
    clearance of radioiodine, 447, 448
    comparison of approaches, 440–443
    internal radiation dosimetry,
        classical dosimetry, 434, 435
        medical internal radiation dose, 435, 440
    iodine contamination impact on studies, 451
    iodine radioisotopes, 223, 439
    Maxon approach, 439, 440, 442, 443
    overview, 434
    recombinant human thyrotropin studies, 447–451
    thyroid remnants, 448, 449
    tumor dosimetry, 449–451

Doxorubicin
    medullary thyroid cancer chemotherapy, 609, 610
    thyroid cancer management, 491

E

E-cadherin, expression in thyroid cancer, 25
Ectopic gastric mucosa, false-positive radioiodine scans, 183, 185
Ectopic thyroid tissue
    embryology, 5
    false-positive radioiodine scans, 180
EMA, *see* Epithelial membrane antigen
Embolization therapy, metastases, 501, 510, 511
Encapsulated variant, papillary thyroid cancer, 267
Epidemiology, thyroid cancer
    distribution by histological type, 10, 55
    incidence, 9
    mortality, 10
    papillary thyroid cancer, 253, 254
    pediatric thyroid cancer, 97–100
    prevalence, 9, 10
    radiation-induced thyroid cancer, *see* Radiation-induced thyroid cancer
    risk factors, 10, 11, 55, 247
    ultrasonography screening, 238
Epirubicin, thyroid cancer management, 491
Epithelial membrane antigen (EMA), thyroid nodule malignancy marker, 217
ErbB1/HER1, thyroid cancer role, 20
ErbB2/Neu/HER2, thyroid cancer role, 20
Ethanol ablation, metastases, 509, 510
Etoposide,
    medullary thyroid cancer chemotherapy, 609
    thyroid cancer management, 492
Extensively fibrotic carcinoma, papillary thyroid cancer, 267
External beam radiation therapy,
    advances in, 653–654
    anaplastic thyroid cancer, 641, 642
    bone metastasis, 501, 502
    chemotherapy combination, 494, 495
    clinical treatment volume, 653
    follicular thyroid carcinoma
        adjuvant therapy, 545–547
        Hürthle cell carcinoma, 547
        palliation, 547
        planning, 547
        radical therapy for gross disease, 545
    intensity modulated radiation therapy, 653, 654

medullary thyroid cancer
  adjuvant therapy, 505
  gross residual disease, 605
  metastatic disease, 606
  planning, 605
nomenclature, 653, 654
papillary thyroid cancer
  adjuvant therapy, 485–488
  dose distribution, 488
  metastases, 488, 489
  radical therapy for gross disease, 485
thyroid lymphoma, 617
toxicity, 654, 655
treatment planing, 653

F

Facial nerve paralysis, radioiodine side effect, 466
Familial adenomatous polyposis, thyroid neoplasms, 575
Fas/Fas L, 57–58
Fermi, Enrico, nuclear medicine contributions, 118
FGF, see Fibroblast growth factor
Fibroblast growth factor (FGF),
  serum marker utilization, 306
  thyroid cancer expression, 50
Fine-needle aspiration (FNA)
  equipment, 211
  Hürthle cell carcinoma, 531, 532
  medullary thyroid cancer, 583
  pediatric papillary thyroid cancer, 378
  technique, 211, 212
  thyroglossal duct carcinoma, 393, 563, 564
  thyroid nodule evaluation, 203, 204, 206, 207, 248
  ultrasound guidance, 236, 237
Fluorescent thyroid scanning, 205
Fluorodeoxyglucose scanning, see Positron emission tomography
FNA, see Fine-needle aspiration
Follicular adenoma, 44
Follicular thyroid carcinoma (FTC), see also Hürthle cell carcinoma
  chemotherapy, see Chemotherapy
  children, 543, 544
  clinical presentation, 518
  external-beam radiation therapy, see External-beam radiation therapy
  follicular variant papillary thyroid cancer differential diagnosis, 266, 519, 520
  mixed medullary-follicular cell carcinoma, 561
  pathology, 527–529
  positron emission tomography, 533, 534, 541
  prognosis
    minimally invasive follicular thyroid cancer, 549
    survival, 521, 537, 549
    therapy effects, 549, 550
  radioiodine therapy, see Radioiodine ablation therapy
  Ras mutations, 22
  scintigraphy, 537
  staging, 91, 92, 520
  surgical management, 520, 523, 524
  surveillance, 539, 540
  thyroid function tests and evaluation, 518–520
Follicular variant, papillary thyroid cancer, 266, 519, 520
FTC, see Follicular thyroid carcinoma

G

Galectin-3, thyroid nodule malignancy marker, 213, 214
Gamma camera, see Radioiodine scanning
Gardner syndrome, 25, 34, 98
Gemcitabine, thyroid cancer management, 493
Gene therapy, prospects, 668
Genetic
  mutations, 43
  syndromes, 25, 33–34
Growth factors, cancer, 16, 19, 35–36
gsp, thyroid cancer mutations, 23, 44, 45

H

Hair loss, radioiodine side effect, 459
Hanford Radiation exposure, 67
HBME-1, thyroid nodule malignancy marker, 216
Hepatocyte growth factor (HGF), thyroid nodule malignancy marker, 218
Hevesy, George, nuclear medicine contributions, 118, 119
HGF, see Hepatocyte growth factor
High-mobility group I (HMGI), thyroid nodule malignancy and transcripts, 216, 217
HMGI, see High-mobility group I
Hürthle cell carcinoma, see also Follicular thyroid carcinoma
  clinical presentation, 532–534, 565–567
  external-beam radiation therapy, 547
  metastasis, 531
  oncogene activation and mutation, 22, 23
  pathology and histology, 531, 565

prognosis, 531, 532, 537
scintigraphy, 533, 534
surveillance, 566, 567
Hyalizing trabecular neoplasms, thyroid, 574, 575
Hypoparathyroidism, radioiodine side effect, 467

I

IGF-1, *see* Insulin-like growth factor-1
Imaging, *see* Radiation scanning; CT; MRI; Ultrasonography
Imatinib mesylate (STI571), thyroid cancer trials, 671, 672
Immune response to thyroid cancer, 36
Immunotherapy, prospects, 669
IMRT, *see* Intensity modulated radiation therapy
Incidence, thyroid cancer, 9
Incidentaloma
    computed tomography, 359
    magnetic resonance imaging, 359
    papillary thyroid cancer, 257
    thyroid nodule features, 205
    ultrasonography, 235
Individualized cancer therapy, prospects, 665, 666
Insular thyroid carcinoma
    clinical characteristics, 556
    demographics, 555, 556
    prognosis, 557
    treatment, 556–558
Insulin-like growth factor-1 (IGF-1), pediatric thyroid cancer expression, 35
Intensity modulated radiation therapy (IMRT), principles, 653, 654
Iodine
    diet restriction, *see* Low iodine diet
    dietary sources, 679
    metabolism, 677, 678
    organification, 6
    pharmacological sources, 678–680
    prophylaxis against radiation exposure, 129–131
    sodium iodide symporter (NIS), 6
Iodine-123 (*see also* Radioiodine scanning), stunning prevention, 340–344
Iodine-124, *see* Radioiodine scanning
Iodine-131 (*see also* Radioiodine scanning),
    ablation therapy, *see* Radioiodine ablation therapy
    scintigraphy, *see* Radioiodine scanning
    stunning, *see* Stunning
Irinotecan, thyroid cancer management, 492, 493

J

Jod–Basedow phenomenon, 6

K

Kidney
    metastasis, radioiodine scanning, 168
    renal failure and thyroid cancer management, 388
Kyphoplasty, spinal metastasis palliative therapy, 511

L

Lacrimal gland, radioiodine side effects, 460, 461
Lactoferrin, thyroid nodule malignancy marker, 218
Lanreotide, medullary thyroid cancer management, 610
Laryngeal nerve, recurrent, 3, 4
Laser thermal ablation, spinal metastasis palliative therapy, 512
Lawrence, Ernest, 119
Leiomyoma, thyroid, 563, 574
Leu-7/CD57, thyroid nodule malignancy marker, 217
Levothyroxine, *see* Thyroid hormone
Lithium
    hyperthyroidism management, 454
    radioiodine therapy adjuvant,
        complications, 455
        patient selection, 454, 455
        prospects, 455, 456, 662
        protocol, 455
        rationale, 454
    thyroid effects, 453, 454
Liver metastasis, radioiodine scanning, 166
Low iodine diet (*see also* Iodine)
    drug avoidance, 678–680
    food avoidance, 679, 680
    recommendations before radioiodine scanning, 679, 680
Lymph node metastasis
    anatomy, 351
    incidence, 352
    intraoperative ultrasonography and lymphadenopathy, 357
    palpation, 352
    pediatric papillary thyroid cancer, 378
    radioiodine scanning, 162
    staging, 360
    ultrasonography
        benign lymph nodes, 352, 353
        biopsy guidance, 357

Index

cervical lymph nodes, 352
characteristics of malignancy, 353
metastatic lymph nodes, 353–355
rationale, 351
surveillance after thyroidectomy, 357
Lymphadenopathy, ultrasonography, 235, 357
Lymphoma, *see* Thyroid lymphoma

M

MACIS system, thyroid cancer staging, 91
Magnetic resonance imaging (MRI)
  advantages and limitations in thyroid cancer, 361
  comparison with other imaging
    techniques, 238, 239, 241, 361, 362
  follow-up of thyroid cancer, 362
  indications, 230, 241
  medullary thyroid cancer surveillance, 587, 588
  neck anatomy, 359, 360
  post-therapy imaging, 363
  preoperative staging of thyroid cancer, 363
  principles, 361
  recurrent thyroid cancer interpretation, 363, 364
  thyroid cancer findings, 362, 363
Manumycin, thyroid cancer trials, 672
Marshall Islands, radiation exposure, 68
Maxon approach, dosimetry, 439, 440, 442, 443
MDM2
  expression in thyroid cancer, 24
  p53 binding, 18
Mediastinal metastasis, radioiodine scanning, 162
Medical internal radiation dose (MIRD), dosimetry, 435, 440
Medullary thyroid cancer (MTC)
  biochemistry, 582
  chemotherapy, 609, 610
  classification, 581, 582
  complications, 586
  external beam radiation therapy
    adjuvant therapy, 505
    gross residual disease, 605
    metastatic disease, 606
    planning, 605
  gene mutations, 25, 47, 48, 581, 582
  genetics, 581–582
  incidence, 10
  markers, 582, 583
  mixed medullary–follicular cell
    carcinoma, 561
  multiple endocrine neoplasia type II
    preoperative studies, 585, 586
    prognosis, 587
    prophylactic thyroidectomy, 584
    screening, 584
  natural course and complications, 586
  pathology, 591–593
  positron emission tomography, 603, 604
  radiation therapy, *see* External radiation therapy
  residual disease management, 588
  RET, 47–48, 50, 51, 203, 581
  scintigraphy options, 599, 600
  screening, 50, 51
  somatostatin receptor scintigraphy
    diagnosis, 599
    dose and distribution, 597, 598
    somatostatin treatment analog monitoring, 599
    uptake of analogs, 597
  sporadic cancer,
    calcitonin testing, 583, 584
    clinical presentation, 583
    fine-needle aspiration, 583
    preoperative imaging, 584
    prognosis, 586, 587
  staging, 92, 587
  surgical management, 595, 596
  surveillance, 587, 588
MENII, *see* Multiple endocrine neoplasia type II
MET, thyroid cancer role, 20, 48
Metastasis, *see also specific metastases*,
  anaplastic thyroid cancer, 630
  bone, 509–512
  embolization therapy, 501, 510, 511
  ethanol ablation, 509, 510
  external-beam radiation therapy, 488, 489
  Hürthle cell carcinoma, 531
  radioiodine therapy
    algorithm, 422–424
    bone metastasis, 415, 418–421, 500, 501
    lithium adjuvant therapy, *see* Lithium
    lung metastasis, 411–414, 417, 418
    prescribed activity
      comparison of approaches, 440–443
      dosimetric determination, 433–440
      empiric recommendations, 421, 433
    thyrotropin stimulation studies, 427–431
  secondary neoplasms to thyroid gland from other tumors, 564, 565, 573
Methotrexate, thyroid cancer management, 493
Microcarcinoma, papillary thyroid cancer, 9, 87, 268

MIRD, *see* Medical internal radiation dose
Mitoxantrone, thyroid cancer management, 491, 492
Mixed medullary-follicular cell carcinoma, clinical features, 561
Molecular markers, 213–219
Molecular pathogenesis of thyroid cancer, 15–25
Mortality, thyroid cancer, 10
MRI, *see* Magnetic resonance imaging
MTC, *see* Medullary thyroid cancer
Mucoepidermoid carcinoma,
   clinical characteristics, 562
   demographics, 561, 562
   pathology, 575, 576
   prognosis, 562
   treatment, 562
Multiple endocrine neoplasia type II (MENII)
   preoperative studies, 585, 586
   prognosis, 587
   prophylactic thyroidectomy, 584
   screening, 584
   types and medullary thyroid cancer, 581, 582
Multistep carcinogenesis, thyroid cancer, 19
Mutations, somatic versus germline, 43

N

Neurilemoma, thyroid, 563
NIS, *see* Sodium-iodide symporter
Nitric oxide synthase (NOS), thyroid cancer expression, 35
NM23, thyroid nodule malignancy marker, 217, 218
Nodules, *see* Thyroid nodules
NOS, *see* Nitric oxide synthase
NTCTCS system, thyroid cancer staging, 91
NTRK1, thyroid cancer role, 20
Nuclear medicine, *see also* Radioiodine ablation therapy
   future approaches, 657–662
   historical perspective, 117–123, 125–128
   scintigraphy, *see* Radioiodine scanning; Somatostatin receptor scintigraphy; Technetium-99m pertechnetate scanning; Technetium-99m sestamibi; Thallium-201 chloride scanning
Nuclear transcription factors, 23–24
Nutrition, *see* Low iodine diet

O

Octreotide, *see* Somatostatin analogs
Oncofetal fibronectin, thyroid nodule malignancy marker, 215, 216
Oncogene (*see also* Proto-oncogene), 41–51
   definition, 43
   mutations, 22, 23
   prognostic value, 51
   screening and diagnostic use, 50, 51
OPG, *see* Osteoprotegerin
Osteoprotegerin (OPG), bone metastasis control, 504, 505
Ovarian cystadenoma, radioiodine uptake, 169
Oxyphilic papillary carcinoma, papillary thyroid cancer, 268

P

p53
   apoptosis, 57
   cell cycle regulation, 58
   MDM2 binding, 18
   mutations in thyroid cancer, 16, 24, 35, 44, 49, 77, 99
   tumor suppressor activity, 18
Papillary thyroid cancer (PTC)
   chemotherapy, *see* Chemotherapy
   children (*see also* Pediatric thyroid cancer), 377–383
      clinical presentation, 377
      fine-needle aspiration, 378
      imaging, 379
      incidence, 377
      lymph node metastasis, 378
      management
         radioiodine ablation therapy, 380, 381
         thyroid hormone replacement therapy, 381, 382
         thyroidectomy, 379, 380
      prognostic factors, 382, 383
   clinical presentation, 253–257
   cytology and pathology
      classical pattern, 263, 264
      clear-cell papillary carcinoma, 268
      columnar-cell carcinoma, 269, 560
      cystic carcinoma, 267
      diffuse capillary carcinoma, 267, 268, 560, 561
      encapsulated variant, 267
      extensively fibrotic carcinoma, 267
      follicular variant, 266, 519, 520
      less well-differentiated papillary carcinomas, 269
      microcarcinoma, 9, 10, 268
      oxyphilic papillary carcinoma, 268

tall-cell variant, 268, 269, 558–560
epidemiology, 9–11, 253, 254
follow-up
    clinical practice guidelines, 290–292
    level of surveillance, 289
    risk assessment, 289
    whole-body radioiodine scanning, 289, 290
gene mutations, 48–49, 75–77
incidence, 253–254
malignant incidentalomas, 257
management
    radioiodine ablation therapy, see Radioiodine ablation therapy
    radioiodine-resistant tumors, 256
    thyroidectomy, 255, 256, 261, 262
microcarcinoma, 9, 87, 268
p53 mutations, 24, 76
pathogenesis, 15–25
prognostic factors
    children, 382, 383
    overview of studies, 375, 376
    treatment type, 376
    tumor subtype, 376
radiation therapy, see External-beam radiation therapy; Radioiodine ablation therapy
RAS mutations, 22
scintigraphy, see Radioiodine scanning; Somatostatin receptor scintigraphy; Technetium-99m pertechnetate scanning; Technetium-99m sestamibi; Thallium-201 chloride scanning
solid variant, 561
staging, see Staging, thyroid cancer,
surgical approach, 261–262
surveillance, 289–292, 309–310
thyroglobulin testing, see Thyroglobulin
thyroglossal duct carcinoma, see Thyroglossal duct carcinoma
thyroid hormone therapy, see Thyroid hormone
thyrosine kinase, 48
PAX8
peroxisome proliferator-activated receptor-γ fusion, 24, 46, 47
thyroid nodule malignancy and PPARγ rearrangement, 217
PDGF, see Platelet-derived growth factor
Pediatric thyroid cancer
clinical presentation, 100
epidemiology, 97–100
follicular thyroid carcinoma, 543, 544

molecular pathogenesis
    BRAF mutations, 34, 35
    growth factor expression, 35, 36
    immune system, 36
    Ras mutations, 35
    RET mutations, 34, 75–76
    sodium-iodide symporter expression, 36
papillary thyroid cancer
    clinical presentation, 377
    fine-needle aspiration, 378
    imaging, 379
    incidence, 377
    lymph node metastasis, 378
    management
        radioiodine ablation therapy, 380, 381
        thyroid hormone replacement therapy, 381, 382
        thyroidectomy, 379, 380
pathologic diagnosis, 100
prognosis, 33
radiation induction, 34, 73–77, 98–100
radioiodine ablation therapy
    complications, 315
    dosing, 314
    endpoints, 316
    long-term risks, 315
    patient selection, 313, 314
radionuclide imaging, 316
staging, 93, 94
syndromes, 33, 34
types, 33, 100
Peroxisome proliferator-activated receptor-γ (PPARγ),
apoptosis induction, 58
PAX8 fusion, 24, 44, 46, 47
therapeutic targeting, 58, 59
PET, see Positron emission tomography
Phospholipase C (PLC), signaling in thyroid cancer, 18
PKC, see Protein kinase C
Platelet-derived growth factor (PDGF), thyroid cancer expression, 20
PLC, see Phospholipase C
Poorly differentiated carcinoma, pathology, 573, 574
Positron emission tomography (PET)
anaplastic thyroid cancer, 631, 639, 640
computed tomography combination, 319, 604, 657
fluorodeoxyglucose imaging in well-differentiated thyroid cancer

false-positive scans, 322, 323
follicular thyroid carcinoma, 533, 534, 541
interpretation, 322
normal findings and variations, 320–322
prognostic value, 324, 325
technique, 320
thyroglobulin-positive, radioiodine-negative thyroid cancer, 323, 324, 369, 370
thyrotropin effects on tracer uptake, 325, 370
incidentalomas, 257
iodine-124 imaging, 142, 177, 325
medullary thyroid cancer, 588, 603, 604
principles, 319
prospects in thyroid cancer, 657–660
radionuclides and tracers, 319, 320
radiotracer development, 659, 660
reporter gene imaging, 659
thyroid lymphoma, 616, 621, 622
Potassium iodide
pharmacology, 129, 130
radiation-induced thyroid cancer prophylaxis
availability and distribution, 131
guidelines, 130, 131
historical perspective, 129
side effects, 130
PPARγ, *see* Peroxisome proliferator-activated receptor-γ
Pregnancy, thyroid cancer presentation and management, 388–390
Prevalence, thyroid cancer, 9, 10
Professional organizations, thyroid cancer resources, 685
Protein kinase C (PKC), signaling in thyroid cancer, 18
Proto-oncogenes
activation, 20, 21
definition, 42, 43
PTC, *see* Papillary thyroid cancer
PTEN tumor suppressor gene, 34, 667
Publications, thyroid cancer resources, 683
Pulmonary metastasis
radioiodine scan interpretation,
macronodular metastasis, 164
micronodular metastasis, 164
patterns, 163
radioiodine therapy
dose estimation, 468, 469
outcomes, 411–414, 417, 418

side effects
presentation, 467, 468
prevention, 469–472

R

Radiation-induced thyroid cancer, 63–67, 98–99
Chernobyl accident analysis
cesium-137 release, 71
children, 73–75
geographical distribution of radioisotopes, 70
population analysis and pediatric thyroid cancer
Belarus, 72–74
children, 99
epidemiology, 77
gene mutations, 75–77
latency, 76
pathology and biology, 75
Russian federation, 72, 74
Tula Oblast, 77
Ukraine, 72–75
radioactivity release, 70
radioiodine release, 71, 72
thyroid dose reconstruction, 72
External radiation exposure
acne patients, 65
atomic bomb survivors, 64, 69, 98
cancer radiation therapy patients, 66
cervical tuberculous adenitis patients, 64
dose response, 69
hemangioma patients, 65
Hodgkin's lymphoma, 99
occupational exposure, 66
prenatal exposure, 66, 67
thymic enlargement patients, 65, 66, 98
tinea capitis patients, 66, 98
tonsillitis patients, 65
incidence, 9
internal radiation studies
children, 68
diagnostic radioiodine, 67
fallout exposure, 67, 68
nuclear facility populations, 67
therapeutic radioiodine, 67
iodine prophylaxis, *see* Potassium iodide
pathology, 63, 64
pediatric thyroid cancer, 34, 98
potassium iodide prophylaxis, *see* Potassium iodide

risk assessment
- dose–response relationship, 69
- modifying factors, 68, 69

Radiation safety
- acceptable dose rates for patient release, 407, 408
- containment, 403, 404
- early release of patients, 404–406
- excreted radioiodine, 406
- forms and instructions, 689–692
- hospitalization for isotope administration, 402
- hygiene, 404
- isolation of patients, 403
- monitoring, 404
- people in contact with thyroid cancer patients, 402
- written instructions for patients, 403, 689–692

Radiation therapy, see External radiation therapy

Radioactivity
- decay pathways, 133–135, 660, 661
- deterministic effects, 400
- Internet resources, 402
- ionizing versus nonionizing radiation, 400
- myths and fears, 406, 408
- radiation types, 133–135, 399, 400
- regulatory agencies, 128, 401
- stochastic effects, 400
- units
  - international system, 400
  - special units system, 400, 401

Radiofrequency ablation (RFA), spinal metastasis palliative therapy, 511, 512

Radioiodine ablation therapy
- children, 313–316
- criteria for successful ablation, 280, 281
- dose selection, 272–281
- dosimetry, see Dosimetry
- enhancers, 662
- forms and instructions, 689–692
- fractionated iodine-131 therapy, 340
- historical perspective, 313
- iodine-123 scanning and stunning prevention, 340–344
- lithium, 453–456
- metastases treatment,
  - algorithm, 422–424
  - bone metastasis, 415, 418–421
  - lithium adjuvant therapy, see Lithium
  - lung metastasis, 411–414, 417, 418
  - prescribed activity
    - comparison of approaches, 440–443
    - dosimetric determination, 433–440
    - empiric recommendations, 421, 433
    - thyrotropin stimulation studies, 427–431
- outcomes
  - primary tumor size effects, 274, 275, 277
  - recurrence, 274
  - survival, 274
- patient forms and instructions, 403, 689–692
- pediatric papillary thyroid cancer, 380, 381
- pediatric thyroid cancer
  - complications, 315
  - dosing, 314
  - endpoints, 316
  - long-term risks, 315
  - patient selection, 313, 314
- posttherapy whole-body scintigraphy, 148, 274, 285
- prescribed activity selection, 277–279
- prospects, 660, 661
- radioiodine-negative thyroid cancer, see Thyroglobulin-positive, radioiodine-negative thyroid cancer
- rationale, 273, 281
- redifferentiation therapy, 661, 662
- regulatory agencies, 128, 401
- renal failure, 388
- side effects
  - bone marrow, 473–477
  - brain, 459
  - cystitis, 473
  - eye, 459–461
  - facial nerve, 466
  - fertility, 477–479
  - gastrointestinal tract, 472, 473
  - hair loss, 459
  - hypoparathyroidism, 467
  - lungs, 467–472
  - nasal effects, 466
  - salivary glands
    - anatomy and physiology, 461
    - frequency, 461
    - management, 465
    - prevention, 463–465
    - signs and symptoms, 461, 462
    - stomatitis, 463
    - xerostomia, 462, 463
  - second primary cancers, 479, 480
  - spinal cord, 459

Index

taste and smell, 466
thyroiditis, 466, 467
thyrotoxicosis, 467
vocal cords, 467
stunning, *see* Stunning
thyrotropin stimulation, *see* Thyrotropin
Radioiodine scanning
Atlas and Primer, 171–197
children, 316
false-positive scans, 151–165
artifacts, 171, 172
ectopic gastric mucosa, 183, 185
ectopic thyroid tissue, 180
gastrointestinal uptake abnormalities, 185–187
importance of identification, 179, 180
inflammation or infection site uptake, 189–191
mammary variations and abnormalities, 188, 189
nonthyroidal neoplasm uptake, 192, 193
physiological secretions, 183, 184
physiological sites of nonthyroidal uptake or biodistribution, 156–161, 180, 182, 183
serous cavity and cyst uptake, 189, 191, 169
unexplained sites of uptake, 193
urinary tract abnormalities, 186
gamma camera
collimator, 136–139
overview, 135, 136
photomultiplier tubes, 139
processing electronics and image display, 139, 140
scintillation crystal, 139
historical perspective, 117–123, 125–128
imaging techniques
acquisition parameters, 142
static planar imaging, 140
whole-body imaging, 140, 141
interpretation of whole-body scans
databases, 151, 190
metastatic disease patterns
bone metastasis, 166
brain metastasis, 167
kidney metastasis, 168
liver metastasis, 166
lymph node metastasis, 162
mediastinal metastasis, 162
pulmonary metastasis, 163, 164
physiological uptake in nonthyroidal tissues
bladder, 161
cardiac blood pool, 158
esophageal, 157
facial area uptake, 156, 157
gastrointestinal tract, 160
liver, 159
thymus, 158
spectrum of thyroid tissue uptake
marked postoperative remnant thyroid tissue, 154
preoperative scan with hypofunctioning area, 153
struma ovarii, 155
thyroglossal tract functioning thyroid tissue, 154
thyroid remnant tissue, 153
systematic approach, 151, 152
tools
anatomic markers, 176
history and physical examination, 173
lateral views, 175
overview, 151, 152
pinhole collimator images, 174
isotope types
comparison for scintigraphy, 135, 136
half-life, 135
production, 135
selection, 144–147
negative results from failure to uptake iodine, *see* Thyroglobulin-positive, radioiodine-negative thyroid cancer
papillary thyroid cancer follow-up, 289, 290
post-therapy scans, utility, 148–149, 274, 285
Primer and Atlas, 171–197
radioiodine uptake
assay, 141, 142
probe, 142
regulatory agencies, 128, 401
stunning of thyroid, *see* Stunning
thyroid nodules
alternative radiopharmaceuticals, 205, 223, 224
clinical utility, 227
dosimetry, 223
hot nodule features, 204
malignancy rates, 226
technique, 223
technetium-99m scan discordance, 227
terminology, 223–226
thyrotropin stimulation, *see* Thyrotropin
whole-body scintigraphy

703

false positive scans, 151–165
metastatic survey, 140, 141
no scan alternative, 147
posttherapy scans, 148, 274, 285
radioisotope selection
  initial ablation, 147, 148
  iodine-123, 145, 146
  iodine-124, 146, 147
  iodine-131, 145
  overview, 144, 145, 147
  pretreatment scans, 148
  surveillance scan, 148, 309, 310
surveillance versus pretreatment scans, 309, 310
thyroid stimulation, 144
time points of scanning, 142–144
radioiodine
  side effects, *see* Radioiodine ablation therapy
  therapy, *see* Radioiodine ablation therapy
  uptake, 141–142
RAF, 15
RANK system, bone metastasis control, 504, 505
Ras
  classification of thyroid malignancies, 85, 86
  isoforms, 16
  mutations in thyroid cancer, 16, 17, 22, 23, 44–46
  pediatric thyroid cancer mutations, 35
  signaling, 15, 16
  therapeutic targeting, 668
Rb, *see* Retinoblastoma protein
Receptor tyrosine kinases (RTKs)
  mutations, 48
  signaling in thyroid cancer, 15–17, 20–22
  therapeutic targeting, 667, 668, 671, 672
Renal failure, thyroid cancer presentation and management, 388
Renal metastasis, *see* Kidney
Reporter genes, imaging in thyroid cancer, 658, 659
Reserpine, salivary gland protection in radioiodine therapy, 464, 465
Resources for the cancer patient, 683, 685–688
RET
  Hürthle cell carcinoma rearrangements, 533
  medullary thyroid cancer, 47–51, 203
  multiple endocrine neoplasia mutations, 581, 582
  pediatric thyroid cancer mutations, 34, 75, 76
  radiation-induced, 75–76
  therapeutic targeting, 667, 672
  thyroid cancer rearrangements, 20–22, 25, 44, 47, 48

thyroid nodule malignancy and PTC rearrangements, 216
Retinoblastoma protein (Rb), cell cycle control, 19
Retinoic acid, redifferentiation therapy, 662, 666
RFA, *see* Radiofrequency ablation
Risk factors, thyroid cancer, 10, 11, 55, 247
RTKs, *see* Receptor tyrosine kinases

S

Salivary glands
  anatomy and physiology, 461
  neoplasms in thyroid, 563, 576
  radioiodine side effects
    cancer, 480
    frequency, 461
    management, 465
    prevention, 463–465
    signs and symptoms, 461, 462
    stomatitis, 463
    xerostomia, 462, 463
Sarcoma, thyroid, 562, 563
Second malignancies, 66
Scintigraphy, *see* Radioiodine scanning; Somatostatin receptor scintigraphy; Technetium-99m pertechnetate scanning; Technetium-99m sestamibi; Thallium-201 chloride scanning
Sestamibi, *see* Technetium-99m sestamibi
Signal transduction, 15, 43, 667
Sialoadenitis, radioiodine side effect, 461, 462, 465
Single-photon emission computed tomography (SPECT), prospects in thyroid cancer, 657–659
Sistrunk procedure, thyroglossal duct carcinoma, 394
Sodium-iodide symporter (NIS), 6
  lithium effects, 453
  pediatric thyroid cancer expression, 36
  physiology, 6
  radioiodine-resistant tumor deficiency, 256, 666, 677
  therapeutic targeting, 666
Somatostatin analogs
  differentiated thyroid cancer imaging, 600, 601
  dose and distribution, 597, 598
  indium-111 octreotide treatment of medullary thyroid cancer, 599
  radiolabels, 599
  uptake of analogs, 597
Somatostatin receptor scintigraphy
  medullary thyroid cancer

diagnosis, 599
dose and distribution, 597, 598
somatostatin treatment analog monitoring, 599
uptake of analogs, 597
prospects, 658
thyroglobulin-positive, radioiodine-negative thyroid cancer, 370
well-differentiated thyroid cancer, 332, 333
SPECT, *see* Single-photon emission computed tomography
Squamous cell carcinoma, thyroid
clinical characteristics, 554, 555
demographics, 553
pathology, 573
prognosis, 555
treatment, 555
Staging, thyroid cancer, 87–94
anaplastic carcinoma of the thyroid, 92, 647
applications, 87
definition, 87
follicular thyroid cancer, 91, 92
lymph node classification, 360
medullary thyroid cancer, 92, 587
pediatric thyroid cancer, 93, 94
prognostic value, 92, 93
scoring systems
AGES system, 91
AMES system, 88
MACIS system, 91
NTCTCS system, 91
Ohio State system, 90, 91
TNM system, 88–90
age impact on staging, 89, 90
distant metastasis, 89
lymph node involvement, 89
multifocality, 89
papillary thyroid cancer histologic variants, 90
tumor size, 88, 89
updates, 90
STI571, *see* Imatinib mesylate
Stomatitis, radioiodine side effect, 463
Struma ovarii
radioiodine uptake, 155
thyroid cancer presentation and management, 390, 391
Stunning
controversies, 349
definition, 337, 346
evidence

against, 346–348
for, 338, 340
interpretation, 349
iodine-131
decay properties, 337
specificity of phenomenon, 337
thyroid radiation dose, 337, 338
prevention
iodine-123 scanning, 340–344
low-dose iodine-131, 343
radioiodine ablation therapy outcomes, 340
Support groups, thyroid cancer resources, 685–687
Suppressor genes, 42–43, 58
Surgical management
anaplastic thyroid cancer, 633, 634
follicular thyroid carcinoma, 520, 523, 524
intraoperative ultrasound, 237, 238
medullary thyroid cancer
preoperative studies, 584–586
prophylactic thyroidectomy in hereditary cancer, 584
recommendations, 595, 596
papillary thyroid cancer thyroidectomy, 255, 256, 261, 262
pediatric papillary thyroid cancer thyroidectomy, 379, 380
thyroglobulin-positive, radioiodine-negative thyroid cancer, 371
thyroglossal duct carcinoma, 394
thyroid nodules, 207, 248, 249

T

Tall-cell variant, papillary thyroid cancer
clinical characteristics, 558, 559
children, 33
demographics, 558
pathology, 268, 269
prognosis, 559, 560
treatment, 559, 560
Technetium-99m DMSA, medullary thyroid cancer imaging, 599, 600
Technetium-99m methylene diphosphate, medullary thyroid cancer imaging, 600
Technetium-99m pertechnetate scanning
postoperative preablation scanning, 147
thyroid nodules, 227
Technetium-99m sestamibi
thyroglobulin-positive, radioiodine-negative thyroid cancer, 369

well-differentiated thyroid cancer imaging, 330–332
Technetium-99m tetrofosin,
  well-differentiated thyroid cancer imaging, 332
Telomerase
  pediatric thyroid cancer expression, 35, 36
  thyroid nodule malignancy marker, 214
Teratoma, thyroid, 563, 576
Tetrofosmin, *see* Technetium-99m tetrofosmin
TGF-α, *see* Transforming growth factor-α
Thallium-201 chloride scanning
  thyroglobulin-positive, radioiodine-negative thyroid cancer, 369
  well-differentiated thyroid cancer, 329, 330
Thymus
  neoplasms in thyroid, 563, 576
  radioiodine uptake, 158
Thyrogen®, *see* Thyrotropin recombinant human
Thyroglobulin, 297–302
  clinical applications in differentiated thyroid cancer
    preoperative levels and prognosis, 301
    thyrotropin stimulation testing, 302
    thyrotropin suppression therapy, 301, 302
  follicular thyroid carcinoma
    surveillance, 540
  immunoassays
    antibodies, 297, 298
    competitive immunoassay, 298
    kits, 299
    laboratory guidelines, 300
    sandwich immunoassays, 298, 299
    sensitivity, 299, 300
  iodine storage, 677
  residual thyroid function analysis, 273, 305
  reverse transcriptase-polymerase chain reaction
    detection of transcripts, 306, 307
  structure, 297
  synthesis induction by thyrotropin, 297
Thyroglobulin antibodies
  assays, 300, 301, 305, 306
  disease monitoring, 307
  interference in thyroglobulin assays, 301, 305
  prevalence
    differentiated thyroid cancer, 300, 301
    general population, 306
Thyroglobulin-positive, radioiodine-negative thyroid cancer
  fluorodeoxyglucose positron emission tomography, 323, 324, 369, 370
  management approach, 367, 368

radionuclide scintigraphy agents, 369
sodium-iodide symporter deficiency, 256
somatostatin receptor scintigraphy, 370, 371
surgical management, 371
Thyroglossal duct carcinoma
  clinical presentation, 563, 564
  epidemiology, 393
  evaluation, 393, 563, 564
  pathology, 574
  surgical management, 394
Thyroidectomy, *see* Surgical management
Thyroiditis, radioiodine side effect, 466, 467
Thyroid gland
  anatomy, 3, 4
  blood supply, 4, 5
  ectopic tissue, 5
  embryology, 5
  histology, 5
  innervation, 3, 4
  lymphatic drainage, 5
  physiology, 5–7
Thyroid hormone
  iodine storage, 677
  levothyroxine therapy,
    combined triiodothyronine therapy, 295, 296
    indications, 293
    papillary thyroid cancer outcomes, 293
    regimens, 293–295
    replacement therapy in pediatric
      papillary thyroid cancer, 381, 382
  thyroid hormone synthesis, 6
  thyroid nodule suppression, 205, 206
  thriiodothyronine (T3) therapy, 295–296
Thyroid lymphoma
  chemotherapy, 617
  classification, 615, 616
  clinical presentation, 616
  epidemiology, 615
  imaging, 616
  management, 616, 617
  pathology, 615, 621
  positron emission tomography, 616, 621, 622
  prognosis, 617
  risk factors, 615
Thyroid nodules, 201–207
  autonomous, 204
  differential diagnosis, 202
  DNA microarray analysis, 218, 219
  evaluation

cost-effectiveness of diagnostic protocols, 207, 230
fine-needle aspiration, *see* Fine-needle aspiration
history and physical examination, 202, 203, 229, 230
laboratory tests, 203
radioiodine scanning, 204, 205, 223–228
ultrasonography, 205
ultrasonography, *see* Ultrasonography
incidentalomas, 205
malignancy rates, 229, 247
management approach, 206–207
markers for malignancy
BRAF mutations, 217
carcinoembryonic antigen, 203
CD30 and ligand, 218
CD44, 215
CD97, 216
ceruloplasmin, 218
CK19, 218
cyclooxygenase-2, 215
epithelial membrane antigen, 217
galectin-3, 213, 214
HBME-1, 216
hepatocyte growth factor and receptor, 218
high-mobility group I transcripts, 216, 217
lactoferrin, 218
Leu-7/CD57, 217
NM23, 217, 218
oncofetal fibronectin, 215, 216
PAX8/PPARγ rearrangement, 217
RET/PTC rearrangements, 216
telomerase, 214
thyroid peroxidase, 214, 215
thyroid-stimulating hormone receptor gene hypermethylation, 218
pathogenesis, 201, 202
prevalence, 201
surgical management, 207, 248, 249
thyroid hormone suppression, 205, 206
Thyroid peroxidase
physiology, 6
thyroid nodule malignancy marker, 214, 215
Thyroid-stimulating hormone, *see* Thyrotropin
Thyroid-stimulating hormone receptor
gene hypermethylation as thyroid nodule malignancy marker, 218
reverse transcriptase-polymerase chain reaction detection of
transcripts, 306, 307
Thyroid stunning, *see* Stunning
Thyrotoxicosis
metastatic thyroid cancer, 387, 388
radioiodine side effect, 467
thyroid cancer presentation and management, 387
Thyrotropin (TSH)
bovine, 104
clinical applications
bovine hormone, 104
human hormone preparations, 104, 105
overview, 103
fluorodeoxyglucose uptake effects, 325, 370
radioiodine ablation therapy stimulation
dosimetry studies, 447–451
metastasis treatment, 427–431
papillary thyroid cancer, 256
rationale, 273, 283
receptor
mutations in thyroid cancer, 22, 45
signaling, 17, 18
recombinant human TSH (Thyrogen®), 103–111
clinical studies
normal subjects, 105
thyroid cancer patients, 105–109
preclinical studies, 105
prospects for study, 109–111, 285, 286
radioiodine ablation therapy, 427–431
dosimetry, 447–451
outcomes, 283–285
thyroglobulin monitoring, 108–110
thyrotropin-releasing hormone for stimulation, 103, 104
Thyrotropin-releasing hormone (TRH), thyrotropin stimulation, 103, 104
TNM system, thyroid cancer staging,
age impact on staging, 89, 90
distant metastasis, 89
lymph node involvement, 89
multifocality, 89
papillary thyroid cancer histologic variants, 90
tumor size, 88, 89
updates, 90

Index

Topotecan, thyroid cancer management, 492, 493
TPO, see Thyroid peroxidase
TRAIL, 59, 668
Transforming growth factor-α (TGF-α), thyroid cancer role, 19
TRH, see Thyrotropin-releasing hormone
Triiodothyronine, see Thyroid hormone
TRK, mutations in thyroid cancer, 48
TSH, see Thyrotropin
Tumor suppressor gene, definition, 42, 43, 58
Tyrosine kinases, see Receptor tyrosine kinases

U

Ultrasonography, 229–243
   comparison with other imaging techniques, 238, 239, 241
   fine-needle aspiration guidance, 236, 237
   follow-up evaluation, 241–243
   gray scale, 230–231
   incidentalomas, 235
   lymph nodes
      benign lymph nodes, 352, 353
      biopsy guidance, 357
      cervical lymph nodes, 352
      metastatic lymph nodes, 353–355
      rationale, 351
      surveillance after thyroidectomy, 357
   lymphadenopathy, 235
   pathology of thyroid nodules and goiters, 234
   principles
      color flow Doppler imaging, 231, 234, 237
      gray-scale ultrasonography, 230, 231
   thyroid cancer
      color Doppler imaging, 237
      enhanced imaging, 238
      epidemiologic use, 238
      intraoperative ultrasound, 237, 238
      percutaneous therapy guidance, 237
      small lesions, 236
   thyroid nodules, 205

V

Vascular endothelial growth factor (VEGF)
   pediatric thyroid cancer expression, 35, 36
   serum marker utilization, 306
   therapeutic targeting, 666, 667
   thyroid cancer role, 19
VEGF, see Vascular endothelial growth factor
Vertebroplasty, spinal metastasis palliative therapy, 511

W

Wagner, Henry N. Jr., reflections on nuclear medicine, 117–123, 125–128
Wolff–Chaikoff phenomenon, 6

X

Xerostomia, radioiodine side effect, 462, 463

About the Editors

Leonard Wartofsky, MD, MPH, MACP

Dr. Wartofsky is a Professor of Medicine, Anatomy, Physiology and Genetics at the Uniformed Services University of the Health Sciences in Bethesda, MD, Professor of Medicine at the Georgetown University School of Medicine, and Clinical Professor of Medicine at the University of Maryland, Howard University, and George Washington University Schools of Medicine. He is Chairman of the Department of Medicine at the Washington Hospital Center, and was Program Director of the Internal Medicine Training Program from 1993-2000. He is a graduate of George Washington University and did his postgraduate training in internal medicine at the Barnes Hospital of Washington University in St. Louis and the Albert Einstein Medical Center in New York, and trained in endocrinology with Dr. Sidney Ingbar in the Harvard University Service, Thorndike Memorial Laboratory, at Boston City Hospital. He is board certified both in internal medicine and in endocrinology and metabolism. Prior to joining the Washington Hospital Center, he was on active duty at the Walter Reed Army Medical Center where he held the positions of Director of the Endocrinology Division and the Endocrinology Fellowship Training Program, then as Chief of the Department of Medicine and Program Director of the Internal Medicine Program. While at Walter Reed, he served as Consultant in Medicine to the Surgeon General.

Dr. Wartofsky has been elected to membership of several prestigious medical societies including the American Society of Clinical Investigation, the Association of American Physicians, The American Federation of Clinical Research, The Endocrine Society, Society of General Internal Medicine, American College of Physicians, and the American Thyroid Association. He is an honorary member of both the Medical Society and Endocrinology and Metabolism Society of Chile, and the Endocrine Society of the Dominican Republic. Dr. Wartofsky is one of only several hundred senior physicians who have been honored with election as a Master of the American College of Physicians out of over 100,000 members. He has also served as a Governor of the College, was President of the American Thyroid Association in 1995, and will be President of the Endocrine Society in 2006. He has been presented with numerous military and civilian awards, and was the 2001 recipient of the Distinguished Educator Award of the Endocrine Society of the United States. He is an internationally known authority on thyroid disorders and is the author or coauthor of over 250 articles or book chapters in the medical literature.

Douglas Van Nostrand, MD, FACP, FACNP

Dr. Van Nostrand is the Director of the Division of Nuclear Medicine at the Washington Hospital Center and has been practicing Nuclear Medicine for 27 years. He received his Bachelor of Science degree from Duke University in 1969 and his Medical degree from Emory University in 1973. He completed his residency in Internal Medicine at Wilford Hall Medical Center in 1976 and his fellowship in Nuclear Medicine at the National Naval Medical Center in 1978. He is board certified in both Internal Medicine and Nuclear Medicine. He was previously the Director of Nuclear Medicine at Malcolm Grow Medical Center (1979-1980), Walter Reed Army Medical Center (1980-1987), and Good Samaritan Hospital (1987-1999). He has been actively involved in training physicians in cardiac nuclear medicine both within fellowship training programs and through computer-based workshops over the last 10 years throughout the east coast with over 1000 cardiologists having attended his programs. He has published more than 70 articles and 7 books.

Printed by Publishers' Graphics LLC
DBZ140510.23.35.5 20140510